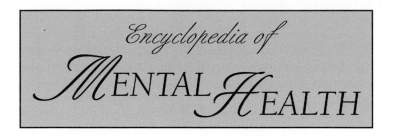

Encyclopedia of
Mental Health

Volume 2   Do–N

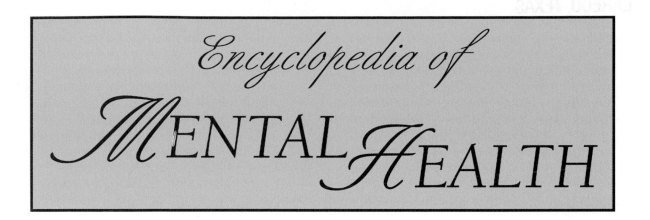

Encyclopedia of MENTAL HEALTH

Volume 2   Do–N

Editor-in-Chief

HOWARD S. FRIEDMAN

Department of Psychology
University of California, Riverside

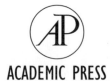

ACADEMIC PRESS

SAN DIEGO   LONDON   BOSTON   NEW YORK   SYDNEY   TOKYO   TORONTO

This book is printed on acid-free paper. ∞

Academic Press
a division of Harcourt Brace & Company
525 B Street, Suite 1900, San Diego, California 92101-4495, USA
http://www.apnet.com

Academic Press Limited
24-28 Oval Road, London NW1 7DX, UK
http://www.hbuk.co.uk/ap/

Library of Congress Card Catalog Number: 98-84208

International Standard Book Number: 0-12-226675-7 (set)
International Standard Book Number: 0-12-226676-5 (volume 1)
International Standard Book Number: 0-12-226677-3 (volume 2)
International Standard Book Number: 0-12-226678-1 (volume 3)

PRINTED IN THE UNITED STATES OF AMERICA
99 00 01 02 03 MM 9 8 7 6 5 4 3 2

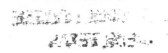

Contents

S

T

U

W

How to Use the Encyclopedia

The *Encyclopedia of Mental Health* is intended for use by students, research professionals, and practicing clinicians. Articles have been chosen to reflect major disciplines in the study of mental health, common topics of research by professionals in this domain, and areas of public interest and concern. Each article serves as a comprehensive overview of a given area, providing both breadth of coverage for students, and depth of coverage for research and clinical professionals. We have designed the encyclopedia with the following features for maximum accessibility for all readers.

Articles in the encyclopedia are arranged alphabetically by subject. Complete tables of contents appear in all volumes. The index is located in Volume 3. Because the reader's topic of interest may be listed under a broader article title, we encourage use of the Index for access to a subject area, rather than use of the Table of Contents alone. For instance, the topic area of recovered/repressed memories is covered under the article title "Standards for Psychotherapy." Because a topic of study in mental health is often applicable to more than one article, the Index provides a complete listing of where a subject is covered and in what context. As an example, the topic of aging and mental health is covered in a number of articles including "Aging and Mental Health," "Assessment of Mental Health in Older Adults," and "Emotion and Aging."

Each article contains an outline, a glossary, cross-references, and a bibliography. The outline allows a quick scan of the major areas discussed within each article. The glossary contains terms that may be unfamiliar to the reader, with each term defined *in the context of its use in that article*. Thus, a term may appear in the glossary for another article defined in a slightly different manner or with a subtle nuance specific to that article. For clarity, we have allowed these differences in definition to remain so that the terms are defined relative to the context of the particular article.

The articles have been cross-referenced to other related articles in the encyclopedia. Cross-references are found at the first or predominant mention of a subject area covered elsewhere in the encyclopedia. Cross-references will always appear at the end of a paragraph. Where multiple cross-references apply to a single paragraph, the cross-references are listed in alphabetical order. We encourage readers to use the cross-references to locate other encyclopedia articles that will provide more detailed information about a subject.

The Bibliography lists recent secondary sources to aid the reader in locating more detailed or technical information. Review articles and research articles that are considered of primary importance to the understanding of a given subject area are also listed. Bibliographies are not intended to provide a full reference listing of all material covered in the context of a given article, but are provided as guides to further reading.

Domestic Violence Intervention

Sandra A. Graham-Bermann

University of Michigan

Domestic Violence   Physical violence committed by one intimate partner against the other with the intention of causing physical pain or injury. Violence ranges from pushing, shoving, and slapping, to punching, hitting with an object, injuring, using a weapon, or threatening someone with a weapon. When such violence results in injury, women are likely to be the victims 95% of the time. Thus, domestic violence is a general term used to describe both woman-abuse and spouse-abuse. But, given the injury statistics, feminists argue that the term woman-abuse is a more accurate one, since it reflects the actual dynamics of domestic violence, and the term spouse abuse is not inclusive of the many abused women who may not be married to their abusive partners.

Emotional Maltreatment   Psychological abuse of women includes repeated verbal assault, for example, threats, name calling, put-downs, and other deprecating remarks, as well as tactics used by the batterer to control and constrict the woman's movement and behavior. Batterers use emotional maltreatment to wear down the woman and isolate her from others so as to subordinate and dominate her in the relationship.

While domestic violence almost always includes the psychological intimidation and abuse of the partner, psychological abuse may or may not include physical assault.

Marital Conflict   Verbal disagreements that range from subtle differences in opinion to heated arguments between married partners. There are several important differences between marital conflict and domestic violence. The first is that marital conflict is limited to verbal interaction, whereas domestic violence includes verbal, as well as mild and/or severe physical assault. Second, domestic violence is distinguished by the psychological maltreatment of the woman with the aim of controlling her actions and behaviors. Other important differences are that domestic violence spans the range of the intimate relationships and can include the actions of couples who are married, cohabiting, separated, or divorced.

Posttraumatic Stress Disorder (PTSD)   A psychiatric diagnosis consisting of behaviors in evidence at least 3 months after witnessing or experiencing extremely distressing events. In this context, physical assault by an intimate partner may result in trauma reactions lasting beyond the violence events themselves. PTSD criteria include having a strong, negative reaction to the event, having nightmares and flashbacks of the event, avoiding people or places associated with the event, and physiological arousal in response to remembering the event. In order to qualify for the PTSD diagnosis, behavioral reactions must be tied to the specific traumatizing event and not reported as general stress symptoms. Delayed onset PTSD occurs when symptoms first manifest themselves at least

6 months following the event. Both battered women and their children who witness the violence can have PTSD symptoms.

Primary, Secondary, and Tertiary Prevention
Public health efforts that address identified problems on the societal level are called primary preventions. Thus, primary prevention against woman abuse would include programs and initiatives designed to change attitudes and behaviors that lead to and support violence against women. Secondary prevention refers to programs designed to help people considered to be at-risk for the identified problem. Secondary prevention against woman abuse would include programs to assist children of battered women, dating violence prevention programs, and educational efforts aimed at teaching social skills to children in the hopes of changing deleterious patterns of interacting with others. Tertiary prevention is reserved for those remedial efforts created to treat individuals after the abuse and/ or harm has been perpetrated. Such interventions are usually referred to as treatment or therapy.

DOMESTIC VIOLENCE is now considered to be a serious public health problem, because one woman is battered every 15 seconds in the United States. The number of emergency room visits by battered women exceeds those caused by accidents and rape, and many battered women are killed by their abusers. Woman abuse refers to the physical and psychological maltreatment of a woman by a partner, usually in the context of an ongoing or recently terminated intimate relationship. Physical abuse to the woman is usually accompanied by acts designed to control her behavior and to intimidate her. These can include humiliating, shaming, threatening, coercing, isolating, and otherwise dominating the woman in order to establish her subordination within the relationship. For most batterers, the acts of physical assault are infrequent. However, verbal abuse, for example, threats to kill or to injure the woman, can have similar devastating effects, particularly for women who have been traumatized by previous assaults.

We know from national surveys that at least 3.3 million children live in homes where the mother is being abused. While children exposed to the battering of their mothers were once considered to be the "unintended victims" of domestic violence, more recent formulations have described woman abuse as also abu-

sive to any child who watches these traumatic events. In addition, many children of battered women are themselves at-risk for abuse and serious injury during a battering incident. Domestic violence is a crime, a social problem, a public health epidemic, and a political issue in this country. Thus, efforts to intervene and to prevent domestic violence take many forms.

I. INTERVENTIONS FOR MEN WHO BATTER

A. Who Are the Batterers?

There is currently considerable debate in the research literature as to whether and how abuse is transmitted from one generation to the next. Retrospective studies have found high rates of transmission; upward of 60% of abusive parents or partner-abusers report having been abused themselves during their childhood. On the other hand, prospective studies have found rates between 18 and 40%. The distinction appears to be that a large majority of currently abusive parents or partners were abused as children, but a lower percentage of abused children grow up to be abusers. In addition, some initial research has indicated that boys who lived in families with violence (either spouse or child abuse) are more likely than are girls to be involved in violent dating relationships as adolescents. Other contextual variables may add to the risk, for example, living in a community with high rates of interpersonal violence, high levels of exposure to violence against women in movies and media, and low arrest and conviction rates of batterers. Although there are clearly other factors that influence whether or not an abused child will be involved in abusive relationships as an adult, the overall evidence shows that the childhood experience of abuse is an important risk factor for problems in relationships in adolescence and adulthood.

The results of studies of the typologies of batterers generally agree on at least three subtypes based on their violent behavior, the family history, as well as the personality characteristics and disorders of the batterer. First are the family-only batterers who show the least severe levels of emotional abuse and violence to their partner. This group of men is least likely to be violent outside the home, is less psychologically abusive, is more likely to report being satisfied in their marriages, and is less likely to have a history of being abused as children than other types of batterers. Substance abuse is associated with their violence only about half of the time. Within-family abusers do not appear to have clinical levels of depression or anger, but do appear to be jealous and to minimize their violent behavior. Approximately half of all batterers who enter treatment programs match the description of the family-only batterer.

The second categorical dimension is the pan-violent or antisocial batterer. Approximately one-fourth of batterers in treatment programs fit this description. Generally, pan-violent batterers have the highest rates of severe physical assault to their partners and are most likely to behave in violent ways in settings outside of the family. Not surprisingly, they have high rates of substance abuse, arrest, and involvement with the legal system. They are likely to have been severely abused as children and show only moderate levels of marital satisfaction, anger, and depression. Yet they are most likely to score high on antisocial personality disorder or psychopathy. That is, they are dominating and bullying, do not feel guilty about their abusive behavior, and lack empathy toward the victim.

The third type are dysphoric or have borderline personality disorders. This group is depressed, psychologically distressed, and emotionally volatile. They engage in moderate to severe levels of psychological and sexual abuse, as well as physical violence toward their partners. They are likely to be dependent on the woman and suspicious of her activities and motives. Intense jealousy characterizes these men. Approximately one-fourth of those who enter treatment are personality-disordered batterers.

Substance abuse may accompany battering, may precede battering, or may not be involved at all. We know that approximately half of all abuse incidents involve the use or abuse of drugs or alcohol but that the two are not inextricably linked. [*See* SUBSTANCE ABUSE.]

B. Range of Programs and Underlying Theoretical Assumptions

The best intervention programs for batterers are those that take a comprehensive and coordinated approach to the problem. That is, communities that offer treatment programs that are tied to the police and judicial systems, as well as to programs that offer services to the victims of abuse, are better able to monitor the progress of the offender from initial arrest through several years of treatment than are services that focus on only one part of the problem. Some communities have antiviolence education campaigns, school-based antiviolence programs, mandatory arrest policies, and judges and probation officers who are sophisticated about the dynamics and patterns of abusers. Clearly, the strong and immediate response of professionals to domestic violence plays a part in reducing the chances that such violence in families will happen again. Psychoeducational intervention programs designed to stop the batterer's violent behavior take a number of forms. Many programs use a combination of strategies, but the unique properties of different types of programs will be explained. [*See* COMMUNITY MENTAL HEALTH.]

Programs that rely on a behavioral learning approach first identify factors that reinforce and maintain the abuser's behavior toward the woman. These behaviors typically include controlling her access to money and resources, monitoring her behavior when outside the home, restricting access to family and friends, verbal abuse aimed at undermining her sense of competence, and, of course, physical assault to reinforce the other forms of intimidation. Hence, in addition to the physical assault, the batterers' behaviors that serve to control and to limit the woman are the focus of treatment. Behavioral programs for batterers are typically group programs that use skills training to teach alternative behaviors. A prerequisite for most programs is to have the abuser take responsibility for his actions and to not blame the woman for his abusive behavior. By focusing on the behavior of the batterer, rather than on his explanations for events, behavioral programs seek to force recognition that the abuser is ultimately responsible for the violence.

Somewhat akin are programs that take a cognitive restructuring approach and recognize that cognitions or thinking processes play an important role in the development of abusive behavior. Many researchers have described cognitive-behavioral models designed to focus on skills training and attitude change. These programs are considered suitable for antisocial and generally violent batterers, in addition to the other batterer types. The assumptions of this model of treatment are that batterers who have been victimized during their childhoods, who hold rigid stereotypes about women, and who have poor social skills need direct teaching and education, rather than interventions that only require the ability to build trust and develop relationships with group leaders and other group members. Men who lacked adequate role models as children may not have learned appropriate interpersonal skills and may continue to rely on distorted cognitions and inappropriate problem-solving techniques in their relationships as adults. Without intervention, these men will continue destructive and hurtful patterns of interacting with the important people in their lives.

Cognitive-behavioral groups typically have 6 to 10 participants, and one or two leaders. They use a teaching and training format that may include homework and specific lessons each week. Cognitive-behavioral practices such as the rehearsal of new thoughts and behavior are standard fare. For example, participants learn to identify and to reinterpret their reactions to stressful events and to think differently about appropriate responses. There is a weekly emphasis on improving communication, building cognitive skills, and consciousness-raising about men's attitudes toward women's roles and violence against women.

Abusive and controlling behaviors toward a partner are reported each week in the group session. With the help of the group leaders, batterers can be confronted about their illogical thinking and reinforced when they take responsibility for their behavior and make a change toward more appropriate ways of relating to the women in their lives. Cognitive-behavioral groups typically discuss managing and expressing anger at women, they discuss alternative ways to express anger and other negative emotions, and they learn to respect the rights and wishes of others, including wives or partners and their children. Change is achieved through feedback, reinforcement from the group, as well as from social learning or modeling one's behavior on other members and leaders. [See BEHAVIOR THERAPY; COGNITIVE THERAPY.]

Another type of program employs relationship-based interventions and is considered to be most appropriate for batterers who experienced trauma during childhood. Psychodynamic theory is used to explain the ways in which the abuser's current behavior is the result of efforts to cope with past experiences of witnessing violence or being abused. It is thought that some men, in their efforts to overcome feeling inadequate and powerless in relationships as a child, have identified with the perpetrator, or currently try to gain control over traumatic memories by venting anger and behaving aggressively. The process-

psychodynamic treatment model is focused on revisiting past relationships in order to work through and overcome the trauma in a supportive group setting. [See PSYCHOANALYSIS.]

These groups are not structured with a teaching agenda but rather they allow each participant the chance to explore the ways in which early abusive experiences have led to unhealthy patterns in relationships today. By uncovering past trauma and discussing it in a supportive group setting, the batterer can then realize the ways in which current violent behavior is an attempt to control past abuse and feelings of inadequacy related to the trauma. The goal is for men to be able to respect and to have empathy for others after having insights and empathy for themselves as children. The relationships of group members to the leaders and to one another are salient here and provide the support needed for this type of self-exploration. This is a relatively new approach to treating batterers and, thus far, it is not widely used.

C. Current Issues in Interventions for Men

1. Individual versus Group Therapy

A variety of treatment modalities exists for most types of psychological and behavioral problems, but group therapy is considered the treatment of choice for abusive men. Group sessions can range from 6 to 32 weeks in design. While individual therapy can focus on the behavioral, psychodynamic, or the cognitive methods described above, most experts in this field consider group therapy to be the most effective. There are several reasons. First, there are distinct benefits in discussing abusive behavior in front of other abusers. Many batterers are in denial about their own abusive behavior yet are able to identify violent behavior in other people. Thus, the group can be used to help break through an individual member's denial of his negative attitudes, or abuse toward his partner. Here the culture of violence is challenged by the group. Second, men can find comfort and support when they discover that others like them have had similarly difficult experiences during childhood, and/or suffer from the same feelings of frustration in dealing with the stress and the women in their lives. Group leaders also serve as living models of nonviolent men who are sensitive to their own and other peoples' needs.

2. Is Couples' Treatment Safe?

There is considerable debate in the field as to whether it is ever acceptable to treat a batterer and abused woman together as a couple. The underlying assumptions of couples' therapy are that both parties are able to participate fully in the treatment, that there are no power differentials supported by an external system, and that each person is free to discuss issues of importance to him- or herself and to the couple. However, when one partner is being abused and dominated by the other, these assumptions are often violated. That is, battered women may not be free to participate fully in the treatment, to disclose their opinions, or to report on the behavior of the abuser. Battered women know that there are serious and often severe consequences for revealing the abuse—they may be reprimanded, beaten, or even killed by their partner. We know from research studies that battered women who go to emergency rooms do not often report on the abuse when asked about it in the presence of the abuser. Similarly, battered women may not be free to discuss the most important and urgent issues in their lives (e.g., their victimization) in couples treatment.

Psychologists have argued that, by treating the couple, the focus of the problems may shift to the interactions between batterer and victim, thus deflecting the batterer's responsibility for his abusive behavior onto features of the woman or of the couple. Obviously, many batterers would prefer to engage in couples' treatment where their actions would be considered as part of a system that includes the personality of the battered woman, her reactions to the violence, and her behavior that could be used to justify the abuse. Batterers regularly use denial and they blame the victim for her plight. The bottom line, however, is that the abuser alone is responsible for his violent behavior and until he receives non-couples' treatment to change his behavior, there is little that can be accomplished in the couples' treatment setting. Given the physical and emotional consequences to the woman, couples' treatment is considered by many to be completely safe only after the batterer has successfully completed an intervention program specifically designed to stop his violence.

Some therapists who endorse couples' treatment for domestic violence argue that not all physical abuse is severe or frequent, that not all violence is the sole responsibility of the abuser, and that battered women want to remain in their relationships, despite the risks

to themselves. Yet many therapists may not be familiar with the dynamics of abusive relationships, may minimize the danger to the woman, and may see battering as an exaggerated form of marital conflict. Just knowing that the woman may be threatened with harm or may be harmed as a result of her participation in couples' treatment renders it particularly risky. Still, we know that when a woman is battered, the physical assault is but one of many forms of domination and control exerted by her partner. Nonetheless, once the batterer has completed a group intervention program, couples' treatment may be appropriate if the therapist has a firm grasp of the dynamics of domestic violence and is vigilant in monitoring the abuser's behavior. [*See* COUPLES THERAPY.]

D. Efficacy of Treatment

Studies of the effectiveness of treatment programs for men who batter show inconsistent results and have many problems. Even so, there is preliminary evidence that some forms of treatment work to reduce recidivism, or additional assaults, for some men when they stay in therapy. More recent studies have tried to sort out which qualities of particular programs are helpful, and for which men various types of programs are best suited.

1. Study Design and Criterion for Success

It is difficult to compare studies because they often measure different things. For example, some treatment programs are based on changing behavior, others on changing thinking, and still others rely on success in exploring childhood trauma. All programs for men work to stop the violence, to change attitudes about women, and in many, to increase the man's feelings of adequacy and reduce his level of anger. Success has traditionally been predicated on whether the program is effective in stopping the violence. Studies currently underway also include outcomes such as reducing the amount of sexual abuse and/or emotional maltreatment, eliminating the woman's fear, and reducing concomitant abuse of the children.

Given the above qualifiers, we can say that there are preliminary findings that some treatment is better than no treatment in reducing violence rates. In well-controlled studies, that is studies that use random assignment to treatment groups, outcomes varied not by the kind of treatment group but by the type of batterer in a particular group. In 1996, Saunders found that the cognitive-behavioral treatment was more effective for generally violent/antisocial batterers than for other types and that process-psychodynamic treatment was more successful for the dependent batterers than for other types. In each group less than half of the participants were violent 2 years following treatment. There is no evidence that programs that treat couples are effective in stopping the violence or are better than those that treat groups of men. Similarly, we have no evidence that individual treatment is more or less effective than group intervention programs.

2. Rates of Retention and Recidivism

A major problem with samples in research studies includes subject attrition, or dropping out of the research program before the end of the study. We do know that batterers who drop out of treatment are more likely to be young, to have substance abuse problems, and to have a longer history of abuse. Yet some offenders are so violent as to be considered untreatable and thus are not referred for intervention by courts, probation officers, or community agencies. They are seldom included in treatment outcome studies. In addition, women may not want to participate initially or to continue in research studies for a number of reasons, including deciding to return to the abuser, lack of interest, or out of fear for their safety.

3. Current Issues in Assessment

In doing program evaluation research it is essential to have more than one source of information about the abuser's behavior. Thus, multimethod studies that include police reports and arrest records, reports from the abusers and the women they assault, as well documentation of injuries from hospitals and doctors, are preferred. In addition, studies that have an extended posttreatment evaluation are more convincing as they give more evidence that the intervention has had a lasting effect. For example, some of the early outcome studies relied on only a 6-month period to test whether the batterer had changed his pattern of behavior. Some studies relied on the batterer's report of the amount of his violence. More recent studies have followed batterers for 2 to 4 years and beyond and have relied on reports from several sources. Finally, assessment of a range of batterer behaviors should be included in efforts to decide whether or not change

has occurred. Studies can go beyond documenting re-arrest (which essentially counts only about one-tenth of physical assaults), to include incidents of stalking, harassment, violating protection orders, as well as rates of psychological maltreatment of the woman.

II. INTERVENTIONS FOR BATTERED WOMEN

A. Impact of Battering on the Woman

Battered women are at high-risk for physical and psychological problems directly related to the violence and to the emotional abuse that they have endured. Battering by an intimate partner is considered to be the primary cause of injury to women ages 15 to 44. Some battered women may suffer contusions, bruises, or broken bones as a result of assault or they may be killed by their assailant. Although the vast majority of battered women do not seek treatment for their injuries, those who do use medical facilities do so for only the most severe injuries and often not after the first incident of abuse.

Many battered women are clinically depressed. They are more likely to have major depressive episodes than women with serious relationship problems that do not include violence. Depression and low self-esteem, in turn, influence the woman's coping, as she may become less active and more avoidant as she feels a loss of personal control. Recall that batterers strive to take control away from the woman so as to more easily dominate her. Several studies of battered women in shelters report that approximately 40 to 60% experience posttraumatic stress disorder related to the threats to their life, repeated physical assaults, and the extent and severity of abuse. However, with more time out of the abusive relationship, the rates of PTSD decrease, depression abates, and women can be helped to feel a sense of control over their lives once more. [See DEPRESSION.]

B. Shelter-Based Programs

1. Goals and Range of Services

The battered women's movement started in the 1970s when the first shelters for women and children were created. Today there are more than 1300 shelters and thousands of service programs in the United States; most are overcrowded and have waiting lists. The immediate goal of most shelters is to provide safety to the woman. Referral for emergency medical care is often provided for those who arrive with injuries. Additional goals including providing legal advocacy for women, help in finding jobs, and social services. Many shelters offer support in the form of group programs and individual advocacy for women and some provide programs for their children. Ultimately, battered women need to find affordable shelter and ways to support themselves should they elect to leave the batterer for good.

2. Support Groups for Battered Women

The primary goals of most support groups are keeping the woman safe from harm and providing education about the dynamics of woman abuse. In addition, support groups are often the source of information about a range of topics from effective childcare methods to obtaining housing. The main topic of conversation in support groups is the abuse that the women have endured. For those who have left the abuser for the first time, or those who have never told anyone about their suffering, it is empowering and eye-opening to hear quite similar stories from other women with a range of educational, economic, and cultural backgrounds. Only women with shared experiences can resonate so strongly to one another's stories. Thus, the chief contribution of support groups within shelters is to provide a format for women to share and to explore what they have endured, and to then get help in becoming safe and avoiding the abuse. [*See* SUPPORT GROUPS.]

3. Shelter Parenting Groups

When battered women elect to come to a shelter, they are often escaping from a severe assault, leaving in the middle of the night, and taking their children and possessions with them to an unknown place. This stream of events often leaves the women and children confused, anxious, and eventually angry. Yet the women must assume complete control over their children, at a time when they may feel least up to the task. In addition, children who have been traumatized by violence are often agitated and aggressive, making the mother's job even harder. The problem is further compounded by having so many children in the same small space. Thus, support for the development of parenting skills

is routinely provided in battered women's shelters. These groups focus on behavior management techniques, on identifying children's feelings, and on children's developmental needs.

4. Substance Abuse

There is currently a debate about whether some women are beaten because their own substance abuse renders them vulnerable to attack or whether they self-medicate in response to being abused over a period of years. These may be two distinct groups of women. Either way, many abused women suffer from addiction to drugs or alcohol. Recent studies have shown that a far greater percentage of substance-abusing battered women did not use or abuse substances before the start of the battering. Some women have reported that the batterer encouraged them to drink or to use drugs. Others have noted that the batterer forced them to use alcohol or drugs along with him. Nonetheless, many shelters address the issues of drug and alcohol dependency in their efforts to help battered women survive. These efforts can take the form of classes, support groups, or transportation to existing programs in the community.

5. Advocacy and Placement

Individual advocacy is an important part of most shelter programs as many battered women must decide whether to file charges, whether to stay out of the abusive relationship, whether to get a job, an apartment, or food stamps—all while recovering from the most traumatic events in their lives. Most battered women face a number of adjustments that require action immediately following assault. Recall, however, that, for some women, the healing process often brings with it renewed energy, less depression, and release from debilitating fears and nightmares associated with the abuse. Yet for others, the healing process takes more time. Many abused women are left with PTSD symptoms and a realistic fear of re-assault for years after separating from the batterer.

C. Coordinated Community Response

The battered women's movement has involved thousands of grass-roots workers and professionals, often battered women themselves, in efforts to combat violence against women. Most cities now have emergency hotlines, information directories, advocacy programs, and victim services. Many shelters and community groups work with law enforcement agencies, judges, and social service agencies to coordinate services from the time of the first emergency call to sentencing, treatment, and follow-up. In many states, volunteers and shelter workers have fought for legislation such as mandatory arrest laws and antistalking laws. The National Coalition Against Domestic Violence was established in 1978 to coordinate the efforts of workers from around the country and to disseminate information on various aspects of domestic violence.

1. Hospital/Emergency Room Interventions

Efforts are underway nationwide to train emergency room staff and medical students in the identification and treatment of violence against women. Currently, few medical schools spend more than a few minutes on evaluating and treating women for abuse injury. Studies of hospital clinics and emergency rooms reveal that many physicians do not recognize the signs of abuse and few ever ask the woman whether she is in a violent relationship or whether her injuries are the result of interpersonal conflict. When the batterer does accompany the woman to the ER oftentimes he may not be separated from the woman when she is questioned about her injuries. Clearly, policies aimed at educating emergency room personnel are needed to protect abused women and to facilitate the prosecution of the abuser. Just as in the case of rape, when a woman's claim of abuse is backed up by medical reports and photographs of her injuries, the case will be stronger in court. Many feminists argue that woman abuse will stop in this country only after men in positions of authority are willing to take a zero-tolerance stand against such violence. This will take primary prevention programs. Thus, coordinated efforts are underway in some communities to train police, physicians, prosecutors, and judges to reduce their tolerance for violence against women.

2. Community Support Groups for Women

Many communities offer free drop-in groups for battered women that have the same goals as those run within a shelter. These groups provide support on an as-needed basis and rely mostly on education, referral to services, and the chance to speak with other women about their experiences. The group leaders may be volunteers, formerly battered women and/or professionals, and the number of participants varies from week to week. Many women go to drop-in groups as a first step in getting help. Thus, they differ from shelter groups in that some women may still reside with their partner, while others may be in the process of leaving, may have already left, or may have returned. Once again, the important contribution of drop-in groups is the opportunity to listen to other women with shared experiences. Most often community drop-in groups are supported and run as part of the shelter program. Very few groups are provided by established clinical settings, such as mental health clinics, social service agencies, or private practice settings.

Some communities do provide longer term, or ongoing, clinical intervention groups for battered women. These are distinguished from drop-in groups by the stability of the group, for example, the same women return each week, and often by the presence of professionally trained group leaders such as social workers or psychologists. Ongoing groups take many forms and can last anywhere from several weeks to several years. Some programs are free, while others charge a nominal fee.

One program which adopts a feminist-ecological model in efforts to help women to overcome the effects of battering on their lives was created in 1985 by Ginette Larouche in Quebec, Canada. Feminists believe that woman abuse originates in a male-dominated society and that the responsibility for ending the violence rests with the community. The aims of the feminist model are to denounce woman abuse, to return responsibility for violence to the man, as opposed to the victim, and to focus on counterbalancing the negative consequences to the woman.

These groups take a social and psycho-educational approach that includes listening to the woman and providing active support, as well as clarification and education designed to explode myths perpetrated by the abuser. For example, many women come to believe that they are the cause of the violence against them, as batterers often cite small infractions by the woman as the reason for their violent behavior. Over time, some battered women come to believe the abuser and work diligently to avoid setting off a confrontation. These efforts are seldom successful and lead to low self-esteem, to self-blame, and to guilt, as well as to the risk of injury. Support groups provide battered women with information about their rights, available resources, and they empower women to endorse a broader range of gender roles. Along the way, it is hoped that tension is reduced, support is provided for reducing victim behaviors, and the woman's sense of autonomy is restored.

3. Individual Treatment

The exact number of battered women who receive individual therapy for their problems is unknown. Clearly, one difference in who obtains individual treatment is socioeconomic status. The ability to pay is associated with private therapy, although some community mental health centers accept low-fee clients that may include battered women. It is interesting to note that the socioeconomic status of women who are abused usually does not reflect the total household income. Many battered women are denied access to money and so must rely on public services. An additional constraint is that of using insurance to obtain treatment. Often insurance companies reimburse the account holder, who is not atypically the abuser. Efforts to keep treatment information confidential and away from the spouse might prove unsuccessful and thus are not worth the risk to some battered women.

Women enter individual therapy for a number of reasons, most often having to do with relationships and emotional disturbances such as depression. Battered women who are able to find a supportive therapist, one who understands the dynamics of woman abuse, can build the therapeutic, bridging relationship needed to explore their current lives.

D. What Works and Why

One of the most frequently heard complaints of care providers and shelter workers is that, despite their efforts, so many battered women elect to return to their abuser. Yet it is essential to note here that most battered women eventually DO leave their abusive partners for good. In one study, 67% eventually separated from or divorced an abusive partner and did not return.

Studies of the efficacy of treatment and intervention programs for battered women are few. The goals of treatment for women usually do not focus on stopping the violence but rather on the degree to which the woman is empowered, has increased her self-esteem, has reduced her depression, and has heightened her

sense of autonomy. Overall results indicate that those women who receive treatment improve more than those who receive no treatment.

Studies of the correlates of violence and women's success at leaving the abuser show that both objective and subjective aspects of the woman's life are important to consider. Objectively, battered women cite fear, lack of money, unemployment, and other economic factors as reasons for returning to the abuser. Subjectively, the loss of friends, loss of intimacy with the batterer, loneliness, facing the anger of other relatives, or a misplaced sense of responsibility for the dysfunction in their relationships are the interpersonal reasons given by battered women for not leaving the abuser. However, we know that many battered women are at highest risk for injury or even death when the batterer becomes convinced that the relationship is over. Thus, treatment programs that address these concerns are most likely to lead to success.

How abuse is treated shows that, for many women, community resources are absent. Without help, many battered women cannot leave the abuser. For example, few men who abuse their wives are arrested and convicted of this crime. In most communities, if the batterer had assaulted someone outside the home, the chances that he would be arrested are much greater than if he elected to assault his partner. Many battered women do not have an extended family who will support them, they do not have police who will come to the home and arrest the perpetrator of violence, they do not have shelters with room for them, they do not have judges who will issue and then enforce restraining orders, and they do not have access to affordable housing, and to treatment for themselves or their children. Programs should evaluate and then address the woman's help-seeking history as part of the treatment she receives.

Just as there are different typologies of battering men, battered women's experiences vary as well. Researchers have shown that the varieties of abuse experienced by the woman are related to her ability to leave the abuser. One-third of the battered women most likely to leave and to stay out have partners who are unstable, explosive, and severely abusive. About one-fifth are rarely physically abused, but experience severe emotional abuse. These women are most likely to have a stable relationship with the abuser and are most likely to stay. Another one-fifth have extensive and chronic abuse but may leave and return several times before being able to successfully live apart from the abuser. Approximately 10% leave only when the abuser starts to abuse the children as well. Those who are least likely to leave, who repeatedly go back to the perpetrator despite severe physical violence, are most likely to have a family history of violence, to have been abused themselves as children, and to think that violence is inescapable and expected. Programs to help battered women could take these typologies into account and tailor their services to the needs of the individual woman. In the future, outcome studies may include the entire community as the sample, to see whether education efforts have had an impact on attitude change, whether there have been fewer repeat offenders, whether arrest rates have increased, and whether the number of women who are abused by a partner each year has decreased.

III. PREVENTIVE INTERVENTIONS FOR CHILDREN EXPOSED TO DOMESTIC VIOLENCE

A. Children's Reactions to Witnessing Domestic Violence

Children whose mothers have been physically and emotionally abused are considered victims of family violence. We know from research studies that individual children respond differently to the violence, from those who evidence major psychological disorders and posttraumatic stress symptoms, to those who appear resilient and unaffected by the trauma. Approximately 40 to 60% of children who witness the abuse of their mothers are above the clinical cutoff level on measures of mood and behaviors. That is, they are in need of clinical treatment for their anxiety, depression, and aggressive behavior. In one study, more than half of the children who witnessed domestic violence had symptoms of posttraumatic stress, and 13% qualified for a full Posttraumatic Stress Disorder (PTSD) diagnosis—the diagnosis first given to returning combat veterans who showed extreme stress reactions to the atrocities witnessed during war.

Most children who observe violence in the family are worried and concerned about the behavior of their father and the welfare of their mother relative to children who have not observed such violence. Many of these children feel anxious because they harbor a ter-

rible family secret—one that they often are unable to share with friends. In this instance, they may avoid or withdraw from social contacts. Other children may behave aggressively with peers and find themselves rejected by others, socially neglected, or avoided. Without some intervention, these lessons and reactions can interfere with a child's social and emotional development. Yet there is often little opportunity for children to discuss their perceptions, worries, and fears, or to get new information. [See CHILDHOOD STRESS; POSTTRAUMATIC STRESS.]

B. Theoretical Assumptions of Programs for Children

Social learning theory tells us that children learn about violence and aggressive tactics as a result of being exposed to the abuse of their mothers. In the process children develop attitudes about violence, and learn lessons about power in relationships. Children are highly likely to believe that at least some of the blame for the parents' conflicts resides within themselves. In some families, the children are directly blamed for the fighting in the family. As children get older, they are much more capable of seeing alternative explanations as causes for the events happening around them. However, children raised in violent families may either attempt to reject the aggressive behavior of the adults in their family, or they may attempt to wholly incorporate this aggressive behavior. Both approaches are problematic. For most children, these conflictual role models hamper the child's efforts to move forward with a clear sense of competence.

Children's reaction to the violence is mediated by their level of cognitive development. Preschool-age children are considered to be egocentric. That is, they understand the world in terms of themselves. Thus, younger children are more likely to blame themselves for their parents' problems and/or to believe many of the threats made by the batterer. They are often frightened yet unable to discuss what is happening. Most children aged 6 to 12 understand that one person may have different feelings than another in response to different situations or events. In terms of understanding domestic violence, the school-age child is able to imagine various causes for the violence. In particular, the child can see the causes of domestic violence as beyond those immediately connected with her- or himself. The child also is able to play out or imagine other possibilities or outcomes to domestic conflict. [*See* Aggression.]

C. Programs for Preschoolers

While many communities have programs designed to aid and support battered women and to treat the batterers, the development of children's programs lags far behind. In many communities there are simply no services available for children of abused women. When services do exist, they often take the form of drop-in groups in shelters. Programs designed for younger children most often have the goals of providing support and building self-esteem. For reasons stated above, younger children are less cognitively mature, and hence, less able to consider and to process the distressing events in their family. Yet they are no less affected by these events. We know from the few research studies on preschool-age children of battered women that they are more likely to have difficulty modulating negative emotions and solving problems in social situations than children who have not been exposed to such abuse. Therefore, programs that emphasize the role-modeling of appropriate social interaction may be very helpful to these children.

It is generally believed that the best way to help young children is to help their mothers. Thus, programs that focus on honing and developing better parenting skills, in addition to keeping the mother safe, indirectly serve to help the young child. Programs that involve both the mother and the child may be the most successful of all, as they focus on interaction and provide an opportunity to enhance and to support parenting efforts. However, many battered women need to have their own support before they can attend to the needs of their youngest children. In this case, child care and groups for preschool children are necessary. Also, many of the youngest children of battered women are often cared for by their older siblings. Efforts to include relief and skill building for these older children may be additional and appropriate ways to provide for the preschool-age child's needs. [*See* Parenting.]

D. Programs for Children Ages 6 to 12

The strategy most widely recommended for working with children of abused mothers is the small group format. These groups can be either ongoing, with the same children meeting over a set period of time, or drop-in, where the participants vary from week to week. Drop-in groups are typically found in shelters whereas ongoing groups for children are best suited for children in the community. Children who come to shelters following the abuse of their mothers are in need of an accepting environment, and of the self-esteem-enhancing activities usually provided by drop-in groups. It is a time when children need to recover and receive support in mastering their anxiety, but not to uncover their deepest fears and worries about the violence in their lives.

Before children can be expected to discuss the trauma in their lives, it is necessary to build trusting relationships. When these relationships are strong, they facilitate disclosure and the child's acceptance of the group leader's support. Thus, ongoing groups that build relationships both with the group leader and with the other group members are considered the most appropriate intervention strategy either before or after the child's stay in a shelter. Efforts by group leaders and therapists to disconfirm negative stereotypes and distorted expectations about family and gender roles focus on experiential exercises, such as those described below for the children in one intervention group program. Strategies such as role playing or puppet play are expected to show greater changes in the children's understanding of the experience of domestic violence over strategies using direct teaching, dialogue, or discussion alone.

"The Kids' Club: A Preventive Intervention Group Program for Children of Battered Women" is a time limited, 10-week clinical program designed by Sandra Graham-Bermann in 1992. This intervention is directed at three levels. The goal at the cognitive level is to improve the child's knowledge base about family violence and conflict resolution. By expressing and identifying feelings, fears and worries associated with fighting in the family, children learn that others their age have similar, negative reactions to the violence. Discussions of safety planning teach children different ways of responding to violence. The goal at the social level is to build skills and to change behavior in interaction with others. Here, discussions of gender roles and practicing alternative problem-solving strategies provide a platform for discussing social behavior and expectations. At the relationship level the focus is on building trust and gaining support from both the group and the group leaders. Relationships with peers in the group are equally important in that there is a special quality of relief and comfort in being with other children who share the "secret" of domestic violence in their own families. This atmosphere allows children to feel less stigmatized and less alone in their distress, to exchange information and impressions, and to validate their feelings of outrage and sadness.

Children between the ages of 6 and 12 are accepted into two groups based on their age. They may or may not be living with the batterer. Each group is led by two therapists who receive weekly supervision of their work. Here, group leaders are master's-level or doctoral-level clinical psychologists and social workers. The curriculum helps children to discuss a specific aspect of domestic violence and how it affects their lives each week, although there is no pressure for children to participate or to disclose anything about themselves or their families. In fact, all activities are designed to use displacement. For example, group leaders seek the child's thoughts, referring to children as "experts on what most kids really think," thus making it both safe and compelling for the child to give his or her advice.

As a result of participating in the group, it is hoped that children learn that the violence between parents is not their fault, that they have a right to feel angry at the perpetrators of the violence, and even at their mothers, and that they can employ a broader range of conflict resolution skills, along with the understanding that physical aggression is not an acceptable way of coping with family stress and conflict.

E. Parenting Support and Education Programs

One program designed specifically to address the needs of battered women through empowering them as parents was designed in 1994 by Graham-Bermann and Levendosky. Many battered women do not identify their own needs and are reluctant to seek help for themselves, but are often quite worried about their children. On the other hand, many battered women cite the children's needs as a primary reason for staying with the abuser. Specifically, the women want to have a family, think it is important for children to have a father, and worry about whether they could manage raising children alone. When society reinforces the importance of having a man as the head of the family, many battered women feel caught in the bind of whether an abusive father is better than no father at all. Further, it is often difficult for women as

mothers to claim power and to take control of their families. Battered women often struggle with asserting themselves as mothers and in handling aggression by their children.

The parenting support program provides basic education about domestic violence, advocacy for women to obtain services in the community, and a support group where the woman can share and process issues related to both the violence and to parenting children under these most difficult family circumstances. Two trained clinicians (social workers or clinical psychologists) serve as leaders for each group of approximately five to eight women. It is essential that the group leaders receive weekly supervision for their work, in order to reduce the potential for secondary traumatization from the many vivid and horrific stories that are heard each week.

The groups begin with each woman telling her story, including her present circumstances and concerns. A list of worries about children and concerns about parenting is kept. Each session emphasizes both the emotional and physical abuse as well as child-rearing issues. Along the way, these parenting topics are addressed—discipline and controlling negative behavior in children, mothers' worries and fears about their children, the impact of woman abuse on the child, understanding children's developmental needs, having fun with children, helping children to identify emotions, and communication in the mother–child relationship. Group leaders make referrals as needed to shelters, lawyers, doctors, and other advocates and community agencies that provide support for battered women.

This program is designed to serve only as a starting point for battered women to think about issues associated with domestic violence and raising healthy children. The aim is not to cover all that can be learned about any subject in a few hours' time, but to provide an opportunity for the women to discover their shared concerns and to learn new strategies for dealing with the very real problems presented by their children. In this way it is hoped that battered women may experience a sense of empowerment as they become more effective mothers to their children.

F. Assessment of Intervention Efficacy

While the best programs are firmly grounded in theory and take into account the results of previous research on children exposed to domestic violence, we know little about whether these programs are effective and for which children they are most effective. Some of the risk variables that should be considered are the duration of the abuse, the number of abusive partners, other stressful family and neighborhood events, the child's role in family violence, and the presence of physical abuse to the child. Protective factors may include the amount of support available to the child and the mother, as well as the response of the community to the violence. The timing of the assessment, relative to the violence events, should also be considered, as many children exposed to domestic violence do not show evidence of dysfunction at the time of assessment. These children may be either resilient or unaffected by the events, or more likely, they may show symptoms later. Finally, children whose mothers join support groups for abused women, or who remove themselves from a violent situation through separation and divorce, may be expected to fare better in treatment programs than those in families with ongoing abuse.

Some fathers successfully complete programs designed to address domestic aggression. Studies have shown a concomitant decrease in child abuse by some graduates of domestic aggression treatment programs. Thus, some children have seen a resolution to the battering, and have witnessed a parent acting in the child's interest. Other children from woman-abusing families have extensive contact with positive male adult figures, such as grandparents or teachers, who may serve as alternative role models. Efforts to test the efficacy of intervention programs for children are underway in several states, with projects funded by the National Injury Prevention Center, Centers for Disease Control in Atlanta, Georgia.

IV. PREVENTIVE INTERVENTIONS FOR ADOLESCENTS EXPOSED TO DOMESTIC VIOLENCE

A. Developmental Strengths and Needs of Adolescents

Teenagers are in an important transitional period in terms of gaining their independence and establishing their identities apart from the family, and in solidifying social relationships with friends. In addition, patterns of relating to others are formed with intimate partners during adolescence. For teens whose mothers are abused, these tasks can be complicated by the deleterious models of male and female adult behavior that they have witnessed and, perhaps, incorporated and taken as their own. Further, teenagers who have witnessed domestic violence are more likely to be depressed, to behave in antisocial ways, and to be physically aggressive and anxious than are teens from nonviolent families. In addition to the psychological scars, teenagers may be recovering from physical abuse and injury, as they are more likely to intervene in parents' fights than are younger children.

The cognitive skills of teenagers vastly exceed those of younger children. At this point, most adolescents can consider many causes for events, can think abstractly, and can entertain a range of possible outcomes to events. They are able to take a longer time perspective and to envision their futures more clearly than are younger children. At the same time, biological changes require the management and regulation of more intense emotions, such as anger and love, as well as sexual urges. Programs designed to address their needs must take into account their longer histories of coping with domestic violence, as well as the developmental tasks of establishing themselves as competent, well liked, and independent from their families.

Research studies tell us that the long-term effects of witnessing domestic violence differ for boys and for girls, with many boys at-risk for repeating violence in relationships with others outside the home. Males who have grown up around men who use power and control tactics need to learn other ways of communicating and they to develop skill in nonviolent conflict resolution. Females who have witnessed their mothers as victims of violence, or have been abused themselves, may need to develop a better understanding of themselves as competent, they may need to learn more about self-protection and about intolerance for various forms of abuse and harassment. While complicated by many developmental changes, adolescence is considered a good time to intervene, as children are forming their own intimate relationships and are beginning to put into practice the models that they have learned.

B. Domestic Violence Intervention Programs for Teenagers

The program "Promoting Healthy, Nonviolent Relationships: A Group Approach with Adolescents for the Prevention of Woman Abuse and Interpersonal Violence" was created by David Wolfe in 1994. It was based on his extensive clinical work and research with children living in abusive homes. The three main elements of the program are information dissemination, skills development, and social action learning. The program is unique as it capitalizes on adolescents' interest in forming and maintaining healthy relationships with members of the opposite sex. It takes a positive view of adolescents' development rather than the "youth as problem" approach that characterizes many other intervention programs designed for this age group. Finally, the program includes the adolescents themselves in finding solutions to the broader problem of woman abuse in their community.

One-third of the program is focused on understanding gender stereotypes, attitudes toward women, and violence in intimate relationships. These concepts are placed in the context of the broader society as each adolescent seeks to expose myths and to learn the ways in which aggression against women is promulgated in the media and in the culture. Group facilitators work with questionnaires, active exercises, video presentations, and group discussion to explode myths and to get at the facts. Discussion of dating violence is included.

The second section focuses on skills development and requires change at the level of the individual. Here each participant works to improve the ways in which he or she interacts with members of the opposite sex. Males learn about noncoercive communication and listening skills, while females learn personal safety skills. Assertiveness training is geared toward empowering youth to take responsibility for their interpersonal signals and actions.

The social action part of the program actively engages group members in working together to identify and to challenge some aspect of violence in their own community. First, there is a series of exercises aimed at teaching group members about resources available to teenagers, men, and women in their community. Next, group members develop a social action or a fundraising activity in which they all participate. Examples include setting up a display about stopping sexual assault in a shopping mall and selling t-shirts to raise funds for a local battered women's shelter. In this way teenagers put their skills to use on the broader community level. Along the way they learn to respect one another and themselves, to think differently about sex roles and family roles, and to develop healthier relationships as they work together to stop violence against women.

V. PREVENTIVE INTERVENTIONS IN COMMUNITY SETTINGS

There is considerable debate in the field as to whether it is better to move intervention efforts into established institutional settings—places that have traditionally not been responsive to abused women—or to focus on community-based services. However, help is needed throughout each community. A similar debate occurs over whether volunteers or professionals are best equipped to bring the most help to battered women and their children. Yet, these labels can be misleading when they dichotomize roles. For example, they do not recognize the number of professionals who are battered women, the number of volunteers who are professionals, and the professional training of shelter workers. Further, many theorists and researchers have taken an ecological perspective and they have conceptualized the problem and hence the solutions to woman abuse on a number of levels. On the societal level primary prevention has focused on national policy to bring attention to the problem and to obtain needed funds. On the community level both professional and volunteer workers share secondary prevention initiatives to provide services and to work on prevention with children. Some of these efforts are described below.

Social skills building and violence prevention programs are now offered in many schools. They are designed to offer education to all children but are considered to be particularly useful to children exposed to violence in the home. Typically, these programs include identifying feelings associated with violence, teaching and modeling alternative problem-solving skills, and demonstrating intolerance for violence at home, at school, and in the community. By addressing the problems early on, rather than waiting until after violent patterns have been established, it is hoped that all children can be empowered to respond to violence, and that those who have witnessed violence at home can get help. Concomitantly, some schools have trained teachers and counselors how to respond to children exposed to domestic violence and how to make referrals to provide for their needs.

Police departments in some communities provide training for dealing with domestic violence, for when and how to make arrests of batterers, for identifying battered women, and for providing for the needs of both women and children in the family following a domestic assault. These training programs include educating officers about the impact of domestic violence on women and children, and teaching them how to handle the often confusing presentation of abused women when asked to file complaints about the assailant, how to inform women of their rights to protection, and how to obtain services for victims of such abuse. Some police departments have developed domestic violence units and have hired social workers and psychologists specifically trained to work with women and children before and during the court process.

In some communities police department and battered women's shelters work hand in hand to track abusers, to identify women at risk for repeated abuse, and to monitor compliance with the conditions of an abuser's probation. Such efforts are sorely needed, as studies of both the training of police officers and the attitudes they hold toward domestic violence cases show that many officers avoid these calls or handle them quickly because they feel uncomfortable dealing with these issues. However, the legal understanding of domestic violence has come a long way from early identification of this as a "family problem" to our current understanding of the social, emotional, and economic costs to individual women, to children, and to the larger community.

Similarly, the legal community has expanded its understanding of domestic violence and what is needed to provide protection to women and children. Hence, many states have enacted mandatory arrest laws and antistalking ordinances with strict penalties and sentencing guidelines. There is currently some debate as to whether mandatory arrest reduces the occurrence of domestic violence or whether it puts the woman at greater risk for abuse. In addition, the cost of arresting all batterers has been a significant burden for some communities. However, research has shown that younger abusers and those with an active criminal history were more likely to abuse after a restraining order was issued than were older and less violent men. In the future, researchers should be able to provide more sophisticated answers to these questions as they move away from gross generalizations of whether mandatory arrest works to deciding for whom it works best. Then, policies and laws can be tailored to the needs of individual perpetrators and victims to provide the most effective, safest, and economical response to domestic violence.

Innovative educational initiatives sponsored by some communities include postering in subways and on buses and using billboards and newspaper advertisements in efforts to stop violence against women. Other cities have started campaigns with easily identifiable slogans and logos, such as "zero tolerance for violence against women." In some areas businesses and other volunteer groups have worked with local shelters to sponsor communitywide events in support of stopping the violence. These efforts reflect the growing knowledge that societal attitudes that condone violence against women need to change. Challenging the culture of violence in communities is another way to protect women and to inoculate children against commiting or tolerating violence in their lives.

VI. CONCLUSIONS

Domestic violence is a serious public health problem in America with far-reaching consequences for women and children. Efforts to stop the violence have taken many forms and include diverse settings such as community shelters, schools, courts, hospitals and clinics, and research institutions.

While treatment outcome research is in its infancy, there is some preliminary evidence that certain kinds of interventions work better for particular batterer types than for others, that some offenders may not be helped by traditional interventions, and that even brief intervention programs are better than no treatment at all. Group treatment is generally preferred to individual or couples' treatment. Those batterers who drop out of treatment, and are therefore hardest to treat, are likely to be young substance abusers with a long history of violence.

Interventions for women generally take the form of shelter programs and group treatment programs. However, few communities offer interventions designed specifically to meet the needs of children exposed to domestic violence. While most battered women eventually do leave their abusive partners, those who have access to social and financial support, and who feel protected in the community and by the police, are more likely to leave.

Current efforts can be seen in communities that take an ecological or multilayered approach to the problem. That is, they offer coordinated responses to domestic violence in terms of primary, secondary, and tertiary prevention. Educational programs aimed at reducing the culture of violence against women and school-based programs that teach nonviolent problem solving and social skills are primary preventions.

Dating violence programs for teenagers and psycho-educational intervention programs for younger children exposed to domestic violence are examples of innovative secondary preventions. It is hoped that in the future communities that take the initiative in pre-empting and combating violence against women will need fewer treatment programs and police units to respond to domestic violence after it occurs.

BIBLIOGRAPHY

Buzawa, E. S., & Buzawa, C. G. (1996). *Domestic violence: The criminal justice response* (2nd Ed.). Thousand Oaks, CA: Sage Publications, Inc.

Edelson, J. L., & Eisikovits, Z. C. (Eds.) (1996). *Future interventions with battered women and their families.* Thousand Oaks, CA: Sage Publications, Inc.

Edelson, J. L., & Tolman, R. M. (1992). *Intervention for men who batter: An ecological approach.* Newbury Park, CA: Sage Publications, Inc.

Graham-Bermann, S. A. (1992). *The kids' club: A preventive intervention program for children of battered women.* Ann Arbor: University of Michigan, Department of Psychology.

Graham-Bermann, S. A., & Levendosky, A. A. (1994). *The moms' group: A parenting support and intervention program for battered women who are mothers.* Ann Arbor: University of Michigan.

Larouche, G. (1985). *A guide to intervention with battered women.* Montreal: Corporation professionnelle des travailleurs sociaux du Quebec.

Saunders, D. (1996). Cognitive-behavioral and process-psychodynamic treatments for men who batter: Interaction of abuser traits and treatment models. *Violence and Victims,* 11(4), 393–414

Dreaming

John S. Antrobus

The City College of the City University of New York

Association Learned connection between two or more items or events.

Cataplexy Sleep–waking disorder in which a waking person suddenly moves into a REM sleep-like state.

Cognition Thought.

Dreaming An imagined, visual, hallucinated event that occurs during sleep.

Frontal Eye Fields A portion of the cortex where the final decision is made about where, when, and how fast to move the eyes.

Hallucination Mental image to which one responds as though it were a perception of a real–world event. An image that is believed to be "real."

Lateral Geniculate Nucleus Group of many nuclei that link the cortex with incoming sensory and outgoing motor neurons.

Lucid Dream Dream in which the dreamer is aware that he or she is dreaming.

Mentation Thought and/or imagery. Mental events of any kind.

Neurocognition The field of study concerned with the relation of cognition to neurophysiology.

NREM Sleep Non-REM sleep: including EEG stages 2, 3, and 4.

Nuclei Clusters of neurons.

Occipital Referring to the visual portion of the cerebral cortex.

Ocular Referring to the eyes.

Parapsychology The study of events, perception, and behavior that cannot be accounted for by psychological relationships. Literally, beyond psychology.

Parietal A portion of the cortex that processes spatial information.

PET Scan Method of obtaining three-dimensional pictures of the brain and estimates of the distribution of brain metabolism. The metabolic measures estimate neural activity or information processing.

PGO *Pontine* (referring to the pons), *geniculate* (referring to the lateral geniculate), *occipital* (referring to the occipital cortex).

Polygraph A multiple-channel-writing device.

Pons A part of the brain stem, below the thalamus.

Psychophysiology The study of the relation between mind and body, or behavior and physiology.

REM Rapid eye movements.

REM sleep Stage 1 EEG marked by REMs and a

waking-like EEG, generally accompanied by more intense dreaming than NREM sleep.

Stressor An event that forces an individual to use his or her resources to adjust, protect, or otherwise respond to that event.

The dramatic, unpredictable, and often bizarre character of **DREAMING** has fascinated or frightened men and women since the beginning of written history. Although dreams are produced by the mind/brain of the dreamer, their strangeness has suggested to many people that they are produced by someone else. Until recent times, the someone else was a god or spirit of some kind. Since life is full of uncertainty, and people who have the most power have the most to lose in unpredictable situations, kings and generals routinely consulted dream interpreters prior to going to war to predict their chance of winning. Interpretations were deliberately ambiguous so that, when the war was over, the interpretation could be judged as accurate, regardless of who won. In this fashion, the business of dream interpretation was kept secure, and the faith in the divine source of the dream was unshaken. Of course, some dream interpreters, such as Joseph in the Bible, were more persuasive than others. Eventually, interpretations became codified so that certain objects in a dream were considered symbols of certain events in life, and they were compiled in dream books that are still in use today.

I. FREUD AND HIS INTERPRETATION OF DREAMS

Although we know that dreams are created by the brain of the dreamer, we are a long way from understanding precisely how that process works. Certainly, no one understands it well enough to predict what a person is going to dream about. But that does not seem to dissuade people from interpreting dreams. In his book *The Interpretation of Dreams,* Sigmund Freud, a Viennese doctor, argued that much of our thought and behavior are caused by desires and feelings about which we are completely unconscious. He believed that these unconscious thoughts could produce disorders such as the hysterical fainting spells of Victorian ladies when they were exposed to something shocking, particularly something sexual. In fact,

Freud believed that all of these unconscious thoughts were driven by sexual drives forced underground by a society that harshly repressed sexual expression. Since dreams are not under control of the conscious mind, they were, for Freud, an ideal place to observe the working of these unconscious processes. He assumed that all neurotic behavior could be attributed to unconscious processes. Unconscious processes could be understood by interpreting the dreams of the neurotic person, and once the unconscious processes were fully exposed and understood the person would be free of neurosis. Although there is little merit in this argument, it nonetheless remains today as the central strategy of orthodox psychoanalysis.

As the science of psychology began to develop, there were many who were unwilling to accept Freud's dogmatic assertion that his theory was correct and did not need to be subject to scientific test. Freud and his followers could always find an explanation for how *any* dream, indeed, any segment of a dream, was consistent with the theory. Since no one could find a way to test the theory, it became essentially a belief. One either believed or did not.

Meanwhile early cognitive psychologists were trying to find the link between dream images and objects in the everyday world. For example, waving perfume under the nose of sleeper on a hot night resulted in a dream of being on a romantic south sea island. The experimenter deduced that the perfume in the presence of the heat had aroused the sleeper's memory of stories of the south seas, and these memories, in turn, had been played out as a dream. This explanation is based on association theory which describes how objects and events with similar, as well as opposite, features tend to activate one another.

Indeed, Freud's theory of dreaming was a special kind of association theory. First, objects and events could be activated because of their previous associations with emotions. Freud believed that dream images were activated by sexual feelings, but sexual images tended to activate fear, and so some form of compromise association took place. For example, sexual feelings might tend to associate to images of sex organs. Since the image of a penis would induce anxiety, the dreamer might dream of a sexual object in a more neutral form, such as a cigarette or a pen. Similarly, any round object might be the compromise association for the unacceptable image of a vagina.

Freud's joining of association and motivational processes created a more sophisticated model of dreaming than that of the early associationists. By restricting the source of motivation to sex, and by discouraging experimental evaluation and revision of his model, however, he established a movement in which his followers were unable to contribute further to our understanding of dreaming. Indeed, nothing of significance to the theory of dreaming occurred in the first half of this century. Constructing theories of what goes on inside the brain when an individual perceives, thinks, learns, and recalls had been of such limited value to early experimental psychologists that they decided to confine the terms of their theories to the publicly observable stimuli, the external stimulus, and the observable behavioral response, the input and the output. This radical behaviorist period of psychology effectively discouraged research on dreaming from 1920 to 1953.

II. THE NEUROCOGNITIVE LINK: ASERINSKY AND KLEITMAN

In 1953, a Ph.D. student in physiology named Aserinsky and his mentor, the father of modern sleep research, Nathaniel Kleitman, stumbled across the Stage I sleep electroencephalogram (EEG) rapid eye movement (REM) association with dreaming. That started an explosion of dream research that extended for over 30 years. Multiple pen-writing amplifiers (polygraphs) had just become available for research purposes. Although sleep had been recorded on the polygraph for about 15 minutes, sleep was regarded as a kind of bland monotonous state so there was no incentive to stay up to record an entire night of sleep. But that is what Aserinsky did. To his surprise he found that the brain waves kept changing from one pattern to another through the night in 90-minute cycles. At one phase of these cycles, the brain waves looked remarkably like those of the waking brain, and the *eyes were moving rapidly under the sleepers' lids!*

He could not resist. He did what any of us would have done. He awakened the subject and asked him what was going through his mind. The subject reported a long dream! Aserinsky repeated the awakenings in many other REM periods and nearly always got long dreamlike reports. But in the non-REM (NREM) periods he generally got very brief reports of mental experience, and often nothing at all.

This dramatic discovery indicated that if one wished to study dreams one should get them right at the source, during REM sleep. It also pointed to a particular brain state, Stage I REM, as the condition under which dreams were most likely produced. Indeed, the discovery helped to launch the field of cognitive neuropsychology where cognitive processes are understood in terms of their associated neurophysiological processes.

III. DEFINING CHARACTERISTICS OF DREAMING, AND REM VERSUS NREM SLEEP MENTATION

The close association of REM versus NREM sleep with dreaming versus not dreaming has created some confusion about whether we are studying the physiological characteristics of dreaming or the cognitive characteristics of brain states. When reports are matched by subject and time of night, 94% of REM reports are more dreamlike than NREM reports. So, while sleepers are generally dreaming in REM sleep, dreaming and REM are not synonymous.

Nevertheless, research focuses on the neurological, REM–NREM variable because the experimenter cannot see a dream, but she *can* see the polygraph evidence of the sleeper's state. Furthermore, REM and NREM brain states have clear discrete boundaries whereas the definition of dreaming is complex and a little fuzzy. Before the Aserinsky and Kleitman discovery, dreaming was defined as the imagery and thought of a sleeping person. After their discovery, it was clear that the dramatic imagery reported by sleepers as dreaming was produced almost exclusively in REM sleep. Consequently, the definition of dreaming has become indistinguishable from a description of the cognitive characteristics that distinguish REM from NREM sleep.

Dreaming may be defined as hallucinatory imagery and thought that occurs during sleep. By hallucinatory, we mean that the dreamer assumes that the images are occurring in the real or public world, and not until awakening does the individual identify the perception-like objects and events as imaginal. "Lucid" dreams are an apparent exception to this definition. In a lucid dream, the dreamer is aware that he is dreaming, can modify the course of the dream, and can even signal with his eyes or fingers that a lucid dream is in progress. During a lucid dream the brain state is somewhat altered from that of normal REM sleep, so that it may be called an altered, *REM-like*, dream like state.

Dream images are primarily visual and in color. Their brightness and clarity is approximately 80% that of waking perception. Dreamers sometimes experience a sequence of images as though watching a movie, but they more typically experience participating in the dream. They act and the images respond. Auditory images occur much less commonly. The sense of body movement, pain, and emotions are noticeably reduced or absent during REM dreaming and may appear only as the dreamer makes the transition to waking, or when she sleeps late and the brain moves back and forth between REM and drowsiness.

Dreams are popularly associated with bizarre objects and events. The most common class of bizarreness is sudden or unexpected changes of scene. Much less common are shapes of objects or creatures that are improbable or nonexistent in real life. The least frequent class is persons whose visual identity is different from their known identity. For example, "It was my brother, but he was a girl (in the dream)."

All of these characteristics are expressed in life-like sequences that are longer and more detailed in REM than in NREM sleep. A typical NREM report consists of one or two persons or objects. They are not clear images, and they tend not to interact. In one-third of NREM awakenings, subjects cannot remember anything. In summary, the length of the mentation report and the number of reported visual images are the sharpest discriminator of REM versus NREM mental life.

IV. DREAM RECALL

The discovery that an individual spends well over an hour, about 21% of his sleep time, in REM dreaming raised the question of what determines whether the individual remembers a dream in the morning. Over a dozen factors influence dream recall. If you are interested in your dreams, you will pay more attention to them, and you will tend to "notice" them *while* you are sleeping. The same holds for persons in psychoanalytic therapy. Some of this noticing may occur in the brief interval of near wakefulness that prevents one from falling out of bed as one shifts body position at the end of a REM period.

You are more likely to remember an interesting dream than a normal one. If, upon awakening, you lie still and try to remember your dreams you will recall more than if you awaken to a radio or phone call. The lack in the waking state of cues that might help recall events in a dream tends to handicap the recall of dreams that are in memory. Sometimes, chance events of the day will trigger the recall of a dream. Above all, dreams that occur while sleeping late in the morning, a weekend habit for many people, are better recalled than those that occur earlier in the night.

V. THE ACTIVATION PARADOX

The association of the rich mental life of the dreamer in REM sleep with the neurophysiological picture of brain waves that are remarkably similar to those of a waking individual makes a certain amount of sense. The bedroom is quiet, the eyes are closed, and the brain is awake in some way. So the brain makes dreams out of its own memories. But if the brain is awake, why is the individual lying limp on the bed instead of walking around and interacting with the real world?

Several investigators found that the sensory pathways that carry information about the outside world to the brain were functionally turned off during REM sleep. The brain could not, even if the eyelids were taped open, know what was going on. Jouvet found the specific nucleus that during REM sleep inhibits not only sensory input but the output of the neurons of the motor system. By disengaging this nucleus in a cat, he showed that the cat ran about hissing as though it were chasing the image in its dream! Imagine what night life would be like if all of us ran about for an hour every night acting out our dreams!

In 1949, Moruzzi and Magoun had shown that a small set of nuclei in the brain stem determine whether the brain is awake or asleep. Hobson and McCarley showed that the same nuclei act in REM sleep to awaken the brain. But in REM sleep they are joined by additional nuclei that essentially turned off the sensory input to the brain and turned off the motor neurons that carry out the commands of the motor cortex. Isolated from the outside world, the brain did the same thing as it did when awake, but with nothing coming in from outside, it was no wonder that its mental output was a little odd at times.

Neurologists and cognitive neuropsychologists

have clearly established that different parts of the brain are dedicated to different cognitive operations. Although the brain, in REM sleep may be cut off from the outside world, one part of the brain may still send information to another part of the brain. Hobson and McCarley identified a pontine part of the brain stem-lateral geniculate nucleus (in the midbrain)–occipital cortex (PGO) wave in the cat that has a dramatically high electrical potential and is unusually frequent in REM sleep. They suggested that it was the origin of dreaming.

The activity of the pontine nuclei not only reaches the cortex in the form of PGO waves, but through its connections to the ocular motor system it is able to drive the eye movements of REM sleep. Although the eyes are quiescent during most of a REM period, PGO activity within the REM period is always accompanied by bursts of eye movements. Hobson and McCarley reasoned that the high voltage of PGO waves would disrupt any ongoing dream sequence and thereby cause the bizarre or improbable sequences described above. They further proposed that since PGO waves carry eye movement information, the brain must interpret this information as evidence that the eyes are looking at something. For example, if the PGO waves move the eyes in a particular pattern, the brain must invent a story that is consistent with the eye movement pattern. In other words, according to this activation–synthesis model of dreaming, the activated brain produces the images of the dream by "synthesizing" the eye movement information implied by the PGO waves. Finally, they argued, that since the PGO waves originate in the brain stem, well below the cerebral cortex where memories are stored, the pattern of PGO is essentially random. Since it is random, the origin of dream images is random and there can be no basis for interpreting dreams!

Although the suggestion that the brain could somehow create a sequence of dream images to fit a sequence of eye movements may seem preposterous, experimental studies of stimulus "incorporation" in REM sleep show that the activated brain is remarkably adept at interpreting any sensory stimulus in such a way that it is consistent with the context of the preceding dream. For example, if the sleeper is dreaming that he is sitting in a chair on a hot day, a light spray of water on his skin may elicit a dream of spilling a glass of water on his clothes. If she dreams she is in a room, the spray of water may become evidence that the roof is leaking. If dreaming that he is reading a book, the sound of a bell may be interpreted as a telephone ringing. In the dream context of walking down the street, a loud clap may be interpreted as a gunshot, particularly in times of warfare or violence in the waking world. In short, the brain in REM sleep interprets whatever information it receives in a way that makes the new information as consistent as possible with the context of the preceding dream. The dream reports that are prefaced by phrases such as "and all of a sudden . . ." may be instances where the brain fails to find a smooth transition from one image to another.

According to the activation–synthesis model, the brain must know in which direction the eyes move even though no external visual information reaches the eyes during dreaming sleep. Several experiments have obtained detailed reports of the time and direction of looking behavior during REM dreaming and measured the degree of association between eye movement predicted from these imaged events and the actual recorded eye movements. Although the evidence is inconsistent from one experiment to the next, the best studies show that many, but not all, sequences of eye movements are indeed associated with the dreamer's experience of looking. For example, one experimenter noticed that the dreamer's eye movements were moving in a continuous fast right–left pattern. Although the experiment was not concerned with eye movements, the pattern was so unusual that the experimenter felt compelled to find out what the dreamer was imaging. The subject reported that she was riding on a subway car looking out of the window watching the supporting columns flash past. The eye movement pattern matched the sequence of dream images very nicely.

All of this evidence applies to sequences of *individual* eye movements, up, down, left, right, etc. When eye movements occur in rapid bursts of several per second, they are too close together to be correlated with the dreamer's subjective impressions. Since PGO waves are reliably associated with eye movement bursts but not discrete eye movements, the correlation of PGO with the ocular orientation in the dream is unknown.

One aspect of the eye movement–dreaming pattern is clearly incompatible with the activation–synthesis model. Although Stage I REM sleep is defined by the occurrence of REMs, and a waking-like EEG within sleep, long stretches of the Stage I REM period are without any REMs. But visual imagery as well as all other characteristics of dreaming continue almost undiminished in the absence of PGO waves or eye movements. If these are not PGO waves, what then, is the input to the brain that is interpreted as a dream?

VI. DREAMING AS A SERIAL MODULAR CONSTRAINT SATISFACTION PROCESS

Antrobus has suggested a neural network, serial constraint satisfaction model of dreaming in which the activated brain in REM sleep behaves in much the same way as the activated brain in the waking state would if all of its sensory input was cut off. For example, in waking perception, the lateral geniculate nuclei in the thalamus and the primary occipital cortex carry out the first in a series of interpretations of the visual information that is registered on the retina. Visual perception is a series of neural interpretations that terminates in different brain regions that recognize the shape, color, spatial position, parts, function, and name of an object or a person. Although retinal information is inhibited in REM sleep, the lateral geniculate nuclei and primary visual cortex and higher regions of the brain are sufficiently well activated to do exactly what they do in the waking state. Even in the waking state these brain areas do not 'see" what the retina sees. They "see," or more correctly interpret, the information they get from other cortical and subcortical regions.

This interpretation process may be represented by the neural network models of constraint satisfaction described by Rumelhart and his colleagues. Constraint satisfaction is a precise mathematical model for how interpretations may be carried out at levels as small as networks of neurons. Each of these neuronal areas or nuclei essentially interprets the pattern of activation in the neurons to which it is connected. The connections may be positive or negative and are learned during the course of waking perception. For example if neurons in the primary visual cortex interpret some random neural activity as two dark spots, and the spatial regions of the parietal cortex interpret them as approximately horizontal, then the more anterior regions of the brain may interpret them as eyes. Since most of the eyes we see are those of people, the brain may go on to construct the rest of the face, and so on.

At the higher levels of constraint satisfaction, the process of dream image construction is precisely like that described above by the incorporation experiments described above. Each segment of the brain makes the best sense it can of what the other segments of the brain tell it. Just as the constraint satisfaction model shows how a fragment of sensory stimuli is sufficient to produce a complete waking perception, so Antrobus shows how nonsensory activity in the visual brain can lead to a complete imagined percept in REM sleep.

How does this model account for the association of dream images with eye movements? Waking eye movements are determined by a large number of neural processes: visual stimuli, auditory stimuli, orientation and motion of the head and body in space, shift in balance, memory, interest, volition, and more. All of these "inputs" are coordinated through the frontal eye fields in a part of the cortex that controls all body movements. In the waking state, a perceptual image would provide one basis for a decision by the frontal eye fields to move the eyes. The execution of the movement would be carried out by a complex subcortical process that ends up in the oculomotor system. The fine tuning of the eye movements is carried out in the cerebellum which is attached to the brain stem by a branch that includes the cells that originate the PGO spikes.

Antrobus proposed that the dream image, coupled with the dreamer's interest, sends the decision to the frontal eye fields to move the eyes just as they would in the waking state. Hong and his colleagues, using a PET scan of the brain has recently shown that the frontal eye fields are, indeed, very active during REM sleep, particularly in the right hemisphere. Obviously, the Antrobus model says that the dream determines the eye movements, rather than the dream being an interpretation of eye movements. Although both the Antrobus and the activation–synthesis models start with a random process, the successive interpretations by different brain regions in the Antrobus model make the dream very much the product of the interests and perceptual styles of the dreamer. Since these motivations and perceptual characteristics are learned in the waking state, they do have potential for representing some of the waking characteristics of the dreamer. Whether such interpretations are accurate or valid, however is another question. The poor agreement by different interpreters of the same dream suggests that the validity of dream interpretations is poor.

The role, if any, of PGO waves in dreaming remains

to be determined. Dreaming can clearly proceed in the absence of PGO waves, and PGO waves may be independent of neural decisions made by the frontal eye fields. There is simply not sufficient neurophysiological evidence at this point to determine their role, if any, in dreaming.

The serial modular constraint satisfaction model says that the brain processes in REM sleep and waking are similar, that the output of the brain in the two states differs only because the input during REM sleep and waking is quite different. Compared to REM sleep and waking, the output of the brain in NREM sleep is impoverished because the cortex receives little activation from the pontine brainstem structures that determine the overall activation of the brain.

For many years, experimenters who studied dreaming sleep ignored waking imagery, apparently because they felt it was too familiar to everyone to warrant study. Furthermore, because waking thought and imagery differ so much from one waking situation to another there did not seem to be a single kind of waking thought that could serve as a basis for comparison with mentation produced in the sleep states. Foulkes, and later Antrobus, Wollman, and Reinsel, decided that for the purpose of comparing imagery and thought across the three states, waking mentation should be obtained from individuals in the same quiet, dark bedrooms that are used for the study of sleep mentation.

If the hypothesis that dreaming sleep is simply the output of an active brain that is cut off from external stimuli is correct, it should be possible to observe dreamlike mentation from awake subjects in this environment. The hypothesis was confirmed. Waking visual imagery was just as clear and bright, and the mentation just as storylike and bizarre as in REM sleep. The two differences that did emerge were that the storylike sequences of waking mentation were less continuous and the images were not hallucinatory. Both of these characteristics could be attributed to the lower sensory thresholds (greater sensitivity) of the brain to external stimuli during waking. No matter how dark and quiet the room, the waking subject is intermittently aware of his external environment and therefore knows that the images are *not* real perceptions. In REM sleep, there is no sensory evidence to compare with the dreamer's images, so the dreamer *knows,* wrongly of course, that the images are real perceptions!

Similarly, the intermittent awareness of external stimuli interrupts the imagery from time to time much as Hobson and McCarley assumed that PGO waves interrupt dreaming. But despite the occasional report of "and all of a sudden . . . ," image and thought sequences during REM dreaming exhibited greater continuity than did waking mentation.

Further support for the position that dreaming is the output of an activated brain that is isolated from the outside world by high sensory thresholds comes from a close look at dreams that occur when an individual sleeps later in the morning. Late morning seems to be the ideal time for dream recall, bizarre dreams, and even lucid dreaming. Antrobus, Kondo, Reinsel, and Fein reasoned that by sleeping late into the morning, the brain was activated by both the rising phase of the wake–sleep, 24-hour diurnal rhythm, and the alternating 90-minute REM–NREM cycle. Therefore, both NREM and REM reports should be longer and their images clearer and brighter in the late morning. In the REM phase, dreams should be longer and more vivid than at any other time during sleep. And that is what they found.

In other words, the pattern of activation that is distributed across the brain in REM sleep and waking, and is controlled by nuclei in the pontine portion of the brain stem, is fairly similar in both states. The primary difference in the two patterns of activation is that, as mentioned earlier, the REM activation pattern includes the active suppression of sensory input and inhibition at the spinal level of execution of the motor commands of the cortex. That is, the motor cortex can say "run," but the command to the skeletal muscles is not carried out. Nor is the expected sensation of moving transmitted back to the brain. And so the dreamer is apt to feel paralyzed. The second difference is that waking imagery is predominantly auditory and often verbal, whereas REM imagery is largely visual. The source of this difference is unknown. By way of further comparison, fever and many drug states are accompanied by visual imagery and hallucinations, whereas schizophrenia is associated with auditory hallucinations.

VII. FUNCTION OF DREAMING SLEEP

It is curious that the inhibitory processes of REM sleep are not active in NREM sleep. Clearly they are unnecessary because the brain is not sufficiently active in

NREM sleep to either interpret the incoming sensory information or to issue motor commands. For reasons that are buried far back in the history of mammalian evolution, the sleeping brain becomes active in 90-minute REM–NREM cycles, but cuts off its sensory input and motor output during the REM phase so that the individual does not get into trouble by chasing its hallucinated demons in the dark. Although many theories have been proposed to account for this intermittent activation, they are so speculative that they do not warrant extended comment here. The most plausible hypothesis is that neurons require stimulation for their survival and growth. But people and other mammals also require rest in the form of sleep so that certain restorative processes can take place. The period of the wake–sleep cycle is determined by the 24-hour rotation to the earth, however, not by the needs of cortical neurons for stimulation. And so, perhaps, the brain stem developed its own internal form of stimulation which it delivers to the cortex intermittently when the individual is cut off from external stimulation. One strong piece of support for this self-stimulation theory is that REM sleep makes up about 70% of the 24-hour day of the fetus when its nervous system is in the process of rapid development.

The reader may wonder whether the sensory and motor systems are also deprived of this intermittent self-stimulation. The answer is that they are not inhibited during the 79% of the night that makes up NREM sleep. In fact subjects are vaguely aware of their environment during about 30% of NREM sleep. But since the cortex is not sufficiently active to fully perceive this sensory information, much less remember it or issue motor commands, there is no reason for the motor system to be actively inhibited.

Perhaps the most widely known hypothesis of the function of dreaming is Freud's suggestion that it is the guardian of sleep. Freud did not know, of course, that most dreaming occurs within the 21% of the night devoted to REM sleep. There would not be much value to a guardian that guarded only 21% of one's sleep. The notion that dreaming protects sleep comes from the remarkable ability of the brain to "incorporate" into an ongoing dream external stimuli that might otherwise awaken the sleeper. Although this process has not been studied systematically, there is little doubt that a ringing bell that is interpreted as a telephone in one's dream excuses the dreamer from getting out of bed to answer one's real telephone. Freud, however, was more concerned about the sleeper being awakened by the perception of raw sexual energy. He proposed that dreaming protected sleep by transforming this sexual threat to sleep into a more benign form. For example, a penis might be rendered as a cigar.

A recent hypothesis about the purpose of REM sleep deserves some comment because it was proposed by Crick, the Nobel Prize–winning geneticist. In his work with mathematical models of neural networks, he found that networks often become in effect gridlocked. So many neurons may become active that the network cannot process any information. He found that if he stimulated such a network with random information, it became essentially unlocked. Assuming that the origin of PGO waves in dreaming sleep is random, he suggested that they might function to free up cortical networks that might be gridlocked by the cumulative information processing of a day's work. This random, PGO-dreaming process, he suggested, would be a form of cleaning out the trivial memories accumulated during the day.

Of course the function or value of REM sleep is not necessarily the same as the function of dreaming. If the function of REM sleep is to stimulate cortical neurons, then those neurons are bound to produce the images and thought that they do in the waking state. But this does not mean that the particular mentation that is produced during REM sleep has a value for the individual. It may mean that the capability to produce that imagery and thought has value for the individual when in her waking environment, and if that ability is not exercised from time to time, even in sleep, its ability to process information will be weakened where it is most needed, namely in the waking state. [*See* SLEEP.]

VIII. REM DEPRIVATION

The discovery that dreaming is closely associated with Stage 1 REM sleep suggested to Bill Dement, another student of Kleitman's, a simple way to determine the function or value of dreaming sleep. He could simply waken the sleeper every time the brain moved into REM sleep. And so he did. And to his surprise, the more often he interrupted an individual's REM sleep the sooner the sleep moved back into REM sleep. That meant that the more often he interrupted the sleeper's dreams, the sooner the brain began to dream again.

Moreover, if Dement deprived a sleeper of an hour of REM dreaming, the brain tended to make up the loss, almost minute for minute, during the following nights.

The immediate conclusion was that everyone has a need to dream. One psychiatrist proposed that if one could not get sufficient dream time, one would become psychotic. When subjects were deprived of an equal amount of Stage 4 sleep, a "deep" NREM sleep stage that predominates in the early part of the night, however, sleepers showed the same tendency to make up stage 4 sleep. In fact, if totally sleep deprived, people tend to make up the lost stage 4 sleep first, and the lost REM sleep second. The obvious question about the consequences in the waking state for the individual who is deprived of Stage 1 REM sleep remain unanswered. It has proved too costly to systematically deprive people of REM sleep over a number of days, study their waking thought and behavior all day long, and then compare this behavior with that of individuals deprived of equal amounts of NREM sleep. And so, the deprivation of REM sleep never did tell us about the function of REM sleep. And if it had, it would not necessarily have told us anything about the function of dreaming. Dreaming is one of many characteristics of REM sleep. Any consequence of REM deprivation might well be due to the loss of some characteristic other than dreaming.

IX. PROBLEM SOLVING IN DREAMS

Our tendency to see reflections of our personal concerns and problems in our dreams prompts the notion that dreams are a form of personal problem solving. The suggestion is so general that it is difficult to confirm or disconfirm. Herbert Simon, one of the fathers of artificial intelligence, the science of simulating the mental processes of the brain on computers, maintains that *all* mental processes are forms of problem solving. Even the automatic process of determining if an eye movement should move 10° or 11° to the right is a complicated problem that takes a very large computer to simulate. We are, of course, much more aware of the big problems of life such as whom one should marry, but they are no different in their neuronal representation than are decisions about eye movements. So, yes, dreams are a form of personal problem solving. When the dreamer imagines a strange person in the kitchen, he "solves" the

problem by imagining an escape. One might then ask whether a solution imagined in one's dreams will generalize to the waking state. People who "solve" threats in their dreams by running away may well also run away from threats in their waking world. But, like the chicken and the egg, it is difficult to determine which comes first.

The strongest support for the notion that large conceptual problems may be solved during dreaming comes from a number of anecdotes by scientists, writers, and creative artists, including Mozart, in which they have imagined substantial scientific solutions or artistic works, while dreaming. Indeed, some poets and surrealistic novelists regularly look to their dreams for images that they could not possibly construe in their waking life. Because sleep removes the individual from the constraints of the waking world, the activated brain of the dreamer should be able to produce images and events that are creative in that they are somewhat free of waking constraints. And if there is sufficient motivation and sufficient preliminary knowledge some of these productions may well represent solutions to real world problems.

Nevertheless, the argument should not be overstated. For example, a screen writer might incorporate features of a bizarre dream image in a film. Although the image might well constitute a solution to the writer's problem, the process of generating the dream image would not be a problem solving process unless the original problem had in some way directed the dream process.

There is no way to know whether these anecdotes of creative dreams were produced in REM sleep or in those less well studied dreams that occur late in the morning, where the brain wanders back and forth between a highly activated REM sleep and a drowsy never-never land between sleep and waking. That the most dedicated dream recaller remembers less than 1% of her dreams each night suggests that whatever the solutions that REM dreams provide, they have little chance of being remembered upon awakening.

X. STRESS, GOALS, AND MOTIVATION

In order for a dream to contribute to the solution of a problem, some representation of the problem must be activated within the brain. Because sleep removes the individual from an external problem for 7 to 9 hours, the only cues that might reactivate the waking problem are imaginal ones. Dream images rarely represent objects, persons, or events from the recent past, so current problems are rarely explicitly represented in a dream. The events of the day do make up a large part of the sleeper's images during the interval of falling asleep, but these are not REM sleep dream images. If a waking problem is going to influence the dream, then, the problem must be both significant and long-standing. The horror of some repetitive life stressors such as child abuse, rape, a traumatic divorce, or warfare are so powerful, and they become associated to so many other events in an individual's life, that any of a large number of images are able to reactivate the memories at any time of the night, and may do so for many years after the original stressor. Weaker stressors may also influence a dream to the extent that they share some of the features of these more severe stressors. [*See* STRESS.]

Outside of these traumatic events, there is very little evidence that the stressors of the day influence one's dreams. For example, systematic study of patients before and after surgery show almost no evidence of cutting or threat of any kind. As might be expected, there are individual differences in the response to stress. A very small number of adults who experience persistent night terrors seem to feel vulnerable to many of the minor life stressors to which most people are indifferent.

XI. EMOTIONS IN DREAMS: NIGHTMARES AND NIGHT TERRORS

Stress is normally associated with powerful emotions as an individual strives to escape or cope from a stressor. But these emotions are rarely experienced with the REM dream. On the other hand there are many instances where individuals wake up screaming from a dream. There are several possible explanations for this paradox, none of them well researched. The most dramatic association of dreaming and panic occurs in night terrors, a nonpathological developmental problem experienced by some children during NREM sleep within the first 2 hours of sleep. The child awakens screaming in terror and continues to hallucinate images of being attacked. Occasionally, the child is able to respond to the parents, but many immediately fall back into the hallucinated terror.

The best current explanation for these terrors is that the neural mechanisms that normally inhibit or modulate the experience of emotional arousal are so deeply asleep that the mechanisms that amplify emotions expand without any neural constraints. Anything that lightens the first hour of sleep, such as awakening the child after 30 minutes of sleep, or a small drink of coffee before going to bed, tends to eliminate the terrors. Because most night terrors spontaneously disappear after a year or two it may be assumed that they are not caused by any personal stressor of maladjustment. A serious problem can develop, however, if the parents mishandle the behavior. Some parents are embarrassed because the neighbors hear the screaming. Others are angered because the hallucinating child appears to be completely ignoring their orders to be quiet. If the child is punished or beaten he will become afraid to go to sleep and a serious sleep problem may develop. At that point the family should seek help at a sleep disorders center.

The experience of emotion in nightmares, which occur primarily in REM sleep, seems to begin as the sleeper moves out of sleep. In that brief transition to wakefulness, the psychophysiological indices of emotion, such as elevated and irregular cardiac and respiratory activity, and increased muscle tonus and body movement, move to dramatic levels. Some investigators assume that the cognitive representation of threat is represented in the images of the dream, but the normal connections to the subcortical mechanisms that participate in emotional experience are inhibited during sleep, especially REM sleep, and becomes active only as the dreamer struggles toward wakefulness.

One reason for our poor understanding of the relation between dreams and emotions is that dreams reported in the laboratory are much less emotional than those reported at home. Although the laboratory setting may put a damper on the expression of emotions, a more likely explanation for the difference is that the home dreams that are emotional are noticed on those mornings when the dreamer sleeps late, where REM dreaming may intermingle with periods of drowsy wakefulness. In other words, the brain is well activated, but the REM sleep processes that normally inhibit the experience of emotion may be weakened by the broad-based activation provided by the rising phase of the 24-hour diurnal rhythm.

XII. SLEEP WALKING AND TALKING

Although sleep talking is popularly associated with dreaming, only 20% of sleep talking occurs in REM sleep. Sleep talking and sleep walking both require activated skeletal muscles. Sleep walking requires vision and balance. Because these processes are not inhibited in NREM sleep they predominate in that state. Although most sleep talking is confined to only words, such as, "good," or "okay," some utterances are long enough to establish that they are related to a concurrent dream. Many people have attempted to carry on conversations with sleep talkers. Arkin shows that the brain must move into a NREM–waking transition state in order for the sleep talker to reply to a question from another person.

XIII. MIXED DREAMLIKE STATES

I have already pointed out that while the characteristics of dreaming are strongest in REM sleep, the most dramatic dreams, the most emotional, bizarre, vivid, and lucid, seem to occur in the late morning when the rising phase of the diurnal rhythm overlaps the REM phase of the 90-minute REM–NREM cycle. Sometimes, fortunately rarely, the REM cycle intrudes into the middle of waking experience. In the disordered state of narcolepsy, an emotional incident may trigger a temporary interval of motor weakness, drowsiness, and even a hallucination. Cataplexy, a related, more severe, but rarer disorder, is accompanied by severe loss of motor tonus. Other evidence of REM sleep intruding into the waking state is the occurrence of a drowsy episode accompanied by penile tumescence. Penile erection is common during REM sleep, particularly following a body movement. But only about 10% of these erections in REM sleep are associated with sexual content in the dream.

XIV. PARAPSYCHOLOGY, DREAM INTERPRETATION, AND SPURIOUS ASSOCIATIONS

There is so much information in a dream, that one can find connections or associations between some dream events and some events in real life. Once the associations have been made, it is tempting to assume that a causal relationship holds between the two. For believers of parapsychology, the association of a dream event with a future real life event seems so strong that the dream seems to predict the future. For the dream interpreter, the association between the dream event and some personality characteristic of the individual seems so compelling that the dream seems to be able to reveal some meaning of the person's mental processes. Scientific evidence for both of these positions is close to zero. Yet both practices continue to flourish.

The article has been reprinted from the *Encyclopedia of Human Behavior, Volume 2*.

BIBLIOGRAPHY

Antrobus, J. (1990). The neurocognition of sleep mentation: Phasic and tonic REM sleep. In "Sleep and Cognition" (R. R. Bootzin, J. F. Kihlstrom, & D. L. Schacter, Eds.), pp. 1–24. American Psychological Association, Washington, DC.

Antrobus, J. (1991). Dreaming: Cognitive processes during cortical activation and high afferent thresholds. Psycholog. Rev. 98, 96–121.

Aserinsky, E., & Kleitman, N. (1953). Regularly occurring periods of ocular motility and concomitant phenomena during sleep. Science 118, 273–274.

Dement, W. C. (1972). "Some Must Watch While Some Must Sleep." Freeman, San Francisco.

Ellman, S. J., Spielman, A. J., Luck, D., Steiner, S. S., & Halperin, R. (1991). REM deprivation: A review. In "The Mind in Sleep: Psychology and Psychophysiology" 2nd ed. (S. J. Ellman and J. S. Antrobus, Eds.), pp. 329–389. Wiley Interscience, New York.

Ellman, S. J., Spielman, A. J., & Lipschutz-Brach, L. (1991). REM deprivation update. In "The Mind in Sleep: Psychology and Psychophysiology," 2nd Ed. (S. J. Ellman and J. S. Antrobus, Eds.), pp. 369–376. Wiley Interscience, New York.

Foulkes, D. (1966). "The Psychology of Sleep." Scribners, New York.

Hobson, J. A., & McCarley, R. W. (1977). The brain as a dream state generator: An activation-synthesis hypothesis of the dream process. Am. J. Psychiat. 134, 1335–1348.

Moruzzi, G., & Magoun, H. W. (1949). Brain reticular formation and activation of the EEG. Electroencephalograph and Clin. Neurophysiol. 1, 455–473.

Reinsel, R., Antrobus, J., & Wollman, M. (1992). Bizarreness in sleep and waking mentation. In "The Neuropsychology of Sleep and Dreaming" (J. Antrobus, & M. Bertini, Eds.), Erlbaum, Hillsdale, NJ.

Rumelhart, D. E., Smolensky, P., McClelland, J. L., & Hinton, G. E. (1986). Schemata and sequential thought in PDP models. In "Parallel distributed processing: Explorations in the microstructure of cognition," Vol. 2 (J. L. McClelland, D. R. Rumelhart, Eds.), pp. 7–57. MIT Press, Bradford, Cambridge, MA.

Wollman, M. C., & Antrobus, J. S. (1986). Sleeping and waking thought: Effects of external stimulation. Sleep 9, 438–448.

DSM-IV

John J. B. Allen

University of Arizona

Comorbidity The co-occurrence of two or more mental disorders in the same individual.

Diagnosis The determination of the nature of a disease. Although in most branches of medicine this implies that the cause of the disorder has been identified, this is often not the case with psychiatric diagnosis using the *DSM-IV,* which involves assigning a diagnostic label on the basis of the observed and/or reported behaviors and symptoms.

Etiology The cause of a disorder.

Heterogeneity The situation where individuals who share the diagnosis of a particular disorder do not share all symptoms in common. A heterogeneous disorder is one where people with the disorder can present with a variety of different symptoms.

Mental Disorder The *DSM* defines mental disorder as a pattern of behavior, or psychological features, occurring in an individual that are currently associated with any of the following: a subjective sense of distress; impairment in important areas of function, such as work, school, relationships; or a significantly increased risk of posing a danger to oneself or others, or of losing an important freedom.

Prognosis Estimating the likely course and outcome for those with a mental disorder.

Reliability Consistency of diagnosis. If diagnoses can be assigned reliably, an individual will be assigned the same diagnosis across differing circumstances (e.g., different diagnosticians).

Validity The extent to which a diagnosis is meaningful. A valid diagnosis allows that individuals with the diagnosis can be distinguished from individuals with other diagnoses and from individuals with no diagnosis. Valid diagnoses should also provide useful information about the etiology, treatment, or prognosis of the mental disorder.

DSM-IV is the abbreviation for the *Diagnostic and Statistical Manual of Mental Disorders,* 4th Edition. The *DSM-IV* details the diagnostic criteria for nearly 300 mental disorders, and nearly 100 other psychological conditions that might be the focus of professional attention, thereby providing a standardized system of classification that is intended to be used internationally. The *DSM-IV* also provides systems for noting medical conditions and stressors that may be related to the psychological conditions, and for noting how the individual's functioning (for example, job performance or ability to care for one's self) may be affected.

I. THE PURPOSE OF DIAGNOSIS

Diagnosis of psychological symptoms using the *DSM-IV* entails classifying observable symptoms, or reports of such symptoms, into discrete categories termed mental disorders. A mental disorder (defined above) represents a pattern of behavior or psychological features that in some way causes the person distress or impairment. Moreover, a mental disorder is conceptualized in the *DSM-IV* as a problem or dysfunction that resides within an individual, rather than a problem that results from a conflict between that individual and society. This caveat is important because it is supposed to prevent the misuse of diagnostic labels for the purpose of social control, applying them to individuals whose values or beliefs differ from those of the majority.

Assigning a diagnosis using the *DSM-IV* does not necessarily suggest that the etiology (cause) of the symptoms is known, but only than an individual's symptoms meet the criteria for the particular mental disorder. For example, two individuals might meet the criteria for a diagnosis of Major Depressive Disorder, but might develop these symptoms after a very different set of circumstances; one person might experience these symptoms only after a series of troubling setbacks (e.g., financial, legal, and relationship problems) while another might experience these symptoms after an apparently unstressful period. Although one might imagine that the etiology of the depression differs for these two individuals, they would both receive the same diagnosis using the *DSM*.

Assigning a diagnostic label may have profound implications for the person receiving the diagnosis. On the one hand, diagnostic labels may allow individuals to receive the treatment they are seeking. On the other hand, such labels may have a stigmatizing effect for the person diagnosed. Consider, for example, how you might think about yourself, and how others might begin to think about you and to treat you, if they learned you had received a diagnosis of a severe psychosis—schizophrenia. Diagnostic labels convey a wealth of information, some of it intended, some of it not. Because assigning a diagnostic label may have profound effects on how people may view the person who receives the label, the diagnosis of mental disorders should be taken seriously, and should have the potential for some clear benefits for those diagnosed.

What, then, is the purpose of diagnosing mental disorders? First, diagnosis should help us identify a homogeneous group of individuals. For example, many different disorders may entail delusions—beliefs that most persons in an individual's culture would regard as false, such as the belief that one can read verbatim another's thoughts. Yet despite similarity in this particular symptom, individuals with delusions may differ in important ways. Delusions are associated in some cases with the ingestion of psychoactive substances (e.g., amphetamines), in others with a disturbance in mood (e.g., mania or depression), and in others with hallucinations and disorganization of thought (e.g., schizophrenia). These different diagnoses, while sharing a symptom in common, may differ in other important ways. By identifying patterns of symptoms that tend to occur together, important differences between individuals with a common symptom may be identified, such as the cause of the disorder, the most effective treatments, or the prognosis for the future.

Second, diagnosis should help in the planning of treatment. For example, the delusional behavior that can be seen in both mania and schizophrenia will typically be treated by different drugs. Similarly, knowing that the delusional behavior results from use of psychoactive substances suggests a different intervention; i.e., stopping use of the substance causing the symptom.

Third, diagnosis can facilitate communication among professionals. A diagnostic label provides a succinct means of conveying information. For example, if, after an assessment interview, a mental health professional determines that an individual needs to be referred to another mental health professional or facility, the diagnostic label can summarize much of the information. Of course the diagnosis does not summarize all relevant information, but can reduce the amount of description required to round out the assessment picture. Another instance in which diagnostic labels facilitate communication is the case of communication between mental health professionals and insurance providers. Given particular diagnoses, insurance providers will authorize reimbursement for particular treatments, without the need to review the entire assessment interview.

II. A BRIEF HISTORY OF THE DEVELOPMENT OF THE *DSM-IV* AND ITS PREDECESSORS

Over the last several thousand years, many systems have existed for diagnosing mental disorders. The *DSM* series is relatively recent, with the first edition of the *Diagnostic and Statistical Manual* (now referred to as *DSM-I*) appearing in 1952. The manual has been revised several times since, with the *DSM-II* appearing in 1968, the *DSM-III* appearing in 1979, a minor revision—the *DSM-III-R*—appearing in 1987, and the current version of the manual—the *DSM-IV*—appearing in 1994. In contrast to the *DSM* series, most earlier systems detailed only a handful of diagnostic categories.

Several categorization systems existed for use in the United States prior to the development of the *DSM*. These systems included: simple systems with between one and seven diagnostic categories to aid in collecting census data concerning mental illness during the nineteenth century; a system for statistically tallying information on patients in mental hospitals in the early twentieth century; a system developed by the U.S. Army, and modified by the Veteran's Administration, for use with servicemen; and several editions of a system developed by the World Health Organization (WHO). Since the latter part of the nineteenth century, the WHO had ben publishing the *International Classification of Disease (ICD)*, a comprehensive listing of medical conditions. With the sixth edition (*ICD-6*), mental disorders were included for the first time. In each revision of the *DSM* series, an attempt was made to coordinate the system with the corresponding revision of the *ICD* system. Each of the disorders listed in the *DSM-IV* has a corresponding code in the most recent versions of the *ICD,* namely the *ICD-9-CM* and *ICD-10*.

The *DSM-I* was the product of The American Psychiatric Association Committee on Nomenclature and Statistics, and contained 106 mental disorders, with an emphasis on being clinically useful. *DSM-II* added 76 new disorders and, unlike its predecessor, encouraged rather than discouraged assigning multiple diagnoses to each patient. Both *DSM-I* and *DSM-II* were similar in format, providing a description of the disorder, but lacking detailed criteria by which to diagnose the disorder. *DSM-III* represented a major change, with each disorder possessing tangible, operational criteria. This change was inspired by research that showed that clinicians using the previous *DSM* versions failed to agree on a diagnosis for a surprisingly large percentage of the patients. Although inconsistency in information provided by the patients, and inconsistencies in the type of information gathered by clinicians could explain some of the disagreement, a vast majority of the problem lay with the diagnostic criteria themselves. The descriptions were overly broad, were often vague, sometimes included reference to unobservable processes, and often overlapped with descriptions of other diagnostic categories. The operational criteria of the *DSM-III* referred to observable or reportable symptoms, with specific numeric criteria for frequency and duration of symptoms. The *DSM-III* for the first time included a *multiaxial* system of diagnosis (see below), a feature that has been retained in subsequent revisions.

In contrast to earlier systems, which contained only a few broad and severe diagnostic categories that were likely to be relevant to governmental and institutional interests, the *DSM* series was designed to be of use to the clinical psychiatrist; *DSM* therefore focused on a broader range of symptoms, including less severe forms of disturbance that might be treated outside of institutional settings. The origins of this trend began a decade prior to the publication of the *DSM-I*, as military and Veterans Administration psychiatrists found a need for additional diagnostic categories to cover the psychiatric conditions resulting from the stress of combat. These conditions were less severe and less chronic than the few severe categories that existed prior to World War II. Moreover, these conditions could be treated in an outpatient setting rather than through institutionalization.

As a diagnostic system was developed to delineate these broader, less severe, diagnostic categories, it became impossible to unequivocally link each diagnostic category to a specific etiology. The *DSM* series, therefore, established diagnostic categories on the basis of the pattern of symptoms and their appearance over time, remaining largely agnostic with respect to etiology (with some clear exceptions). This *descriptive categorical approach* defines discrete categories of mental illness, based primarily on observable symptoms. In contrast to an etiologically based system, where each diagnostic category is included because a cause has been scientifically established, the decision to include a diagnostic category in the descriptive system must be based on informed judgments of experts as to whether the symptoms co-occur in such a manner to merit the inclusion of a discrete category defining those symptoms. Although such judgments will ideally be influenced by scientific research, some subjectivity is inevitable.

The development of *DSM-IV,* in particular, involved many individuals chosen for their expertise in a variety of areas. A 27-member *DSM-IV* Task Force worked with 13 Work Groups, each comprised of up to a dozen members. Additionally, each task force relied on the advice of committees of up to 100 people. Members of these committees represented many different specializations and professions, with medical doctors having the largest representation. Over the course of 6 years, a three-step process was followed to increase the likelihood that changes would be based on the basis of research findings, rather than the whim of committee members. This three-step process involved literature reviews, reanalysis of previously collected data sets, and field trials to assess the reliability of several alternative criterion sets. New diagnostic categories were included when the Task Force considered that sufficient evidence existed to justify the addition of a new category in terms of antecedent indicators (e.g., family history or precipitating situations), concurrent indicators (e.g., physiological and psychological symptoms that co-occur), and predictive indicators (e.g., response to treatment, prognosis). Conversely, in a few instances, a category from the *DSM-III-R* was removed when insufficient evidence existed to merit retaining it.

The *DSM-IV*, therefore, ideally represents the informed scientific judgment of many experts in the mental health field. On the other hand, these judgments are inevitably shaped and limited by the current scientific knowledge base, the previous diagnostic systems that form the basis for scientific research, the particular composition of the Task Force and Work Groups, and the idiosyncratic preferences of these various committee members. The *DSM-IV*, therefore, may best be viewed as one more chapter of a work in progress.

III. ORGANIZATION AND CONTENTS OF THE *DSM-IV*

The *DSM-IV* details a *multiaxial* system of diagnosis, meaning that individuals are assessed in multiple areas, or along multiple dimensions or *axes*. Axis I contains 15 major classes of mental disorders. Axis II contains personality and developmental disorders. Axis III contains medical conditions. Axis IV provides for the notation of psychological, social, and environmental stressors that may affect diagnosis. Axis V provides for a measure of the individual's function in

areas such as work, social activities, and self-care. The multiaxial system is designed to encourage a comprehensive evaluation of biological, social, and psychological factors relevant to each person's presenting symptoms. The multiaxial system also provides a means for detailing differences between those with identical diagnoses. With respect to the example provided at the beginning of the chapter—two depressed individuals who developed symptoms after different life events—Axis IV would provide a way of summarizing that one individual developed depression only after a series of troubling setbacks while another developed depression in the absence of such events.

A. Axis I: Clinical Disorders and Other Conditions That May Be a Focus of Clinical Attention

Almost all mental disorders or conditions that may be a focus of clinical attention appear on Axis I, with a few exceptions that appear on Axis II. Axis I organizes mental disorders into 15 major groups of disorders, as presented in Table I. Most of the groups in Table I were created based on the similarity of symptoms of disorders within that group, although in some cases disorders are grouped together because of the typical age at which symptoms first appear (Disorders Usually First Diagnosed in Infancy, Childhood or Adolescence), or because of common etiology (Mental Disorders due to a General Medical Condition, Substance-Related Disorders, Adjustment Disorders). In many cases, an individual may receive more than one Axis I diagnosis, although some diagnoses by definition will preclude another diagnosis.

Each disorder on Axis I includes a set of diagnostic criteria, which are typically a combination of *monothetic* (i.e., all conditions of the criterion must be met) and *polythetic* (i.e., only some from among a larger set of conditions must be met) criteria. For example, to diagnosis Attention Deficit/Hyperactivity disorder, an individual must meet the following criteria: (a) either 6 or more symptoms (from among 9) of inattention, *or* 6 or more symptoms (from among 9) of hyperactivity-impulsivity (*polythetic*); (b) some symptoms are present and causing impairment before age 7 (*monothetic*); (c) impairment is seen in at least two settings, such as school and home (*monothetic*); (d) the symptoms clearly cause impairment in functioning (*monothetic*); and (e) the symptoms are not

Table I Examples of Disorders in Each of the 15 Major Groups Listed on Axis I of *DSM-IV*

Group	Examples of Disorders
Disorders Usually First Diagnosed in Infancy, Childhood, or Adolescence	Attention Deficit/Hyperactivity Disorder, Autistic Disorder
Delirium, Dementia, and Amnestic and Other Cognitive Disorders	Dementia of the Alzheimer's Type, Vascular Dementia
Mental Disorders Due to a General Medical Condition	Mood Disorder Due to a General Medical Condition (e.g., stroke, hypothyroidism)
Substance-Related Disorders	Alcohol Abuse, Nicotine Dependence, Caffeine Intoxication, Cocaine Withdrawal
Schizophrenia and Other Psychotic Disorders	Schizophrenia, Delusional Disorder, Schizoaffective Disorder
Mood Disorders	Major Depressive Disorder, Bipolar I Disorder (aka Manic Depression), Dysthymic Disorder
Anxiety Disorders	Agoraphobia, Social Phobia, Panic Disorder, Obsessive-Compulsive Disorder, Posttraumatic Stress Disorder
Somatoform Disorders	Somatization Disorder, Hypochondriasis
Factitious Disorders	Factitious Disorder
Dissociative Disorders	Dissociative Identity Disorder (*formerly* Multiple Personality Disorder), Dissociative Amnesia
Sexual and Gender Identity Disorders	Sexual Dysfunctions (e.g., Male Erectile Disorder), Paraphilias (e.g., Exhibitionism, Pedophilia), Gender Identity Disorder
Eating Disorders	Anorexia Nervosa, Bulimia Nervosa
Sleep Disorders	Primary Insomnia, Narcolepsy, Sleep Terror Disorder
Impulse-Control Disorders Not Elsewhere Classified	Kleptomania, Pyromania, Pathological Gambling

better accounted for by another mental or physical disorder (*monothetic*). Polythetic criterion sets have advantages and disadvantages. The primary advantage is that polythetic sets reduce the number of diagnostic categories required, since people with highly similar but nonidentical symptoms can receive the same diagnosis. If, by contrast, each and every criterion were required, such highly similar people would require different diagnoses. The primary disadvantage to polythetic criterion sets is symptom heterogeneity, where people with the same diagnosis may be quite different in terms of their symptoms. In fact, in the case of some disorders, it is possible that two individuals with the same diagnosis may not share a single symptom in common. [*See* ATTENTION DEFICIT HYPERACTIVITY DISORDER (ADHD).]

There are also disorders that appear on Axis I that do not have such clearly defined criterion sets. There are over 40 disorders that include "NOS" in their name, an abbreviation for Not Otherwise Specified. These disorders are diagnosed if the symptoms resemble those of another diagnosis but fail to meet the full criteria required for diagnosis. For example, Anxi-

ety Disorder NOS is a diagnosis for cases in which there is "prominent anxiety or phobic avoidance that do not meet the criteria for any specific Anxiety Disorder" (p. 444) or meet criteria for Adjustment Disorder. [*See* ANXIETY.]

Also found for each disorder (other than NOS disorders) listed on Axis I are other sections providing more detailed information that may be of use to clinicians. The *Diagnostic Features* section provides an overview of the essential features of the disorder, along with examples and definitions of criteria and terms that are part of the criterion set for that disorder. The *Subtypes and/or Specifiers* section delineates subtypes of the disorder (e.g., Catatonic Subtype of Schizophrenia) or specifiers of the disorder (e.g., Postpartum Onset for Major Depressive Disorder), where applicable. The *Recording Procedures* section includes information to assist in reporting the correct name of the disorder and the associated five-digit code that corresponds to the disorder. These five-digit codes correspond to the codes listed in the *International Classification of Disease* (9th edition, with clinical modification), the diagnostic system of the

World Health Organization that includes both medical and mental disorders.

The *Associated Features and Disorders* section describes symptoms that, while not necessary for the diagnosis of the disorder, are often seen in persons with the disorder. This section also includes a listing of other mental disorders that are commonly comorbid (likely to co-occur) with the disorder, and includes a listing of laboratory findings, clinical findings from examination, and medical conditions that may be associated with the disorder. The *Specific Age, Culture, or Gender Features* section details information concerning how the symptoms of a disorder may differ as a function of these demographic variables, including how symptoms may present differently in children and the elderly, how particular symptoms of the disorder may present differently in different cultures, and the proportion of women and men among those with the disorder. The *Prevalence* section provides information estimating how common the disorder is thought to be. These estimates are taken from large-scale epidemiological studies when possible, and include estimates of point prevalence (prevalence at any point in time) as well as lifetime prevalence (the proportion of people that in their lifetimes will experience the disorder). The *Course* section details information concerning onset and progression of symptoms, as well as the prognosis for remission and for relapse. In this section are included the typical age (or ages) of onset, factors that may predispose one to develop the disorder, and information concerning whether symptoms may worsen or improve with age. Also included in this section are estimates of whether a disorder is likely to involve one episode, multiple episodes with symptom-free periods between episodes, or chronic unremitting symptoms. The *Familial Pattern* section summarizes evidence concerning whether the disorder and related disorders are more common in the first-degree biological relatives of those with the disorder than members of the general population. This section also summarizes the results of twin or adoption studies, when available. Finally, the *Differential Diagnosis* section provides information to assist the diagnostician in distinguishing the disorder from other disorders that may appear similar or that may share symptoms in common. This section highlights the differences between disorders that could possibly be confused (e.g., Major Depressive Disorder versus Adjustment Disorder with Depressed Mood or, in the elderly, Dementia). [*See* Depression.]

B. Axis II: Personality Disorders and Mental Retardation

On Axis II are listed Personality Disorders and Mental Retardation. These disorders, by definition, are present for a substantial period of time (i.e., years). Although Axis I disorders may also be present for similar lengths of time, enduring symptoms are fundamentally part of these Axis II disorders. Also listed on Axis II are other traits or prominent features of a person's personality that a clinician deems maladaptive (e.g., frequent use of denial, excessive impulsivity).

In addition to the Personality Disorders, Mental Retardation appears on Axis II and is defined by (a) significantly below average intellectual abilities; (b) significant problems with adaptive functioning, defined as serious problems in carrying out duties expected for the person's age (e.g., self-care, interpersonal skills, work); and (c) an onset of these symptoms before the age of 18. Mental Retardation is placed on Axis II because of its pervasive and persistent effects on a person's function. It is worth noting that in the previous version of the *DSM* (*DSM-III-R*), other developmental disorders such as Autism and learning disorders were also listed on Axis II; these disorders, however, are listed on Axis I in *DSM-IV*. [*See* Autism and Pervasive Developmental Disorders; Mental Retardation and Mental Health.]

As the term Personality Disorder implies, people with these disorders have characterological features that create difficulties. *DSM-IV* defines a Personality Disorder as follows:

> A Personality Disorder is an enduring pattern of inner experience and behavior that deviates markedly from the expectations of the individual's culture, is pervasive and inflexible, has an onset in adolescence or early adulthood, is stable over time, and leads to distress or impairment (p. 629).

Upon a casual reading of the criteria for the various personality disorders, one may see many descriptions that may seem applicable to oneself or others at times. Symptoms of various personality disorders include, as examples, emotional lability, feelings of emptiness, bearing grudges, lacking close friends, suspiciousness, impulsivity, suggestibility, feeling envious, concern with criticism or rejection, difficulty in making everyday decisions, and perfectionism. In fact, many writers have criticized the *DSM* series' Personality Disorders for pathologizing anyone who simply may be different, or difficult. A Personality Disorder, however, can (in theory) be distinguished from what might be considered normal variation in personality because a Personality Disorder is *persistent, pervasive,* and *pathological.* [*See* PERSONALITY.]

By persistent, it is meant that the pattern of behavior in Personality Disorders is consistent over time. Whereas people without personality disorders may from time to time, after a bad day or following certain triggering events, display some of the features of certain personality disorders (e.g., difficulty controlling anger), such persons do not do so often or with any consistency.

By pervasive, it is meant that the behavior in Personality Disorders is seen across many different situations in the person's life. Whereas people without personality disorders may demonstrate some features of certain personality disorders in restricted situations (e.g., one is extremely suspicious of a difficult coworker; e.g., one doubts the fidelity of a spouse or sexual partner after a previously difficult and unfaithful relationship), such persons do not do so across situations (e.g., with coworkers, with spouse or partner, and with neighbors).

By pathological, it is meant that the severity of the symptom in Personality Disorders exceeds that which would be considered acceptable or normal by most people. Hot tempers, while not well-liked, are not necessarily pathological, but repeatedly getting into physical fights could be considered excessive. Daydreaming of a life more fantastic than one's own may be an occasional brief escape, but losing hours lost in fantasy could be considered excessive. Impulsive spontaneity can be fun, but impulsivity that results in overextended spending sprees, sexual indiscretions, or reckless driving could be considered excessive. Feeling empty and lonely are a part of the human condition, but suicide attempts that result from these feelings could be considered excessive. In each of these examples, what makes the behavior pathological in Personality Disorders involves the intensity of the subjective feeling, an impairment in judgment, and the degree to which the subjective feeling is translated into unacceptable or problematic behavior.

The personality disorders are organized by their apparent similarity into three clusters. Cluster A, the odd and eccentric cluster, includes the Paranoid, Schizoid, and Schizotypal Personality Disorders. Cluster B, the dramatic, emotional, and erratic cluster, includes the Antisocial, Borderline, Histrionic, and Narcissistic Personality Disorders. Finally, Cluster C,

the anxious and fearful cluster, includes the Avoidant, Dependent, and Obsessive-Compulsive Personality Disorders. In addition to general criteria for Personality Disorders, each disorder has its own polythetic criterion where an individual must have some minimum number (ranging from 3 to 5 for various disorders) from among a larger number (ranging from 7 to 9 across disorders) of symptoms. [*See* OBSESSIVE-COMPULSIVE DISORDERS; SCHIZOPHRENIA.]

C. Axis III: General Medical Conditions

On Axis III are listed general medical conditions that may be relevant to the disorder(s) listed on Axes I and II. The presence of Axis III should not be taken to suggest a mind–brain dualism, with Axes I and II representing problems of the mind in the absence of a physiological basis. On the contrary, mental experience is rooted in the function of the brain. Axis III is included in the *DSM* to encourage a comprehensive evaluation and a consideration of the various ways in which a general medical condition may be related to mental disorders.

There are several ways in which medical conditions may be related to mental disorders. First, the medical condition may be the direct cause of the mental condition. For example, hypothyroidism (Axis III) can lead to a syndrome of depressed mood known as Mood Disorder due to Hypothyroidism (Axis I). Similarly, Alzheimer's Disease (Axis III) produces Dementia of the Alzheimer's type (Axis I), and systemic infections (Axis III) can produce a Delirium (Axis I). [*See* ALZHEIMER'S DISEASE; DEMENTIA.]

The second manner in which a general medical condition may be relevant to a mental disorder is that the medical condition may be related to the development of the mental disorder, but not through direct physiological means. For example, an Axis I disorder such as Major Depression or Adjustment Disorder with Depressed Mood might follow in reaction to learning of one is diagnosed with a malignant melanoma (Axis III).

Finally, an Axis III medical condition, while not related to the appearance of the symptoms of a mental disorder, might be relevant in the treatment of a disorder. For example, certain antidepressant medications might be ill-advised in the presence of certain cardiovascular conditions. Alternatively, someone with a severe psychosis (Axis I) might have a medical condition (Axis III) that needs careful monitoring or treatment (e.g., diabetes), and might be unable to adhere to the treatment without assistance.

D. Axis IV: Psychosocial and Environmental Problems

Axis IV is included for detailing psychological, social, and environmental problems that may be relevant to the presenting mental disorder. Such problems may have influenced the development of the disorder, may have developed as a consequence of the disorder, may be relevant to the selection of an appropriate treatment, or may influence the prognosis for recovery. Although both positive (e.g., job promotion) and negative (e.g., job loss) life events can be perceived as stressful, typically only the negative events are detailed on Axis IV unless the positive event is clearly related to the mental disorder. Moreover, only events during the last year are typically noted, unless remote events still appear to be a significant influence on the mental disorder. Examples of problems that could be listed on Axis IV include death of a loved one, divorce, problems with school, unemployment or other job problems, homelessness or a difficult living situation, financial troubles, lack of insurance, legal troubles, or experiencing a natural disaster. [*See* BEREAVEMENT; DIVORCE; HOMELESSNESS; UNEMPLOYMENT AND MENTAL HEALTH.]

A careful assessment of the problems listed on Axis IV may suggest that, in some cases, the most appropriate intervention will not focus on the individual (as is the case with psychological counseling or the prescription of psychotropic medication), but rather on the broader social environment in which the individual must exist. In such cases, the primary intervention could involve not only mental health professionals (e.g., providing family therapy), but teachers, landlords, lawyers, insurance companies, and so on. On the other hand, some mental disorders may arise in the relative absence of psychosocial and environmental problems and suggest that the treatment might most fruitfully focus on the individual.

E. Axis V: Global Assessment of Functioning

Axis V provides a scale for the assessment of a person's overall level of functioning. Ratings reflect a continuum of mental health to mental illness and range from 100 (exemplary) to 1 (inordinately poor). Taken into account in making the rating are the person's psychological, social, and occupational functioning. Limitations due to purely physical limitations (e.g., spinal cord injury) are not considered when making the rating. The severity of psychological symptoms and the potential for suicide or violence are important determinants of the person's functioning rating. Global functioning is typically rated for the period surrounding the current evaluation, although it may be useful to rate, in addition, previous time periods to provide an indication of how well or poorly the individual may function at other times.

At the top end of the scale (81–100) are people who are models of mental health. These scores are reserved for those fortunate individuals who not only are without impairment, but exhibit many of the traits considered to be mentally healthy (superior functioning, wide range of interests, social effectiveness, warmth, and integrity). Just below this range (71–80) are individuals with no significant symptoms or impairment, but who lack the positive mental health features. Below this range are scores that will likely characterize a majority of individuals in need of psychological or psychiatric treatment. Those in the upper range (31–70) will most likely be capable of receiving outpatient treatment, whereas those in the lower range (1–40) will most likely require inpatient treatment.

F. Appendices to the *DSM-IV*

Included in the *DSM-IV* are 10 appendices. The appendices include a guide to facilitate differential diagnosis, a glossary, alphabetical and numerical listings of the diagnoses described in the manual, a summary of changes between the *DSM-IV* and the previous version of the *DSM*, comparisons of *DSM-IV* codes to the codes in two editions of the International Classification of Diseases, and a listing of contributors.

Worth special mention are two other appendices, *Criteria Sets and Axes Provided for Further Study*, and an *Outline for Cultural Formulation and Glossary of Culture-Bound Syndromes*. The first of these lists entries that were considered for inclusion in the *DSM-IV*, but were not included due to insufficient evidence. The disorders or axes are listed in the appendix to encourage research that will provide sufficient evidence to include or exclude these entries from future editions of the *DSM*. The appendix encourages researchers to study refinements in these sets of criteria. Examples of entries in this appendix include Caffeine Withdrawal, alternative descriptions of Schizophrenia and other disorders related to Schizophrenia, other variants of depressive disorders, Premenstrual Dysphoric Disorder, Mixed Anxiety-Depressive Disorder, a series of Medication-Induced Movement Disorders, and Passive Aggressive Personality Disorder (which appeared as an Axis II disorder in the previous edition of the *DSM*). The proposed Axes include a scale to measure strategies for coping with emotional states, termed the Defensive Functioning Scale, and two scales modeled after Axis V to measure functioning in specific areas (relationships, and social/occupational).

The appendix covering cultural variations in the presentation of mental disorders provides information that might be of assistance in evaluating individuals from cultures other than one's own. One could mistakenly label as mental illness behaviors that appear abnormal from one's own culture, but that would not be regarded as aberrant by members of the culture from which the individual originates. For example, hearing voices is typically considered a psychotic symptom by members of the mental health community, although within some religious groups the experience is supported and interpreted as an experience that is to be heeded or revered. When diagnosing, one needs to take into account how such symptoms would be viewed by fellow members of an individual's culture, which may be include religious, ethnic, racial, and geographic influences.

IV. EVALUATION OF DIAGNOSTIC SYSTEMS: RELIABILITY AND VALIDITY

A discussion of the validity of a diagnostic system must first assume that diagnoses can be assigned reliably. Reliability of diagnosis simply means that the same diagnoses will be assigned to individuals across different circumstances. Such different circumstances might involve the passage of time (in the case of test-retest reliability) or different diagnosticians (in the case of inter-rater reliability). Because symptoms of mental illness often wax and wane, test-retest reliability may not be the most appropriate means of assessing the reliability of diagnosis, since we might

expect diagnoses to change over time. The standard method of assessing the reliability of the diagnosis of mental illness, therefore, is inter-rater reliability, or the extent to which two (or more) independent raters agree on the presence or on the absence of a mental illness.

A. Calculation of Inter-Rater Reliability

In assessing inter-rater reliability, one could simply calculate the overall proportion of agreement between two independent raters. This approach, however, fails to account for the proportion of time that two raters would agree merely by chance. For example, imagine that two raters agree on the presence or absence of depression 70% of the time. Although this might appear promising, one needs to compute the likelihood that they would agree by chance alone. To illustrate, imagine that these two diagnosticians each "diagnose" 100 individuals for depression with the flip of a coin. Each diagnostician therefore labels 50 individuals depressed, and 50 nondepressed. Of the 50 individuals labeled depressed by the first diagnostician, half (25) will also be diagnosed as depressed by the second diagnostician (since the second diagnostician is independently "diagnosing" by a coin flip). Similarly, among the 50 individuals labeled nondepressed by the first diagnostician, 25 will be similarly labeled by the second diagnostician. Therefore, by chance alone, these two diagnosticians would agree for 50 (25 + 25) of the 100 individuals.

Of course diagnosticians do not diagnose by coin flips, but the calculation of chance agreement follows in a similar fashion. Assume that in a particular clinic, based on the observation of symptoms, each diagnostician identifies half of the patients as depressed. Also assume, for the moment, that the diagnosticians' ratings agree only for reasons of chance. The raters would agree that 25 of the patients merit a diagnosis of depression, and would agree that 25 do not, yielding an overall agreement of 50/100 cases, or 50%. The actual agreement of 70%, while higher than that expected by chance, is not as promising as it initially appeared.

To account for chance agreement, a corrected estimate of agreement, termed *Kappa*, is often calculated:

$$\kappa = \frac{p_o - p_c}{1 - p_c}$$

Kappa reflects the extent to which the observed proportion of agreement (p_o; e.g., 70%) exceeds the proportion of agreement expected by chance (p_c; e.g., 50%), expressed as a proportion of the difference between perfect agreement (1.0) and chance agreement (e.g., 50%). Stated differently, Kappa reflects the improvement beyond chance actually obtained by the diagnosticians, expressed as a proportion of the maximum possible improvement beyond chance. Kappa therefore ranges from 0 (chance agreement) to 1.0 (perfect agreement). A Kappa of .50, for example, would indicate that the agreement of the diagnosticians fell midway between chance and perfect agreement. In the hypothetical example above, where 70% agreement was obtained, but 50% was expected by chance:

$$\kappa = \frac{p_o - p_c}{1 - p_c} = \frac{.70 - .50}{1 - .50} = \frac{.20}{.50} = .40$$

For *DSM-III* diagnoses, Kappas range from near 0 to near 1. Reliability data, while provided as an appendix in *DSM-III,* have been conspicuously absent from *DSM-III-R* and *DSM-IV* manuals. The reliability data from the *DSM-IV* field trials is promised to appear in Volume V of the *DSM-IV Sourcebook,* a compendium of the literature reviews and empirical research on which *DSM-IV* is based. Two years after the publication of the *DSM-IV,* however, only Volumes I and II of the *Sourcebook* have appeared in print. It is reasonable to assume that Kappas will again span a broad range, but on average be slightly higher than those associated with earlier versions of the *DSM.*

While Kappa provides a simple metric for summarizing agreement beyond chance, Kappa is not a panacea. Kappa is influenced by base rates of diagnosis, and Kappa provides no direct evidence of validity. The base-rate problem results when diagnoses are assigned very frequently or virtually never. In such cases, even small increases beyond chance can result in an appreciable value of Kappa. This can be problematic since the rate of many mental disorders in the general population is rather low. Imagine that two diagnosticians agree on only 4% more cases than would be expected by chance for a disorder that affects 5% of the population. If each of these diagnosticians label 5% of the sample with the diagnosis, they will agree that 90.25% (.95 * .95) of the people do not have the disorder, and will agree that fewer than 1% (.05 * .05 =

.25%) of the people have the disorder. In other words, by chance alone, they would agree 90.5% of the time. If their actual agreement exceeds this by 4% (94.5%), Kappa would be .42. As can be seen from the preceding examples, it required agreement that was 20% higher than that expected by chance to achieve a Kappa in the range of .4 when the baserate of diagnosis was in the range of 50%, but it only required agreement that exceeded chance by 4% to achieve a similar Kappa when the base rate was quite low. The interpretation of Kappa is not absolute, as Kappa is considerably influenced by the base rate of diagnosis.

A second form of the base-rate problem stems from the fact that the base rate of disorders may vary dramatically by setting. For example, while schizophrenia is quite rare in the general population, it is considerably more prevalent among patients in a psychiatric hospital. Because the value of Kappa is influenced by the baserate of the diagnosis, Kappa can vary by setting even when raters apply criteria consistently across these settings.

The second caveat to consider is that Kappa provides no direct evidence of the validity of diagnosis. High values of Kappa merely indicate agreement. In fact, independent of any correspondence to the actual symptoms, perfect agreement ($\kappa = 1.0$) would be obtained if both diagnosticians agreed that every individual had the diagnosis in question. Therefore, while high values of Kappa may be necessary to ensure validity, they are by no means sufficient. Moreover, it is possible to alter diagnostic criteria to improve interrater agreement as indexed by Kappa, but to sacrifice validity in the process. For example, by making the criteria for a disorder increasingly tangible, one might increase agreement at the expense of making the criteria so narrow that many individuals no longer meet the criteria, despite having symptoms that many people would consider to be essential features of the disorder.

A final caution to keep in mind when considering the reliability of diagnosis, whether it be measured by Kappa or some other index, is that two raters can disagree for a variety of reasons, only some of which may reflect a poor system of diagnostic classification. For example, the particular method used to assess the symptoms (e.g., a standardized interview versus an unstructured interview) can determine what symptoms are elicited. Moreover, poor training of the diagnosticians can also lead to poor reliability. Research studies of mental illness, therefore, typically employ highly trained diagnosticians who use a standard structured interview to inquire about each of the symptoms of the disorder under study.

Reliability, therefore, should not be the sole standard by which the adequacy of diagnostic criteria are judged. Although this sounds obvious, there is a tendency for researchers to use high reliability as evidence of the adequacy of diagnostic criteria; this may be tempting since a single number can provide a summary of reliability whereas establishing validity is considerably more complicated.

B. Validity

When considering whether a set of diagnostic criteria have validity, one is asking whether assigning the diagnostic label provides valuable information—beyond the specific symptoms that begot the diagnosis—about a person with a particular diagnosis. There may be many such *external indicators* of validity, but three of the most important would include etiology, treatment, and prognosis. Additionally, and perhaps most primary, a valid system of diagnosis should allow one to clearly make distinctions between one disorder and another, and between a disorder and the absence of a disorder. Individuals who share a diagnosis should be similar to one another (in terms of symptoms, etiology, response to treatment, or prognosis) and should be clearly different than individuals with other diagnoses or individuals with no diagnosis. If such a clear delineation is not possible, then there is insufficient evidence to justify the existence of the diagnostic category. The *DSM-IV* in particular has been criticized for inadequately distinguishing between mental disorders and normal variations in behavior. For example, although significant depressive symptoms that follow the death of a loved one are considered a normal reaction (for a period, incidentally, of up to 2 months), depressive symptoms following other major losses or setbacks (e.g., divorce, diagnosis with a terminal illness) are considered evidence of the mental disorder Major Depression.

In terms of etiology, a valid system would ensure that people with the same diagnostic label would share a common etiology. In some instances in the *DSM-IV,* this is clearly the case (e.g., Alcohol Withdrawal Delirium, also known as "delirium tremens"); in other instances, it is likely that people with the same

diagnosis may have different etiological influences (e.g., Major Depressive Disorder).

In terms of treatment, a valid system should suggest particular treatments that are likely to be effective for a particular disorder. Alternatively, since no treatments are 100% effective, a valid system should inform us of the likelihood that different treatments may be effective for the disorder. For example, given an episode of Major Depression that has lasted less than 2 years, there is a 50 to 70% chance that an individual will experience remission using one of several antidepressant medications, or by receiving one of two varieties of psychotherapy.

In terms of prognosis, a valid system should provide an indication of what is likely to happen in the future given that a person has a particular diagnosis. For example, given that a person has experienced one episode of Major Depression, there is approximately a 50% chance that the person will experience another at some point in life. Given that one has a personality disorder diagnosis, it is likely that the pattern of behavior will continue for quite some time, if not indefinitely.

V. CHALLENGES TO VALIDITY AND FUTURE DIRECTIONS IN DIAGNOSIS

The *DSM-IV,* like its predecessors, has adopted a *descriptive categorical approach* to diagnosis, which assumes that there exist *discrete categories* of mental illness that can be defined—for most diagnoses—primarily on the basis of observable symptoms. Discrete categories of illness dichotomize individuals into those who do, and those who do not, have the illness; borderline cases are categorized into one or the other category (or given one of the may NOS diagnoses). When the etiology of an illness is known, the categorical approach is defensible and is likely to provide useful information. For example, people either do or do not have a history of a stroke. Within the category of those with strokes, there are certainly gradations in severity, but there is a clear delineation between those who have, and those who have not, experienced a stroke. In the case of most mental disorders, by contrast, there are not such obvious distinctions between the presence and the absence of the condition. For example, *DSM-IV* requires that five of nine symptoms be present in order to make the diagnosis of a Major

Depressive Episode. Certainly people who meet four of the nine symptoms are not free of depression, yet they would not be categorized as having a Major Depressive Episode.

Strictly speaking, a categorical approach assumes that there exist necessary and sufficient features for categorical membership. Although the *DSM-IV* adopts a categorical approach, there are many instances of disorders that do not have necessary or sufficient criteria. Consider for example, the case of Obsessive-Compulsive Personality Disorder, for which an individual must meet at least four of eight possible criteria to receive the diagnosis. None of the individual criteria are necessary and, moreover, two individuals could both meet criteria and share not a single one of the criteria in common. In other words, there can exist considerable heterogeneity in symptoms among those who share a common diagnosis.

Strictly speaking, a categorical approach also assumes that categories are either nested, or mutually exclusive. For example, a square is a special (nested) case of a rectangle, but is mutually exclusive with the category of circle. For diagnoses of mental illness, by contrast, there exists considerable overlap (comorbidity) of diagnoses. A recent large-scale community study found that, across the life span, about one-sixth of the population had three (or more) diagnoses, and that this group accounted for over half all diagnoses. Such high comorbidity certainly raises questions as to whether the categorical approach to diagnosis is justified. When comorbidity of diagnoses is observed, it is unclear whether the different disorders reflect different manifestations of the same underlying cause, whether one disorder served to facilitate the development of another, or whether the disorders resulted from different underlying causes and merely co-occurred by chance. Comorbidity can also present an enigma in terms of treatment, as it can be unclear which disorder to treat, or how to coordinate treatments for different disorders.

A modification to the classical categorical approach is the *prototype* approach, in which exemplars (also known as prototypes) of a given diagnosis become the standard for comparison. Each individual is compared to the diagnostic prototypes, and assigned the diagnosis associated with the best-fitting prototype. Such a system has several advantages. Such a system eliminates the problem of borderline cases, since such cases will receive a diagnosis if they are more similar to the diagnostic prototype than to any other prototype. Such a system also virtually eliminates the need for the NOS categories, which in the *DSM* seem to have become the "wastebasket" for many borderline or unusual cases. On the other hand, a prototype system has its drawbacks. Prototypes stem from the perceptions of the diagnosticians, and therefore may fail to reflect important features of a disorder that are not easily observable (e.g., lab findings). Moreover, the use of prototypes may make the identification of new disorders more difficult, and instead simply reify the implicit theories that people have about forms of mental illness. Finally, to distinguish mental health from mental illness, one would presumably require a prototype of mental health. Although it could be difficult to define a single prototype for each diagnostic category, it might be even more challenging to define the prototype(s) for mental health.

Other modifications to the categorical approach of the *DSM-IV* have been proposed, including eliminating categories entirely. The dimensional approach involves assessing individuals along a set of relevant dimensions. Under such a system, an individual would receive a quantitative rating along each dimension in the diagnostic system. Although the conceptual simplicity of a category may be lost using such a system, such a system could possibly convey more information about each individual, would eliminate the problem of classifying borderline cases, and would have no problems of comorbidity. On the other hand, many diagnosticians prefer the yes-or-no simplicity of categorical diagnosis, and may be likely to establish idiosyncratic cutpoints on the dimensions, such that those individuals scoring above a certain value would be considered to have a particular categorical diagnosis. Additionally, it is no trivial matter to determine the relevant set of dimensions to use in such a system.

In the final analysis, there may exist some types of problems for which a categorical system is well-suited, and others where a dimensional approach may hold greater utility. The *DSM-IV* is already an amalgam of different approaches to categorization, with some diagnoses clearly defined by etiology, and others defined solely by the presence of particular symptoms. This may reflect the nature of different forms of mental illness. Some forms may have a single causal factor that is more potent than all other contributing factors, and have a homogeneous set of symptoms that appear. Others, by contrast, may have multiple determinants, and may present with a heterogeneous set of symptoms that differ for each individual.

The *DSM-IV* is the current version of the most widely-used diagnostic system for mental disorders. If history provides an accurate indication, many other revisions—some major, and some minor—are likely to follow, with considerable controversy and debate surrounding each.

BIBLIOGRAPHY

American Psychiatric Association (1987). *Diagnostic and statistical manual of mental disorders* (3rd ed., revised). Washington, DC: American Psychiatric Association.

American Psychiatric Association (1994). *Diagnostic and statistical manual of mental disorders* (4th ed.). Washington, DC: American Psychiatric Association.

Cantor, N., Smith, E. E., deSales French, R., & Mezzich, J. (1980). Psychiatric diagnosis as prototype categorization. *Journal of Abnormal Psychology, 89*, 181–193.

Clark, L. A., Watson, D., & Reynolds, S. (1995). Diagnosis and classification of psychopathology: Challenges to the current system and future directions. *Annual Review of Psychology, 46*, 121–153.

Kessler, R. C., McGonagle, K. A., Shanyang, Z., Nelson, C. B., Hughes, M., Eshlemen, S., Wittchen, H., Kendler, K. (1994). Lifetime and 12-month prevalence of *DSM-III*-R Psychiatric Disorders in the United States: Results from the National Comorbidity Study. *Archives of General Psychiatry, 51*, 8–19.

Kirk, S. A., & Kutchins, H. (1992). The selling of DSM: The rhetoric of science in psychiatry. New York: Walter de Gruyter, Inc.

Robins, L. N., & Barrett, J. E. (1989). The validity of psychiatric diagnosis. New York: Raven Press Ltd.

Rosenhan, D. L. (1973). On being sane in insane places. *Science, 179*, 250–258.

Wakefield, J. C. (1996). DSM-IV: Are we making progress? *Contemporary Psychology, 41*, 646–652.

Dying

Robert Kastenbaum

Arizona State University

Brain Death A condition in which vegetative processes of the body may continue, although the capacity for thought, experience, and behavior has been destroyed.

Dying The progressive and irreversible loss of physical function that ends in death.

Hospice An alternative to traditional medical care of dying people that gives highest priority to relief of pain and other symptoms (also known as the palliative care approach).

Persistent Vegetative State The continuation of vital body functions over a period of weeks, months, or even years despite the individual's lack of responsiveness (a condition often maintained through the use of a ventilator and/or other life-support devices, but that may also exist spontaneously).

Terminal Illness An incurable condition that will lead to a person's death within a relatively short period of time (usually defined as within 6 months or a year). The period immediately preceding death is known as the end phase or end stage.

DYING is a progressive and irreversible loss of physical function that ends in death. The duration, personal experience, and social impact of this process differ markedly from person to person, but it is commonly a period of stress, loss of control, and discontinuity. There are often episodes of anxiety and depression and alterations of consciousness. Nevertheless, dying is a universal experience, not a psychiatric disorder. Many clinicians and humanists agree that it is possible to have a "good," "appropriate," or "healthy" death, but there is a continuing need for reflection on precisely what should be meant by these terms. One must also reflect on the basic concept of mental health when it is applied to the situation of dying people and their interpersonal support network. It is necessary therefore to examine attitudes, values, and the ever-changing health care system as well as the biomedical facts of dying.

I. KEY QUESTIONS AND ISSUES

A. What *Is* Dying?

More than 600 years ago a virulent plague swept through much of the world. It has been estimated that the Black Death took the lives of a third of the population as it moved in a broad swath through much of Asia, Europe, and the Middle East. A person apparently in good health would experience the sudden onset of agonizing and disfiguring symptoms that often found no relief until the cessation of life. It was within the context of this widespread catastrophe that a word previously unfamiliar to most people became prominent. *Die* was first spoken in Old Frisian, a Low German dialect used by people exposed to the terror of the plague in northern Holland. Soon this word in slightly variant forms entered English and other European languages.

The word that became part of our cultural heritage in the plague-stricken fourteenth century is still in use today. However, this familiar term is becoming less reliable as a practical guide for understanding, decision making, and care giving. There are still many situations in which it is evident that a person's life will soon come to an end. In these situations there is no serious doubt that the person is experiencing "a progressive and irreversible loss of physical function that ends in death." Nevertheless, health care providers are encountering an increased incidence of situations in which neither "dying" nor any other familiar term seems adequate. It is not only that reasonable people may have different interpretations of the status of a particular person whose life is in jeopardy. The concept of dying has itself become subject to ambiguity and uncertainty. Understanding the mental health implications of the dying process therefore requires recognition of the complex and transitional status of "dying" and its companion concept, "terminal illness." Following are some of the biomedical and societal developments that are unsettling the familiar concept of "dying":

• Advances in medical technology have outraced society's ability to identify and conceptualize states of being for which the terms "living" and "dying" (or "alive" and "dead") do not seem to be adequate. For example, the nonresponsive person who is maintained in a persistent vegetative state through life-support devices might be regarded variously as living, dying, or dead. The situation becomes further confused when it is said that a "brain dead" person is dying. It is not surprising that family members, the general public and the Supreme Court have all found themselves with troubling issues to resolve regarding the status and rights of a person who exists on the tenuous border between life and death.

• Deaths from virulent diseases and rapidly disseminating infections are much less common than in the past. "Dying" usually referred to a relatively brief period of acute distress followed by death, as during the plague years. Today many people live for extended periods of time with preterminal or terminal conditions, and during this time they continue to participate in meaningful relationships and activities. The same term—*dying*—does not seem to apply equally

well to a person in acute distress and decline and to a person with a progressive and apparently nonreversible physical condition who is not at immediate risk for death.

• A person may be experiencing a progressive loss of physical functioning that has all the features associated with dying. This pattern may be halted or even reversed, however, with a new treatment modality. Furthermore, there are occasional spontaneous remissions. Although the odds may be against successful treatment or spontaneous remission, even the occasional example raises questions about traditional assumptions. In retrospect it can be asked: was this person really "dying" if there was recovery? Perhaps the defining specification that dying is a nonreversible process should be postponed until death has actually occurred. From the mental health standpoint this ambiguity could make it more difficult for patient, family, and caregivers to cope with the situation: should one prepare for death or fight for life? At present there is no established concept or term for the person who is experiencing the progressive debilitation consistent with dying, but who may still have a real, although small chance of recovery. Every hint of a new "medical miracle" brings more people into this zone of ambiguity. Physicians today, with an unprecedented array of biomedical resources to draw upon, may contribute significantly to this ambiguity with the attitude that "This patient is not dying if there is one more thing we can try!"

• Both the government and the insurance industry are attempting to control the costs of health care. Costs tend to increase significantly during the period of physical decline that precedes death. These bureaucracies are devising their own definitions in the effort to limit entitlements and costs. For example, federal agencies have defined a terminal illness as one that will end in death within 6 months. Physicians have been required to certify that a person will be dead within 6 months in order to become eligible to select the hospice alternative for terminal care under federal health care entitlements. Many physicians have been reluctant to participate in this certification process because they recognize that the course of an illness can vary from person to person. The 6-month requirement eventually may be modified in response to criticism. However, it has already established the precedent that the concept of dying can be transformed into a number (of entitlement days) for purposes of bureaucratic and fiscal control. All such bureaucratic definitions have consequences for the management of the terminal phase of life.

• Technological advances have made organ donation a significant part of the health care system, offering hope to many people with life-threatening conditions. Law and public opinion require that organs not be removed until the death of the donor. Successful transplantation requires the removal of the organ before it has deteriorated. A tension system exists in which there is a built-in conflict between those who are dedicated to preserving life and those who are dedicated to organ transplantation to save another person's life. In this uncomfortable situation there is temptation to define dying and death in ways that favor either preservation of life or timely organ transplantation. Furthermore, there is also pressure to define "dead" in such a way that it delays or hastens the opportunity for organ removal.

What are the implications of these developments for understanding the dying process from a mental health perspective? One general implication is that we do not have to completely abandon tradition. There *is* a period of physical decline that immediately precedes death, and we might as well continue to designate this distinctive and crucial phase of life as *dying*. Alterations of mood, thought, and behavior that occur within the context of the dying process can have markedly different implications than similar changes occurring for a person in good physical health.

However, this familiar term, dying, does not provide adequate information to guide understanding and care. There is a tendency to regard dying people as a homogenous class. This tendency is expressed in such statements as, "Dying people feel. . . ." and "Dying people want. . . ." Such statements are built on the assumptions that dying is essentially the same process and generates essentially the same responses in all individuals. The mental health needs of the dying person may then be approached with a predetermined set of concepts and interventions. The classification "dying patient" becomes the dominant consideration, leading to insufficient consideration of the individual's personality, life history, and present circumstances.

These assumptions are at variance with the facts. Some of the difficulties with a fixed and monolithic definition of dying have already been noted. These include: (a) people who are in a prolonged vegetative or other nonresponsive state; (b) the possibility of remission from an apparently terminal condition; (c) growing bureaucratic influence over the definition of dying; and (d) the biopolitics of organ donation that influence the definition of death as well as dying.

There are other difficulties as well. The individual's experiences during the last phase of life depend much upon the particular life-threatening condition, the type of care being received, and the setting in which it takes place. Some people experience a long debilitating process in which fatigue and slow, progressive loss of function are the primary concerns. Others experience a terminal process in which there are alarming episodes, such as an acute struggle for breath. Still others have multiple symptoms that profoundly affect all realms of functioning. One person may require hospitalization for a variety of medical and nursing interventions to control pain and other symptoms; another person may be at home, gradually drifting toward death with little fear or anguish and with the support of caring family members. One person may be mentally alert throughout the process; another person may be disoriented. All of these people are dying, but their experiences are so varied and distinctive that we must go well beyond their proximity to death if we are to understand their situations. Note, for example, the 10 most common causes of death in the United States (Table I). The experiences of people terminally ill with

Table I 10 Most Common Causes of Death in the United States

Rank	Cause	Number	Percentage of total deaths
1	Heart disease	739,860	32.6
2	Cancer	530,870	23.4
3	Stroke	149,740	6.6
4	Chronic obstructive lung disease	101,090	4.5
5	Accident	88,630	3.9
6	Pneumonia and influenza	81,730	3.6
7	Diabetes melitus	55,110	2.4
8	AIDS-related	38,500	1.7
9	Suicide	31,230	1.4
10	Homicide	25,470	1.1
	All causes	2,268,000	

Data are based on a 10% sampling of U.S. deaths in 1993 by the National Center for Health Statistics.

heart disease (#1 cause) and cancer (#2 cause) generally differ in such important respects as symptomatology and duration of end-phase. Other significant differences are typical for most of the other major causes of death. These differences encompass not only the individual's experience, but also the type and setting of care and the impact of the course of death on family and friends.

We might also follow the lead of health care professionals who have learned to distinguish between the general course of a terminal illness and the *end-stage* with its collapse of the organ systems that support life. The end-stage varies in duration and form. Often it is a matter of days or weeks. There may be conscious symptoms, or the person may gradually spend more and more time in a non- or low-responsive state. The final moment may be a quiet slipping away while in a sleeplike state, or following a brief and lucid conversation.

The following example is not uncommon. A terminally ill man was receiving care at the home of one of his daughters and her family. He was not in pain nor was he anxious. Each day he could do a little less physically and spent more time lying in bed with his eyes closed. One afternoon the daughter asked if there was anything he needed or wanted. "A glass of water—please." He sipped the water, then, smiled slightly and said, in his characteristically quiet and appreciative way, "Thank you." A moment later he closed his eyes again, and the father's body stiffened and froze at the touch of death. In this instance, a peaceful final phase of life was the outcome of a fortunate configuration of individual personality, a caring environment, and a terminal condition that proceeded in an almost gentle manner from the first diagnostic signs through the end-stage.

It would be simplistic and misleading, however, to overgeneralize from the journey of any one person from health to illness, from illness to terminal illness, and from terminal illness through the end-stage. The mental health challenges depend much on the particularities of person, type and phase of illness, treatment and management strategy, and interpersonal support.

B. Mental Health Issues

Mental health issues do not stand alone. There are as many possible mental health issues as there are particular individuals and circumstances. The selected issues identified here should be taken only as a current sampling.

- *Living with uncertainty.* It is well established that uncertainty about the future course of events increases anxiety and stress. A person with a life-threatening condition may have to cope with uncertainty in many forms: *Will I die from this condition? When? How? How should I and how will I respond to the risks and challenges? How will my illness and death affect my family?*

- *Loss of control.* Anxiety, stress, and depression are also frequent corollaries of a perceived loss of control over one's life. The dying process tends to diminish the individual's ability to exercise control in all spheres of life, including one's own body functions.

- *Loss of relationships.* Emotional pain and depression are often experienced when a valued relationship is threatened or lost. Stress, illness, substance abuse, social withdrawal, and suicide attempts are among the problems that may develop in response to the loss of a crucial relationship. The dying person may feel abandoned or rejected by others, or she may be apprehensive about the eventual loss of support and companionship.

- *Disturbance of body image and self-concept.* People sometimes respond with anxiety to even small violations of their body image, for example, that first gray hair or wrinkle. Any progressive illness has the potential to have a devastating effect on the person's body image and, therefore, the total self-concept. The dying process confronts some people with such extensive physical changes that they may find it difficult to relate to their own bodies. Denial-type responses often represent an attempt to distance one's self (concept) from its damaged abode. [*See* BODY IMAGE.]

- *Loss of communication.* Physical disabilities associated with the dying process may interfere with the ability to share one's thoughts and feelings with others. Some treatment modalities also inhibit communication. Moreover, both family members and health care professionals may avoid, limit, or distort their interactions with the dying person because of their own anxieties. Whatever contributes to the failure of communication is also likely to contribute to stress, anxiety, and despair.

- *Unfulfilled dreams, uncompleted projects.* There may be tension, frustration, and disappointment because the dying person has not seen the fulfillment of his or her goals, whether person-oriented (e.g., seeing the graduation of a favorite grandchild) or achievement-oriented (e.g., writing a book or bringing a new product to market). The physical stress of dying and the realization of a foreshortened life expectancy can intensify the tensions associated with unfulfilled dreams and provoke rage, confusion, or despair.

- *Loss of meaning.* All of the foregoing challenges can lead dying people to question the meaning of their lives as death approaches. There may be a pressing need to "validate" one's life through meditation and supportive conversations. There may also be a heightened need to reaffirm one's guiding beliefs. As many insightful observers have noted, the concern that one's life may have been meaningless or "inauthentic" can be the source of profound despair. Whatever protects a person from experiencing the despair of perceived meaninglessness will do much to enable that person to cope with the other stresses of the dying process.

These are examples of issues that may or may not be salient for a particular person as he or she moves through the dying process. Furthermore, an issue may become salient or lose its saliency at various points in the process. Those who are available to help the dying person should not assume that a particular issue must be crucial to that person but, rather, maintain open and effective communication that will improve their abilities to recognize issues as they arise.

II. ATTITUDES TOWARD DYING AND THE DYING PERSON AND THEIR IMPLICATIONS FOR MENTAL HEALTH

Attention has been focused on the dying person. However, the mental health of the dying person depends much on the attitudes and behaviors of the people in his or her life. The substantial literature on attitudes toward dying and the dying person offers several major findings.

A. Keeping the Dying Person at a Distance

Avoiding contact with the dying person has been a conspicuous feature of American society for many years. This phobia has also been characteristic of many other societies as well, a point that has emerged clearly with the on-going establishment of hospice (palliative) care programs beyond the Euro-American orbit.

Early studies quickly demonstrated that physicians and nurses engaged in systematic patterns of avoiding contact with the dying person. One very simple study clearly delineated the situation. Unknown to themselves, hospital nurses were timed by a psychologist as they responded to calls from the patients on their floor. It was found that the nurses took much longer to go to the rooms of patients who were terminally ill as compared with other patients. There is an (unpublished) epilogue to this research story. The nurses were surprised and dismayed when this finding was shared with them. They had not been aware of this behavior pattern. The nurses spontaneously vowed to quicken their response to terminally ill patients. After a few weeks the psychologist repeated his little stopwatch experiment: same result! Despite their conscious intention to serve terminally ill patients without hesitation or delay, the nurses were still being influenced by the cultural attitude of avoiding contact with dying people.

Subsequent studies by other investigators using other methods have confirmed both the avoidance pattern and the difficulties encountered in attempting to break away from it. Physician-avoidant behavior was found to be even more ubiquitous and persistent than was the case with nurses. It was repeatedly observed that physicians spent less time and engaged in less eye contact with terminally ill patients. They were also reported as unresponsive to the questions raised and the needs expressed by these patients. The higher status and greater mobility of physicians were seen as making it relatively easy for them to avoid contact with dying people, while nurses were under more obligation to provide direct (primary) care.

Some of the most effective criticism mounted against physicians from the 1960s onward came from physicians. These insider analyses included such points as the following:

- Medical school reinforced the cultural belief that dying is a failure—therefore, physicians become failures when their patients die, and it is best to have as little involvement as possible with these patients.
- Medical school also provided almost no training in human relations; in fact, it presented a model of

"objectivity" and distancing rather than building a physician–patient alliance. Young physicians were therefore ill-prepared to understand and cope with the dynamics and emotional complexities involved with dying people and their families—another good reason to keep such contact to a minimum.

- Physicians, so much exposed to human vulnerability, often were anxious about their own mortality and yet prohibited by the rules of the game from discussing their fears openly. Contact with dying people therefore had the potential of stirring up the physician's own unresolved problems.
- The belief that there was little one could do to help dying patients contributed much to avoidance. Not only was the physician confronted by failure to cure, but also by the failure to provide relief from pain and other symptoms. "There is nothing more I can do for you," followed by a brisk walk away from the patient's bedside was a type of interaction frequently reported by patients and confirmed by the physician-reformists.

Hospital administrators, social workers, psychologists, pharmacists, respiratory therapists, and clergy were also documented as engaging in avoidance attitudes and behaviors. Although the details varied with the particular field, these service providers often shared the same characteristic: personal anxiety and lack of preparation for communicating with—even for *being* with—terminally ill people and their families.

Avoidance was also documented as a family characteristic. It was discovered that dying and death had been taboo subjects in most family circles. This rule of silence left each family member in his or her own compartment of isolation and fear. Effective communication was difficult to achieve when a family member became terminally ill because of the "let's not talk about it" tradition. Many observers (including those commenting on their own family experiences) lamented that the people who should provide the most intimate and significant support for each other were often in their own separate worlds of confusion and pain as a member of the family moved through the dying process.

The behavioral avoidance of dying people was closely related to semantic avoidance. Tactful people did not speak of dying or death, either in the general or the specific. Cancer was a word to be avoided whenever possible because of its associations with death.

People seldom actually died of cancer, however; newspaper obituaries would refer to a "long illness." The reluctance to speak openly of death and dying was a major barrier to learning and exchanging information. The fear of speaking about death contributed to a general anxiety about interpersonal communication. *Perhaps somebody would say the wrong thing. Perhaps one would be at a loss for words. Perhaps one would be caught in a deception.* The rule of silence about dying and death distorted interpersonal communication and therefore undermined social solidarity.

B. Reducing the Social Value of the Dying Person

Ideally, gender, age, place of origin, race, ethnicity, religion and socioeconomic status do not bear on a person's value. In the real world, though, all of these factors and more do affect the attribution of value. Aging and dying are unusual among these conditions. Most of the attributes that affect social value are fixed and mutually exclusive. For example, a person who begins life as an African-American female is not likely to become a White male, or vice versa. By contrast, all people are mortal and everybody who lives long enough will experience the aging process. There is a normative (expected or expectable) transition from youth to age and from life to death. This transition also represents, in general, a decline in attributed social value. The angle of decline is sharper when socioeconomic status also diminishes with age (e.g., as a consequence of retirement, inflation, or widowhood).

Gerontologists have documented the prevalence of negative stereotypes about older adults. It is widely believed that people become less important, competent, and useful as they enter the later adult years. The veracity of this belief is vigorously contested by gerontologists as well as by a great many active and flourishing elders. Even though seriously flawed, the belief is consequential. Elders report being angered and frustrated when treated as though incompetent—or invisible—people. Self-doubt and social withdrawal are among the other responses that develop when exposed regularly to negative stereotypes.

Elderly men and women are in double jeopardy for social value because of their perceived proximity to death. Avoidant attitudes toward dying and death are often coupled with dysvaluation of elders. In fact, many people barely distinguish between "elderly" and "dying." Some of the most popular theories of human development play into this mindset. These widely taught theories assert that the "developmental task" of the older adult is to prepare for death. This attitude configuration offers the subtle reassurance that younger adults do *not* need to concern themselves about dying and death: elders will do all of the death work for society. It also conveys the implicit message that elders should move outside the mainstream of social, political, and economic activity, the better to prepare themselves for death. Advocates for elder rights counter that this attempt to assign elders to the margins of society "for their own good" actually is motivated by the desire to disempower the older generation.

It has been found repeatedly that the death of an elderly man or woman is regarded as much less than a social loss by Americans than the death of a younger person. There is a syncretic effect between the dysvaluation of aging and the dysvaluation of dying. This effect can be summarized in this blunt formulation: *Older people have smaller, less important lives, so they also have smaller, less important deaths. It is shocking and disturbing when death takes a young person, but disposing of the aged is the routine and approved task of death.*

In examining a broad spectrum of human service activities and settings it has been found that elders generally receive lower priority assistance than younger people, and that terminally ill people receive lower priority assistance than those with more favorable prognoses. The person who is both elderly and terminally ill has often been the most neglected. For example, some dying elderly men and women have been placed in mental institutions because no other care setting was available to them. They were given diagnoses of senile dementia and/or clinical depression although, in fact, they were just lonely, frightened, and suffering people without economic or social resources at their command.

The tendency to equate "aging" and "dying" contributes to misdiagnoses and mismanagement in both the mental and physical health spheres. Specialists in geriatric medicine have discovered that many conditions previously considered untreatable can be managed effectively when physicians have educated themselves and re-oriented their attitudes toward elderly patients. Unfortunately, only about 1% of American

physicians have become qualified in geriatric medicine, although elders comprise more than 12% of the population (taking age 65 as the conventional marker) and are steadily increasing in number. Many elders who receive prompt and knowledgeable medical care can be rescued from a trajectory that would otherwise have become terminal. The mental health parallel has included the failure to recognize that anxiety, depression, and confusion may be prodomal manifestations or accompaniments of terminal illness. Medication—all too often the primary or the only intervention offered to elderly clients—can be counterproductive when it is based on the premise that the terminally ill person's difficulties are primarily mental or emotional. Along with more geriatric specialists in medicine, there is also a need for more nurses, psychologists, social workers, and clergy who are qualified and motivated to enter into helping relationships with elders.

This dismal picture started to improve with the emergence of the death awareness movement and the establishment of hospice programs (see Section VI, below). It should also be noted that not all individuals and families have followed society's practice of distancing the dying and dysvaluating the aged. At the same time that society at large considers the death of elders to be relatively inconsequential, there are people who are intensely involved with a terminally ill family member or client, and who will grieve deeply when that person dies.

It is not just the elderly person who becomes further dysvalued when death is in prospect. Dysvaluation of the dying person is a possibility at any age: *"This person cannot help me in the future." "I no longer have to meet this person's standards and expectations." "This person is no longer in the game, and so, no longer matters." "This person is no longer fun . . . sexy . . . attractive . . ." "This person is now a loser, a failure."* These are among the negative responses to people who are perceived as dying, although seldom expressed as bluntly. Dying is viewed as the nemesis or undoing of dominant social values. The dying person is not a young, attractive, sexy, active, and powerful winner in the game of life—so what good is this person?

Are there other values in a person that are *not* destroyed by the dying process? Helping to identify and protect these values would be a major contribution from mental health specialists, although this would require moving well beyond routine thinking, assessment, and treatment.

III. THE EXPERIENCE OF DYING

It has already been observed that (a) the circumstances and even the definition of "dying" are being altered through sociotechnical change; (b) there are marked differences in the way people experience the last phases of life; and (c) societal attitudes of distancing and disvaluing often increase the isolation and vulnerability of the dying person. We have also identified a set of mental health issues that often are salient: *living with uncertainty, loss of control, loss of relationships, disturbances of body image and self-concept, loss of communication, unfulfilled dreams and uncompleted projects, and loss of meaning.* With these observations in mind we now consider mental health perspectives on the overall experience of dying.

A. Basic Considerations

A realistic perspective on the experience of dying requires acknowledgement of the following facts:

- *The process is dynamic.* We must expect the individual's physical condition to change over time and, accordingly, the cognitive and emotional response to these changes as well.
- *The process is interactive.* Events in one sphere of functioning can have immediate and significant effects on other spheres. For example, a woman expected to die within the day vowed that she would live long enough to congratulate her parents on their 50th anniversary, almost 2 weeks away. She did.
- *Interpretations and coping strategies are likely to change throughout the process.* Changes in physical condition affect comfort level, body image, and functional ability. It is therefore difficult to maintain a fixed self-concept and interpretation of the situation. Furthermore, the dying person often receives changing and mixed signals from other people as they respond to his or her condition. Much of the person's energy may be devoted to working out new interpretations of the situation. These interpretations are expressed verbally and nonverbally in their interactions, and are also subject to modification through the interactions.
- *Awareness of dying is likely to vary throughout the process.* Although a facet of the individual's overall interpretation, the awareness of dying deserves special consideration. Psychiatrist Avery D. Weisman's concept of *middle knowledge* calls attention to the often elusive and shifting state of dying awareness. A person who seems to be "in denial" on one occasion may clearly express awareness of the terminal prognosis on another occasion—or to another person. Even a person who is well aware of the outcome may suspend this knowledge from time to time. "I get awfully tired of dying," said a retired school principal, "so I give myself a little recess once in a while—I think I'm entitled to fool myself, don't you?"

- *There is a profound need for what might be called either "security" or "safe passage."* Dying people often express the desire to be at home or in some other familiar setting with the companionship of a few treasured people. Predictability and reliability of services is also much appreciated. Many dying people feel more secure when they know that they will be kept adequately informed about procedures to be used and new developments in their condition. There is apprehension about being separated from or abandoned by the significant people in their lives, not receiving the right medications at the right time, and being confronted with new people, new procedures, or new choices without advance preparation. Over and above these factors, the dying person is better able to weather the multiple stresses if there is confidence that one has lived a good life and is valued by the people who matter to him or her. Anxiety, anger, depression, and confusion often arise from the uneasy feeling that one cannot trust others to safeguard the passage from life to death.

B. Stages? Tasks?

Attempts have been made to conceptualize the experience of dying within a mental health perspective. The first model to be offered portrayed the dying process as movement through a series of stages. A more recent model has extended the developmental task approach to include the dying process.

C. Stage Theory

Scientists and scholars in many fields of learning have found it useful to organize their information in the form of stages. Historians, for example, have delineated stages of industrial development, and biomedical researchers have delineated stages of cancer growth. Stage theories have several features in common: (a) a progression through time (b) from one level or quality of phenomena to the next (c) in a fixed sequence. Furthermore, each stage is distinctive and clearly discernible from the other, and the number and nature of the stages is fixed. It is not assumed that there will always be development from stage 1 to the end-stage, but it is assumed that development will always be in that direction. A departure from the stage sequence becomes noteworthy and the stimulus for further inquiry.

Buddhist teachings have long included a description of the stages through which a person passes from life to death. This is both a physiological and a spiritual transformation that continues beyond the point of certifiable death when some people reach *the clear light of death,* an unique visionary state of consciousness. More familiar and influential in the Euro-American world is the stage theory offered by Elizabeth Kubler-Ross. She identified five stages in the dying process, although not all people advance through the entire set. These well-known stages are:

- *Denial and shock.* The first response to awareness of dying.
- *Anger:* Rage and resentment: "Why me?"
- *Bargaining:* The attempt to make a deal with fate, to somehow escape death (e.g., by promising to become a better person).
- *Depression:* Withdrawal and decreased responsiveness as it becomes evident that bargaining will not work and the physical condition continues to deteriorate. Fear of dying and other painful feelings rise to the surface.
- *Acceptance:* This stage is actually described as more of a *detachment.* In Kubler-Ross's words: "It is as if the pain had gone, the struggle is over, and there comes a time for 'the little rest before the long journey' as one patient phrased it."

This stage theory of dying has been found useful by many people in overcoming their anxieties about approaching dying friends, family members, or professional clients. Perhaps the most helpful facet of stage theory is its reminder that the dying person is not a species apart who we cannot understand and comfort. Rather, the dying person is still a living person who is attempting to cope with exceptionally stressful circumstances. It is easy to recognize ourselves in "denial," "anger," and the other responses identified by Kubler-Ross; therefore, it also becomes easier to relate to dying people.

Unfortunately, despite its quick acceptance in popular culture, stage theory has not proved an adequate guide to the dying person's experience. The major assertion of stage theory has not been confirmed, namely that dying people pass in sequence through the five steps described by Kubler-Ross, nor is there evidence for this proposition in her own reports. Instead, it has been found that people have a variety of interpretations and responses to their condition, and that these may be expressed at various points in the illness. All of the responses described by Kubler-Ross do occur, but not universally, and not necessarily in the given sequence. There are numerous other interpretations and responses as well, including vicarious engagement and transcendence. The stage theory is also limited in scope, with little attention given to the specific physical condition and its management, the individual's life history and personality, ethnic, racial, and religious factors, and the interpersonal and environmental setting within which the individual experiences the dying process.

There have also been criticisms of the way stage theory has been used by some who accept its premises. These criticisms include the neglect of each dying person's uniqueness and a corresponding rush to judgment on the part of the observer. In the worst examples, the dying person becomes the object of a classification procedure ("Is he in stage 2 or 3?") and is treated like a product moving along an assembly line. Ironically, a theory that was intended to improve care of dying people has sometimes become a barrier because of the emphasis on the stage rather than the total person–environment interaction. For example, a dying person's anger has sometimes been dismissed as "Stage 2!" instead of considering it as a possible response to a pattern of avoidance, neglect, and misinformation. The erroneous assumption that stage theory has been confirmed by scientific research has also had the unfortunate effect of discouraging inquiry that might lead to more adequate conceptualizations. Those who focus on Kubler-Ross's central message—recognizing the dying person as a living person—are more likely to be helpful than those who use stage theory in a literal, narrow, and mechanistic manner.

D. Developmental Task Theory

Social and behavioral scientists have been giving increased attention to the total course of human life from cradle to grave. This is a promising approach, but one that requires new methods and theories that can encompass such a broad spectrum of time and change. Several of the most influential life-course theories have emphasized the need for individuals to complete a set of "developmental tasks," each of which becomes salient at a particular point in life. These tasks resemble stages in that they occur in a fixed temporal order. There is a significant difference with respect to the individual's role and responsibilities, however. The individual is regarded as an active, coping problem solver who has decisions to make and goals to reach. This contrasts with the more reactive and passive status of the individual as usually conceived in stage theory.

It has already been noted that life-course theories have tended to assign "preparing for death" as the primary developmental task for elderly people. More recently preliminary efforts have been made to apply the developmental task approach to the course of the dying process itself or to any life-threatening illness whether or not it results in death. The developmental task approach to the dying process may be particularly useful to those who have already accepted this perspective on the general course of life. It also has the advantages of calling attention to (a) the particular phase of the illness (acute, chronic, and terminal) and (b) the active role of the individual in coping with a variety of physical, interpersonal, and symbolic challenges.

The developmental task approach may prove valuable if it is taken as a general guide to the world of the dying person, helping us to appreciate the continuity between the individual's previous life experience and the daunting problems that are now being encountered. Although there is a terminal illness, the *person* is not sick. One tries to cope with life's tasks in one's long-established style. Developmental task theory also emphasizes the individual's attempt to resolve existential and spiritual issues that become more salient with the near prospect of death.

This approach, like stage theory, can be counterproductive if used in a rigid and mechanistic way instead of as an invitation to explore the thoughts and feelings of the individual patient. It is also subject to criticism from the cultural bias standpoint. "Tasks" that one must accomplish throughout life smack of middle-class, salvation-and-achievement-oriented industrial society. If some people believe that life is a series of tasks, then this may be their truth and, therefore, an important theme in understanding their interpretation of dying and death. However, it is not an objective, scientifically established fact that the life course, including the dying process, is comprised of a series of developmental tasks that must be accomplished. Insensitive use of developmental task theory could impose rules and expectations upon dying people and their families instead of learning the rules and expectations by which they have been living through the years.

E. Narrative-Construction Theory

Another emerging perspective on the dying process does focus on the individual and family's own interpretations. Knowledge of the biomedical facets of terminal illness is strongly encouraged, but the main emphasis is on the narrative or story that is developed by the dying person and each family member and friend. These stories are not fictions. They represent systematic attempts to make sense of a varied, shifting, discordant, and disturbing set of phenomena, an attempt to discover or create meaning. These stories or narrative constructions represent the individual's own theory.

The dying person is not approached with a fixed set of ideas about what is most important to that person or what rules that person should follow to move from stage to stage or task to task. Instead, one observes, listens, and encourages the communication of the individual's implicit theory or story. The process as well as the outcome of narrative sharing could be valuable to all concerned. Early applications of this approach have had some encouraging results, including an enhanced sense of mutual support and understanding, and the resolution of conflicts and uncertainties. By sharing their individual constructions of the dying process, the patient, family members, and friends can correct misunderstandings and affirm relationships and meanings.

The narrative-construction approach is being used with some success in a variety of interpersonal situations. These include other normative developmental situations such as the comparison of mothers' and fathers' stories of their children's birth, and problem-solving situations, such as psychotherapy and counseling. As with the other theoretical perspectives on the experience of dying, the narrative-construction approach requires of the users nonjudgmental attitudes, emotional sensitivity, and cognitive flexibility. The "tell-me-your-story" approach has potential for discovering the major themes, values, and rules of each unique dying person; by that same token, however, it may not easily yield a simple general model. This lack of a standard model could prove to be a blessing in disguise. We would need to improve our ability to communicate with dying people to understand each individual's own frame of reference, instead of taking a one-size-fits-all model down from the shelf. Eventually, we should be able to distinguish several types of models within which a particular individual's version could be better comprehended without losing its distinctive characteristics. Perhaps it is time to replace the rush toward a simple and universal model of the dying process with a patient and careful "reading" of each individual's life and death narrative.

IV. DYING AS AN INTERPERSONAL CHALLENGE

Dying occurs between as well as within people. Family, friends, and colleagues are affected by the suffering and incapacity of the dying person, and concerned about how life will go for them after the death. As these people respond with their own needs, feelings, and interpretations, they also influence the dying person's experiences in various intended or unintended ways. Furthermore, their own lives may be affected. Involvement in events surrounding the death of a loved one can have either a positive or a negative effect on recovery from grief, depending on the circumstances of that death. The death of a loved one can also serve as an implicit rehearsal that increases or decreases anxiety about how one's own life will end. It is useful, then, to consider the entire interpersonal context of dying from the mental health perspective.

A guide to evaluating the interpersonal context of dying is presented in Table II. Six dimensions of the family interpersonal context prior to the advent of a terminal illness are identified here. One can also apply this checklist to friends, colleagues, and, with some modification, professional service providers. The first point commanding our attention is one so obvious that it is sometimes neglected: there is usually a well-established pattern of interpersonal communication in place *before* a family member becomes terminally ill. Taking the characteristics of this pattern into account is a valuable first step in making accommodations for the care and comfort of the dying person and anticipating areas in which interpersonal problems are most likely to arise.

The usefulness of this checklist can be illustrated with the first dimension, *general family communication pattern*. Families differ markedly in the implicit rules that govern their interactions. In some families almost all communicational interactions are tense and

Table II A Guide to the Interpersonal Context of Dying: Family Characteristics Prior to Terminal Illness

1. *General family communication pattern:*
   Open-spontaneous _____   Cautious-channeled _____   Anxious-conflicted _____
2. *Communication pattern for intense emotional issues:*
   Open-forthright _____   Guarded-evasive _____   Denying-resisting _____
3. *General decision making process:*
   Shared-consensual _____   Individualistic _____   Laissez-faire _____
4. *Expression of affection and support:*
   Spontaneous-frequent _____   Limited-occasional _____   Rare-awkward _____
5. *Level of preexisting family conflicts and stresses:*
   Under control _____   Some anxiety and dysfunction _____   Out of control _____
6. *Experience with previous life-threatening illnesses and deaths:*
   Little or none _____   Coped and recovered _____   Stress continues _____

Based on material presented in R. Kastenbaum: *Death, Society, & Human Experience*, 6th edition, Boston: Allyn & Bacon, 1998.

stressful. The extra pressure of coping with a dying family member can lead to destructive and divisive episodes, much reducing the ability to provide security and emotional support. In other families there are fairly rigid lines of communication that dictate who is allowed to speak to whom in what way under what circumstances. This type of pattern often is challenged by the uncertainties and ambiguities associated with the dying process and may become even more resistant to change. Families whose communications have been free and easy for the most part—everybody talks, everybody listens—usually are in the most advantageous position to support one of their members through the dying process.

When *intense emotional issues* arise there may be a significant shift in the family's communication patterns. At the extremes are the families who fragment and those who come together with renewed commitment during adversity. Knowing the particular family's history of responding to difficult situations (e.g., unwanted pregnancy, stormy divorce, elder losing the ability to do self-care) can be helpful in anticipating the response to coping with a dying person. The *general decision-making process* can also be a significant factor. Many decisions arise during a terminal illness. These include redistribution of roles and responsibilities and resources, funeral and memorial arrangements, as well as those decisions that directly affect the care of the dying person. A family that has preferred to "let decisions make themselves" may miss opportunities to safeguard the comfort and security of the dying person and to reduce their own stress by failing adequately to inform themselves and review their value priorities. Both individualistic and shared-consensual modes of decision making can be effective, but each has distinctive advantages and vulnerabilities that are likely to come to the surface during the terminal process.

There are families in which people spontaneously touch and hug each other and in which there is a regular flow of supportive nonverbal communication (smiles, winks, touches). There are other families for whom *expression of affection and support* is reserved for special occasions. Both of these patterns can make positive contributions to the experience of the dying person, although families in which the expression of affection has been rationed may have difficulty in acknowledging the dying process as one of those special occasions because of their doubts and anxieties. This problem is intensified in families where a warm smile, a comforting touch, and affectionate words have been virtually unknown. Grief counselors have often heard the lament that "I never did tell her how much I loved her!" Expression of affection is perhaps best received when delivered in "the family style," but a style that very nearly precludes open expression of affection may increase the dying person's sense of abandonment, regret, or unworthiness.

The difference between a sense of "safe passage" and a troubled and apprehensive experience for the dying person may hinge on the nature of *preexisting family conflicts and stresses*. The family may already be fully engaged in coping with a demanding situation and therefore they may have relatively little emotional energy to devote to care of the dying person. Effective and comforting attention to the dying person is even more problematic in seriously dysfunctional families. Unlike the competent family that is confronted with multiple stressors, the dysfunctional family has not learned how to cope adequately with the everyday challenges of life, and so has little to offer in the terminal illness situation.

Families also differ markedly in their experience with *previous life-threatening illnesses and deaths*. There are families that literally do not have a clue about what to do and how to do it when a member becomes terminally ill. They may be highly dependent at first on what the popular media happen to be saying about death and dying at the moment, and whatever information or misinformation they pick up from friends. Other families have already come through experiences with a life-threatening illness or bereavement. Not all of these experiences are helpful in responding to the needs of the dying family member. They may have observed another dying person becoming socially isolated, exposed to invasive medical procedures, or given inadequate medication for relief of pain. One of the most valuable contributions of the hospice movement is that more people are becoming aware that the dying person can be given sensitive and competent care through a team effort of family members, community volunteers, and professional health service providers.

The family system approach is now well appreciated by many mental health workers. This approach could be applied more frequently to understanding characteristics of the family and general interpersonal context that will either comfort or fail the dying person. [*See* FAMILY SYSTEMS.]

V. THE DYING CHILD AND ADOLESCENT

All that has been discussed up to this point applies to children and adolescents as well. There are additional considerations, however, when the dying person is young.

Family support must be direct, reliable, and continuous. Fear of being uprooted from the home and family circle is one of the major concerns of children with life-threatening illnesses. It is often necessary for separations to occur in the interest of medical management. There are also the more subtle separations that can occur when family, friends, teachers and others back off from the dying child because of their own discomfort. The most effective support is the actual physical presence of family members and, when that is not possible, the knowledge that one can count on being with them at predictable times. Separation, loneliness, and concern about being rejected can be as demoralizing to a child as the physical condition with which they suffer.

It is often very difficult for families to be with terminally ill children. The death of a child—in prospect and in reality—constitutes a severe, often overwhelming stress for families and siblings. The anguish of watching a child lose function and vitality is intensified by the realization that the lives of the survivors will never be the same. The death of a child may threaten to be the death of the family dream. To be with their children—emotionally as well as physically—the parents often must overcome their anxiety and sense of helplessness.

Children often know more about their condition than adults realize. Adults generally tend to underestimate children's powers of observation. Additionally, it may be comforting to assume that a dying child does not understand death. Research offers a rather different picture. Dying children are usually well aware that they are in a vulnerable and dangerous condition. Although they may not understand death in the abstract sense, young children know the difference between a lively fish and one that floats on the surface of the tank, and the fact that a fallen leaf does not return

to the branch. They recognize "dead," even if the concepts of universal, personal, and irreversible death have not yet matured in their minds. Children who are suffering from the pain, decline of function, and medical interventions of a life-threatening illness are adept at learning about the dying process. Often they also become aware that adults, including doctors and nurses as well as parents, have a hard time in talking to them honestly about their condition. Dying children have been known to "put on a happy face" for their parents out of fear that they would drive others away if they expressed their true feelings.

Pain too often is not controlled. It has taken the effort of many physicians, nurses, and community advocates to make pain control the highest priority in managing the care of a dying person. Hospice leaders had to overcome ingrained attitudes that (a) nothing really could be done to mitigate pain associated with terminal illness and or that (b) any drug that might actually provide relief would also turn the dying person into an addict. There is now much better control of pain for most patients with terminal cancer (the most common condition in hospice care programs). However, there is still a lingering tradition that children do not experience as much pain as adults and therefore do not need much in the way of analgesics. This demonstrably erroneous assumption is often joined with the underestimation of the pain caused by diagnostic and treatment procedures. At present the medical management of terminally ill children is divided between physicians who are current in their knowledge and motivated to reduce pain and those who have persuaded themselves that pain is not a major problem for children.

Severe and unrelenting pain is one of the conditions most likely to ravage a person's quality of life, including the ability to think coherently and relate well to others. Making sure that dying children do not suffer pain when there are means for relief available is one of the best safeguards of mental health for the children and their family members. [*See* PAIN.]

Children as decision makers? Traditionally, children are excluded from health services decision making. This exclusion is consistent with legal codes that have long maintained that persons under a specified age (usually 18 or 21) cannot enter into a wide variety of contracts and agreements without adult sponsorship. "Coming of age" is based both on social ritual and an assumption that cognitive and moral responsibility reaches an acceptable level at a particular age point. There is now a children's rights movement that challenges this tradition. Any reconsideration should include the situation of the dying child. Here the issue is not so much whether children do or do not have natural rights to make health care decisions, but whether it is humane and realistic to deny them the opportunity to *participate* in decision making. Some physicians and families have successfully worked together to involve children in the decision-making process to the extent of their individual ability and inclination to do so. Case histories reveal that some dying children have been exposed to invasive procedures, social isolation, and inadequate pain relief despite their desperate protests. Those who have witnessed these proceedings without the power to intervene are dedicated to preventing others from having to undergo such experiences at the most vulnerable time in their lives.

What about the brothers and sisters? It is natural for the family's focus to be on the dying child. The siblings have their own lives and needs, however, and are also deeply affected by the illness. There is heightened risk for emotional and behavioral disturbances as the siblings find themselves on the periphery of the family and have less time to interact with their parents (who are also more stressed and exhausted). Recent studies have confirmed the value of educing the siblings' interpretations of the situation. Some siblings, for example, blame themselves for the illness; others feel they have to get themselves ready to replace the dying child by taking on his or her ways if they hope to be cherished by their parents. Often stretched to their maximum effort, parents may welcome assistance in providing companionship and support to the siblings.

The dying adolescent. Almost anything that is said about the inner world of adolescents can be quickly contradicted. It is for many young men and women a time of rapid intellectual growth, sexual awakening, horizon broadening, and experimentation with a variety of attitudes and life-styles. Amidst all this ferment there often is a multifaceted interest in death that is likely to subside or be suppressed during the middle adult years. Most forms of risk-taking behavior are at a peak during the teen and early adult years. Furthermore, the leading causes of death in adolescence are associated with actions rather than diseases: accident,

murder, suicide. Studies indicate that at least half of the youth (ages 15 to 24) population has thought about suicide, although most do not act upon these thoughts. Death themes permeate much of teen-culture music while interest in graphic and bizarre depictions of death in movies is at a peak. If there is a "typical" adolescent attitude it is the attempt to think of oneself as immortal while at the same time feeling quite vulnerable.

It is a terrific jolt to learn that one is dying at the very moment when everything important seems just about ready to begin. Dying adolescents often express profound concerns about the loss of their futurity. There are also strong concerns about becoming socially isolated, and losing the sense of personal identity they had been so arduously cultivating. Along with quality palliative care, dying adolescents need the opportunity to maintain peer as well as family interaction as long as possible. Sensitive caregivers also respect the adolescent's need to stay in control of at least some aspects of the situation and to keep their hard-earned identity as a maturing individual while at the same time feeling comfortable in accepting assistance in their increasingly dependent condition. Adolescents are more likely than older adults to desire some additional taste of the life they will miss (as in the controversial Make a Wish Foundation sponsorship of a bear-hunting trip by a terminally ill teenager). Because they were already on a powerful personal growth trajectory, dying adolescents are sometimes able to integrate their stressful experiences and achieve a remarkably trenchant understanding of life and death.

VI. THE ART OF DYING: A CONTEMPORARY PERSPECTIVE

We cannot evade death, but we can die in a serene and dignified manner. This was the message of the *ars moriendi* tradition that started in the late middle ages, drawing added impetus from the experience of the Black Death. Religious faith and a moral, responsible life were keys to passing safely through the final crisis.

The social and technological context of dying is much different today, but the concept of a "good death" has been revived as part of the palliative care and death education movements. Both the development of hospice care programs and the establishment of academic courses and research programs on death-related matters gained their foothold in the United States through the 1970s and 1980s. Modern hospice care was pioneered by Dame Cicely Saunders and her colleagues in the London area in the late 1960s and soon was emulated in the United States and elsewhere.

The present scene is a mix of three conflicting attitudes and practices:

1. *Fearing, distancing, and rejecting.* This configuration has already been described. It is the residue of a tradition once dominant and virtually without challenge. The characteristic scenario centered around a physician who had no further interest in a patient who had failed to be cured. The rule for all people in the situation was to avoid speaking of dying and death ("That would destroy hope! Patients can't take it!"). It was also a rule to remain securely within one's role as a quasi-scientific professional ("Don't get involved with your patients!"). Where this pattern still prevails there is tension and distrust in the network interpersonal relationships that includes the dying person, health service providers, family, and community. Anxieties and misunderstandings about the dying process and the dying person continue to flourish in this atmosphere. The dying person is the most immediate and direct victim: at risk for social isolation and inadequate management of symptoms. Mental health workers are also at risk for misunderstanding the emotional and behavioral responses they observe in a particular individual, especially the dying patient and family members. These responses may be incorrectly construed as individual disorders and pathologies instead of being recognized as an attempt to cope with a system of neglect, dysvaluation, and torment.

2. *Accepting, sharing, palliating.* This configuration has also been described. It is one line of development within a larger movement to restore a sense of caring and belonging to a mass, high-tech society in which individuals are at risk of feeling "processed" and alienated. Parallel movements include those for consumer rights, natural childbirth, flex-time schedules, and the varied manifestations of "do-it-yourself." Hospice programs constitute perhaps the most successful introduction of what might be called "humanity backlash" within the health services domain. Both the dying process and the dying person are accepted. In this view, life is a journey in which both the exit point and the entry point are natural and the individual is valuable every step of the way. Health service professionals who have become expert in the relief of pain and other symptoms form an alliance with community volunteers and family members. The dying patient is not put through the system; rather, a system is developed around that person to meet his or her special wishes and needs. Close relationships are encouraged, their form and intensity depending on the dying person's own inclinations. Decisions are made and care provided on a team basis, with concern present for the emotional well-being of family members and service providers as well as the dying person. Although each terminal course is distinctive, there is a greater likelihood in hospice care that dying people will spend much of their time at home with the companionship of the people who are most important to them.

3. *Controlling, processing, prospering.* Both of the traditions noted above are becoming under increasing pressure from new economics-driven trends. The physician following his or her own best judgment in private practice has been going the way of the corner grocery store. The push toward larger and larger corporations with larger and larger profit margins is matched in the public sector with hierarchies of bureaucracies and regulations. In announcing his unexpectedly early retirement, one physician said simply: "It's not much fun being a doctor any more!" Many nurses have also left the field because they felt that the new-style health services system does not allow them to provide care as they believe care should be provided.

The bureaucratic approach to health services does not take sides in the continuing conflict between the two opposing traditions. It functions instead in a pragmatic manner: what is the most cost-efficient method to provide services? The dying person is therefore neither feared and rejected nor given special consideration. This approach was already evident when the Health Care Finance Administration provided financial support for the National Hospice Demonstration Study (1979–1985). The burning question for the agency was not: "Does hospice help people to weather the dying process with less suffering?" The question was: "Will hospice save us money?" (The answer was sufficiently in the affirmative direction to establish a federal entitlements program for hospice care.)

The core values of the hospice movement are threatened by the same bureaucratic forces that provide limited support. There is constant pressure for hospice organizations to become more like the rest of the health services system. Some of this pressure represents legitimate demands for accountability and quality assurance. There are also pressures, however, for hospice programs to abide by the general practices of hospital systems with which they may be associated, and to turn a profit for the parent organization. It is not unusual for a local pioneer of hospice care to leave the organization because it is perceived as becoming too bureaucratic, and to be replaced by an administrator who has no background or feel for what is distinctive about hospice care.

The art of dying today often requires making one's way through a labyrinth of competing attitudes and practices as well as corporate rules and governmental regulations. Faith and good works may still be the key. People who believe in the intrinsic value of the person have amply demonstrated through hospice care programs that this value can be safeguarded through the perilous final journey. The implications for mental health go far beyond the immediate circle of dying person, family, and caregivers. Fear of dying and death and unresolved grief are among the major sources of anxiety in the general population. Some penetrating observers, such as Ernest Becker, have concluded that death-related anxiety is *the* primary cause of what ails us as a society. One does not have to accept this extreme statement in order to recognize that whatever we can do to afford the dying person "safe passage" is also likely to dissipate the cloud of dread that floats above many a head long before one's personal encounter with mortality.

BIBLIOGRAPHY

Becker, E. (1973). *The denial of death.* New York: The Free Press.

Callanan, M., & Kelley, P. (1992). *Final gifts: Understanding the special awareness, needs, and communications of the dying.* New York: Poseidon Press (Simon & Schuster).

Glaser, B. G., & Strauss, A. L. (1965). *Awareness of dying.* Chicago: Aldine Publishing Co.

Kastenbaum, R. (1998). *Death, society, and human experience* (6th ed.). Boston: Allyn & Bacon.

Kastenbaum, R. (1995–1996). "How far can an intellectual effort diminish pain?" William McDougall's journal as a model for facing death. *Omega, Journal of Death & Dying, 32:* 123–164.

Kastenbaum, R. (1992). *The psychology of death* (Rev. ed.). New York: Springer Publishing Co., Inc.

Kubler-Ross, E. (1969). *On death and dying.* New York: Macmillan.

Nuland, S. B. (1994). *How we die: Reflections on life's final chapter.* New York: Knopf.

Quill, T. E. (1993). *Death and dignity.* New York: W. W. Norton & Co.

Weisman, A. D. (1972). *Death and denial.* New York: Behavioral Publications.

E

Eating and Body Weight: Physiological Controls

B. Glenn Stanley, Elizabeth R. Gillard, and Arshad M. Khan

University of California, Riverside

Conditioned Taste Aversion A powerful learned aversion to a novel taste paired with subsequent nausea.

Glucostatic Hypothesis The theory that declines in the levels of glucose in the blood or in cellular glucose utilization are key factors signaling hunger and food intake. The ingested food ultimately provides glucose to normalize blood glucose levels.

Lateral Hypothalamus A large region located laterally in the hypothalamus that contains many neurons whose activity precedes and predicts the behavioral response to food. Glutamate acts in this region to elicit eating.

Lipostatic Hypothesis The theory that eating behavior is regulated so as to maintain body lipid levels at a "set point."

Long-Term Satiety Satiety that results mainly from a substantial excess of body fat.

Metabolism The chemical processes within cells that are necessary for the maintenance of life.

Neuropeptide Y A peptide believed to be utilized as a neurotransmitter/modulator by some neural components of eating control neurocircuitry. It is an extremely powerful stimulant of eating behavior.

Paraventricular Nucleus of the Hypothalamus A small paired hypothalamic nucleus bracketing the third cerebroventricle that acts to integrate the eating stimulatory and inhibitory effects of numerous neurotransmitters.

Perifornical Area of the Hypothalamus A paired hypothalamic area surrounding the fornix. Neuropeptide Y acts in this area to elicit eating and dopamine acts there to inhibit eating.

Short-Term Satiety Satiety that lasts for a few minutes to several hours after the ingestion of a single meal.

I. INTRODUCTION

The evolution from unicellular organisms, typically bathed in nutrient-rich sea water, to animals with multiple organ systems, effectively separated cells from the external environment. This separation required the evolution of physiological mechanisms for obtaining the substances needed to maintain normal cellular function and for disposing of cellular waste products.

Most cells require a tightly controlled environment for optimal function; perturbations in extracellular levels of oxygen or carbon dioxide, in ion concentrations, in pH, or in levels of metabolic fuels, rapidly lead to abnormal cellular function or even death. To provide relatively constant extracellular conditions despite a highly variable external environment, various homeostatic systems, through behavioral, autonomic and endocrine mechanisms, act to regulate respiration and body temperature (in homeotherms), as well as fluid intake and excretion. All animals are heterotrophs, which means that they cannot synthesize their own essential nutrients, but must obtain them from other organisms. To provide uninterrupted supplies of required metabolic fuels, vitamins, electrolytes, and micronutrients, neural systems have evolved to regulate eating behavior in animals, and to coordinate the autonomic and endocrine subsystems that control the disposition, storage, and metabolism of ingested food.

The choices of what, when, and how much to eat are controlled by complex, hierarchically organized neural systems that integrate multiple internal stimuli related to body lipid content, gastrointestinal distention and nutrient contents, circulating levels of metabolic fuels (chiefly glucose and free fatty acids) and their regulatory hormones (chiefly, insulin, glucagon and glucocorticoids), with circadian factors and with external factors, such as the taste and smell of food, to produce well-organized and appropriate feeding responses. Since eating occurs in the form of discrete meals, it is important to understand the factors that lead to meal initiation (frequently equated with hunger) and the different factors that lead to meal termination (usually associated with satiety). Additionally, the effects of these short-term factors are modulated by long-term factors that act to enhance or suppress eating in order to maintain body weight.

The study of these factors by neuroscientists is founded on evidence that the influences on a behavior like eating, be they genetic, environmental, developmental, social, or cognitive, are mediated through the nervous system, and that similar behaviors in related species are typically produced by neural control systems with similar features and properties. Thus, studies of feeding behavior conducted with rodents and other animals should provide key insights into eating control mechanisms in people. Indeed, studies of feeding in rodents and monkeys have successfully predicted the effects of drugs, brain pathology, hormonal imbalances, gastrointestinal and various other manipulations on eating and body weight in humans.

II. DIGESTION AND ABSORPTION

Since a major function of eating is to provide cells with metabolic fuels and since these fuels also provide afferent signals that influence eating behavior, it is important to understand how complex foods are broken down into the simpler nutrients utilized by cells. The principal nutrients from which cells extract energy are glucose, amino acids, and free fatty acids, which are obtained initially from ingested carbohydrates, proteins, and fats, respectively. Before being absorbed, the food must be broken down into simpler components, a process called *digestion*. The carbohydrates are digested into simple sugars (glucose, fructose and galactose), the proteins into amino acids, and the fats into small droplets of lipids. Subsequently, these simplified components enter the blood from the intestines, a process called *absorption*. Ultimately, these fuels are oxidized by cells to obtain energy, a process termed *catabolism*. Any excess fuels obtained from this process are shuttled to storage depots through energy-requiring synthetic pathways, a process called *anabolism*.

The digestion of carbohydrates and fats begins in the mouth. Saliva, secreted as a parasympathetic reflex response to food, contains the enzymes *α-amylase*, which digests starchy carbohydrates, and *salivary lipase*, which preferentially attacks lipids. After being chewed, the partially digested food travels down the esophagus into the stomach.

The digestion of proteins begins in the stomach. Proteins are preferentially digested by the gastric enzyme *pepsin*, which is secreted in the inactive form, *pepsinogen*. Hydrochloric acid in the stomach converts pepsinogen to pepsin. The release of both hydrochloric acid and pepsinogen within the stomach is triggered by the hormone *gastrin*. Gastrin is released from the gastric mucosa in response to the arrival of amino acids and partially digested protein, and by gastric distention, which reflexively stimulates firing by the vagus nerve innervating the stomach. Digestion is aided by the mixing of food caused by peristaltic waves of stomach contractions. These contractions also assist in the passage of food through the pyloric sphincter into the duodenum, the first part of the small intestine.

Food then enters the small intestine and encounters *bile*, which is secreted by the liver and stored in the gall bladder before passing to the intestines via the bile duct. The bile emulsifies lipids, converting them into tiny fat droplets suitable for absorption. Lipids are additionally digested by pancreatic enzymes: *pancreatic lipase, cholesteryl esterase,* and *phospholipases A_1 and A_2*, which digest neutral fats cholesteryl esters, and phospholipids, respectively. Carbohydrates enter the small intestine primarily as dextrins and maltose, starches and glycogen, or as sucrose or lactose. An *amylase* selected by the pancreas converts the starches, dextrins, and glycogen into maltose. Intestinal enzymes break down maltose and other disaccharides into molecules of glucose, fructose, and galactose. Proteins are also further digested in the small intestines by enzymes, including: *trypsin, chymotrypsin, carboxypeptidases A and B,* and *elastase.* All are first secreted into the small intestine by the pancreas as inactive proenzymes and are activated by intestinal enzymes.

The small intestine also secretes the peptide hormones: *secretin, cholecystokinin,* and *gastric inhibitory peptide.* Secretin, released into the blood in response to the entry of gastric acid in the intestines, causes the pancreas to release bicarbonate to neutralize this acid. Cholecystokinin, which is released from the intestines in proportion to the entry of fats and amino acids into the intestines, enhances the actions of secretin, stimulates the emptying of bile from the gall bladder, and inhibits gastric emptying. Finally, gastric inhibitory peptide is released in response to glucose in the gut. It is a potent inhibitor of gastric acid secretion, gastric motility, and gastric emptying. The primary effect of this hormone, however, is to stimulate insulin release by the pancreas. Insulin allows the uptake of circulating glucose by cells, resulting in a decrease in blood glucose. Thus, it can be seen that each of these hormones acts by negative feedback to regulate the levels of substances that cause their release. Once digested, food is absorbed across the wall of the small intestine into the hepatic portal vein (carbohydrates, proteins, and small free fatty acids), or assembled into complex macromolecular complexes called *chylomicrons* for entry into the lymphatic system (all other lipids). Carbohydrates are absorbed in the form of glucose, fructose, and galactose; proteins in the form of amino acids, and fats in the form of free fatty acids or triacylglycerols (glycerol combined with fatty acids). Some of this absorbed fuel is utilized immediately and the rest is stored as glycogen in liver and muscle tissue, or as lipids in adipose tissue.

III. THE FLUX OF METABOLIC FUELS IN RESPONSE TO ENERGY DEMANDS

There are two distinct phases of energy utilization: the *absorptive phase* and the *postabsorptive phase*. In the absorptive phase, during the hours immediately after eating, metabolic fuels are obtained from the food absorbed through the intestines, with the excess stored as glycogen and fat. In the postabsorptive phase, after the intestinal source is depleted, the metabolic fuels come from bodily stores of glycogen and adipose tissue. The approximately 900 kcals of energy stored as glycogen by the human body can supply energy needs for about 7 hours at a normal resting metabolic rate of about 125 kcals/hour. Subsequently lipids, the long-term source of metabolic fuels, are catabolized. Because 1 kg of fat supplies 9400 kcals of energy, the 15 kg of fat in the body of a normal weight (70 kg) man is calorically sufficient to support his existence for well over 2 months without food, and extremely obese individuals may survive for 1 year. (This is based on the basal metabolism in adult humans, typically in the range of 2000–3000 kcals/day, being reduced to about 1800 kcals/day during starvation). Once lipids are depleted, the body begins to rapidly catabolize protein from muscles and other sources and death typically ensues within days.

These fluxes of metabolic fuels in the absorptive and postabsorptive phases are largely regulated by the hormones *insulin* and *glucagon*. When the body needs energy, glucagon is released to promote the catabolism of stored fuels (glycogen, triacylglycerols) for usable energy (glucose and free fatty acids); and when the body has an excess of usable energy, insulin is released to facilitate the storage of this excess. Specifically, after food within the digestive tract has been absorbed, the levels of blood glucose gradually begin to fall. This fall causes the peptide hormone glucagon to be secreted into the blood by the *α cells* in the pancreas in response to a reflexive increase in the firing of sympathetic neurons innervating the pancreas. Glucagon facilitates the breakdown of glycogen within the liver and muscle into glucose, thus reversing the decline in blood glucose levels. Glucagon also induces adipocytes to break down their triacylglycerol stores into free fatty acids. The glucose is preferentially used by brain cells, with free fatty acids supplying energy for most other tissue.

When eating occurs, the increase in absorbed glucose from the food will reduce glucagon production by the pancreas, and instead promote the release of insulin from pancreatic β cells. Insulin facilitates the conversion of glucose back into glycogen, and free fatty acids back into triacylglycerols in adipose tissue. Insulin is also necessary to permit the use of glucose by all cells except those of the nervous system, which can use glucose independently of insulin. Except for the use of ketone bodies produced by the liver during prolonged starvation, glucose is virtually the only metabolic fuel that can be used by the nervous system.

The heightened cellular need for metabolic fuels during stress and exercise is met by the actions of two other hormones that regulate metabolic fluxes. These are *epinephrine* and *norepinephrine,* which are released from the adrenal medulla in response to stress-induced increases in sympathetic input, and act to increase heart rate and blood pressure. In terms of regulating metabolic fuel consumption, epinephrine acts on muscle, adipose, and hepatic tissues. It increases glucose availability by activating the enzyme *glycogen phosphorylase,* which catalyzes the breakdown of glycogen into glucose, and by inactivating the enzyme *glycogen synthase,* which catalyzes the synthesis of glycogen from glucose. The adrenal cortex also releases hormones that influence metabolism. The most common of these *glucocorticoids* are *cortisol* and *corticosterone,* which affect the metabolism of carbohydrate, protein and lipid in a manner nearly opposite to that of insulin.

IV. SHORT-TERM FACTORS ASSOCIATED WITH HUNGER AND MEAL INITIATION

While bodily stores can provide needed metabolic fuels for extended periods, eating is required to maintain these stores and to provide the types of fuels and other substances needed for optimal function. Much of the research on the physiological controls of eating has focused on the sources and nature of the peripheral afferent signals involved in initiating eating behavior, and this will be emphasized in this section.

A. Evidence from Meal Patterns

The reduction or depletion of gastrointestinal contents and associated or consequent factors appears to be a major determinant of when a meal begins. Some evidence for this comes from studies of meal patterning in freely eating rats. These studies show that meal size is positively correlated with the duration of the postmeal interval but not with the duration of the premeal interval: Large meals are followed by long periods without eating and small meals are followed by shorter periods without eating, but long periods without *spontaneous* eating are not followed by large meals. This suggests that hunger is delayed in proportion to the amount of food eaten in the previous meal. The logical but so far unproven explanation is that eating begins when the contents of the gastrointestinal tract or other short-term fuel stores decline to some critical level. This interpretation is supported by work showing that the onset of spontaneous feeding can be delayed in proportion to the amount of nutrients infused into the stomach. Since the stomach typically empties at a relatively constant caloric rate, large or calorically dense meals or infusions take longer to empty than small or calorically dilute meals, thus delaying the onset of the next meal and accounting for the relationship between meal size and postmeal interval. Accordingly, the size of meals may be unaffected by the time interval since the preceding meal because all the meals should begin under the same conditions, when the gastrointestinal contents decline to a critical level. Although the size of a meal is independent of the duration of the premeal interval in freely feeding individuals, it must be emphasized that meal size can be increased by an imposed fast. This may occur in order to compensate for the depletion of metabolic fuels occurring during the fast. Similarly, when the timing of meals is experimentally or socially fixed, then meal size does increase with increasing time since the previous meal.

B. The Role of Stomach Contractions in Hunger

Hunger in humans is apparently made salient by the inception of strong rhythmic contractions of the stomach. Between 1912 and 1916 Walter Cannon and Anton Carlson showed that the empty stomach of humans exhibits strong contractions that become more intense as the time since the last meal increases. These rhythmic gastric contractions reliably precede and predict the inception of "hunger pangs" and also predict their intensity. Gastric contractions that are induced experimentally are followed by hunger pangs, suggesting that the sensation is causally related to the stomach contractions. Evidence suggests that the contractions may be triggered by a decrease in blood glucose utilization. Although the source(s) of the gastric contractions has yet to be identified, they are apparently generated within the enteric nervous system, a semi-autonomous neural component of the gastrointestinal system, because they continue even when the stomach is deprived of innervation by cutting the vagus and splanchnic nerves. The sensation of the hunger pangs is apparently conveyed to the central nervous system from the stomach by the vagus nerve, as severing this nerve abolished the sensation of but not the gastric contractions themselves. Neither vagotomy nor complete gastric deafferentation, nor removal of the stomach prevents eating, however. Thus, hunger pangs are but one of many factors involved in the initiation of eating behavior.

C. The Role of Glucose

Hunger can also be produced by decreased levels or utilization of metabolic fuels, the best understood of which is glucose. Anton Carlson first suggested that reduced blood glucose levels or utilization might produce hunger, based on his observations that gastric "hunger" contractions in dogs were abolished by intravenous injections of glucose, whereas these contractions were enhanced by insulin injections, which produce hypoglycemia. In contrast, in the diabetics he examined, who were hyperglycemic and insulin deficient, glucose was ineffective and insulin actually reduced gastric contractions. He proposed that the reduced glucose levels and utilization acted directly on stomach tissue to trigger these gastric "hunger" contractions. Whether the stomach is the actual locus of action is currently unknown; however, it is well established that low levels of glucose or its utilization do produce eating.

It should be emphasized that hunger is associated with both unusually low or high circulating levels of glucose. As mentioned above, insulin, in amounts sufficient to produce hypoglycemia, elicits eating in animals and hunger in people. Conversely, the hyperglycemia in people with insulin-dependent (Type I)

diabetes is associated with a ravenous appetite, which can be reduced with insulin injections. In both cases, as popularized in the *glucostatic hypothesis* proposed by Jean Mayer (1953), hunger is believed to result when glucose *utilization* drops below some critical level. This occurs in some diabetics because they lack insulin, which is essential for glucose utilization by most tissues. Additional evidence for the importance of glucose utilization is that eating may be elicited by injection of various glucose analogues, like 2-deoxyglucose, that inhibit glucose utilization. Further support for a decline in glucose utilization as a trigger for spontaneous feeding comes from measures of changes in metabolism with respect to the timing of meal initiation. These measures suggest that immediately prior to the beginning of a spontaneous meal there is a switch from carbohydrate to fats as the primary source of metabolic fuel.

Despite this, no premeal declines in blood glucose were observed for many years. The problem, as first demonstrated by J. Le Magnen and then L. A. Campfield and associates, was that the premeal declines in blood glucose had escaped detection because of their small size and duration. In spontaneously feeding rats, meals are invariably predicted by "V" shaped declines in blood glucose levels, with a nadir of about 12% and a total duration of less than 20 minutes. After the nadir, blood glucose levels normalize rapidly and completely even if eating is prevented. Eating begins after the nadir, when glucose levels are actually increasing. Interestingly, the signal to eat is itself transient: If eating is prevented until just a few minutes after the glucose decline is over, the food is ignored until after another transient decline in blood glucose levels occurs much later.

That the glucose declines actually cause eating was established by intravenous injection of glucose, which effectively blocked the eating response when they counteracted the spontaneous glucose decline. The specificity for glucose is illustrated by the failure of other metabolic fuels to block the spontaneous eating response. Further, similar declines in blood glucose have been shown to occur prior to the inception of hunger in humans that were isolated from social and timing cues. Thus, declines in blood glucose are well established as a signal for feeding initiation. What causes the transient decline in glucose is unknown, but a sharp transient peak in blood levels of insulin occurs just prior to the glucose decline. This may contribute to the decline since insulin would be expected to decrease blood glucose levels by increasing the rate of its utilization and storage. It is also possible that a reduced rate of intestinal nutrient absorption also participates in inducing the glucose declines. The glucose sensors that detect these glucose declines to produce eating are apparently located in the liver, as well as in several brainstem areas, including one near the *area postrema*.

D. The Role of Circadian Factors

Timing can also powerfully affect eating behavior. Like many other behaviors it has a *circadian* rhythm, a cycle of about 24 hours. Diurnal animals, like humans, eat primarily during the light portion of the day and nocturnal animals, like rats, eat mostly at night. These cycles are endogenous; they do not depend on the rising or setting of the sun. Humans and other animals will eat in cycles of about 24 hours for weeks or months when isolated from time cues, even when kept in constant light or darkness. Normally however, these cycles are reset by sunlight or other bright lights so as to remain synchronized with the solar cycle. Without the solar timing cues, the circadian cycle gradually drifts away from the solar cycle, such that after prolonged isolation, sleep and eating cycles become completely out of phase with the solar cycle. Upon reexposure to the solar cycle, the endogenous rhythm synchronizes with the natural cycle over a period of days, a process somewhat like "jet lag."

Most circadian rhythms depend upon a paired cluster of cells in the base of the hypothalamus, namely the *suprachiasmatic nucleus*. This nucleus is believed to be the brain's major clock. Neurons there generate action potentials with a period of 24 hours, even when isolated from the rest of the brain; this is due to rhythmic cycles of gene expression by these cells. Destroying this nucleus disrupts virtually all circadian cycles, and transplanting these cells into the hypothalamus of a lesioned animal reinstates circadian cycles. The circadian activity of these cells and of behavior is reset to the solar cycle by the direct neural input from subsets of retinal ganglion cells. These cells convey information from the eyes to the suprachiasmatic nucleus about changes in the intensity of ambient light, for instance at sunrise and sunset.

How suprachiasmatic nucleus neurons regulate circadian feeding cycles is unknown; however, direct modulation of feeding control neurons is likely to play a role. Additionally, numerous hormonal and autonomic systems exhibit circadian cycles in response to input from suprachiasmatic nucleus neurons, and these may provide an indirect method for the regulation of circadian feeding cycles. For example, circadian cycles exist in rates of gastric emptying, in blood levels of insulin, corticosterone and glucose. Any or all of these would be likely to influence the pattern of eating behavior. For example, the increased eating of rats at night may be due, in part, to the more rapid rate of gastric emptying that is present at that time.

Finally, eating within different portions of the solar cycle may be functionally and mechanistically distinct. Rats, for example, have large peaks of eating just after dusk and just before dawn. The eating at dusk is apparently due to the immediate metabolic need for nutrients caused by the minimal intake during the preceding light phase. At dusk their gastrointestinal tracts are nearly empty and hepatic stores of glycogen are at their lowest. In contrast, the predawn eating apparently occurs in anticipation of the subsequent light-phase anorexia. In this predawn period, rats eat frequent meals despite the large quantity of undigested food already present in their stomachs and intestines, and the quantity of stored glycogen in their livers. These short-term stores from food eaten before dawn seem to permit the anorexia during the following light-phase, because rats prevented from eating just during this predawn period then eat substantially during the following light-phase. Moreover, the timing of this predawn eating is tightly coupled to sunrise, because advancing the time of the apparent dawn causes an almost immediate equivalent advancement in the timing of the predawn peak of feeding. [*See* BODY RHYTHMS/BODY CLOCKS.]

E. Unlearned Sensory Factors

Taste plays a variety of roles in feeding. The four basic taste submodalities (sweet, sour, salty, and bitter) are represented by receptors in different but overlapping locations on the tongue. Sensitivity to each of these taste categories is present at birth and there are characteristic motor responses to these tastes at that time. Typically, sweet tastes are most avidly consumed and bitter tastes are rejected. It is also known that there is an innate "salt appetite" that can become very powerful in sodium-depleted animals and humans. These innate preferences and aversions function in guiding our ingestive behavior toward nutritious foods with a high sugar content and away from bitter-tasting foods, which frequently contain toxins.

F. Learned Cues

Learned cues can trigger eating even in the absence of a metabolic need. Satiated rats will start eating within seconds of hearing an auditory cue that has previously been repeatedly paired with food delivery. Learned taste factors can also stimulate eating. Rats develop strong preferences for flavors repeatedly paired with gastric infusions of nutrients, and weaker preferences for flavors paired with direct intravenous nutrient infusions. Thus, increases in gastric or circulating levels of metabolic fuels can be detected, associated with immediately preceding tastes (which would normally be of the food that produced the change in metabolic fuels), and these tastes can then act to induce or maintain subsequent eating behavior. This ability to associate the tastes of a specific food with the postingestive consequences (i.e., caloric yield) of eating that food, may be critical to learning how to meter the intake of various foods so as to replenish low stores of metabolic fuels.

Food selection, even in rats, can be markedly affected by learned social cues. Single rats, when given a choice of several nutritionally deficient diets and one that is adequate, frequently fail to choose the appropriate diet and die. However, when exposed to rats that have previously solved the diet selection problem, the naive rats perform much better and typically choose the nutritionally adequate diet. Olfactory cues are critical to this social learning.

V. SHORT-TERM FACTORS ASSOCIATED WITH THE INDUCTION OF SATIETY

Satiety, as used here, is defined as the physiological condition that acts to terminate a meal. As with hunger, the physiological mechanisms underlying satiety are multifaceted and largely unidentified. However, eating itself is what causes the termination of eating. Thus, signals for satiety must arise from the areas of the body that come in contact with food. These are the mouth, which provides information about the orosensory qualities of the ingested food, the stomach, and the intestines (first the duodenum, then the ileum, followed by the jejunum and colon). The nutrients are absorbed from the intestines into the blood, and then pass through the liver, followed by other organs, such as the brain. Each of these areas contributes in some way to the development of postprandial satiety.

A. Orosensory Factors in Satiety

Orosensory factors such as taste and smell can produce satiety of a very short duration. These influences on satiety have been studied in sham feeding preparations, where the actions of the ingested food are restricted to the mouth and esophagus by having the food exit the body via a surgically exteriorized esophagus or by a gastric fistula. When mildly food deprived, these sham eating rats eat a larger meal than control rats, but they do stop eating and show signs of normal satiety. That they stop eating clearly demonstrates that orosensory factors can produce satiety. That they begin to eat again shortly after exhibiting satiety demonstrates that the satiety is short lived. That they eat larger meals than their controls demonstrates that other factors, in addition to those from the orosensory region, are important in satiety.

Particularly important is that, with experience, the tastes of foods are associated with their nutritional value, such that the taste alone will produce satiety even when digestion is prevented. This was demonstrated by David Booth who arbitrarily paired selected tastes with two diets. One taste was paired with a calorically dense diet and the other was paired with a less dense diet. When tested with a diet of intermediate density, less was eaten (i.e., satiety occurred sooner) when food was flavored with the taste previously paired with the rich diet, than when it was flavored with the taste paired with the dilute diet. Thus, animals learn to associate the specific taste of a food with its caloric value and to meter intake so as to consume only the calories needed.

Satiety can also be affected by the variety of foods available. Animals, including humans, will eat substantially more as a function of the variety of foods available. That is, satiety rapidly develops when only one food is available; however, eating will resume if a food with a different flavor is offered. This is called "sensory specific satiety," and it serves to increase the variety of foods eaten. Moreover, it can result in a substantially increased food intake, as demonstrated by the enormous overeating by rats given nutritionally identical diets flavored with four different tastes. It is likely that the current prevalence of obesity in Western society is due, in large part, to the presence of such an unusually large variety of available foods that can be obtained with so little effort.

Animals may also learn to associate the taste of a novel food with an illness or gastrointestinal distress occurring soon after the food is eaten. After eating an unfamiliar food, animals injected with a compound that makes them nauseous will subsequently refuse to eat the food. This so called, "conditioned taste aversion" is very strong after only a single association, even if the illness occurs as late as several hours after the food is eaten. Many people have developed lifelong aversions to foods eaten before they became ill, even when the illness was unrelated to the food eaten. Such a mechanism ensures that humans and other animals learn to avoid sampled foods that have contained toxins. Such a mechanism is particularly important for omnivorous animals like ourselves who may sample a wide variety of different foods during a lifetime. While the capability to eat a variety of foods has been essential to our ability to populate most of the planet, to survive we must also be able to identify the foods that are potentially injurious. Conditioned taste aversion learning provides one such mechanism. Additionally, avoidance of poisoned foods is facilitated by cues acquired in social contacts. Rats are resistant to forming a conditioned taste aversion to novel foods that have been ingested by other rats. The key stimulus for this appears to be an olfactory cue. Rats are resistant to forming aversions to the diets that they have smelled on the snouts of healthy rats.

Conditioned taste aversion learning is also of major clinical importance for many cancer patients. These patients frequently refuse to eat adequately and die of malnutrition, well before the cancer itself would be fatal. Some forms of cancer and many forms of chemotherapy and/or radiation therapy for the treatment of cancer produce severe nausea. There is strong evidence to suggest that these patients form overwhelmingly powerful taste aversions to foods, because after eating they frequently become ill. With time, the aversions become so powerful and widespread that the patients essentially starve themselves to death. In addition to these learned effects, some tumors appear to secrete substances that act directly to suppress appetite. Research is being conducted to determine whether having patients abstain from eating before their scheduled chemotherapy or radiation-therapy decreases the formation of taste aversions and promotes recovery.

B. The Role of the Stomach in Satiety

In contrast to the brief satiety produced by orosensory factors, satiety cues derived from the stomach can be powerful and long lasting. Gastric mechanisms also confer the ability to accurately meter nutrient intake, as animals will reduce food intake to precisely compensate for the number of calories infused directly into the stomach during a meal. This occurs across a wide range of diet concentrations and with various types of nutrients. There appear to be at least two gastric satiety mechanisms. One transmits information via the release of hormones to produce satiety in response to gastric nutrient load, as opposed to gastric volume. Another acts via sensory afferents traveling in the gastric branch of the vagus nerve to produce satiety in response to excessive gastric volume. The latter mechanism seems to act mainly as a fail-safe mechanism that puts an upper limit on the amount of food eaten, when particularly large volumes of food are contained within the stomach. The former presumably acts to ensure that adequate nutrients are ingested during a meal, whether the particular food being eaten is calorically dilute or calorically rich. Foods of low caloric density are less satiating and thus more will be eaten during a meal.

The role of the stomach in satiety has been illustrated by Anthony Deutsch, who showed that rats with closed pyloric cuffs, which block the flow of food from the stomach to the small intestines, stopped eating at the same point in a meal as animals with an opened pyloric cuff. Thus, orosensory and gastric cues in combination can produce normal satiety even when food does not enter into the intestines. Except when the meals were very large, gastric infusions of normal saline did not reduce the amount eaten, showing that volume *per se* is not the crucial factor. However, the removal of nutrients from the stomach during a meal caused overeating in amounts that rather precisely compensated for the lost nutrients, even when saline was infused to replace the volume removed. This satiety signal is most likely conveyed by a hormone, perhaps released from the stomach or small intestines in proportion to gastric nutrient load. Hormonal mediation was suggested by persistence of the eating in compensation for removed gastric nutrients in animals with a transected vagus nerve. Further support is that intakes were reduced by infusions of nutrients into a transplanted supernumerary stomach, which would presumably be lacking neural innervation but not a blood supply, even if the transplanted stomach was cuffed at the pylorus. In contrast, cutting the vagus nerve blocked the satiating effects of intragastric infusions of large volumes of saline, illustrating the role of the vagus in this fail-safe mechanism.

C. The Role of the Intestines in Satiety

Food entering the intestines can also contribute to satiety. This is evidenced by the overeating in humans and animals having upper intestinal fistulas that interfere with intestinal retention of food. Additionally, in animals that have been surgically joined (parabiosis), such that food eaten by one animal passes from its stomach to the duodenum of their partner, the food eaten by one animal inhibits intake by the partner, presumably because it enters the partner's intestinal tract. Conversely, the partner beginning a meal first overeats, presumably because the food entering its partner's intestines is no longer satiating. Although their nature has not yet been specified in detail, three types of satiety signals appear to operate at the intestinal level: delivery of nutrients, exposure to hyperosmotic liquids, and intestinal distention. Numerous studies have shown that eating is reduced by intestinal infusions of nutrients (i.e., carbohydrates, amino acids, or lipids) or nonnutritive hyperosmotic stimuli. Direct intestinal nutrient infusions are typically more effective than matched hepatoportal injections, suggesting that the nutrients actually act on the intestines rather than just in the bloodstream to reduce eating. The satiating effects of glucose and amino acids are apparently conveyed to the brain from sensory receptors in the intestinal wall that respond to those nutrients via the vagus nerve. Thus, the satiating effect of intestinal infusions of glucose and amino acids, but not lipids, are lost in vagotomized rats.

D. The Role of Blood-Borne Factors and the Liver in Short-Term Satiety

Meal-related increases in levels of blood-borne nutrients and hormones can induce satiety; however, there is substantial controversy about the roles of specific hormones, and little consensus about the mechanisms of their action. Powerful evidence for the existence of short-term blood-borne satiety factors comes from blood transfusion studies which show that the blood from a satiated rat markedly suppresses eating in a

fasted recipient rat. The circulating satiety factors are short-lived, because the satiating effect of the transfusions is lost with donor rats that have been fasted for only four or five hours. Further evidence comes from parabiotic animals, which share a common blood supply (but where their intestines are uncrossed). In parabiotic rats, feeding by one member of the pair suppresses subsequent intake by the partner.

Measures taken near the end of meals have shown that levels of various blood borne factors increase at this time. Among these are glucose and amino acids absorbed from the intestines, as well as insulin and glucagon released from the pancreas, and cholecystokinin (CCK) released from the small intestines. Intravenous injections of each of these compounds consistently suppress eating under some conditions. Conversely, eating is stimulated by treatments that block the actions of several of these compounds. For example, eating is increased by injections of antibodies or antagonists to insulin, glucagon and CCK, as well as by injection of the glucose antimetabolite, 2-deoxyglucose. Thus, all are potential satiety factors.

The liver is the first organ reached by blood from the intestines, and thus it is uniquely situated to monitor blood levels of absorbed nutrients. The liver contains sensors that project satiety information via the hepatic branch of the vagus nerve to the brain. The activity of these sensory fibers is markedly inhibited by physiological levels of glucose infused into the liver. A role for the liver in satiety was suggested by evidence that infusions of amino acids, glucose, or glucagon are each much more effective in suppressing eating in the hepatic circulation than in other portions of the circulation. Additionally, the satiating effects of intravenous glucose and glucagon are absent in vagotomized animals. However, the virtual absence of effects of complete hepatic denervation on meal patterns, shows that neural input from the liver is not essential for normal patterns of spontaneous eating. Additionally, several of these compounds may act directly within the brain to produce their effects on eating.

VI. LONG-TERM MODULATION OF EATING BY BODY FAT

A. Mechanisms

When food is freely available, body weight, and therefore body fat is highly stable and resistant to change in most adults: Humans and animals typically regain precisely the body weight lost during imposed food restriction or dieting, and lose precisely the weight gained during forced overfeeding. Also, animals markedly increase eating to compensate for the higher energy demands imposed by cold ambient temperatures, high levels of exercise, or lactation. There are both behavioral and metabolic components to this regulation of body weight. As weight is lost below the "body weight set point" not only does the motivation to eat increase, but metabolic efficiency also increases, so that weight loss is slowed even with stable caloric intake. Likewise, body weight gain above the "set point" results in decreased appetite and can lead to a lowering of metabolic efficiency; however, the control of weight above the "set point" is frequently not as strong as the control of weight below the set point.

This has led to the concept, introduced and termed the *lipostatic hypothesis* by G. C. Kennedy, that food intake is largely regulated so as to maintain constant stores of body lipids. Over long periods, this regulation is extremely precise, as illustrated by the observation that overeating only 3 to 4% of the approximately 3000 kcals needed to maintain a stable weight, the mere 100 or so kcals per day contained in a single pat of butter, would result in a fat gain of about 3.9 kg (8.6 lb) per year, a relatively uncommon occurrence except after a food restriction diet. However, that well over 30% of Americans in recent surveys were obese by medical and societal norms, demonstrates that the level at which body weight is regulated by physiological mechanisms may be very different from the level considered ideal by the individual. That this body energy balance is long-term rather than short-term, is suggested by studies in people showing that the energy acquired by eating is uncorrelated with that lost in energy expenditure over 1 day, whereas there is a strong correlation between these variables over a period of 1 week. Thus, energy intake and utilization are balanced over the long term but not over the short term.

What are the mechanisms of body fat regulation? One possibility is that hormones released by fat cells in proportion to total body lipid or to the size of fat cells provide information about levels of body fat to brain mechanisms controlling eating behavior. The involvement of hormones has been strongly supported by studies of parabiotic rats and mice, which share a common blood supply. These studies show that weight gain in one member of the pair, whether by forced feeding or by brain stimulation or lesions that cause overeating, results in reduced eating and body weight loss by the other member of the pair. The strength of this appetite suppressive effect increases as a function of the weight gain by the fat member of the pair.

Insight into the mechanisms of body weight regulation has come from genetically obese mice. Two of these are the *ob/ob* (for obese) and *db/db* (for diabetic) mice. *ob/ob* is an autosomal recessive disorder resulting from a single gene mutation on chromosome 6, while *db/db* results from a gene mutation on chromosome 4. Despite the difference in the genotype, the *ob/ob* and the *db/db* are phenotypically almost identical. Both become extremely obese, overeat, are hyperinsulinemic and hyperglycemic, and are highly metabolically efficient. When parabiosed with normal mice, the obese *db/db* mice continue to gain weight while the normal member of the pair stops eating and starves to death. In contrast, normal mice gain weight and the *ob/ob* mice lose weight when parabiosed, and when *ob/ob* and *db/db* are parabiosed the *ob/ob* lose weight and the *db/db* mice continue rapid weight gain. Based on these findings, Doug Coleman suggested that the *ob/ob* mice were deficient in a weight-related satiety hormone and the *db/db* mice produced this hormone but were insensitive to its satiating effects. Thus, the *db/db* mice gain weight when parabiosed to either normal or *ob/ob* mice because they are insensitive to the satiety hormone, and the *ob/ob* mice lose weight when parabiosed to normal or *db/db* mice in response to the satiety hormone from those animals.

Recently the *ob* and the *db* genes have been cloned, confirming and specifying Coleman's hypothesis. The *ob* gene is responsible for producing the hormone *leptin,* which is released into the blood from fat cells. Thus, the level of blood leptin could act as an index of body fat mass. In contrast, the *db* gene appears to encode the leptin receptor. Thus, the *ob/ob* mice are deficient in producing normal leptin and the *db/db* mice are deficient in producing the leptin receptor. Leptin acts as a powerful satiety hormone. When injected into *ob/ob* or normal mice, leptin suppresses food intake and causes body weight loss. It is ineffective in the *db/db* mice, presumably because they lack the leptin receptor. Although the precise mechanisms by which leptin produces satiety have yet to be established, evidence suggests that leptin released from fat cells into the blood acts directly on hypothalamic feeding control circuits to suppress eating.

B. Obesity in Humans

What factors are responsible for the growing prevalence of obesity in our society? Animal studies suggest that a major factor in the sensory quality of the food we eat. Access to a variety of highly palatable diets causes weight gain in animals and it is almost certain that the easy access to a wide variety of highly palatable, calorically dense diets contributes to weight gain in many people, especially when combined with a sedentary life-style. A much less common factor is exposure to certain drugs or hormones. Increased eating and weight gain is a frequent side effect of taking synthetic glucocorticoids, or of ingesting antipsychotic drugs that block dopamine receptors. Similarly, Cushing syndrome, which is characterized by an excess in circulating levels of glucocorticoids, is frequently associated with weight gain and overeating. The effect of many of these compounds on body weight is due to their actions on brain mechanisms controlling eating behavior and energy metabolism. In rare cases, weight gain is due to an organic neuropathology. Some people with damage to the portions of the medial hypothalamus, which contain elements of neurocircuitry controlling eating, become ravenous overeaters and hence, massively obese. Genetic mutations may, in rare cases, also lead to obesity. People with Prader-Willi syndrome, a genetic anomaly caused by an unspecified mutation on chromosome 15, are typically ravenous eaters and extremely obese. Body weight is also strongly influenced by the normal genotype. This is exemplified by the strong concordance in the body weights of "identical twins," even when separated at birth and reared in different homes. [See OBESITY.]

VII. NEURAL CONTROLS OF EATING

Eating behavior arises as a result of the hierarchical interactions between a variety of functionally specialized brain areas. The brainstem and spinal cord contain the motor neurons whose activity produces contractions of the muscle groups active during eating behavior, as well as the upper motor neurons of the parasympathetic and sympathetic nervous system that produce the autonomic responses that accompany eating behavior. Additionally, some brainstem neurons generate the complex temporally sequenced activity that drives motor neurons to fire in a pattern that yields the complex movements characteristic of eating behavior.

These brainstem neurons are stimulated and/or inhibited by the previously described food-related visceral sensory afferents from the gastrointestinal tract, by blood-borne metabolic fuels and their regulatory hormones, and by afferents from the oral region conveying food-related sensory information, such that major components of eating behavior and the associated autonomic responses can be appropriately elicited in animals without a forebrain. These brainstem control mechanisms and their responses to sensory inputs are powerfully modulated by descending projections from the hypothalamus. These feeding regulatory hypothalamic neurons, in addition to the visceral, taste, and hormonal inputs, receive food-related visual, auditory, olfactory, and circadian inputs, and their activity is also modulated by inputs from subsets of cortical neurons that process food-related taste, olfactory, auditory and visual information. Some of these relationships are illustrated in Figure 1.

A. Brain Stem

The brainstem consists of the *midbrain, pons* and *medulla oblongata*. These regions contain the basic neural circuitry for the discrimination of taste and the motor programs that produce chewing, swallowing, or rejection responses to food. The motor outputs of the brainstem are mediated by several nuclei. These include the *trigeminal nucleus,* which contains motor neurons controlling the muscles of mastication; the *nucleus ambiguus,* those that deal with the motor act of swallowing, and the *dorsal motor nucleus of the vagus (DMNX),* which contains the motor neurons of the vagus nerve that controls parasympathetic activity in the gastrointestinal system and liver, and the secretion of insulin by the pancreas. The brainstem also contains the *area postrema,* which is believed to directly detect toxins in the blood and to produce consequent vomiting, and other sensory regions which will be described later.

In rats that have had the neuronal connections between the brainstem and forebrain severed, the autonomic responses such as cephalic phase insulin release and the sympathoadrenal response to low glucose availability remain undisturbed. These decerebrate rats show normal facial and mouth movements characteristic of ingestion when pleasant tastes are applied directly into the mouth, and they show characteristic rejection responses such as gaping and head shaking

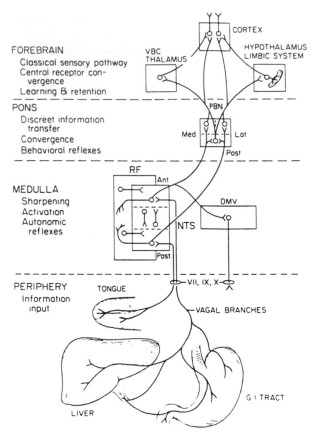

FOREBRAIN
  Classical sensory pathway
  Central receptor con-
    vergence
  Learning & retention

PONS
  Discreet information
    transfer
  Convergence
  Behavioral reflexes

MEDULLA
  Sharpening
  Activation
  Autonomic
    reflexes

PERIPHERY
  Information
    input

Figure 1 A highly schematized diagram of the neural networks by which gustatory and visceral inputs modulate feeding behavior. VBC Thalamus, ventrobasal complex of the thalamus; PBN, parabrachial nucleus; RF, reticular formation; DMV, dorsal motor nucleus of the vagus; NTS, nucleus of the solitary tract. [Reprinted by permission of the *Western Journal of Medicine* (Novin, 1985).]

when unpleasant foods are tasted. More strikingly, these animals also crudely regulate their food intake; deprived animals ingest liquid food injected directly into the mouth, while satiated rats reject it. Thus, the basic motor programs for food ingestion, and some mechanisms for regulating intake based on physiological needs, reside in the caudal brainstem.

B. Taste Pathways

Taste is important for food selection and rejection, as well as for influencing the amount of food eaten. Taste information from receptors on the tongue reaches the brain through *cranial nerves* VII (facial nerve), IX

(glossopharyngeal nerve) and X (vagus nerve, laryngeal branch). The first relay for these gustatory afferents is in the anterior portion of the medullary *nucleus of the solitary tract* (*NTS*) (see Figs. 1 and 2). The anterior NTS sends fibers relaying gustatory information to several brain nuclei. The parasympathetic targets are the DMNX, a medullary motor nucleus that controls parasympathetic autonomic activity related to eating and digestion (as described earlier); the nucleus ambiguus, which controls the muscles of swallowing in the pharynx and esophagus (as described earlier); and the *salivatory nuclei,* which control salivation. These sensory-motor loops mediate some of the normal reflex responses to food that persist in decerebrate rats. In the rat, neurons in the anterior NTS also project to the posterior and medial *parabrachial nuclei* (*PBN*) in the *pons;* this is the second relay in the taste system of the rat (see Fig. 2). The PBN then relays gustatory information to several different brain areas. One is the thalamic taste area, the *ventral posteromedial nucleus* (*VPM*) of the thalamus, which relays gustatory information to the *primary taste cortex.* The PBN also projects to the *lateral hypothalamus* (*LH*), the *central nucleus of the amygdala* (*CNA*), and the *bed nucleus of the stria terminalis* (*BNST*) in the forebrain.

The taste system of primates is similar, except that taste information is relayed directly from the anterior NTS to the thalamic taste area, bypassing the PBN. There are two primary taste areas in the primate cortex: the frontal opercular cortex and the insular cortex. These project to a secondary cortical taste area, the *orbitofrontal cortex* (*OBF*). This is actually a *multimodal* area, with neurons responding to taste, smell, and taste-related visual inputs. The OBF has mutual interconnections with the amygdala, which receives gustatory information from the primary taste cortex. The OBF projects to the LH, providing a means for the hypothalamus to receive gustatory information.

C. The Coding of Feeding-Related Taste and Visceral Sensory Information in the Nucleus of the Solitary Tract

The NTS is the first central relay for sensory information from the oral cavity and gastrointestinal tract, and therefore is in a position to have an important in-

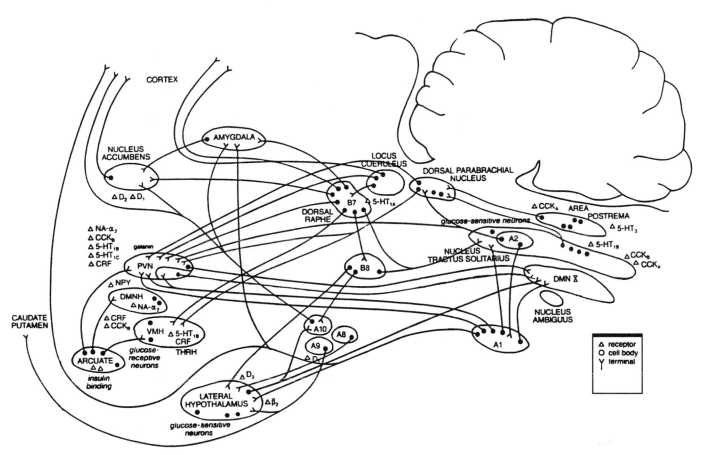

Figure 2   Some of the brain areas, and their interconnections, believed to participate in the neural control of eating. PVN, paraventricular nucleus of the hypothalamus; DMNX, dorsal motor nucleus of the vagus; DMNH, dorsomedial nucleus of the hypothalamus; VMH, ventromedial nucleus of the hypothalamus. D, dopamine; NA, noradrenaline; CCK, cholecystokinin; 5-HT, serotonin; CRF, corticotropin-releasing factor; NPY, neuropeptide Y; THRH, thyrotropin-releasing hormone. Modified from *Trends in Pharmacological Sciences,* 12:147–157, 1991.

fluence on eating behavior. The cranial nerves that convey taste information also carry *somatosensory* information from the oral cavity to the NTS and *spinal trigeminal nucleus* of the pons; these inputs allow discrimination of the texture of food. The NTS is also the first brain relay for sensory information from the *viscera*. Visceral afferent fibers originating in the intestines, stomach and liver project in the vagus nerve to neurons in the posterior NTS. These visceral afferents relay food-related information to the brain about the extent of gastrointestinal distention, intestinal nutrient content, and blood glucose levels, all of which reflect the level of nutrients available for metabolic processes.

The processing of taste and visceral sensory information by the NTS is an integral component in the neural controls of food intake. Because the NTS is the first brain area to receive taste information, it is here that this sensory modality is first "coded" by the brain. Tastes are classified as either sweet, sour, bitter, or salty. These tastes are coded by distinct *patterns* of activity across anterior NTS neurons. For example, the subset of NTS neurons activated, and their degree of response, varies for salty or sweet tastes. Interestingly, this coding is influenced by prior experience. For example, the rat NTS coding of saccharin is altered in rats that have developed a taste aversion to that substance. Specifically, the NTS response to saccharin, instead of resembling the pattern of response to a sweet taste, comes to resemble that of a bitter aversive flavor after a taste aversion to saccharin has developed. That the behavior of the animal toward a flavor changes in parallel with the neural coding for that flavor, suggests that the coding of taste information may be critical in determining the ability to discriminate between different foods and to choose foods based on past experience. However, areas of the brain outside of the brainstem are also required for the expression of conditioned taste aversion.

In the rat, the responsiveness of gustatory NTS neurons to taste stimuli on the tongue is modulated by hunger and satiety. For example, experimental distention of the stomach (to simulate the stretching that occurs when the stomach is full of food) or hyperglycemia are both associated with reduced responses of anterior NTS neurons to taste stimuli in rats. These findings suggest that the acceptance responses to food in hungry rats and rejection responses in satiated rats may, in part, be due to the integration of taste and visceral information in the NTS. More specifically, progressively reduced neural responses to positive taste stimuli during a meal may contribute to the development of satiety. It should be noted that in primates, as opposed to rats, the taste responses of NTS neurons do not appear to be readily modulated by experience. Instead, modulation appears to occur primarily at cortical and hypothalamic levels.

Additionally, the NTS and nearby area postrema contain some neurons that show alterations in electrical activity during direct application of glucose. Typically direct application of glucose reduces the rate of firing of these neurons. These NTS and area postrema glucose-sensitive neurons may detect brain glucose levels, which can be influenced by blood glucose levels, and act to stimulate or suppress eating. Evidence suggesting this is that central application of compounds that cause glucoprivation elicit eating only when they have access to the caudal brainstem. The glucose-sensing neurons in the brain region may also be involved in the natural initiation of eating in response to low blood glucose.

D. Hypothalamic Sites and Feeding Stimulation

Various hypothalamic sites act in response to afferent information relayed from brainstem nuclei to initiate and terminate eating behavior, in part, by their projections to brainstem sensory and motor nuclei.

1. The Paraventricular Nucleus

The *paraventricular nucleus of the hypothalamus* (PVN) lies on either side of the third ventricle in the anterior medial hypothalamus. That this nucleus participates in the control of eating is suggested by the finding that electrolytic lesions of the PVN result in overeating and obesity, while electrical stimulation in this region inhibits eating. Additionally, several neurotransmitters act within the PVN to stimulate eating. Studies conducted by Sarah F. Leibowitz have shown that *norepinephrine* (NE) microinjected into the PVN of satiated rats acts on α_2 receptors to elicit a robust, normal appearing, short-latency eating response that is relatively selective for carbohydrates. That NE is involved in the physiological control of food intake is suggested by the findings that acute blockade of α_2 receptors or destruction of NE-containing afferents to the PVN suppress natural eating, particularly of carbohydrates, and may also cause loss of body weight. In addition, extracellular NE in the PVN rises sharply just after the onset of the dark cycle, when rats normally eat a large, carbohydrate-rich meal. Thus, it is likely that the release of endogenous NE within the PVN mediates spontaneous eating, particularly of carbohydrates. Another neurotransmitter, *serotonin*, is released in the PVN as rats eat at the beginning of the dark cycle, and it acts antagonistically to NE in the PVN to inhibit carbohydrate appetite.

The PVN has anatomical connections with the NTS, and autonomic nervous system (to the DMNX and sympathetic preganglionic neurons) as well as to the pituitary gland, so it is well positioned to modulate taste, autonomic and endocrine activity in relation to feeding. In relation to this, it is known that the feeding stimulatory effect of NE in the PVN is partially dependent on intact projections to the NTS and DMNX, as well as on intact vagal projections to the pancreas, the source of insulin, and on circulating levels of the adrenal hormone, corticosterone. The sources of endogenous NE in the PVN are the *locus coeruleus* in the pons, as well as noradrenergic input from the NTS and the *A1 cell group* in the medulla. Disruption of these noradrenergic fibers to the PVN reduces spontaneous eating and causes body weight loss.

The PVN is also sensitive to the feeding-stimulatory

effects of another neurochemical, *neuropeptide Y* (NPY). This neuropeptide is composed of 36 amino acids and is contained in afferents to the PVN that arise from the *arcuate nucleus* of the hypothalamus and from nuclei in the brain stem. That NPY in this brain area is involved in the natural control of eating is supported by the finding that food deprivation causes increased expression of NPY in the arcuate nucleus and increased levels of extracellular NPY in the PVN. This peptide is the most powerful stimulant of eating behavior known, capable of causing satiated rats to gorge food until their stomachs are extremely distended. Like NE-injected rats, animals injected with NPY in the PVN preferentially consume carbohydrates. The PVN also appears to be the locus of many autonomic and endocrine responses to hypothalamic NPY. Specifically, the administration of NPY directly into the PVN results in an array of autonomic and endocrine responses that collectively result in the mobilization of stored energy and the utilization of stored and circulating fuels for energy. These include increased circulating insulin, glucagon, and corticosterone, and inhibition of the sympathetic nervous input to thermogenic brown adipose tissue. These responses to NPY, combined with increased food intake, result in a positive energy balance. Indeed, chronic daily injection of NPY results in massive overeating and a dramatic increase in body weight gain, which appears to depend in part upon increased metabolic efficiency.

2. The Perifornical Hypothalamus

The *perifornical hypothalamus*, (PFH) a small cylindrical area surrounding the portion of the *fornix* running from the caudal end of the PVN to the posterior end of ventromedial nucleus of the hypothalamus, also appears to play an important role in control of eating and body weight. For example, NPY in the PFH is more effective in eliciting eating than in the PVN, and the PFH is believed to be the primary locus for the eating-stimulatory effects of this peptide. Similarly, electrical stimulation in the area of the PFH and adjacent lateral hypothalamus (LH) is especially effective in eliciting eating.

This area receives brain stem projections containing epinephrine, from the *C1 cell groups* and norepinephrine from the A1 cell groups in the ventrolateral medulla, from the *A2 noradrenergic cell groups* in the NTS, and from the midbrain dopamine containing *A8*

cell group. Lesions of any of these ascending catecholamine pathways to the PFH results in overeating and obesity. The catecholamine neurotransmitters norepinephrine, epinephrine and dopamine, when microinjected into the PFH, markedly reduce food-deprivation induced eating. The PFH is also the locus for the appetite-suppressive effects of amphetamine, a chemical which causes release of catecholamines from axon terminals. Conversely, dopamine antagonists applied to the PFH stimulate eating. Moreover, the levels of some of these catecholamines increase during eating or infusion of glucose into the duodenum. Taken collectively, the above findings suggest that the catecholamine neurotransmitters contribute to satiety when they are released in the PFH in response to peripheral satiety factors. Dopamine in the PFH may act to produce satiety in part by counteracting the eating stimulatory effects of NPY.

Although it is not known which efferent connections of the PFH are essential in eating control, projections from the PFH to areas of the cerebral cortex, amygdala, nucleus accumbens, PBN, NTS, superior salivatory nucleus, and the C1 cell group in the medulla have been demonstrated. Polysynaptic connections also connect the PFH with masticatory neurons in the trigeminal motor nucleus, which control the muscles of chewing. The PFH has descending projections to the spinal cord, through which it may be able to modulate motor and autonomic activity during eating.

3. The Lateral Hypothalamus:

The *lateral hypothalamus (LH)* (see Fig. 2), an area just lateral to the PFH, appears to play a major role in stimulation of eating. Classic studies demonstrated that bilateral lesions of the lateral hypothalamus cause aphagia in rats, and conversely that satiated animals eat in response to electrical stimulation of the LH. Although some of these effects were due to actions on axons passing through the LH, more recent work strongly suggests that neurons originating within the LH mediate natural eating. Specifically, neurotoxic lesions of the LH, which spare fibers of passage, also suppress eating behavior, and stimulation of LH neurons by the neurotransmitter glutamate and glutamate receptor agonists induces an intense eating response in satiated rats. These feeding stimulatory LH neurons appear to express glutamate receptors of the NMDA subtype, because LH injections of NMDA elicit eating and blockade of NMDA-type glutamate receptors suppresses natural eating and causes body weight loss.

Neurons in the LH are responsive to a variety of food-related stimuli. Their activity is correlated with spontaneous eating and has a circadian periodicity that parallels the circadian periodicity of eating in the rat. Many LH neurons are responsive to internal signals related to the nutritive state of the animal. For example, the rat LH contains neurons whose activity is modulated by circulating levels of the metabolic fuel glucose and by direct application of glucose and other metabolites. In addition, some neurons responding to direct glucose application also receive convergent input from peripheral glucoreceptors in the liver via the NTS. Inputs to the LH from the NTS may also modulate LH neuron activity following distention of the stomach, a well-known satiety signal.

LH neurons also appear to be responsive to external food-related stimuli when animals are hungry. The LH receives gustatory and olfactory information from the central nucleus of the amygdala (CNA), with which it has mutual interconnections. The LH also receives input from other brain areas involved in gustatory and visual processing. In an elegant series of studies, Edmund T. Rolls and colleagues have shown that subsets of LH neurons respond with a change in firing rate to the sight, smell and/or taste of food or food-related objects in the hungry monkey. These responses both precede and predict the behavioral responses of the animal to food. As the hungry monkey is fed to satiety on a particular food, the response of an LH neuron (inhibition or excitation) to that food declines progressively, until the response disappears at the same time that the monkey no longer accepts the offered food but rejects it (a sign of satiety). The loss of LH responses, and the monkey's satiety, are selective for the food that has been eaten. This may account for the previously mentioned "sensory-specific satiety."

The LH projects to several brain areas which may be involved in responses to food. Among these areas are the NTS, PBN, the DMNX, nucleus ambiguus and hypoglossal nucleus, *reticular formation* of the brainstem, and the spinal cord. Projections to the nucleus ambiguus and hypoglossal nucleus provide a means of influencing jaw and mouth movements necessary for eating. The projections of the LH to the salivatory nuclei may participate in the salivation that occurs in feeding and LH electrical stimulation. Projections to the reticular formation and spinal cord may facilitate locomotion and motor responses used in obtaining food. The LH also has reciprocal connections with the amygdala, a forebrain site that is involved in learning about foods.

E. The Amygdala

The amygdala is a forebrain structure that is essential for the formation of conditioned taste aversion. The amygdala receives visceral, taste, auditory, olfactory, and visual information from many brain areas, and has interconnections with the limbic system. Lesions of the amygdala can disrupt normal feeding, causing hyperphagia or anorexia and food rejection, depending on the site of the lesion.

F. Cortical and Other Forebrain Areas

Areas involved in the processing of sensory information in the forebrain are also involved in the identification of food items. In primates the olfactory bulb relays olfactory information to the *septal nuclei in the medial olfactory area,* which have connections to the *limbic system,* including the hypothalamus. The medial olfactory area is responsible for appetitive responses to olfactory stimuli such as salivation and licking of the lips. Olfactory information is also relayed to the thalamus, which projects to the *orbitofrontal cortex* (OBF). The OBF in the monkey is a multimodal area in which neurons respond to taste, visual, and/or olfactory stimuli. The OBF projects to the LH and to the amygdala. Like LH neurons, the OBF neurons respond to the stimuli associated with food in a hunger-dependent manner. The OBF neurons respond to these stimuli when they are associated with reward. Thus the OBF may be involved in directing the animal's response to food with which it has had beneficial past experience. That the OBF and other cortical visual areas are important in the selection of foods is suggested by the finding that lesions of the OBF of inferotemporal cortex (an area involved in object recognition) cause inability to discriminate food from non-food objects.

BIBLIOGRAPHY

Booth, D. A. (Ed.). (1993). *Neurophysiology of ingestion.* New York: Pergamon Press.

Cooper, S. J., & Clifton, P. G. (Eds.). (1996). *Drug receptor subtypes and ingestive behaviour.* London: Academic Press.

Le Magnen, J. (1992). *Neurobiology of feeding and nutrition.* New York: Academic Press.

Martin, R. H., White, B. D., & Hulsey, M. G. (1991). The regulation of body weight. *American Scientist,* Vol. 79, 528–541.

Ritter, R. C., Ritter, S., & Barnes, C. D. (Eds.). (1986). *Feeding behavior: Neural and humoral controls.* New York: Academic Press.

Stricker, E. M. (Ed.). (1990). *Neurobiology of food and fluid intake: Handbook of behavioral neurobiology,* Vol. 10. New York: Plenum Press.

Westerterp-Plantenge, M. S., Fredrix, E. W. H. M., & Steffens, A. B. (Eds.). (1994). *Food intake and energy expenditure.* Boca Raton, FL: CRC Press.

Emotional Regulation

Sandra Losoya and Nancy Eisenberg

Arizona State University

Attention Focusing   The capacity to willfully maintain and hold the attentional focus on a desired channel (resisting the urge to become attentionally distracted).

Attention Shifting   The capacity to willfully shift attention from channel to channel (thereby avoiding unintentional focusing on particular channels).

Behavioral Inhibition   A self-regulatory characteristic associated with the inhibition of action or approach responses to novelty.

Emotionality   Defined as individual differences in the dynamic characteristics associated with the expression and experience of emotion. Relevant characteristics include threshold and intensity levels as well as latency, duration, and recovery from peak emotion.

Emotion Regulation   Processes involved in the initiation, maintenance, and modulation of internal emotional and physiological states.

Externalizing Disorders   A category of psychopathology in children that includes outwardly expressed behaviors such as aggression, impulsivity, hyperactivity, and conduct problems.

Internalizing Disorders   A category of psychopathology in children that includes inner-directed problems such as anxiety, extreme shyness, depression, and tendencies to withdraw.

Temperament   Constitutionally based individual differences in emotionality, attention, activity levels (personal tempo) and self-regulation (which includes behavioral inhibition and effortful control).

EMOTION REGULATION, a capacity believed to be central to the development of quality of social functioning, is a construct that implies that emotions are both regulatory (such as for the regulation of emotionally driven behavior or the emotion-eliciting context) and regulated (i.e., the regulation of one's own emotional experiences). In this article, we will present work on the development of emotion regulation in infancy and childhood and current findings on the relations between emotion regulation and both social competence and childhood psychopathology.

I. OVERVIEW OF EMOTION REGULATION

In recent years, there has been a striking increase in interest among psychologists in the topic of emotion. Although early in the century many psychologists were interested in emotions (e.g., in Freudian theory), the study of emotion was considered to be unnecessary or even worthless by many psychologists for nearly 50 years. Early behaviorists, who studied only overt behavior, felt that there was no need to examine internal states; all human and animal behavior varied as a function of external factors such as rewards and punishment. In the 1960s and 1970s, many psychologists reacted against the limited view of humans held by behaviorists and focused on the development and elicitation of internal cognitive states. However, emotions still were not an issue of concern to most researchers focusing on cognition.

It has been only in the last decade or two that interest in emotion has reappeared as a focal theme in psychology. In fact, the topic of emotion has become central to the study of social development, personality, and clinical psychology. There has been an increasing appreciation of the interrelatedness of emotion, motivation, and behavior, and of the role of emotion in normal development and social functioning. Emotion currently is viewed as both a product of, and a process in, social interaction.

A natural accompaniment of current interest in emotion is concern with the regulation of emotion and the development of such regulation. Consider the role of emotion regulation in everyday conceptions of normal social behavior and psychopathology. An individual who expresses unusual amounts of negative emotion in public likely is thought to lack social skills whereas the person who expresses emotion in the culturally expected manner is more likely to be viewed as socially competent. Moreover, individuals who frequently lose control of their behavior due to emotions such as sadness, anger, frustration, or exhilaration tend to be labeled as having psychological or behavioral problems. Specifically, people who express their emotion in behaviors such as verbal and physical aggression are likely to be viewed as having conduct disorders whereas those who feel excessive amounts of sadness, anxiety, fear, and hopelessness may be labeled as having internalizing problems such as depression.

Thus, emotion and its regulation are highly relevant to quality of everyday social functioning, as well as to psychological and behavioral problems. Nonetheless, research and theory pertaining to the role of emotion and its regulation in normal social functioning still is somewhat limited. For example, there is a dearth of research on the relation of the ability to regulate emotions effectively to social competence with peers. Moreover, much of the existing work on emotion and its regulation concerns early socioemotional functioning (e.g., temperament in infancy and emotion in early relationships); empirical study and theory on the development of emotion regulation during childhood, adolescence, and adulthood, and on the variables that affect the course of development, are modest in both quantity and scope.

In this article, several aspects of the research on the regulation of emotion are summarized. We begin by presenting the conceptualization of types of emotion-relevant regulation that emerges from research on coping and infant temperament and early socioemotional functioning. This discussion is followed up with a consideration of some of the factors that influence the development of emotion regulation, namely, age, individual difference characteristics, and socialization processes (e.g., parenting). First, what is known about the development and stability of emotion-relevant regulation is summarized. Next, we provide a model of emotionality and regulation that serves as the foundation for a discussion on individual differences in emotion and regulation and how these differences interact to predict social functioning. We then move to the topic of the socialization of emotion and its regulation. Finally, the social/psychological costs and benefits associated with the regulation of emotion are considered. Thus, the role of emotion-relevant regulation in social competence is reviewed, followed by a discussion of emotional regulation and psychopathology in children. The focus of this article is primarily on emotion and its regulation in infancy and childhood, although many of the issues covered likely pertain in adulthood.

II. CONCEPTIONS OF EMOTION REGULATION

Emotion regulation has been defined in a variety of ways, some of which are person-centered, such as those that consider physiological changes and person-related feeling experiences as primary and others that expand the boundaries of emotion regulation to include interactions with the environment. Consistent with the latter view, we believe that the regulation of emotion-related processes pertains to more than merely suppressing or expressing emotion. As suggested by Joseph Campos and his colleagues, emotion-relevant regulation can occur on three levels: input regulation (involving sensory receptors), central regulation (information or cognitive processing), or output regulation (at the response selection or behavioral level). Moreover, emotion has direct effects on behavior and people's overt behavior (e.g., coping behavior) has a regulating effect on emotion. Thus, it is necessary to consider several types of regulation when discussing emotion and its regulation.

Nancy Eisenberg and Richard Fabes proposed that there are at least three types of emotion-relevant regulation germane to the development of quality of social functioning and intrapsychic emotional development: regulation of internal (experienced) emotion, regulation of emotionally driven behavior, and regulation of the emotion-eliciting context/factors.

Regulation of experienced emotion refers to the process of initiating, maintaining, or modulating the occurrence, intensity, or duration of internal feeling states and emotion-related physiological processes. Thus, it pertains to the regulation of the experience, not expression, of emotion. Cognitive and attentional processes frequently are used to regulate the experience of emotion: for example, people can shift their attention from an emotion-arousing stimulus, focus their attention on issues or things that elicit or suppress emotion, or cognitively restructure events in their minds so as to alter their emotion (e.g., think about a bad experience in a more positive light). Other ways to regulate emotion include moving oneself physically closer or further from events or objects that may elicit emotion, and seeking comfort from others to reduce an aversive internal state.

Researchers and theorists studying temperament (constitutionally based individual differences among people) frequently have discussed the use of attentional control as a means of regulation. Indeed, Mary Rothbart, a leading temperament theorist, considers attention shifting and focusing as aspects of temperament that are central to the regulation of emotion. Cognitive (e.g., attentional) methods of managing emotion also have been the focus of coping theorists who are interested in how people manage stressful situations. Richard Lazarus, a leader in theory and research on coping, defines coping as changing cognitive and behavioral efforts to manage specific external or internal demands that are appraised as taxing or exceeding the resources of the individual. One type of coping is the regulation of emotional distress (i.e., emotion-focused coping), which can be considered regula-

tion in particularly stressful contexts. Of course, regulation also occurs in situations that are not particularly stressful. [*See* Coping with Stress; Personality.]

The second type of regulation, the regulation of emotionally driven behavior, also is relevant to understanding emotion and its regulation. Behavior, including overt actions toward others as well as facial expressions, often is an expression of internal emotional states. The construct of behavioral regulation has been discussed by several groups of theorists. For example, temperament theorists assess constructs such as impulsivity and behavioral inhibition (the ability to inhibit action); Rothbart considers these types of regulation to be central components of temperament. In addition, other developmentalists have been interested in the control of behavior (e.g., ego control), and in highly inhibited behavior (e.g., very constrained behavior with new people or novel situations). Similarly, personality theorists have studied behavioral disinhibition and constraint in adults, and clinical researchers have examined impulsive, undercontrolled behavior.

The third type of regulation, regulation of the emotion-eliciting context, has been discussed most often by coping theorists. A major type of coping delineated by Richard Lazarus is problem-focused coping—efforts to modify the source of the problem. For example, if a girl tries a new approach to entering a peer group such as offering to share a toy, she is using problem-focused coping. Such coping frequently is used when trying to deal with stressful situations and, except in situations over which the child has no control, generally is considered constructive.

III. EMOTION-RELEVANT REGULATION IN INFANCY AND EARLY CHILDHOOD

All of the three aforementioned types of regulation can be used to manage emotion and the behavioral expression of emotion. However, only rudimentary strategies designed to reduce the experience of negative arousal are evident in early infancy. Claire Kopp, who is noted for her work on self-regulation, suggested that during the first few years of life, strategies that enable the regulation of emotion and arousal are acquired slowly.

Kopp proposed a model of emotion regulation from birth to toddlerhood that outlines a progression from innate, hard-wired types of regulation to levels of regulation dependent on learning and cognition. For instance, in early infancy, self-soothing behaviors such as looking away and nonnutritive sucking help to regulate arousal by limiting the intake of, or reducing the distress associated with, external and internal stimulation. After about 3 months, advances in attentional processes and motor maturation result in the management of arousal and emotion through the ability to distract oneself. Infants exposed to distressing stimuli are able to escape by rotating the head, shifting attention, and attending to visually interesting sights that they are now able to see with some clarity.

Although young infants employ simple emotion regulation strategies such as looking away to reduce the experience of negative arousal, they greatly rely on the management of emotions provided by caregivers. Parents help reduce negative internal states by separating an infant from a stressor and by providing emotional comfort and nurturing in times of infant distress. Moreover, parents begin teaching early lessons about the regulation of emotion when 2- to 3-month-old infants become more aware of their social environment. It is at this time that infants suddenly begin smiling and laughing in response to caregiver solicitations. Indeed, infants and their caregivers frequently engage in an emotion-based form of communication that leads to the expectation of reciprocal emotional interchanges (e.g., parent smiles and vocalizes to the infant who reciprocates with smiles, gurgles, and excited body movements; parent continues positive stimulation until one or the other disengages). These interchanges assist the infant in discovering associations between her or his actions, others' responses, and changes in feeling states.

By late in the first year, advances have been made in the infant's motor, cognitive, social, and emotional domains. Infants are much more coordinated in their ability to reach and grasp objects; indeed, they are adept at crawling toward or withdrawing from objects or persons. They have improved memories, are able to discriminate among faces, and have developed expectations regarding caregiver behaviors.

Moreover, infants have begun to reference and communicate needs to caregivers. By 9 months, they appear to be checking on their caregivers' continuing presence. However, by 12 months of age, infants actively seek and are influenced by parental emotional communication. Social referencing, as it is commonly referred to, is a process whereby infants seek out emo-

tional signals of caregivers to determine how to react to novel situations or objects. Several researchers have demonstrated that infants refer to and use facial and vocal emotional expressions of their caregivers to inform them of the safety of an object or event. In one study, 12-month-old infants touched toys that parents expressed positive emotion toward almost twice the number of times in a short period than when the parents' message was fearful. In another study, mothers who showed positive expressions or vocalizations had infants who moved closer to a novel object or stranger. In contrast, mothers who showed expressions of fear or made negative vocalizations had infants who moved closer to the mother. Thus, it is clear that caregivers' emotional signals affect infants' behavioral regulation through the process of social referencing and may foster learning of emotional responses.

By the third year, children's control and influence over their emotional states increase markedly with the onset and growth of language skills and their understanding of others' behavior. Moreover, symbolic representational capacities, recall memory, and notions of cause and effect allow the child to exhibit planful behavior and focus on a goal while inhibiting other inappropriate responses. Strategies used in the regulation of emotionally driven behavior have been the focus of research on children's ability to delay gratification. Walter Mischel and his colleagues demonstrated that preschoolers who were successful in the ability to delay gratification when rewards (e.g., food) were present during a waiting period used a variety of self-distraction techniques, including verbal and motor strategies. The most frequently used strategy in one delay of gratification task was active engagement with substitute objects. Other studies (with mostly older children) indicate that there is an age-related increase in children's use of cognitive strategies, although children's use of behavioral strategies remains relatively constant throughout childhood.

Thus, in the early years of life into childhood, several broad developmental trends are evident. First, with increasing age, regulation of emotion and behavior is shifted gradually from external sources (e.g., parents) in the social environment to self-initiated, intraindividual (i.e., child-based) resources. At a young age, caregivers soothe children, manage the young child's emotion by selecting situations that children are in, and provide children with information to help interpret the environment. With age and cognitive development, children are better able to allocate attention, control their own behavior, and use cognitive strategies to manage emotion. Second, mentalistic strategies such as thinking about situations in a positive light and shifting and focusing attention increase with use in age. The use of such strategies is, no doubt, fostered by the development of children's understanding of the nature of emotion, including factors that elicit, maintain, and modulate emotion. Third, with age, children increasingly develop the capacity to modulate the course of their emotional arousal, for example, the intensity and duration of arousal. The development of attentional strategies and an increased understanding of emotion undoubtedly play a role in this trend.

In summary, there is a clear progression in the regulation of emotion that occurs in the context of important cognitive and behavioral changes in the developing child. Moreover, these new developments offer expanded possibilities for regulating the experience of emotions, emotionally driven behavior, and the emotion-eliciting context. We turn now to a discussion of age-related stability and change in the regulation of emotion.

A. Stability and Change with Age in Emotionality and Regulation

Data on age-related stability and change (rather than interindividual consistency) are sparse and mostly pertain to the first 8 years of life. One group of researchers found that children became more persistent (often considered evidence of regulation), as well as more active/cheerful/sensitive, from age 3 to 7. Other researchers have found that parents view their children as becoming less intense, more positive, more persistent, but more sensitive/reactive from age 3 to 5. Crying also decreases in frequency from infancy into the preschool years. However, some investigators have obtained no clear age changes in temperamental emotionality and regulation in middle childhood. In brief, children usually appear to become more regulated in the early years as well as in elementary school, although the data are not entirely consistent.

In early to mid adolescence, children experience puberty, transitions in schools, and a host of stressors related to changes in others' expectations and in the need to start preparing for adulthood (e.g., in terms of preparing for economic independence and family life, and developing an ethical code). These stressors might

be expected to be associated with increases in negative emotion, although young adolescents do not consistently report more stressors than do younger children. At least in interactions with parents, adolescents' pubertal status (and age in late childhood/early adolescence) has been correlated with increases in negative emotion or decreases in positive emotion. Although this increase in negative emotion often has been noted in the context of interactions with parents, which seem to become increasingly conflictual around puberty, there also may be a mild increase in negative emotionality in early adolescence. In a study of children aged 4 to 16 years, researchers found that although younger children were perceived by parents to be more sullen and irritable, older children were viewed as more unhappy, sad, and depressed than younger children. Overall, then, children appear to become somewhat more negative in early adolescence, although it is not very clear whether children change in degree of regulation or simply become more negative in their emotionality (intensity or frequency of same negative emotions) from mid-elementary school into adolescence.

IV. A MODEL OF EMOTIONALITY AND REGULATION

Individuals differ in both degree and kind of emotions they regularly experience. People who are emotionally intense, that is, who experience their emotions intensely, have a greater need to regulate their emotion and emotionally driven behavior. Similarly, individuals prone to experience negative emotions would be expected to behave in relatively nonadaptive ways (e.g., engage in more anger-driven behavior or withdraw from social interactions).

Based on this line of reasoning, Nancy Eisenberg and Richard Fabes proposed that whether individuals become overaroused in social situations varies as a function of at least two person variables: (1) the person's dispositional level of reactivity, particularly intensity of emotional responding and quantity of negative and positive emotions (aspects of temperament or personality), and (2) individuals' abilities to regulate their emotional reactions, their emotionally driven behavior, and the evocative situation.

Emotional arousability and regulation—although separate constructs—are interrelated. People's temperament and personality, including arousal components, may influence the style that characterizes their regulation (including coping) and vice versa. However, emotionality and regulation also are distinctive and may be associated in a variety of different ways. For example, some people who are easily overaroused may exhibit behavioral inhibition and fear in response to a stressful stimulus whereas others seem to become undercontrolled in their behavior (e.g., display inappropriate disruptive or aggressive behaviors). Thus, it is useful to study individual differences in both emotionality and regulation.

Eisenberg and Fabes proposed that individual differences in emotionality and regulation jointly contribute to the prediction of numerous aspects of social functioning, including socially appropriate behavior, problem behavior such as aggression, popularity with peers, shyness, sympathy and prosocial behavior. In some cases the contributions of emotionality and regulation are additive; in other cases, one would predict interactive or moderating effects. For example, individuals prone to intense emotions (particularly negative emotions) who also are low in the various modes of regulation would be expected to be relatively disruptive, aggressive, inappropriate socially, and generally out of control. In contrast, people high in emotional intensity, high in behavioral regulation, and low in emotional regulation and problem-focused coping appear to be shy, anxious, and behaviorally inhibited in novel contexts. Individuals who are emotionally regulated, able to manage emotion-eliciting contexts, and able to inhibit their behavior (but not to an extreme degree) would be expected to be appropriate in their social behavior and well adjusted, regardless of their level of emotional intensity. Further, numerous researchers have noted that socioemotional functioning is fostered by regulation that is flexible—that changes in an adaptive manner to the demands in a given context. Evidence relevant to these predictions is reviewed later after a consideration of the work on individual differences in emotionality and regulation and the socialization of emotion and regulation.

A. Individual Differences in Emotionality and Regulation

Investigators interested in temperament and the developing personality have found that infants differ in tendencies to express positive and negative emotions.

Some infants, for instance, tend to express more positive emotions and are perceived by caregivers as being easy to rear. Similarly, other infants who are perceived as emotionally challenging by their parents tend to experience and express greater levels of negative emotion. Individual differences are also seen in manifestations of emotional reactivity. Some infants who express more negative emotion also tend to react negatively quickly, are relatively emotionally intense, and are slow to recover from distress when confronted with arousing information. Thus, constitutionally based biases in emotionality and reactivity have implications for the development of emotion regulation as they can and do influence the infant's own behavior and that of caregivers.

Individual differences in infants' behavioral regulation also have been found. One such difference is referred to by temperament theorists as the tendency to approach a novel object. Latency to reach for and grasp the object is considered an index of approach and has been found to be related to children's smiling and laughter in the laboratory. Infants who quickly and frequently reach for a novel object tend to smile and laugh more. In contrast, infants who are easily overaroused tend to withdraw from novelty; for example, they are slower to reach for the new object and may turn away and avert their gaze.

Withdrawal from novelty is related at later ages to the development of behavioral inhibition and fearfulness. Infants younger than 6 months of age tend to reach for and grasp both familiar and unfamiliar objects. By about the age of 8 months, however, individual differences appear in the relative strength of approach versus inhibition. Some infants, for instance, who tend to be more irritable and easily distressed, inhibit behavior fairly consistently when confronted with strange or new objects and situations (i.e., are behaviorally inhibited). By preschool age, it appears that the temperamental construct of behavioral inhibition represents a constellation of behavioral coping strategies used by a child who is temperamentally prone to overarousal.

Individual differences in attentional capacities (e.g., attention focusing and shifting), which, as noted earlier, are an important component of emotion regulation, also are evident in infancy and are related to behaviors of interest. In newborns, measures of orienting responses (e.g., average looking time and duration of orienting to visual stimuli) tend to be negatively related to expressions of distress and positively related to soothability. Also, ability to shift attention, which occurs sometime after 3 months of age, has been found to be positively related to smiling and laughter as measured in the laboratory and with questionnaires. Indeed, caregivers make use of this new development in their efforts to manage the arousal of distressed or bored infants by redirecting their attention to interesting objects. Later, individual differences in the ability to focus and sustain attention predict individual differences in the regulation of emotionally driven behavior. In situations requiring the delay of gratification, for instance, sustained attention was found to be positively related to preschoolers' ability to delay gratification in the presence of an attractive toy.

In summary, individual differences in emotionality, behavioral regulation, and attention are apparent in infancy and are important influences on the development of the regulation of emotion. These differences are related to behaviors of interest and may influence individual coping styles. Moreover, biases in emotional expression and reactivity, for instance, affect caregiver responses, which in turn, affect what children learn about emotion and regulation. Evidence relevant to social agent influences on the development of emotion regulation is considered after a brief summary of what is known about consistency of individual differences in emotion-relevant regulation. [See INDIVIDUAL DIFFERENCES IN MENTAL HEALTH.]

B. Consistency of Individual Differences

In general, little is known about consistency in emotionality and regulation from infancy to childhood and adolescence. Most of the available data indicate that there is moderate consistency in children's temperamental emotionality and regulation in childhood (relative to that of other children) and into adolescence and early adulthood.

Individual differences in two aspects of emotionality and regulation show strong evidence of continuity throughout infancy and into childhood: proneness to distress or irritability and behavioral inhibition. With regard to irritability, researchers find high stability in neonatal irritability and irritability or negative emotionality at 4, 9, and 24 months of age. Aspects of temperament reflecting positive and/or negative emotion and regulation were stable in structure (i.e., in how components grouped together) in another study

of children from 3 to 8 years of age. Other researchers have found modest to relatively high stability in emotional responding from age 4 to 7 to early adolescence. Thus, it appears that aspects of children's temperamental emotionality and regulation are somewhat stable over time, at least in terms of children's standing relative to other children.

Studies of the consistency of behavioral inhibition over time also are impressive and emerge primarily from longitudinal studies conducted by Jerome Kagan and his colleagues. Twenty-one month-old infants who were extreme in their scores on behavioral inhibition were found to be relatively timid, inhibited and quiet at the age of 7 years. Similar findings were obtained in three additional cohorts of children.

Other aspects of temperament related to the regulation of emotion such as approach behavior and attentional capacities also have shown stability. For instance, some investigators have found the tendency to approach to be stable from 4 to 8 months to 1 to 3 years; others have shown moderate stability in approach from 6 months to 2 years of age. In studies of attentional capacities in early infancy, stability of duration of looking has been found from 3 through 4, 7, and 9 months of age; others have found stability from 10 to 13.5 months in rates of attention shifting and duration of orienting. Moreover, investigators have reported stability of attention span, attentional control, or distractibility in infancy, from infancy over several years' time, and during childhood.

Thus, individual differences in emotionality and regulation appear to have a constitutional basis and are somewhat stable over time. However, it also is clear from the existing research that social agents' (particularly parents') practices and behaviors are linked to children's socioemotional responding. We turn now to a discussion of the socialization of emotion regulation.

V. THE SOCIALIZATION OF EMOTION AND ITS REGULATION

There are a number of ways that parents may influence how children respond to, or cope with, emotionally evocative situations. For example, Ross Parke noted that parental influence generally can be divided into direct and indirect influences, which differ in regard to parents' intent or objective in socializing the child. Direct socialization influences are intentional attempts by parents to influence children's emotional behavior; for example, parents may take an instructive or organizing role with the child. Indirect socializing influences are those in which parents are not explicitly or intentionally trying to modify their children's emotional behavior; an example is parental displays of their own emotions. Of course, parental influences on children's emotion-related regulation and competence consist of both direct and indirect types.

Parental emotion-related practices would be expected to influence both the degree to which children express their emotions and their ability to appropriately regulate their emotion and emotionally driven behavior. Parents teach children how and when to express emotion and ways to manage their emotion so that they are able to behave in a socially acceptable manner. Most likely, the direction of causation is bidirectional: children's dispositional emotionality probably affects the emotion-relevant practices used by socializers, as well as vice versa.

Ross Buck hypothesized that children who are punished for the expression of negative emotion learn over time to hide or inhibit expression of these emotions. He suggested that such children are likely, as they age, to become more physiologically aroused than other people in situations likely to involve negative emotions because of the association between negative sanctions and situations involving negative emotions. Consistent with Buck's theorizing, how parents respond to children's displays of negative emotions has been linked to children's displays and reports of vicariously induced emotion. For example, Eisenberg and her colleagues found that parental encouragement to control one's emotions was correlated with children's self-monitoring behavior and boys' reports of low levels of dispositional sympathy (i.e., concern for others). Similarly, boys whose mothers reported restrictive reactions to their sons' displays of negative emotion tended to become physiologically distressed (overaroused) by exposure to others' negative emotions but denied feeling distressed. The fact that the aforementioned findings were primarily for boys is likely due to the cultural norms regarding emotion and suggest that males may be more likely than females to express their emotions internally rather than externally.

The effects of discouraging the expression of emotion vary with the specific emotion and the context. Although restrictiveness of children's expression of their own negative emotion has been associated with negative outcomes, in one study parents who were relatively restrictive of inappropriate and potentially hurtful emotional displays had same-sex, school-aged children who reported high levels of sympathy. Presumably parents who are restrictive teach their school-aged children when it is inappropriate to display emotions that are hurtful, although the restrictiveness involved in such teachings may cause anxiety in younger children.

Parental responses to children's negative emotions are linked to aspects of children's social functioning beyond their vicarious emotional responding. Children whose parents respond to their children's anger appropriately appear to be relatively well adjusted and happy. Parental encouragement of children's emotional expressiveness when they are distressed has been related to children's popularity and low use of socially inappropriate methods of coping with anger provocations. In contrast, parental efforts to minimize children's emotional responses (e.g., to tell them not to make such a big deal out of things that bother them) sometimes have been related to low levels of children's social competence. Moreover, there is initial evidence that mothers who are supportive and sensitive to children's attempts to cope with negative emotion tend to have children that are prosocial and sympathetic toward others, presumably because their children are able to deal with others' negative emotion without becoming overwhelmed.

There may be an optimal level of parental encouragement of the expression of emotion. One group of researchers found that a moderate level of parental encouragement of the expression of negative affect was linked to preschoolers' social competence. However, the decline in children's social competence at high levels of parental encouragement (in comparison to moderate levels) was small. Moreover, experiences involving negative emotion and conflict, when used by parents as a context for teaching about emotion, may facilitate the development of emotional and social competence.

Some parental reactions in stressful or emotional situations are problem focused (i.e., aimed at modifying the source of the problem) rather than designed to deal directly with children's emotion. A few studies suggest that parental modeling and encouragement of problem-focused coping may foster children's emotional and social competence.

Parental discussion of children's emotion has been linked to children's understanding of emotion and their social competence. For example, Judy Dunn and her colleagues reported that mother–child discussions about feelings and their causes and consequences were associated with later success on affective perspective-taking tasks (assessing the ability to understand others' emotional states). By 2 years of age most children talk with their mothers about feelings and mothers seem to use these conversations to guide the child's behavior or explain another's emotions. Moreover, frequency of mothers' discussions of emotions with their children predicts children's popularity with peers.

Some theorists have suggested that children's emotion regulation is associated with quality of the parent–child relationship. Specifically, attachment styles and relationships have been viewed as reflecting strategies for regulating emotion in interpersonal relationships. The securely attached infant whose parent is consistently and appropriately responsive to the infant's distress signals is believed to learn that it is acceptable to exhibit distress and to seek out the assistance of others for comfort when distressed. The infant with an avoidant attachment is believed to experience parental nonresponsiveness to his or her distress, with the consequence that the infant learns to inhibit emotional expressiveness as well as other-directed self-regulatory strategies (e.g., contact-seeking behavior). In fact, maternal responsiveness to the child's interactive behaviors has been associated with infants' increasing positive emotionality and socially competent behavior, both of which likely reflect, in part, regulatory capacities. Moreover, maternal support has been correlated with children using a variety of coping behaviors, as well as the use of relatively appropriate strategies (e.g., avoidant strategies in uncontrollable situations). Similarly, young adults who were classified as secure in their attachment style were viewed by peers as ego-resilient and low in anxiety; they also reported little distress and high levels of social support. Those classified as avoidant or dismissive (i.e., insecure) in their attachment style were rated by peers as relatively hostile. The overall pattern of results suggests that a positive, secure parent–child relationship is associated with optimal emotional and behavioral regulation whereas children whose parents are punishing or nonresponsive to their negative emotional states and condition have difficulty regulating their emotion.

As noted previously, it is likely that parents' emotion-related socialization practices are in part a reaction to their children's emotion-related tendencies. At this time, there is relatively little research on this topic. Nancy Eisenberg and Richard Fabes found that mothers tended to be relatively punitive and avoidant in response to children's negative emotions if they viewed their children as high in negative affectivity and low in their abilities to regulate their attention. In contrast, mothers tended to report more supportive and constructive socialization practices rather than punitive strategies if they viewed their children as able to regulate their attention. Moreover, they found that mothers tended to try to buffer their young children from experiencing too much negative emotion by using positive emotion when discussing negative events, particularly if they viewed their children as relatively vulnerable to such emotion. Thus, mothers' actions appeared to be influenced by their perceptions of their children's vulnerability to become dysregulated as a consequence of exposure to negative emotion. [See PARENTING.]

From the previous discussions it is clear that both intraindividual and environmental variables can affect the course of the development of emotion regulation. Given these sources of influence, we turn to the discussion of the relations of emotion regulation to social competence. The following review provides evidence that skills as well as deficits in the ability to regulate emotions influence the quality of social and psychological functioning.

VI. THE RELATIONS OF REGULATION AND EMOTIONALITY TO SOCIAL COMPETENCE

A. Normative Samples

Evidence that quality of children's social competence is related to the regulation of emotion, regulation of emotionally driven behavior, and the regulation of stressful context is accumulating. Relations between regulation and social functioning have been noted not only for diagnosed or at-risk children (see below), but also for groups of nondiagnosed children, for whom major problems with regulation would not be expected.

In general, even in normative samples of children, undercontrol or low behavioral regulation has been associated with a rapid personal tempo and restlessness; aggression and acting out behavior; inability to delay behavior and overly high reactivity to frustration; low levels of prosocial and cooperative behavior; susceptibility to negative emotionality and personal distress (a self-focused vicarious emotional reaction to others' distress); lack of obedience, compliance, and planfulness; and regression under stress.

Although behavioral regulation generally is related to positive social functioning, unusually high levels of behavioral inhibition seem to be associated with deficits in social functioning. Behaviorally inhibited children, in comparison to less-inhibited children, tend to be shy with unfamiliar peers and adults, fearful, cautious in situations involving mild risk, and socially withdrawn.

As noted previously, attentional control—often viewed as a mechanism for emotional regulation—has been linked to low levels of negative emotionality in infants, children, and adults. In studies of preschool and school-aged children, there is evidence that the ability to manage attention is linked with coping with stress, delay of gratification, social competence and popularity, management of anger, sympathy, and, when combined with behavioral regulation, with a proneness to empathy and guilt.

Individual differences in coping behavior have been studied primarily in regard to dealing with significant stressor (e.g., divorce), although research on coping among normal children in everyday situations is increasing in quantity. In general, instrumental problem solving (i.e., trying to resolve the problem situation) has been linked with positive outcomes, particularly if the stressful context is perceived as controllable. Although theorists frequently have argued that social support or instrumental assistance from others reduces stress, the very limited evidence pertaining to a link between children's seeking of support and social (rather than psychological) functioning is somewhat equivocal.

There is some evidence that emotional intensity and regulation interact in regard to the prediction of social functioning. In one study, low levels of school children's regulation were related to problem behavior at all levels of negative emotion; however, the relation was strongest for children high in negative emotionality. Thus, regulation was most important for predicting low levels of problem behavior for children prone to negative emotion. Similarly, young children

low in intensity of negative emotion and high in regulation (i.e., attentional control and constructive coping) are higher in sociometric status and teacher-rated social skills than are other children, and regulation has been found to be a stronger predictor of socially appropriate and prosocial behavior for children prone to negative emotion than for children who are lower in negative emotionality. Further, recent data suggest that unregulated children are low in sympathy regardless of their level of general emotional intensity whereas, for moderately and highly regulated children, sympathy increases with increasing level of general emotional intensity (i.e., the general tendency to feel emotions strongly, without reference specifically to valence of the emotion). Thus, children who are likely to be emotionally intense tend to be sympathetic if they are at least moderately well regulated whereas children low in regulation are unlikely to be sympathetic toward others.

In summary, in studies of typical populations of children, regulation has been associated with a variety of aspects of socially competent functioning. These relations sometimes vary with children's dispositional negative emotionality. Moreover, young children who are particularly high in behavioral regulation are withdrawn, fearful, and behaviorally constrained—behavior that later is associated with internalizing disorders. The topic of emotion and emotion-relevant regulation in psychological disorders is now considered in more detail.

VII. EMOTION REGULATION AND PSYCHOPATHOLOGY IN CHILDREN

There is a growing body of evidence for the links between emotionality and regulation and two primary categories of psychopathology in children: internalizing and externalizing disorders. Internalizing disorders are those that include problems that are inner-directed such as anxiety and extreme shyness. They also include depressed behaviors and tendencies to behave in a withdrawn fashion. In contrast, externalizing problems include outwardly expressed behaviors such as aggression, hyperactivity, impulsivity, and conduct problems. Internalizing and externalizing symptoms frequently co-occur and are often substantially correlated. Indeed, there is a subset of children characterized by aspects of both disorders such as depression, aggression, and social withdrawal. [*See* Ag-gression; Conduct Disorders; Depression; Impulse Control.]

The defining characteristics of internalizing and externalizing disorders are suggestive of over- or under-regulation of behavior, respectively, and heightened experience and expression of emotionality. For instance, characteristics of externalizing disorders include aggression and impulsivity, both of which suggest a diminished ability to control emotion-related impulses, an inability to inhibit socially prohibited behavior, and perhaps a tendency to express anger/frustration and a lack of fear (fear serves to inhibit behavior in some situations). In contrast, internalizing disorders appear to involve negative emotionality (i.e., anxiety and sadness or despair), underregulation of the experience of negative emotion, and overregulation of behavior (i.e., extreme levels of behavioral inhibition).

A. Internalizing Disorders

Overall, there is little research on the roles of dispositional emotionality and regulation in internalizing problems. However, in a few studies that span early childhood to young adulthood, researchers have demonstrated links of early attentional problems and/or overcontrolled behavior with depression and anxiety. For instance, some investigators found that elementary school children with internalizing disorders were intense, prone to negative moods and anxiety, and were unable to focus attention. In another study, negative moods (e.g., sadness, anger, shame, shyness, guilt, and self-directed hostility) were reported by depressed youths aged 10 to 17 years. These youths also reported less joy than nondepressed youths who were diagnosed with other nonpsychotic conditions. Investigators also have found that depressed mood in 18-year-old women (but not men) tended to be related to a measure of overcontrolled behavior in childhood, including anxiety and rigid, self-focused thinking. In contrast, undercontrolled, aggressive tendencies in childhood have been found to be related to depression in young men. Among young adults, depression also has been linked to low attentional control (distractibility).

In other studies, extreme behavioral inhibition appears to be a risk factor associated with the onset of anxiety in childhood. Jerome Kagan and his colleagues demonstrated that the rates of childhood onset anxiety disorders were significantly higher in children with behavioral inhibition than those without. In addition, they found that children of parents with agoraphobia and/or panic disorder had higher rates of behavioral inhibition than children of adults who had other psychological conditions unrelated to agoraphobia.

Relations between behavioral inhibition and the onset of anxiety were also demonstrated in a longitudinal study of the temperamental origins of adolescent behavior problems. In this study of more than 800 children, Avshalom Caspi and his colleagues found that for girls, high rates of sluggishness, a composite of measures of behavioral inhibition and low positive emotion, were related to the development of anxiety over the course of 12 years (from ages 3 to 15) and attentional problems in adolescence. For boys, internalizing problems were weakly predicted by low ratings on approach-type measures (including adaptability to new situations, self-confidence, self-reliance, and friendliness) and higher ratings on lack of control (e.g., emotional lability, negativity, restlessness, and impulsivity in childhood).

In summary, there is support for the link of emotionality and regulation with the development of later disorders such as anxiety and depression. Internalizing disorders in children tend to be associated with anxiety, negativity or low positive emotion, low emotion regulation, and sometimes highly inhibited behavior (for girls) and impulsivity (for boys). [*See* Anxiety.]

B. Externalizing Disorders

Studies of the relations of emotionality and regulation with externalizing disorders are relatively sparse. Moreover, different types of problem behaviors (e.g., aggression, impulsivity) that might be differentially related to emotionality and regulation have not been examined separately; nor has the status of children with externalizing problems (e.g., if they were diagnosed and what they were diagnosed with) been consistently controlled within or across studies. Nevertheless, problem behaviors have been linked to characteristics such as high intensity or reactivity, negative emotionality, and low adaptability.

For instance, in an 8-year longitudinal study, three groups of children who were either hyperactive but not aggressive, aggressive but not hyperactive, or hyperactive and aggressive were rated by parents, teachers, and nurses as being more negative, emotionally intense, and overreactive than children without externalizing problems. Behaviorally, the three groups of children showed attentional deficits and also were rated as lacking in persistence, adaptability, and flexibility. Further, the results of this study demonstrated that the onset of problems with aggression was associated with high ratings of unregulated behavior and temperamental difficultness in early childhood.

Similar results also were found in another longitudinal study of children from infancy to 13 years. Measures of individual differences in approach and response to novelty were derived from examiners' ratings of behavior of children at ages 3, 5, 7, and 9. The results showed that a factor that included measures of emotional lability, restlessness, distractibility, and negativity predicted parents' and teachers' reports of inattention, hyperactivity, and antisocial behavior at ages 9, 11, and 13. Other investigators have found that parental reports of preschoolers' aggression-noncompliance and hyperactive-distractable behavior have been related to teachers' reports and independent raters of preschoolers' impulsivity and hostility; moreover, parental reports of undercontrolled and impulsive behavior at age 5 predict later antisocial outcomes.

Finally, type of expression of emotion (which reflects the ability to regulate emotionally driven behavior) in positive social situations has been found to be associated with diagnostic status. In one study, children aged 7 to 14 years were complimented by same-sex, same-age confederate peers in another room (the peer was observed through a monitor). Although the children in the diagnosed group reported positive reactions to the compliments of the confederate, they displayed more facial expressions of hostility and surprise, suggesting an inability to regulate facial emotional expressions, as well as inappropriate emotional reactions. The two groups did not differ on their appraisals of emotions; however, the diagnosed children demonstrated less sophistication in their understanding of their own emotions.

As is evident from the previous review, there is a growing literature on the link between children's externalizing problems and low regulation or high emotionality. In general, findings have held even when reporters or observers of problem behaviors and emotion regulation differed (such as in studies with parents', teachers', and nurses' reports, as well as independent raters of child behavior). In summary, the findings support the view that individual differences in regulation and emotionality predict externalizing problems in later childhood and early and late adolescence.

VIII. SUMMARY

We have outlined some of the important variables involved in the development of emotion regulation. These include age, individual differences in emotionality and regulation, and agents of socialization (i.e., parents or primary caregivers). Regarding age, rudimentary abilities relevant to the regulation of emotion are present at birth or shortly thereafter. The development of language and cognitive capacities broadens the child's ability to regulate emotions, emotionally driven behavior, as well as the emotion-eliciting context. Individual differences in emotionality and regulation add a degree of complexity to the development of emotion regulation; these differences appear to influence the course of development by providing an intraindividual checkpoint for the likelihood of becoming over- or underaroused in a given situation. Individual differences in emotionality and regulation also influence caregivers, which, in turn, result in caregiver behaviors that teach children about emotion and its regulation. An important question is the degree to which a mismatch, in terms of child temperamental tendencies (e.g., emotionality and reactivity) and caregivers' coping skills is associated with emotional and behavioral regulation and disregulation. Longitudinal data on the interaction of individual differences in emotionality and regulation, as well as the moderating effects of socialization, should yield exciting new insights into the development of children's ability to regulate emotions.

ACKNOWLEDGMENTS

This research was supported by a grant from the National Science Foundation (DBS-9208375), a Research Scientist Award from the National Institute of Mental Health (K05 MH801321-01) to Nancy Eisenberg, and a postdoctoral fellowship in prevention research from the National Institute of Mental Health (MH18387-07), which supported Sandra Losoya.

BIBLIOGRAPHY

Caspi, A. (in press). Personality development. In W. Damon (Series Ed.) & N. Eisenberg (Vol. Ed.), *Handbook of child psychology:*

Vol. 3. Social, emotional, and personality development. New York: Wiley.

Eisenberg, N., & Fabes, R. A. (1992). Emotion, regulation, and the development of social competence. In M. S. Clark (Ed.), *Review of personality and social psychology: Vol. 14. Emotion and social behavior* (pp. 119–150). Newbury Park, CA: Sage.

Eisenberg, N., Fabes, R. A., Carlo, G., & Karbon, M. (1992). Emotional responsivity to others: Behavioral correlates and socialization antecedents. In N. Eisenberg & R. A. Fabes (Eds.), *New Directions in Child Development, 55,* 57–73.

Fox, N. A. (Ed.) (1994). The development of emotion regulation: Biological and behavioral considerations. *Monographs of the Society for Research in Child Development, 59,* No. 2–3 (Serial No. 240).

Garber, J., & Dodge, K. A. (Eds.). (1991). *The development of emotion regulation and dysregulation.* New York: Cambridge University Press.

Kopp, C. B. (1989). Regulation of distress and negative emotions: A developmental view. *Developmental Psychology, 25,* 343–354.

Lazarus, R. S., & Folkman, S. (1984). *Stress, appraisal, and coping.* New York: Springer.

Rothbart, M. K. (1989). Temperament and development. In G. A. Kohnstamm, J. F. Bates, & M. K. Rothbart (Eds.) *Temperament in childhood* (pp. 187–247). New York: John Wiley & Sons.

Rothbart, M. K., & Bates, J. E. (in press). In W. Damon (Series Ed.) & N. Eisenberg (Vol. Ed.), *Handbook of child psychology: Vol. 3. Social, emotional, and personality development.* New York: Wiley.

Thompson, R. (1994). Emotion regulation: A theme in search of definition. In N. A. Fox (Ed.), *The development of emotion regulation: Biological and behavioral considerations* (pp. 25–52). *Monographs of the Society for Research in Child Development, 59* (2–3, Serial No. 240). Chicago: Chicago University Press.

Emotion and Aging

Monisha Pasupathi and Laura L. Carstensen
Stanford University

Susan Turk-Charles
University of Southern California

Jeanne Tsai
University of California, Berkeley

Cormorbidity The co-occurrence of two separate diseases or disorders, in this case, of depression and medical illnesses.

Convenience Samples The use of volunteers or easily recruited populations (e.g., introductory psychology students) rather than representative or random samples.

Cross-Sectional Design Comparisons among multiple age cohorts at the same time; confounds age differences with generational differences.

Rumination Repetitive and emotion-focused thinking pattern in response to sadness, which exacerbates the intensity of depression.

This article reviews the literature on emotional experience and **EMOTION REGULATION IN LATER LIFE.** We focus on three broad areas in which age has been examined: (1) specific emotion processes (viz., physiology, expressive behavior, and subjective experience), (2) the regulation of emotional experience, and (3) the relationship between emotional experience and health.

I. INTRODUCTION

The research literature on adulthood and aging that has accumulated over the past 50 years documents widespread deleterious changes associated with the aging process, ranging from greater vulnerability to disease and disability to a generalized slowing in cognitive processing. Indeed, "slowing" is widely viewed as the hallmark of aging in the second half of life.

The extent of the losses associated with aging is compelling. Researchers in the social sciences, however, are beginning to realize that an emphasis on loss in old age may have obscured a potential for gains; clearly, a complete picture of aging must encompass both. Recent research suggests positive change in some domains, even into very old age. Emotional functioning appears to be one such domain. Not only does emotional functioning appear to be largely spared from declines in late life, there is growing evidence that it may improve.

In the following sections we review theoretical perspectives and empirical evidence on emotion and aging, focusing on emotional responding, emotion regulation strategies, and the interaction between emotional functioning and physical and mental health. We begin, however, with a definition of emotion.

What is emotion? This deceptively simple question is the subject of considerable intellectual debate in the fields of psychology, anthropology, sociology, and philosophy. In psychology, emotions are generally viewed as short-lived responses to environmental events, comprised of concomitant changes in physiology, subjective experience, and expressive behavior.

Research on emotion suggests that there are a handful of basic emotions, such as anger, disgust, and happiness, which are characterized by specific physiological, subjective, and behavioral profiles. Anger, for example, is typically evoked by environmental events that trigger a subjective sense of being thwarted, demeaned, and offended, and involves an increase in heart rate and a furrowing of the eyebrows. Disgust, on the other hand, typically occurs in response to events that trigger a subjective sense of being too close to a contaminated object, and involves a slowing of heart rate and wrinkling of the nose. These core emotions are believed to be relatively consistent across cultures, although there may be considerable cultural variation in the appropriateness of displaying emotions, or even in the specific events that elicit particular emotions.

Core emotions are distinguished from other aspects of emotional functioning, such as subjective well-being or life satisfaction, as well as other aspects of emotional dysfunction, such as clinical depression, anxiety, and other affective disorders, by their time course (relatively brief) and by specificity in component processes (e.g., physiological responding, facial expression, subjective experience). Because emotional functioning more broadly defined is related to the everyday experience of emotions, we also address life satisfaction and affective disorders.

Three main questions emerge from the literature on emotion and aging. First, does emotional experience change with age, and if so, in what ways? Second, does the ability to effectively regulate emotion change with age? And, finally, because age-related changes in emotional functioning occur along with other age-related changes, particularly declines in physical health, what is the relationship between health and emotion over the life span?

II. DOES EMOTIONAL RESPONDING CHANGE OVER THE LIFE SPAN?

There are clear developmental changes in emotional functioning. The literature, however, has focused primarily on changes in early life. Emotional development in childhood is conceptualized as a process of increasing differentiation, complexity, and competence. Nathan Fox and Richard Davidson at the University of Wisconsin, Madison, propose that during infancy, infants appraise stimuli as "appetitive" or "aversive," and respond to those stimuli by simply approaching or withdrawing. As the children mature, experiencing more of the world, they acquire more differentiated emotional states such as anger, sadness, fear, and contentment. By the age of 4 or 5, children have acquired even more complex, socially relevant emotions such as shame and guilt. Similarly, in facial expressive behavior, infants acquire the ability to make increasingly complex emotional facial expressions with increasing age. Infants also demonstrate increasing sophistication in their understanding of environmental stimuli. At birth, for example, hungry infants cry until the moment a breast or bottle is placed in their mouths. Eventually, they are calmed by the appearance of the mother or bottle, having come to understand that mother and/or bottle indicate the imminent satisfaction of their needs.

Emotion regulation also changes with age. Parents pay considerable attention to their children's emotions, teaching them to express emotions in culturally appropriate ways (e.g., in European-American culture, children are taught to calm themselves, and to talk about their internal emotional states). Throughout the early years, children come to regulate their emotions more effectively, suppressing facial expressions and disguising displays of internal states. Emotional control is considered a mark of maturity. By adulthood, individuals who fail to modulate their emotions well are viewed, at best, as "immature," and at worst, as "psychopathological."

Thus, the early part of life is characterized by the acquisition of greater emotional specificity and differentiation and proficiency in emotion regulation. The bulk of basic research on emotional functioning is concentrated on young adult college populations, leaving great gaps in our knowledge about the development of emotional functioning from early childhood until young adulthood, and beyond early adulthood. Researchers have paid some attention, however, to emotions in later life.

Until a decade or so ago, the view of emotional functioning toward the end of the life span according to popular lore and social science theory has been quite negative. Older adults have been viewed as emotionally rigid and disengaged from life. Early in the century, Jung wrote that older people turn away from the social world, engaging increasingly in introspection. In the 1960s and 1970s, proponents of disengagement theory argued that older adults become emotionally quiescent, withdrawing from other people in a symbolic preparation for death. The notion that emotional responding declines in later life is consistent with biomedical models of aging, where decrement and decline reign, as well as psychoanalytic models of aging, which focus on the defense mechanisms employed to cope with the inevitability of death.

An understanding of emotion in old age is only beginning to be informed by empirical evidence, thus the picture we paint in this chapter may change. However, at present, there is little evidence that emotional quiescence is typical of old age. Although negative emotions appear to grow more infrequent, positive emotions do not. Moreover, when negative emotions do occur, older people's subjective experience is indistinguishable from younger peoples' experience, a picture more consistent with improved emotion regulation than with a general emotional dampening. [*See* AGING AND MENTAL HEALTH.]

Below, we consider findings from some of the research questions that have been put to empirical test. We first review some common methods used to examine emotional experience in the laboratory, and then discuss what these methods reveal about aging and emotion.

A. Emotional Responding in the Laboratory

Given that organic deficits are the presumed root of cognitive decline in old age, such deficits could also influence emotional functioning. For example, it is conceivable that older people experience fewer negative emotions because general deterioration of the central and autonomic nervous systems lessens the physical impact of such emotions. In order to investigate these issues, researchers have examined the physiological aspects of emotional responses. Specifically, the magnitude and the specificity of autonomic nervous system activity associated with emotions has been studied.

Much of the research examining the psychophysiology of emotion in later life has been conducted by Robert Levenson, at the University of California at Berkeley, and his colleagues. In the laboratory, research participants engage in experimental tasks designed to elicit specific emotions. These tasks include viewing emotional films, making emotional facial expressions, or vividly remembering emotional events in the past. As subjects engage in these tasks, their physiological activity (i.e., autonomic nervous system response) is continuously monitored and their facial expressions videotaped. Either during or after they complete the task, participants report how intensely they experienced a number of different emotions (e.g., anger, sadness, happiness) during the tasks. These tasks produce measurable emotional responses in younger and older participants, males and females, and European Americans and Chinese Americans.

Levenson and colleagues have identified emotion-specific patterns of autonomic nervous system responding. For example, in response to making emotional facial configurations and imagining past emotional events, changes in heart rate are distinguished for the emotions of anger, fear, sadness, and disgust. If emotional functioning decays in later life, one result might be that these emotion-specific patterns are less differentiated in older people. This is not the case; older people exhibit the same emotion-specific patterns as younger people. The magnitude of autonomic nervous system response, however, is somewhat lower in older people. It is unclear whether this reduction in autonomic arousal is specific to emotional functioning, or is a reflection of overall physiological changes that accompany age. In short, research has shown that emotions can be elicited in older people in the same way they are elicited in younger people. Physiologically, the pattern of emotional responding is similar in older and younger adults, although the magnitude of response is lower for older adults. Moreover, the age similarities and differences are consistent in European-American and Chinese-American groups.

Facial expressiveness might also show age changes.

Paul Ekman of the University of California at San Francisco and his colleagues, have demonstrated that predictable facial muscle movements are associated with specific emotions. For example, anger is characterized by lowered brows and a tight mouth; fear by raised brows and widened eyes. Paul Ekman and Wallace Friesen developed a highly sophisticated system called the Facial Action Coding System to help identify muscle-by-muscle movements in the face as people experience a variety of emotions. Work by Levenson, Carstensen, Ekman, and Friesen revealed no differences between facial expressiveness in older and younger people. That is, older and younger people use similar facial movements to express the emotions they are feeling. In other laboratory studies of facial expressivity, by Carol Malatesta-Magai at Long Island University and her colleagues, older adults appear more emotionally expressive than younger adults. Research subjects were videotaped while they were asked to recall times when they experienced particular emotions. In this case, older research subjects expressed more emotion via the face during the experimental task. Research subjects were also asked about their expressiveness in everyday life. Older adults reported that they were more expressive than younger adults.

Despite being equally or more facially expressive than younger adults, older adults' facial expressions may be more difficult for others to decode, particularly others of different ages (e.g., younger adults). Malatesta-Magai and her colleagues provided evidence that there may be static changes (e.g., wrinkling) in the faces of older people that reflect individual personality traits. These changes may obscure the expression of more transient emotion states. Older adults completed emotional trait measures and were then asked to pose various emotional expressions. Those posed faces were photographed and then shown to naive judges, who were asked to identify which emotion the person was expressing. The traits that characterized a person (e.g., depression), predicted which emotions were easy for judges to identify (e.g., sadness) and which were more difficult (e.g., joy).

Finally, older adults may be less skilled at decoding others' emotional faces. Malatesta-Magai and colleagues showed videotapes of subjects experiencing different emotions to people of various ages, and asked them to judge which of 10 emotions the person on the tape was feeling. Older adults showed slightly lower accuracy at this task than younger adults. Other researchers have used photographs of people posing facial expressions, and have documented similar deficits. However, such deficits might have multiple causes that have little to do with emotional functioning. For example, age-related declines in facial recognition ability, visual ability, or even a differential need for practice at the task might all contribute to elderly adults' lowered performance. When researchers have equated young and old adults for the ability to recognize faces, age-related deficits in recognizing emotional facial expressions disappear, suggesting that this deficit is related to nonemotional aspects of cognitive aging. Moreover, there is no clear relationship between the ability to identify emotional facial expressions in the laboratory and everyday emotional functioning.

Perhaps most important are age differences in the subjective experience of emotion during laboratory inductions. Here the findings are clear. Older and younger people do not differ from each other in the intensity of emotions induced in the laboratory, regardless of how the emotion was induced. Thus, when the emotional stimuli are tightly controlled, older and younger people respond to the same degree.

In summary, experimental studies of emotional responding suggest far more similarities than differences between younger and older adults. As compared to younger adults, older adults respond to emotional stimuli similarly, and report a comparable intensity of emotional experience. They show similar patterns of autonomic arousal and are at least as emotionally expressive as younger adults (perhaps more so). The magnitude of physiological arousal is somewhat reduced, however. This difference is difficult to interpret because it is unclear whether the reductions are specific to the emotion domain or instead are due to more general changes in physiological functioning in later life. At any rate, this difference does not influence reports of subjective experience.

B. Emotions in Everyday Life

In contrast to examining emotions "on-line" while they are experienced in the laboratory, other studies have used surveys to assess the ways that older and younger people judge their experience of emotions in everyday life. Here again, researchers have asked questions about the kinds of emotions people experience, as well as the intensity with which they are experienced. Responses to such surveys are important in that they tap the ways that people view their own emotional functioning. These methods are limited, however, by demand characteristics and simple miscalculations or biases that can distort people's self-assessments.

Nevertheless, results from such research suggest that in everyday life, older and younger adults experience specific emotions at different frequencies. Compared to younger adults, older adults report that they experience sadness and anger less often, and contentment more often. Older and younger adults do not differ in the intensity with which they report feeling particular emotions.

Powell Lawton and his colleagues at the Philadelphia Geriatric Center suggest that the structural dimensions underlying emotional experience may also be different for older and younger adults. Most notably, younger adults' conceptions of positive emotional experience include more arousing emotions, like excitement, whereas older adults' conceptions of positive emotional experience include more subdued emotions like contentment.

Whereas laboratory investigations of emotionality show substantial stability in emotional experience across the life span, survey studies show that older adults may experience more positive emotions and fewer negative emotions, suggesting that emotional functioning may be improved in later life. Overall, the most robust changes in emotional functioning seem to involve decreased physiological arousal and surgency. Table I summarizes the findings on basic aspects of emotional experience in older versus younger adults.

Laboratory and survey investigations of emotion

Table I

Aspect of emotional functioning	Findings
Subjective responsiveness to laboratory stimuli	Age stability
Physiology	
Pattern	Age stability
Magnitude	Age declines
Facial expression	
Amount of expression	Age stability/ increase
Pattern of expression	Age stability
Decoding others' expressions	Age declines
Subjective experience	
Intensity	Age stability
Type of emotions experienced	More positive Fewer negative

reveal much about emotional experience, but such investigations also leave much ground uncovered. Emotion does not occur in a social vacuum, independent of other mental processes. Rather, it influences and is influenced by cognitive and social processes.

C. Emotion, Cognition, and Social Behavior

Although emotions serve very adaptive purposes, they can also disrupt logical reasoning, memory, and other cognitive processes. Gisela Labouvie-Vief, of Wayne State University, and her colleagues have argued that a developmental task of childhood and early adulthood is to learn to separate "emotional" from "objective" aspects of experience, and to approach problems encountered in everyday life with "reason" rather than emotion. In order to learn the language and social rules of a culture, children must learn to distinguish between abstract, collectively shared meanings and idiosyncratic private meanings. The task of later adulthood is to reintegrate emotional or subjective aspects of experience with objective aspects, leading to what is called synthetic, or "dialectical" reasoning. Such reasoning might be portrayed as the dialogue between the self and the external world. For example, a person might understand that lying is immoral but simultaneously appreciate the necessity to lie on certain occasions.

One prediction that this theoretical model makes is that younger adults reason more poorly about emotion-laden topics because it is difficult to separate emotional from objective information for such topics. For example, younger adults might have difficulty reasoning about situations that contrast objective regulations with their own subjective desires. The emotionality of the topic should not interfere with the reasoning of older adults, as they have learned to distinguish and make use of private, subjective, or emotional information as well as objective information. This prediction has been supported with adolescents, young adults and middle-aged adults. Middle-aged adults reason equally well about emotional and nonemotional topics, while adolescents and younger adults perform more poorly when reasoning about emotional topics. [*See* EMOTION AND COGNITION.]

Labouvie-Vief and her colleagues also suggest that older adults think differently about emotion than do younger adults. When they asked adults of various ages to describe emotional experiences, they found that older adults had more cognitively complex representations of emotion than did younger adults. In particular, older adults describing emotional experiences used language that was oriented toward inner feelings, and that suggested more variability of emotional experience over time and across situations. Older adults also report a more reciprocal understanding of emotional encounters, in which the people involved and the situation are seen as exerting influence on one another.

Laura Carstensen and her colleagues at Stanford University argue that emotion is more salient for older as compared to younger adults. They propose that this difference should be reflected in memory for emotionally relevant information, with older adults showing better memory for emotional versus nonemotional information. They tested the prediction by having older and younger adults read prose passages excerpted from novels. Later, when asked to recall the passages, older adults remembered proportionally more emotional information than did younger adults.

So far we have maintained a focus on emotional experiences or cognition–emotion relationships that are assessed in a solitary context. Yet emotion is clearly a social phenomenon. The experience of emotions often has social antecedents and social consequences. Even our emotional expressions are fundamentally social, fulfilling communicative functions. Researchers have shown that emotional expressions occur with far greater frequency in social settings, functioning to communicate emotions to others. Consequently, we might see age-related changes in emotion by looking at age-related shifts in social behavior and social functioning.

According to Carstensen's socioemotional selectivity theory, emotion becomes more important whenever people approach social endings. Because old age is inextricably confounded with the ultimate ending, namely death, older people are more motivated by emotional aspects of experience, including increased efforts to regulate and optimize their emotional experience. Experiments rooted in this theory have shown that older adults differ from younger adults in the type of social partners they choose, and in the ways that they mentally represent social partners. Older adults, relative to younger adults, are more likely to choose emotionally meaningful social contacts, like family members or long-term friends. Moreover, older adults' representations of social partners tend to em-

phasize the emotional implications of spending time with those partners, rather than the potential to gain new information, or the likelihood of future contact. Finally, emotionally close social partners represent increasingly larger proportions of people's social networks as they age. Older adults' greater investment in emotionally important relationships can be viewed as one way of controlling their social environments to achieve positive emotional goals, a point to which we return below.

In a collaborative effort, Robert Levenson, Laura Carstensen, and John Gottman studied marital conflict in middle-aged and older couples in order to investigate age differences in the ways that couples negotiate emotionally negative social situations. Married couples came into the laboratory and were asked to engage in conversations about the events of the day, an important, mutually selected marital conflict, and a topic both spouses enjoy talking about. The conflict-related conversations were analyzed for the kinds of emotions experienced and expressed by both spouses. Older adults were able to express more affection and less hostility during a conversation about marital conflict, regardless of whether they were happily or unhappily married. This work, like the work on social networks, also suggests that older adults are relatively adept at managing their social environment to regulate their own emotional outcomes, perhaps more so than younger and middle-aged adults.

Emotion, then, is more cognitively salient to older adults, and plays a much larger role in perceptions of and choices about social partners. Moreover, there is evidence that changes in the relationship between cognition and emotion (e.g., dialectical reasoning) and in the relationship between social functioning and emotion (e.g., selective investment in emotionally close partners) are adaptive.

III. DOES EMOTION REGULATION CHANGE WITH AGE?

The positive nature of everyday emotional experience in later life contrasts sharply with popular views of old age as a time of loss and grief. Gerontologists have coined the phrase "the paradox of aging" to capture the nearly ironic profile of findings on social and emotional aging. Old age is fraught with physical illness and social losses (e.g., due to deaths, retirement, illness, etc.). Yet, despite the greater likelihood of experiencing stressful events in old age, coupled with heightened constraints on everyday activities due to physical and financial changes that typically accompany old age, older adults' life satisfaction is indistinguishable from that of younger adults. Thus, life circumstances are objectively poorer in old age for most people, but emotionally, older people are faring as well as younger people.

Improvement in emotion regulation may account for this paradox. Better able to regulate emotion, older adults may encounter the negative events common to old age with greater resilience than younger adults confronted with similar life circumstances.

As mentioned above, socioemotional selectivity theory contends that older adults are more motivated by emotional aspects of experience. Evidence for the theory suggests that not only is emotion regulation more important for older adults, older adults make effective use of their social environments to regulate emotions. They do so by choosing familiar and intimate social partners, with whom emotional experience is predictable, usually positive and meaningful. They also manage "risky" interactions, like conversations about marital conflict, with greater skill. Clearly, older adults demonstrate greater investment and skill in managing the emotional side of their social lives.

A good deal of evidence suggests that as people grow older, they become more skilled at regulating their emotions through social means, by choosing to engage in social interactions that will yield predictable positive emotional experience. Other aspects of emotion regulation may also improve with age, including strategies that are aimed at managing an emotion while it is being experienced. For example, people may become sad and try to feel better. While there are few studies on age differences in managing emotions, older adults report that they are better able to manage their emotions than younger adults, and that they are less likely to engage in rumination, a process known to increase the duration and severity of sadness.

Another aspect of emotion regulation involves coping with the constraints of later life, and with the negative events that are more likely to occur in later life. We will first look at some specific ways that older adults might cope with age-related constraints on their resources, whether physical or financial, and then explore the ways that older adults might cope more effectively with negative life events.

Many theorists, including Richard Lazarus at the University of California at Berkeley and his colleagues, suggest that emotions occur in response to the attainment or loss of people's chosen goals, with positive emotions associated with reaching or maintaining a selected goal. In later life, because age-related constraints (e.g., physical, financial) may make some goals difficult to attain or to maintain, it is important to be flexible in one's commitment to a given goal. Jochen Brandtstädter and his colleagues at the University of Trier and Jutta Heckhausen, at the Max Planck Institute for Human Development, and her colleagues have explored the ways that adults of different ages manage their goals. They find that older adults tend to be more flexible about their chosen goals, giving up goals that are clearly unattainable, and selecting goals that will be attainable given current resources. Flexibility increases the likelihood that people will succeed at the goals they do select, thus experiencing fewer negative emotions, and more positive emotions.

A second strategy for maintaining positive affect in the face of age-related constraints involves comparing one's own circumstances with those of others. Shelley Taylor, at the University of California at Los Angeles, and her colleagues argue that comparing oneself to others who are worse off allows people to feel better about their own life. Ironically, negative stereotypes about aging may actually allow older people to evaluate their own situations favorably despite troubles they encounter. If most older people are seen as lonely, depressed, and ill, older people who experience none of these things can feel fortunate. Most older people, when asked, report that they are doing better than the average person their age. This does not mean negative stereotypes about aging are inherently good; rather, older adults may make adaptive use of ageist beliefs.

However, it is not simply that old age is associated with declines in physical capacity or reduced financial circumstances. Old age is also associated with negative life events, including the deaths of close friends and loved ones. Research on coping with such events suggests that older adults may be more skilled at this aspect of emotion regulation as well.

Susan Folkman, at the University of California at San Francisco, along with Lazarus and their colleagues have explored responses to negative life events and have classified coping behaviors as either instrumental or emotional. Instrumental coping activities are those that directly influence a person's circumstances—for example, seeking medical care, or avoiding dangerous behaviors, or eating healthier foods. Although such strategies do not directly influence emotion, engaging in active instrumental behaviors may restore an individual's sense of control and well-being in spite of the negative life event. Most research suggests there are no age differences in the use of these strategies. Lazarus and Folkman have outlined a second broad class of coping strategies that are aimed at emotion regulation in the face of negative events. They find that older adults use more emotion-focused coping strategies than do younger adults. In particular, older adults use more distancing responses (going on as if nothing had changed), more acceptance of their own responsibility for events, and more positive reframing of the negative event. As Folkman and Lazarus argue, these strategies are effective ones. [See COPING WITH STRESS.]

Thus, although older adults encounter more age-related constraints and negative life events, there is good evidence that older adults have strategies for coping with them. Further, they may be more skilled at emotion regulation in general. This gain in emotion regulation partly demystifies the paradox outlined at the beginning of this section. However, there are other possible resolutions. All of the above explanations for the paradox retain the tacit assumption that emotional well-being is threatened in old age and that elderly adults do something to compensate for the threats, resulting in stability of well-being across the life span. The assumption of threat is based upon the notion that negative life events are associated with decreases in well-being and the objective fact that such events are more likely in old age (e.g., death of a spouse, serious physical illness). There are two other possibilities: one is that such events are better anticipated in old age, and thus older adults are actually less distressed by those events than younger adults in comparable circumstances. A second possibility is that negative life events themselves are not as clearly associated with negative emotions and subjective distress as is typically assumed.

Does the "predictability" of a negative life event matter in terms of its impact on emotional responses? Research on control and depressive mood suggests that knowing when a negative event will occur lessens the negative impact associated with it, at least for animals who are being shocked either randomly (unpre-

dictably) or on a regular schedule (predictably). There is some evidence that human beings operate similarly. The loss of a spouse produces an immediate drop in well-being for people of all ages. Up to 2 months after the loss of a spouse, both men and women report higher levels of depression and psychological distress compared to same-aged adults who have not lost their spouse. These differences diminish 1 to 2 years after the death of the spouse. However, compared to older adults, middle-aged adults report higher levels of anxiety and hopelessness/helplessness 2 and 6 months after the death of their spouses. In later life, spousal bereavement is both more likely and may be more predictable. Thus the "expectedness" of a death may influence the relationship between bereavement and distress. [See ANXIETY; DEPRESSION.]

Caregiving for an infirm relative is a common event in middle and old age. Elizabeth Clipp and Linda George at Duke University report that younger caregivers also fare more poorly than older caregivers, especially when emotional outcomes are measured. Regardless of whether the family member who requires care is suffering from cancer or from dementia, younger caregivers are more likely to be depressed than older adults. Again, this difference may have to do with the differential impact of expected caregiving versus unexpected caregiving on emotional distress.

A second possibility is that negative life events do not, in and of themselves, influence emotional well-being. Despite the intuitive appeal of the idea that life events are related to well-being, few empirical findings support this hypothesis. With the exception of spousal bereavement and caregiving, most life events examined in the literature do not have a strong relationship to emotional well-being in the long-term. Thus, for those older adults who are not mourning the recent loss of a spouse or caregiving for an ill relative, there may be little threat to their well-being. This is not to deny, of course, that some individuals are quite distressed by specific events, like retirement. The findings simply suggest events like retirement are not experienced as negative and stressful for *most* individuals. Given the individualized nature of many life events, then, it is problematic to suggest that old age is fraught with negative life events that necessarily have a strong impact on well-being or everyday emotional experience.

The low prevalence of affective disorders in later life also suggests the possibility of gains in emotion regulation. Fewer older adults are clinically depressed or anxious, and fewer older adults experience clinical depression for the first time in old age, compared to younger adults. Much of the available evidence suggests that older adults are actually less vulnerable to these clinically significant failures in affect regulation. Below, we briefly review the cases of depression and anxiety.

A. Affective Disorders

Both depression and anxiety (and indeed, all psychiatric disorders except the dementias) have lower incidence and prevalence rates in elderly populations. In other words, fewer elderly than young are depressed or anxious at any given time, and far fewer elderly adults become depressed or anxious for the first time in their later life. In fact, some evidence suggests that older adults who have a history of clinical depression are at lower risk for relapse in old age than in young and middle adulthood.

Despite lower rates of affective disorders, older adults do report more depressive symptoms than middle-aged adults. These symptoms are likely to correspond to a decrease in energy and a lack of interest in activities, but do not meet the diagnostic criteria for clinical depression. In other words, older adults do experience negative feelings, but they do not become depressed.[1] This is true despite age-related increases in risk factors for depression and anxiety, particularly disease and disability. In fact, physical illness is strongly associated with negative affect, particularly sadness, anxiety, and depression. In the next section, we explore the relationship of health to emotion in later life.

IV. HOW DOES HEALTH INFLUENCE EMOTION?

Older adults are clearly at greater risk for ill health than younger adults. As we noted above, many physical conditions common in old age can create symptoms that mimic affective disorders. These disorders include metabolic deficiencies, endocrine disorders, cardiovascular disease, and nutritional problems. Strokes, dementia, Parkinson's disease, and Huntington's disease are highly likely to co-occur with depression. Many medications used to treat common disorders have side effects influencing mood. High prevalence rates of chronic health conditions and subsequent drug treatment may make infirm older adults particularly vulnerable to depression.

It is hardly surprising that chronic health problems can lead to high levels of negative affect. Physical illnesses impair people's ability to live independently and undermine their sense of control over their lives. Much evidence shows that having a sense of control is related to feeling positive about one's life, and is a protective factor against affective disorders. Thus, even when an illness does not cause depression-like symptoms or induce negative affect, physical illness and depression may be indirectly related.

In fact, an estimated 15% of elderly people who are hospitalized meet the criteria for major depression. Nursing home populations also have high rates of depression and depressive symptoms. Much of the literature on the relationship between health and emotions has focused on clinical depression or on symptoms of depression, rather than on everyday emotional experience. While clinical depression encompasses a range of symptoms, one of the major aspects of clinical depression is the frequent experience of sadness and related emotions. In this chapter, we consider findings on depressive symptoms to reflect, in part, emotional distress.

One question is whether older adults are actually more likely to experience depression in response to physical illness than are younger adults. Linda George, at Duke University, and her colleagues point out that in absolute numbers there will be more depression co-occurring with physical illness among older adults simply because there are more older adults who are ill.

In fact, when George and her colleagues examined the risk of developing an affective disorder given that one has a physical condition, they found that this risk was high for all age groups. Regardless of age, everyone who is physically ill is more vulnerable to depression. Moreover, the elderly are relatively less at risk than members of other age groups. That is, although

---

[1] In general, findings about affective disorders in later life are controversial, and it would require an entire article to adequately address even the current state of knowledge about geriatric depression. For our purposes, it is simply interesting to note the epidemiological findings, and their consistency with other findings about emotion and aging.

being physically ill increases risk for everyone, those with the lowest increase in risk are the elderly. Depression is associated with physical illness and disability; but this association is not stronger in older adults. Rather, the rates of physical illness and disability rise disproportionately in old age, making it appear that older adults are more vulnerable to depression in conjunction with physical disabilities.

One reason for the relative invulnerability of frail elderly to depression may be the coping strategies that they use in response to illnesses. Older adults may cope with illnesses more effectively than do young adults, especially with respect to emotion. Folkman and colleagues have not concentrated on coping with illnesses specifically, but other researchers have applied their model (of instrumental and emotion-focused coping) to the specific problem of coping with later life illnesses.

Barbara Felton, at New York University, and her colleagues find that older adults are less likely to vent their frustration, anger, or hostility about their illness on family and friends. This does not mean that older adults suppress their emotional responses, but it does mean that they do not express those emotional responses in a problematic way. Similarly, in the work of Carolyn Aldwin, at the University of California at Davis, and her colleagues, older adults are less likely than younger adults to use hostile, blaming, or other emotionally negative coping strategies, which are among the least effective ways to cope with stress.

For example, cancer is an illness that is far more likely in later life, and one that is also associated with twice as much depression as are general medical conditions. In fact, emotional distress in cancer patients can remain higher than in control groups for as long as 5 years. Here, too, older adults appear to be at an advantage. Vincent Mor, at Brown University, and his colleagues have examined the impact of cancer on patients of varying ages. They interviewed patients repeatedly over the period just following diagnosis, and up to 2 years after the diagnosis of cancer was made. Their findings show that older patients are less distressed from the time at which diagnosis is made, through the follow-up period. Moreover, the lower emotional distress of older patients is consistent across varying types of cancers, and when dependency and severity of symptoms are statistically controlled. [*See* CANCER.]

Just as the literature on coping with life events suggested, older adults appear to cope better with physi-

cal disability than do younger adults. Again, this may be partly due to the anticipation of disability in later life, partly due to the smaller number of competing demands for older adults' time and resources, partly due to the existence of social institutions like Medicare that are designed to help older adults with medical care, and partly due to improved abilities to regulate emotion. The overall picture, however, is quite positive.

Emotions do influence physical health, as well, and this is one area in which the elderly may be at greater risk than the young. The specific ways in which emotional experiences can influence physical functioning are largely unspecified, but most researchers think that the mechanism involves immunological functioning. Steven Schliefer, at Mount Sinai School of Medicine, and his colleagues have been examining the impact of clinical depression on immunological functioning in adults of various ages. They recruit people of various ages who are clinically depressed, and assess their immunologic functioning in a variety of ways. Regardless of how they assess immunological functions, older adults who are clinically depressed show lowered immune functioning. Suppressed immune functioning can render older adults susceptible to a variety of illnesses, and Schliefer and his colleagues have evidence that bereavement can produce suppressed immune functioning similarly to depression.

In short, research on the impact of health conditions on emotional functioning suggests that older adults are functioning better than younger adults—coping better with illnesses and, relative to infirm younger adults, are less vulnerable to depression in response to illness. On the other hand, emotional distress, at least from bereavement, can have a more serious impact on the immunological functioning of older adults than on younger adults.

V. SUMMARY AND CONCLUSIONS

In this article, we have examined different aspects of emotional functioning—including the component processes of emotion—in search of age differences. The vast majority of findings suggest that emotional functioning in adulthood is characterized by either stability or modest gain. Although older adults do show lowered physiological arousal in response to laboratory emotional stimuli, the cause of this reduced arousal is unclear. It is likely that reduced physiological arousal in response to negative emotions represents a more global trend toward reduced autonomic responsiveness, rather than a decline in emotional functioning, given that there are no age differences in the subjective experience of emotion.

Despite optimistic beginnings, far more research is needed in the area of emotion and aging. Much of what is known about affect and aging relies on self-reports. Most is based on cross-sectional age comparisons. Much of the research has been based on convenience samples and has not adequately addressed issues of ethnicity, class, or gender, not to mention cultural differences. Yet the potential for improved functioning in the emotion domain is clear from the research literature. Aging is not simply a time of loss, rather, accumulated life experiences may, in fact, help us cope well with the challenges of our increasing longevity.

BIBLIOGRAPHY

Carstensen, L. L. (1995). Evidence for a life-span theory of socioemotional selectivity. *Current Directions in Psychological Science*, 4(5), 151–156.

Ekman, P., & Davidson, R. J. (1994). *The nature of emotion: Fundamental questions*. Oxford: Oxford University Press.

Folkman, S., Lazarus, R. S., Pimley, S., & Novacek, J. (1987). Age Differences in Stress and Coping Processes. *Psychology and Aging*, 2(2), 171–184.

George, L. K., Landerman, R., Blazer, D., & Melville, M. L. (1989). Concurrent Morbidity between Physical and Mental Illness: An Epidemiologic Examination. In L. L. Carstensen & J. Neale (Eds.), *Mechanisms of psychological influence on physical health* (pp. 9–22). New York: Plenum.

Labouvie-Vief, G., Hakim-Larson, J., DeVoe, M., & Schoeberlein, S. (1989). Emotions and self-regulation: A life-span view. *Human Development*, 32, 279–299.

Powell Lawton, M., Kleban, M. H., & Dean, J. (1993). Affect and age: Cross-sectional comparisons of structure and prevalence. *Psychology and Aging*, 8(2), 165–175.

Levenson, R. W., Carstensen, L. L., Friesen, W. V., & Ekman, P. (1991). Emotion, Physiology, and Expression in Old Age. *Psychology and Aging*, 6, 28–35.

Malatesta-Magai, C., Jonas, R., Shapard, B., & Culver, L. C. (1992). Type A behavior pattern and emotion expression in younger and older adults. *Psychology and Aging*, 7(4), 551–561.

Mor, V., Allen, S., & Malin, M. (1994). The psychosocial impact of cancer on older versus younger patients and their families. *Cancer*, 74(7) (Suppl.), 2118–2126.

Schleifer, S. (1989). Bereavement, depression, and immunity: The role of age. In L. L. Carstensen & J. M. Neale (Eds.), *Mechanisms of psychological influence on physical health* (pp. 61–80). New York: Plenum.

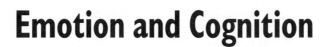

Emotion and Cognition

Anthony Scioli

Keene State College

James R. Averill

University of Massachusetts, Amherst

Cognition In the classical sense, the term "cognition" refers to the acquisition of knowledge. Among contemporary psychologists, cognition is often interpreted more broadly to include all forms of information processing, from the transduction of sensory input to complex problem solving.

Common-Process Theories Theories of emotion that assume that cognition and emotion involve the same underlying processes.

Emotion A heterogeneous class of responses (e.g., anger, fear, grief, love, hope) by which a person relates to events that facilitate (positive emotions) or hinder (negative emotions) important goals; emotional concepts also imply that the response is intense, immediate, or beyond personal control, thus contrasting emotional with more deliberate, rational behavior.

Emotional Creativity The acquisition of new emotions or the application of standard emotions in novel and adaptive ways.

Emotional Intelligence A set of interrelated skills that encompasses the regulation and monitoring of one's personal feelings and the emotions of others, and the ability to use emotional experiences for motivational and planning purposes.

Emotional Memory The process of storing and retrieving material of an emotional nature, for example, events that involve physiological arousal or trauma.

Special-Process Theories Theories of emotion that assume that cognition and emotion involve different underlying processes.

A thorough exploration of **EMOTION AND COGNITION** would require excursions into perception, attention, memory, language, imagination, and other "higher" thought processes—in short, about the whole of psychology. To help organize such a wide range of issues we first clarify some ambiguities in the concept of "cognition." We then explore theories of emotion with an emphasis on underlying processes. Finally, we examine five issues where the interface between emotion and cognition is particularly salient or relevant to mental health, namely, the nature of emotional feelings, unconscious emotions, emotions and memory, emotional intelligence, and emotional creativity.

I. THE CONCEPT OF COGNITION

In the classical tradition "cognition" referred to the acquisition of knowledge, of which rational, logical thought is a prime example. We will call this "cognition in the narrow sense." Among many contemporary psychologists, cognition is interpreted more broadly, to include all information processing beyond simple sensory input. In this broader sense, "cognition" is roughly equivalent to "mentation," that is, any kind of mental activity.

In the narrow (classical) sense just described, a proper contrast can be made between cognition and emotion. Emotions are concerned not with the acquisition of knowledge, but with the implications of an event for a person's well-being. In anger, for example, an incident is appraised as an affront; in fear, as a danger; and so forth. Moreover, as traditionally conceived, emotions are interpreted as beyond personal control, that is, as passions (things that happen to us) rather than as actions (things we do). Colloquially speaking, we are "overcome" by anger, "seized" by fear, and so forth. By contrast, rational (cognitive) behavior is the paradigm of an action, and hence contrasted with emotion.

However, when used in the broadest sense of mentation, the contrast between cognition and emotion loses much of its meaning. Emotional behavior requires information processing, from the appraisal of eliciting events to the organization of responses.

Obviously, the stance theorists take on the relation between emotion and cognition depends on whether they conceive of cognition in a narrow or broad sense. And, needless to say, the concept of emotion is also vague and subject to differing interpretations. In view of these ambiguities, it might seem that a simple solution to the emotion–cognition debate would be to agree on the definition of terms. That, however, is not as easy or as unproblematic as it might seem. As psychological constructs, "emotion" and "cognition" do not stand in isolation, but derive their meaning, in part, from the role they play in broader theories of human behavior.

In short, the emotion–cognition debate is not simply a debate about words; it cannot be dismissed simply as a matter of semantics. Rather, the controversy reflects deeper divisions in scientific and even philosophical assumptions, including questions about the mind–body relationship, and the nature of the mind as a receiver of raw inputs to be later synthesized (a realist view) or an interpreter of complex stimuli that relies upon meaning systems and preestablished rules of judgments and perception to organize complex stimuli (an idealist view).

II. THEORIES OF EMOTION

Most theories of emotion can be categorized as either common-process or special-process theories. Special-process theorists tend to interpret cognition narrowly and conclude that emotions and cognitions must therefore involve different underlying processes. By contrast, common-process theorists take a broader view of cognition and conclude that emotions, like more rational and deliberate forms of behavior, are ineluctably cognitive.

A. Special-Process Theories

The idea that emotion and cognition involve separate processes has a long and distinguished history, dating back at least to Plato's tripartite division of the psyche into reason, spirit, and appetite, each located in a separate part of the body. But perhaps the historically most famous special-process theory is that proposed by the seventeenth-century philosopher, Renè Descartes. Descartes attributed the emotions to bodily mechanisms, the activation of which was presumably impressed upon the soul via the pineal gland and hence experienced as passions rather than as actions.

Echoes of Descartes can be heard today in the theory of emotion proposed by William James and its contemporary offshoots (e.g., Stanley Schachter). According to James, emotional experience arises when perception of bodily changes, mainly from the viscera, is added to the "cold" perception of an exciting event.

Special-process theories were also given impetus by Charles Darwin, who viewed the emotions (or at least many expressions of emotion) as remnants of our biological past. Darwin's influence can be seen in theories that postulate a series of basic emotions that presumably are biologically primitive and hence distinguishable from those cognitive processes (rational, symbolic thought) that are most characteristically human.

Carroll Izard's "differential-emotions" theory provides a good illustration of a contemporary special-process model. Reflecting the tradition of both James and Darwin, Izard postulates that emotions are experienced when cognition is combined with feedback from bodily responses, especially the facial musculature. He further postulates a small set of biologically basic emotions, each accompanied by a unique facial expression. More complex emotions arise when expressive reactions become associated with different modes of cognition or ways of interpreting events.

Robert Zajonc is another staunch defender of the special process view. Emotion and cognition, he contends, are partially independent systems that operate in parallel. Zajonc draws on two main sources of evidence to support this contention. First, there is experimental evidence that suggests that people can state a preference for or against a stimulus before they can state (know) what the stimulus is (e.g., subjects can state whether they like or dislike a particular tone or brand of cigarette before they are able to state exactly which tone or brand is presented to them). Second, Zajonc and his colleagues have explored a controversial variant of the facial-feedback hypothesis in which emotional experience (defined broadly as pleasant and unpleasant affect) is thought to be due to the role of facial musculature in regulating blood flow to the brain and hence brain temperature.

Another type of special-process theory focuses on cerebral lateral asymmetries. In popular psychology magazines, the left hemisphere is often depicted as analytic (cognitive), and the right hemisphere as holistic (emotional). For most people, linguistic functions, which help mediate analytic thought, are localized primarily (but not exclusively) in the left hemisphere. Emotions, however, are not so readily localized in any one hemisphere. For example, research suggests that approach-related positive affect is correlated with left anterior activation whereas withdrawal-related negative affect appears associated with right anterior activation. To complicate matters further, most emotions cannot be classified easily in terms of simple approach or avoidance tendencies.

Not all special process theories have an explicit physiological emphasis as in the above examples. Some postulate two different modes of thought, without linking either mode to specific physiological mechanisms. The Freudian distinction between primary- and secondary-process thinking is perhaps the best example of this approach. Primary process originates in the Id (a caldron of biologically based impulses) and is presumably immune to the laws of logic; secondary process, by contrast, is conceived as a later acquisition, both phylogenetically and ontogenetically, and is characteristic of the ego rather than the Id. Another way of stating the difference is that primary process thought follows the pleasure principle, whereas secondary process thought follows the reality principle.

Epstein has attempted to bridge the gap between classic Freudian conceptions and modern views of information processing. He postulates two interacting but separate modes of thought: A rational system that is analytical and logical, mediated by conscious appraisals, and used to manipulate abstract symbols, words, and numbers; and an experiential system that is automatic, intuitive, unconscious, and that processes information holistically via associations, images, narratives, and metaphors. The latter (experiential) system is primarily involved in emotion, according to Epstein.

As a final example of a special process theory, we may cite Oatley and Johnson-Laird. Stemming from the tradition of artificial intelligence and computer simulation, Oatley and Johnson-Laird offer a computationally oriented model that depicts the emotions as part of an elaborate system (the mind) that must reach decisions, often under conditions of inadequate or conflicting information. Two kinds of information are postulated: "Control signals" communicate the need to rearrange priorities within the system, much as a fire alarm would rearrange priorities in a school or business; "semantic signals," by contrast, reflect an evolutionarily more advanced mode of information processing that operates when everything seems to be going "as planned." Oatley and Johnson-Laird further postulate a small number of basic emotions (anger, fear, sadness, happiness, and possibly others), each with its unique control signal. Emotions are aroused, and hence control signals are emitted and priorities rearranged, whenever there is a conscious or unconscious evaluation of a change in the probability of achieving a particular goal, and more standard, deliberate (rational) modes of coping are inadequate.

B. Common-Process Theories

Common-process theorists do not recognize any isomorphic relation between cognition and emotion, on the one hand, and separate physiological or psychological mechanisms, on the other. Rather, they believe the same set of mechanisms (which may involve more than one type of information processing) helps mediate emotional and nonemotional behavior, albeit perhaps in varying combination and emphasis.

Common-process theories also have a long history. In ancient times, they were best represented by the Stoics, who conceived of emotion as a form of false judgment. Since judgments, whether true or false, are necessarily cognitive, emotions are also necessarily cognitive. It follows that the management of emotion involves replacing false with accurate judgments. In this regard, there is little difference between the advice offered by the Stoics and the recommendations given by modern cognitive therapists (e.g., rational emotive therapy).

Among contemporary theorists, Robert Solomon is perhaps the most radical in treating emotions as a form of judgment. To be sure, many theorists recognize that emotions *influence* judgment. But for Solomon, as for the Stoics, emotions *are* judgments. The idea that emotions are passions, or events over when we have little control, is a myth, according to Solomon. Rather, we choose which emotions (judgments) to make, and hence we are responsible for our emotions. More specifically, emotions are means by which we project our values, ideals, and beliefs onto the world, indeed, by which we construct our world.

If emotions are judgments, as Solomon suggests, the question arises: On what bases are emotional judgments made? There is a whole class of psychological theories specifically devoted to this question, namely, appraisal theory. Richard Lazarus is perhaps the best-known appraisal theorist. Lazarus distinguishes between primary and secondary appraisal. The former involves assessments of the meaning of an event for the welfare of the individual, and the latter involves an assessment of coping options. For example, if the primary appraisal indicates danger and the secondary appraisal suggests that flight is the most viable option, then fear will be the emotion experienced. Lazarus also postulates a set of presumably universal "core relational themes" that help distinguish among certain emotions. For example, the core relational theme for anger is "a demeaning offense against me or mine," and for jealousy, "resenting a third party for loss or threat to another's affection."

A more clinical example of an appraisal theory is offered by Aaron Beck, who links various affective disorders to specific negative thought processes. For example, Beck views depression, not in biochemical terms, but as a cognitive set composed of a triad of negative appraisals concerning the self, the world, and the future. Like the Stoics of antiquity, Beck believes that many affective disorders can be treated by challenging and modifying distorted automatic thoughts. [*See* DEPRESSION.]

Appraisal is a dynamic not a static process, more like a motion picture than a still photograph. To capture this temporal dimension, Scherer has postulated a sequence of rapid, hierarchically organized "system evaluation checks." First, the novelty or lack of novelty of the stimulus is checked, then its pleasantness/unpleasantness, then its goal relevance (will it hinder or advance attainment of goals or satisfaction of needs), and finally, its coping implications. This last check has four subchecks: (a) a check to identify the responsible agent and motive, or cause; (b) a control check to determine if the individual can affect consequences; (c) a power check with respect to obstacles or adversaries; and (d) an adjustment check to assess how easy or difficult it will be to make needed changes.

The cognitive mediation of emotion does not stop at the level of appraisal. After a stimulus has been evaluated and response options are assessed, but before an actual response is made, a good deal of information processing can occur, much of it unconscious. Freudian defense mechanisms (e.g., projection, denial, reaction formation) illustrate some of the ways in which an emotional experience can be cognitively transformed to better fit a person's motives, goals, and self-concept.

The fact that such cognitive transformations can occur below the level of awareness, and frequently do so for defensive purposes, is viewed by some theorists as a major factor underlying the experience of passivity during an emotional response. Standard emotions, from this perspective, are like hysterical conversion reactions that are legitimized by society.

C. Levels of Information Processing

Neither common- nor special-process theories assume that there is only one or two kinds of information processing. For example, Leventhal describes three levels of information processing. The levels include a basic or core sensory-processing system that encompasses autonomic arousal, facial expressions, and elementary overt responses. At the next level, a schematic processing system stores memories of emotion-eliciting situations, the resulting feelings, and a motor memory of expressive and autonomic reactions. Finally, the most abstract system is the conceptual system that stores information about past emotional episodes in a propositional fashion for reflection and analysis of emotional experiences.

Johnson and Multhaup propose a modular common-process theory that includes two perceptual subsystems for processing external stimuli and two reflective subsystems that deal with internal stimuli or self-generated processes such as occur in fantasy, imagination, or problem solving.

The levels are presented in terms of an interacting chain of four levels, arranged in a hierarchy beginning with a simpler and then more advanced perceptual subsystem and ending with a simpler and then more advanced reflective subsystem. All four subsystems may contribute to emotion. For example, an episode of anger might be discussed in the following terms. At a party a person hears a comment (level 1 perception). The individual clarifies that this comment was in fact directed toward them (level 2 perception). The person judges this comment as an affront or attack (level 1 reflection). The individual processes this comment further and decides it was unjustified (level 2 reflection) and that in fact they are angry.

Johnson and Multhaup suggest that this particular model may be useful in clarifying a range of phenomena including: emotion responses that may occur without awareness of the source, variations in emotional responsiveness to the same environmental cues presented over time, and instances whereby it appears an individual is having an emotion of which they are unaware. The authors speculate that such events may be explained by the differential impact of emotional stimuli upon the perceptual and reflective subsystems and the degree of complexity involved in the interactions among the subsystems.

Multilevel formulations appeal to cognitively oriented psychologists and philosophers who believe consciousness is not a unitary phenomenon. At present some of these approaches are more memory focused than emotion focused (in terms of the degree of conceptual development completed on memory structures and processes versus emotion components and processes). Moreover, further work is needed to specify the role of serial (sequential) as opposed to parallel (simultaneous) processes, and the relationship of cognitive to noncognitive components. Finally, while serializing the emotion eliciting process may be necessary to account for particular observations, this strategy alone is not likely to resolve deeper philosophical issues (e.g., whether to view the mind from a realist or idealist perspective).

D. Range of Convenience

Special- and common-process theories are not incompatible alternatives, each type of theory has its "range of convenience," that is, phenomena to which it is best suited. Two factors, in particular, help determine the appropriateness of each type of theory, namely, the kind of emotion to be explained (simple versus complex) and the principles of explanation adopted (biological, psychological, or social).

I. Kinds of Emotion

The concept of emotion covers a wide range of phenomena, from very simple, reflex-like reactions (pain, pleasure, startle) to highly complex states (e.g., love, pride, grief). Whether one adopts a special-process or common-process theory depends in part on the kinds of emotion emphasized. Consider, for example, the implications of centering one's theory around sudden fright as opposed to hope.

In the case of fright there is clearly a biological and adaptive basis for the presence of reflexive reactions to sudden and potentially dangerous stimuli. Little cognitive elaboration is required and might even be harmful if it produced too long a delay in response. Fright reactions can be recognized in human infants, across cultures, and even across species, which suggests that very primitive mechanisms are involved. A special-process theory, one that distinguishes between emotional and cognitive ("higher-order") processes would seem to be appropriate here.

By contrast, hope requires the ability to conceive of alternative futures, which presumes a highly developed cognitive capacity. In one study, Scioli found that the nature of hope varied with cognitive development, from primarily a problem-solving advantage in younger children, to a time-conception bias in adolescence. Hope also varies across cultures, not just superficially but in its underlying nature, so that even to use the same word "hope" is somewhat misleading. Such developmental and cultural alterations demonstrate the highly cognitive nature of hope and suggest that a common-process theory is more appropriate in the case of this emotion. [*See* HOPE.]

The trend in psychology is away from grand unifying theories and toward minitheories. With regard to emotion, there has been a slow evolutionary process whereby emotions were initially ignored, then subsumed under prevailing grand theories of behavior, and most recently approached at the level of general "emotion theories." As a result, we have developed a better appreciation of the complexity inherent in emotions. Perhaps it is time to acknowledge a need to develop more specialized and complementary mini-theories, each appropriate to a subclass of emotions.

2. Explanatory Preference

Another source of disagreement in the emotion–cognition debate involves the perspective from which theorists seek to explain the origins and functions of emotional behavior. Three possibilities exist: biological evolution, psychological development, and social history. Needless to say, all three perspectives are necessary, but theorists differ with regard to the relative importance placed on each. For example, biologically oriented theorists typically adopt a special-process approach, psychologically oriented theorists may adopt either a common- or special-process approach, and socially oriented theorists tend to favor common-process theories.

The reasons for the above associations are readily apparent. Biologically oriented theorists are concerned with commonalities between humans and other animals and hence tend to focus on processes that are distinct from "higher" (cognitive) thought processes. Socially oriented theorists are concerned with the influence of culture on behavior, an influence that is primarily exerted only through cognitive processes. Finally, psychologically oriented theorists can go either way, sometimes emphasizing the biological and sometimes the social in human nature.

Although common, the association between explanatory principles and theoretical orientation is by no means invariant. For example, some social psychologists look to the emotions as the biological foundations for society. Conversely, some biologically oriented theorists view the emotions as later evolutionary developments, much like the emergence of language. But these are the exceptions.

To further complicate matters, within the realm of any explanatory approach (biological, psychological, or social), there are multiple sublevels of components and processes that one can choose to focus upon. For example, a biologically oriented theorist interested in emotion and memory might focus on the role of general arousal, or the role of the amygdala, or the anterior portion of the amygdala, or the electrochemical processes moving through cells within the amygdala. The further down the sublevels one descends, the more difficult it may become to maintain a special-process view, for at the level of elementary processes, the

same mechanisms often help mediate many different behaviors.

III. ISSUES ON THE INTERFACE BETWEEN EMOTION AND COGNITION

However one conceives of the relation between emotion and cognition in terms of underlying mechanisms (e.g., in terms of special- or common-processes), at a more surface level, there are a number of topics that lie on the interface between emotion and cognition that need to be addressed. We will consider briefly five issues that have particular relevance to mental health: the nature of emotional feelings, unconscious emotions, emotions and memory, emotional intelligence, and emotional creativity.

A. The Nature of Emotional Feelings

Colloquially, and in some psychological theories, the concepts of "feeling" and "emotion" are used interchangeably. This is particularly true of special-process theories, where presumably "raw" feelings, unmediated by higher (cognitive) thought processes, are considered the sine qua non of emotion. However, the term "feeling" is one of the vaguest in the English language. A person can feel simple sensations (the touch of velvet, the color red), a variety of different aches and pains, pleasures of all sorts, and numerous other physical and mental conditions (feelings of fatigue, confusion, excitement, curiosity, etc.).

If we restrict feelings to simple sensory experiences, then they are not limited to the emotions. The sweet taste of ice cream, for example, or the discomfort of a toothache, are not usually considered emotional. Conversely, the "pleasures" of love and the "pain" of grief cannot be reduced to simple sensory experiences.

A more fruitful way to think about emotional feelings is to conceptualize them as sources of information coming from both inside and outside the person, that when combined, lend an emotional quality to experience. In this approach, feelings are viewed as derivatives of information processing rather than as pure inputs and as such are analogous to other complex perceptual experiences. The perception of depth, for example, also involves the synthesis of bodily and situational cues, as well as information about possible responses afforded by the environment. To be more specific, the way we appraise a situation in relation to our goals determines, in part, the way we feel. Feedback from physiological arousal and facial expressions also plays a role in generating feelings, and so do instrumental acts, whether actual or only desired. Information from these diverse sources is integrated into a coherent whole when interpreted within a folk-theoretical system symbolized by such concepts as anger, fear, and so forth.

In short, emotional feelings are not precognitive, on the contrary, they are as much a product of cognition as are other complex subjective experiences. This does not mean, of course, that emotional feelings are epiphenomena or inconsequential byproducts. Rather, as outputs of earlier stages of information processing they can serve as inputs to subsequent stages. Emotional feelings can thus inform a person of facts that he or she might otherwise overlook or not fully realize. This is the principle that underlies the hackneyed phrase, "Get in touch with your feelings."

B. Conscious and Unconscious Emotions

A perennial debate is whether emotional states can ever be unconscious. A common view, adopted since the time of Freud, is to assume that while eliciting conditions and mediating mechanisms may be nonconscious, the resulting emotion—qua feeling—must be conscious, as in "free-floating" anxiety. (See the earlier discussion on levels of information processing.) To speak of feelings as unconscious does involve a contradiction of terms, for part of the meaning of feeling is that it be felt. But in spite of their overlapping meanings and frequent interchangeableness, "emotion" and "feeling" are not synonymous concepts; attributions of feelings, whether to oneself or others, are based on different kinds of information than are attributions of emotion.

Therefore, one can say without self-contradiction that a person is in an emotional state but has no corresponding feeling. It is commonplace in everyday affairs, not to mention clinical practice, to attribute anger, jealousy, envy, love, or whatever, even though the person might deny harboring any such feelings. Succinctly put, feelings are not necessary conditions for emotion.

Neither are feelings sufficient conditions for emotion. For example, a person may feel angry but not be in an angry state. In this respect, emotional feelings may be compared with other complex perceptual experiences, such as hearing voices or having visions. The vividness of an experience does not guarantee its veridicality. Emotional feelings can be illusory.

C. Emotions and Memory

The relation between emotion and memory has received a great deal of attention in recent years. Three phenomena are of particular interest: state-dependent memory, mood congruent memory, and memory for traumatic experiences.

In the movie *City Lights,* Charlie Chaplin befriends a drunken millionaire and saves him from attempted suicide. Later, when sober, the millionaire no longer recognizes Charlie and treats him with disdain. But the millionaire does not remain sober for long, and when again drunk, he recognizes Charlie and takes him into his home, only to throw him out when sobriety returns. This is an illustration of state-dependent memory, that is, events that happen in one state (e.g., a drunken stupor) are remembered when the person is again in that state but not while in another state (e.g., sober). The state need not be drug-induced, as in *City Lights,* but may be emotional in the ordinary sense. For example, if you study for a test while in a happy mood, you may do better if you also take the test while in a happy mood, even though the test material itself is affectively neutral.

While state-dependent memory appears to be a real phenomenon, it is not particularly robust, at least when mild emotional states are involved. Evidence is stronger for mood-congruent recall. This refers to the recollection of events consistent in affective tone with one's present emotional state. For example, when happy, people are more likely to recall happy events, and when sad, negative experiences come more readily to mind.

Currently, there is no satisfactory explanation for state-dependent and mood-congruent recall. Bower has suggested that stimuli presented while an individual is in an emotional state becomes linked in memory with that state. Later recall of the stimuli presumably is facilitated if the person reenters the same emotional state, since this activates a network consisting of the emotion and associated events. One difficulty with this type of explanation is that it leaves unclear how the emotional state is itself encoded in memory. As discussed earlier, emotions are complex; it is not reasonable to assume that they are encoded as a unit.

Nor are emotional experiences recalled as a unit. Try to remember a time when you were in an emotional state—anger, say. Most likely, you can recall aspects of the situation that made you angry, but you cannot easily recapture the quality of the experience itself—the anger is somehow lost in memory. This is true even of "flashbulb memories," that is, detailed and seemingly precise recall of very important, often emotionally arousing events. There are several potential explanations for the vivid recall of emotionally arousing (particularly traumatic) events.

From an evolutionary perspective, it would be adaptive for an organism *not* to forget events that carry implications for its survival, directly or indirectly. Physiologically, there is evidence that increased release of neurotransmitters and neuropeptides during arousal may play a role in enhancing the encoding process. On the psychological level, emotionally significant events may be attended to more carefully and subsequently reprocessed or repeatedly "mulled over."

But not all traumatic events are easily remembered. We can all call to mind experiences that we would prefer to forget. At the extreme, the memory may be "repressed," a kind of motivated forgetting. Lift the repression (change the motivation), and the memory may return. For example, a child who is sexually abused may subsequently repress the memory, only to recall it years later, perhaps under the guidance of a therapist. Not all memories, however, are accurate. When allegations of child abuse have been retracted or invalidated by other sources of evidence, a diagnosis of "false memory syndrome" may be invoked.

Based on case studies and retrospective narratives, many clinicians support the idea that memories of traumatic experiences may be lost and recovered years later. Experimentally oriented psychologists tend to be more skeptical. Their doubts are based on two grounds: First, memory is quite vulnerable to suggestion, as might occur during psychotherapy or under hypnosis; second, memory is not a direct readout of prior experience, but is largely a constructive and reconstructive process. That is, memories are impacted by present needs, goals, and emotions; they are not unadulterated prints or traces of actual events.

From their perspective, clinical advocates of repressed memory do not believe one can extrapolate from laboratory studies, which for obvious reasons cannot easily simulate traumatic events. Perhaps the fairest assessment of the available evidence is that memories can sometimes be "repressed" and later recovered, but that without independent verification, reports of childhood abuse should be treated with extreme caution, especially if such abuse purportedly occurred at a very early age or was repeated over many years.

In those cases where recall of previously forgotten traumatic events can be verified, how might we account for the lapse in memory? At the physiological level, one set of theories, which could be considered special-process theories, is based on the assumption that the peculiarities of memories for traumatic events are due to a separate physiological process that is activated in the presence of a highly charged emotional stimulus. Specifically, these theories assume the amygdala is selectively involved in the processing of emotional memories, while the hippocampus, (which some believe normally plays an integrative role in the memory process), is essentially left out of the process. Other theories hypothesize that the structure and/or functioning of the hippocampus is altered by biochemical changes that accompany stress reactions and that this alteration may explain some of the dissociative and amnestic events seen in traumatized patients. Lastly, from a psychological perspective, Erdeyli considers the possibility of viewing memory in terms of multiple systems with multiple functions. "Forgetting," he suggests, may not mean that a unitary trace has been lost from a unitary system. Rather, it is possible that elements of the emotional memory, for example, the narrative or declarative aspects, may be unavailable, while the procedural elements are retained, in the form of ongoing behaviors, fears, and dreams that reflect retention.

Taken together, the literature on "repressed memory" is difficult to evaluate at this time. It is a heated topic and has generated some spirited debates among memory researchers and clinicians—as well as lawsuits brought by people accused of abuse that later proved to be the result of "false memories." Few studies of trauma have been conducted to support clinical case records, but the relevance of laboratory studies is understandably questioned by clinicians who work with clients who have been raped, tortured, or subjected to other unimaginable forms of cruelty and abuse.

D. Emotional Intelligence

Large individual differences exist, not only in the ability to recall emotional events, but also to express emotions adaptively. Some people appear emotionally "limited" in their experiences and expressions, whereas others always seem to know just how much anger, concern, or pride to experience and express in any given situation. Salovey and his colleagues have coined the term "emotional intelligence" to refer to such individual differences. Emotional intelligence is a set of interrelated skills that encompasses the recognition and monitoring of one's own feelings as well as the emotions of others, the ability to express and/ or regulate appropriate emotions across varied situations, and the ability to use one's emotional experiences as a source of motivation, or to assist in decision making, or long-term planning.

Emotional intelligence, like the older concept of social intelligence, is dependent upon higher thought processes, including memory, attention, perception, and language. However emotional intelligence is more narrowly defined and hence easier to distinguish from intellectual ability in general.

From a practical point of view, one of the most intriguing aspects of emotional intelligence concerns emotion construction and regulation across levels of consciousness. Mayer and Salovey suggest that emotions may be constructed and regulated (with more and less skill) at a nonconscious level, at a low level of awareness, or at a metalevel where the individual engages in deliberate and extensive efforts to understand, define, and develop their emotional lives (cf. earlier discussion of levels of information processing). Furthermore Mayer and Salovey suggest that the degree of emotional intelligence realized at one level may be independent of the degree of emotional intelligence achieved at another level. One example they cite is the person with great expert knowledge about depression (perhaps gleaned from the self-help literature) but who nevertheless remains depressed as a result of a lack of emotional development that was shaped long ago at a nonconscious level. [See INTELLIGENCE AND MENTAL HEALTH.]

E. Emotional Creativity

In popular stereotypes creative individuals are often depicted as unusually emotional. Whether accurate or not, the stereotype contains a paradox: Whereas creativity is ranked among the highest and most esteemed of the "higher" thought processes, emotions are often viewed as primitive, noncognitive responses, closely associated with physiological activity (cf. the special-process theories discussed earlier). One way around this paradox is to treat the emotions only as antecedents (e.g., as facilitators or inhibitors) or as consequences of creativity, but not as creative products in their own right. There is, however, another alternative. If emotions involve many of the same cognitive mechanisms (broadly conceived) that help mediate nonemotional behavior, as common-process theories suggest, then the possibility exists that emotions themselves are subject to innovation and change.

Like creative behavior in other domains, an emotionally creative response can be assessed according to three major criteria: novelty, effectiveness, and authenticity (originality). An emotional response that is novel, but also ineffective or phoney, is liable to be classified as neurotic. The conversion reactions of a hysteric would be one example; the superficial displays of a con artist would be another. Conversely, mental health presumes the ability to respond in ways that are out of the ordinary, yet effective and genuine, when meeting challenges for which socially prescribed responses are inadequate.

To some extent there is overlap between emotional creativity and emotional intelligence. Both concepts address the process of making careful and accurate appraisals, the monitoring of one's emotions and those of others in a variety of situations, and the assimilation of emotional experiences to achieve a better understanding of life events and to derive greater meaning.

But emotional creativity is also concerned with the acquisition of new emotions, as well as the application of standard emotions in novel ways or to new and unusual situations. In the highest sense, emotional creativity refers to a transformative process whereby one develops entirely new and different types of emotion. [See CREATIVITY AND GENIUS.]

IV. CONCLUSIONS

As used in ordinary language the concepts of emotion and cognition have contrasting connotations. Cognition is concerned with how we come to know the world, dispassionately and objectively. A cognition may thus be judged true or false. Emotions, by contrast, are passionate and subjective; that is, they are concerned with how a person evaluates the world in relation to his or her own goals and concerns. Thus, emotions such as anger, say, or joy are not typically judged true or false, but appropriate or inappropriate.

Contrasts such as the above are based on molar behavior interpreted within a social context. Whether or not a similar contrast applies on the molecular level (i.e., to mediating mechanisms on either the physiological or psychological level) is an open question. Special-process theories assume that distinctions made with respect to molar behavior can be applied *mutatis mutandis* to mediating mechanisms; common-process theories assume that the same (albeit multiple) mechanisms mediate both emotion and cognition. The appropriateness (range of convenience) of each kind of theory depends, in part, on such metatheoretical issues as the kind of emotion considered basic (e.g., fright versus hope) and the explanatory principles emphasized (biological, psychological, social).

But on two things most theorists agree: First, mental health implies an integration of psychological functions, just as physical health implies an integration of bodily functions, and second, in a rapidly changing social environment, emotional adaptability is as important as cognitive flexibility. The nature of emotional feelings, unconscious emotions, emotions and memory, emotional intelligence, and emotional creativity—these are some of the issues that lie at the interface between emotion and cognition, where problems of integration and adaptability are most acute.

BIBLIOGRAPHY

Averill, J. R., Catlin, G., & Chon, K. K. (1990). *Rules of hope.* New York: Springer-Verlag.

Averill, J. R., & Nunley, E. P. (1992). *Voyages of the heart: Living an emotionally creative life.* New York: Free Press.

Bower, G. (1994). Some relations between emotions and memory. In P. K. Ekman & R. J. Davidson (Eds.), *The nature of emotion* (pp. 303–305). New York: Oxford University Press.

Davidson, R. J. (1994). Complexities in the search for emotion-specific physiology. In P. K. Ekman & R. J. Davidson (Eds.), *The nature of emotion* (pp. 237–242). New York: Oxford University Press.

Ellis, A. (1982). *Rational-emotive therapy and cognitive behavior therapy.* New York: Springer.

Epstein, S. (1994). Integration of the cognitive and the psychodynamic unconscious. *American Psychologist, 49,* 8, 709–724.

Erdelyi, M. (1993). Repression: the mechanism and the defense. In D. M. Wegner & L. W. Pennybaker (Eds.), *Handbook of mental control* (pp. 126–148). Englewood Cliffs, NJ: Prentice-Hall.

Izard, C. E. (1991). *The psychology of emotions.* New York: Plenum.

Johnson, M. K., & Multhaup, K. S. (1992). Emotion and MEM. In S. A. Christianson (Ed.), *The handbook of emotion and memory: Current research and theory* (pp. 36–66). Hillsdale, NJ: Lawrence Erlbaum.

Laird, J. D., & Apostoleris, N. H. (1996). Emotional self-control and self-perception: Feelings are the solution, not the problem. In R. Harre & W. G. Parrot (Eds.), *The emotions: Social, cultural, and biological dimensions* (pp. 285–301). Thousand Oaks, CA: Sage.

Lazarus, R. S. (1991). *Emotion and adaptation.* New York: Oxford.

LeDoux, J. E. (1994, June). Emotion, memory, and the brain. *Scientific American,* 50–57.

Leventhal, H. (1984). A perceptual motor theory of emotion. In K. Scherer & P. Ekman (Eds.), *Approaches to emotion* (pp. 271–291). Hillsdale, NJ: Lawrence Erlbaum.

Loftus, E. F. (1993). The reality of repressed memories. *American Psychologist, 48,* 2, 518–537.

Mayer, J. D., & Salovey, P. (1995). Emotional intelligence and the construction and regulation of feeling. *Applied and Preventive Psychology, 4,* 197–208.

Oatley, K., & Johnson-Laird, P. N. (1987). Toward a cognitive theory of emotions. *Cognition and Emotion, 1,* 29–50.

Scherer, K. R. (1988). *Facets of emotion: recent research.* Hillsdale, NJ: Lawrence Erlbaum.

Scioli, A. (1990). The development of hope and hopelessness: Structural and functional aspects. Doctoral Dissertation, University of Rhode Island, Kingston.

Solomon, R. C. (1993). *The passions: Emotions and the meaning of life* (rev. ed.). Indianapolis: Hackett.

Zajonc, R. B., Murphy, S. T., & Inglehart, M. (1989). Feeling and facial inference: Implications of the vascular theory of emotion. *Psychological Review, 96,* 396–416.

Emotions and Mental Health

Carroll E. Izard, David Schultz, and Karen L. Levinson

University of Delaware

Discrete Emotions An approach to the study of emotions that assumes categorically distinct emotions such as joy, sadness, and anger, and assumes that each emotion has a unique effect on cognition and action.

Emotionality Traditionally, the intensity and frequency of experiencing negative emotions. Some authorities now divide the concept into two parts: positive emotionality and negative emotionality. Others divide it into the more specific patterns of emotions that, for example, characterize anxiety and depression.

Emotion Components The neural component includes brain structures and neurotransmitters that function in emotion activation, emotion expression, and emotion experience. Emotion expression is the facial, bodily, and vocal signals that communicate one's emotional state to others. Emotion experience, described as feeling, motivational state, or action readiness, is the quality of consciousness associated with an emotion.

Emotion Reactivity The extent to which a person's autonomic, neuroendocrine, and behavioral systems are activated in response to stimuli.

Emotion Recognition The ability to recognize and label emotion expressions and experiences.

Emotion Regulation The processes of moderating emotions, including traits of temperament or personality, cognitive and behavioral skills, and relationships with others, especially with one's parents.

Empathy To assume the role and vicariously experience the emotional response of a person being observed.

Temperament A person's characteristic physiological and behavioral responses to stimuli; for example, characteristic activity level, mood, or adaptability. Temperament is influenced by both genes and environment.

An **EMOTION** consists of activity in the brain and nervous system that is reflected in bodily changes and in a particular subjective experience typically described as a feeling or mood. To understand the part that emotions play in coping and mental health, one must view emotions in the larger context of biosocial systems. To this end, we describe the components of an emotion, the emotions system, and personality as a set of systems that has emotions as the primary motivational system. We include an overview of the anatomy and neurophysiology of emotions. An understanding of these processes helps us appreciate how readily emotions play a direct role in physical and mental health. We conclude with emotion regulation and the role of emotions in relationships and in specific psychological disorders.

I. INTRODUCTION

Emotions are important factors in the development of a healthy personality and social competence, and in the development of psychopathology. It has been noted that a person's skills in understanding and regulating emotions are more important to overall competence than IQ.

Because emotions are compelling motivational forces, they have a pervasive influence on perception, thought, and action. Each of the discrete emotions of human experience has unique motivational characteristics, and their motivational power is stable across the life span. For example, fear motivates protective behavior and the search for safety and security at all ages.

Studies of the effect of emotions on behavior suggest that the motivational functions of emotions are inherently adaptive. Emotions become maladaptive when they are not effectively connected to appropriate thought and action. Thus, fear helps ensure our well-being whenever our security is threatened, but unrealistic fear may lead to an anxiety disorder. Sadness over the loss of a loved one can bring a family together and strengthen social bonds, but unrelieved sadness and grief can lead to depression.

As a result of evolutionary processes through thousands of generations, our genes give us emotion-response predispositions that are relatively specific to each emotion. Thus, a particular emotion predisposes us to think and act in a particular manner that facilitates coping with the situation, as when fear generates protective behavior in a dangerous situation. The evolutionary processes that put so much adaptive information in our genes required millions of years and proceed at a very slow pace. [See EVOLUTION AND MENTAL HEALTH.]

By comparison, cultural evolution is rapid; it has greatly increased the number, variety, and complexity of emotion-eliciting events and situations in daily life. The number and variety of responses required to adapt to contemporary life circumstances is far greater than that provided by biological evolution. Genetic predisposition to respond to natural clues to danger has worked well in keeping us from stepping off precipices or from exploring the recesses of a strange and dark cave alone, but it does far less well in protecting us from the multitude of culturally derived dangers of contemporary urban culture. In our complex society, we are required to learn a new array of protective be-havior. Thus, the development of a healthy personality and the avoidance of mental health problems demands that we learn many new connections between a wide variety of cultural artifacts and emotions and between emotions and coping skills.

II. EMOTIONS, EMOTIONS SYSTEM, AND PERSONALITY

Some scientists think that emotions can be studied in terms of broad dimensions, such as pleasantness and arousal. In this view, it is important to know the valence (positivity, negativity) and intensity of an emotional state. Others take a discrete emotions approach in which it is important to distinguish specific emotions, such as interest, joy, sadness, anger, and fear. This type of theory is based on the premise that each emotion has unique motivational functions and hence differential effects on thought and behavior. We adopt a discrete emotions approach but recognize, as do others, that both approaches have merit. Emotions often occur in clusters or patterns, which makes it difficult to distinguish single-emotion effects. In some cases, it is possible to identify distinct clusters or patterns of negative emotions that relate differentially to depression and anxiety.

A. Components of an Emotion

Each emotion has three components: neural, expressive, and experiential. The neural and experiential components are essential in defining an emotion state. The role of expressive behavior in defining emotion is more complex because it is observable, socially communicative, and, even in early development, it begins to yield to voluntary control.

1. Neural Component

This component is defined in terms of the brain structures and neurotransmitters that function in emotion activation, emotion expression, and emotion experience. As described in the next section, neuroscience has provided considerable information on the substrates of the first two components but much less on the experiential component. The first function of the neural component is to evaluate the ongoing stream of information from our sense organs (e.g., eyes, ears) and to activate a change in emotion state when the situation requires it. In many circumstances, incoming sensory information demands no new emotion, and the neural substrates can continue their work of sustaining the emotion state already present in consciousness. In a person of positive mental health, the ongoing state is typically the emotion of interest, the emotion that motivates most of our constructive and creative endeavors, including play, the learning of abstract knowledge, and the acquisition of the skills that lead to mental and social competence.

In some cases, the information we obtain through our senses from internal and external events requires the activation of a new emotion. We know most about what happens in the brain when we perceive danger and the incoming information elicits fear. Neuroscientists have not yet explained the brain activities involved in the activation of other emotions. At present we can only speculate that processes similar to those in fear occur when a situation calls for joy, sadness, anger, or some other emotion.

Three things are important in evaluating the role of the neural component of emotion in mental health; however these things are not altogether independent of other systems. First, misperceptions and misinterpretations can fool the brain and cause it to generate an inappropriate or unnecessary emotion. Misperceiving a garden lizard as a poisonous snake or an innocuous remark as threatening will activate needless fear. Second, because the brain has separate pathways for spontaneous (involuntary) and intentional (voluntary) facial expressions of emotions, a person can intentionally deceive the observer. All that is required for deception is to learn to exert voluntary control over facial expressions of emotions, a skill which begins in toddlerhood. Use of the voluntarily controlled smile may be inconsequential in a social greeting, but deleterious as a sign of innocence after antisocial behavior. Third, genetic defects or injuries in certain brain structures can create dysfunction in the emotions system, and this can lead to serious deficits in social competence and to mental health problems.

2. Expressive Component

The face, body, and voice provide observable signals of emotion states. A facial expression of an emotion consists of a configuration of movements or any one of the several components of this configuration. Vocal expression of a given emotion changes several acoustic characteristics of the vocalization, and these are heard as changes in intonation or tone of voice. Bodily expressions produce changes in posture and gesture.

Of these three types of expressive behavior, facial expression has attracted the most research. Scientific interest in the face owes much to Charles Darwin. He made careful observations of facial expressions, inquired about them in many different cultures, and declared that facial expressions of the emotions were innate and universal. Although this view was questioned on the basis of psychological experiments and debated by proponents of the evolutionary and social-constructivist views, most behavioral scientists agree that Darwin made a valid conclusion—the facial signals of several of the emotions are products of evolutionary–biological processes.

Some scientists believe that expressive behavior consists not only of externally visible movement, but of internal activity as well. The most studied internal activities are those governed by the autonomic nervous system, such as heart rate, blood pressure, respiration, and the electrodermal response. Some evidence suggests that people differ in the extent to which they externalize or internalize emotion-related behavior. Externalizing is associated with extroversion and sociability, internalizing with introversion. In deviant development, externalizing is associated with antisocial and aggressive behavior, internalizing with depression and withdrawal.

Appropriate emotion expressions are critical to social communication and mental health from infancy throughout the life span. Either undercontrolled or overcontrolled emotion expression can be associated with the development of behavior problems and psychopathology. The mental health consequences of expression undercontrol or overcontrol vary across the different discrete emotions. For example, undercontrolled and frequent expressions of anger may be associated with aggressive conduct disorder, whereas frequent undercontrolled expression of sadness may be associated with depression. [*See* ANGER.]

3. Emotion Feelings: Experiential Component

Spontaneous or involuntary emotion expression is associated with underlying changes in particular brain structures and pathways that result in a change in the quality of consciousness. This new state of consciousness can be described as feeling, action readiness, and motivational condition. As already noted, this does not mean that a specific emotion expression and the corresponding specific emotion feeling are locked together. Biological maturation and social learning make for congruent and incongruent expression–feeling combinations. Voluntarily controlled, intentional emotion expressions are used for deception, manipulation, and symbolic communication.

Nevertheless, people's mental health and well-being demand that they maintain a reasonable degree of regularity in emotion expression–feeling congruence. Such congruence is the basis of trust and respect, crucial elements in the development and maintenance of social relationships. Each person in a relationship must feel confident in the assumption of a veridical association between a specific expression and a corresponding feeling. If a person continually invalidates this assumption through deceptive and manipulative emotion expressions, she destroys her relationships and jeopardizes her mental health. Because we make the assumption that spontaneous expressions are associated with corresponding emotion feelings, the implications of expressions and feelings for mental health are discussed together in a later section.

B. Emotions System

The concept of the emotions operating as a system provides insight into the roots of human behavior. A biological or biosocial system is a set of interrelated and interacting elements, and its level of complexity ranges from that of protein molecules, the building blocks of organisms, to human personality and social relationships.

Each discrete emotion functions as a system in that the three components are normally interdependent, interrelated, and interactive. The neural component functions as the proximal cause of emotion expression and emotion feeling. However, both of these latter components can influence the brain activity in emotion through feedback loops. Since Darwin, we have known that suppressing expression can dampen feeling, and we now know that this process is mediated by particular brain mechanisms.

In similar fashion, discrete emotions exert influence on each other. Sustained interest fosters children's play and the achievements and goal attainments that bring joy throughout life. Either acute shame or prolonged sadness sometimes leads to anger, and in some cases the sadness–anger pattern becomes a symptom

of depression and the shame–anger pattern produces aggression. The activation of anger decreases or eliminates fear. Dynamic relations between emotions account for important aspects of behavior and personality, including facilitation of emotion regulation.

C. Personality System

All of our biological and biosocial systems participate in the formation of the self-system and the supersystem termed personality. The emotions system and the cognitive system manifest themselves most prominently. The forming of connections and relations between emotion feelings and thoughts constitutes a major part of personality development. These feeling–thought or affective–cognitive structures reveal themselves as attachments, values, and goals. Through biological and social development, they also become organized as traits of personality. A number of studies have shown robust relationships between specific emotions or patterns of emotions and particular traits or broad dimensions of personality on the one hand and personality disorders on the other. For example, social interest and joy are part of extroversion, and the apparent absence of shame and guilt is a characteristic of antisocial personality disorders. [*See* PERSONALITY.]

III. NEUROPHYSIOLOGY OF EMOTIONS

Colloquial expressions are often used to describe emotional experiences. When one is angry, one's "blood boils"; when one is disgusted, one may be "sick" to one's stomach; or, when one is sad, one may develop a "lump" in one's throat. These metaphors all describe bodily activities that are concomitant with emotional experiences. Research into the neurological, hormonal, and autonomic nervous system processes involved in emotional experience has given us a greater understanding of these bodily changes and their implications for mental health.

A. Neural Networks in the Brain

The left and right hemispheres of the brain are involved differently in emotional processes: The right is more involved with the negative emotions such as fear and disgust, and the left is more involved with the positive emotions of interest and joy. Measurement of electrical activity within the left and right prefrontal and anterior temporal regions of the brain provides an indicator of both a person's emotional responsiveness to aversive situations and prevailing mood. People who have greater resting state activation in the right hemisphere than in the left hemisphere report (a) greater negative affect in response to watching fear-provoking and disgusting film segments, and (b) increased negative mood in general. This pattern of activation appears to be stable regardless of current emotional experience. People who had been previously depressed but who did not exhibit symptoms of depression for at least a year still showed greater right-hemisphere than left-hemisphere activation.

In addition to the left–right hemisphere distinction in positive and negative emotions, researchers agree that at least a few emotion-specific neural pathways exist within the brain. Most of the studies of neural circuits have been limited to experimental work with animals. Recent developments in brain imaging techniques make it possible to examine complex neural networks within the living human being and should usher in a period of discovery concerning emotions and the brain.

The one neural pathway that has been mapped well, at least within the rat's brain, is that for fear. The findings from the animal research on the neural pathways in the learning of a fear response are suggestive for understanding the fear process in humans. The results of this research are consistent with findings from work with brain-injured patients.

The fear response has two components: (a) conditioned neural networks that when confronted by particular stimuli activate an innate response, and (b) an innate response syndrome that entails mobilization of bodily resources. Processing of a sensory stimulus, such as a loud noise, first transmits information to the thalamus. From there, the neural message is transmitted to the amygdala (in the temporal lobe) along one of two pathways: an indirect path through the cerebral cortex, or a direct path through the thalamo-amygdala pathway. Neural messages travelling to the cortex are made more comprehensible there by more extensive information processing and evaluation. Neural projections from the cortex then carry this information to the lateral nucleus of the amygdala. The direct route from the thalamus to the amygdala does not require cortical processing of the neural message and is faster. It is rapid, automatic, and unconscious. Simple conditioning can be mediated along this pathway. Such conditioning is based on rudimentary assessment of the emotional significance of a stimulus by the amygdala. As with the thalamo-cortico-amygdala pathway, the direct thalamo-amygdala pathway involves the lateral nucleus of the amygdala.

The fact that the thalamo-amygdala pathway does not require cortical processing suggests that at times people may feel a response to threat without understanding the origins of their fear. Research with animals has shown that it is difficult to extinguish a conditioned fear response that was acquired through subcortical pathways without neocortical involvement. This suggests that some phobias that are difficult to extinguish may be based on inadequate cortical processing of the stimulus and its context.

Whereas the lateral nucleus is the input center of the amygdala, the central nucleus is responsible for output. If a stimulus is deemed emotionally significant, messages from the central nucleus are sent to trigger bodily responses. Neural pathways from the central nucleus to the bed nucleus of the stria terminalis and paraventricular nucleus within the hypothalamus control neuroendocrine responses (e.g., increased adrenaline output) that are involved in the body's response to stress. Neural pathways from the central nucleus to the lateral hypothalamus stimulate sympathetic autonomic nervous system activities (e.g., increased heart rate). Finally, neural pathways from the central nucleus to the central gray activate freezing and other defensive behaviors for coping with danger.

B. Neuroendocrine Response

Whereas researchers agree that mechanisms specific to particular emotions have been and will continue to be found in the neural networks of the brain, the bodily responses of hormone release and autonomic nervous system (ANS) reactivity do not seem as clearly linked to specific emotions. For example, the hypothalamic-pituitary-adrenal (HPA) axis, which produces corticotropin-releasing hormone, functions in both fear/anxiety and sad/depressive reactions. Abnormal regulation of this axis is a trademark of affective disorders pertaining to both anxiety and depression. The more general activation of neuroendocrine (i.e., hormonal) and ANS systems reflects the fact that a major function of emotional arousal is to prepare the body to respond to challenging or threatening stimuli. This state of preparedness includes similar physiological responses across different emotions.

Hormones associated specifically with negative emotions, and especially with emotional dysregulation, are corticotropin-releasing hormone (CRH) and adrenocorticotropic hormone (ACTH), both of which are involved in the production of another hormone, cortisol. A stimulus assessed as threatening can stimulate increased activity of the HPA axis and, in particular, can cause an increase in the production of CRH in the central amygdala and in the hypothalamus. The CRH produced in the amygdala increases sympathetic nervous system activity of the ANS, elevating attentional capacities and behavioral arousal. The CRH produced in the hypothalamus, along with other hormones, activates the production of ACTH in the anterior pituitary gland, Once circulated, ACTH then activates cells in the adrenal cortex to generate cortisol. Cortisol affects bodily functioning in multiple ways, such as elevating glucose (blood sugar) levels in circulation, increasing blood volume, and by interacting with the immune system. Prolonged stress and elevated cortisol level increases susceptibility to high blood pressure and autoimmune disease. In turn, these medical problems increase the risk of emotional dysregulation.

The release of cortisol, as measured in assays of saliva, is a reliable index of stress. For example, the greater the amount of time 18-month-old infants take to quiet after being inoculated, the higher the level of cortisol found in their saliva. Prolonged stress has multiple effects on HPA axis functioning: CRH production in the hypothalamus becomes less sensitive to paraventricular infusions and ACTH production in the pituitary becomes less sensitive to CRH infusions, but cortisol production in the adrenal cortex becomes more responsive to ACTH. This last effect is normally counterbalanced by a negative feedback system that inhibits the production of ACTH when increased levels of cortisol appear, allowing the gradual return of normal HPA axis activity. This negative feedback loop is suppressed in 40 to 70% of people hospitalized with depression, allowing for the hypersecretion of cortisol, and their adrenal glands tend to be abnormally large as well. After successful therapy for depression, however, HPA axis activity returns to normal, suggesting that the dysregulation of HPA activity within clinical populations is not a stable or innate trait. [See Psychoneuroimmunology.]

C. ANS Activity

The ANS activity in emotion-eliciting situations provides support for behavioral response. The ANS consists of the sympathetic nervous system, which is responsible for exciting most—but not all—visceral organs (e.g., the heart muscle), and the parasympathetic nervous system, which is responsible for inhibiting most—but, again, not all—visceral organs. Most research on emotion-specific physiology has involved the peripheral ANS, but, as mentioned previously, this research has produced limited results. A few studies have shown distinct patterns of activity in the sympathetic nervous system for some negative emotions but none for positive emotions. The positive emotions of joy and interest are not concomitant with readiness for physical action in the same way as negative emotions and, therefore, one might not expect as much differentiated ANS activity. Furthermore, negative emotions often involve similar types of behavioral readiness. For example, increased heart rate is found in both anger and fear because both emotional states require increased blood in the skeletomuscular system (e.g., the arm and leg muscles) and increased circulation of certain hormones (e.g., adrenaline).

Nevertheless, a few studies have found that under certain conditions some negative emotions can be differentiated by a complex pattern of several ANS responses. For example, whereas anger, fear, and sadness all entail heart rate acceleration, reflecting increased circulation of blood and oxygen to organs, disgust involves either no heart rate change or possibly even deceleration. Disgust often entails an orienting response, searching the environment for the aversive stimulus, and orienting is known to cause a heart rate deceleration. Compared with fear, anger creates greater diastolic blood pressure, less vasoconstriction, and greater blood flow to the periphery (e.g., the fingers) than fear. The phenomenon of "blood boiling" during anger is a result of this increased blood flow to the periphery, which subsequently increases the temperature of the peripheral region.

Differences relating to emotional responsiveness in general are related to differences in a person's parasympathetic nervous system activity. Stimulation of the vagus nerve decelerates heart rate (a parasympathetic function). Vagal tone is a measure of rhythmic fluctuations in heart rate related to respiration. Infants with higher vagal tone (i.e., greater heart rate variability) are more likely to be emotionally expressive and to sustain interest in stimuli. Furthermore, by 5 months of age, infants with higher vagal tone are more likely to respond to distress by regulating their emotions through processes such as looking at their mothers, at themselves in a mirror, or simply by vocalizing. Compared with infants of normal mothers, infants of depressed mothers show lower vagal tone (and thus higher heart rate) and increased cortisol levels as early as 3 months of age. Vagal tone amplitude is stable in the early years of life. The data suggest that because of dysfunction in the parasympathetic regulation of their heart rate, infants of depressed mothers may be at risk for symptoms related to sustained autonomic arousal. [*See* REACTIVITY.]

IV. EMOTIONS AND INTERPERSONAL FUNCTIONING

Human beings are social by nature, and a large part of our sociability relies on the expression and communication of emotions. Emotion regulation and the management of emotion expressions are critical to establishing satisfying and rewarding relationships and to good mental health. Emotion expressions give meaning and significance to social communication, and the quality of any relationship depends on the frequency and quality of expressed emotions. Emotion expressions especially influence the development and quality of a child's first relationship, that is, the attachment to the mother or primary caregiver. Children who have an easy temperament and readily express positive emotions elicit positive emotions from the caregiver. The mother's sensitivity and responsiveness to the child's emotion expressions and repeated and mutually satisfying reciprocal expressions of positive emotions foster the development of a secure attachment. The latter becomes a secure base from which the child can explore the social and physical environment. Easy temperament, positive emotionality, and a secure attachment to the primary caregiver serve as protective factors or buffers against the development of mental health problems. [*See* ATTACHMENT.]

In the context of any social relationship, expressions of emotions can be contagious and cause another person to respond with a similar emotion. The reciprocal activation of positive emotions strengthens a relationship and increases the satisfaction derived

from that relationship. The reciprocal activation of negative emotions has opposite effects. For example, the frequency of expressions of negative emotions helps predict marital satisfaction and the quality of family life. Similarly, the frequent expression of negative emotions has particularly deleterious effects when occurring within a family with members who have been diagnosed as mentally or physically ill. For example, in families with a member who is schizophrenic, the level of expressed negative emotion and criticism when this member lives at home plays a major role in his or her recovery and ability to remain free of symptoms. The most successful treatment of schizophrenia includes a combination of medications for the patient and family training to control the level of negative expressed emotion. After being hospitalized, patients with schizophrenia who return to families who express high levels of negative emotion show the highest rates of relapse.

A. Emotion Regulation

Emotion regulation is a broad term for the mechanisms and processes that enable people to keep their emotions from running out of control. Emotion regulation is realized in three ways through the development of (a) traits of temperament and personality, (b) specific cognitive and behavioral skills for managing emotions in challenging and stressful situations, and (c) a network of caring family members and friends who provide emotional support by sharing emotional experiences. The first of the three is relatively more influenced by genes and biological predispositions. A person with a "built in" easy temperament and positive emotionality has a head start in any situation that requires emotion regulation.

Regulation of negative emotions is important for the development of social competence and for the avoidance of behavior problems in children and adolescents. Uncontrolled expression of negative emotions is linked to a variety of clinical problems, including delinquency and drug abuse. Temper tantrums in the toddler are a pretty good predictor of behavior problems in later childhood and adolescence.

Emotion regulation can also be viewed in terms of its adaptive function, helping an individual to cope with self-doubt or stressful life events. When caught in a cycle of chronic expression of negative emotions, people become less able to solve problems and are more likely to jeopardize their relationships with others. With appropriate emotion regulation, attention may be focused on possible solutions to problems rather than on the experience of negative emotion expressions. [*See* EMOTIONAL REGULATION.]

At different points in development, the goals of emotion regulation are somewhat different. The following sections describe some of these differences within early development.

B. Emotional Development in Infancy

Infants have different emotional dispositions. Some people are highly reactive to stimuli, others are not as reactive. In a person's emotional development, one of the first goals is control over emotional reactivity or arousal. Three common behaviors infants use to regulate affective arousal, especially in response to aversive events, are (a) orienting toward their caretakers, (b) shifting their attention away from the stimulus, and (c) engaging in self-stimulation. Concerning the first behavior, when confronted with a novel stimulus, such as when a stranger enters a room, infants are likely to orient toward their mothers. By looking at their mother's facial expressions or by listening to their mother's vocal tones, they obtain information that enables an appropriate emotional response to a new stimulus. Similarly, once able to crawl, an infant's arousal is often attenuated by the infant distancing himself from the stimulus and seeking proximity to his caregiver. Second, when presented with an aversive stimulus, an infant's heart rate increases initially, but then decreases if and when the infant averts his or her gaze from the stimulus. Not surprisingly, an attenuated ability to avert attention from a stimulus in infancy relates to an increased susceptibility to experience negative emotions. This relationship between attentional ability and negative emotional experience holds true in adulthood as well. Finally, self-stimulation—such as sucking or rhythmic behaviors such as rocking or hand clasping—regulates emotional arousal. Sucking on a pacifier, for example, reduces both an infant's motoric and physiological arousal.

Although these three emotion regulation techniques are used by almost all infants, depending on the infant's disposition toward regulating his or her emotional reactivity, they are used to differing degrees. Some infants who are highly reactive to a novel stimulus (e.g., a stranger) are classified as *inhibited* (shy, fearful), and others who are less reactive are classified as *uninhibited*. Those who are classified as inhibited are more likely to engage in the previously described emotion regulation procedures of proximity-seeking to their caretakers, self-stimulation, and long periods of gaze aversion from aversive stimuli. Those who are classified as uninhibited are more likely to sustain attention to stimuli, especially if it is aversive, and are more likely to approach a novel stimulus. Inhibited infants also show more negative emotional expressions in response to novel stimuli, and uninhibited infants show more positive emotional expressions. From the earliest months of life these dispositions can be distinguished by the electrical activity in infants' right brain hemispheres relative to their left, their cortisol output, and the variability in their heart rate (e.g., vagal tone).

C. Emotional Development in Childhood

The inhibited and uninhibited patterns of response are important for understanding early mental health. Depending on the infant and young child's ability to regulate their emotional arousal, these early dispositional differences may lead to different childhood behavior problems. The inhibited preschooler who can regulate her emotional arousal well, especially by self-soothing, may be more reticent within social groups than other children but still be able to engage in constructive and exploratory behaviors and not exhibit socioemotional difficulties. The inhibited child who is not good at emotion regulation, however, is more likely to show anxiety within a social group and may even have difficulty engaging in constructive individual play activities. These inhibited young children are later more likely to show signs of anxiety and depression. Uninhibited infants also can develop behavior problems in early childhood. Uninhibited young children who are poor at emotion regulation are more likely than others to show impulsiveness and aggression toward playmates.

D. Stressful Environments and Emotional Development

Infants and children raised in stressful environments show deviations from more typical emotional development. Research has focused on two types of stressful situations in particular: infants and young children with depressed caretakers, and maltreated children. Concerning the first of these, early in life, infants depend on their caretakers to help with their regulation of emotion, for example, by eliminating stimuli such as loud noises that are stressful to the infant. Infant emotional expressions (e.g., crying) are the primary means by which the infant communicates these needs to the caretaker. When an infant's emotion expressions continually fail to be met by reparative actions by the caretaker, the infant's emotional assertions change. Because depressed caretakers are in general less interactive with their infants, these infants are at risk for maladaptive emotional functioning. This altered functioning includes a lack of interest in communicating with adults, a limited range of emotional experience, and irritability.

Second, children raised in homes with recurring conflict between parents become more sensitive to cues related to impending conflict and show increased negative reactions. This phenomenon is found especially among physically abused children. In response to interadult anger, physically abused children show greater fear, heightened arousal and aggression, and are more likely to focus on the distressful stimuli. This hypervigilance in attention can be protective, as children are more able to anticipate situations that are beneficial to avoid, but it also leads to an overreaction to other, nonthreatening, stimuli. For example, maltreated children are often found to respond with anger and aggression to signs of distress from peers. This hypersensitivity to mildly negative emotions seems to be an integral link between parental maltreatment and the peer rejection experienced by many abused children. Maltreated children may seem "cold" to peers because they react negatively to somewhat ambiguous situations. Compounding this hypersensitivity, maltreated children are also less able to identify correctly others' emotion expressions, are less verbal about their own emotions, and are more likely to attribute hostile intentions to other children's behaviors and statements. [See CHILD MALTREATMENT.]

V. EMOTION AND PSYCHOPATHOLOGY

As the primary motivating forces for cognition and action, emotions figure prominently in normal and abnormal behavior. In one sense, the real source of men-

tal health problems is not the emotions but the poor or missing connections between emotions, thoughts, and deeds. Anger can become strongly linked to interpersonal violence, but typically this is not the case. A little anger can facilitate appropriate self-assertiveness without leading to any form of aggression. A similar argument can be made for an adaptive function in each of the basic emotions. Extreme emotional states can become maladaptive, and such states can be caused by extremely stressful conditions or a brain malfunction from a genetic defect or injury. On the other hand, under a wide range of conditions, emotions motivate and organize adaptive thought and action and are forces for positive mental health.

In any case, in normal and abnormal behavior, emotion and cognition and action affect each other in a reciprocal fashion. In disorders where thoughts and perceptions are dysfunctional, the appropriate emotion information processing and emotion expression are also disordered, causing a breakdown in social communication. In disorders characterized by extreme emotion feeling states, processes that are normally adaptive become disordered, causing behavioral dysfunction.

Lack of emotion feelings and inappropriate emotion expressions have been implicated in several types of psychopathology. These problems relate to dysfunction in the ability to evaluate the emotional significance of events (emotion information processing ability), an inability to modulate emotion expressions in accord with social norms, an abnormal need for stimulation, and an excessively high or low threshold for the activation of emotion feelings. Emotions play a role in a variety of disorders, including schizophrenia, personality disorders, and alexithymia, and in those designated as affective disorders (e.g., depression, manic-depressive disorder).

A. Emotions and Schizophrenia

Schizophrenia is a disorder of perception and cognition that may be largely inherited. Because emotions are frequently activated by perceptual and cognitive processes such as appraisal and comparison, it follows that a dysfunction in cognition may result in emotional disturbance. Some individuals suffering from schizophrenia appear emotionally unresponsive. Their emotion is said to be "flat" or "bland." This suggests a defect in information processing or in the neural mechanisms (particularly the amygdala and hippocampus) that evaluate the emotional significance of an event and enable memory of its context. The deficiency in appropriate emotion expression does not mean that the schizophrenic is always devoid of emotional experience. Their cognitions may result in their being very emotional, but their cognitions are quite different from those that activate emotions in normal individuals.

Disturbances of emotion in the schizophrenic can also take a different form. A schizophrenic may perceive a person or situation in qualitatively different ways. Two opposite feelings may arise simultaneously and produce intense ambivalence. In this case, the individual may act in bizarre ways to try to resolve the emotional battle raging within. Conversely, these opposite feelings may lead to a paralysis of action, leaving the individual unable to react to the stimuli.

These dysfunctions in emotion information processing relate not only to the experience of emotion within the schizophrenic individual but also to an inability to recognize emotions that other people are expressing. As part of their general disordered perceptual ability, schizophrenics are less able to discriminate faces and decode the emotions that are being facially communicated. This adds to the difficulty the schizophrenic experiences in trying to communicate with others. The lack of shared symbols and meaning attributed to facial expression and situations prevents meaningful exchange in interpersonal relations. [*See* SCHIZOPHRENIA.]

B. Emotionality and Personality Disorders

It has been observed that individuals diagnosed with antisocial personality disorder are suffering from a chronic level of underarousal in the brain and nervous system. This may manifest itself in the appearance of being emotionally flat. "Emotional poverty" is one of three broad categories that have been used to describe the sociopathic personality. Sociopathic individuals do not experience emotions in the same way as normal people do. In contrast to the schizophrenic, who may experience inappropriate emotions, sociopaths seem to lack the capacity to sustain emotions such as sadness, anger, and complex emotional experiences such as love and grief. Because they are chronically underaroused and deficient in their ability to empathize with others, the emotion feelings that ordinarily inhibit sociopathic behavior (guilt, sadness) are not sufficiently activated to inhibit the antisocial behavior. This may cause a sociopath to commit crimes that would be regulated in the normal person by the appropriate emotion feelings.

Because of their lack of emotion, sociopaths do not usually commit "crimes of passion." They are not driven to action by intense emotion such as anger, but rather commit "cool" crimes such as burglary, forgery, and fraud. These crimes rely more on cunning and calculation than on a surge of emotion. When sociopaths are involved in violent crimes, it is more a result of impulsive behavior uninhibited by the appropriate emotion and with no anticipation of moral guilt. Indeed, a sociopath's lack of conscience and continual failure to behave according to societal expectations is most likely a direct result of his or her inability to experience and understand the normal range of human emotions.

C. Emotions and Alexithymia

Alexithymia is a disturbance that affects one's ability to identify and describe one's own feelings. It is associated with illnesses affecting both physical and mental health. The incidence of alexithymia is associated with somatic complaints in both clinical and normal populations. It is also more commonly found in patients with cancer and diabetes, and in individuals suffering from substance abuse and post-traumatic stress disorder, than in the nonclinical population.

Persons who report having grown up in emotionally restrictive families that did not permit free expression of emotions are at greater risk for developing alexithymia than the general population. The best predictor of alexithymia is growing up in a home where positive communication is minimal. The more uncomfortable and ambivalent individuals are about expressing emotion, the higher their levels of alexithymia.

D. Emotions and Affective Disorder

Affective disorder describes the disorders of mood, which include depression and manic-depression (which is also called bipolar disorder). Clinical depression encompasses a variety of symptoms, including those that are designated as primarily emotional. The most salient symptom of depression is the experience of sadness. Common adjectives associated with the depressive state are feeling sad, miserable, blue, hopeless, lonely, and unhappy. All of these words refer to the overwhelming sense of sadness that characterize a depressed person.

Another emotional symptom of depression is called anhedonia. This state describes a loss of interest and pleasure in life experiences. Even activities that were once enjoyed are made dull and uninviting by depressive mood. Depression also affects biological drives— food no longer tastes as good, and sexual activity is undesirable. Loss of interest and enjoyment may be initially limited to only a few areas of life, but as the severity of the depression increases, the individual's sense of inability to experience positive emotions pervades all areas of life. Interest in the pleasures derived from hobbies, recreation, and relationships diminishes so that in some cases there seems to be no reason to get out of bed and face another day.

Eighty to 95% of depressions are unipolar, meaning they involve symptoms of only one pole of the affective spectrum, depression. However, the 5 to 20% of depressed individuals who suffer from bipolar disorder have symptoms of depression and mania. Although the dysfunctional emotional symptoms are the same in the depressed phase of manic-depression as in unipolar depression, there are new mood symptoms that appear during the manic phase. These symptoms include a highly elevated positive mood that may be accompanied by periodic irritability. The positive mood is traditionally described as euphoria, suggesting enjoyment, but "highly intense interest" or "extreme excitement" may be better descriptions. [*See* MOOD DISORDERS.]

There are underlying patterns of emotions that relate to temperament and personality and, consequently, to psychopathology. For example, the phenomenology of depression includes far more than sadness. Continued and unrelieved sadness often evokes anger, and, in the depressed person, the anger may be turned inward. A sense of failure and inadequacy may elicit shame. Shame can also elicit anger, and the anger may be turned on the self because the depressed person perceives the self as incompetent. Thus, on average, depressed people describe their emotional experience in terms of sadness, anger, shame, and inner-directed hostility. The latter may include inner-directed disgust and contempt as well as anger. [*See* DEPRESSION.]

The phenomenology of anxiety, like that of depression, also includes a pattern of emotions. Whereas sadness is the key emotion in depression, fear is the dominant emotion in anxiety disorders. The anxiety pattern may also include shame, shyness, and guilt. There is some overlap in the phenomenology of anxiety and depression in terms of the discrete emotions in the two patterns. Responses to self-reported measures of emotion feeling states in these two types of disorders overlap each other. The distinguishing feature of each is its key emotion—sadness in depression and fear in anxiety. [*See* ANXIETY.]

VI. EMOTION AND PSYCHOTHERAPY

Because emotions are essential for adaptive cognition and behavior, they also play a significant role in psychotherapy. Individual psychotherapists' conceptualizations of emotion will influence the choice of which specific aspect of a client's current functioning and past life he or she will focus on during the therapy session. Theories of emotion suggest that emotion results from interactions between several systems, including cognitive, behavioral, perceptual, and neurophysiological, but many therapists choose to focus on only one of these aspects in their treatment of disorders.

A. Rational–Emotive Therapy and Emotion

Rational–emotive therapy deals with the interrelationship of emotion and thought. Consistent with cognitive theories of emotion activation, the founder of rational–emotive therapy, Albert Ellis, proposes that emotions result from an individual's internal dialogue. As a person conducts an internal dialogue, even irrational phrases and sentences about the self that are frequently repeated can become beliefs that elicit negative emotions. For example, a person who repeatedly questions her or his own abilities comes to believe those internal musings and becomes insecure and doubting of those abilities when there is no real basis for doubt. Ellis believes disorder stems from a set of common incorrect beliefs that inevitably lead to disappointment and failure and the accompanying negative emotions. An irrational belief system might lead a person to think that she needs to be loved and approved of by everyone in her community and that she needs to be competent and capable in every aspect of life. It may include the beliefs that unhappiness is a result of external and uncontrollable forces, past events are determinants of present functioning without the possibility of change, a perfect solution to life's problems exists, and that not finding this solution is catastrophic. The aim of therapy is to identify and extinguish the irrational and illogical beliefs.

B. Cognitive Therapy and Emotion

Another cognitive model, mainly attributed to Aaron T. Beck, postulates that maladaptive schemas (cognitive structures) result in negative emotional and behavioral responses. These schemas cause a person to make consistently negative conclusions about themselves, the world, and the future. Thus an emotional disturbance is maintained and fueled by these negative attributions. Therapy tries to identify and extinguish these distorted cognitions through cognitive and behavioral exercises designed to reduce negative symptoms. [See COGNITIVE THERAPY.]

C. Client-Centered Therapy and Emotion

Carl Roger's client-centered therapy stands in sharp contrast to cognitive behavioral therapies. Rogerian therapy relies heavily on the technique of reflecting the client's feelings. The therapist attempts to empathize with the client. Empathy enables the therapist to reflect the client's true feelings. In addition, the therapist uses verbal and nonverbal expressions of emotion as the primary tool for showing the client unconditional positive regard, an essential element in client-centered therapy. The theory postulates that if the client feels unconditionally accepted within the therapeutic relationship, emotions, feelings, and events will be more comfortably and willingly examined and understood.

VII. EMOTION AND PREVENTION

The evidence for the primary role of emotions in mental health and social competence points to the need for interventions to prevent emotion-related disorders and the consequences which may occur from unhealthy experiences and expressions of emotions. Programs have targeted at-risk children to help them develop appropriate emotion regulatory skills that may lessen the manifestations of problem behavior. As noted earlier, interventions have also been directed at families of patients with schizophrenia or bipolar disorder. Other types of interventions help people recover from and control the stress-related aspects of cardiac disease and also to recover from being victims of crime.

A. Intervention and Parenting

Dysfunctional parenting often involves expression of inappropriate levels of emotion (either too high and abusive, or too low and neglectful). As a result, children show behavioral problems and may perform poorly in school. Prevention can be effectively directed to the parents to help them understand their roles in teaching their children the skills for appropriately expressing and regulating emotions, especially negative emotions. [See PARENTING.]

B. Intervention and Expressed Emotion

Intervention programs aimed at families of schizophrenic patients significantly help to reduce relapse of symptoms when the patients return home. Returning home to a dysfunctional family environment, in which negative emotions and criticisms are expressed at a high level, serves as a risk factor for relapse and reemergence of the symptoms associated with schizophrenia. Similarly, key relatives of bipolar patients have an effect on relapse and rehospitalization, depending on the relatives' level of expressed negative emotions. An intervention program that reduces the relatives' expressed negative emotions reduces the relapse rate in the patients.

C. Intervention and Cardiovascular Disease

Other areas of research have shown a relationship between emotion and cardiovascular disease in which people who experience more stress, anxiety, and hostility are more prone to heart disease. Preventive programs try to help individuals change their lifestyles to reduce their levels of stress-related emotions, particularly hostility. Conclusions suggest that maintaining mental health through emotion regulation and healthy levels of expression may prevent cardiovascular disease.

D. Intervention and Coping with Crime

A Dutch intervention program highlights the role that appropriate emotion expression can play in enabling a crime victim to cope with burglary. Police officers were trained to administer an interview that was aimed at facilitating emotion and problem-focused coping. Victims felt greater positive regard for the police, a greater sense of being protected, and less concern about the crime.

Because emotions are so central to our functioning as human beings, there are many ways that improving the experience of emotions, enhancing the ability to regulate emotions, or changing the level of emotions expressed in the family can improve a person's psychosocial functioning. Mental health professionals can help teach the skills of emotion regulation and problem solving to improve mental health and social competence.

BIBLIOGRAPHY

Berenbaum, H., & James, T. (1994). Correlates and retrospectively reported antecedents of alexithymia. *Psychosomatic Medicine, 56,* 353–359.
Ekman, P., & Davidson, R. J. (Eds.). (1994). *The nature of emotion: Fundamental questions.* New York: Oxford University Press.
Izard, C. E. (1991). *The psychology of emotion.* New York: Plenum.
Lazarus, R. (1991). *Emotion and adaptation.* New York: Oxford University Press.
Plutchik, R., & Kellerman, H. (Eds.). (1990). *Emotion: Theory, research, and experience: Vol. 5. Emotion, psychopathology, and psychotherapy.* San Diego: Academic Press.

Epidemiology: Psychiatric

Ronald C. Kessler

Harvard Medical School

Shanyang Zhao

Temple University

AXES The *Diagnostic and Statistical Manual of the American Psychiatric Association* system uses a multiaxial method of evaluating psychiatric disorders to elicit information for planning treatment and predicting outcomes. The only axes discussed here are Axis I, pertaining to mental disorders, and Axis II, pertaining to developmental and personality disorders.

DSM *Diagnostic and Statistical Manual of the American Psychiatric Association*. Version III (*DSM-III*), published in 1980, and Version III-R (*DSM-III-R*), published in 1987, are the systems used to operationalize the disorders in the recent epidemiologic surveys presented here.

ICD The World Health Organization's International Classification of Diseases, a diagnostic system that is used in most parts of the world. The *DSM* system, used in the United States, has many features in common with the ICD classification scheme for psychiatric disorders, but the two systems also differ in a number of important respects that hamper cross-national comparative epidemiologic studies.

EPIDEMIOLOGY is the study of the patterns and correlates of illness in a population. Descriptive epidemiology is concerned with the distribution of illness onset and course. Analytic epidemiology uses nonexperimental data to elucidate causal processes involved in illness onset and course. Experimental epidemiology is concerned with the development and evaluation of interventions aimed at modifying risk factors in order to prevent illness onset or modify illness course. Most epidemiologic studies of psychiatric disorders are either descriptive or analytic. Experimental studies are, for the most part, limited to preventive interventions for children, although there are also a small number of preventive interventions for high-risk adults.

I. HISTORICAL OVERVIEW

Descriptive psychiatric epidemiologic studies comparing admission and discharge rates of asylums were carried out as early as the seventeenth century. However, it was not until the beginning of the nineteenth century that analytic epidemiologic studies of psychiatric disorders began to appear. These early studies typically documented associations that were interpreted as showing that environmental stresses can lead to psychiatric disorders. For example, in 1820, in one of the best known of these early studies, Burrows documented an association between admission rates to British mental asylums and crop failures. Later in the century, in the most famous psychiatric epidemiologic study conducted in nineteenth century America,

Jarvis documented a relationship between poverty and insanity in the 1850 Massachusetts Census.

Most of these early studies were hampered by the fact that they focused on treatment statistics, which confounded information about help-seeking with information about illness prevalence. In the few cases where they relied on population data rather than on treatment statistics, as in the Jarvis study, concerns existed about accuracy of assessment. Indeed, the initial data collected by the Massachusetts Census takers for Jarvis' study were so clearly biased by underreporting that Jarvis had to carry out a second census of more than 1700 physicians, clergy, and other key informants who were enlisted to identify the insane people in their communities. This key-informant method continued to be the mainstay of psychiatric epidemiologic studies from the time of Jarvis until the beginning of World War II. Although this method was useful in avoiding the help-seeking biases associated with treatment studies and the concealment biases associated with self-report studies, key informants tended to miss people whose disorders were characterized more by private distress than public acting out. This led to an underestimation of disorder as well as to a distorted picture of disorders being much more prevalent among men than women.

The end of World War II brought with it the beginning of modern psychiatric epidemiology, in which studies were carried out with direct interviews of representative community samples. Sometimes these studies were carried out by clinicians and at other times by lay interviewers. In some cases, these studies combined interview data with record data and used clinician evaluations of all available data to arrive at caseness designations. In later studies, clinical judgment was abandoned in favor of using objective self-report symptom rating scales that assigned each respondent a score on a continuous dimension of nonspecific psychological distress. Research based on these continuous measures of distress had an advantage over research based on the assessment of dichotomous measures of caseness in that the former dealt more directly with the actual constellations of signs and symptoms that existed in the population than with the classification schemes imposed on these constellations by clinical raters. Another advantage was that the clinical raters typically used poorly specified criteria, whereas the rating scales were based on clearly defined criteria.

There were also disadvantages to working with distress measures. The most important of these was that there was nothing in these measures themselves that allowed the researcher to discriminate between people who did and did not have clinically significant psychiatric problems. This discrimination is important for purposes of making social policy decisions regarding such things as the number of people in need of mental health services. Researchers who worked with measures of nonspecific psychological distress often dealt with this problem by developing rules for classifying people with scores above a certain threshold as psychiatric "cases." However, considerable controversy surrounded the decision of exactly where to put these cut points.

It was not until the 1970s that the field was able to advance beyond this controversy with the establishment of clear research diagnostic criteria and the development of systematic research diagnostic interviews aimed at operationalizing these criteria. The early interviews of this type required administration by clinicians, which yielded rich data but limited their use in epidemiologic surveys because of the high costs associated with large-scale use of clinicians as interviewers. These interviews led to advances in epidemiologic studies of patient samples. However, as it is enormously expensive to carry out clinician-based epidemiologic surveys of this sort, it is not surprising that only a handful of such studies were carried out during the past two decades and that these studies were either quite small, based on samples that were not representative of the general population, or were conducted outside the United States.

Two responses to this situation occurred. The first was the development of two-stage screening methods in which an inexpensive first-stage interview carried out by lay interviewers could be administered to a very large community sample, followed by a more expensive second-stage clinical interview administered only to a subsample of the initial respondents who screened positive and a subsample of those who screened negative. The hope was that this two-stage design would substantially reduce the costs of carrying out clinician-administered community epidemiologic surveys. However, there were problems with reduced response rates and increased logistic costs that resulted in this approach not being widely used.

The second response was the development of research diagnostic interviews that could be administered by lay interviewers. The first instrument of this type was the Diagnostic Interview Schedule (DIS), which was developed with support from the National Institute of Mental Health (NIMH) for use in the Epidemiologic Catchment Area (ECA) Study. The ECA was a landmark study in psychiatric epidemiology in which more than 20,000 adult respondents from catchment areas within five U.S. communities, including not only those living in households but also those in institutional settings such as nursing homes and hospitals, were interviewed in an effort to establish the lifetime and recent prevalences and correlates of common psychiatric disorders. The enormous amount of information provided by the ECA study has led to a great many replications in other parts of the world, to the development of more elaborate and valid structured diagnostic interview schedules, and to a more recent nationally representative survey of psychiatric disorders in this country.

This entry provides a brief overview of the results regarding the descriptive epidemiology of psychiatric disorders among adults in the United States based on these recent studies. No attempt is made to review research on child or adolescent mental health, mental health problems of the elderly, or the mental health of special populations such as the homeless and residents of nursing homes. The reader interested in these more focused populations is referred to recent reviews cited in the bibliography. Also excluded is a review of the substantial literature on the analytic epidemiology or experimental epidemiology of psychiatric disorders. The focus here is on measures of psychiatric disorder as assessed in the *Diagnostic and Statistical Manual* (*DSM*) of the American Psychiatric Association (APA) as operationalized in the DIS and in the more recently developed Composite International Diagnostic Interview. Most of the results reported here are based on the *DSM-III-R* because this is the system that has been the basis for most recent general population research on the prevalence of psychiatric disorders.

II. MODERN SURVEYS

Modern data on the general population descriptive epidemiology of psychiatric disorders among adults in the United States are based largely on two sources. The first is the ECA Study. The ECA has been the main source of data in the United States on the prevalence of psychiatric disorders and use of services for these disorders for the past decade. However, an important limitation of the ECA Study for purposes of providing representative data is that it was carried out in nonrepresentative catchment areas in only five communities around the country: New Haven, Baltimore, Durham, St. Louis, and Los Angeles. Although the ECA investigators used after-the-fact weighting procedures to combine these local data into a consolidated data file that was representative of the country as a whole on the distribution of age, sex, and race, no attempt was made to adjust the sample for the distributions of such important variables as socioeconomic status or health insurance coverage. Furthermore, it was impossible to apply any type of weighting or adjustment procedure to compensate for the fact that the five ECA sites were all in urban areas that contained large university-based hospitals. As the interviews were conducted entirely within the metropolitan areas containing these hospitals, the results tell nothing about areas of the country that have low access to specialty mental and addictive services, including rural areas that are not contiguous to a major metropolitan area. Twenty percent of the U.S. population live in such rural areas.

This problem was subsequently addressed when the NIMH funded a second major epidemiologic study, the National Comorbidity Survey (NCS), a household survey of more than 8000 respondents in the age range of 15 to 54 that was carried out in a widely dispersed (174 counties in 34 states) sample designed to be representative of the entire United States. The NCS interview used a modified version of the DIS known as the Composite International Diagnostic Interview (CIDI). The CIDI expands the DIS to include diagnoses based on *DSM-III-R* criteria. World Health Organization (WHO) field trials of the CIDI have documented adequate reliability and validity for all diagnoses. However, it is important to recognize that most of the WHO field trials were carried out in clinical samples. Previous research has shown that the estimated accuracy of diagnostic interviews is greater in clinical samples than in general population samples. Therefore, caution is needed in interpreting the results of the ECA and NCS.

III. LIFETIME AND RECENT PREVALENCES OF AXIS I *DSM-III-R* DISORDERS

We focus in this section on descriptive results from the NCS because this is the only nationally representative survey in the United States to have assessed the prevalences of a broad range of *DSM-III-R* disorders. The NCS is based on a national household sample of respondents in the age range of 15 to 54. The results in Table I show NCS/*DSM-III-R* prevalence estimates for the lifetime and 12-month disorders assessed in the core NCS interview. Lifetime prevalence is the proportion of the sample who ever experienced a disor-

der, and 12-month prevalence is the proportion who experienced the disorder at some time in their lives and who also reported an episode of the disorder in the 12 months prior to the interview. The prevalence estimates in Table 1 are presented without exclusions for *DSM-III-R* hierarchy rules. Standard errors are reported in parentheses.

The most common psychiatric disorders assessed in the NCS are major depression and alcohol dependence. Seventeen percent (17.1%) of respondents reported a major depressive episode in their lifetime, and 10.3% had an episode in the past 12 months. Fourteen percent (14.1%) of respondents had a life-

Table I Lifetime and 12-Month Prevalences of CIDI/*DSM-III-R* Disorders in the NCS

	Male				Female				Total			
	Lifetime		12-Month		Lifetime		12-Month		Lifetime		12-Month	
Disorders	%	(SE[a])	%	(SE)	%	(SE)	%	(SE)	%	(SE)	%	(SE)
A. Affective disorders												
Major depressive episode	12.7	(0.9)	7.7	(0.8)	21.3	(0.9)	12.9	(0.8)	17.1	(0.7)	10.3	(0.6)
Manic episode	1.6	(0.3)	1.4	(0.3)	1.7	(0.3)	1.3	(0.3)	1.6	(0.3)	1.3	(0.2)
Dysthymia	4.8	(0.4)	2.1	(0.3)	8.0	(0.6)	3.0	(0.4)	6.4	(0.4)	2.5	(0.2)
Any affective disorder	14.7	(0.8)	8.5	(0.8)	23.9	(0.9)	14.1	(0.9)	19.3	(0.7)	11.3	(0.7)
B. Anxiety disorders												
Panic disorder	2.0	(0.3)	1.3	(0.3)	5.0	(1.4)	3.2	(0.4)	3.5	(0.3)	2.3	(0.3)
Agoraphobia without panic	3.5	(0.4)	1.7	(0.3)	7.0	(0.6)	3.8	(0.4)	5.3	(0.4)	2.8	(0.3)
Social phobia	11.1	(0.8)	6.6	(0.4)	15.5	(1.0)	9.1	(0.7)	13.3	(0.7)	7.9	(0.4)
Simple phobia	6.7	(0.5)	4.4	(0.5)	15.7	(1.1)	13.2	(0.9)	11.3	(0.6)	8.8	(0.5)
Generalized anxiety disorder	3.6	(0.5)	2.0	(0.3)	6.6	(0.5)	4.3	(0.4)	5.1	(0.3)	3.1	(0.3)
Posttraumatic stress disorder	4.8	(0.6)	2.3	(0.3)	10.1	(0.8)	5.4	(0.7)	7.6	(0.5)	3.9	(0.4)
Any anxiety disorder	22.6	(1.2)	13.4	(0.7)	34.3	(1.8)	24.7	(1.5)	28.7	(0.9)	19.3	(0.8)
C. Addictive disorders												
Alcohol abuse	12.5	(0.8)	3.4	(0.4)	6.4	(0.6)	1.6	(0.2)	9.4	(0.5)	2.5	(0.2)
Alcohol dependence	20.1	(1.0)	10.7	(0.9)	8.2	(0.7)	3.7	(0.4)	14.1	(0.7)	7.2	(0.5)
Drug abuse	5.4	(0.5)	1.3	(0.2)	3.5	(0.4)	0.3	(0.1)	4.4	(0.3)	0.8	(0.1)
Drug dependence	9.2	(0.7)	3.8	(0.4)	5.9	(0.5)	1.9	(0.3)	7.5	(0.4)	2.8	(0.3)
Any substance abuse/ dependence	35.4	(1.2)	16.1	(0.7)	17.9	(1.1)	6.6	(0.4)	26.6	(1.0)	11.3	(0.5)
D. Other disorders												
Antisocial personality	4.8	(0.5)			1.0	(0.2)			2.8	(0.2)		
Nonaffective psychosis[b]	0.3	(0.1)	0.2	(0.1)	0.7	(0.2)	0.4	(0.1)	0.5	(0.1)	0.3	(0.1)
E. Any NCS disorder	51.2	(1.6)	29.4	(1.0)	48.5	(2.0)	32.3	(1.6)	49.7	(1.2)	30.9	(1.0)

Note. Reproduced from Kessler et al. (1994). *Archives of General Psychiatry 51*, 8–19. Copyright 1994, American Medical Association.

[a] SE, standard error.

[b] Nonaffective psychosis includes schizophrenia, schizophreniform disorder, schizoaffective disorder, delusional disorder, and atypical psychosis.

time history of alcohol dependence and 7.2% continued to be dependent in the past 12 months. The next most common disorders are social and simple phobias, with lifetime prevalences of 13.3% and 11.3%, respectively, and 12-month prevalences of 7.9% and 8.8%, respectively. As a group, addictive disorders and anxiety disorders are somewhat more prevalent than affective disorders. Approximately one in every four respondents reported a lifetime history of at least one addictive disorder and a similar number reported a lifetime history of at least one anxiety disorder. Approximately one in every five respondents reported a lifetime history of at least one affective disorder. Anxiety disorders, as a group, are considerably more likely to occur in the 12 months prior to interview (19.3%) than either addictive disorders (11.3%) or affective disorders (11.3%), suggesting that anxiety disorders are more chronic than either addictive disorders or affective disorders. The prevalence of other NCS disorders is quite low. Antisocial personality disorder (ASPD), which was only assessed on a lifetime basis, was reported by 2.8% of respondents, while schizophrenia and other nonaffective psychoses (NAP) were found among only 0.5% of respondents. It is important to note that the diagnosis of NAP was based on clinical reinterviews using a clinician-administered interview rather than on the CIDI alone.

As shown in the last row of Table I, 49.7% of the sample reported a lifetime history of at least one NCS/*DSM-III-R* disorder and 30.9% had one or more disorders in the 12 months prior to the interview. Although there is no meaningful sex difference in these overall prevalences, there are sex differences in prevalences of specific disorders. Consistent with previous research, men are much more likely to have addictive disorders and ASPD than women, while women are much more likely to have affective disorders (with the exception of mania, for which there is no sex difference) and anxiety disorders than men. The data also show, consistent with a trend found in the ECA, that women in the household population are more likely to have nonaffective psychoses than men. [*See* Alcohol Problems; Anxiety; Depression; Substance Abuse; Mood Disorders.]

IV. COMORBIDITY AMONG AXIS I DISORDERS

The sum of the individual prevalence estimates across the disorders in each row of Table 1 consistently exceeds the prevalence of having any disorder in the last row. This comorbidity is quite important for understanding the distribution of psychiatric disorders. Although it is beyond the scope of this entry to delve into the many different types of comorbidity that exist in the population, some aggregate results are important to review. The results in Table II document that these patterns are important. Fifty-two percent of respondents never had any NCS/*DSM-III-R* disorder, 21%

Table II Concentration of Lifetime and 12-Month CIDI/*DSM-III-R* Disorders among Persons with Lifetime Comorbidity in the NCS

No. Lifetime Disorders	Sample		Lifetime disorders		12-Month disorders		Respondents with severe 12-month disorders[a]	
	%	(SE[b])	%	(SE)	%	(SE)	%	(SE)
0	52.0	(1.1)						
1	21.0	(0.6)	20.6	(0.6)	17.4	(0.8)	2.6	(1.7)
2	13.0	(0.5)	25.5	(1.0)	23.1	(1.0)	7.9	(2.1)
3 or more	14.0	(0.7)	53.9	(2.7)	58.9	(1.8)	89.5	(2.8)

Note. Reproduced from Kessler et al. (1994). *Archives of General Psychiatry 51*, 8–19. Copyright 1994, American Medical Association.

[a] Severe 12-month disorders includes active mania, NAP, or active disorders of other types that either required hospitalization or created severe role impairment.

[b] SE, standard error.

had one, 13% had two, and 14% had three or more disorders. Only 21% of all of the lifetime disorders occurred to respondents with a lifetime history of just one disorder. This means that the vast majority of lifetime disorders in this sample (79%) are comorbid disorders. Furthermore, an even greater proportion of 12-month disorders occurred to respondents with a lifetime history of comorbidity. Close to 6 out of every 10 (58.9%) 12-month disorders and nearly 9 out of 10 (89.5%) severe 12-month disorders were reported by the 14% of the sample with a lifetime history of three or more disorders. These results show that although a history of some psychiatric disorder is quite common among persons 15 to 54 years old in the United States, the major burden of psychiatric disorder in this sector of society is concentrated in a group of highly comorbid people who constitute about one sixth of the population.

V. MAJOR DEPRESSION

Although it is impossible to discuss all of the disorders in depth here, it is of interest to examine more detailed results about some of these disorders. This section focuses on major depression (MD). Epidemiologic research has documented a number of consistently significant correlates of MD, including stressful life events, low social support, personality, and a range of demographic variables such as low socioeconomic status, and being female and young. Studies of twins have also documented powerful genetic influences on depression. Current research based on genetically informative designs is attempting to combine information about environmental and genetic risk to construct a more complete picture of their joint effects, which includes the possible influence of gene–environment interactions in which genetic factors influence sensitivity to environmental risks.

The higher prevalence of MD among women has been of special interest. This sex difference has been found consistently in community epidemiologic studies throughout the world using a variety of diagnostic schemes and interview methods, with a prevalence among women between 1½ and 3 times that found among men. Research on the sex difference in MD has emphasized the importance of stresses associated with adult sex roles based on the observation that the sex difference is most pronounced among middle-aged

married men and women. However, recent research has shown that this is an inadequate explanation because while women are more likely than men to become depressed, they do not remain depressed longer than men once onset has occurred. This is inconsistent with an argument that chronic sex-role stresses lead to the sex difference. Furthermore, research has shown that the sex difference in onset risk first emerges before full adult sex role differentiation, usually shortly after the onset of puberty, and decreases near the end of midlife, a pattern that is inconsistent with adult sex role theories of depression. This last observation raises the possibility that sex hormones are somehow implicated in the sex difference in depression. This possibility is being explored in studies that are collecting data on sex hormones in the context of developmental epidemiologic surveys.

VI. POSTTRAUMATIC STRESS DISORDER

It has long been known that pathological stress response syndromes can result from exposure to war, sexual assault, and other types of trauma. However, research on the prevalence of these disorders was unsystematic prior to the codification of diagnostic criteria in *DSM-III* under the diagnosis of Posttraumatic Stress Disorder (PTSD). A number of traumas have been studied in detail since that time. The empirical information and conceptual refinements generated by this research have significantly advanced our understanding of posttraumatic stress responses and have led to revisions of the diagnostic criteria for PTSD in *DSM-III-R*. These criteria require (a) exposure to a traumatic event that is "outside the range of usual human experience"; (b) reliving the experience in either nightmares, flashbacks, or intrusive thoughts; (c) numbing or avoidant symptoms; and (d) hypersensitivity, either as indicated by general signs and symptoms of autonomic arousal or by hypersensitivity to cues reminiscent of the trauma. These symptoms must persist for at least 1 month.

Several epidemiologic surveys have found results consistent with the NCS that 10 to 12% of women and 5 to 6% of men have a lifetime history of PTSD. Estimates of the lifetime prevalence of trauma exposure in the NCS are that more than 60% of men and more than 50% of women experienced at least one traumatic event in their life; the majority of people with some type of lifetime trauma actually experience two or more traumas. The existence of multiple traumas in the lives of many people has been found in other research as well. A significantly higher proportion of men than women experience physical attacks and combat, or being threatened with a weapon, held captive, or kidnapped. A significantly higher proportion of women than men experience sexual molestation and rape. The probability of a trauma leading to PTSD varies substantially across trauma types, with research on this issue consistently finding that rape is the trauma most likely to provoke PTSD among women and combat experience to provoke it among men.

What little is known about the course of PTSD suggests that it is typically a very chronic disorder. In the NCS, survival curves based on retrospective reports suggest in the estimate that the median time to remission is 3 years among those who seek professional treatment and more than 5 years among those who do not. Somewhat more than one third of persons with PTSD fail to remit even after many years. [*See* POST-TRAUMATIC STRESS.]

VII. PERSONALITY DISORDERS

As with PTSD, the concept of personality disorder can be traced back to the beginnings of nineteenth century psychiatry. However, it has only recently become the subject of epidemiologic research because standardized diagnostic criteria only became available for the first time in the 1970s. Unfortunately, it has proven to be difficult to develop reliable and valid measures of personality disorder. Furthermore, there are a number of differences among contending diagnostic systems that add to the complexity of synthesizing the available epidemiologic evidence.

All classification schemes recognize three broad clusters of personality disorder, each defined by a series of traits that must be manifest habitually in a number of life domains to qualify as a disorder. These three are the odd (e.g., paranoid or schizoid personality disorders), dramatic (e.g., histrionic or borderline personality disorders), and anxious (e.g., avoidant or dependent personality disorders) clusters. A recent comprehensive international review of the epidemiology of personality disorder found only four fairly small community studies that assessed personality disorder in all three of these clusters using valid

assessment methods. These four studies yielded very consistent lifetime prevalence estimates for overall personality disorder ranging from 10.3% to 13.5%. A prevalence of 11.0% was found in a subsequent nonpatient survey of personality disorder. Caution is needed in interpreting these results, however, as previous research has shown that prevalence estimates vary substantially depending on whether, as in these surveys, full diagnostic criteria for personality disorder are required or respondents are counted if they manifest some traits of personality disorder on dimensional scales.

There have also been a number of community surveys that included assessments of one or more specific personality disorders without attempting to assess the full range of personality disturbances. By far the most commonly studied of these has been antisocial personality disorder, a disorder characterized by persistent evidence of "irresponsible and antisocial behavior beginning in childhood or early adolescence and continuing into adulthood." Irritability, aggressiveness, persistent reckless behavior, promiscuity, and the absence of remorse about the effects of this behavior on others are cardinal features of antisocial personality disorder. A number of epidemiologic surveys, including both the ECA and NCS, have found lifetime prevalences of antisocial personality disorder to average about 1% among women and 4 to 5% among men. Much less is known about the prevalences of other individual personality disorders, although the available evidence suggests that none of them alone has a prevalence greater than about 2% in the general population. [*See* PERSONALITY.]

VIII. OVERVIEW

The results reviewed here show that psychiatric disorders are highly prevalent in the general population. Although no truly comprehensive assessment of all Axis I and Axis II disorders has ever been carried out in a general population sample, it is almost certainly the case that such a study would find that the majority of the population met criteria for at least one of these disorders at some time in their lives. Although such a result might initially seem remarkable, it is actually quite easy to understand. The *DSM* and ICD classification systems are very broad. They both include a number of disorders that are usually self-limiting and not severely impairing. It should be no more surprising to find that half the population has met criteria for one or more of these disorders than to find that the majority of the population has had the flu or measles or some other common physical malady at some time in their lives.

The more surprising result is that even though many people have been touched by mental illness, the major burden of psychiatric disorder in the population is concentrated in the relatively small subset of people who are highly comorbid. This means that having a pileup of multiple disorders is the most important defining characteristic of serious mental illness, a result that points to the previously underappreciated importance of research on the primary prevention of secondary disorders. It also means that epidemiologic information about the prevalences of individual disorders is much less important than information on the prevalences of functional impairment, comorbidity, and chronicity. This realization has led to interest concerning functional impairment in changes to the diagnostic criteria in *DSM-IV*.

This emphasis is also evident in the focus of the NIMH National Advisory Mental Health Council on what it defined as "severe and persistent mental illness" (SPMI) and of the Substance Abuse and Mental Health Service Administration on what it defined as "serious mental illness" (SMI). Joint methodological analyses of the ECA and NCS suggest that the 1-year prevalences of *DSM-III-R* SPMI and SMI are approximately 3% and 6%, respectively, compared with 1-year prevalences of any *DSM-III-R* disorder, which is in excess of 30%.

It is likely that epidemiologic research on adult mental disorders over the next decade will focus on these severe disorders rather than on overall prevalence. To the extent that the prevalences of particular disorders are emphasized in this research, it will likely be to study the underlying pathologies associated with ongoing impairment in functioning. An increased interest in the part played by personality disorders in the creation of ongoing role impairment is likely to emerge over the next decade in light of recent advances in conceptualization and measurement. There is also likely to be a considerable expansion of research on the epidemiology of child and adolescent disorders due to new initiatives, which have not yet advanced far enough to be reviewed here. In addition, epidemiologic

research based on genetically informative designs (e.g., twin and adoption samples) is likely to grow in importance. Important new risk factor results, such as the evidence that Apoliprotein E alleles are risk factors for Alzheimer's disease, will continue to be explored. Finally, with the growth of managed care it is likely that a new emphasis on maintaining wellness will evolve. This, in turn, will likely lead to an increase in experimental epidemiologic research aimed at developing preventive interventions for people at high risk of psychiatric disorders. [*See* ALZHEIMER'S DISEASE; MANAGED CARE.]

ACKNOWLEDGMENTS

Preparation of this article was supported by the National Institute of Mental Health (grants R01-MH46376, R01-MH49098, K05-MH00507, and T32-MH16806), the National Institute of Drug Abuse (through a supplement to R01-MH46376), and the W.T. Grant Foundation (grant 90135190).

BIBLIOGRAPHY

Burrows, G. M. (1820). An Inquiry Into Certain Errors Relative to Insanity and Their Consequences, Physical, Moral, and Civil. London: Thomas & George Underwood.

De Girolamo, G., & Reich, J. H. (1993). *Epidemiology of mental disorders and psychosocial problems: Personality disorders*. Geneva: World Health Organization.

Dryfoos, J. G. (1990). *Adolescents at risk: Prevalence and prevention*. New York: Oxford University Press.

Fischer, P. J., & Breakey, W. R. (1991). The epidemiology of alcohol, drug, and mental disorders among homeless persons. *American Psychologist, 46*, 1115–1128.

Henderson, A. S. (1994). *Dementia: Epidemiology of mental disorders and psychosocial problems*. Geneva: World Health Organization.

Jarvis, E. (1855). Report on Insanity and Idiocy in Massachusetts, by the Commission on Lunacy, under resolve of the Legislature of 1854. Boston: William White, printer to the state.

Kessler, R. L., McGonagle, K. A., Zhao, S., Nelson, C. B., Hughes, M., Eshelman, S., Wittchen, H. V., & Kendler, K. S. (1994). Lifetime and 12-month prevalence of DSM-III-R psychiatric disorders in the United States: Results from the National Comorbidity Survey. *Archives of General Psychiatry, 51*, 8–19.

Mazure, C. (Ed.). (1995). *Does stress cause psychiatric illness?* Washington, DC: American Psychiatry Press.

Robins, L. N., & Regier, D. A. (Eds.). (1991). *Psychiatric disorders in America: The Epidemiologic Catchment Area Study.* New York: Free Press.

Roses, A. D. (1996). Apoliprotein E alleles as risk factors in Alzheimer's disease. *Annual Review of Medicine, 47,* 387–400.

Strahan, G. W. (1990). Prevalence of selected mental disorders in nursing and related care homes. In R. W. Manderscheid & M. A. Sonnenschein (Eds.), *Mental Health, United States.* (DHHS Publication No. (SMA) 94-3000. Washington, DC: U.S. Government Printing Office.

Tsuang, M. T., Tohen, M., & Zahner, G. E. P. (Eds.). (1995). *Textbook in psychiatric epidemiology.* New York: Wiley & Sons.

Verhulst, F. C., & Koot, H. M. (1992). *Child psychiatric epidemiology: Concepts, methods, findings.* Newbury Park, CA: Sage.

Epilepsy

Henry A. Buchtel

Ann Arbor Veterans Administration Medical Center and University of Michigan

I. Overview
II. Prevalence and Incidence
III. Classification of Epileptic Seizures
IV. Impact on the Individual with Epilepsy
V. Causes and Diagnosis
VI. Nonepileptic Seizures
VII. Effects of Epilepsy on Cognition
VIII. Personality Changes and Behavioral Problems
IX. Treatment Options
X. Epilepsy Advocacy Groups
XI. Future Directions

Antiepilepsy Drug (AED) Medication prescribed to control seizures.
Aura A feeling or sensation that frequently precedes the seizure.
Electroencephalogram (EEG) Recording of electrical activity of the brain, usually with small flat electrodes glued to the scalp.
Epilepsy Surgery Surgical removal of brain tissue that has been identified as responsible for the seizures, or cutting of the neural band connecting the two hemispheres (surgery is generally sought when the seizures cannot be controlled by antiepilepsy medication).
Febrile Seizure A seizure that occurs during a high fever, experienced by about 5% of children.
Ictal Discharge Abnormal firing of neurons in synchrony during a seizure, frequently consisting of a repetitive "spike and wave" pattern.
Pseudoseizures Nonepileptic episodes that otherwise resemble real ("organic") seizures (the term is

considered pejorative and the term psychogenic seizures is preferred).
Seizure An episode of abnormal activity in the brain that causes a disturbance of consciousness or of sensory/motor functions.
Seizure Focus A defined area in the brain that is the origin of an epileptic seizure.

EPILEPSY is a behavioral manifestation of a brain disturbance that causes synchronous firing of large numbers of neurons. Its incidence in the population and the severity of the disability in millions of individuals makes this a serious health problem worldwide. Diagnosis depends on a careful analysis of the person's behavior and the pattern of neuronal activity in the brain, sometimes supplemented by brain imaging studies. In some individuals, there is no discernible physiological cause of the seizures and a diagnosis of psychogenic seizures will be made, often with the help of someone in the mental health field. Psychologists and social workers often play a role in the choice of treatments and their implementation. Another role of the mental health worker is to point the person with epilepsy or that person's family to groups in the community and national groups that are dedicated to helping persons with this disorder.

I. OVERVIEW

Unlike most medical conditions, epilepsy is entirely defined by and diagnosed on the basis of publicly ob-

Encyclopedia of Mental Health
Volume 2

137

Copyright © 1998 by Academic Press.
All rights of reproduction in any form reserved.

servable behavior: the epileptic seizure. Purists will argue that epilepsy is not a disease but rather the symptom of an underlying neurological condition. Usually the seizure disorder is accompanied by an obvious abnormality in the electroencephalogram (EEG), but the presence of abnormal brain waves in the EEG is not a necessary condition for diagnosis. The condition has serious consequences for schooling, psychosocial development, and employment. Life expectancy is also reduced for persons with epilepsy, with mortality rates 2 to 4 times those of matched nonepilepsy persons. Treatment options have increased markedly in the past 50 years, and strictly behavioral treatments have been developed. Opportunities for a normal life with epilepsy are greatly improved compared with even a generation ago, and persons with seizures and their families are being involved increasingly in choosing treatments.

The earliest known descriptions of epilepsy are in the writings of Hippocrates (ca. 460–ca. 377 BC), most notably in his essay titled "On the Sacred Disease," so named because in ancient Greece, the inexplicable cause of seizures had led to the common belief that the person with epilepsy was periodically possessed by spirits (in more recent times, demons). Hippocrates denounced such interpretations as charlatanism and argued that this was a human disease with physical causes. In this interesting essay he also refers to the shame that is felt by those who have seizures, although it is clear from the following quote that he thought children would seek comfort whereas adults would choose to be alone during the seizure:

> But such persons as are habituated to the disease know beforehand when they are about to be seized and flee from men [to a place] where as few persons as possible will see them falling. . . . This they do from shame of the affliction, and not from fear of the divinity, as many suppose. And little children at first fall down wherever they may happen to be, from inexperience. But when they have been often seized, and feel its approach beforehand, they flee to their mothers, or to any other person they are acquainted with, from terror and dread of the affliction, for being still infants they do not know yet what it is to be ashamed. (¶15)

Many extraordinary individuals have had epilepsy, and writers have for centuries suggested a connection between genius and epilepsy. Although some of the early cases may be better classed as having episodes of insanity (Aristotle, who compiled a list of ancient epileptics, agreed with the Hippocratic view of a close relationship between epilepsy and insanity, which at

that time was attributed to black bile), the behaviors described often sound very much like seizures. Intriguingly, some have suggested that an aggressive drive needed for success may be caused by temporal lobe epilepsy. A partial listing of early famous persons with behaviors that may have been epileptic include Pythagoras (b580 BC), Socrates (b470 BC), Alexander the Great (b356 BC), Caesar (b100 BC), Caligula (b12 AD), and Mohammed (b569). Some later figures for whom epilepsy is clearly established or very likely include Petrarch (b1304), Charles V of Spain (b1500), St. Teresa of Avila (b1515), Cardinal Richelieu (b1585), Louis XIII (b1601), Moliere (Childhood; b1622), Pascal (b1623), Peter the Great (b1672), Handel (b1685), Napoleon (b1769), Paganini (b1782), Byron (b1788), Shelley (b1792), Dickens (Childhood; b1812), Edward Lear (b1812), Dostoyevski (b1821), Flaubert (b1821), Nobel (b1833), William Morris (b1834), Swinburne (b1837), Tchaikovsky (b1840), de Maupassant (b1850), and van Gogh (b1853). Interestingly, epilepsy among Queen Victoria's relatives in the late nineteenth century led to the founding of the internationally renowned National Hospital for the Paralysed and Epileptic at Queen Square, London (now known as The National Hospital for Neurology and Neurosurgery). It is probably obvious that these famous individuals are mentioned frequently in essays and articles for the general public in order to demythologize the illness and to provide inspiration for persons with epilepsy by showing that a normal or even extraordinary life can be led by persons with the disorder.

II. PREVALENCE AND INCIDENCE

Estimates of the prevalence of epilepsy in the general population, that is, the ratio of individuals affected to those unaffected, have varied from 2 per 1000 to 50 per 1000. The variability reflects the different definitions of what constitutes epilepsy (e.g., Does the diagnosis require a minimum seizure frequency? Are febrile seizures included? How accurate is the diagnosis?). On average, the most accurate estimates suggest that the prevalence is around 5 per 1000, meaning that in a city of 1,000,000 there would be 5000 individuals with seizures. Thus in the United States, with a population of around 250,000,000, there are approximately 1.5 million individuals with a seizure disorder. Twenty percent of these will have intractable seizures (uncontrollable using current treatments). Over a lifetime, 1 in 20 individuals (5%) will have at least one seizure; of those that have a seizure, 12% will develop chronic epilepsy (this suggests that the prevalence should be .12 × .05 or 6/1000 rather than 5/1000—the discrepancy probably reflects the increased death rate among persons with epilepsy, which is described in more detail in the next section.

The incidence of epilepsy (new cases in a particular time period) has been estimated to be about 0.5 to 1.0 per 1000 per year, meaning that in a group of 1,000,000 individuals there would be about 500 to 1000 new cases each year. Data from studies in Great Britain indicate that most seizure disorders begin in the age range of 0 to 4 years (.75/1000). The next most common ages of onset are 15 to 19 years (.53/1000), 10 to 14 years (.44/1000), and 5 to 9 years (.33/1000). All other age groups have incidence rates below .23/1000. Males and females appear to be equally affected; there are more left-handers with epilepsy than would be expected by chance.

III. CLASSIFICATION OF EPILEPTIC SEIZURES

In 1970, an international group established a classification scheme according to the **type of seizure**, consisting of four general classes, each with several subcategories, as shown in Table I.

IV. IMPACT ON THE INDIVIDUAL WITH EPILEPSY

Seizures are not just unpleasant and embarrassing experiences for the person with seizures. Epilepsy entails a significant increase in morbidity and mortality. Particularly important for the mental health clinician is the increased risk for serious depression (around 5% across all kinds of epilepsy and 3 to 4 times the national average; among persons with epilepsy, suicide is listed as cause of death in 7 to 22% of deaths). Studies since the turn of the century have consistently shown that the life expectancy of persons with epilepsy is shorter than in the rest of the population; the death rate of children with epilepsy 0 to 5 years of age is 1.3 times greater

Table I International Classification of Epileptic Seizures

I. Partial seizures (seizures beginning locally)
   A. Partial seizures with elementary symptomatology (generally without impairment of consciousness)
      1. With motor symptoms (includes Jacksonian seizures)
      2. With special sensory or somatosensory symptoms
      3. With autonomic symptoms
      4. Compound forms
   B. Partial seizures with complex symptomology (generally with impairment of consciousness); temporal lobe or psychomotor seizures
      1. With impairment of consciousness only
      2. With cognitive symptomology
      3. With affective symptomology
      4. With "psychosensory" symptomatology
      5. With "psychomotor" symptomatology (automatisms)
      6. Compound forms
   C. Partial seizures secondarily generalized
II. Generalized seizures (bilaterally symmetrical and without local onset)
      1. Absences (petit mal)
      2. Bilateral massive epileptic myoclonus
      3. Infantile spasms
      4. Clonic seizures
      5. Tonic seizures
      6. Tonic–clonic seizures (grand mal)
      7. Atonic seizures
      8. Akinetic seizures
III. Unilateral seizures (or predominantly)
IV. Unclassified epileptic seizures (owing to incomplete data)

than that of the general population; from 5 to 24 years of age, the rate is 6.6 times greater; and from 24 to 25 years of age, the rate is 3.7 times greater. During the period when persons with epilepsy were typically institutionalized, as many as 50% of them died of causes either directly or indirectly associated with their seizures. Among those whose deaths were directly attributed to seizures, about 12% died of status epilepticus (a continuous and uncontrollable seizure); many others died of the accumulative effects of multiple injuries sustained during seizures.

Still important but not directly life-threatening, childhood epilepsy also negatively affects educational achievement and, regardless of the age of onset, has an impact on the person's eventual employment level. About one third of children with epilepsy receive special educational support, and IQ increases linearly as a function of age of onset (from 83 for adults whose seizures began in infancy to 102 for those with adult onset). Equally serious, and probably not unrelated to the person's educational experiences, a person's ability to find employment is greatly reduced by epilepsy. In a 1973 survey, almost one half of persons with epilepsy reported that they had been turned down for a job because of their epilepsy, and 30% reported that they had lost at least one job because of seizures. Various studies over this century have shown that the unemployment rate among working-age persons with epilepsy is between 2 and 7 times the rate of unemployment in the general population. In general, an employer has the right to ask a prospective employee if he or she has any medical condition that will interfere with successful carrying out of the duties, so the reduction in employment opportunities may not be entirely the product of a prejudice against epilepsy itself. Loss of the ability to drive a car is mentioned by most persons with epilepsy as a major loss (the period of being seizure-free before driving again differs from place to place; e.g., in Michigan, it is 6 months, in Ontario, Canada, 1 year).

There have been reported cases of birth defects for women who use antiepileptic drugs (AEDs). In the overall population, the rate of birth defects is 2 to 3%, and the rate is slightly higher (0.5%) for women with epilepsy who are not taking medication. Women taking a single AED have a risk of about 6 to 7%, with some medications being more problematic than others. Taking several AEDs increases the risk even more. Unfortunately, seizure frequency may go up during pregnancy, so the need for AEDs may even increase. In some cases, the person's physician may feel that the risks of pregnancy are too great for the mother and child, and recommend that pregnancy be avoided. Finally, some AEDs reduce the effectiveness of oral birth control pills. As discussed later, the genetics of epilepsy suggest that children may inherit a predisposition to epilepsy, but not epilepsy itself. This means, for example, that a head injury would more likely lead to a seizure disorder if the person has close relatives with epilepsy.

Persons with epilepsy frequently suffer consequences when bystanders do not know what to do when they see a seizure occur. It was once believed that a soft object should be inserted between the person's teeth to prevent biting the tongue during a seizure. This is now highly discouraged. The proper response, if any, depends on the kind of seizure. In general, only a person having a generalized tonic–clonic seizure (grand mal) needs attention, and in this case the greatest help consists of remaining calm, helping the person gently to the floor, and loosening any tight clothing. Hot or sharp objects that could cause harm should be moved away. Placing a cushion or folded piece of clothing beneath the person's head can reduce the chance of a head injury, and turning the head to one side so the saliva can escape is a good idea. It is useless to try to interrupt the seizure; when the seizure is over, the person may need to rest or sleep. Seizures usually stop within several minutes, but if the seizure continues for 10 minutes or more, or if seizures follow in succession without a period of complete recovery, then medical attention should be sought (this could signal the beginning of status epilepticus). Focal (simple partial) seizures do not require any action on the part of observers. A person having a complex partial seizure should not be restrained unless the person is placing him/herself in danger. As in the case of a generalized seizure, hot or sharp objects should be removed. Partial seizures sometimes progress to a generalized seizure (secondarily generalized), so further precautions may be necessary.

V. CAUSES AND DIAGNOSIS

When classified according to the known or putative origin of the seizure disorder, there are three etiological categories.

1. *Symptomatic Epilepsy.* Symptomatic epilepsy comprises cases in which the seizures are one of the clinical manifestations of a neurological disorder, such as tuberous sclerosis, Sturge-Weber syndrome, and cerebral degenerative diseases. Alcohol withdrawal seizures would also fit into this category.

2. *Secondary or Organic Epilepsy.* This type of epilepsy results from nonspecific cerebral changes or damage that is permanent and nonprogressive, such as head trauma or perinatal anoxia (i.e., temporary lack of oxygen during a difficult delivery).

3. *Idiopathic Epilepsy.* This epilepsy is also referred to as cryptogenic, essential, pure, primary, or true. These are cases in which the cause is unknown; genetic factors may be involved in the etiology. About 75 to 80% of all cases of epilepsy are of this type.

An enormous amount of work has been dedicated to uncovering the biochemical events that are responsible for an epileptic seizure. It is likely that seizures are caused by a lack of inhibition in the region of the epileptogenic focus rather than by an increase of excitation of the neurons in that area, but both factors may need to be present for the initiation of many if not most seizures. An important factor thought to be involved in the development and expansion of an epileptogenic seizure focus is the so-called "kindling" phenomenon. This was discovered by Goddard at McGill in the 1960s while testing Hebb's theory of synaptic changes in learning and memory. Goddard found that if a restricted subcortical brain region of a rat was stimulated electrically over many days, an initially innocuous stimulus would eventually lead to seizures, presumably because of the establishment or strengthening of pathways that convey the excitation of the stimulus from a localized area to a more widespread region, and thereby eventually synchronous activity of the whole brain (a seizure). Although the causal connection is still controversial, the development of an epileptogenic focus in another part of the brain has been attributed to this kindling effect, with the "mirror focus" in the homologous position of the opposite hemisphere being a special candidate for this designation.

There are two distinct steps in the process of diagnosing epilepsy. First, the neurologist or general physician has to be convinced that the spells, which are almost always described secondhand by someone not well trained in observation, are characteristic of epilepsy and not some other illness, organic or otherwise (Table II). Abnormal EEGs are very helpful in confirming that the seizures probably have a physiological (organic) rather than psychogenic cause, but epileptiform brain activity (i.e., EEG abnormalities characteristic of epilepsy) can also be found in indi-

Table II   Distinguishing Characteristics of Epileptic and Nonepileptic Seizures[a]

Epileptic seizure	Nonepileptic seizure
Usual onset <12 years	Onset >12 years
Emotional but adequate description	Patient evades direct questions
No "shortage of breath" as aura	Shortage of breath or hyperventilation

Table II   *Continued*

Epileptic seizure	Nonepileptic seizure
Seldom visual aura	Often visual aura (twinkles/colors)
Cannot resist beginning of seizure	Often lengthy fights against the seizures
Often rising epigastric sensations in aura	No rising epigastric sensation
Status epilepticus not frequent	Often very long seizures (up to hours)
Bilateral synchronous tonic and clonic jerks	Alternating left and right jerks
Seldom turning of head	Alternating turning of head, often quick
Incontinence occurs	Incontinence very rare
Bystanders not often hit	Bystanders often hit or kicked
With bilateral jerks, unconsciousness	Can remember bilateral jerks
Short period of atonia after falling	Long periods of atonia
Understandable injuries, biting of tongue	Automutilation, strange injuries
With bilateral tonic–clonic seizure, no speech	Massive jerks together with speech
No rapid shivering	Rapid shivering
More flexion of trunk than extension	Arching of back
Neurological signs often present	No neurological signs on examination
After tonic–clonic seizures, minutes of coma	Consciousness after massive jerks
Seldom crying afterward	Often crying afterward
Malaise and passive afterward	Either relieved or complaining afterward
In focal epilepsy, seizures in sleep	No seizures during sleep
Usually some benefit from anticonvulsants	No or inconsistent reaction to AEDs
Bystanders worried	Bystanders often irritated by patient
Seizures usually not seen by doctor	Doctors often see seizures
Patient speaks about epilepsy only	Patient speaks of all kinds of complaints
Seldom non-anticonvulsant co-meds	History of many other drugs taken

[a] The presence of characteristics in the nonepileptic seizure column does *not* constitute sufficient evidence that the spells have a psychogenic origin. However, a preponderance of characteristics in this column would certainly raise the question that at least some of the person's spells may be nonorganic in origin.

viduals without seizures, and some persons with epilepsy have an apparently normal EEG between seizures. In rare cases, the seizure focus is too deep in the brain to be discerned by scalp electrodes, and the EEG will remain normal even during a seizure. If the spells are determined to be epileptic in nature, their cause needs to be found as that will dictate the appropriate treatment (e.g., medication or surgery). Sometimes the seizure is the first manifestation of the presence of a brain tumor. In this case, the malignancy of the tumor will need to be determined so the benefits of surgery can be weighed. If the seizure occurs in childhood, both the child and the family will need to be educated about epilepsy and the importance of following a medication regimen. In some patient groups, the cessation of seizures under medication control for 2 to 5 years may mean that the medications can be safely stopped without a return to seizures (stopping the medication too soon can lead to a resumption of seizures, which may now be harder to stop, possibly because of kindling effects as described earlier).

VI. NONEPILEPTIC SEIZURES

The vast majority of seizures have an organic basis, and mental health workers should assume that a patient or client with seizures has no control over their frequency, duration, or form. However, some seizures are nonorganic in origin and will need to be treated by nonmedical therapies. Nonepileptic seizures may be under conscious control (malingering), presumably because of secondary gain, or they may be outside the patient's control (e.g., Munchausen syndrome) and difficult to understand in terms of a supposed "reward" for the behavior. When the seizure is believed to be nonorganic in origin, it has been called a pseudoseizure or hysterical seizure, although these terms are generally discouraged because their pejorative connotations may interfere with effective communication with the individual and his or her family. One should also be aware of the fact that the majority of nonepileptic seizures occur in individuals who also have organically determined seizures (this probably explains why they are so good at mimicking the seizure behavior).

Withdrawal symptoms from alcohol dependency may occur for several days after abstinence. It is thought that postsynaptic supersensitivity is caused by alcohol's prolonged inhibition of a particular trans-

mitter system in the brain (the glutamatergic system). With alcohol withdrawal, approximately 15% of individuals will experience seizures, which can be successfully treated or prevented with anticonvulsants and/or sedatives (e.g., diazepam [Valium] or chlordiazepoxide [Librium]). The seizures in such cases are not expected to continue beyond the acute withdrawal period. Of course, individuals with a history of frequent falls during intoxication are at increased risk of seizures from brain damage, and in such cases, seizures may occur as a consequence even without the added effect of withdrawal. Recurrent hospitalization and detoxification appears to lead to increased risk for seizures at a subsequent detoxification, suggesting a kindling effect. [See ALCOHOL PROBLEMS.]

VII. EFFECTS OF EPILEPSY ON COGNITION

The performance of epilepsy patients on cognitive tests has been of great help in exploring the brain organization involved in perception, thinking, and reasoning. Memory functions of patients who have a seizure focus in the temporal lobe (or who have had an excision of part of their temporal lobe) have been particularly informative in breaking down memory functions into their component parts. A small number of patients have focal motor seizures that leave consciousness and cognitive abilities intact, but the vast majority of persons with epilepsy lose consciousness and are subsequently amnesic for the events that occurred during the episode. However, unlike the case of most psychiatric illnesses, these effects are discrete in time and the person can be entirely normal between seizures. Of significance for the mental health professional is that there can be lasting behavioral effects of the seizures (especially episodes of continuous seizure activity) and/or the effect of the brain damage that is the cause of the seizures in the first place. Factors to be considered when deciding whether a person is showing effects of a time-related decline in abilities include age of onset, the site of the focus or foci, treatment side effects (medication, surgery), effects of injuries sustained during a seizure (especially head injuries), and effects of status epilepticus or prolonged seizures with inefficient breathing. Age of onset has obvious effects on the acquisition of knowledge and on interpersonal relationships. Sometimes the effects of a seizure focus are direct (lowered attentional abilities), sometimes indirect (missing school for a school-age child). Overall, significant brain reorganization is much more likely if the brain damage and seizures onset occurs before the age of 6 years than after that age, with puberty providing a likely upper limit for the period of useful plasticity.

VIII. PERSONALITY CHANGES AND BEHAVIORAL PROBLEMS

There has been much written about the so-called "epileptic personality," some sensible and some bordering on the ridiculous. Lennox and Lennox in their 1960 book, *Epilepsy and Related Disorders,* point out that many of the personality characteristics supposedly associated with epilepsy are actually frequently seen in many institutionalized patients suffering from a variety of debilitating chronic physical illnesses. Therefore they cautioned against an overarching assumption that the epilepsy itself may cause a personality disorder. Nevertheless, the particular characteristics of epilepsy (sudden loss of consciousness and other bodily functions, uncertainty about when a seizure will occur and what danger it may engender, the attendant problems dealing with family and friends, etc.) make it likely that individuals with seizures will be at increased risk for psychological problems. Joseph A. Schwartz, a psychiatrist who often works with epilepsy patients, has found that consultation requests by neurologists mention personality disorders about 10 times more often for epilepsy patients than for patients with other neurological disorders. He has proposed that the problems experienced by persons with epilepsy be referred to as "social apraxia" in order to remove the moral opprobrium usually associated with the term personality disorder.

The auras themselves may resemble a psychotic experience (25% of auras involve a feeling or sensation; 15% involve a change in mood). It is not uncommon to become fearful before, during, and after seizures. These emotional concomitants are naturally associated primarily with temporal lobe seizure foci (because of the connection with the limbic system), with mood disturbances being more associated with left-sided foci than with a right-hemisphere foci (approximately 65% vs. 45%). Interestingly, depressed mood is sometimes alleviated after a seizure in these patients, much as electroconvulsive shock has been shown to be helpful in cases of severe intractable depression. Rarely, patients will experience a delayed psychotic episode 12 to 48 hours after a seizure. [*See* Depression.]

For these reasons and others, personality testing is often requested and may be used to help determine the origins of the various facets of the person's problem (especially in cases of possible nonorganic origins). Psychological assessments of epilepsy patients will naturally be tailored to reflect the needs of the patient and referral question. If the patient is being considered for epilepsy surgery, the assessment will include a full neuropsychological battery, with a focus on memory functions, but also assessing frontal, parietal, and occipital functions (prognosis for successful outcome is greatly improved if the neuropsychological findings point to a disturbance of functions of a single region of the brain). For psychosocial assessments, a commonly accepted instrument is Dodrill's 1977 Washington Psychosocial Seizure Inventory, a yes/no questionnaire of 132 questions about the epilepsy patient's feelings and attitudes concerning his or her seizure disorder (e.g., Do your seizures keep you from driving? Are you generally free from depression? Are you concerned people won't like you or want you around after a seizure?). There are 29 "Critical Items" that may suggest the need for further discussion or action (e.g., Do you often wish you were dead? Do you need vocational counseling?) and eight clinical scales assessing seven psychosocial areas and an overall index of adjustment:

1. Family Background (questions about relationships with family members, happiness, and security in the home, etc.)
2. Emotional Adjustment (questions about depression, feelings of hopelessness, fatigue, worry, etc.)
3. Interpersonal Adjustment (questions about the patient's relationships with people outside the family)
4. Vocational Adjustment (questions about problems at work)
5. Financial Status (questions about the patient's financial resources and feelings of financial security)
6. Adjustment to Seizures (questions about attitude toward the seizures, dread of the seizures, etc.)
7. Medicine and Medical Management (questions about the patient's perception of his or her doctors, compliance with medication regimen, etc.)
8. Overall Psychosocial Functioning

After scoring the responses, the clinician plots the scores on each of the clinical scales, noting where the major concerns are focused and taking appropriate action if indicated.

IX. TREATMENT OPTIONS

In the fifth century BC, when Hippocrates wrote "The Sacred Disease," epilepsy was treated by purifications, incantations, and magical spells. Certain foods were forbidden, as were particular kinds of clothing (e.g., goat skin) and fabric colors. Hippocrates thought such "treatments" were fraudulent and argued convincingly (largely on philosophical grounds) that the disease should be treated as any other physical illnesses. He concluded that the disease was hereditary (as discussed earlier, a predisposing hereditary component is in fact present in some cases). Hippocrates' explanation for the onset of epilepsy seems absurd today, being based as it was on his theories on the effect of phlegm as it moves within the body and the brain (the weather, southerly winds in particular, also played a role in Hippocrates' explanation, mainly insofar as they affect the production of mucus). His prescribed treatment was vague and appears internally inconsistent:

> And in this disease as in all others, he [the physician] must strive not to feed the disease, but endeavor to wear it out by administering whatever is most opposed to each disease, and not that which favors and is allied to it. For by that which is allied to it, it gains vigor and increases, but it wears out and disappears under the use of that which is opposed to it. But whoever is acquainted with such a change in men, and can render a man humid and dry, hot and cold by regimen, could also cure this disease, if he recognizes the proper season for administering his remedies, without minding purifications, spells, and all other illiberal practices of a like kind. (¶21)

It is likely that further relevant details of treatment were passed from physician to student during medical apprenticeship (some have even suggested that the Hippocratic writings were meant only for lay people and were therefore purposefully uninformative, with treatment secrets reserved for one-on-one training).

The prescription of treatments that are considered useless today continued well into this century. For reasons that are no longer clear, at the turn of the century even reputable physicians tried the so-called Corsican treatment, cauterization of the ears. Institutionalization of persons with epilepsy was common until the 1940s and they made up as much as 25% of the residents in institutional settings. This was at least in part the consequence of prejudice against the person with epilepsy, both by physicians and by the general public.

A. Medication (Drug) Therapies

Anticonvulsant medications are numerous and trials of new medications are common. Early attempts to find effective treatments do not sound very scientific by today's standards (Galen preferred mistletoe, reasoning that it is a plant that grows on oak and therefore resistant to falling, thus useful for the "falling disease," epilepsy). Bromides (sedatives made of compounds of bromine and another element, such as potassium) gained popularity in the second half of the nineteenth century and helped approximately half the patients, although side effects of long-term use (mental torpor) were unacceptable. The popularity of this drug was so great that around the turn of the century, over a ton of bromides were being delivered yearly to the main hospital treating epilepsy in London, England. In 1912, phenobarbital was found to control seizures better than any substance before it, and many of the current effective medications are variations on the molecular structure of this substance.

All anticonvulsants will cause side effects if the dose is high enough, but none of these medications should have unacceptable side effects in the vast majority of patients if the serum levels are kept within the therapeutic range. Around 4% of pediatric patients will need to switch to another anticonvulsant because of the severity of the side effects of the medication. Table III gives common antiepileptic medications and

Table III Common Antiepileptic Drugs (AEDs), Typical Effectiveness, and Relevant Common Side Effects (Registered names are for the United States unless otherwise noted)[a]

Carbamazepine (1,2,3)[b] (Tegretol): Especially effective for partial seizures; behavioral side effects in approximately 30% of pediatric cases; useful in posttraumatic seizure disorders. Many cause mild sedation, ataxia, disequilibrium, and visual blurring.

Clonazepam (4) (Klonopin, Rivotril): A benzodiazepine, often used as adjunctive therapy for absence seizures or generalized seizures; rarely the first choice except for myoclonic seizures (muscle jerks). May cause mild to severe sedation; rarely may cause ataxia, increased depression, or personality change.

Ethosuximide (5) (Zarontin): Particularly effective for absence seizures; sedative and gastrointestinal side effects are common.

Table III *Continued*

Gabapentin (1,2,3) (Neurontin): Well tolerated; usually used as adjunctive therapy with other AEDs. May cause mild sedation, ataxia, and disequilibrium.

Lamotrigine (1,2,3) (Lamictal): Usually used as adjunctive therapy with other AEDs. Side effects are less common than with carbamazepine and phenytoin. May cause mild sedation, ataxia, disequilibrium, and visual blurring.

Phenobarbital (1,2,3) (Luminal) Inexpensive, relatively safe. Previously used commonly with children, less commonly used with adults; behavioral side effects such as sedation or cognitive interference seen in up to 60% of pediatric cases. Rarely may cause increased depression and memory impairment.

Phenytoin (1,2,3) (Dilantin): Especially effective for partial seizures; behavioral side effects in approximately 15% of pediatric cases. May cause mild sedation, ataxia, disequilibrium, visual blurring, and sometimes gingival hyperplasia (swollen gums).

Primidone (1,2,3) (Mysoline): Behavioral side effects in approximately 20% of pediatric cases. May cause mild to severe sedation, especially initially; rarely may cause increased depression and memory impairment.

Valproate (1,2,3,4,5) (Depakene, Depakote, Epival in Canada, Epilim in Great Britain): Gastrointestinal side effects at the beginning of therapy are common; behavioral side effects are seen in approximately 15% of pediatric cases. May cause mild sedation, appetite stimulation (weight gain), and hair breakage.

Less Common AEDs

Clobazam (1,2,3) (Frisium in Canada and Great Britain): May cause mild to severe sedation; rarely may cause ataxia, increased depression, or personality change.

Diazepam (7) (Valium): A benzodiazepine. May cause mild to severe sedation; rarely may cause ataxia, increased depression, or personality change.

Felbamate (1,2,3,6) (Felbatol): May cause anorexia and weight loss, vomiting, and insomnia. Associated with unacceptably high incidence of aplastic anemia and hepatic failure.

Nitrazepam (4) (Mogadon in Canada and Great Britain): See Clonazepam.

Oxycarbazepine (1,2,3) Closely related to Carbamazepine, but with fewer interactions and possibly fewer side effects.

Vigabatrin (1,2,3) (Sabril in Canada and Great Britain): May cause sedation and weight gain; rarely may cause encephalopathy and personality change.

Zonisamide (1,2,3,4,6) (Excegran in Japan): May cause mild sedation and weight loss; rarely may cause memory impairment.

[a] The author thanks Linda Selwa and Thomas Henry for help in constructing this table.

[b] Typically used for: 1, simple partial; 2, complex partial; 3, tonic–clonic; 4, myoclonic; 5, absence; 6, atypical absence; 7, convulsive and nonconvulsive status epilepticus.

descriptions of some of their side-effects. [*See* PSY-CHOPHARMACOLOGY.]

B. Surgery

Surgical removal of brain tissue or the cutting of intrahemispheric commissures (corpus callosotomy) to eliminate a seizure disorder may seem an extraordinary treatment, but as it has become clear that the origin of the seizure lies in the brain, it has in some cases become the most viable option. Because in most cases epilepsy surgery is elective (i.e., not necessary to preserve life), psychological and neuropsychological findings assume an unusual importance in the decision-making process. Psychologists, social workers, and others in mental health provide essential input into the decision about whether or not to proceed to surgery. For surgery to be considered, the following six conditions should be met:

1. The seizures are uncontrollable even with high doses of anticonvulsants. Or if the seizures *are* controllable with high doses of medication, the side effects at these levels are unacceptable or dangerous. A watershed decision is made at this step to establish candidacy for surgery. Even if condition 1 is satisfied, some patients and their families may not want to proceed further toward brain surgery because of the possible dangers of surgery or in the hope that an effective medication will be developed in the near future.

2. The seizures are intolerable to the person experiencing them (sometimes this means that the person may be unemployable or the seizures may be dangerous or extremely unpleasant).

3. All or most of the seizures arise from a single focal brain region (i.e., removal of the focus—usually scar tissue within the gray matter of the brain—is likely to eliminate or reduce the seizures because there is no other potential source of seizures).

4. This seizure focus is accessible (i.e., it is in a part of the brain that can be exposed during surgery without undue risk to the patient).

5. The tissue that would need to be excised can be removed without intolerable consequences for the person with epilepsy (i.e., surgery would not lead to severe loss of cognitive abilities, such as speech or memory).

6. The individual has the internal psychological resources and a support network in place to help with postsurgery recovery and a successful transition to nonepilepsy status.

When the first two conditions are met, the patient begins a lengthy process to establish the remaining four conditions. Psychologists (usually neuropsychologists) are involved in conditions 3, 5, and 6. Condition 4 is the province of the neurosurgeon or neurologist. Condition 6 usually requires contributions from a social worker as well as the psychologist and nurse clinician working with the individual. On occasion, a patient will be told that before he or she can progress further toward surgery, an improvement in mood or a strengthening of the support network is needed. Different epilepsy surgery teams may differ in their threshold for this kind of problem.

Condition 3 usually includes a neuropsychological evaluation designed to pinpoint which brain areas are functioning at levels below expectation. This is important because if the pattern of cognitive strengths and weaknesses indicates bilateral involvement or damage to areas outside the region thought to harbor the epileptogenic focus, the prognosis for seizure control after surgery is worse. In the case of temporal lobe epilepsy, the memory functions for verbal and pictorial materials are tested (tapping speech- and nonspeech-hemisphere functions, respectively). Other examinations are usually done at the same time: EEG localization, brain scans, including computerized tomography (CT) or magnetic resonance imaging (MRI), and metabolic positron emission tomography (PET) or single-photon emission computerized tomography (SPECT). The ideal candidate for surgery has findings from all of these examinations that point to the same area of the brain as the probable origin of the seizures. Magneto-encephalography (MEG) is being developed as an alternative to EEG; it is reported to have a localizing accuracy of approximately 8 mm, compared with 10 mm for EEG. The test measures the magnetic field generated by cortical activity by using extremely sensitive detectors (strength of the field is about one billionth that of the earth's gravitational field). [See BRAIN SCANNING/NEUROIMAGING.]

If conditions 3 and 4 are satisfactorily answered, condition 5 is evaluated by using one or both of the following methods: (1) the Intracarotid Amobarbital Procedure (IAP; sometimes called the Wada Test, after Juhn Wada, the neurologist who introduced the technique at the Montreal Neurological Institute in the 1950s), or (2) speech mapping if the hemisphere to be operated on makes a contribution to normal language production and comprehension.

1. The Intracarotid Amobarbital Procedure

This test is designed to determine the hemispheric organization of speech abilities and to prevent post-surgery amnesia by eliminating candidates whose memory abilities depend on the tissue in the area to be respected. Typically, a small amount of sodium amobarbital (Amytal) is injected into the internal carotid artery, which serves most of the cerebral hemisphere on the same side. After the injection, the neuropsychologist has approximately 5 minutes to test cognitive functions of the nonaffected hemisphere. Language abilities are tested and new information is presented to determine whether memory mechanisms of the noninjected hemisphere are capable of forming new memories. If the person can speak and learn new information after the injection, the noninjected hemisphere is considered able to support language and memory functions.

2. Speech Mapping

If the epileptogenic focus is near regions of the brain that are required for language, the area near the proposed surgical removal needs to be mapped (mapping may also be needed for motor and sensory functions if the removal is near the primary sensory or motor cortices). Electrical stimulation is applied to the brain surface, usually during the surgery in the awake patient, although in some cases it may be preferable to stimulate the region using an implanted electrode array over an extended period before surgery. In the case of language functions, an interruption of speaking or comprehension during stimulation indicates that the underlying cortex should be left intact.

C. Nonmedical Therapies

Physicians rely primarily on medication or surgery to treat their epilepsy patients, but nonmedical treatments of seizure disorders have played at least a peripheral role throughout the history of the illness. On the most superficial level, patients themselves often feel that something in their environment or a modification of their behavior can affect the frequency, duration, or severity of their seizures, both positively and negatively. This knowledge, either because it is accurate or through a superstitious process, leads to modifications in behavior. Rarely, patients actually like the feeling of the aura or seizure and so find ways to trigger one. Visual stimulation, such as passing the fingers back and forth in front of the eyes, can elicit seizures, and flashing lights (photic driving) are used as part of the diagnostic workup, because they can frequently produce abnormalities in the EEG or actual seizures. Patients with visually evoked seizures learn to avoid visual conditions with flashing lights (e.g., strobe-illuminated dance halls) or repetitive moving patterns (e.g., a picket fence). Some people have their seizures elicited by any sudden stimulus that causes a mild startle reaction. Although it is difficult for a person to eliminate entirely the possibility of being startled, those around the patient can learn to reduce unexpected loud noises or sudden movements.

Other non-medication/non-surgical treatments include:

1. Behavioral approaches, often used adjunctively. These treatments work best when the activities of the neurologist treating the patient are carried out in concert with the behavioral work. Three types are most common: (1) behavior modification, reward management or reinforcement-based strategies; (2) therapy, self-control or cognitive and psychodynamic-based strategies; and (3) conditioning, psychophysiological methods (desensitization and classical conditioning extinction, of greatest use in reflex epilepsy).

2. Biofeedback using the EEG (e.g., individuals with seizures having a motor component may be able to learn to normalize the cortical neural firing patterns and thereby dramatically reduce seizure frequency); biofeedback using exhaled CO_2 (hyperventilation, which will cause a seizure in susceptible individuals, leads to a decrease in the CO_2 in exhaled breath; learning to increase CO_2 levels by means of biofeedback training may act in the opposite direction and decrease the frequency of seizures). [See BIOFEEDBACK.]

3. Special diet. One of these is the ketogenic diet, which is high in lipids (fats) and low in proteins and carbohydrates. This causes a condition in the body called ketosis, which appears to cause a rise in the threshold for seizures. This diet needs to be supervised closely by the person's physician. Fasting in the short term has the same effect. [See FOOD, NUTRITION, AND MENTAL HEALTH.]

4. Unconventional and as yet poorly studied treatments include the application of magnetic fields to the scalp over the seizure focus (applying to the brain a magnetic field within the same characteristics as seen when recording over the epileptogenic focus).

X. EPILEPSY ADVOCACY GROUPS

The Epilepsy Foundation of America (EFA) is an active group with hundreds of chapters and tens of thousands of members. The Foundation supports research into the causes and treatment of epilepsy and is a resource for professionals and patients and their families concerning new knowledge about epilepsy, treatment options, local experts, and support groups. Its Web Site contains much useful information for both professionals and lay persons. The National Tuberous Sclerosis Association also helps persons with epilepsy from tuberous sclerosis.

Epilepsy Foundation of America (EFA)
4351 Garden City Drive
Landover, MD 20785-2267
Local Phone: (301) 459-3700
Toll Free: (800) EFA-1000
Fax: (301) 377-2684
Web Site: http://www.efa.org

National Tuberous Sclerosis Association
8181 Professional Place, Suite 110
Landover, MD 20785-2226
Phone: 1-800-225-NTSA or 301-459-9888
FAX: 301-459-3094
E-mail: ntsa@ntsa.org or ntsa@aol.com
Web Site: http://www.ntsa.org

In Canada, contact:

Epilepsy Canada
1470 Peel Street, Suite 745
Montreal, Quebec, Canada
H3A 1T1
(514) 845-7866

The International League Against Epilepsy publishes *Epilepsia*, a scientific journal containing articles on basic and applied research into causes and treatment of seizure disorders. The American Epilepsy Society (AES) has yearly meetings for its members, with scholarly presentations on all aspects of epilepsy.

Additional information on the Ketogenic diet can be obtained from The Johns Hopkins Pediatric Epilepsy Center (410) 955-9100 or The Charlie Foundation to Help Cure Pediatric Epilepsy (800) 367-5386.

Books for the general public include:

Devinsky, O. (1994). *A guide to understanding and living with epilepsy*. Philadelphia: Davis.

Evans, M. (1953). *A ray of darkness*. New York: Roy. Possibly the most readable description of the experience of an epileptic attack.

Gumnit, R. J. (1990). *Living well with epilepsy*. New York: Demos.

Gumnit, R. J. (1995). *The epilepsy handbook: The practical management of seizures* (2nd ed.). New York: Raven.

Gumnit, R. J. (1995). *Your child and epilepsy: A guide to living well*. New York: Demos.

Lechtenberg, R. (1984). *Epilepsy and the family*. Cambridge, MA: Harvard University Press.

XI. FUTURE DIRECTIONS

At the time of this writing, efforts are underway in a number of domains of importance to mental health workers concerned with epilepsy. Persons with epilepsy, after a long history of being fairly passive in their treatment, are beginning to be asked to play a more active or even a central role in the management of their illness. Toward this end, they and their family members are being asked about the impact of their illness with established questionnaires such a the WPSI and the Quality of Life in Epilepsy Inventory; similarly, families are being given a larger role when the physician considers the advisability of discontinuing antiepileptic medication after an interval without a seizure (usually more than 2 years). In cases of epilepsy, as well as other illnesses in which the person's behavior may modulate the progression of the disease process, the increasingly active role that members of the public are playing in determining the nature of their medical care is a positive one that should be encouraged by mental health professionals.

BIBLIOGRAPHY

Dam, M. & Gram, L. (Eds.). (1991). *Comprehensive epileptology*. New York: Raven.

Epilepsy Foundation of America (1975). *Basic statistics on the epilepsies*. Philadelphia: Davis.

Hippocrates (1964). The sacred disease. In *The theory and practice of medicine* [reprint of Francis Adams (1849) translation] pp. 356–357. New York: Philosophical Library. Also available at http://www.mit/techclassics.html.

Lennox, W. G. (1960). *Epilepsy and related disorders* (with the collaboration of Margaret Lennox). Boston: Little, Brown.

Mostofsky, D. I., & Løyning, Y. (1993). *The neurobehavioral treatment of epilepsy*. Hillsdale, NJ: Lawrence Erlbaum.

Sackellares, J. C., & Berent, S. (Eds.). (1996). *Psychological disturbances in epilepsy*. Boston: Butterworth-Heinemann.

Sands, H. (1983) *Epilepsy: A handbook for the mental health professional*. New York: Bruner/Mazel.

Temkin, O. (1971). *The falling sickness: A history of epilepsy from the Greeks to the beginnings of modern neurology (2nd ed.)*. Baltimore: Johns Hopkins.

Internet Resources (accurate as of 10/97):

Frequently asked questions about epilepsy: http://debra.dgbt.doc.ca/~andrew/epilepsy//FAQ.txt

Massachusetts General Hospital information about epilepsy surgery: http://neurosurgery.mgh.harvard.edu/epil-nih.htm

Information Guide from the National Institute of Neurological Disorders and Stroke: http://www.ninds.nih.gov/healinfo/disorder/epilepsy/epilepfs.htm

On-Line questions and answers from persons with epilepsy: http://dem0nmac.mgh.harvard.edu/neuroweb-forum/EpilepsyMenu.html (the "0" in the first part of this URL is a "zero", not the letter "O")

For an up-to-date listing, search for "Epilepsy" using one of the Web Search pages.

Ethics and Mental Health Research

Diane Scott-Jones and Ralph L. Rosnow

Temple University

Confederate   Someone who is presented as a research participant but who is surreptitiously working with the investigator in some manner to set up the study.

Confidentiality   The protection of the participant's disclosures against unwarranted access.

Debriefing   The investigator's interaction with each participant at the end of the research for the purpose of revealing the true nature of the study, removing any misconceptions, and allaying any negative emotions, attitudes, or thoughts of the participant.

Ethics   The rules of conduct by which the morality of a study or the investigator's behavior is judged.

Informed Consent   A procedure in which prospective participants (or their legal guardians) voluntarily agree to participate in the research after being told about the purpose of the study, including the nature of the instruments to be used and any anticipated risks and benefits.

Institutional Review Board (IRB)   A designated regulatory body mandated by federal regulations that is maintained at every institution that applies for federal funding of research. It is responsible for assessing whether proposed and ongoing studies meet ethical standards.

Minimal Risk   A designation for research in which the likelihood and extent of harm to the participants are no greater than that typically experienced in everyday life or in routine physical or psychological examinations or tests.

Placebo   A procedure intended to have no effect, but represented as a treatment, usually given to a control group to provide a comparison with an experimental treatment intended to have an effect.

Privacy   The freedom of individuals to claim protection against unwarranted access to information about themselves.

Protocol   The written plan of a proposed study describing its purpose, procedures (including the procedure of recruiting participants and obtaining their informed consent), and any projected risks and benefits to the participants.

Volunteer Bias   Systematic error that results when individuals who volunteer for research participation respond differently from persons in the general population.

ETHICAL ISSUES IN MENTAL HEALTH RESEARCH, along with scientific requirements, guide the investigatory process from beginning to end. From the conceptualization and implementation of a study to the analysis, interpretation, and dissemination of findings, both ethical and scientific considerations provide standards for the way in which the researcher should proceed. Sometimes a conflict arises between these standards. Researchers must resolve such conflicts, as they are accountable for both the ethical and scientific merit of the study. The occurrence of conflicts may provide an opportunity to expand knowledge and build a stronger science. Thus, the successful resolution of ethical conflicts may serve a scientific as well as a moral purpose.

I. ETHICAL PRINCIPLES UNDERLYING MENTAL HEALTH RESEARCH

The goal of the mental health researcher is to produce valid and generalizable knowledge to improve mental health. While engaged in the scientific pursuit, the researcher is required to protect the health and well-being of individuals who agree to participate in the research. The efficient progress of scientific understanding may at times be in conflict with the ethical treatment of individual participants in research studies, such as when prospective participants have a limited capacity to understand details about the nature of their participation or when informed consent may lead to volunteer bias. Researchers must be aware of basic principles underlying ethical issues that can arise and resolve conflicts responsibly while maintaining high standards of scientific integrity.

Three enduring ethical principles—beneficence, respect, and justice—guide researchers through changes in research topics and research methods that can give rise to new ethical issues. Beneficence refers to the ethical ideal that the potential for harm to participants will be minimized and any benefits to them will be maximized. Respect refers to the researcher's responsibility to protect the rights, freedom, and dignity of participants. Justice refers to the idea that, insofar as possible, benefits of research will accrue equitably to different segments of society; conversely, risks of research should be borne equitably across groups. These three principles, which underly all ethical guidelines in research on mental health, originally were presented in the Belmont Report, which is discussed in the next section.

II. ENCOURAGING AND MONITORING THE ETHICAL CONDUCT OF RESEARCH

Because ethical principles cannot always be easily translated into clear courses of action, systems must be set up to educate and encourage individual researchers to give constant, careful consideration to ethical issues. Systems to monitor the ethical conduct of research are necessary so that researchers benefit from the airing of ethical issues among both competent peers and community representatives.

A. The Belmont Report

Safeguards to protect the rights and welfare of participants in medical research have existed as part of Public Health Service (PHS) policy since 1966. In 1969, Surgeon General Philip Lee issued a statement extending PHS policy to all research studies involving human participants, including behavioral research, and reviewed the meaning of consent. This policy was expanded in 1971 to include all grants and contracts within the Department of Health, Education, and Welfare (DHEW, now the Department of Health and Human Services, DHHS). During this period, concerns were voiced regarding abuses in medical studies, some resulting in the death of human participants, and the issue of scientific misconduct was aired in hearings in 1973 before the Senate Health Subcommittee, chaired by Senator Edward Kennedy. Among the prominent cases of abuses was the 40-year Tuskegee syphilis experiment.

From 1932 to 1972, the PHS studied the course of untreated syphilis in more than 400 low-income African American men in Tuskegee, Alabama. The men were not told they had syphilis, and when a cure (penicillin) was discovered in 1943, it was not made available to them. Consequently, over the years, the men experienced the well-known effects of syphilis: damage to the skeletal, cardiovascular, and central nervous systems and, in some cases, death. The Tuskegee experiment did not yield any new knowledge or new treatment for syphilis. No formal protocol existed for the study; research procedures were established as the study was implemented. The men were given free health care, including a free annual examination, as an incentive to participate in the study. They were told, however, that if they sought treatment from other sources, they would be dropped from the study and lose their free health care. After details of the study were made public by an Associated Press reporter in 1972, the study was terminated. Some researchers defended the Tuskegee study, but public opinion held that society should be protected from ethical transgressions made in the name of science.

In 1974, the National Research Act (Public Law 93–348) was passed, requiring the establishment of Institutional Review Boards (IRBs) and creating the National Commission for the Protection of Human Subjects in Biomedical and Behavioral Research. The National Commission conducted hearings over a 3-year period, culminating in recommendations and a two-volume report, issued in 1979, *The Belmont Report: Ethical Principles and Guidelines for the Protection of Human Subjects in Research*. The report concluded that beneficence, respect, and justice should provide the foundation for research ethics. Also proposed in the report were norms for scientific conduct in six major areas: (a) valid research design, (b) competence of the researcher, (c) identification of consequences (risks and benefits), (d) appropriate selection of participants, (e) voluntary informed consent, and (f) compensation for injury.

Hearings on these recommendations were conducted by the President's Commission for the Study of Ethical Problems in Medicine, Biomedical, and Behavioral Research. Drawing on this information and on other sources of advice, the DHHS issued a set of regulations in the January 26, 1981, issue of the *Federal Register*. Current DHHS regulations governing the implementation of the National Research Act and subsequent amendments, such as the Health Research Extension Act of 1985 (Public Law 99–158), are set forth in the Code of Federal Regulations, Title 45, Part 46—Protection of Human Subjects, 1991.

In addition to the propositions in the Belmont Report and DHHS regulations, professional groups in the United States and abroad have promulgated ethical guidelines. In 1966, the American Psychological Association (APA) created a task force to develop a set of ethical principles for research with human participants. From these deliberations came a 1971 draft report, a 1972 revised version based on feedback from the APA membership, and the 1973 *Ethical Principles in the Conduct of Research with Human Participants*. *Ethical Principles* was updated by another APA task force and reissued in 1982 and is currently undergoing a third revision in which the APA has been joined by the American Psychological Society in a collaborative effort. In the initial statement and in all of its subsequent revisions, these principles have been based on actual ethical problems that researchers experienced, and extensive discussion throughout the profession has been incorporated in each edition of this manual. Ethical principles for research have also been developed and adopted by other, more specialized professional societies, such as the Society for Research in Child Development, and by organizations of psychologists in other countries, such as the Canadian Psychological Association and the British Psychological Society.

B. Institutional Review Boards (IRBs)

As required under the National Research Act of 1974, any institution that applies for federal grant funds is responsible for maintaining an IRB for the purpose of evaluating grant proposals and monitoring ongoing federally funded research. Using a protocol that the researcher submits, the IRB decides whether the study complies with standards for ethical treatment of participants. For example, the IRB judges whether the recruitment process is fair, the procedure for obtaining informed consent is appropriate, and steps to maintain the confidentiality of the data are in place. The IRB evaluates the risks and benefits of the research and once an approved study is underway, the IRB will request a periodic update on the work.

Some categories of research are exempt from IRB review. Examples of these categories are research in normal educational settings on normal educational processes; research involving educational tests, surveys, interviews, or observations of public behavior, as long as individuals cannot be identified; and research involving existing public data in which individuals cannot be identified. In practice, however, university IRBs typically require the review of all research; at minimum, the researcher would be expected to submit a research protocol to allow the IRB to determine whether the study falls into a category that is exempt from review.

IRBs may conduct expedited reviews if the research involves only minimal risk and involves participants in standard methods in one or more of 10 categories, such as research that uses existing data, documents, or records, and studies in which the researcher does not manipulate the participants' behavior and the procedures do not involve stress. Expedited reviews are conducted by the chairperson of the IRB or by one or more experienced members of the IRB, instead of the full complement of IRB members. The reviewer, however, cannot disapprove the research in the expedited review; the research protocol must be reviewed again in the regular meeting of the IRB if the decision is disapproval.

Because IRBs have substantial responsibility and control in the research process, their decisions must be made carefully and without social, political, or disciplinary bias. The IRB consists of five or more members who, ideally, reflect both the range of expertise in the research conducted at the institution and the cultural and ethnic diversity of the local community; both men and women should be included. At least one member must be included whose primary concerns are not scientific, plus at least one member who has no affiliation with the institution. The oversight of IRBs occurs in the DHHS, in the Office for Protection from Research Risks (OPRR), which is part of the National Institutes of Health (NIH). The OPRR provides assistance to local IRBs and has the authority to investigate charges and to recommend sanctions (including the withdrawal of all federal funding) against institutions that do not comply with regulations. An additional source of information regarding the functioning of IRBs is the bimonthly journal *IRB, A Review of Human Subjects Research*.

In practice, IRBs may vary considerably from the ideal of consistent, objective judgments. Prominent researchers in the field of mental health have described the frustrations of seemingly capricious or overly conservative decisions from IRBs. Evidence exists that a protocol approved by one IRB may not be approved in that form by another IRB. One explanation for this variability is that state laws can influence what IRBs allow from one location to another. In addition, ethical standards are not clear-cut and local community standards may prevail in IRB decisions. Researchers also have suggested that individual characteristics or interests of IRB members may be related to decision making and have documented that IRBs take into account the sociopolitical content of studies, independently of ethical standards.

The risk–benefit assessments made by IRBs are often routine, but decisions may be particularly difficult if the research is of a sensitive nature. Especially troublesome are proposed studies that carry some widely recognized risk but also offer the possibility of great societal benefit. Figure 1 shows a decision-plane model proposed by Rosenthal and Rosnow in 1984 to represent the process by which IRBs usually reach their decisions. In theory, studies falling at A will *not* be approved, because the risks are high and the benefits are low; studies falling at D *will* be approved, because the risks are low and the benefits are high. Studies falling along the B–C axis appear to be too difficult

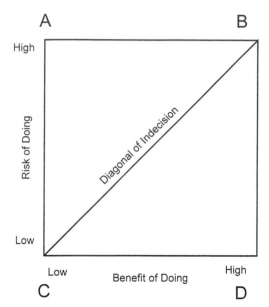

Figure I   Decision-plane model of risks and benefits of research.

to decide because the risks and benefits are in equal opposition. In the case of low risk, low benefit research, the IRB may be reluctant to approve a study that is harmless but is likely to yield little benefit. High risk, high benefit research will cause the greatest concern. In the decision process, the IRB should weigh the consequences of the obstruction of risky but potentially beneficial research against the costs of conducting such research. Researchers who are attentive to this risk–benefit analysis will maximize the benefits and minimize the risks as they design studies and protocols.

With a properly constituted IRB, ethical issues in research are assessed from a variety of perspectives. The researcher's perspective will be tempered by the IRB's analysis and by views solicited from others; however, the researcher is ultimately responsible for ensuring that ethical standards are upheld. The researcher cannot circumvent a difficult ethical decision by passing on responsibility to the IRB or to another person or group.

III. ETHICAL ISSUES AND METHODOLOGICAL OPPORTUNITIES

Ethical issues have provided the backdrop for the development of innovative procedures that will meet both scientific and ethical standards. Progress in research methodology and advances in the ethical treatment of participants are interconnected and, indeed, strengthening both aspects of research simultaneously may be possible. Opportunities to improve the ethics and methodology of research have been examined within several contexts. A discussion of some specific issues follows, with the proviso that the resolution of ethical issues generally is not permanent and is not formulaic. Standards for resolving ethical issues in mental health research can change over time, and new ethical issues can arise as new areas of research are identified.

A. Competence of Researchers

Researchers are obligated to develop their scientific skills and to conduct research as well as it can be done within ethical limitations. Researchers are also ethically bound to use their abilities to advance knowledge and, ultimately, to contribute to the well-being of individuals in society. Researchers who lack the relevant background or skills to perform good research may inadvertently produce spurious results with possibly harmful consequences. Researchers must not undertake projects for which they are not properly trained or skilled and must acccept responsibility for the training and supervision of all members of their research team. Researchers must therefore recognize and concede the boundaries of their own and others' expertise, and not exceed those boundaries.

It has been argued that the scientific validity of research design should also be viewed as an ethical issue. Poorly designed research cannot yield benefits and may actually be harmful. Asking people to participate in poorly designed research is not respectful and is also not just. Although many researchers construe ethics to be in a separate domain from research strategies, the ethical treatment of participants and the development of valid research methods are considered by many as integral, inseparable components of sound research practice.

B. Risks and Benefits of Research Participation

The avoidance of physical and psychological harm as a standard for ethical research emanated from the Nuremberg code of 1946–1949, developed in conjunction with expert testimony against Nazi physicians at the Nuremberg Military Tribunal after World War II.

The researcher is responsible for protecting the participants from physical or psychological harm that could arise from participation in the research. Where specific risks are known to exist, the prospective participants must be informed of those risks as part of the consent procedure. If the risks to mental or physical health are substantial (i.e., the potential harm could be very serious or even permanent), then the study should not be undertaken without the full understanding and consent of the participants or (in some cases, such as when participants are mentally incapacitated) their proper advocates or surrogates. Informing prospective participants or legal surrogates must go beyond the mere ritualized presentation of the consent form to ensure that the risks of participation are understood and accepted.

Risks cannot be completely anticipated, however, and sometimes estimating the likelihood of adverse consequences is difficult or impossible. Federal regulations use the concept of "minimal risk" to denote an acceptable level of risk in research. Minimal risk is defined as the level of risk at which the likelihood and extent of harm expected in the study are no greater than that experienced in everyday life or in ordinary psychological or physical tests. Applying the idea of minimal risk may be difficult because potential participants may vary greatly in the risks of their everyday lives. For example, some individuals live in dangerous neighborhoods in which their physical safety is a constant concern. Minimal risk defined on the basis of these individuals' everyday lives would be substantial risk for those who live in safer environments. The notion of minimal risk is not intended to justify greater risk for some participants than for others; this concept needs to be augmented by a recognition of the wide variation in the probability of harm in individuals' everyday lives.

Ethical standards require not only the absence of harm in mental health research but also some benefit from research participation. As is the case in the assessment of risk, benefits may be obvious in some research studies but unclear in other studies; research may have long-term benefits that are not foreseen. Researchers are expected to produce and disseminate careful, meaningful reports of their research. Benefits may occur when research findings are reported in professional outlets and also when the findings are applied appropriately to real-life settings and to policy decisions. Researchers may prepare nontechnical reports to be distributed to participants after the study is completed. A long-standing program of research may result in relationships with community organizations or schools, for example, which become beneficiaries of the research. Responsible researchers share their findings cautiously, however, and are reluctant to publicize their work prematurely, especially if the findings have negative implications for individuals or groups.

The risks of research participation sometimes are judged to be offset by the benefits of research. Such a determination is difficult because risks and benefits to the individual participant ordinarily cannot be quantified and easily compared to one another. In addition, the risks of research participation occur for the participants themselves; in contrast, the benefits of research may be to society in general with little or no direct benefit to the participant. Given the problems inherent in creating a risks-to-benefits ratio for individual participants, researchers remain ethically bound to minimize risks and maximize benefits.

In mental health research using a treatment-control design, participants are randomly assigned to treatment and control conditions. The ethical use of this design requires that researchers be able to entertain reasonably the null hypothesis that no difference exists between the treatment and control conditions. In practice, however, differential benefits are expected to accrue to participants assigned a presumably beneficial treatment. This design, then, is susceptible to the criticism that it violates the principle of justice, which requires that risks and benefits of research be shared equally across the population. If participants who receive the treatment gain from it as hypothesized, then they have received a benefit not available to the control group. If the treatment involves physical or psychological risk, then the treatment group faces a possibility of harm to which the control group is not exposed. Confronted with either alternative, researchers can adopt strategies to cope with such a situation. For example, the control group can be scheduled to receive the beneficial treatment after the study is completed; this procedure is effective except in instances in which timing the presentation of the treatment is critical. Another approach is to provide the control group with a different experience that is known to be beneficial; this alternative not only avoids the ethical problem of depriving control participants of beneficial effects but it also focuses the comparison between the groups on a question of practical importance (i.e.,

whether the tested treatment is more beneficial than an existing treatment). An additional option is to discontinue the treatment–control comparison and provide the beneficial treatment to the control group, once the treatment is clearly shown to be effective.

Although the treatment–control design is generally preferred in many areas of research, this design can lead to problems of interpretation in some cases. For example, participants who are randomly assigned to a no-treatment control group after agreeing to participate and completing the screening assessment necessary to determine their eligibility for the research, may react negatively to their exclusion from the treatment group. Participants would have been forewarned of the likelihood of control group assignment but may become demoralized once they learn they will not receive treatment that they were previously told could be beneficial. Demoralized participants are not then a neutral control group. In drug trials using a placebo-control group, participants are not told whether they are assigned to the treatment or control group. Researchers, however, may inform potential participants of the possible benefits of the experimental medicine and of the possibility of participants' not receiving the medicine but instead the placebo. Participants who believe the procedure is unfair may surreptitiously share doses in an attempt to increase the likelihood that each person will get at least some access to the experimental medicine. If it is essential to use a placebo-control condition (i.e., rather than providing the control group with an alternative treatment that is known to be beneficial), then it is advisable to enlist the support of prospective participants and provide some option for the control group after the study is completed. In this way the researcher practices beneficence, respect, and justice as required by ethical standards and also increases the likelihood of a valid research design.

Because the benefits of research should extend throughout society, researchers are expected to conduct studies that will provide information about both genders and the range of American ethnic groups. The inappropriate generalization of research findings from one gender or ethnic group to another may have harmful effects. The most damaging effects of restricted samples occur not when one or a few studies are limited, but when the body of research in an area has sampled mainly one gender or one ethnic group. Guidelines established by the NIH in 1994 require that women and diverse ethnic groups be included as participants in NIH-supported biomedical and behavioral research unless there is compelling justification for their exclusion. According to NIH guidelines, the inclusion of these groups also requires attention to socioeconomic status, including education, occupation, and income. The requirement of inclusivity affords opportunities for researchers to advance knowledge about gender and ethnic groups that have been underrepresented in many research areas in the past. Because of the huge gaps in the knowledge base, studies of a single underrepresented group are sometimes appropriate. Researchers are expected to engage in outreach efforts to recruit and retain inclusive samples. The NIH urges involvement of individuals and organizations in the communities of interest so that mutual trust and cooperation are established.

C. Selection of Research Participants

In general, researchers aim to select research participants who are representative of the population to which generalizations will be made. A random sample (i.e., a sample chosen by chance procedures and with known probabilities of selection) satisfies the requirement of representativeness, but random sampling is seldom possible in mental health research. The researcher's obligation to respect people's privacy usually requires that participation in research be voluntary, in which case the right of prospective participants to refuse will jeopardize the chances of obtaining a representative sample. Even if researchers could draw a random sample and have everyone verbally agree to participate, not everyone will likely keep appointments to participate. Research has found that volunteers who fail to keep their appointments tend to be more like the nonvolunteers than the volunteers who participate in the research. Not only might the use of volunteer participants produce biased results (volunteer bias), but volunteers who actually participate might not be representative of all volunteers. Research also has shown that volunteers who are paid substantially for their participation differ from unpaid volunteers. The problem of volunteer bias has been studied and procedures have been suggested to stimulate participation within the boundaries of ethical principles and also to estimate the direction and amount of volunteer bias that may occur in a given research situation.

Individuals not only have the right to refuse to participate but also retain the right to withdraw without penalty at any point after their participation has begun. In longitudinal research, researchers should periodically repeat the consent procedure, documenting that participants remain aware of the purposes of the study and that they wish to continue to participate. Furthermore, researchers must refrain from using any coercive tactics in recruiting participants. Although monetary or other compensation often is offered to prospective participants, such compensation may be deemed coercive if the amount is excessive. Ethical problems arise when the incentive for participation is so great or so highly valued that the individual is unable to make a wise decision about the risks and benefits of participation. Excessive rewards are considered to be coercive because the potential participant is motivated by the desire for the reward and not by the value of the research. Coercion can be subtle as well as direct. In the absence of excessive rewards, researchers may make coercive appeals to the potential participants' sense of obligation to science, society, a particular ethnic group, or other important reference group. The researcher must strike a balance between enthusiastically promoting the research and respecting the right of the individual to decline to participate.

D. Voluntary Informed Consent

Before agreeing to participate, individuals must have a clear understanding of the purpose of the research and the procedures they will experience. Prospective participants have a right to accurate information about the research so that they can make an informed decision about participation. The usual procedure to indicate one's agreement to participate in research consists of signing a written document that outlines the purpose of the research and the procedures to be used. Although some exceptions may be allowed, the consent document first conveys clearly that research (in contrast to therapy, education, etc.) is occurring. Statements regarding risks and benefits expected, confidentiality, and the voluntary nature of participation also are included and potential participants are told who to contact with questions about the research. Additional statements may be necessary depending on the nature of the research. IRBs may decide to alter some or all of the elements of informed consent if the research involves no more than minimal risk, the departure from informed consent will not affect the welfare of the participants, the research could not reasonably be carried out under the requirement of informed consent, or the participants are provided with appropriate information after their participation.

The consent document should be free of technical jargon and written in a style that prospective participants will find easy to understand. In some cases, consent forms can be so detailed and cumbersome that they are not easy to comprehend, thereby defeating the purpose of informed consent. Researchers in several areas of investigation are studying consent procedures, with an eye toward identifying persons who might have difficulty in understanding (e.g., participants who have some mental or emotional impairment) and the problematic aspects of the details communicated to them (e.g., abstract vs. concrete details). In signing the consent form, the participant does not relinquish the right to take legal action against the researcher if harm results from participation. Additionally, signed consent forms do not release the researcher from ethical responsibility for the participant's well-being.

In some instances, fully informing potential participants of the purpose of a study may jeopardize its scientific validity. For example, participants may experience anxiety about the possibility of being negatively evaluated (called evaluation apprehension) if they are told the purpose of the research and the nature of the instruments to be used. In such an instance, the researcher may instead propose to withhold some information (called passive deception) or to represent the study in a way that is not directly connected with its true purpose (called active deception). Deception in research is problematic because it can be seen as violating the principle of respect for participants; furthermore, once deceived, the participants may become distrustful not only of researchers but of other people. Although active and passive deceptions are common in society, researchers are expected to consider alternative procedures carefully before deciding on the use of deception. In some research areas, deceptive procedures have been used with some frequency, such as observing people in a public setting without telling them they are being studied, using confederates, and using projective tests and other measurement techniques without disclosing their purpose to the participants.

Ethical guidelines call for debriefing if deception is used in the research. The purpose of the debriefing is to remove any misconceptions that the participants have about the research (sometimes called dehoaxing) and to leave them with a sense of dignity, knowledge, and a perception of time not wasted. Furthermore, the debriefing serves to reduce any negative emotions or thoughts the participant may have developed during the deception (sometimes called desensitizing). The debriefing session can also be an opportunity for the researcher to learn what participants thought the research was about, thus providing the researcher with an experiential context within which to interpret the results. The use of debriefing after deception has been criticized on the grounds that it could spawn skepticism when participants learn that they have been tricked by an authority figure. The researchers, therefore, must be prepared to explain the reason for the deception and the benefit of the research to the participant as well as to the field. In clinical research, for example, many participants may have volunteered in order to learn something about themselves, and debriefing can provide an opportunity to receive information regarding their performance or responses. In this way, the participants can benefit in a personal sense, just as the researcher has benefited from their willingness to participate.

E. Use of Confidentiality

Maintaining confidentiality in psychological research is often justified on the basis of three assumptions: (a) that respect for the participants' privacy requires confidentiality, (b) that researchers have a professional obligation and right to keep participants' disclosures confidential, and (c) that the use of confidentiality results in more open and honest disclosures. Research evidence supports this third assumption. For example, evaluation apprehension appears to be alleviated when participants believe their disclosures will be held in strict confidence.

To maintain confidentiality, the researcher must set in place procedures for protecting the data, such as those stored in written records, videotapes or audiotapes, or computer files. Any anticipated possibility of departure from the standard of confidentiality must be explained to the prospective participants as part of the procedure of informed consent. Complications can arise in some situations. For example, the Child Abuse Prevention and Treatment Act of 1974 and its revisions and amendments mandate that each state pass laws to require the reporting of child abuse and neglect. Thus, researchers in mental health may be pressed to report child abuse, which implies violation of the confidentiality of disclosures. In some research in which illegal or unethical behavior of participants may be known to the researcher, the researcher may seek a special exemption providing protection from subpoena. The NIH can issue a "certificate of confidentiality" to researchers, but the extent of legal protection actually attained has not yet been established in the courts.

IV. RESEARCH WITH SPECIAL POPULATIONS

Some populations may require special ethical considerations in the research process. In some populations, individuals are particularly vulnerable to the possibility of harm. The individual may not be able to make a reasoned judgment about the merits of participating or declining to participate in the research. In other populations, coercion or the perception of coercion may be especially likely.

A. Children and Adolescents

Research with children who have not reached the age of majority typically requires written informed consent of the parents. Often, parental consent is sought by mailing to or sending through school children a letter to the parents describing the purposes of the research and outlining the procedures the child would experience. The use of written informed parental consent may lead to smaller and more select samples than would be the case if consent were not sought. Researchers attempt to increase the sample size by telephoning parents who do not return consent forms and by speaking to groups of parents to enlist their support. For children who do not live with their parents but who are wards of the state or other agencies, the Federal Regulations, Title 45, Part 46.409, requires that an advocate be appointed to act in the best interests of the child in the consent process.

Researchers should not make direct appeals to children for participation before parental consent is obtained. For example, researchers must not use the promise of rewards to entice children to participate. In some instances, the researcher may have contact with the children before contact with the parents. Researchers may visit a school classroom, for example, to distribute the consent forms to be taken home to the parents. The researcher, or a classroom teacher acting on behalf of the researcher, must not convey that the appeal is directly to the student rather than to the parents. In addition, the researcher (or teacher) must not suggest that the research is part of the regular curriculum, or is an enhancement of the existing curriculum, unless that is entirely true.

Under federal regulations, the categories of exempt research apply to children as well as to adults, with the exception of survey and interview procedures and observations of public behavior; these categories are not exempt from review in research with children. Categories of research with children that are exempt from review include research on normal educational processes in normal educational settings. The IRB can decide to waive the requirement of parental consent under certain conditions. For example, if parental consent does not seem relevant to the protection of the child, as in the case of abused or neglected children, the IRB can waive parental consent and require that consent be requested of an advocate for the children. The IRB's authority is superseded by federal law in researchers' access to children's school records. The Buckley Amendment, the 1979 Family Educational Rights and Privacy Act, requires written parental consent for the release of personally identifiable information from children's school records.

Using a strategy called passive consent, some researchers bypass the requirement of parental consent by asking parents to respond only if they do not want their children to participate in the study. The researcher then assumes that all parents who do not return a signed form refusing to grant permission have in fact consented. The researcher, however, has no documentation that parents have actually agreed to allow their children to participate and thus has not actually obtained parental consent. The use of passive consent is acceptable only if the IRB agrees and waives the requirement of parental consent, as is allowable in some cases, but its use may raise legal questions that have not been resolved.

A bill passed by the House of Representatives in 1995 (H.R. 1271), but not brought to a vote in the

Senate, would have required that parents provide written informed consent for minor children's participation in research on any "socially sensitive" topic. Some in the research community feared that such a strong federal requirement of parental consent might prevent the study of certain sensitive but important issues for children and adolescents. With such a mandate, researchers would need Herculean efforts to reach out to communities and convince parents of the value of research on sensitive issues. Here, ethical obligations appear to be in conflict with the scientific need to conduct research efficiently. Current federal regulations focus on risks and benefits to children and do not make explicit reference to the sensitivity of the research topic as a limiting feature of the research.

Once parental consent is obtained, the child's assent also is sought on the day of the study, if the child is old enough or mature enough to be asked about participation. Children may still refuse to participate, even after parents have signed consent forms. The child's assent is more than the lack of refusal; the child must actively agree to participate. The child's assent is not required in research judged to be important to the child's health or well-being, if parents have consented. Researchers should watch for indications that a child is uncomfortable and may not wish to continue a procedure. Furthermore, researchers who become aware of any situation that may place the child's well-being in jeopardy are obligated to report the information to parents or guardians and appropriate experts so that assistance may be sought for the child.

In sum, the risk associated with research participation needs to be considered carefully when children are participants. Risk may be difficult to assess; children, like adults, are not a homogeneous population. Some children are exposed to danger in their everyday lives, whereas other, more fortunate children are reared without substantial likelihood of harm. The notion of minimal risk, in which the risks of a child's everyday life are allowable in research, may need to be replaced with a less variable concept of risk. In addition, children's vulnerabilities may change with age; risks may be greater or less for children of different ages. To assist the researcher who studies children, the Society for Research in Child Development has formulated ethical standards for research with children, expressed in a set of 14 ethical principles, which provide an excellent guide for ethical research with children.

B. Persons Confined to Prisons or Mental Institutions

For prisoners (i.e., individuals confined involuntarily to penal institutions), special requirements are outlined in the 1991 Federal Regulations, Title 45, Part 46.301–306. Prisoners exist in an environment of limited choices; however, researchers are still guided by principles of beneficence, respect, and justice. Safeguards are necessary so that prisoners, who by definition have limited choices, are not coerced and do not feel coerced into participating in research. Treatment and control groups must be randomly selected from prisoners possessing the characteristics required in the study; prison authorities may not arbitrarily select participants. Participation in research cannot have an effect on parole decisions. The possible benefits of participation or incentives to participate, such as changes in medical care, food, earnings, or general living conditions, cannot be so great that prisoners are unable to make an informed decision based on risks and benefits of the research. The risks to which prisoners are exposed in research must be no greater than the level of risk that would be acceptable to voluntary participants who are not prisoners. The IRB that reviews research to be conducted with prisoners must have at least one member who is a prisoner or who has the background to act as a representative of prisoners.

For research participants who are mentally disabled, consent to participate in research should be obtained from a legal guardian or from some other person who is acting in the potential participant's interest. Insofar as possible, however, the agreement of the participants themselves should be obtained. Efforts should be made to convey the purpose of the research in an understandable manner and to respect the wishes of the disabled person. For persons who are confined to mental institutions, the general lack of choices may suggest that the right to refuse to participate in research is diminished as well. As is the case with prisoners, however, the broad ethical principles of beneficence, respect, and justice still apply. Research that assesses the institutional arrangements in the mental institution is more easily justified than are other kinds of research, such as research assessing different therapies or research that is irrelevant to the disabilities of the mentally disabled participants. Federal regulations do not provide additional protections, beyond the basic policy, for mentally disabled persons, although DHHS does specify additional federal regulations for children, for prisoners, and for fetuses and pregnant women.

C. Clients of Researchers

Potential participants in research may bear a "client" relationship to the researcher, as in the case of patients or students of the researcher. In these situations, the researcher is responsible for the well-being of the participant but also has some authority over the participant. Researchers studying their own patients or students have dual, potentially conflicting roles. Patients deserve the best treatment possible from their therapists or physicians. Similarly, students deserve the best educational experience possible from their professors. Researchers' goals, however, may not include the best treatment or the best learning experience for each participant. Furthermore, patients and students may feel pressured to participate. A partial preventive to the possibility of coercion or perceived coerciveness would be not to allow researchers to recruit their own patients or students.

Universities commonly allow student subject pools for researchers. Undergraduate students are samples of convenience for many researchers. With a ready supply of students to participate in research, the recruitment process is made relatively easy for many researchers. Participation in research typically is presented to the student as a course requirement. Guidelines are necessary to prevent coercion or the appearance of coercion in the use of student subject pools. The students' participation should be educational; student subject pools must be justified on the basis of the educational value of participation in research. Students may learn about the research process by participating in an actual study, in addition to reading about research in classroom texts. Students' participation, however, must be voluntary. Students, like all other research participants, must be allowed to end their participation at any point during the study without penalty. Therefore, students must have a choice of research projects and must be able to choose an alternative to participating in research, such as reading a journal article or attending a lecture on research. The alternatives must not be more difficult than is research participation.

The research requirements tied to enrollment in a particular course should be carefully detailed in the course advertisement and in the course syllabus distributed to students in class. Thus, students should be informed of the research requirement prior to enrollment and should receive the details immediately after the class begins. In some classes, research participation affects the students' grades for the course. This linking of research participation to class grades is difficult to justify from an ethical standpoint. A low grade or a grade of Incomplete for failure to participate in research is coercive unless alternatives of equal difficulty and educational value are possible.

D. Employees in the Private Sector and in the Military

For employees in business and industry and for military personnel, research participation may involve benefits not available to those who do not participate. Furthermore, those who do not participate may suffer some penalty or may not be judged favorably by their supervisors or others in positions of authority. Not only are issues of coercion, benefits, and penalties important, but so are the beliefs that may exist among the employees and military personnel about their obligation to participate and the consequences of participation. Researchers must exercise great care to communicate explicitly that participation is voluntary. Research conducted in these settings should have some bearing on the functioning of the organization and should be accompanied by a plan to use the research findings. Ideally, a statement regarding the expectation of research participation should be provided to individuals before they become part of the organization or the military unit.

V. ETHICAL ISSUES IN RESEARCH SPONSORSHIP

Organizations that sponsor research may be able to affect the manner in which studies are conducted and may exercise control over the dissemination and application of the findings. Conflicts can arise when the sponsor of research has a vested interest in the outcome of the research. For example, a foundation may have a particular point of view on mental health research and may support only like-minded researchers who will validate the foundation's beliefs. Similarly, an organization may commission an evaluation of its treatment program and may be loath to publicize any results that do not present the treatment in a favorable light. An egregious instance of conflict occurred when tobacco companies allegedly funded research on the impact of nicotine. Instead of disseminating findings widely to benefit individuals and to prevent harm to them, the companies are said to have used the information to alter the levels of nicotine so that individuals would become more addicted to cigarettes and would be more likely to continue to buy them. Researchers are obligated to prevent the misuse of their findings, as much as is possible, and to encourage appropriate application of the results.

VI. SUMMARY

Ethical issues, as well as scientific considerations, are used to determine the course of programs of mental health research. Although specific ethical issues may change as new research topics and research methods become prominent, three basic principles—beneficence, respect, and justice—remain as the foundation of ethical research. Easy solutions are not typically available for ethical issues in research; therefore, researchers are urged to give careful consideration to the various perspectives on ethical issues and are expected to use IRBs as a mechanism to foster ethical research. Ultimately, researchers themselves are responsible for maintaining ethical and scientific standards and must constantly strive to integrate the two successfully in their work.

BIBLIOGRAPHY

American Psychological Association. (1982). *Ethical principles in the conduct of research with human participants.* Washington, DC: American Psychological Association.

Bersoff, D. N. (Ed.). (1995). *Ethical conflicts in psychology.* Washington, DC: American Psychological Association.

Blanck, P. D., Bellack, A. S., Rosnow, R. L., Rotheram-Borus, M. J., & Schooler, N. R. (1992). Scientific rewards and conflicts of ethical choices in human subjects research. *American Psychologist, 47, 959–965.*

Fisher, C. B., & Tryon, W. W. (Eds.). (1990). *Ethics in applied developmental psychology: Emerging issues in an emerging field.* Norwood, NJ: Ablex.

Kimmel, A. J. (1996). *Ethical issues in behavioral research: A survey.* Cambridge, MA: Blackwell.

Koocher, G. P., & Keith-Spiegel, P. C. (1990). *Children, ethics, and the law.* Lincoln, NE: University of Nebraska Press.

Rosenthal, R. (1994). Science and ethics in conducting, analyzing, and reporting psychological research. *Psychological Science, 5, 127–134.*

Rosenthal, R., & Rosnow, R. L. (1975). *The volunteer subject.* New York: Wiley.

Rosnow, R. L., & Rosenthal, R. (1997). *People studying people: Artifacts and ethics in behavioral research.* New York: Freeman.

Rosnow, R. L., Rotheram-Borus, M. J., Ceci, S. J., Blanck, P. D., & Koocher, G. P. (1993). The institutional review board as a mirror of scientific and ethical standards. *American Psychologist, 48, 821–826.*

Schuler, H. (1982). *Ethical problems in psychological research.* (M. S. Woodruff & R. A. Wicklund (Trans.). New York: Academic Press. (Original work published 1980)

Scott-Jones, D. (1994). Ethical issues in reporting and referring in research with minority and low-income populations. *Ethics and Behavior, 4, 97–108.*

Sieber, J. E. (1992). *Planning ethically responsible research.* Newbury Park, CA: Sage.

Stanley, B., & Sieber, J. E. (Eds.). (1992). *Social research on children and adolescents: Ethical issues.* Newbury Park, CA: Sage.

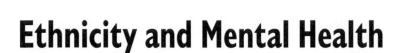

Ethnicity and Mental Health

Jonathan S. Kaplan, Doris Chang, and David Takeuchi

University of California, Los Angeles

Jennifer Abe-Kim

Loyola Marymount University

Bias In the context of psychological assessment, bias may be characterized as either overpathologizing (in which culturally normative behavior is judged to reflect more psychopathology than is the case) or underpathologizing (when abnormal behavior is judged to reflect more culturally appropriate behavior than is actually the case).

Cultural Sensitivity The careful consideration of the applicability of universal (etic) norms versus culture-specific (emic) norms in the diagnosis, assessment, and treatment of a particular patient or client.

Ethnic Group A group that is socially distinguished by itself or by others on the basis of nationality, language, or cultural characteristics.

Ethnicity A multidimensional psychological construct that includes such components as cultural characteristics, ethnic identity, particular linguistic capabilities, and experiences of racism and discrimination.

Quality of Care A tripartite entity that includes the structure, process, and outcome of service delivery.

In this entry the relationship of **ETHNICITY TO MENTAL HEALTH** is explored in terms of psychiatric epidemiology, psychological assessment, psychotherapy outcome, and health care policy. Theoretical and practical issues confronting investigations of eth-

nicity and mental health are examined. The terms African American, Asian American, Hispanic American, and Native American simultaneously highlight the unique attributes and commonalities of these ethnic groups. Collectively, these groups are referred to as ethnic minorities. This designation reflects the traditional, White-population-based reference to these groups. However, this term is no longer applicable in some cities, such as Los Angeles, New York, and Washington, D.C. Furthermore, our use of ethnic minority is not meant to suggest any inferiority of these groups. In the text, White, Caucasian and European American are used interchangeably to represent the dominant group in American society. It should be noted that much heterogeneity exists within each ethnic group. Differences in age, generation, immigration history, religion, gender, and class all contribute to intraethnic diversity. For immigrant groups, acculturation is another important factor that describes the adoption of American cultural norms and the maintenance of values that are associated with their country of origin. Although typically designated as being high or low, acculturation is actually a complex concept that includes many different dimensions, such as attitudes, language use, ethnic identity, social networks, and even food preferences. Thus, the reader should be aware that many significant differences exist both between and within ethnic groups.

I. DEFINITION OF ETHNICITY

The term "ethnicity" was originally derived from the Greek word for nation, *ethnos*. Over time, the term has been transformed to have many different meanings. In psychology, an ethnic group is typically defined as a group that is socially distinguished by itself or by others on the basis of nationality, language, or cultural characteristics. Although outward physical similarities may exist within certain ethnic groups, it is important to note that this definition is a social one—not a biological one. Research has shown that there is more physical and genetic heterogeneity within ethnic groups than between them.

To date, ethnicity has been treated typically as a categorical variable in psychology. It is useful for delineating ethnic differences and testing the generalizability of mainstream theories. However, ethnicity by itself cannot provide explanations for research findings. That is, if ethnic differences are discovered along a particular variable, there is little explanation as to why that difference exists. Thus, many authors have argued for a closer examination of the multiple dimensions that comprise ethnicity. Cultural characteristics, a sense of ethnic identity, bilingualism, socioeconomic status, and experiences of racism and discrimination are components of ethnic group membership that are more useful in providing explanations for research findings. Furthermore, ethnicity and its dimensions may be determined objectively by "outside" observers, such as research psychologists, or subjectively by the research participants themselves. In the future, researchers will be encouraged to delineate specifically the source of ethnic group data and measure the components of ethnicity that are theorized to relate to the other variables under investigation.

In psychological research, as well as in everyday society, ethnicity is often confused with race and culture. Essentially, culture is a collection of subjective norms which could apply to any kind of group, not only to different ethnic groups. Race, on the other hand, is typically defined in terms of shared physical characteristics, such as skin color, hair type, and facial structure, that evolved from geographically isolated in-group breeding. The traditional anthropological distinctions consist of Mongoloid, Negroid, and Caucasoid.

II. PREVALENCE OF MENTAL DISORDERS

The prevalence of mental disorders (psychiatric epidemiology) is typically determined by clinical records or community surveys. Both methods have been used in the past to assess the rates and types of psychiatric problems associated with different ethnic groups. Once discovered, ethnic differences in prevalence rates have been explained by a variety of perspectives.

A. Clinical Records

Statistics on people admitted into mental hospitals and outpatient clinics have often been used to draw conclusions about ethnic differences in the rates of mental illness. In many instances, especially before World War II, clinic records represented the best data available to estimate the prevalence of mental disorders. Because African Americans tended to be overrepresented in mental hospitals in the early 1900s, it was concluded that they suffered from more mental disorders than Whites. Data on hospital admissions were also used to conclude that immigrants, primarily from Europe, suffered from poorer mental health than native-born residents. Explanations for these differences ranged from racist (i.e., ethnic minorities and immigrants were believed inferior) to social (e.g., ethnic minorities and immigrants faced discrimination or other adjustment problems in American society). A second prevailing theme was that mental health services were a coercive form of social control that disproportionately defined ethnic minority behavior as deviant.

Prevalence estimates based on treatment data have built-in biases, such as the assumption that all people who have a mental illness eventually receive treatment. This assumption is unwarranted, as more recent evidence shows that people who suffer from some form of mental health problem, regardless of race or ethnicity, are unlikely to seek professional help. When comparisons are made, however, ethnic minority group members are less likely to use mental health services than Whites. For example, some data suggest that the use of mental health services is quite distinct for African Americans compared with Whites. Although African Americans and Whites are equally likely to seek some source of professional help (e.g., social services, clergy, mental health services) for their emotional problems, Whites are more likely than African Americans to contact voluntarily a mental health professional. This pattern seems consistent for other ethnic groups as well, and has led to the notion that ethnic minorities are less likely to use mental health services than Whites because of limited access to clinics, cultural stigma against mental illness, and culture-specific, help-seeking behaviors that help reduce hospital admissions.

In addition to sociocultural factors, some ethnic minority groups may be financially constrained from seeking professional help. One such constraining factor in seeking care for a mental health problem is the absence of or limited health insurance coverage. Because the United States has the costliest health care system among developed nations, quality health care is unaffordable for a large segment of the American population. Although health insurance is intended to assist Americans in paying for health care, it is estimated that 37 million Americans are not covered by public or private health insurance. Ethnic minorities are a large segment of the uninsured. In a 1995 national survey sponsored by the Commonwealth Fund, 14% of White adults reported no health insurance coverage. This proportion is lower than the uninsured rates for African Americans (26%), Latinos (38%), and Asian Americans (23%).

B. Community Surveys

Beginning in the 1940s, survey research became a more prominent means of data collection, which led to innovative ways to gain access to community samples for estimating the prevalence of mental disorders, a trend that continues into the present. In the latter part of the 1970s and the early part of the part of the 1980s, the Epidemiologic Catchment Area (ECA) study pioneered the use of the Diagnostic Interview Schedule (DIS) in large community samples. It could be administered by lay interviewers, and, through a series of computer algorithms, psychiatric diagnoses could be obtained for discrete mental disorders (e.g., depression, anxiety, schizophrenia). The project was conducted in five geographic sites across the country (Durham, North Carolina; New Haven, Connecticut; Baltimore, Maryland; St. Louis, Missouri; and Los Angeles, California). At the time, the ECA provided the most comprehensive assessment of the prevalence of mental disorders for different ethnic categories.

The ECA included relatively large samples of African Americans from Durham, New Haven, Baltimore, and St. Louis. The Los Angeles ECA site included a large Hispanic sample composed largely of Mexican Americans. Analyses of the ECA data generally found few race or ethnic differences in the lifetime and current (12-month) prevalences of various disorders. Among the differences that were uncovered was that

African Americans had lower prevalence rates of affective disorders and substance abuse and dependence. Young African Americans also had a lower prevalence of drug and alcohol abuse and dependence than young White Americans. The ECA did find that African Americans had nearly double the lifetime prevalence of simple phobia and agoraphobia. Hispanics in the ECA had elevated rates of alcohol use disorders and lower lifetime rates of affective disorders compared with Whites.

In response to a need for an estimate of the prevalence of mental illness that reflected American demographics, the National Comorbidity Study (NCS) was specifically designed to develop a nationally representative sample of people aged 15 to 55. Conducted nearly 15 years after the ECA, the NCS found a higher prevalence of mental disorders than the ECA; nearly one in two persons in the NCS sample had experienced some type of mental disorder in their lifetime compared with 30% in the ECA study. Moreover, the prevalence comparisons for race also departed from the ECA results. African Americans in the NCS did not have a higher rate on any disorder when compared to Whites. Hispanics, on the other hand, had a higher prevalence of current affective disorders than did Whites. Unlike the ECA study, the NCS did not show any differences between Hispanics and Whites on alcohol use disorders. [See ALCOHOL PROBLEMS.]

The study of prevalence among ethnic minority categories such as Asian Americans and Native Americans poses a number of methodological issues. One problem is that the ethnic categories are quite diverse and heterogeneous, which constrains the ability of researchers to make generalizations. A second problem is that these ethnic categories are relatively rare in many geographic settings, which makes data collection from a representative sample extremely costly. Despite these problems, some evidence suggests that the American Indians have elevated rates of depression compared with Whites. Estimates for Asian Americans tend to be more mixed, depending on the Asian ethnic group, geographic location, and type of instrument that is used to derive estimates.

C. Explanatory Perspectives

When ethnic or racial differences are found in the prevalence of mental illness, considerable debate has ensued over the meaning of these differences. Three perspectives are usually advanced to explain ethnic minority–White differences in psychological distress and psychopathology. The *minority status* argument contends that society, in part, stratifies people according to their ethnic or racial background. Institutional obstacles prevent some groups from achieving educational and occupational parity in American society. Economic differentials between minorities and Whites represent a social "tax" on minorities for not being White. The discrepancies between minorities and dominant group members create a social environment characterized by alienation, frustration, and powerlessness. Distress, demoralization, and more serious forms of psychopathology are likely to result from this environment.

The *social class* argument holds that race differences in psychopathology disappear when social class is controlled. This argument is based on the fact that in many communities, members of some ethnic minority groups have lower incomes than Whites. Because they cannot access the economic and social resources to cope with the debilitating effects of their physical and social environment, members in the lower social classes exhibit higher levels of distress regardless of their ethnic minority status. [*See* SOCIOECONOMIC STATUS.]

The final perspective suggests that ethnic differences may reflect *cultural variations* in the reporting and expression of distress, as well as different help-seeking behaviors. Rates of major depression, for example, show a wide range of estimates in different countries. It is also recognized that social structure can shape the cultural forms that the expression of distress takes. The Hutterites, for example, a religiously orthodox communal society, expected individual rights to be secondary to the welfare of the group. Interpersonal conflicts were seen not as resulting from social interaction, but rather as problems that resulted from individual imperfections. Thus, confrontations and transgressions against others were discouraged and more internalized means of resolving problems were sanctioned. The Hutterites did not approve the use of substances such as alcohol and cigarettes as a means of tension relief. Instead, the Hutterites have a very high rate of depression—an internal, individual form of expressing distress. In much the same way, ethnic groups may have cultural forms of expressing their tensions and distress that are uniquely shaped by their social organizations.

Obviously, these three perspectives are not mutually exclusive. For example, some researchers argue that race and class intersect to explain psychological problems. That is, African Americans in the lower socioeconomic levels have higher rates of psychological distress than Whites at the same socioeconomic level. The adoption of different perspectives tends to be group-specific. Studies on African Americans typically focus on the issue of race and class. Research on American Indian communities tends to focus on minority status and cultural explanations that emphasize the understanding of risk factors for alcohol abuse, suicide, depression, and the co-occurrence of disorders—problems that have had a devastating impact in American Indian and Alaskan Native communities. Research on Asian Americans and Hispanic Americans has tended to concentrate on "cultural" issues revolving around immigration and refugee status, such as acculturation, ethnic identity, and adaptation. However, despite these tendencies to emphasize certain perspectives over others, it is clear that future studies must consider various explanations to "unpackage" systematically the meaning of ethnic differences in mental health areas.

III. ASSESSMENT OF ETHNIC MINORITIES

In recent years, the problem of clinical assessment of ethnic minorities has generated considerable discussion in both research and clinical arenas. At the heart of this discussion is how ethnicity affects the reliability and validity of the assessment process. As mentioned, some epidemiological and clinical studies have revealed race differences in rates of diagnosis for a variety of psychiatric disorders. Although these rates may reflect "true" differences in psychiatric morbidity, they may also be influenced by biased assessment procedures applied to ethnic minorities. Many investigators have suggested that cultural biases may affect therapists' interpretations of the psychological functioning of ethnic minority clients. The purpose of this section is to examine theoretical, methodological, and clinical issues related to the assessment and diagnosis of ethnically diverse individuals. In addition, some practical guidelines are offered for conducting culturally valid assessment research and practice.

A. Clinical Judgment Bias

The psychologist working with ethnically diverse patients is faced with the challenge of conducting psychological assessment in a culturally sensitive manner.

Cultural sensitivity has been defined as the careful consideration of the applicability of universal (etic) norms versus culture-specific (emic) norms in the assessment of a particular patient or client. An overreliance on either standard without consideration of the other may have negative consequences for the client. For example, practitioners and researchers may err in their assumption that certain behaviors have the same meaning for all populations, when in fact their significance and meaning may vary across ethnic and cultural groups. For example, some researchers have argued that Latinos' scores on personality measures are often interpreted as indicative of low verbal fluency, less emotional responsiveness, and more pathology. However, the same scores may also be interpreted as reflecting culturally appropriate restraint and respect for authority.

In contrast, practitioners may also make the opposite error by applying culture-specific norms to a particular client or group, when in fact more general or universal norms may be more appropriate. For example, symptoms and behaviors such as hallucinating, extreme grandiosity, or even ingestion of sharp objects by African American children have been viewed by therapists as culturally appropriate or manipulative. Others suggest that the African American juvenile offender is more often seen as exhibiting behavior characteristic of his or her culture and frequently receives inadequate psychological counseling.

Failures to consider alternative interpretations of clinical material, particularly in the case of ethnic minorities, have been discussed in the research literature as evidence of bias. In 1989, Lopez described two main types of bias that may occur in the clinical judgment setting. The overpathologizing bias refers to findings that minority group members are perceived as more disturbed or as requiring more treatment than is actually the case. Conversely, the minimizing or underpathologizing bias occurs when practitioners minimize symptoms of actual pathology. In other words, they judge symptoms of pathology as normative for a given minority group. [See RACISM AND MENTAL HEALTH.]

In reviews of the literature, consistent evidence of bias was found by a number of investigators who studied the accuracy of assessments of ethnic minority clients. Data from one study suggest that being African American is predictive of a diagnosis of schizophrenia, even after controlling for mental health service usage, diagnoses from standardized interviews,

and clinical ratings of adjustment. In another study, analyses of the records of 76 bipolar patients from different ethnic groups revealed that more than two thirds of the patients had been previously misdiagnosed with schizophrenia. These data suggested that Hispanic Americans and African Americans were previously misdiagnosed with schizophrenia significantly more often than were White Americans. [See SCHIZOPHRENIA.]

Clearly, these clinical judgment biases toward ethnic minorities have significant consequences for the client being assessed. Misassessment may lead to clients' failure to receive appropriate treatment and services and fair consideration in educational and employment settings. In addition, the overdiagnosis of schizophrenic disorders in bipolar ethnic patients may result in long-term exposure to antipsychotic medication, thereby increasing the patients' risk of developing tardive dyskinesia. The substantial risks involved underscore the importance of testing hypotheses generated by both universal and culture-specific norms, rather than accepting a priori a particular interpretation.

B. Barriers to Clinical Assessment

Several reasons have been posited to explain evidence of bias toward ethnic minorities, most of which are related to the amount of social and cultural distance between the therapist and client, which in part is dependent on race. One such barrier to accurate assessment is the effect of racial stereotypes elicited by both clinician and patient. For example, it is a popularly held stereotype that Asian Americans, including recent immigrants and refugees, are well-adjusted and psychologically resilient. However, recent studies have found that Indochinese refugees and other immigrant groups may be more at risk for psychological and physical complaints than the general population. The misperception of Asians as well-adjusted may lead practitioners to overlook clinical material that might suggest psychological distress. Conversely, it is also possible that a patient from an ethnic minority race may react to a clinician from a majority race with feelings of suspicion and resentment, which in turn may be interpreted by the clinician as paranoia, lability, or avoidance.

In addition to racial stereotypes elicited in the therapist–client interaction, cultural differences may also influence the diagnostic practices of clinicians.

In 1980, Li-Repac instructed Caucasian and Chinese American therapists to evaluate Chinese and Caucasian clients during a videotaped interview. Caucasian clinicians described Chinese clients as anxious, awkward, confused, nervous, quiet, and reserved, whereas Chinese clinicians described the same clients as adaptable, alert, dependable, friendly, and practical. In evaluations of Caucasian clients, Caucasian clinicians rated them as affectionate, adventurous, and capable, whereas Chinese clinicians used terms such as active, aggressive, and rebellious. In general, Caucasian raters saw Chinese patients as more depressed and inhibited, socially unskilled, and having less capacity for interpersonal relationships. Conversely, Chinese clinicians rated Caucasian clients as more seriously disturbed than did Caucasian clinicians. The results suggest that culture affects the therapists' impressions of mental health as well as mental illness.

Third, because most assessment procedures rely on verbal communication in English, conducting an accurate assessment of a patient with limited English skills may be especially difficult. Many immigrants and refugees speak little or no English, thereby increasing the risk of misdiagnosis. For example, it has been suggested that the disproportionately high reported rates of schizophrenia among Puerto Ricans in New York City may be due to the patients' use of their nondominant language. Puerto Ricans (as well as other foreign language speakers) with limited English proficiency often speak with a limited vocabulary, with a high rate of repetition, misconstructed sentences, and a vocabulary that appears to be idiosyncratic. Schizophrenic speech is also characterized by repetitions, individualized vocabularies, and atypical sentence construction.

Although the presence of bilingual therapists may facilitate rapport and communication, some studies have questioned which language (primary or secondary) conveys the true nature and extent of pathology. Additional problems may arise when in the absence of bilingual therapists, family members or interpreters are used during the assessment interview. The introduction of a third party may lead to distortions, inaccuracies, and embellishments in the translation which may interfere with the assessment process.

It is important to note that although these language difficulties are especially pervasive in clinical assessment of recent immigrants and refugees, linguistic differences among native English-speakers may also

occur. For example, several researchers studied the linguistic compatibility of Caucasian counselors and African American and Caucasian high school students. Lists of the common words used by each of the three groups were created and used to develop three vocabulary tests that were administered to the groups. Results revealed that the counselors knew less than one fifth of the words the African American students knew and used. Conversely, the African American students knew less than one third of the words the counselors knew and used. The Caucasian students on the other hand, showed more knowledge and usage of the words used by both the African American students and the Caucasian counselors. These results suggest that linguistic differences even among native English-speakers may significantly impact the assessment process by impairing effective communication and understanding of the client's experience.

Fourth, in addition to language and linguistic differences, different styles of communication may also jeopardize the assessment of ethnic minority clients. Particularly among Asian groups, a reliance on nonverbal communication may lead to diagnostic bias in the clinical setting. For example, nonverbal signs such as infrequent eye contact and a downward angling of the head are often viewed as signs of depression. However, in many Asian cultures, these nonverbal cues are normative ways of communicating respect for authority. Although this difference in meaning of nonverbal behaviors may lead to overdiagnosis, underdiagnosis may also result. Because Chinese people rarely use excessive gestures, a Western therapist may overlook the degree of distress experienced by Chinese clients due to their more restrained style.

Fifth, the practice of using assessment tools and strategies that have been developed, standardized, and validated in nonminority, middle-class, English-speaking populations may contribute to biased assessments of ethnic minority clients. Although efforts have been made to provide reliable multilingual translations of popular pen-and-paper tests of intelligence tests, personality measures, and mental health surveys, independent data demonstrating their translation, conceptual, and metric equivalence have rarely been established. Perhaps the most widely used and translated self-report inventory used in clinical assessment is the Minnesota Multiphasic Personality Inventory (MMPI). However, reports of ethnic differences in MMPI and MMPI-2 score profiles have raised questions about possible biases inherent in the tests. These differences have been interpreted in several ways. Some researchers argue that culture bias in the MMPI results in the pathologizing of ethnic minorities when compared to the primarily Caucasian standardization sample. Metric nonequivalence of the scores or different response sets may also account for ethnic differences. Finally, it is possible that these differences in score profiles may reflect higher levels of pathology in ethnic minority individuals. In short, the lack of conclusive empirical studies pertaining to the intellectual, personality, and mental health assessment of ethnic minorities suggests that one must exercise caution in interpreting test scores of minority clients. Cultural background and racial identity should also be assessed to provide additional information that may clarify test results.

A final consideration when assessing ethnic minority clients is that symptom expression may also be influenced by culture. For example, it has been suggested that Chinese Americans and other Asian American groups initially tend to present more somatic complaints than do Caucasian patients, and tend to hold back information or not report symptoms that may cause themselves or their families shame (e.g., marital conflict). Psychological distress related to adjustment difficulties may also be communicated through the discussion of difficulties in family relationships. Because of these tendencies, clinicians should specifically inquire about psychological symptoms, because Chinese patients are not likely to volunteer them.

In summary, the assessment and diagnosis of ethnically and culturally diverse clients is complicated by a variety of factors such as stereotypes held by the client and therapist, cultural background, language and linguistic issues, modes of communication, lack of culturally equivalent assessment tools, and differences in symptom expression. These factors suggest the need for clinicians working with ethnic minorities to act as scientists—carefully generating hypotheses based on universal and culture-specific norms, collecting "data" through various methodologies, and testing them before formulating a clinical decision. In addition to being able to provide appropriate clinical services, an openness to exploring ethnic and cultural variation in behavior may yield a broader understanding of psychological constructs in general and lead to advancements in psychological theory and practice.

IV. ETHNICITY AND TREATMENT OUTCOME

Research on the relationship between ethnicity and the outcome of psychotherapy has been growing in recent years. The basic question has been, Do non-White ethnic groups benefit from psychotherapy? Most researchers theorize that ethnic clients will fare worse than Whites in treatment because of a variety of factors, including diagnostic bias, racism, cultural differences, linguistic barriers, and so on. Unfortunately, the evidence available to answer this question is scarce and often contradictory. In fact, there are almost no studies that compare treated and untreated groups of ethnic clients. Conceptual and methodological limitations in outcome research, coupled with the scarcity of suitable research subjects, have restricted psychological research thus far.

A. Research

Investigations into the mental health outcomes of ethnic clients have typically relied on indirect measures of treatment outcome derived from community samples. Psychotherapy utilization rates, length of treatment, premature dropout, and global measures of functioning (e.g., Global Assessment Scale or GAS) have been used as dependent variables in this research. In general, results have indicated that psychotherapy is helpful for ethnic clients. That is, all clients—regardless of ethnicity—show some improvement over time as a result of receiving psychological treatment. Studies differ in the relative size and ranking of therapeutic progress across different ethnic groups, however.

A number of studies have found that ethnic minorities fare worse than European Americans in mental health treatment. In a study examining the services received by minority clients in Seattle mental health centers over a 3-year period, the four groups of minority clients (African Americans, Asian Americans, Hispanics, and Native Americans) had a significantly higher dropout rate than European American clients. Minority clients also averaged significantly fewer sessions than European Americans. These results were not explained by systematic differences between Whites and minority clients in the following areas: diagnosis, staff seen at intake, staff seen during therapy, type of program, or type of service. When differences in socioeconomic status (SES) were statistically controlled, all of the minority groups, except

Hispanics, remained significantly more likely to drop out of treatment than White clients.

A similar study of the Los Angeles County mental health system found ethnic differences in dropout rates and GAS scores. Specifically, African Americans had a significantly higher percentage of dropouts than did Whites and Mexican Americans. In contrast, the percentage of Asian Americans who dropped out of treatment was significantly lower than the percentages for Whites and Mexican Americans. That is, African Americans were the most likely, and Asian Americans were the least likely, to terminate treatment after just one therapy session. Using discharge GAS scores adjusted for the clients' GAS rating at admission, results indicated that Mexican Americans were the most likely to improve after treatment. At the other extreme, African Americans were the least likely of all four groups to improve after treatment. The difference between Whites and Asian Americans was not statistically significant.

Other studies have found no relationship between ethnicity and treatment outcome. For example, a 1989 follow-up to the 1977 study in Seattle found that dropout rates had decreased over time for all ethnic groups. Furthermore, ethnicity was not a statistically significant predictor of GAS scores at discharge. In 1978 and 1982, respectively, Jones conducted two studies that also found no ethnic differences in client and therapist ratings of treatment outcome.

In addition to the aforementioned large-scale community studies involving thousands of minority clients, several researchers have investigated the effects of culturally sensitive psychotherapies. To date, these studies have focused exclusively on Hispanic clients. Preliminary evidence suggests that the use of folktales and biographical modeling are effective interventions with Hispanic children and teenagers, respectively. Incorporating cultural practices into psychotherapy promises to be a fertile area of future investigation.

B. Guidelines

On the basis of past research on ethnicity and treatment outcome, there are concerns that need to be addressed in subsequent studies. First, there is a lack of agreement concerning meaningful evaluatory criteria for outcome studies in general. In other words, researchers disagree about the methods, standards, and instruments used to measure the effectiveness of psychotherapy. Once these criteria are determined, it is necessary to establish their applicability to the assessment of different ethnic groups. Second, researchers need to study dimensions of ethnicity that may explain ethnic differences in outcome. Given the current use of ethnicity as a categorical variable, psychologists are unable to explain why ethnic clients have negative or positive results from psychological treatment. Finally, there is a lack of information about the treatment process itself. Variables that are closely aligned to the dynamics of therapy—called proximal variables—need to be identified to understand how ethnicity affects the therapy process. For example, research on the effects of an ethnic match between the client and therapist is gaining popularity. Regardless of the results, the specific mechanisms of how ethnic match may or may not affect therapy will be undetermined. Proximal variables, such as rapport, empathy, and knowledge of the client's culture, may provide better descriptions of the therapy dynamics involving ethnic clients.

In conclusion, ethnic minority clients benefit from psychological treatment. Studies vary about how much or how little minority clients benefit relative to European American clients. As these empirical investigations continue, researchers will ask *what treatment* conducted *by whom* is effective for *which client* with *what problem* in *what setting?* How and why questions will naturally follow. Future studies will undoubtedly provide many answers to these questions and most assuredly generate even more questions.

V. MENTAL HEALTH SERVICE DELIVERY: IMPLICATIONS OF MANAGED CARE

Studies of treatment outcome typically focus on the relationship of ethnicity to the client–therapist relationship. However, a critical examination of ethnicity at a broader level of analysis is also required. Specifically, the characteristics and dynamics of mental health delivery systems (e.g., community mental health centers) contain important information relevant to the care of ethnic clients. Treatment in the context of managed care offers unique challenges for clients, therapists, and researchers alike.

A. Quality of Care

Ethnic variations in rates of service utilization and in the measurement of related outcomes (e.g., premature termination, global assessment of functioning, etc.) may be conceptualized as reflecting differential *quality of care* levels across these populations. Similarly, to the extent that systematic variations in psychotherapy and other modes of mental health service delivery occur across populations, quality of care may be differentially distributed as well. Quality has been defined in various ways, but most notably as a tripartite entity that includes the structure (or the environment of care), process (or the content), and outcome (or the results of care) of service delivery. The structural component, the most indirect measure of quality, focuses on the resources that are necessary to provide care, whether in terms of facilities, types of services offered, or staffing requirements. Understanding the process component requires a comparison of the actual service delivery with explicit criteria or normative standards. Finally, an assessment of outcome entails an evaluation of the effects of treatment, or the effect of process variables on patient outcome. In addition, some researchers have called for an expansion of this definition to include factors beyond the site of service delivery, such as aspects of the community context in which service delivery occurs.

B. Cultural Competence

This expanded quality of care framework is instructive for conceptualizing mental health services delivered to ethnic minority populations for several reasons. First, recommendations to make services more "culturally responsive" to ethnic minorities imply that such services would require improved structure (e.g., bilingual/bicultural staffing, parallel services, location of service, and hours that allow for greater access, etc.), process (e.g., greater cultural sensitivity among therapists, appropriateness of services provided, etc.), and outcome (e.g., less premature termination, better overall functioning, increased satisfaction with services, etc.). In other words, such services would promote higher quality. This indicates that cultural responsiveness or "cultural competence" is a critical underlying dimension of high quality of care. Some researchers note that all therapy, regardless of the ethnicity of the client, is culturally contextualized, and that positive therapeutic outcomes depend on the ability of the therapist to incorporate successfully cultural factors into the treatment intervention. From this perspective, cultural responsiveness is a necessary component of quality for clients of all ethnic backgrounds; for European American clients, however, there is a greater likelihood that a therapist may share in a client's cultural context, thus permitting greater cultural sensitivity in the therapeutic process.

Most of the research on cultural sensitivity focuses on the structure, process, and outcomes associated with interventions that occur within the context of a dyadic counseling relationship, that is, interventions at an interpersonal level. Issues of cultural competence in delivering mental health care tend to be neglected at an institutional or systemic level. However, with the emergence of new systems of health and mental health service delivery (i.e., managed care), an examination of the potential impact of these systems on the delivery of services to ethnic minority populations is crucial. In addition to examining potential deficiencies in mental health service delivery to ethnic minorities within managed care contexts, better descriptions are needed concerning what culturally competent service delivery would actually look like within managed care settings.

C. Managed Care

As a generic term, managed care simply refers to a range of practices designed to regulate the utilization of services, and where a major focus is to reduce health care costs through eliminating unnecessary treatments and procedures. Judgments regarding the necessity and appropriateness of care provided are made at various points in treatment through utilization management (UM) programs. For instance, preadmission certification occurs before care is actually provided, and concurrent review and discharge planning occur while the patient is undergoing treatment. In contrast, retrospective review and denial of payment policies occur after a patient has completed treatment. These programs operate in a wide variety of managed care systems (i.e., group or staff HMOs, PPOs, POSs, etc.), which must balance the competing demands of cost, access, and quality in the provision of services.

A primary mode of cost containment is to limit access to services. One way in which access may be limited is by managing the demand for services. Restructuring insurance benefits and co-payment structures, for example, is an effective means of controlling help-seeking behavior and service utilization. The implications of these demand-based payment structures for service delivery to ethnic minorities are not adequately recognized in the mental health literature. For many ethnic minority populations, for instance, *demand* for services may not accurately reflect the actual *need* for services in the community. In epidemiological studies of utilization of mental health services, Asian American and Latino populations have been found to underutilize services, whereas African Americans tend to overutilize services relative to Whites. These utilization patterns may be used by third-party payors (e.g., insurance companies) to target ethnic populations in at least two ways. First, because insurance companies commonly target membership to desirable (e.g., low-risk) communities, ethnic groups with traditionally low utilization rates (e.g., low demand) may be targeted as desirable populations to cover. Thus, insurance companies may maximize their profits by providing coverage to Asian American and Latino populations, particularly if they do not engage in any outreach activities to promote utilization of services. Nevertheless, some evidence suggests that low initial demand for services may be misleading, as these individuals may not present for treatment until their symptoms are fairly severe, resulting in a later demand for more intensive and expensive services.

Second, ethnic populations that display patterns of overutilization of services because of such factors as chronic poverty, immigration stress, racism, and so on, may be labeled as "high risk" by insurance companies. Consequently, insurance companies may be motivated to avoid or exclude these populations (i.e., adverse selection) because they may include a disproportionate enrollment of individuals who are poorer or more prone to suffer more loss or make more claims than the average risk, which would raise the costs of providing care. Not only are a significant proportion of ethnic minorities located in the lowest level of the socioeconomic status strata, but evidence suggests that they are indeed less likely to be covered by insurance relative to White Americans. Insurance coverage has emerged as a significant predictor of mental health care use, so differential rates of coverage across ethnic minority and White groups are of significant concern. Ethnic minority populations may be more likely to experience inequities in health and mental health outcomes, not only because of potentially greater vulnerability to negative outcomes, but also because of lowered availability and access into systems of care. [*See* MANAGED CARE.]

D. Access to Appropriate Care

Even with adequate insurance coverage, however, many ethnic minorities may find it difficult to access needed services within a managed care system. Many managed care systems are structured so that specifically designated primary care physicians, called gatekeepers, determine whether a patient's condition meets criteria for "medical necessity." If medical necessity for services is established, gatekeeper physicians may refer patients to specialists, including psychiatrists, psychologists, and other mental health service providers. The inappropriateness of this criterion for people with mental and addictive disorders (because much necessary and effective treatment for mental illness is not strictly "medical" in nature) is being highlighted by mental health field leaders and researchers. Compounding this problem, primary care physicians serving as gatekeepers often demonstrate limited diagnostic and referral skills for mental health problems. Ethnic minority patients with mental health concerns thus face a dual barrier. First, gatekeepers in current systems are not yet adequately trained to recognize reliably mental health problems; the use of mental health specialty services appears to decrease when gatekeeping systems are in place. Second, reliance on medical necessity criteria may block ethnic minority access to treatment because of language barriers, misdiagnoses, cultural limitations of current diagnostic criteria, and inadequate recognition of cultural determinants in the expression of symptoms of mental illness.

With various utilization management programs in place, treatment of an ethnic minority client by a culturally responsive therapist may not necessarily result in greater treatment effectivenes, because a therapist has relatively limited authority in many managed care systems. Instead, treatment is managed by case managers and concurrent utilization reviewers (many of whom are not mental health professionals), and the therapist–client relationship is invariably subject to these "intrusive" influences. Consequently, culturally responsive treatment requires that *all* individuals in the managed care hierarchy, not just the therapist, be sensitive to cultural factors that might influence access into treatment, the treatment process itself, as well as evaluation of the outcomes of treatment for ethnic patients.

Quality of care for mental health service delivery requires cultural competence, whether in traditional service delivery or in evolving managed care systems. At the same time, attaining some level of cultural competence requires an evaluation of service delivery at a system-wide level, in terms of structures, processes, and outcomes of care. Traditional conceptions of cultural sensitivity as an examination of therapist–client dynamics are still useful, but not sufficient for understanding the impact of culture and ethnicity on service delivery within these systems. Access to care may serve as an important starting point for examining cultural competence from a systemic perspective, particularly within the context of the larger community in which treatment occurs. Equal access exists when services are distributed on the basis of need rather than on demographic variables (e.g., race, family income, place of residence, etc.). Such a community-based framework facilitates an exploration of the role cultural and racial factors may play in treated (or treatment-eligible) versus untreated (or treatment-ineligible) individuals' ability to access mental health care and obtain appropriate and effective mental health services. Indeed, it will become increasingly clear that cultural competence, beginning with access to care, is a critical dimension in the provision of quality services to ethnic minority populations within managed care settings.

VI. CONCLUSIONS

To date, psychological research on the relationship of ethnicity to mental health has been a search for ethnic differences. Studies on the prevalence of mental disorders, psychological assessment, and psychotherapy outcome have all yielded significant findings. These results suggest careful scrutiny of the treatment of ethnic clients by mental health delivery systems such as managed care.

In terms of psychiatric epidemiology, both clinic records and community surveys have been used to assess the prevalence of mental disorders across ethnic groups. Clinic records often indicate that ethnic minorities are underrepresented in the mental health care system. However, these findings do not indicate lower rates of psychopathology, because access barriers, financial constraints, discrimination, cultural stigmas against psychological treatment, and other factors may reduce the likelihood of ethnic minorities using existing services. Community-based studies, such as the ECA and NCS, found few ethnic differences. For ethnic clients, the ECA reported the following rates of psychopathology relative to Whites: African Americans had lower rates of affective disorders and substance abuse, but higher rates of anxiety disorders. Hispanic Americans had lower rates of affective disorders, but higher rates of alcoholism. The NCS revealed even fewer ethnic differences: Hispanic Americans showed a higher rate of affective disorders relative to Whites. Otherwise, the NCS did not reveal any significant ethnic differences in psychiatric diagnosis.

Research on the assessment of ethnic minorities suggests that clinicians may be biased in their evaluations of minority clients. This bias may result in the overpathologizing of the client, such as an increased likelihood to diagnose an African American client as being schizophrenic, or the underpathologizing of the client in which actual psychiatric symptoms are minimized by the therapist.

Research concerning the outcome of psychotherapy with ethnic minority clients indicates that most clients—regardless of ethnicity—benefit from therapy. However, relative to Whites, ethnic minorities may benefit significantly less. A lack of consensus on evaluation strategies and the therapy process have hampered investigations on psychotherapy outcome.

At a systems level of analysis, research on ethnicity involves a different set of variables to evaluate the quality of care for ethnic minorities. For example, the gatekeeping system of managed care may involve structural impediments that prevent some ethnic clients from receiving appropriate mental health care.

In conclusion, many studies have revealed ethnic differences in a variety of areas of mental health. The next step is to explain these differences. Although many different hypotheses have been proposed, ethnicity has typically been treated as a categorical variable, thus bereft of any conclusive, explanatory power. Psychologists will advance society's understanding of ethnicity by systematically examining its components (i.e., cultural characteristics, ethnic identity, socioeconomic status, and racism and discrimination), which theoretically may explain ethnic differences.

BIBLIOGRAPHY

Lopez, S. (1989). Patient variable biases in clinical judgment: Conceptual overview and methodological considerations. *Psychological Bulletin, 106*(2), 184–203.

Phinney, J. (1996). When we talk about American ethnic groups, what do we mean? *American Psychologist, 51*(9), 918–927.

Sue, S., Zane, N., & Young, K. (1994). Research on psychotherapy with culturally diverse populations. In A. E. Bergin & S. L. Garfield (Eds.), *Handbook of psychotherapy and behavior change* (4th ed., pp. 783–8 17). New York: John Wiley & Sons.

Takeuchi, D., & Uehara, E. (1996). Ethnic minority mental health services: Current research and future conceptual directions. In B. Lubotsky Levin and J. Petrilla(Eds.), *Mental health services: A public health perspective* (pp. 63–80). London: Oxford Press.

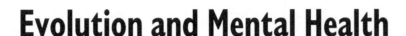

Evolution and Mental Health

Alfonso Troisi

University of Rome Tor Vergata

Michael T. McGuire

University of California, Los Angeles

Evolutionary Biology   The collective disciplines of biology that study and explain evolution.

Fitness   A measure of the contribution of a given genotype to the subsequent generation relative to that of other genotypes.

Genotype   The set of genes possessed by an individual.

Natural Selection   The nonrandom and differential survival and/or reproduction of classes of entities (alleles, genotypes, populations) that differ in one or more hereditary characteristics.

Trait   Any character (e.g., behavior) or property of an organism.

Organic **EVOLUTION** is any gradual change or, more specifically, any genetic change in organisms from generation to generation. Natural selection is the process most responsible for such changes. Traits that are influenced by genetic information track with genetic changes.

I. HISTORY

Historically, two trends in psychology and psychiatry have contributed to the concept of mental health. The

first attempts to understand and define mental health in a positive sense. Examples include: (1) The optimum of growth and happiness combined with the capacity to participate in the reproduction of society. (2) Emotional maturity, strength of character, capacity to deal with conflicting emotions, a balance between inner life and adaptations to reality, and a successful welding into a whole of the different parts of the personality leading to an integrated self-concept. (3) The adjustment of human beings to the world and to each other with a maximum of effectiveness and happiness. These definitions, which emphasize a harmonious view of mental life (without necessarily stating how harmony can be evaluated or measured), and which are largely the work of psychoanalysts, describe mental health as an *ideal* that embodies strong social values and utopian ambitions. They are consistent with the definition of health adopted by the World Health Organization: "Health is a state of complete physical, mental and social well-being and not merely the absence of disease and infirmity."

The second trend is more pragmatic and consonant with current psychiatric practice, which has made the control and treatment of mental disorders its primary objectives. Based on the application of the medical model to psychiatry, this approach characterizes mental health as the absence of mental disease. There is less concern with definitions of health and disease; more concern with strategies for thinking about, studying, and taking care of people with mental disorders; and an assumption that the meaning of mental disorders is understood. Within the medical model framework, mental disorders are not different from somatic illnesses, and the presence of either anatomical or physiological pathology, or both, is the necessary condition for defining morbidity. One of the primary aims of those advocating this approach is to purge mental diagnoses of social and utopian values and to fit mental disease into the objective and empirical structure of modern biological science.

How does an evolutionary model of mental health relate to these competing approaches? The basic view encapsulated in the medical model of mental health and disease is that psychiatry is a branch of medicine, which in turn is a form of applied biology. Because evolutionary theory is the bedrock of modern biology, it is reasonable to expect that the evolutionary concept of mental health will overlap with the view expressed by the advocates of the medical model. This does not turn out to be the case, however. To explain this paradox, it is essential to explore the different meanings that the term *biological* has in medicine, psychiatry, and evolutionary biology. In the medical literature, the term is synonymous with physiological, organic, or nonenvironmental, and its present use in psychiatry signifies the physical–chemical approach to the study of mental processes and behavior: biological psychiatry has been defined as the science examining the physical–chemical basis of abnormal mental processes and behavior. But the biology of behavior is more than the study of brain anatomy and physiology. Findings from different evolutionary disciplines focusing on human psyche and behavior, such as human ethology, Darwinian anthropology, and evolutionary psychology have demonstrated that adaptive function, phylogenetic origin, and genotype–environment interactions are biological phenomena that are as deserving of study as those on which the neurosciences focus. Given this perspective, the biological definition of mental health cannot be reduced to the absence of psychopatological manifestations reflecting disordered processes in various brain systems.

The evolutionary view of mental health also differs in important ways from that described in the psychoanalytic literature, even though the two views agree that the efforts to understand health in a positive sense are legitimate and scientifically acceptable. From an evolutionary perspective, introducing the concepts of efficiency, viability, and happiness into discussions about mental health does not imply that health equates with perfection. Natural selection does not achieve perfection largely because there are costs associated with every beneficial genetic change preserved in evolution. The process of evolution is the process of trade-offs and compromises. Natural selection favors traits that give an overall adaptive advantage, even if those same traits increase vulnerability to specific symptoms. A state of mental health conceptualized in terms of biological adaptation may in fact be incompatible with individual happiness and social armony.

II. THE EVOLUTIONARY CONCEPT OF MENTAL HEALTH

The evolutionary concept of mental health builds from two basic ideas: (1) The capacity to achieve short-term biological goals is the best single attribute that characterizes mental health, and (2) the assessment of functional capacities cannot be properly made without consideration of the environment in which the individual lives. These two ideas reflect a concept of mental health that is both functional and ecological.

Natural selection is strictly an a posteriori process that rewards current success but never sets up future goals. It is the observation that certain traits have advantageous *consequences* for their possessors in certain environments that accounts for their being favored. However, the a posteriori for the species is the a priori for the individual. In an evolutionary context, individuals can be viewed as strategists employing a variety of tactics to achieve biological goals. When we say that a behavioral trait is functional or adaptive, we mean that it enhances the survival or reproductive success of the individual. But these ultimate goals may be achieved through long chains of events consequent upon the behavior in question. For this reason, ultimate goals are of limited value in analyzing the details of behavior. Focusing on short-term goals can facilitate the process of assessing the functional efficiency of individual behavior. For example, to achieve the ultimate goal of enhancing one's own reproductive success, a person must correctly execute a variety of adaptive behaviors including identifying, selecting and acquiring a partner, accurately interpreting his/her needs and desires, and arousing his/her sexual interest. Each of these activities is a short-term goal that may be primarily rewarding, not simply secondarily rewarding because of its contiguous relationship to the ultimate goal. Functional capacities are the means of executing adaptive behaviors. They are essential for achieving short-term biological goals that increase the probability of survival and reproductive success.

The study of interactions between individuals and their environments (the ecological perspective) is essential to evaluate the efficiency of functional capacities. No trait is adaptive in all environments. The same trait can be highly adaptive in one environment and minimally adaptive in another. The classical example of this point is found in sickle-cell anemia. The sickle-cell gene occurs mostly in people from regions where malaria is prevalent because, in its heterozygous state, it confers some resistance to malaria. Homozygotes, however, are anemic and seldom reach reproductive age. In populations that carry such genes but are no longer exposed to malaria, the sickle-cell trait is minimally adaptive.

The preceding discussion underscores two important points. (1) The evolutionary concept of health and disease is consequence-oriented: what makes a condition pathological are its consequences, not its causes or correlates. And (2), the degree of efficiency of functional capacities is dependent on features of the environment. Adverse environments can compromise the efficiency of optimal capacities, just as favorable environments can offset or mitigate the inefficiency of suboptimal capacities.

Although the evolutionary analysis of functional capacities differs in important ways from that described in psychiatry's diagnostic systems, the category of Mild Mental Retardation in *DSM-III-R* (the *Diagnostic and Statistical Manual-III-Revised* of the American Psychiatric Association) provides an example of the application of the functional and ecological concepts. The diagnosis of Mild Mental Retardation requires both a significantly subaverage general intellectual functioning (an IQ between from 50 to 55 and 70) *and* concurrent deficits or impairments in adaptive functioning (e.g. compromised social and daily living skills, personal independence, self-sufficiency). The description of this disorder in *DSM-III-R* goes on to state that: "Some people with Mild Mental Retardation develop good adaptive skills and maintain jobs in competitive employment. For such people the diagnosis of Mild Mental Retardation may no longer be justified, even if it was appropriate when they were of school age and their intellectual deficits limited their academic functioning." The description has been re-phrased in the most recent (1994) version of the *Diagnostic and Statistical Manual (DSM-IV)*: "Individuals who had Mild Mental Retardation earlier in their lives manifested by failure in academic learning tasks may, with appropriate training and opportunities, develop good adaptive skills in other domains and may no longer have the level of impairment required for a diagnosis of Mental Retardation." Such a seemingly minor modification in *DSM-IV* puts more emphasis on rehabilitation, and, therefore, takes a step backward from the context-dependent conceptualization of the disorder in *DSM-III-R*. [*See* MENTAL RETARDATION AND MENTAL HEALTH.]

III. ADAPTATION AND MENTAL HEALTH

Definitions of health (or, conversely, of disease) similar to evolutionary-based definitions have been suggested by a number of authors. For example: (1) A disease is composed of phenomena which are not only abnormal by their species norm, but also place the living organisms displaying the disease at a biological disadvantage. (2) A person is healthy if his body functions with at least species-typical efficiency. And (3), disorders are the results of things that have gone wrong with evolved structures that allow for adequate functioning. These definitions reflect functional views of mental health and disease. However, they have attracted many criticisms, such as the concept of biological disadvantage is too vague and that it is seldom possible to demonstrate that a difference in behavior affects fertility or mortality. Critics emphasize that defining as abnormal anything that does not function according to its design is useful in instances of somatic illness; however, it is less helpful in behavior disorders because the function of many behavior pattern is unknown.

These criticisms, which reflect the fact that the problem of measuring adaptation in the study of human behavior has proven to be difficult, may be addressed in the following ways: (1) The achievement of short-term biological goals is a valid measure of behavioral adaptation. And (2), the assessment of functional capacities is the best predictor of future goal achievement. The focus on functional capacities and short-term biological goals allows clinicians to make cross-sectional functional assessments of individual patients that would be impossible to make by applying the lifetime criteria of fertility and mortality. In addition, it excludes from the category of mental disorders those conditions that involve the failure to achieve ultimate biological goals even if a person's functional capacities are intact (e.g., infertility due to rational use of birth-control measures).

Another concept requiring explanation is the word *adaptation,* which has different uses in psychiatry and evolutionary biology. From a psychiatric viewpoint, adaptation is a process of conforming or reacting to the environment in such way as to fulfill one's wishes and needs. Efforts at self-change through insight constitute the autoplastic pattern of adaptation. Efforts at environmental change constitute the alloplastic pattern of adaptation. In evolutionary biology, the process of adaptation is the long-term modification of a character under selection for efficient or advantageous functioning in a particular context, not the short-term adjustment by a phenotypically plastic individual. While there is a positive correlation between evolutionary adaptation and the capacity of individuals to adjust, adjustment is not synonymous with adaptation. For example, adjustment to a pathological family environment may reduce intrafamily conflict, yet it may also diminish the chances to achieve biological goals in the person who adjusts.

IV. THE CLINICAL ASSESSMENT OF FUNCTIONAL CAPACITIES

Apart from the points discussed in the preceding section, the clinical application of the evolutionary view of mental health and disease would lead to changes in perspective and methodology relative to current clinical practices. These changes are summarized by the following points: (1) Give less weight to symptoms. (2) Move out of the office. And (3), observe behavior.

Give less weight to symptoms means that the clinician should be aware that the severity of psychiatric symptoms is often a poor predictor of the degree of functional impairment. For example, many studies have documented that schizophrenic patients have pronounced deficits in social competence. These impairments in social functioning are largely independent of the signs and symptoms currently used to diagnose schizophrenia. By directly observing schizophrenic patients' behavior, investigators have found

only weak correlations between positive and negative symptom ratings and social skills required for effective functioning. Other studies have shown that social competence deficits manifest many years before the onset of psychiatric symptoms among adolescents at risk for schizophrenia. Yet other studies of depressed patients have failed to reveal a relationship between memory complaint and impairment: the more depressed an individual, the more complaints of memory the individual is likely to report; however, there is no significant relationship between the degree of depression and actual performance on memory tasks.

Move out of the office acknowledges the fact that the artificial setting where mental health assessments generally occur (e.g., clinicians' offices) may give a distorted picture of what happens to patients in their natural environment. For example, depressed individuals can engender negative mood and rejection in those with whom they interact; roommates of depressed college students like their roommates less and tend to reject them more than do roommates of nondepressed subjects; and, spouses of depressed partners report feeling more depressed, hostile, and critical following interactions with their partners. However, studies focusing on interactions of depressed people with strangers have failed to replicate these findings. Thus, the negative quality of depressed persons' interactions will fully emerge only in specific social environments, namely, those in which there is a close relationship among participants.

Observe (and measure) behavior highlights the fact that the objective and quantitative recording of patients' behavior may yield different results from those obtained using psychiatric rating scales or clinical evaluations. For example, the nonverbal behavior of depressed patients has been studied to determine whether their behavior predicts response to antidepressant drugs. In one study, prior to drug treatment, responders and nonresponders did not differ with respect to sex, age, education, *DSM-III-R* diagnosis, and severity of depression. In contrast, ethological profiles at baseline differed, with drug nonresponders showing significantly more assertive and affiliative behaviors. Other studies have employed ethological techniques to monitor the behavior of hospitalized patients suffering from acute schizophrenia. The behavioral profiles of patients were compiled without access to what subjects said. Such studies demonstrate that, compared to unimproved patients, improved patients have fewer pathological behaviors and are more responsive to others' social-participation signals.

The preceding points illustrate the differences in approach and the importance placed on the types of data to be gathered when an evolutionary approach is compared with psychiatry's official nosological systems, which emphasize symptoms over functional capacities. For example, *DSM-III* Axis V (the axis for the assessment of adaptive functioning) failed to achieve widespread clinical use and, therefore, was revised in *DSM-III-R* to explicitly include symptoms. The inclusion of symptoms in the Axis V has been retained by *DSM-IV*, even though there is evidence of poor correlations between various symptom dimensions and Axis V ratings as originally conceptualized in *DSM-III*.

V. PSYCHOLOGICAL WELL-BEING AND MENTAL HEALTH

The concepts of happiness and psychological well-being have been often proposed as indicators of mental health (see History), largely because the majority of psychiatric disorders are associated with unpleasant emotions and mental distress at some stage of their course. This association invites the following question: What is the evolutionary meaning of the frequent association between mental illness and mental suffering? [*See* HAPPINESS: SUBJECTIVE WELL-BEING.]

In the evolutionary view, emotions have evolved to provide information about costs and benefits of past, present, and future behavior. Under minimally adaptive circumstances, individuals experience mental suffering (e.g., depression). Emotions function in part as a warning system that one's goal-seeking efforts are failing and in part as a social signal to others to elicit their assistance in achieving goals. Unpleasant emotions mold subsequent behavior by reducing the likelihood that one will behave in the same way again. Conversely, pleasant emotions associated with adaptive behavior are experienced as beneficial and increase the probability that one will engage in similar behavior in the future. In this context, it is clear why mental suffering and mental illness are so frequently associated: the conditions that are currently classified as psychiatric disorders are usually minimally adaptive (with some exceptions; see the section on Individual Variability), and minimal adaptation elicits suffering.

Further, it is possible that the brain reward systems that mediate pleasure can be intrinsically malfunctioning (as in manic states) or artificially manipulated (as in substance abuse intoxication), and such malfunctions may explain why some mental disorders are associated with pleasurable mental states. [*See* EMOTIONS AND MENTAL HEALTH.]

An evolutionary analysis of mental suffering is also useful for understanding individual differences in response to stressful events. Individuals become anxious or depressed when their efforts to achieve biological goals continually fail even though their motivations to achieve specific goals remain intense. However, the relative importance of biological goals varies as a function of age and sex. For example, studies of the stressful effects of infertility reveal a near 30-fold difference in the response of women and men to infertile marriages, with women being the most affected. These differences can be explained by the fact that women see reproduction as a more central component of their identity. Cultural indoctrination only in part explains such a difference. From an evolutionary perspective, male relative indifference to infertility may be a consequence of paternity uncertainty. Because males cannot be sure of paternity, natural selection should not favor the evolution of male emotional responses to fecundity as a means for assessing reproductive success. Rather, men are expected to value more indirect clues of reproductive success such as control of resources and sexual satisfaction. As a consequence, men should show poorer psychological adjustment to sexual dysfunction. Studies of attendees of marital clinics have found that for men there is a much closer relationship between sexual dysfunction and marital distress than for women. For men, their own sexual dysfunction was able to predict about 25% of the variance of their scores on marital discord, while sexual dysfunction in their partner had no relation whatever to their own satisfaction with the marriage. For women, the level of marital discord was higher when their partner had a sexual problem than when they had a problem themselves. [*See* INFERTILITY.]

VI. INDIVIDUAL VARIABILITY AND MENTAL HEALTH

In ordinary medical usage *normal* has two meanings. The first, *that which is common*, is based on the statistical concept of normality. The second, *that which is compatible with health,* is based on the clinical concept of normality.

The fact that the two meanings are often confused suggests that the relationship between the statistical norm and the clinical norm is anything but simple. On one hand, it is clear that the two connotations do not always coincide. From a clinical perspective, it is not inconsistent to assert that a sizable proportion, even the majority, of individuals in a given population are abnormal. In fact, there are diseases (e.g., malaria in some regions of Africa) that are extremely frequent or normal in the statistical sense, yet abnormal for an individual from a clinical viewpoint. On the other hand, it is possible to find many instances in which statistical and clinical observations are positively and strongly correlated. For example, in laboratory medicine, the statistical mode is often identical with optimal function, as in the count of blood cells or in various chemical titers of plasma substances. Evolutionary theory can improve our understanding of the complex relationship between health and statistical norm.

Individual variability is important to evolutionary processes. Natural selection occurs only when differences in some phenotypic characteristic result in consistent differences in rates of survival and reproduction. There are different modes of selection, however, and they produce different types of interindividual variation. Continuous variation in physical and mental traits is the most common situation in nature. If intermediate phenotypes are most fit, selection is stabilizing and the resulting variation is continuous. In continuous variation, the individuals do not fall into sharp classes but are almost imperceptibly graded between wide extremes. Because the phenotypes that deviate in either direction from an optimal value are selected against, the extremes constitute only a small percentage of the total population with the far larger percentage clustering around the middle. Thus, if a trait is subject to stabilizing selection, it is not surprising that health (to the extent that it depends on the optimal functioning of that specific trait) coincides with the statistical norm.

Psychometric studies have demonstrated that some mental capacities (e.g., intelligence) have a normal distribution in the population. However, this does not mean that all psychological or behavioral traits must necessarily be distributed on a continuum. Variability between individuals can be discontinuous: if two or more phenotypes have high fitness, but intermediates between them have low fitness, selection is diversifying; that is, it acts in favor of two or more modal phenotypes and against those intermediate between them. Diversifying selection produces discontinuous variation, which divides the individuals of a population into two or more sharply distinct forms. Not only may this occur at the anatomical and physiological levels, but also at the behavioral level.

In many species, individuals in a population behave in different ways in order to cope with the adaptive challenges posed by the environment. Formerly, if an animal was seen behaving in a different way from the majority of the population, it was thought to be abnormal. Presently, whenever behavioral ecologists see an animal engaging in atypical behavior, they first explore the possibility that it is employing an alternative strategy to compete successfully with its rivals. Different factors can favor the evolution of alternative strategies within a species. The best strategy may depend on the environment. For example, if nutrition sources are patchy in space or changes frequently in time then different food-gathering strategies may evolve and persist. Or, consider the example of the field cricket *Gryllus integer,* where males adopt one of two strategies for mating with females. They either call frequently to attract females or they call infrequently or not at all and intercept females attracted by calling males. The louder crickets attract more females but they also incur higher costs because calling attracts a parasitic fly whose larvae consume the male crickets within a few days. Because the frequency of fly parasitism varies year by year, both strategies may persist because each does better in a different environment: calling when parasitic flies are scarce and satellite behavior when parasites are abundant.

Making the best of poor circumstances is yet another strategy. Because of their small body size, young male elephant seals have no hope of defending a harem themselves and instead they attempt to sneak copulations by pretending to be a female and joining a large bull's harem. Even though this strategy is not very successful, it is the best chance for young males for copulating with a female. Alternative strategies may also exist as a mixed *evolutionary stable strategy* (ESS), an evolutionary equilibrium where different behavioral strategies enjoy equal success. A mixed ESS is the product of frequency-dependent selection, in which the fitness of a behavioral phenotype increases as its frequency within the population decreases, that is, which behavior is optimal depends on what the other individuals in the population are doing.

How do these findings relate to human behavior? There is of course nothing new either inside or outside of psychiatry about the fact that people differ. However, what may be new is that these differences are far more important than is usually appreciated, and particularly so in considering mental syndromes or symptoms as attempts to adapt. Said differently, an evolutionary analysis suggests that a statistically deviant psychological or behavioral profile may be an alternative strategy. Antisocial personality is a possible example of an alternative, high-risk strategy associated with resource acquisition and reproduction that is currently regarded as a psychiatric disorder. Criminologists estimate that greater than 50% of the persons who could meet the criteria for this disorder go through life undiagnosed and undetected, and they are successful by evolutionary criteria. The earlier discussion of evolutionary stable strategies provides an explanation for how disorder-related traits may be favored by selection. Nonreciprocation or cheating is a central feature of antisocial personality disorder. In a society made up primarily of reciprocators, genes for cheaters can enter the population and remain, provided persons with such genes reproduce.

Chronic somatization is another example of a disorder that can be reinterpreted as an alternative strategy. For this disorder, the alternative strategy would be to make the best of a bad job. Clinical assessment of somatizing patients indicates that they have a limited number of alternative social-interaction strategies and that they view themselves as lacking in social status. Deliberate deception of others and self-deception would allow such persons to manipulate their interpersonal environments. By simulating a disease and displaying care-eliciting behavior, a person can evoke predictable reactions from others that are likely to be phylogenetically related with invalid care behavior observed in several nonhuman species. [*See* DECEPTION; SOMATIZATION AND HYPOCHONDRIASIS.]

It is worth noting that the findings of neurobiological changes in subjects with antisocial personality disorder or chronic somatization do not contradict the hypothesis that these personality traits may be alternative strategies. What are currently interpreted as abnormalities in the brains of persons with these deviant behavior patterns may merely reflect the normal operation of adaptive mechanisms. An example from general medicine can clarify this point. Sideropenia (iron deficiency) is common during infectious disease. In the presence of infection, the body releases a substance called leukocyte endogenous mediator, which greatly decreases the availability of iron in the blood. In addition, iron absorption by the gut is decreased. And finally, there is an increased production of transferrin, a glicoprotein that binds iron and favors its withholding in the liver, the spleen, and the bone marrow. The low iron levels could be interpreted as a pathological defect caused by the infectious disease. However, an evolutionary explanation of iron deficiency calls our attention to the fact that iron is a crucial and scarce resource for bacteria, and their hosts have evolved a wide variety of mechanisms to keep them from getting it.

VII. NOVEL ENVIRONMENTS AND MENTAL HEALTH

From a genetic standpoint, humans living today are Stone Age hunter-gatherers displaced through time to a world that, for certain aspects, differs from that for which our genetic constitution was selected. The Late Paleolithic era, from 35,000 to 20,000 B.C., may be considered the last time period during which the collective human gene pool interacted with bioenvironmental circumstances typical of those for which it had been originally selected. The rapid cultural changes that have occurred during the past 10,000 years have far outpaced any possible genetic adaptation, especially since much of this cultural change has occurred only subsequent to the Industrial Revolution of 200 years ago. The mismatch between our psychological and behavioral design and the current environment may be responsible for some dysfunctional emotional reactions or behavioral patterns that are currently classified as psychiatric disorders. Phobias and substance abuse are two examples of these conditions.

By holding to the apparently rational assumption that the only situation that should properly arouse fear in a human is the presence of something likely to result in pain or physical damage, psychiatrists have often considered common infantile fears, such as the fear of being alone or in the dark or with strangers, as not easily intelligible. The psychoanalytic theory postulated that fear of each of these commonplace situations is to be equated initially with fear of losing the object and ultimately with fear of physical helplessness in the face of mounting instinctual stimulation. However, psychiatrists familiar with evolutionary ideas have argued that being alone or in the dark were conditions statistically associated with an increased risk of danger (e.g., predation) in the natural environment. Because of their crucial biological functions, fear responses elicited by naturally occurring clues to danger are a part of humans' basic repertoire of behavior, and they should be viewed as genetically determined biases that result in a preparedness to meet real dangers. Other investigators have demonstrated that the prevalence of various types of phobias in adults reflects fears of dangers common throughout our evolutionary history (e.g., darkness, snakes, or heights) rather than those typical of modern environments (e.g., knives, cars, or electrical appliances.)

Substance abuse can be viewed as an example of minimally adaptive manipulation of adaptive mechanisms through the use of artificial means made available by cultural evolution. People abuse drugs mainly to seek pleasure and to avoid pain. The evolutionary utility of the pleasure mechanism derives from the fact that it is regularly aroused by adaptive situations. Experiences that are likely to increase fitness stimulate brain reward systems and free neurochemicals (opioids, dopamine) that cause pleasurable emotions. Psychoactive drugs short-circuit these evolved mechanisms. However, direct activation of the brain reward systems through drug use may have catastrophic effects because execution of adaptive behaviors is no longer necessary to experience pleasure. (The behavior of some drug addicts resembles findings from studies of rats that stopped drinking, eating, and mounting estrous females because they continuously engaged in bar pressing to receive electrical stimulation in certain areas of the brain.) [See SUBSTANCE ABUSE.]

VIII. ETHICAL AND THERAPEUTIC IMPLICATIONS

A major problem with the application of evolutionary theory to human behavior is the risk of misinterpretation and abuse. When human behavior is analyzed from an evolutionary perspective, the concept of naturalness often enters into the discussion, and the question as to what is natural and unnatural usually turns

out to be a question about what is good and bad in social terms. In the field of ethics and morality, the term *naturalistic fallacy* has been used to denote the erroneous translation of evolutionary explanations of human behavior into normative or prescriptive terms. The naturalistic fallacy consists in offering some supposedly neutral descriptive statement about what is allegedly natural, as if it could by itself entail some conclusion about what is in some way commendable.

As the unreflecting moral philosopher might take the identity between *natural* and *ethical* for granted, so the unreflecting mental health professional might conclude that all human behaviors evolved by natural selection are *healthy*. If by healthy it is meant that evolved behaviors should never be the target of preventive efforts and therapeutic intervention, then such a conclusion is another instance of the naturalistic fallacy. Evolved human behaviors may sometimes be a source of considerable individual distress and social concern. Because one of the basic aims of medicine is to alleviate human suffering, an understanding of the evolutionary roots of human psyche and behavior should translate into more effective ways for promoting individual and social well-being, not into the search for natural laws determining what is therapeutically right or wrong. Evolutionary theory does not legitimate. Rather, it explains and suggests mechanisms and pathways. Child abuse and neglect can serve as an example.

Sociobiologists have hypothesized that child abuse and neglect could be viewed as an adaptive form of parental discrimination against offspring in circumstances in which confidence of parenthood is low, parental resources are scarce, or offspring quality is poor. Assuming that parents have at their disposal limited resources that can be translated into reproductive effort and that parental care is subject to optimization by natural selection, it is reasonable to hypothesize that parental investment can be adaptively diminished or terminated under circumstances predicting reduced fitness payoffs. The evolutionary hypothesis fits well with data concerning child maltreatment perpetrated by stepparents, by parents with scarce resources, or suffered by children with physical or mental handicaps. Assume for the moment that this hypothesis is correct. An evolutionary understanding of the psychological and behavioral mechanisms that modulate parental care by no means questions the legitimacy of the efforts to prevent child abuse and neglect. On the contrary, by allowing a better identification of the risk factors associated with child maltreatment, evolutionary theory may increase the efficacy of preventive and therapeutic strategies. [*See* CHILD MALTREATMENT.]

The pursuit of conceptual clarity regarding the concept of mental health is not simply an intellectual exercise. The concept of disease acts not only to describe and explain, but also to enjoin to action. For this reason, labeling a psychological condition or a behavior pattern as either sick or healthy may have serious individual and social consequences. The evolutionary approach to mental health and illness takes into account these ethical considerations. The goal of medicine is to help the sick, not to promote biological adaptation. What is natural should not be regarded as necessarily ethical and immune from therapeutic interventions.

BIBLIOGRAPHY

Alexander, R. D. (1987). *The biology of moral systems.* New York: Aldine de Gruyter.

American Psychiatric Association. (1987). *Diagnostic and Statistical Manual of Mental Disorders, DSM-III-R.* Washington, DC: American Psychiatric Association.

American Psychiatric Association. (1994). *Diagnostic and statistical manual of mental disorders, DSM-IV.* Washington, DC: American Psychiatric Association.

Barkow, J. H., Cosmides, L., & Tooby, J. (1992). *The adapted mind.* New York: Oxford University Press.

Bowlby, J. (1969). *Attachment.* London: Hogarth Press.

Eibl-Eibesfeldt, I. (1989). *Human ethology.* New York: Aldine de Gruyter.

Futuyma, D. J. (1986). *Evolutionary biology* (2nd ed.). Sunderland, MA: Sinauer Associates, Inc.

Guze, S. B. (1992). *Why psychiatry is a branch of medicine.* New York: Oxford University Press.

Kendell, R. E. (1975). *The role of diagnosis in psychiatry.* Oxford: Blackwell.

Klein, D. F. (1978). A proposed definition of mental illness. In R. L. Spitzer & D. F. Klein (Eds.), *Critical issues in psychiatric diagnosis,* pp. 41–71. New York: Raven Press.

Hamilton, W. D. (1964). The genetical evolution of social behaviour. I, II. *Journal of Theoretical Biology, 7,* 1–52, 1964.

Marks, I. M. (1987). *Fears, phobias and rituals.* New York: Oxford University Press.

Mayr, E. (1982). *The growth of biological thought.* Cambridge, MA: Harvard University Press.

Nesse, R. M., Williams, G. C. (1994). *Why we get sick: The new science of Darwinian medicine.* New York: Times Books.

Scadding, J. G. (1967). Diagnosis: the clinician and the computer. *Lancet, ii,* 877–882, 1967.

Wilson, E. O. (1975). *Sociobiology.* Cambridge: Harvard University Press.

Wulff, H. R., Andur Pedersen, S., & Rosenberg, R. (1986). *Philosophy of medicine. An introduction.* Oxford: Blackwell.

Exercise and Mental Health

Larry M. Leith

University of Toronto

Distraction Hypothesis Suggests the positive effects of exercise on mental health can be attributed to "time-out" from troubling thoughts and situations.

Endorphin Hypothesis Supports the notion that exercise improves mental health by causing the release of peptides called endorphins, which produce a "feel better" phenomenon.

Exercise The performance of physical activity for the purpose of training or developing the body or mind.

Mental Health The state of psychological and emotional wellness, not merely the absence of disorders.

Monoamine Hypothesis Maintains the improved affect associated with exercise can be explained by changes in one or more of the brain monoamines (i.e., dopamine, serotonin, and norepinephrine).

Psychotropic Medication The use of drugs to treat mood disorders such as depression and anxiety.

Self-Efficacy Theory Suggests that a person's belief that he or she can successfully complete a demanding task (e.g., exercise) affects that person's emotions in a positive manner.

Thermogenic Hypothesis Maintains exercise improves mental health by stimulating the release of pyrogens, which result in body warming.

This chapter will demonstrate the potential of **EXERCISE** to impact positively on mental health. Extant research has portrayed exercise as a viable alternative, or adjunct, to the more traditional treatments such as medication and psychotherapy. This article will identify those areas with potential for improvement, and outline specific exercise guidelines to produce the best results. Explanations for this relationship will also be provided.

I. STATEMENT OF THE PROBLEM

A landmark study from the National Institute of Mental Health provides a comprehensive overview of mental illness in America. At a cost of $15 million, this investigation involved individual interviews with more than 17,000 people in five communities. As a source of diagnostic categories, the interviewers used the *Diagnostic and Statistical Manual of Mental Disorders.*

A major finding of this study indicated that during any 6-month span, 20% (29 million) of the adult population experienced some form of mental disturbance. In addition, it has been estimated that 29% to 38% of American adults can expect a significant psychiatric problem sometime during their lifetimes. However, only one in five of these individuals will seek professional help, usually in the form of a family physician rather than a psychiatrist. Finally, another recent study reveals that stress has been estimated to be a factor in up to 50% of all visits to medical practitioners. Statistics such as these effectively portray the fact that mental health problems are pandemic in modern society. They also highlight the need to develop self-help techniques to prevent and/or eliminate these problems.

II. TRADITIONAL TREATMENTS

Over the years, a variety of techniques have evolved for treating the most common mental disorders. Depression, for example, which afflicts approximately 6% (9.4 million) of the American population, is most often treated by psychotherapy and psychotropic medication. While psychotherapy represents one of the earliest treatments for depression, its efficacy has often been questioned. Most experts now agree that it is at least moderately helpful, and that all forms of psychotherapy appear equally effective. Psychotherapy is probably most effective with mild to moderate depression. Even so, it is often supplemented with antidepressive medication. Severe depression almost always requires medication. The most widely prescribed antidepressant drugs have traditionally been the tricyclic antidepressants (TADs). Common TADs include Surmontil, Elavil, and Tofranil. Although drugs of this nature are usually effective within about 3 weeks, they often cause side effects such as blurred vision, dry mouth, and orthostatic hypotension. Recently, Prozac has become the drug of choice for many psychiatrists, since it has been associated with fewer side effects. [See DEPRESSION; PSYCHOPHARMACOLOGY.]

The National Institute of Mental Health has reported that anxiety represents the most common mental health problem, afflicting almost 8% (13.1 million) of the American population. Traditionally, anxiety has been treated by psychotherapy, cognitive behavior modification, and drug therapy. While the first two treatment categories have experienced reasonable success, their use has been limited by two factors. First, it is often difficult to determine if the anxiety is conditioned (cognitively learned) or biologically based. In the former case, psychotherapy and cognitive behavior modification will prove effective, but in the latter case it will not. Second, it has proved to be very difficult to maintain behavior therapies in everyday life, away from the mental health practitioner. It is for this reason that drugs have been employed as the frontline treatment for anxiety. Drug therapy for anxiety typically involves the use of minor tranquilizers. The benzodiazepines (e.g., Librium, Valium, Dalmane,

Xanax, and Lorazepan) represent the most common family of minor tranquilizers. Although highly effective and fast-acting, these drugs are not without their down side. First, this drug category has been widely abused through legal prescriptions as well as on the streets. As recently as 1988, Xanax was the third most widely prescribed drug in the United States of America. Second, prolonged use of these drugs can produce physical and/or psychological dependence, resulting in severe withdrawal symptoms upon discontinuation. A final problem with these drugs involves frequent side effects, such as skin reactions, dizziness, fainting, blurred vision, headache, nausea, disorientation, and disturbed sleep. In spite of these problems, tranquilizers remain a popular choice among both therapists and patients alike, because of their anxiety-reducing qualities. [See ANXIETY.]

In addition to depression and anxiety, traditional treatments for problems associated with self-concept/self-esteem, personality, and mood have included group therapy, behavior therapy, Gestalt therapy, transactional analysis, marital therapy, medication, and cognitive therapy. It therefore appears that a wide variety of techniques has been employed to treat the most common mental health problems. What is obviously needed is a common treatment and/or adjunct treatment, free of side effects, that is equally effective across a variety of psychological problems. Fortunately, evidence is now available that suggests exercise has the potential to meet this need. [See BEHAVIOR THERAPY; COGNITIVE THERAPY; COUPLES THERAPY; FAMILY THERAPY.]

III. THE EXERCISE ALTERNATIVE

Extant research now indicates that exercise may provide a viable alternative to the more traditional treatments. For example, physical exercise has been shown to compare favorably with other methods used to reduce state anxiety. Acute exercise now appears equally effective to traditional treatment interventions including meditation, relaxation, cognitive behavioral methods, or time-out therapy that includes quiet rest. In a pioneer study conducted in the United States of America, 75 adult male exercisers were randomly assigned to exercise, meditation, and control groups. The exercise group walked on a treadmill at 70% maximum heart rate, and the meditation group engaged in Benson's relaxation technique. The control group merely rested in reclining chairs. The results from this experiment indicated that exercise, meditation, and quiet rest all resulted in significant reductions in state anxiety. An interesting corollary finding was that all three groups experienced comparable reductions. A later study replicated these findings, employing an aerobic dance exercise group, an autogenic relaxation group, and a quiet rest control. Once again, exercise was found to produce comparable results to a more traditional treatment option.

Exercise has also been demonstrated to provide a viable treatment option for depression. The earliest study looking at this relationship compared the effects of a walk/jog program to two different forms of psychotherapy in a 12-month follow-up of randomly assigned psychiatric outpatients. At the conclusion of the exercise program, the results indicated that the reduction in depression associated with exercise was equivalent to time-limited psychotherapy and superior to time-unlimited psychotherapy. In addition, at the 12-month follow-up, 11 of 12 patients treated with exercise were still asymptomatic, whereas approximately one-half of those individuals receiving the more traditional psychotherapy had returned for treatment. These results have been replicated in later studies.

Perhaps the strongest argument for using exercise as an alternative to other treatment options is provided by a study conducted in Norway. In this particular experiment, 43 patients who had been treated in the hospital for major depression were assessed 1 to 2 years after discharge. These individuals were asked to evaluate the different therapeutic treatments they received while at the mental health clinic. These various interventions included medication, community meetings, contact with other patients, group psychotherapy, physical exercise, individual psychotherapy, and contact with the milieu staff. Patients were asked to indicate which intervention they found most helpful and to rank the top three by means of a 3-point scale (with 3 being most helpful). Results of the survey data collected 1 to 2 years after discharge revealed that patients retrospectively ranked physical exercise as the most important element in their comprehensive treatment program. Psychotherapy and contact with other patients ranked second and third, respectively. The authors of the study interpreted these findings to suggest that physical exercise may be a viable alter-

native treatment for depressed patients who do not respond adequately to the more traditional treatments.

In summary, the studies that have been conducted to date suggest that exercise is a valuable treatment option that compares favorably to the more traditional forms of therapy. It would be valuable for future studies to continue to explore the efficacy of exercise compared to a variety of other treatment modalities.

IV. PSYCHOLOGICAL BENEFITS

An accumulating body of research now reveals that exercise has the potential to impact positively on a variety of psychological states and traits. The most commonly reported improvements involve the psychological constructs of depression, anxiety, self-concept, personality, and mood. A brief summary of research findings follows.

A. Depression

The first empirical study investigating the effect of exercise on depression was performed in 1905. In this particular study, physical exercise was reported to have a "retarding" effect on depression. Although this study was indeed a pioneer effort, it appeared to have limited impact on future research. The experiment was seldom cited and served a minimal heuristic function. The early literature reviews on exercise and mental health focused almost exclusively on general mental health rather than on specific psychological constructs. During the past two decades, however, this focus appears to have changed. As a result, a substantial body of research has evolved suggesting that exercise is associated with reductions in psychometrically assessed symptoms of depression.

Significant reductions in depression have been reported following participation in exercises such as running, walking, aerobic dance, cycling, weight lifting, karate, racquetball, jumping rope, and several unspecified aerobic activities. Research has not yet identified one particular type of exercise as being superior in terms of its potential to reduce depression in the participant. In one particular study, running and weight lifting were compared to a waiting-list control group in terms of their depression-reducing effects. Results indicated that both the running and weight lifting groups experienced significant decreases in depression, and that both appeared equally effective. This study has been replicated several times, with the results remaining the same across experiments. It therefore appears that both aerobic and anaerobic exercise sessions are equally effective.

A meta-analytic review performed in the United States sums up completed research by concluding that (a) exercise significantly decreased depression, and the antidepressant effects continued through follow-up measures; (b) subject populations experiencing similar decreases in depression included all age groups, both males and females, as well as clinical populations and nonclinical populations; and (c) all modes of exercise, including anaerobic exercise, were effective in decreasing depression.

Finally, to provide a frame of reference for the aforementioned conclusions, it is important to consider the extent of research conducted. In 1994, Leith reported that 42 empirical studies had been conducted to date that investigated the exercise and depression relationship. The same author revealed that 34 of the 42 studies (81%) reported significant reductions. This relatively high percentage of research studies reporting the same beneficial effects can only strengthen the position that exercise has excellent potential to impact positively on depression in the participant.

B. Anxiety

Research that has investigated the exercise and anxiety relationship has evolved in two distinct directions. On the one hand, an attempt has been made to examine the psychophysiological correlates of anxiety. This growing body of research has documented decreased levels of anxiety by means of several objective physiological measures, including muscle tension, blood pressure, resting heart rate, and cortical activation. A second research focus has concerned itself primarily with psychometric measurement of state and trait anxiety. For some reason, this latter measurement technique has received greater research attention. Therefore, the following summary will be limited exclusively to psychometrically assessed measures of anxiety.

Significant reductions in anxiety have been reported following a variety of exercises, including running, walking, cycling, swimming, aerobic dance, weight lifting, and jumping rope. As was the case with

depression, research has failed to identify the "ideal" exercise to reduce anxiety. It appears that all exercises have the potential for an anxiolytic effect. No differences have been found between aerobic and anaerobic exercises. To date, research studies have compared jogging, walking, swimming, yoga, weight lifting, and fencing. No consistent differences have been found between or among exercise modes.

The most recent research in this area is now attempting to differentiate between components of anxiety, especially cognitive versus somatic anxiety. Early studies reported that exercise reduced both cognitive and somatic anxiety. Later experiments, however, suggest that the introduction of competition into the exercise setting may produce different results. For example, one state-of-the-art study required 24 male and female undergraduates to perform a cycle ergometer task across three conditions: noncompetitive, competitive-success, and competitive-failure. The results of this study indicated increases in somatic anxiety in both success and failure conditions, whereas cognitive anxiety increased following failure and decreased following success. This study suggests that competitive state anxiety changes across time and different competitive conditions, supporting the notion that anxiety is a multidimensional concept, and that the exercise and anxiety association may not be as straightforward as originally suggested.

One final contentious issue is worthy of mention. It was originally believed that exercise would prove effective against state anxiety and not trait anxiety. A review of all completed research, however, indicates that exercise can also be very effective in reducing trait anxiety provided the exercise program lasts a minimum of 9 weeks.

In summary, to once again provide a frame of reference for the aforementioned conclusions, in 1994, Leith reported that 56 empirical studies had examined the exercise and anxiety relationship. Of these 56 studies, 41 (73%) reported significant improvements in anxiety following participation in an exercise program. It therefore appears that exercise has excellent anxiolytic potential when used correctly.

C. Self-Concept

Self-concept has been identified as the variable with the greatest potential to reflect psychological benefit derived from regular exercise. Because body image has been found to be intimately connected to self-image, it is not surprising to find that when an individual's body image improves through participation in physical exercise, there is frequently an improvement in self-concept as well. [*See* BODY IMAGE.]

A wide range of physical exercises have been examined in terms of their potential to impact on self-concept. Significant improvements have been reported following participation in running, cycling, swimming, weight lifting, tennis, basketball, and a variety of unspecified exercise programs. When one examines all of the completed research, it appears that running and weight lifting are the two types of exercise most often associated with significant improvements in self-concept. Studies attempting to compare the relative effectiveness of running and weight lifting have found that both appear equally effective. It is interesting to speculate, however, that the appropriate exercise will be dependent on the participant's initial physical appearance. For example, running may prove to be more effective for individuals wishing to lose weight or improve their overall level of cardiovascular fitness. Weight lifting, on the other hand, may be more effective for people who are slight of build or seek to improve their musculature, and thereby their body image.

Recent research suggests the practitioner may be well advised to avoid including a competitive element in the exercise session. Competitive conditions, especially those resulting in losing outcomes, appear to have a negative effect on the participant's self-concept. For example, a recent study assigned 24 male and female college students to a noncompetitive group, a compete-win group, or a compete-lose condition. At the conclusion of the exercise sessions, participants in the compete-lose condition actually demonstrated worsened self-concept as measured by an appropriate psychometric instrument. It therefore appears that certain qualitative aspects of the exercise session may prove as important as the actual mode of exercise itself.

In summary, an examination of the 52 empirical studies investigating the exercise and self-concept relationship reveals that only 30 of the 52 studies (58%) reported significant improvements in self-concept following exercise. So, while early researchers suggested self-concept was the psychological construct with the most potential to improve with exercise, completed research does not confirm this hypothesis. Having

said this, however, an alternate explanation may be that the results have not been as consistent as was the case with depression and anxiety because self-concept is a more multidimensional construct. In other words, with self-concept, it is probably very important to "match" the type of exercise to the initial problem area involving the person's self-concept. People wishing to lose weight should be placed on exercise programs that are slower paced and longer in duration. This will result in the maximum weight loss. Others wishing to improve their cardiovascular fitness would benefit little from the same program. They would need more intense, shorter duration activities. To date, research has not attempted this type of matching of activity to the goals of the participant. Once this is done, it is likely that self-concept will improve with exercise to the same extent as the other psychological constructs.

D. Personality

Some evidence now exists suggesting exercise may have potential for affecting changes in personality. The majority of research investigating the exercise and personality relationship occurred in the 1960s and 1970s, with few experiments conducted after 1980. This probably reflects the recent trend toward analyzing specific psychological states rather than longer lasting personality traits, which are far more resistant to change. At this point in time, the best that can be said is that the research examining the exercise and personality relationship has produced conflicting results. Because personality represents global and relatively stable traits, the positive benefits of exercise appear to be less consistent across studies.

An examination of completed research reveals that exercise has been associated with participants becoming more reserved, intelligent, emotionally stable, assertive, happy-go-lucky, expedient, shy, trusting, suspicious, imaginative, forthright, placid, experimenting, group-dependent, controlled, relaxed, and self-sufficient. Although exercise has been associated experimentally with changes in a variety of personality variables, only self-sufficiency emerges in a relatively large number of independent studies. This would suggest it is possible that adherence to an exercise program results in the participant's feeling he or she is able to successfully complete a project independent of outside help.

These improvements in personality have been associated with participation in a variety of exercise programs, including jogging, weight lifting, and aerobic conditioning. The majority of studies utilized jogging as the exercise of choice. In act, few studies employed an exercise mode other than jogging. For this reason, it is not possible to speculate as to which type of exercise is most effective in affecting personality changes. More research is needed with different exercise modes before generalizations and conclusions can be generated.

In summary, 20 empirical studies have specifically examined the exercise and personality relationship. Of these 20 studies, 13 (65%) reported significant improvements in at least one personality subscale. While this percentage of improvement is lower than some of the other psychological constructs, it still provides grounds for optimism that exercise may indeed result in personality changes over time. The success rate of exercise may prove even higher if researchers focus more exclusively on "surface" personality traits instead of "source" traits. The surface traits of introversion–extroversion, anxiety, tough-mindedness, and independence represent a superficial cluster of source traits and are believed to be related more to learned behavior. As such, it is reasonable to assume exercise could impact more effectively on these learned personality traits than would be the case with the source traits that are fundamental structures of personality. This hypothesis awaits further research. [*See* PERSONALITY.]

E. Mood

The *Webster Dictionary* defines mood as a conscious state of mind or predominant emotion. Mood is also viewed as transient, fluctuating affective states. We have already seen how exercise has been associated with significant improvements in depression and anxiety, two very common mood states. In fact, depression and anxiety are the two most frequently reported mood changes following participation in exercise programs. Other elements of mood, however, also appear to improve with exercise. Most notably, the moods characterized as confusion–bewilderment, anger–hostility, fatigue–inertia, and vigor–activity are all reported to improve following exercise. In addition to these psychometrically measured mood changes, par-

ticipants frequently report a subjective "feel better" phenomenon following exercise.

The majority of research investigating the exercise and mood relationship utilized jogging and/or walking. However, a variety of other exercises have been consistently associated with improvements in mood. These include swimming, cycling, yoga, tai chi, rowing, weight lifting, aerobic dance, as well as a variety of unspecified exercise programs. To date, no one exercise has been found to be superior in terms of its mood-enhancing effects.

To date, 34 empirical studies have examined the exercise and mood relationship. Twenty-six (77%) of these studies reported significant improvements in some aspect of mood. This relatively high percentage suggests exercise can be very effective in improving mood on a day-to-day basis.

V. PREVENTION VERSUS TREATMENT

In the early years of research on the exercise and mental health relationship, the experts believed exercise was effective only as a treatment for a variety of psychological disorders. For this reason, most of the initial studies involved individuals who were clinically symptomatic. In these experiments, the results consistently portrayed exercise to be effective in treating a variety of disorders, especially depression and anxiety. In fact, some studies reported that patients rated aerobic exercise as the single most important component of their comprehensive treatment programs.

At this point, the research focus shifted to include individuals who were asymptomatic. These experiments were performed on male and female college students, male and female healthy adults, and healthy older adults. At the conclusion of their respective exercise programs, an interesting finding emerged. These individuals also showed significantly improved scores on their respective psychometrically measured constructs. In other words, individuals who were assessed to be in the normal range of depression, anxiety, mood, and self-concept also improved significantly. This outcome is very important. It indicates that participants may actually be able to improve their mental health, even in the absence of troubling symptoms. For example, in the case of depression, even people not experiencing symptoms of depression may lower their "baseline" depression by participating in a regular exercise program. By starting from a lower baseline, they are going a long way toward preventing depression from occurring in the first place. This same argument also holds for the other psychological constructs. Future studies should employ longitudinal designs to follow these individuals, then compare their incidence rate of mental disorders with similar samples that did not participate in the regular exercise. It is tempting to speculate that the exercisers will have a lower rate of mental problems. Some epidemiological studies support this notion.

VI. THE MECHANISMS

Several hypotheses have been advanced as possible change mechanisms to explain how mental health can be improved by participation in a chronic exercise program. In this section, the most frequently cited explanations will be briefly discussed.

Despite the absence of compelling scientific evidence, the endorphin hypothesis represents the most popular explanation of how exercise impacts on mental health. According to this viewpoint, when a person exercises, this causes the release of endorphins into the bloodstream. Endorphins are actually a peptide, and are chemically very similar to morphine. For this reason, it is believed that increased levels of endorphins produce a "feel good" phenomenon, hence improving our mood. A good deal of animal research supports this position. For example, it has been documented that the brain tissue of rats revealed significant increases in opiate-receptor-site occupancy after they had been forced to run in an activity wheel or swim in cold water. A variety of replication studies produced similar results. For the obvious ethical reasons, research with humans has been restricted to peripheral measures of endorphins and their metabolites. Even so, these studies on human subjects, taken cumulatively, provide reasonable support for the endorphin theory of improved mental health following exercise. However, more research needs to be conducted before we can state unequivocally that endorphins are the change mechanism.

A second popular argument is called the monoamine hypothesis. This theory suggests the improved affect associated with exercise can be explained by changes in one or more of the brain monoamines (i.e., dopamine, norepinephrine, and serotonin). It has now been established that certain areas of the brain and particular neural pathways form systems that are associated with mental processes such as anxiety, depression, pleasure, pain, and even organized thought. Each system utilizes particular neurotransmitters (chemical messengers) that transmit signals across synapses between neurons making up the system. If enough neurotransmitters bind onto receptor sites, the message is transmitted. If a sufficient number are not present, the message is not transmitted. Of special interest to this publication is the finding that the number of these neurotransmitters available at synapses along particular neural pathways has been related to our moods, which in turn are affected by such things as drugs and exercise. Because of this established association, the monoamine hypothesis appears a reasonable explanation to explain the positive effects of exercise.

A somewhat different view of the exercise and mental health relationship is termed the thermogenic hypothesis. This idea is by no means a new one. The therapeutic effect of elevating body temperature can be traced back to A.D. 800 in Finland, where sauna baths were popular for their physical and mental benefits. This practice appears to possess a fair degree of merit, since research has shown that whole body warming (e.g., warm shower, sauna bathing, or fever therapy) reduces muscle tension. Researchers have further shown that our bodies respond to exercise in the same manner as when they are invaded by bacteria or viruses. The release of pyrogens (endogenous leukocyte mediators) results in reductions in zinc and iron concentrations in our blood, an increase in white blood cells, and an increase in our body temperature (a fever). This combined effect serves to kill off the bacteria and/or virus. It also results in a relaxation effect, just like a sauna or hot shower. Exercise, then, by producing body warming, may actually serve an anxiolytic effect, thereby improving our mental health.

So far, all of these explanations can be termed biochemical in origin. But it appears there may also be psychological reasons for the effect of exercise on mental health. An alternative explanation, termed the distraction hypothesis, suggests that exercise may improve mental health by providing a "time-out" from daily routine activities and stressful stimuli. Exercise, by giving the participant something else to do and think about, removes the individual from the daily pressures that are bothersome. In its simplest form, then, exercise can improve mental health by providing a temporary "escape" from psychological problems.

A final explanation for the way exercise can improve mental health is called self-efficacy theory. It has been suggested that a person's perception of his or her ability to perform in demanding situations (e.g., exercise) affects that individuals emotions. The basic tenet of this viewpoint is that as a person engages in a regular exercise program, he or she experiences fitness gains or bodily changes. This in turn results in improved self-efficacy, or situation-specific self-confidence. Successful participation in an exercise program, then, results in the person feeling better about him or herself. This may partially explain the positive benefits of exercise on mental health.

In summary, a variety of explanations has been provided. At present, research has been unable to determine if one hypothesis is better than the others. Perhaps the most logical conclusion is that several of these processes may occur at once, possibly combining their effects to produce the improvements in mental health. [*See* PHYSICAL ACTIVITY AND MENTAL HEALTH.]

VII. EXERCISE PRESCRIPTION

Having established that exercise can indeed result in significant improvements in mental health, it is now important to consider qualitative aspects of the exercise program. More specifically, the practitioner needs to know what type of exercise is best, as well as how hard, how often, and how long the client needs to exercise to achieve maximum results. Fortunately, a synthesis of related literature, as well as several meta-analytic reviews provide some general answers to these important questions.

A. What Mode of Exercise Is Best?

Although we have pointed out those exercises most often associated with improvements in each of the psychological constructs, it is possible to provide some general observations. Although no one exercise has been found to be superior, it appears that exercises that involve the large muscle groups and are rhythmic (e.g., walking, jogging, swimming, cycling, and aerobic dance) appear to be most often associated with improvements in mental health. In addition, weight lifting has consistently been associated with improvements across a variety of studies. An important implication for the practitioner is to ask the client which of these exercises he or she prefers, rather than prescribing a particular exercise without consultation. Research indicates that this approach will lead to greater exercise compliance.

B. How Often, How Hard, and How Long Should the Exercise Be Performed?

As general guidelines, exercise should be performed at least three times per week, at mild to moderate intensity, for periods of 20 to 30 minutes per session. These numbers are consistent with the American College of Sport Medicine (1991) guidelines for exercise prescription, as well as the specific prescription guidelines outlined in Leith's *Foundations of Exercise and Mental Health*.

Obviously, the number of exercise sessions per week will be determined by the choice of physical activity and the exercise intensity. For example, if a client chose walking as the preferred activity, it would be entirely appropriate to walk for 20 to 30 minutes five, six, or even seven times per week without undue strain. If the chosen activity was running, or aerobic dance, it would be better to limit participation to three times per week. This caveat is mentioned to guard against overuse injuries, and ultimately exercise program dropout.

C. How Long Must the Exercise Program Be to Produce Results?

It is interesting to note that significant improvements have been documented after only one exercise session. Mood states, for example, can be altered within one bout of exercise. However, a good rule of thumb that can be gleaned from the literature suggests exercise programs of 10 to 12 weeks or more will result in the best mental health benefits. Programs with this minimal length also result in greater stability of psychological improvements at follow-up measurement sessions. Even so, there is nothing wrong with a client going for a walk instead of taking a Valium. In other words, exercise can also be viewed as an appropriate "band-aid" approach to daily mood variations. Best results can still be expected, however, when exercise is incorporated into the client's life-style activities. In this manner, exercise will probably serve as a preventative as well as a treatment technique.

D. Are Fitness Gains Necessary?

The answer to this question is an unqualified "no." Mental health improvements are experienced in the same magnitude even if the participant does not improve his or her fitness levels. Remember, we are dealing with psychological, not physiological benefits. As such, it is important to stress that fitness gains are not necessary prerequisites to improved mental health. The biochemical and psychological change mecha-

nisms appear to occur independent of changes in physiological fitness.

BIBLIOGRAPHY

American College of Sports Medicine. (1991). *Guidelines for exercise testing and prescription.* Philadelphia: Lea & Febiger.

Leith, L. M. (1994). *Foundations of exercise and mental health.* Morgantown, WV: Fitness Information Technology Inc.

Leith, L. M. (1997). *Exercising your way to better mental health.* Morgantown, WV: Fitness Information Technology, Inc.

Martinsen, E. W. (1993). Therapeutic implications of exercise for clinically anxious and depressed patients. *International Journal of Sport Psychology, 24,* 185–199.

North, T. C., McCullagh, P., & Tran, Z. V. (1990). Effects of exercise on depression. *Exercise and Sport Sciences Reviews, 18,* 379–415.

Petruzzello, S. J., Landers, D. M., Hatfield, B. D., Kubitz, K. A., & Salazar, W. (1991). A meta-analysis on the anxiety-reducing effects of acute and chronic exercise: Outcomes and mechanisms. *Sports Medicine, 11,* 143–182.

Extended Family Relationships

Toni C. Antonucci, Elizabeth A. Vandewater, and Jennifer E. Lansford

University of Michigan

Demographics Characteristics such as age, income, education, race, sex, and so on, which can be used to describe individuals or populations.

Extended Family All members of a kin network as defined by either biological or legal (e.g., marriage, adoption) connections.

Family Structure Characteristics used to describe families such as the number of people in a family, their relationships to each other (e.g., spouse, biological child, adopted child, etc.), who lives in the household, and so on.

Interindividual Differences Differences between individuals.

Intraindividual Change Developmental changes over time within a single individual.

Multigenerational Family A family characterized by multiple generations living at the same time.

The role of **EXTENDED FAMILY RELATIONSHIPS** in the mental health of the individual is complex. In this article we outline the need to consider the family within a life-span and multigenerational context. We review the extended family in American history and examine demographic and social changes influencing the extended family in the present. We also consider different characteristics of the family, including individual, race, ethnic, and cultural characteristics, and the changing structure of the family and of the social roles of its members. We emphasize that the influence of the family can be both positive and negative. We conclude that although many aspects of family life and family structures have changed in the twentieth century, the role of the family in determining the mental health and well-being of its members remains central.

I. EXTENDED FAMILIES IN AMERICAN HISTORY

The term extended family conjures up notions of close-knit farm families in America's past, in which multiple generations of family members worked together to produce household goods and food, guided by the benign (but firm) authority of a household elder. In such families (the story goes), family cohesion and community connection were a part of everyday life, with adults performing "gender appropriate" labor and children learning responsibility and values through hard work, chores, and respect for their elders.

The reality of extended family life in the past, however, was far from the attractive picture just painted. The pressures of household production left little time for family closeness or personal development. Mothers engaged in home production generally relegated child care to older children or servants; they could not stop work to savor a baby's first steps or discuss with their husbands how to facilitate a grade-schooler's self-esteem. Children who worked in family production seldom had time for the extracurricular activities that "Wally and Beaver" recounted to their parents over the dinner table—often they did not even go to school full time. Extended families in America's past were harnessed together in household production and held together by dire necessity.

Regardless of this, both social analysts and the popular press have long mourned the passing of this family form. As early as the 1920s and 1930s, social theorists suggested that urbanization and industrialization had weakened the "traditional family" by taking the means of production out of the home, thereby destroying kinship and community networks. This analysis sounds remarkably similar to present day laments about the general loss of respect for elders, ties to family and community, and commitment to "good old hard work" in American society. The assumption behind such laments is that these ideals and values were rooted in our family forms, specifically the extended family.

It may be true that modern American society is lacking in such values. What is less clear, however, is that these values (or lack thereof) are indeed connected to the extended family. In point of fact, extended family households have never been the norm in America. The highest figure for extended family households ever recorded in American history is 20%. In addition, contrary to the popular belief that it was industrialization that destroyed traditional extended families, this high point occurred between 1850 and 1885, during the most intensive period of early industrialization in America.

II. CURRENT DEMOGRAPHIC AND SOCIAL FORCES

Clearly, when people do live in extended family households today, it is not because they are required to produce their own food and household goods. People of different generations live together today for reasons that are more specific to modern American

society. Significant social and demographic changes have taken place in America—some starting at the beginning of this century, others only in the last two decades or so. The combined impact of these changes has led to a recent increased interest in the influence of extended families on the development and well-being of family members.

First, the American population is an aging population. Over the course of the twentieth century, life expectancy (or longevity) in America has increased dramatically. In 1900, the typical white newborn in the United States had a life expectancy of 47 years; the typical African American, a life expectancy of only 29 years. By stark contrast, the average white newborn in the United States today can expect to live about 75 years; the typical African American, about 65. Partly because of this increase in longevity, the American population is aging at an increasingly rapid pace. In 1900, only 1 in 25 Americans was 65 years old or older. By the mid 1980s, about 1 in 9 was at least 65 years of age. Moreover, in the next two decades, the proportion of Americans aged 65 and over will skyrocket, largely because of the aging of the baby boom generation (those born in the post-World War II era between 1946 and 1959). This demographic change is sometimes referred to as "the graying of America."

As the largest cohort of individuals in the history of the United States, the baby boomers have strained local and federal resources as they have aged. Elementary schools, then high schools, were built to educate them and then closed for lack of students as the cohort moved on to college and the workforce (which were also strained to the limits of their capacities). Although many people in this coming senior cohort will need help in a variety of areas (financial help, medical care, mental health services, etc.), it is commonly acknowledged that our social and health care institutions (e.g., Social Security, Medicare) will be unable to accommodate the needs of the vast numbers of aging people (who also live longer than ever). Because of this, much of the responsibility of caring for older generations will rest within the family itself. Many families will soon face the choice of whether to take in elder relatives who need their help. Thus, the need to care for an aging population is one important demographic force affecting the formation of extended family households in modern America.

Along with the increased life expectancy and the large number of aging individuals, the birthrate in America has been decreasing over the past 40 years. It is no longer unusual for families to have one child. This particular demographic combination means that the shape of the family has changed. Social scientists refer to this phenomenon as the "beanpole" family structure, because the shape of the family is one in which many generations of roughly the same number of people are "stacked" on top of one another. Because more and more generations of family members are alive at the same time, it is no longer an anomaly for a child to know his or her great-grandparents.

At the same time that changes in life expectancy have fundamentally altered the demographic structure of society, *social norms* regarding appropriate family structures have also changed dramatically. Families now exist in many varied forms, including the nuclear two-parent family, single-parent families, multi-generation families, divorced families, and remarried/blended/step families. The various types of families may contribute to the increased importance of extended families. As various forms of the immediate, nuclear family show less and less stability, the role of extended family members may take on increased importance.

Families must also negotiate the effects of the widespread economic restructuring which has taken place over the last two decades in the United States. Partly because of such restructuring, many families are now facing a fairly new phenomenon. Because of the difficulties for younger workers in finding entry level jobs that pay a living wage, more and more families find themselves with adult children living at home.

Thus, these particular social and demographic changes have combined to affect the form families are taking today and will take in the near future. In modern day America, families may bond together to make various extended family forms, not because of the necessity to produce goods for survival, but because of an ethic of care that does not allow them to let family members in need go unaided. One of the most pressing questions for families in America today is how best to negotiate the caring for three generations at once that will be required of them in the very near future. For these reasons, it has now become essential that scholars undertake a serious consideration of the influence of extended family relationships (both posi-

tive and negative) on the mental health and well-being of individual family members.

III. A LIFE-SPAN PERSPECTIVE

To understand the role of extended family relationships in mental health, it is critical to recognize that all family relationships are lifelong and developmental in nature. The nature of family ties is such that they usually exist throughout a lifetime, extending, therefore, through infancy, childhood, and adulthood, and into old age. Family members know each other well, and in most cases have a shared history. As we seek to understand how social relationships can influence mental health, these long-term relationships take on special meaning.

To understand the development of individual family members, it is also important to acknowledge that their interactions are shaped by both their individual life stages (intraindividual development) and their shared life history. For example, a young child will have a different perception and reaction to interactions with her or his grandparents than will the grandparents themselves because they are at very different intraindividual developmental stages. Because of these interindividual differences in life stage, the influence of their interactions on individual development will be different. For young children, interactions with their grandparents have the potential to shape their interactions with other older people in the future, as well as their feelings about what kind of grandparent they themselves want to be. For grandparents, however, the interaction with grandchildren may have relatively less influence on the developmental trajectory their lives will take from that point.

Similarly, each interactive relationship has a developmental sequence. A long-term relationship between age-mates such as cousins has a well developed shared history that is both cumulative and potentially influential. These cousins might have a 50-year history of sharing each other's sorrows and helping each other in times of crisis, instead of never being available to help and creating most of the family's crises. A cousin who served as the witness at your wedding, who helped you cope with the serious illness of your infant child, or who shared the heartbreak of a family tragedy is someone you would feel comfortable turning to with a problem in adulthood or old age. On the other hand, the cousin who missed every family event, who had trouble with the law as a young adult, or who was unavailable to help during previous personal or family tragedies is not the person you would call on first in times of crisis.

Obviously, extended family relations that provide the individual with a feeling of warmth, belongingness, and support are most likely to promote mental health. On the other hand, a family that is characterized by hurtful, vindictive, unsupportive or even abusive relationships is less likely to promote mental health and, in fact, may contribute in significant ways to mental illness. However, over time, most family relationships are rarely so unidimensional. For example, the same family that is supportive and nurturing to a young child may have great difficulty providing the particular support needed by an adolescent. Families can even be both supportive and unsupportive at the same time (e.g., supporting a child's achievement strivings while discouraging the same child's attempts at social autonomy).

Because of this, it is essential to take into account the shared, cumulative history of most family members when considering the role of extended family in mental health. Previous and ongoing relationships can contribute both positively and negatively to mental health. When faced with a crisis, individuals might feel able to cope because of the perception that their family will offer support or react with hopelessness because they feel they are facing the crisis alone.

IV. A MULTIGENERATIONAL MODEL

The intraindividual life-span perspective is best complemented by a multigenerational model of the family. As people live longer, and each family bears fewer children, the family comes to take on a beanpole rather than a triangular form. As mentioned previously, in the beanpole family, more generations of each family are represented. This is increasingly the case as we see four- and five-generation families with only one, two, or three members of each generation. This stands in contrast to our historical family structure which was more triangular in nature: each family included only two or three generations with the largest number of generational members present in the youngest generation. A family might have five, six,

or more children, two parents, and only one surviving grandparent. This was the more common family structure when people did not live very long and families had many children.

The new structure of the family suggests that a multigenerational model is essential to conceptualize the modern extended family. This extended family, it should also be noted, has the potential to be horizontally expansive as well. With fewer siblings, each sibling relationship might be more critical, but, similarly, other extended family relationships, such as cousins, uncles, great-aunts, in-laws, and even former in-laws, might take their place as people occupying influential roles in the development and maintenance of the psychological well-being, quality of life, and mental health of the individual.

Multigenerational families can be distinguished from extended families more generally by their vertical rather than horizontal structure. As the name implies, this means that different generations of a lineage are the focus, rather than relationships between age-mates such as cousins or siblings. The most common form of multigenerational family includes members of three generations—a child, parent, and grandparent—who are living together.

The coming together of a multigeneration household raises the question of shared resources. Examination of generational relationships within families suggests that resources can flow linearly (i.e., from old to young or young to old) or curvilinearly (i.e., from the middle to both the older and the younger generations simultaneously). Generational researchers report that although there appear to be differences in cultural and perhaps racial and ethnic expectations, socioeconomic status often determines the directional flow of resources. Thus, among families with many economic resources, the flow is from old to young. In these families, the old have had a lifetime to accumulate wealth (or have inherited it), which they are then willing to redistribute to their young. Among less economically advantaged families, especially families marked by upward mobility or recent immigration, the direction of resource flow often moves from the young to the old. In such families, the youngest family members have had the opportunity to achieve the highest levels of education, the best job opportunities, and the greatest upward mobility. Among families in which all generations have few economic resources, no particular linear pattern appears to be viable. In these families, resources are so scarce that whoever has them is expected to share with others in need. [*See* SOCIOECONOMIC STATUS.]

There are a variety of advantages as well as disadvantages to living in a multigenerational family. Economically, it is easier to maintain only one household, and there are additional adults to help with housework, child care, and other family responsibilities. There is also another adult present (besides one's spouse) to provide companionship and emotional support. However, there may also be overcrowding, a loss of personal space and privacy, and less leisure time available. It is important to consider the health status of family members, because some of the advantages of having additional adults in the house can be outweighed by the burdens of having to provide extensive care for them.

In fact, much of the research on multigenerational families focuses on caregiving to an aging parent or grandparent. This type of family structure is increasing in prevalence as individuals live longer and social entitlement programs are cut. The middle generation appears to have the most responsibility, because these individuals are likely to be providing more support to the younger generation (their children) and to the older generation (their parents) than they are receiving from either of these generations. This is potentially stressful for the middle generation because they are "sandwiched" on all sides by those in need of help from them. However, it can also be stressful for members of the older generation, who may feel they are not upholding their end of the exchange and that support from their children is only given because of a sense of obligation.

A different type of multigenerational family includes younger members or those whose ages are "condensed" because of adolescent childbearing. In these families, adolescent mothers and their infants typically live with the adolescent's mother. Adolescent mothers who continue to live with their own mothers tend to have better educational outcomes (i.e., complete high school), and their infants may benefit from the material resources and help with caregiving their grandmothers can provide. If there is a pattern of adolescent childbearing in a family, an age-condensed structure may result, in which there is a distance of only 12 to 17 years between generations so that many generations may live or interact with one another. In these families, the caregiving pattern typically flows from older generations to younger ones (e.g., the infant's grandmother caring for the infant), rather than from younger generations to older ones (e.g., adult children caring for their aging parents).

The research on women's roles in multigenerational families far exceeds the research on men's roles. It has been documented that women are more likely than men to be caregivers for their aging parents, and mothers rather than fathers of adolescent mothers have been most involved in caring for their grandchildren. In some instances, even daughters-in-law are more likely to care for their aging parents-in-law than are the parents' own sons. Additional research is needed to understand how men fit into multigenerational families.

V. POSITIVE AND NEGATIVE COMPONENTS OF EXTENDED FAMILY

Although examples of positive and negative aspects of the extended family have already been alluded to, we now address the issue directly. We feel it is important to represent both sides of the extended family coin. Although extended families can have a positive influence on well-being and quality of life, the opposite can also be true. Some extended families provide the supportive base from which to reach out and explore new challenges, whereas others can be restricting and confining, chastising any individual family member's interest in doing anything different. Two common proverbs illustrate these respective points: "The squeaky wheel gets the oil" or "The nail that sticks out gets hammered down." Extended families can either provide the oil or the hammer. Depending on the individual family member and the consistency of these viewpoints in the broader societal context, this can either promote or threaten mental health.

Specific characteristics or customs within an extended family framework can also be positive or negative. A family can encourage physical and mental health promoting attitudes on the one hand, or behaviors and attitudes that endanger the health of its members on the other. For example, one can have drinking buddies or drug buddies, running buddies or diet buddies.

Although these are examples of behaviors affecting physical health, the logical extension to mental health is not far. In families, individuals learn how to deal with anger, aggression, crises, and intimate relationships. The influence of extended families on the ways in which individuals handle such issues may be even greater than that of nuclear families, because several generations of individuals are modeling such coping styles at once. Thus, extended families can empower an individual to cope with both normal developmental challenges and significant threats to mental health by providing an anxiety-free environment and a safe zone within which to consider alternative coping strategies. On the other hand, they can encourage maladaptive behavior or even add to crises by exposing the individual to threats generated within the family itself. [*See* COPING WITH STRESS.]

VI. RACE, ETHNICITY, AND CULTURE

No examination of the family in general or the extended family in particular should omit a serious consideration of race, ethnicity, and culture. Each of these characteristics fundamentally shapes the nature of family (and indeed all) relationships. Their consideration is necessary if one is to truly understand roles, resources, expectations, and limits of the family. Race, ethnicity, and culture each have unique qualities that contribute to the experience of an individual family member. These can be positive, offering the individual an identity that focuses both on uniqueness and on belonging to a group with shared values, histories, and traditions in a truly celebratory manner. However, when much of that shared identity has had (or continues to have) negative implications, it can also influence mental health in negative ways.

It has been proposed that racism limits the viability of minority families. Continued discrimination in educational and workforce opportunities certainly contributes to a general lack of economic resources among minority families in the United States. Minority status may strengthen family ties because of the need for aid to survive in a hostile environment. Research indicates that in times of crisis, individuals traditionally tend to turn to their families as sources of material, social, and emotional support. For example, institutions such as the police, government agencies, and the educational system may be viewed as supportive by white families but as exploitative and threatening by minority families. Minority families may therefore depend on each other instead of on nonfamilial

institutions that may provide more support to white families.

The African American family has a long history of external examination by researchers, educators, and policy makers. Unfortunately, many of these examinations have been fairly hostile—emphasizing the dysfunctionality of African American families rather than focusing on the ways in which they have adapted to extremely difficult situations. In 1965, the well-known *Moynihan Report* expressed the view of the traditional two-parent father-as-breadwinner family (which was mostly white and middle-class) as being the normal and healthy family type to which other families should be compared. Because more black families than white families are headed by females, they were characterized in this report as both fragmented and deviant. These views notwithstanding, it is interesting to note that although Americans (including Daniel Moynihan) share a cultural myth that for most of our history, the "traditional" nuclear family form (two-parent, never divorced, breadwinning father) predominated, when in fact this is not true. In actuality, this family form described the majority of families for only a short period of time in American history (between 1956 and 1960), and even then, it only described roughly 60% of American families.

The *Moynihan Report* sparked a great deal of research and debate, much of it aimed at refuting its claims. Examination of the African American family did indeed indicate a strong reliance on the extended family. Far from indicating fragmentation, however, such reliance can be viewed as a healthy adaptation to very difficult circumstances. To offset constraints placed on individuals or nuclear families, African Americans have often turned to the extended family to help provide for the needs of its members. Resources are often shared where they are most needed. Thus, instead of being viewed as fragmented, the black family could be regarded as simply being involved with a wider range of its members.

It appears that there are cultural differences in both the extensiveness of the extended family network and in the intensiveness of their interactions. African Americans, for example, tend to interact with and help a wider variety of kin and to engage in these interactions more frequently than do European Americans. It is common for African Americans to name cousins, aunts, uncles, grandparents, and other relatives as people who provide them with instrumental support such as financial aid or help with housework, as well as emotional support in terms of offering advice and encouragement. Many African Americans have relationships with cousins that are similar to sibling relationships, and parenting responsibilities may be distributed to a range of kin. Hispanic Americans demonstrate similar family patterns.

These alternative family forms seem to be especially useful for children when resources and parental time are limited. In terms of developmental outcomes of children, there is a growing body of evidence that the presence of a supportive adult, not necessarily a parent, in children's lives, regardless of whether they live in the same household, is protective. Extended family members often function as this "supportive adult." In fact, child rearing has been proposed to be one of the most important functions of minority extended families. Nonmaternal child rearing has received the most attention in the context of the children of adolescent mothers. These children are often cared for jointly by the adolescent mother and her extended family, particularly the adolescent's own mother. Support from extended family members can contribute to the well-being of adolescent mothers by allowing them the opportunity to stay in school or get advice and help with child care as they negotiate their transition to parenthood. This support can contribute to the well-being of infants by providing a stable network of care providers.

Although more research has focused on African American families than on families of other racial and ethnic backgrounds, specific issues have been identified that are additionally and perhaps uniquely important for other groups. The research that has been conducted on other ethnic minority families has highlighted the importance of geographic considerations and length of time of residence in the United States. For example, there is some evidence from work with Mexican immigrants that the extended family becomes less important with increased urbanization, acculturation, and contact with the dominant American culture. Acculturation can strain the extended family by contributing to a divergence in attitudes and beliefs between more and less acculturated family members. This often occurs when the youngest generation becomes "Americanized" in the school system while their parents, grandparents, and other older family members maintain a stronger sense of their own cultural heritage. On the other hand, the extended family can also act as a stabilizing force in preserving native cultural backgrounds for family members of all ages. Extended families can maintain traditions through storytelling, celebrations, and rituals that involve participation by all members.

It is recognized that extended families of minorities can have many positive influences on the lives of their members, including providing instrumental and emotional support and helping to preserve the families' cultural heritage. It should also be recognized that for minority as well as majority individuals there may also be disadvantages to having extensive and intensive family ties. For example, individuals from economically disadvantaged backgrounds who obtain well-paying jobs may be expected to provide economic support to extended family members. This may make it difficult for individuals to escape poverty because there are many drains on their resources. Whereas among middle class multigenerational white families, elders often provide resources to younger generations (e.g., buying a car, making a down payment on a house); middle and younger generation family members of poor minority as well as *majority* families often find that they must provide support to their elders. Thus, the importance of the influence of socioeconomic status on extended family relationships should not be confused with the different influences of race and ethnicity, nor should it be underestimated.

VII. FAMILY VALUES AND WOMEN'S ROLES

Over the past 40 years or so, the structure of American family life has changed dramatically, so much so that we have become a nation obsessed by what we view as "the breakdown of family values." The major evidence pointed to for the existence of this "breakdown" is the increasing prevalence of divorce. Although the exact figures are a matter of some debate, it is commonly acknowledged that as many as 50% of marriages today end in divorce. Interestingly, however, Americans are also as committed to marriage as they ever were. The majority of those who divorce will remarry within 5 years. [See DIVORCE.]

Clearly, living through a divorce can have negative consequences for all family members (including both parents and in-laws of the divorcing couple). However, there is also evidence that the level of continuing conflict between the divorced couple may be a more important determinant of mental health than the actual divorce itself. Nonetheless, divorce and remarriage certainly increase the complexity of extended family relationships. Because people are living longer than ever before, it follows that grandparents and great-grandparents will develop fairly long-standing relationships with both their grandchildren and relatives by marriage.

The major question is how will these relationships be negotiated when divorced couples are no longer living (and sometimes no longer even speaking) with one another, when one's daughter or son-in-law gets custody of one's grandchildren, or when children have three or even four sets of parents and/or grandparents. The concerns facing divorced families, remarried families, and issues of step-parenting and grandparenting in such families are all topics of study in and of themselves. What is clear, however, is that the changes in what constitutes the most prevalent family structures must be taken into account when considering the pressures on American families to form extended family households.

One of the most dramatic social changes over the past 30 years has been the increase in women's participation in the workforce. Although women have worked in the paid labor force throughout the course of America's history, in much larger numbers than prevailing notions would have us believe, many of these women left the paid labor force for at least some period of time when their children were young. In recent times, however, the participation of women with very young children (those under 2 years old) has increased dramatically.

This increase is not necessarily by choice. In part because of widespread economic changes and a decrease in jobs that pay a family wage, few families can afford to do without women's wages. In 1970, roughly 70% of families in America could afford an average priced home; by the mid-1980s, the percentage of families who could afford such a house dropped to a mere 15%. Put simply, most families today need the money that two wages provide just to maintain a lower-middle to middle class standard of living.

Changes in women's work roles have brought about changes in the family as well. However, even the most recent research has shown that regardless of their work status, women still perform roughly 90% of child care and household tasks. Moreover, in extended and multigenerational families, it is women who provide most of the caregiving for both younger and older generations. Given the current social and demographic forces shaping extended families in America, researchers must examine the crucial roles men can have in supporting and nurturing their family members.

VIII. METHODOLOGICAL CONCERNS

A great deal of research has focused on the family, including both the nuclear and extended family. Although empirical evidence is always useful, it is also crucial to examine contextual issues that influence the interpretation of research findings. For example, consider the question of how best to examine the role of extended family members and their effects on the mental health of individual family members when the families live in very different contexts.

Although all families certainly share some important characteristics, they are also clearly quite different from one another. Although families in both Iowa and Brooklyn may have mothers, fathers, and children, the fundamental issues influencing their mental health might be quite different. The farm family may be most concerned about losing the family farm; the family raising children in an urban setting will have quite different concerns. We now have excellent research that attests to the significant mental distress families have experienced as a result of the farm crisis in the last decade. However, these concerns do not affect the family in Brooklyn, which may be more concerned with the quality of life in their neighborhoods and the rising costs of living in an urban area. These families, too, may be experiencing crises. However, the manifestation of such crises and their influence on mental health in the two settings will be very different.

Similarly, if the concern is about mental health, it may be tempting to begin with a sample of people with serious mental illness. Once again, the nature of the sample will influence the results of the study. Consider the example of a study on the influence of extended family relationships on severe depression. A sample of severely depressed individuals drawn from the larger community (who can still function fairly independently) is likely to be quite different from one dawn from an inpatient unit (who can no longer function independently). The role of extended family members in the depression of these two groups is likely to be quite different, yet a study including either sample could be described as a study of the influence of extended family on people with severe depression.

Another important issue to consider in the study of mental health is the recent recognition of differential diagnoses by race, culture, or ethnic background. Clearly, such diagnoses have important implications for extended family relationships. Despite the apparent objectivity of criteria for the diagnosis of mental illness, it has now been clearly established that certain diagnoses can vary by sociodemographic characteristics of the patient. For example, there is evidence that an African American presenting exactly the same symptoms as a white American is more likely to be diagnosed as schizophrenic. Moreover, particular diagnoses have an important impact on the ways in which extended families interact with diagnosed family members. These issues should be taken into consideration when examining how families of different backgrounds cope with serious mental illness. [*See* RACISM AND MENTAL HEALTH.]

IX. DISCIPLINARY PERSPECTIVES

The study of the extended family and mental health has been undertaken by psychologists, sociologists, anthropologists, psychiatrists, public health researchers, and biomedical researchers. We believe that mutual respect among people from different disciplines and appreciation for different approaches to the same issues are essential for a comprehensive understanding of the influence of extended families on mental health, because each discipline focuses on different aspects of this relationship. For example, sociologists might be most interested in how sociodemographic characteristics are related to the extended family structure and to the presence of mental health. Psychologists, on the other hand, might focus on the psychological mechanisms that explain the effect of extended family members on mental health and vulnerability to mental illness. Each of these disciplines offers an insight on a particular piece of the puzzle, all of which are required to understand the influence of extended family rela-

tionships on mental health. Each approach, therefore, deserves respect and attention as significant contributors to our knowledge in this area.

X. SUMMARY AND CONCLUSIONS

Although it is true that the structure of the family has changed dramatically in the recent past and will continue to change in the near future, it should be noted that there has been some fundamental consistency in the function of the family. The function of the family, both nuclear and extended, is to provide individuals with basic instrumental and emotional support as well as to contribute to their socialization as productive, healthy members of society. These are major developmental tasks that face all people, tasks that are profoundly influenced by family life. The current increase in the role of extended family in the lives of individuals may be an adaptive strategy adopted to cope with dramatic changes in family structure and in demographic and social forces shaping life in modern America. As the structure of the nuclear family changes, children, adolescents, adults, and old people will increasingly turn to others, specifically, to others whom they consider to be members of their extended family. In essence, extended families remain critical to the health and well-being of family members and may become increasingly important as American families face the future.

BIBLIOGRAPHY

Coontz, S. (1992). *The way we never were: American families and the nostalgia trap.* New York: Basic Books.

Jackson, J. S., & Antonucci, T. C. (1994). Survey methodology in life-span human development research. In S. Cohen & H. Reese (Eds.), *Life-span developmental psychology: Methodological contributions.* Hillsdale, NJ: Lawrence Erlbaum.

Skolnick, A., & Skolnick, J. (Eds.). (1992). *Family in transition: Rethinking marriage, sexuality, child-rearing, and family organization.* New York: Harper Collins.

F

Family Systems

Lee Combrinck-Graham

Oxford Health Plans

Community Interpersonal context including families, affected by politics and culture, where individuals establish membership and identity through reciprocal contributions.

Competence Capacity, ability, mastery.

Family Collection of individuals usually of at least two generations, sometimes connected by marriage or biology, sharing the functions of providing shelter, food, mutual support, culture, and sometimes raising children.

Health A state of systems organized for the mutual benefit of the component parts.

Mental Health The capacity to relate to and make a contribution to one's community.

Reciprocity Give and take between individuals or groups of individuals, a process that connects through generosity, obligation, and commitment.

Resilience Adaptability, elasticity.

The **FAMILY** is the primary context of individual mental health. In the family, individual identities are formed, and from the family individuals are launched into the wider society. A number of principles and processes help to define how families can form a healthy environment in which individuals develop, adapt, and learn to make a loving contribution to their communities.

I. WHAT IS MENTAL HEALTH?

The World Health Organization (WHO) defines health as "a state of complete physical, mental, and social well-being and not merely the absence of disease or infirmity." Health is not simply the absence of illness or distress, and mental health is not simply the absence of mental illness or distress. The vocabulary emphasizing the word "health" in medicine and psychiatry precedes an understanding of what health care really is, because medicine is practiced to fight illness and disease. Doctors and mental "health" professionals are trained to identify, classify, and treat illnesses. Particularly in the last several decades with the development of more sophisticated technology for detecting disease, "healthcare" professionals are not trained specifically to define, recognize, and promote health. The long-time exception to this generality has been well-baby care and immunizations that are a routine part of pediatric practice. And yet pediatricians, too, often see their regular visits with babies and young children as an opportunity to scan for illnesses or developmental deviations.

Another question that arises in thinking about health and mental health is where is it located? In a person with one gangrenous toe, one might refer to the "healthy" toes as those not affected. Yet, would one say that the person is healthy if he or she is suffering from a gangrenous toe? On the other hand, a person could be suffering from a gangrenous toe, but have a "healthy" mental outlook, and even though the toe will have to go, it might be said that this condition exists in an otherwise healthy person. Health and mental health, then, refer to aspects of being besides the presence or absence of pathology. The person with the gangrenous toe could be said to be unhealthy, because he or she has diabetes; or healthy, because he or she has high energy, a positive outlook, and is otherwise fit. Health and mental health are more abstract notions than disease, especially disease that is defined by Koch's postulates (that is, one can identify a pathogen associated with a diseased condition and then cause diseased condition by introducing the pathogen). Clearly this definition of disease works within a closed system and does not consider factors such as virulence of the pathogen, susceptibility of the host, and so on. A concept of health, however, does consider all of these factors. Health exists in a context and the health of individual units in a context are intricately defined by the relationships between themselves and others.

This leads to two definitions of health and mental health: a first is that health exists in a system organized for the benefit of all of its parts. The second is that a mentally healthy individual is one who participates in and makes a contribution to his/her community. Neither definition requires that health be recognized only in the absence of disease. This requires that health care continues and that a healthy status can be achieved even in the face of chronic or terminal illness. Both definitions require attention to the context, including socioeconomic conditions, culture, work, outlook for the future, and primary interpersonal relationships.

II. THE FAMILY AS A CONTEXT FOR MENTAL HEALTH

The family is the most easily identifiable locus of mental health for most people. When there is no family, loneliness, despair, self-destructive behavior, and maladaptive forms of emotional coping may flourish. Several researchers, notably psychiatrist pioneer in community mental health Milton Greenblatt and colleagues, have demonstrated that mental health is associated with a social network, and that morbidity is increased in individuals without a social network. The family is the primary social network. Families are the most important social locus of individual health and mental health, even though many describe families as disintegrating, overtaxed, exploitative, and toxic. It is in the family that individuals forge their identities as children, parents, partners, collaborators, transmitters of traditions and rituals, interpreters of culture. It is through the mediation of experience in a family that most individuals find their places in communities, establishing mental health in relation to the second definition, as members of and contributors to a community. [*See* SOCIAL NETWORKS; SOCIAL SUPPORT.]

Because of the importance of community, the family cannot be treated or studied as a free standing unit because to do this would ignore the systems in which families are embedded, just as to regard the individual without observing interaction with family members gives insufficient information about that person's life, character, style, and resources. Family life is sustained and refreshed by its members' participation in the communities of their own education, vocation, and avocation, as well as the neighborhood and religious organizations in which the family participates. The family unit, or household unit, may be conceived as a relatively stable structure, evolving and elaborating itself over time, but representing a familiar and often dependable retreat from a less predictable larger world. Yet the family's stability is ballast for its members' capacity for creativity and exploration. If one thinks of health as a balance between variety and constraint, the constraint of family tradition, the constancy of its ties, provides a platform for elaborating variety and filters and modifies the variety of experiences and ideas introduced through family members' daily forays into larger society.

When the family is examined in a search for what is wrong with individuals or with societal trends, negative influences can be found. And because our misnamed mental "health" system has been predisposed to identify pathology, the family has been found guilty of causing and sustaining it. To some extent identifying the family as the most essential environment contributing to its members' mental health is only a point of view. However, if one sets out to define mental health and describe its evolution and the resources that support it, then the family's influence will be found to be just as potent in health as it was found to be in malfunction. Because most "mental health" professionals have been trained to define, detect, and treat mental illness, identifying the elements of family interaction that support mental health is not an easy task.

III. FAMILY SYSTEMS PRINCIPLES OF MENTAL HEALTH

Family systems theory contributes several principles that can assist with a focus on mental health.

1. There is no one true version of a story, but multiple versions, each containing truth.

2. Events can be understood to occur in patterns, and these patterns are often recurrent and identifiable at multiple levels of a system.

3. Equifinality and equipotentiality are principles that describe the bifurcating nature of evolution, whether it be development, history, or response to an event.

4. There is competence in all systems, and this competence contributes to survival and adaptation.

5. Similarly, all systems have resilience that enables the system to rebound from various assaults.

6. All systems have resources that can be tapped for sustenance as well as extra support to manage greater demands.

7. Reciprocity, or give and take, is a fundamental interaction in healthy systems.

8. Healthy systems achieve a balance between variety and constraint.

Each of these principles, elaborated, identifies characteristics of mental health.

The first two principles address how a system is observed and described. Principle one, that there are multiple versions of a story, notes that the perspective of the observer is only one of many possible viewpoints. This requires that an observer of family functioning be familiar with the influences on his/her own perspective as well as open to gathering information about the perspectives of others, particularly of family members. This, in turn, leads to a complex multiocular view of any situation that is being reported or experienced by more than one person. To appreciate not only one's own point of view but that of several others has been called "multilateral partiality" by family psychiatrist Ivan Bozsormenyi-Nagy. Multi-

ocular examination permits taking the sides of each participant to achieve a fair and balanced view of that person's contribution and response as well as an integrated overview of the functioning of the entire system. Furthermore, the process of multiocular or multilateral examination encourages other participants to actively consider each other's contributions. For example, a mother of a preverbal toddler was asked, "Who is in your family?" She named several individuals, including her children and her siblings. She was then asked, "If your daughter could talk, who would she tell me is in her family?" The mother then placed herself in her daughter's position, and proceeded to name other individuals, particularly some cousins with whom she played frequently.

The second principle, that there are discernible patterns that describe family functioning and response to events, helps to organize and manage experiences. The principle is represented in the observation that healthy families have traditions, diurnal, weekly, and anniversary occasions. Some researchers on family life in which one of the parents is an alcoholic, for example, observed that children raised in families who had rituals, such as a family gathering for Thanksgiving, or a regular dinnertime, were less likely to became alcoholic.

Patterns provide an esthetic and operate to maintain stability and coherence in interpersonal life. Patterns of behavior may be seen as linear causal, recursive, oscillating, or evolving spirals. Patterns may be identified by an outside observer who then inquires whether the family is aware of such patterns, and whether these are familiar or only manifested at this time? Family members may describe patterns in response to questions that evoke this kind of consideration of their experience. For example the observer might ask the family, "What do you usually do at the children's bedtime?" Such a question focuses the family members on bedtime as an event in daily life, and it asks for identification of the consistent elements of bedtime, regardless of the possible inconsistencies.

When family members become conscious of some of their patterns, they can then decide whether they like things the way they are, or want to change them. Changing patterns affects the relationships between all the elements, and, as in the kaleidoscope, a closed system containing a fixed number of pieces of colored glass, the patterns, once changed, can never be re-established in quite the same way, again, but the new patterns have new esthetic.

The third principle, about equipotentiality and equifinality, notes that a present set of events may result in a variety of outcomes. Thus, a traumatic experience for a family may lead to continuous mourning and a perpetual sense of loss, or it may strengthen family relationships as they face the adversity together. Families with children who have died of cancer after several years of illness and treatment have been observed to have many different outcomes. Among the many adjustments are the following three: some remain fixed on the lost child, creating a shrine of the child's room; some break up entirely; and some reflect on the privilege of having had this child and this experience. This is the principle of equipotentiality. The observer of healthy family functioning will note that the family's response to events is uniquely adaptive given their own history and patterns. While there may be common responses and dangers resulting from certain events, these will not necessarily be the ones experienced by particular individuals or a particular family.

Equifinality describes the observation that a current set of experiences may have arisen from a variety of different sources. This is different from Koch's principles. Psychosis, for example, is not always caused by schizophrenia. Indeed, schizophrenia is not always characterized by psychosis. Psychosis may be an outcome of a variety of different antecedents, such as drugs, overwhelming stress, isolation, brain damage, brainwashing, and so on.

As one examines the patterns involving present events, it is possible to identify how certain matters may have come about and what possibilities there may be for how matters may occur in the future.

Principles four through six refer to inherent or latent facets of family systems that must be identified to identify and promote healthy functioning. Highlighting these elements of family functioning shifts the focus of clinical assessment from scanning for pathology to including health in the assessment process.

For more than 20 years a list of strengths has been required in standard record keeping in many areas. Examples include the individual education plans (IEP) for special education students and many problem lists in the problem oriented records in hospitals and clinics. Generally there is not as much emphasis placed on the usefulness of these lists in the clinical process, and often they are listed more pro forma than as a significant contribution to the overall treatment outcome. Typical examples of strengths on a student's IEP might be "interested and supportive parents," "attractive child." More substantive examples would include some characterization of family competence, resilience and resourcefulness. But to habitually identify these and integrate them into a full picture of family and individual functioning takes some specific training.

All families have competence. When a family experiences many disadvantages, such as poverty, lack of education, and homelessness; or has many negative behaviors, such as abuse and neglect of children; parental substance abuse, or delinquency of the children, clinicians may be distracted and coopted to label the family as "dysfunctional" and "multiproblem" and not ask critical questions relating to how the family survives, what holds the family together, what qualities of coping and problem solving have they identified among themselves? The labels may be accurate and useful, but insufficient to involve this individual family in working toward a more healthy adjustment, because no basis for health has been identified within the family.

Resilience is a specific characteristic of competence. It refers to the capacity to bounce back, to withstand the onslaught of misfortunes. There have been many efforts to characterize resilience, particularly in children who survive trauma, abuse, and illness of parents and who seem to do well in adulthood. Some writers, determined that without certain critical elements, no one could be a healthy adult, might say that the apparent resilience and health of some of these individuals is a facade, and that they suffer from limitations in the capacity to relate fully to others, or from constricted emotional expression. Others have identified relationship factors in supporting resilience in children, noting that with all of the hardship and relational disruptions, there appears to have been a secure attachment or a reliable relationship that carried the child through. Resilience can be facilitated in clinical situations through the examination and recruitment of resources in the patient system, the envisioning of realistic directions and outcomes, and following plans to effect these outcomes.

Resourcefulness is also an aspect of competence. As

with identifying competence, it may be difficult to see a besieged family as having resources. Here it is necessary for the clinician and the family to identify and credit even small things, so that they can be consciously recognized when resources are needed or solutions need to be formulated. For example, a single mother with three young children under 4, one of whom is developmentally disabled, relies on many social services. The social services, themselves, have been resources for this family, but in addition, there is a neighbor who often comes in to chat with the mother, providing brief respite from her maternal duties, and offering adult company. This relationship is a resource, a source of renourishment and resilience to the mother, and an example of the mother's competence to sustain a significant relationship. In another example, a child was referred because of aggressive behavior. His family had been investigated for neglect, and the social service department was offering "family preservation" services, in the form of frequent visits to the home of a case worker. When the child was evaluated by a therapist, he was shy and very polite. Despite the reports of his behavior, this youngster had learned and practiced respect and courtesy. From whom had he learned this? Apparently he had learned this from his mother, who despite her trials had managed to teach manners to her children.

Principle seven highlights the importance of interpersonal discourse in the process of evolving experience and narrative description. Many family systems theorists propose that psychological substance occurs, not within an individual, but in the interactional space between individuals. To some extent this interactional flavor is captured by describing or discovering patterns of interaction (as in principle two). Reciprocity describes several crucial processes that shape and modify experience.

One aspect of reciprocity is the way one person's response is modified by others' responses. British psychiatrist Ronald Laing wrote of elusive experience as he described one observing another observing the first person observing the other's observations, and so on. What is "really" happening? What are the true observations? They are the endless adjustments in the process of registering and responding. One aspect of reciprocity, then, is self-correction.

Another aspect of reciprocity is loyalty and obligation, crucial components of the relational ethics, conceptualized by family systems psychiatrist Ivan Bozsormenyi-Nagy and his colleagues. Human relationships are shaped through give and take. Children are given life by their parents, and, therefore owe their parents filial loyalty. As children are nurtured, civilized, and educated, parents' investment in their children increases, and children's sense of security and value is established. Additionally, however, the children's obligation to repay the investment is established. Repayment may be accomplished by giving back to parents; but direct "repayment" will usually not satisfy the obligation, because usually parents remain more able to give to their children than the reverse. Children, therefore, may invest and repay their obligations through giving to others, investing in their societal obligations, and raising their own children. In this system of give and take, a nexus of relationships both horizontal (through contemporaries) and vertical (across generations) is bound together by loyalty and obligation. Relational ethics describes situations where people are not given their due, for example, not adequately acknowledged for their accomplishments or contributions. These people may become "entitled," demanding from new relationships what has not been forthcoming in past relationships. Some who have been indulged or perceive themselves to be unworthy of good fortune while viewing others' misfortune may feel "unentitled." One man who had many material advantages and a warm and loving family was constantly worried about his health, often seeking medical attention because of his worry about life-threatening illnesses. When asked why he might not be entitled to enjoy the benefits of his life, he was able to reflect on the losses in the Holocaust of many family members in his grandparents' generation. This man felt that he owed something to these lost individuals who had never been properly celebrated and mourned.

A third implication of reciprocity is accountability. Accountability is responsibility in relationships. A child may have a responsibility to feed his pets and help his sister get to school. He is accountable to his family members for his contributions to the family as a whole, how he represents the family in his behavior outside the family, and to acting in a loyal fashion. In families, everyone has roles and responsibilities. In some families roles and responsibilities are clearer than in others. It may be easy for family members to be accountable in some families, because the expectations are evident. At the very least, there are common generation accountabilities. Parents are responsible for nurturing children; children are responsible for being guided by their parents. When children disobey or ignore their parents, they are not being accountable. When parents neglect or abuse their children, they are not being accountable. Accountability, the practice of responsible reciprocity, is a crucial relational function of mental health.

Principle eight addresses variety and constraint. Variety characterized the capacity for creativity and novelty. Variety is generally viewed to be renewing, refreshing, allowing interest to be sustained. Constraint refers to limits or boundaries. As reciprocals, constraint contains and limits, providing a center and grounding, while variety elaborates. Constraints may be imposed on a family system from the outside or the inside. Outside constraints include limitations of socioeconomic status, education, geographical location, and physical capacity. Internal constraints include rules and regulations and rigidity and how status is defined and maintained. A family's ability to explore and to experience variety may be severely affected by constraints from both without and within. Although there may be undisputed obstacles (constraints) to accomplishing certain objectives, tapping into individual capacity for imagination and creativity may make some things possible. An example concerned a family where because of the necessity to have medical assistance to cover the hospital bills of a seriously ill child, the father believed that he could not get full employment, because if he did he would jeopardize the medical coverage. That is, he was constrained by the combined circumstances of his son's illness and the means of paying for his treatment. Accepting the reality of these constraints, the father was invited to imagine what kind of job he might get, if he were not so constrained. Within a very short time he had arranged to work informally, a situation that got him out of the house everyday and brought in some additional money to the family.

In a similar vein, many who work clinically with families with young children find that the unique contributions of the children, when appreciated, often add a creative twist that offers a unique solution to what had appeared as an insoluble problem. Strategic therapist Chloé Madanes uses "pretending" with families, where she had the families enact scenes pretending that something is happening, or pretending a

relationship. Family systems educator Evan Imber Black and associates use rituals. Inventing ritualistic exercises to engage the family both contains (constrains) emotion, anxiety, and nonproductive behavior, and involves them in a fanciful, metaphorical activity, together.

IV. FAMILY FORMS AND FUNCTIONS

There are varying ways to define a family. Flexibility within a structure is associated with health and adaptation. This must be true, too, of the definition of a family. Basically a family defines itself and its functions and covers the conjoint conduct of daily life activities (e.g., shared living, eating, financial, and social arrangements) to the more traditional family functions of bearing and raising children. The most significant aspect of family identification is how its members identify themselves. To the extent that they have a consensual view of family membership they should be regarded as a family for the purposes of looking for mental health.

For the family, then, a significant feature of health is *membership*. Membership in a family entitles one to the family benefits of social relationships as well as giving access to resources and providing significant aspects of personal identity. For social relationships are associated with a greater health and resistance to illness as well as an overall improved sense of well-being. Resources available in the family range from emotional support, assistance with daily tasks, advice and problem solving, and care and sustenance. Personal identity of a sustaining nature arises often out of family relationships. For example, I am someone's daughter, mother, sister, aunt, cousin, and wife. Additionally, these identities are associated with functions in which I am vested by my family relationships and upon which they rely upon me, because I am competent, and those are my roles and responsibilities.

In modern and postmodern times, the traditional nuclear family household of 2 parents and 2 + children has to take its place among the many different recognized family forms, including stepfamilies, adoptive families, single-parent-headed families, grandparent-headed families, teen-headed families, divorced families, gay or lesbian families, communal families, non-married families, extended families, and more. These families provide the supportive and identifying contexts for their members. How they function contributes to the health of their members not whether or not they have the socially condoned hallmarks of family. For example, "family values" is a moral lens through which nontraditional families are seen as pathological. In this view, "father absence" is a deficit likely to cause damage in children growing up without a father. Children who grow up with a mentally ill parent are vulnerable, so that those who turn out well, in spite of these deficits, are called "invulnerable." A study of varying family forms and performance of third graders suggested that there are many combinations of adults and children that are associated with competence in the children, indicating that there are no strictly pathological family forms. Rather there are demands for coping that are met with flexibility and resourcefulness by most families. Families find a way.

A family's functioning and capacity to contribute to the health of all of its members, then, is a function of the members' sense of inclusion/membership, experience of the family relationship system as a support system, and forging of some reliable identities within the family. In this way the family performs its healthy function of providing a stable stage from which other social roles and functions can be assayed and evaluated. Other features of family health are regulation of closeness and distance (proximity) and establishing status.

It is tempting to regard families as strange attractors. As described in the science of Chaos, strange attractors are curvilinear mathematical abstractions of infinite variety within an overall set of limitations. For example, snowflake patterns are strange attractors. They are hexagonal, but the varieties are infinite. Families have some boundaries defining internal membership, but the varieties of repertoires, customs, and relationships within are infinite. Thus it is impossible to arbitrarily say that a family's behaviors are pathological. The strange attractor model, however, allows for a notion of when a family is not acting like a family — as its behavior goes out of the bounds that define it as a family. While this may appear to be a tautology it is not. Let's take a defining family function, for example, producing, nurturing, raising, and civilizing children. The function is a condition that must be satisfied in order for the group to be that strange attractor called family. The varieties of accomplishing these tasks are infinite as well as the family constellations who may be involved in doing so. But if the tasks are perverted,

if the children are exploited instead of nurtured, then the group is acting nonfamily, beyond the boundaries.

V. PARAMETERS OF FAMILY FUNCTIONING

There have been many ways of defining family functioning. In the mental health or psychotherapy literature family characteristics associated with dysfunction and the family's contribution to individual pathology have usually been the object of study. True to the form of the development of the mental "health" field, early studies of family functioning reported negative characteristics, such as "refrigerator mothers," pseudomutuality, schism and skew, the undifferentiated family ego mass, rigid triads. As often happens when the point of an investigation is to discover the cause or explanation of a problem, the findings do not necessarily suggest a solution. Indeed the models of psychopathology that operate from explanations of genetic origins of troubles hold out little hope for treatment, because of the implicit damage. For example, a group of child clinicians were discussing the case of a 6-year-old girl who had undergone a traumatic experience when her major caretaking parent had died suddenly of a heart attack in her presence, when she was 2 years old. The child was brought by the surviving parent for an evaluation, when she was 6. The complaints were that the child was clinging to the parent and was unable to be alone. Further exploration revealed that the parent appeared to have been clinging to the child, but had recently begun to date and was now ready for more distance from her. The child was found to be a bright, curious, articulate, and creative youngster, and as adjustments in the household were made, and as she began to interact with her peers in school, she settled in well, developed good friendships, was able to go for overnights at friends houses, and otherwise demonstrated good health. The clinicians in the discussion could not believe that the child was healthy, because no one could survive the loss without being damaged, they opined.

One approach to define and measure family functioning is the identification of dimensions. Dimensions appear in three general areas: inclusion/membership, status, and proximity. Inclusion is associated with various functions, such as organization and predictability. Status is reflected by decision making, power hierarchies, and negotiation. And proximity is associated with enmeshment/disengagement, or centripetal and centrifugal forces.

Other names for these same general dimensions include structure, communication, adaptability, cohesion, problem solving, and emotional tone. The research group led by psychiatrist researcher David Reiss has named three qualitatively different dimensions: configuration, coordination, and closure.

In their attempts to operationalize family dimensions, different researchers have defined them differently, usually to identify characteristics that address research questions. For example, the Beavers-Timberlawn assessment instrument was developed in the early 1970s to identify what differentiated nonclinical families from families of disturbed adolescents. For the original Beavers-Timberlawn evaluation, samples of family interaction are rated on a scale assessing the dimensions of adaptability and cohesion. Adaptability refers to the ability to accommodate to changes, both from within (due to development) and from outside (due to social or economic forces).

The Circumplex Model of family functioning was theoretically derived, and family data are gained from a self-report instrument, the Family Adaptability and Cohesion Evaluation Scale (FACES). The dimensions of cohesion and adaptability are common to FACES and to the Beavers-Timberlawn assessment models, but FACES expresses adaptability as curvilinear with both rigidity and flexibility being dysfunctional extremes, while the Beavers-Timberlawn assesses rigidity as more adaptive than chaotic flexibility, suggesting that rigidity is a step closer to good adaptation on a linear continuum that extends toward the infinite variety of creative adaptability.

David Reiss developed a different approach to assessing families. Rather than answering questions about themselves, the family members perform a neutral card-sorting task that involves interaction among them. The parameters of configuration, coordination, and closure represent different dimensions of how the task is handled, and the task yields information about the way a family defines and organizes experience, which is called the family's "paradigm." With high configuration, the family views the world as ordered and itself as capable of mastery, as opposed to low configuration, where the family sees the world as disordered and itself as helpless and threatened. With high coordination, the family sees itself being treated

as a unitary group, and views itself as a cohesive entity, while with low coordination, the family experiences itself as loosely connected. With delayed closure, the family sees the world as interesting and itself as evolving and changing with experience, while with early closure, the family views the world as familiar and views itself as continuous with its past traditions. Particular paradigms are not associated with dysfunction or pathology; they provide useful information about the family's style.

An example of the descriptive quality of Reiss's card sort assessment is his portrayal of families of delinquents contrasted with families of schizophrenics and normals. Called "environment-distance-sensitive," delinquent families were distinguished by their tendency to view the environment as if it were disjointed; family members were emotionally separated from each other and seemed to lack knowledge about each other's motives and perspectives; family members appeared to view the interactions during the card-sorting test as an opportunity to express individual interest and to establish independent recognition; they were low on intrafamiliar coordination and had poor problem-solving skills as a family.

A. Typologies

Typologies are constellations of characteristics. One approach to family typology is to name families by the disorders of individual family members (e.g., "schizophrenic" families). Another is to name families by characteristic relationship patterns (e.g., "enmeshed" families).

Many efforts have been made to define a one-to-one relationship between patterns of family interaction and specific disorders. The family field's failed attempts to show how families caused schizophrenia is illustrative of the problems involved in trying to establish such causal connections. Patterns of interaction that have been described in families of individuals with certain disorders (such as anorexia nervosa, schizophrenia, or manic-depressive disorder) probably reflect the complex process of adaptation and adjustment that occurs continuously in families. Recognizing this, the finding of family characteristics associated with certain disorders is useful, not because the families cause these illnesses, but because these observations have provided a useful guide to assist families in managing an ill family member.

VI. DEVELOPMENT IN FAMILY SYSTEMS

How do families change through the life cycle? Are there common processes to family adjustments to the developmental accomplishments of their members? One proposal is that the elements of family structure are first rearranged at a "first order" level (i.e., by increments of adaptation and mastery achieved by one member of the family) followed by a "second order" change (i.e., the transformations of status and meaning within the system as it adjusts to the first order change). These transformations, or second order changes, may appear to evolve continuously or may appear as discontinuous leaps in the nature of family organization, like the kaleidoscope analogy suggested earlier. An additional notion is that systems are always oscillating between states and that development occurs through oscillations between states of greater and lesser competence, with oscillations widening during "developmental transitions" and finally settling on an integrated level of functioning at a higher level. Conventional wisdom that families are more prone to unravel during developmental transitions is explained by noting that the family in transition experiences the widest variations in the level of functioning of its members, and this strains its ability to accommodate as a system.

A. The Individual and Significant Others

The relationship between mothers and infants has been the center of studies of early child development, and descriptions of dyadic processes studied in mother–child relationships recognize reciprocity and recursion in the unfolding of behaviors of both mother and infant and leading to the development of a rich data base on the important relationship between the child and primary caretaker. How the mother–infant relationship is shaped by relationships with others, however, is a study that requires a special framework for including such relational information as patterns of triadic functioning, as well as the influence of larger sociocultural patterns on focal relationships.

Longitudinal studies of marital functioning and the relationship between marital functioning and parenting around the birth of the first child have been performed by several researchers. One group proposed an epigenetic model of family development built on the structure of marital interaction confirming that marital stability through the events of the first child's birth and the first year is variable, depending upon the structure of the marital system prior to the birth. Importantly, however, this group concluded that the impact of the inclusion of a third member of the family cannot be evaluated on the basis of the marital dyad, alone. Another group studied changes in the family environment when a second child is born, expanding the nexus of relationships from a triad to a tetrad. They describe the formation of an autonomous sibling relationship in addition to dyads of each parent with each child and the couple's relationship, a total of six dyads. These studies of the impact of adding new members to the family demonstrate that family formation and development is probably not a straightforward epigenetic process built upon rules established in the marital system. The introduction of new individuals requires the establishment of new structures, new tasks and many new relationships.

B. The Family Life Cycle

Models of the family life cycle have been described that offer several different areas of emphasis: stages of evolution, changing emotional processes, and changing dimensions of family relatedness.

Sociologists such as Evelyn Duvall were among the first to articulate stages of family life, and these, at first, were conceptualized as a series of family stages which correlated with stages in individual's development. Family therapists Elizabeth Carter and Monica McGoldrick proposed six stages: 1. leaving home: single young adults; 2. the joining of families through marriage; 3. families with young children; 4. families with adolescents; 5. launching children and moving on; 6. families in later life. They also described critical emotional issues for the family at different stages. For example, for their stage 3 the critical emotional issue for the family is "accepting new members into the system." For stage 4 the issue is "increasing flexibility of family boundaries to include children's independence and grandparents' frailties." This provides a clinical guide to the usual preoccupations of family members in different stages of the life cycle.

Moving from stages defined by individuals to stages defined by relational development, psychiatrist Lyman Wynne proposed an epigenetic model of relational processes in the family. He suggested that individuals develop relational complexity in the family context in an orderly sequence, as follows: 1. attachment-caregiving; 2. communicating; 3. joint problem solving; 4. mutuality; and sometimes, 5. intimacy.

Child psychiatrist Joan Zilbach defined stages using the family's own history, rather than that of its individual members, as markers for the stages. She proposes seven stages: I and II, forming and nesting; III, IV, and V, family separation processes, beginning when the first family member participates in an extra-familial system (e.g., a child attending school) and ending when the first family member actually exits from the nuclear family; and VI and VII, late stages, one defined by the exit of the last dependent family member, the second defined by the death of one of the spouses.

These stages are marked by movement of individuals into and out of the family system, and they define characteristic issues for the family, regardless of the developmental concerns of the individuals. For example, families in stage I have similar issues, whether it is a first marriage or a remarriage. This scheme focuses on fundamental family tasks rather than the individual's developmental motifs.

Child and family psychiatrist Lee Combrinck-Graham devised a Family Life Spiral model that depicts overlapping developmental issues at three generational levels (such as grandparenthood, childbearing and birth, or retirement, midlife reevaluation and adolescence). She observed that different relational processes seemed to characterize the developmental issues of each generation simultaneously and proposed that instead of an epigenetic unfolding of relational processes (such as in Wynne's model) there was an oscillation from periods of closeness, favoring intimate experiences to periods of differentiation, favoring individuation. When individual developmental issues in three generations of a family are stacked upon each other as they might occur simultaneously, a spiral develops that shows the relationship of these generational events to the internal forces in the family. For example, the simultaneous events of childbirth, becoming a parent, and becoming a grandparent are associated with strong centripetal forces within the family. These events usually stimulate closeness, intimacy, and a functional enmeshment among participants in the family. The often overlapping events of adolescence, the "40s crisis," and retirement or change of life-style of grandparents appear to be responding to centrifugal forces pulling members out of the center of the family and into a larger sphere of peers and new opportunities. An individual who lives three generations in a family may experience three cycles of centripetal and centrifugal family forces. In the centripetal family, intimacy in relationships is favored over autonomy; in the centrifugal family, it is the reverse. From the perspective of these evolving family relationship shapes, many negotiations of status, membership, and proximity may be understood in their overall effect on the shape of the family.

This model of family evolution does not define normal family functioning. Instead it proposes a template upon which family adaptation may be assessed. Many families do not have three generations pursuing life events "on-time." For example, in many two-career families, childbearing may be postponed until the parents are in their mid-to-late thirties. The centripetal shape of a family around childbirth may correspond with ordinarily centrifugal events surrounding career points for adults in career midpoints. Where such a time might have been an opportunity for a working adult to take a new job, move to a new location, or make another work transition, the focus on family life with young children may stimulate altogether different decisions, such as working half-time to share child care, sharing a job with the spouse, fathers staying home with the children while the mothers pursue their careers, and many other possibilities. The "off-time" events of teenage parenthood presents another version of a "centripetal" stimulus occurring during a centrifugal experience. The challenge to family adaptation is how to continue the evolution of the adolescent-parent through the experiences of individuation and autonomy while still providing the intimate, enmeshed environment necessary for caring for young children. A third example of an "off-time" challenge is in remarried families with children of different "generations" as when a parent of teenagers marries and has a new set of children.

As "off-time" family development can be stimulated by births, so, too, can it be stimulated by deaths. Death of an older person that is anticipated, either because of frailty or illness, is generally less challenging to family members than the untimely death of a child or the parent of young children. The latter frequently stimulates a widening family definition as new members are recruited for comfort and assistance. This may include only members of the extended family, or it may involve bringing in new members, such as finding an adult to replace the lost one to care for the children. It may also result in conceiving or adopting a child to replace a lost child. These are family attempts to cope with "off-time" challenges to their sense of consistency and coherence, even as they are developing and changing.

VII. ASSESSMENT OF FAMILY FUNCTIONING

Having a framework for observing mental health in families, such as that provided by the eight principles, having some dimensions through which to classify organizational and relational functions, and having some models of family organization evolving through time and in response to the personal development of family members makes it possible to perform a family assessment that helps both interviewer and family members to evaluate strengths and resources, assess how they are coping with internal and external challenges, define where and how they would like to be as a family, and determine some actions they may take on their own behalf. An interview protocol is a semistructured approach to involving the family in the process of assessing itself. Thus, instead of the standard approach of interviewer asking questions to gather information that later is formulated into diagnoses, the mental health interview is designed to stimulate family members' curiosity about themselves and their functioning so that they are assessing themselves. Through this process both family and interviewer come to know the family in novel ways, increasing variety in conception and understanding and therefore expanding options and resources. Critical processes of the interview address four of the eight

principles particularly: 1. that there are no correct answers; everyone in the family has a valid version of the story; 2. that there are patterns of interaction that can be observed and that have some relevance to the family's stability, cohesion, and, sometimes to where the family gets stuck; 3. that the family has competence, a fact that is highlighted in the way the interview process asks for their expertise; and 4. that the mental health of the family is dependent on the family and surrounding systems being organized for the mutual benefit of all of its members.

Numerous experiences of conducting interviews with families in this way have confirmed that families gain momentum, hope, and energy from having their mental health recognized and brought to the forefront. Even families with severe problems and longstanding dependence on welfare and other systems find sources of pride and independent action through this process.

VIII. CONCLUSION

The family is a most important source of and resource for mental health. Viewing families and family functioning from a health perspective supports families' functions to nurture, civilize, and assist with the formation and evolution of healthy personal identities of their members. The views of family membership, dimensions of family functioning, and family development illustrate some of the many ways that families operate and adapt to care for their members and survive the many challenges and changes experienced through the life cycle.

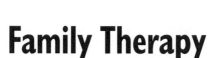

Family Therapy

Philip Barker

University of Calgary and Alberta Children's Hospital

Circular Causation A causal chain in which there is a series of events, each influencing another, the process continuing in a circular manner.

Disengagement The opposite of enmeshment (see below).

Enmeshment The close emotional involvement of two or more people.

Family Structure The ways in which the different family members, or groups of members, are allied, and the nature and strengths of the alliances.

Family System The parts of a family and the ways in which they interact to make up a functioning entity that is more than the sum of the parts.

Linear Causation One event causes another but the second event does not affect the first event.

Strategic Therapy A therapeutic method that uses a carefully planned, usually indirect, approach to promoting changes in families.

FAMILY THERAPY is a treatment approach that takes the family unit as its focus. Family therapists understand the emotional and behavioral problems of individuals as often being related to problems in the family systems of which they are part. They believe that by working to promote change in the family, the symptoms and problems of the family's members will be resolved, or at least ameliorated. Sometimes, but less often, it is the family as a group that presents with problems. An important feature of the family therapy approach is an emphasis on the concept of *circular,* rather than *linear* causation. Family therapists are reluctant to regard events or behaviors in families as due to single, isolated causes, but tend to see them as parts of, usually complex, chains of events.

I. THE DEVELOPMENT OF FAMILY THERAPY

The family therapy approach to the treatment of mental health problems was developed during the years that followed the Second World War. Psychotherapists of various mental health disciplines, together with researchers from other disciplines, began to look at their patients' families as possibly contributing to the disorders they were treating. The idea that families might have a part in the genesis of psychiatric disorders was not new. Freud and others from the early days of psychoanalysis had postulated that the early childhood family relationships of their patients had caused the neurosis with which these patients presented. In those early days, however, the response was to separate the patients from their families for treatment. This was accomplished either by seeing patients for treatment on their own while having minimal or no contact with their families; or by admitting them to psychiatric hospitals or other institutions where they could be cared for and treated away from the supposed adverse influences of their families. What *was* new was the idea that it was possible to work with families, in the here and now, to change their ways of functioning; and that this might be a quicker and more effective approach than individual psychotherapy with individual patients.

One of the first to point out the importance of the family was Christian Midelfort whose book, *The Family in Psychotherapy,* was published in 1957. Despite its promising title, however, this was not truly a book about family therapy. More important was Nathan Ackerman's *The Psychodynamics of Family Life,* published the following year. Like many of the pioneers of family therapy, Ackerman came from a background of psychoanalytic training, and his first book reflects this. But he pointed out that while psychiatrists had become adept in the retrospective study of mental illness and in the careful examination of family histories, they had not yet cultivated an equivalent skill in the study of current family processes. Ackerman went on to suggest that, by acquiring skills in working with whole family groups, we would add a new dimension to our understanding of mental illness as an ongoing process—and one that changes with time and the conditions of group adaptation.

By 1966 Ackerman's thinking had developed further and his second book, *Treating the Troubled Family,* was probably the first true single-author family therapy book published. By the mid-1960s many groups, several of which had commenced their studies and treatment of families in the 1950s, were publishing their findings. Among the other early pioneers in family therapy were Murray Bowen, Don Jackson, John Elderkin Bell, Don Jackson, Jay Haley, John Weakland, Virginia Satir, Lyman Wynn, Salvador Minuchin and Ivan Boszormenyi-Nagy. Each therapist, or group of therapists, developed a particular approach and theoretical framework. While these often differed substantially, they had in common their focus on the family group and how it functioned. The enthusiasm of some of these pioneers was unbounded, and extreme claims for the effectiveness, or at least the potential, for family therapy were sometimes made. All, or almost all, psychiatric problems came to be seen by some as residing, not in individuals, but in the processes of interaction going on in the person's family or other social group or groups.

Over the years, most of these extreme views have become modified. Family therapy has come to be regarded as a useful therapeutic option and the treatment of choice in many cases. But it is not a cure-all

and it may need to be used along with other treatments. The almost religious zeal of some of the early pioneers has been toned down by the harsh reality of clinical experience and the results of research. Many of the pioneers paid particular attention to patients with schizophrenia, the origins of which, they believed, lay in the family. However the failure of family therapy to prove effective as a primary treatment, combined with increasing knowledge of the neurochemical and biological correlates of the condition and the greater effectiveness of pharmacological treatments, has resulted in a shift of focus toward other disorders. Nevertheless, more recent research has shown that family factors are by no means irrelevant in schizophrenia, and may determine whether relapse occurs after patients return home following treatment in hospital. [*See* SCHIZOPHRENIA.]

II. THEORETICAL CONCEPTS

A. Systems Theory

A way of thinking about families that was seized on early in the development of family therapy was that of *general systems theory.* This theory, originally developed in the 1950s, is concerned with how parts are organized into wholes. Although it was not designed with families in mind, systems theory was found to fit in well with the thinking of many of the early family therapists. The idea that families are open systems has continued to be central to the work of virtually all family therapists. The task of the systems-based therapist thus becomes that of first determining how the family system is functioning, and then facilitating any changes that appear to be required in the way it functions. The systems-oriented therapist expects that once the needed changes in family functioning have been achieved, the symptoms of the member(s) who have been experiencing difficulties will be resolved, or at least ameliorated.

What exactly are the basic principles of systems theory that family therapists have found useful? In summary, they are that:

- Families, and other social groups, are systems that have properties that are more than the sum of the properties of their parts.

- Certain general rules govern the functioning of such systems.
- Every system has a boundary. The boundaries of family systems are permeable in varying degrees, so that some families are more readily, and to a greater extent, influenced by what is going on around them than are others.
- Family systems typically reach relatively steady states; that is, each family settles down to function in its own characteristic way, although change can occur; indeed growth and evolution are usual as the composition of the family changes, its members age, and changes occur in the wider systems of which it is a part.
- The amount and quality of the communications between the parts of the system, are important features.
- The concept of *circular causality* is preferred to that of *linear causality*.
- Family systems, like other systems, appear to be purposeful. They serve such purposes as the rearing of children; the provision of mutual comfort and a context for the expression of the marital partners' sexuality; and the promotion of the economic security of the family group.
- Systems are made up of *subsystems* and are parts of larger *suprasystems*.

Many individuals and families come to therapists asking to be told the "cause" of the problem that is concerning them. They tend to see causality in linear terms. An example of linear causality is the action of a man who puts up his umbrella when it starts to rain. The cause is clear—it is raining—and so is the result—up goes the umbrella. It is not usually believed that putting up the umbrella affects the weather. But in families things are seldom, if ever, that simple. If person A tells person B to do something, and B does it, this in turn will affect the behavior of A, who may, for example, be more likely to ask B to do the same task again when the need arises. There may also be similar, or perhaps opposite, effects on the behavior of other family members.

Let us consider a family in which there is a boy who is anxious about going to school. When it is time to leave for school, the boy cries, clings to his mother, and refuses to leave the house. The mother turns for help to her husband. He fails to give her support and

even blames her for not being firm enough with the boy. Instead he speaks angrily to his son. This increases the boy's anxiety and his tears flow even more freely. This leads to the mother becoming yet more worried and upset; she comforts the boy and then turns with even greater force to her husband who gets even more angry with the boy, and perhaps with the mother also. So whose problem is it? Is it the mother's anxiety about her son that results in her being unable to support her son calmly in the task of separating from her to go to school? Or is the basic problem that of a boy who is (for whatever reasons) emotionally immature and constitutionally prone to react anxiously in situations perceived as threatening? Or is the real problem a dysfunctional parental or marital relationship? Or maybe the cause of it all is an angry, dominating, verbally abusive father? And so on. In other words, who or what is causing the problem? Considering this scenario, some might try to answer these questions in a straightforward way. The family therapist interested in circular causality, however, would not consider it useful to do so. All the problems implied in the questions might indeed exist but none is "the cause." They are all simply—or perhaps not so simply—part of a circular process. To put it another way, they all reflect characteristics of the way the family systems works.

B. Learning Theory

Many other theoretical concepts are used by family therapists. Therapy, whether or not it is addressed to the family system, may be looked on as a teaching and learning process. When we are treating families there is nearly always a need for the family to learn such things as new ways of relating to each other; new approaches on the part of the parents to rearing their children; new ways of allocating the tasks the family members must, between them, ensure are done; perhaps a new type of marital relationship.

While few family therapists would regard themselves simply as teachers, and family therapy is much more than telling people what they should do, learning must happen during the treatment if change is to occur. Learning is conceptualized to occur in several ways:

a. In *respondent conditioning,* a behavior is learned when a rewarding stimulus is paired with a desired behavior. Pavlov's much quoted dogs learned to associate the ringing of a bell with the presentation of food. After a while they salivated in response to the ringing of the bell, without the presentation of any food.

b. In *operant conditioning* the circumstances following a behavior are altered either to reinforce the behavior or to extinguish it. In other words it consists of the systematic, and, ideally, carefully planned, application of positive and negative responses (or, in everyday language, rewards and punishments).

c. *Modeling* is the process by which people acquire behaviors by imitating others. It need not be, and usually is not, a conscious process. Therapists can, and regularly do, model behaviors during their sessions with their clients. The respectful way the therapist addresses family members; how the therapist talks or plays with a child; or how the therapist reacts to things family members do or say—all these and many other behaviors carry messages.

d. *Learning by cognition* occurs when a person thinks something through and comes to a conclusion as a result. In lay terms, it is the process of "figuring things out."

All of these learning processes may occur during family therapy. The therapist must devise ways of tapping into the potential all people have to learn new behaviors, concepts, and ways of viewing things.

C. Communications Theory

The processes of communication within families are of great interest to family therapists. In many families with problems, communication is deficient in some way. It may be insufficient, unclear, indirect or contradictory, or the information communicated may be just incorrect. Also important is the process of communication between therapist and family. Much attention has therefore been given to communication theory by family therapists.

Therapists are concerned with *syntax,* the grammatical rules of a language; *semantics,* the meaning of words and how they are put together to convey meaning, including the clarity of language and how it is used in particular situations; and *pragmatics,* the study of the behavioral effects of communication. These latter effects are related as much to the nonverbal communications that go along with the words spoken, as to the words themselves. Indeed sometimes the nonverbal is the essence of the communication—a laugh, perhaps.

Many other aspects of communication have been studied by family therapists. Communications can define relationships; how we talk to our bosses may be very different than how we talk to our employees, our children, or our spouses. Also it is impossible, if one is in the presence of another person, not to communicate. Simply remaining silent, or looking away or busying oneself with someone or something else can carry powerful messages.

Family therapists are interested in whether communications between family members are *symmetrical* or *complementary*. In symmetrical communication the participants are on an equal footing. Complementary interaction occurs when the participants are not on an equal footing; examples would be many (but not necessarily all) doctor–patient, penitent–confessor, teacher–student, and master–servant interactions.

Two other types of communication merit mention here. One is the paradoxical statement. A simple example is the sentence, "I am lying." Another would be, "I will call you when you least expect me to." Related to this is the much written about "double-bind." This is a rather more sophisticated way of giving contradictory messages simultaneously. The double-bind occurs when there are two people in an intense relationship. Two injunctions are given that are incompatible, but the person concerned feels a strong need to obey them both. The subject cannot discuss the conflict (in other words metacommunication—that is, communication about the communication—is not possible), and cannot escape from the situation. Cinderella was placed in a double-bind when her stepmother told her that of course she could go to the ball at the palace, but she must finish the work allocated to her before she could get ready. This was impossible in the time available and only the intervention of her fairy godmother and the latter's magic spell enabled Cinderella to attend.

The double-bind has been frequently observed in the families of patients with schizophrenia, and in the early days of family therapy it was thought by some that it played a part in the causation of the condition. The idea was that, after repeated "double-bind" experiences over a long period of time, a person might be driven to forsake reality for a psychotic world. In due course, however, it was discovered that the double-bind was common in many other families and it is no longer generally considered to be an important etiological factor in schizophrenia. Much the same applies to the concept of "communication deviance," a form of aberrant communication described during the early studies of schizophrenic patients. More recently, evidence has emerged that "expressed emotion" is important. While a high level of expressed emotion in the family is not thought to be a *cause* of schizophrenia, it does seem that it may lead to relapse after treatment away from the family has been successful in producing a remission.

D. Family Structure

The concept of *family structure,* either overtly expressed or implied, is common to many schools of family therapy. It was well described by Salvador Minuchin in his 1974 book, *Families and Family Therapy.* It is related to systems theory concepts in that the perceived "structure" in a family system consists of the various subsystems in the family and the nature—that is strength and permeability—of the boundaries between them.

A typical, well-functioning family might have quite a simple structure: a parental subsystem and a child subsystem. In two-parent families some would distinguish the parent subsystem from the marital subsystem, since the way a couple relate as a marital pair is often distinct from how they function as parental couple. There might be expected to be a well-defined, but not overly rigid and impermeable boundary between the parental and the child subsystems. [*See* FAMILY SYSTEMS.]

The nature of the boundaries that exist between the subsystems in families is of great interest to the structural family therapist. Related to this are the concepts of *enmeshment* and *disengagement.* Enmeshment is said to exist when the boundaries between family members or subsystems are weak and readily permeable; it implies an overclose involvement of those concerned. When families members are enmeshed, their behaviors and, often, emotional states have marked effects on each other. In contrast to this, if members are disengaged, the behavior of one member will have little effect on those with whom the member is disengaged.

In a less well-functioning family one might find a different subsystem pattern. For example, there might be a subsystem consisting of the mother in an enmeshed relationship with one or two children, and another comprising the father. The boundary between the two subsystems might be robust, with little interaction or communication of feeling between them.

Many other family structures may be encountered; indeed the possibilities are limitless. In larger families there may be more than one child subsystem; for example, an older child subsystem and a younger child one, or male and female subsystems. And the structural problems may not be confined to the nuclear family. The extended family—grandparents, uncles, aunts, and other relatives—may be involved. So may friends, school staff and others, depending on the boundary between the family and its suprasystems.

E. Family Development

Families are not static entities. They change and develop. Among the considerations the therapist working with a family must take into account and is where the family is in its life cycle, for families have life cycles, just as individuals do. Moreover, many family problems prove to be associated with difficulties in proceeding from one stage of the life cycle to the next.

The family life cycle has been described and subdivided in a variety of ways. In summary, however, it is generally as follows. The starting point is arbitrary:

- The single adult person.
- Two single adults get together as a couple. Traditionally they get married, but in many societies nowadays a formal marriage ceremony is not required. This may be termed the childless couple stage.
- The couple have a child, often going on to have several more. We now have the couple with young children.
- The oldest child starts school. The family enters the stage of the couple with school-age children.
- The oldest child enters adolescence.
- The first child (it need not be the oldest) leaves home. This is the family launching its children into the wider world.
- The last child leaves home. This is the start of the "empty nest" stage.
- Retirement, aging, and grandparenthood.

The above is necessarily an oversimplification. Clearly, a family can be, and indeed will often be, in several stages at the same time. Some children may be in school while others have not started; some will have reached adolescence and others will not have. The parents may even have retired before all the children have left home. An additional complication is that many families do not follow the above course. We see, for example, family groups that have only contained one parent from the start; others disrupted by divorce or the death of one parent; blended families of various types; homosexual couples, with or without children; families in which it is the grandparents who are caring for the children.

What the family therapist must do, with every family that presents, is determine where the family is in its life cycle, and whether it is encountering any difficulty in moving from one stage to the next. It is often found that a family has functioned well at one stage, perhaps before the arrival of children, but does less well at the next, for example, when a third member, in that case a newborn child, is added. But any transition can present a challenge, as can single parenthood, blended family situations, and other special circumstances—for example, the incarceration of a family member.

The family therapist's work becomes even more complex when families have become split up because of separation or divorce, an increasingly common scenario in many contemporary societies. The children's time may be divided between the separated parents, whose conflicts and disagreements may persist despite the separation or divorce. Emotional problems, conflicts of loyalties, financial hardship and disputes, and custody and access issues may be sources of stress to all concerned. Often the children suffer most, and they sometimes come to play the role of pawns in ongoing "battles" between their parents. One or both parents may be in new relationships, which can complicate matters further. [See DIVORCE.]

In these situations the therapist may come to play the role of mediator, maintaining a neutral stance and being careful not to become overidentified with the point of view of any party. At the same time the well-being of all concerned, especially the children (who tend to be most at risk), must be the primary concern of the therapist. In these often unfortunate, even tragic, situations therapists may need to cast their nets wide and involve more than just the specific family grouping that has initially sought help—regardless of who is paying.

III. SCHOOLS OF FAMILY THERAPY

Many different approaches have been, and continue to be, used by therapists in their efforts to promote change in families. As the field developed, most of the pioneers became identified with particular methods, and so "schools" of family therapy came to be identified. Nevertheless, there was, from the start, much overlap between the methods of different therapists and schools. It can also be difficult to know how far the success of a particular approach is due, on the one hand, to the theoretical underpinnings and the methods used and, on the other hand, to the personality and charisma of the therapist. Many of the pioneers were powerful personalities, with well-developed interpersonal skills and great powers of persuasion. Even today, the ability of therapists to establish rapport with the families they treat, and to be convincing in the interventions they offer, is probably at least as important as their theoretical persuasion or the school of therapy to which they subscribe. Subject to the above provisos, here are brief descriptions of some of the main schools of family therapy.

A. Structural Family Therapy

We have seen how this approach looks at the subsystem pattern within the family and the nature and strength of the boundaries between the subsystems. Structural therapists first assess the existing family structure and how this may be related to the problems the family is experiencing; and then they set out to assist the family in making the changes that seem to be needed. The following are considered:

- The arrangements, or unwritten "rules," that govern the interactions between family members.
- The flexibility of the family's way of functioning, and how easily it can change.
- The family's "resonance." This is the extent to which family members are enmeshed or disengaged.
- The family's life context, that is, the relevant suprasystems.
- The family's developmental stage.
- How the symptoms of the family member(s) who are presented for treatment fit into the family's transactional patterns.

B. Approaches Using Communications Theory

Here the emphasis is on the patterns and styles of communication in the family. It was observed, from the earliest days of the family therapy movement, that families with symptomatic members often had major communication problems. These may involve:

- The cognitive understanding of what the members are saying to each other. What one member intends to convey to another is not correctly understood.
- The communication of feeling. It is often important, if a family is to function well without any members developing symptoms, for the members to be able to communicate effectively to each other how they feel.
- Communication and power. Jay Haley has eloquently pointed out that when one person communicates with another, that person is maneuvering to define a relationship. This probably does not apply to every communication. Some are simply intended to provide needed information, such as what time it is. Yet if one person has persistently to ask another one—the same other one—for the time this may say something about the relationship between the two.

Distinguishing one school of family therapy as particularly concerned with communication should not be taken to mean that therapists of other schools are not interested in family communication. It is merely a matter of emphasis. Indeed, Haley, who has been described as being of the "communication and power" school, also emphasizes the importance of establishing appropriate hierarchical arrangements within families—a concept that has much in common with structural therapy.

C. Behavioral Family Therapy

Therapists who take a behavioral approach lean heavily on learning theory. They understand the dysfunctional or deviant behaviors occurring in the families they treat as learned responses that can be replaced by more functional behaviors and ways of reacting by the use of behavioral techniques such as those outlined above. A prominent practitioner of and researcher in behavioral interventions with families is Gerald Patterson. Like most behaviorists he tends to be precise in his definition of problem behaviors, carrying out

a careful analysis of what is happening—especially what appears to be maintaining the undesired behaviors—before devising interventions in the family system designed to produce behavioral change. [*See* BEHAVIOR THERAPY.]

D. Extended Family Systems Therapy

The extended family systems approach is sometimes referred to as the "three generational approach." Therapists of this school pay particular attention to the extended families of their patients. They are impressed by the way behaviors and ways of relating seem to be handed down from one generation to the next. They emphasize the role of the families of origin of the family members in influencing current family functioning; and they play close attention to the ongoing relationships the families they treat have with their extended families. Many of their therapeutic interventions take into account, or actually involve, the extended family. [*See* EXTENDED FAMILY RELATIONSHIPS.]

Murray Bowen has often been included among the ranks of the "extended family systems" school, and rightly so, but his own theory differs from that of most others. He has maintained that many family problems arise because the family members have not differentiated themselves psychologically from their families of origin, a problem he saw himself having before he made a "voyage of discovery" to his family of origin. He also described the "undifferentiated ego mass," later preferring the term "nuclear family emotional system." A major aim of the therapist using Bowen's theory is to assist family members in differentiating themselves from the "undifferentiated ego mass." This, he asserts, enables them to function independently and autonomously, for example, as members of their own newly created families.

Whether there is a true *school* of extended family therapy may be questioned. Indeed it is probable that none of the schools we are discussing here exists in pure form. What we are describing are the points, the aspects of therapy, to which each school pays particular attention.

E. Experiential Family Therapy

Therapists who come under the "experiential" rubric tend to eschew theory. Instead, they join the family system and allow themselves to become involved in the intense interactions between the family members. Carl Whitaker and Walter Kempler are the best-known proponents of this approach. They do not offer us a consistent theory, but rather trust their instincts, or what Whitaker called, "The accumulated and organized residue of experience, plus the freedom to allow the relationship to happen, to be who you are with the minimum of anticipatory set and maximum responsiveness to authenticity and to our own growth impulses." This school of therapy is probably best experienced; if you cannot do that, the next best thing is to read the writings of Whitaker, Kempler, and their ilk.

F. Psychodynamic Family Therapy

In a sense, this is a contradiction in terms, since family therapy is concerned with family systems, and not primarily with the psychopathology of family members. But many of the figures who played major roles in the early development of family therapy came to it from a psychoanalytic background. As far as there is such a thing as psychodynamic family therapy, it seems to be therapy that aims to help family members gain insight into themselves and how they react with each other. [*See* PSYCHOANALYSIS.]

Psychoanalytic thinking informed the early work of Nathan Ackerman, as well as that of Virginia Satir. However, Satir was a therapist of many parts who seemed to draw her ideas from a wide variety of sources.

G. Strategic Family Therapy

The "strategic" school of therapy is less well defined than some of the other schools. Cloe Madanes, in her 1981 book, *Strategic Family Therapy,* suggested that it is the "responsibility of the therapist to plan a strategy to solve the client's problems." She saw strategic therapy stemming from the work of Milton Erickson, who often used indirect means of promoting change in his patients. These means are discussed below in the section "Indirect Interventions and Injunctions." A problem with the term "strategic therapy," however, is that presumably every effective therapist uses strategies of some sort in attempting to assist families make the changes they seek. It is thus somewhat imprecise.

This brief overview comes nowhere near to covering all the schools of, or approaches to, family therapy. It is presented to make the point that there are many possible approaches to the task of helping families change.

IV. ASSESSING FAMILIES

Regardless of their theoretical orientation, all therapists must first come to an understanding of the changes in the family system that need to be made to resolve the problems that therapy is to address. This involves some sort of assessment, although how detailed it is varies from therapist to therapist. The experiential therapists probably emphasize assessment least. Therapists of most other schools have systematic ways of assessing families along a variety of parameters. As an example, we will consider the Process Model of Family Functioning, which resembles and was in part derived from McMaster Model of Family Functioning. This considers six aspects of family functioning:

A. Task Accomplishment

Task accomplishment is similar to the "problem solving" of the McMaster model. It involves:

- Identifying the tasks to be accomplished;
- Exploring what approaches might be used and selecting one;
- Taking action;
- Observing the results of the action and making any necessary adjustments.

Both models consider three categories of tasks: *basic, developmental,* and *crisis.* Basic tasks are such things as the provision of food, clothing, and shelter. Developmental tasks are those required as the family moves from one developmental stage to the next. Crisis tasks are those presented by such events as the death or serious illness of a family member, job loss, natural disaster, or migration from one culture or another.

B. Role Performance

In a well-functioning family each member has a role, or habitual pattern of behavior. Together, these ensure that everything that needs to be done is done, and each family member's role is an appropriate one. In dysfunctional families it may be found that members, often those with symptoms, have assumed "idiosyncratic" roles, such as family scapegoat, "parental" child, sick member, or disturbed or "crazy" member.

C. Communication, Including Affective Expression

We have seen how important communication is in families, and what some of the main communication problems tend to be. In many families, problems in communication are among the main issues that need to be addressed in therapy.

D. Affective Involvement

This is the degree and quality of family members' interest in and concern for one another. The following types of involvement have been distinguished:

- Lack of involvement. The family members occupy the same house but behave rather like strangers.
- Interest or involvement devoid of feelings.
- Narcissistic involvement. In this case, one family member is involved with another to bolster his or own feelings of self-worth, not because of any real concern for the other person.
- Empathic involvement. Here there is real caring and concern for the needs of the other person. This results in responses which meet the needs of that person.
- Overinvolvement, or enmeshment. This was described above.

E. Control ("Behavior Control" in the McMaster model)

This is a measure of he influence the family members have on the behavior of other family members.

F. Values and Norms

This dimension appears only in the Process Model.

The above is but one of many schemata that are used by therapists of differing schools to understand the families that seek their help. It is quoted to give a flavor of the types of information that interest family therapists.

V. HELPING FAMILIES CHANGE

Promoting change is, of course, the essence of family therapy. To achieve this the therapist must have a coherent theory of change. This can be based on any of the theoretical schemes outlined above, or on others that exist. The therapist's theory of change is then the basis for the interventions he or she employs. The actual techniques used vary widely, but certain stages are required:

a. The establishment of rapport. As rapport develops, the participants become intensively involved with each other; trust also develops. The process has been given other names; some therapists refer to it as "joining" the family or "building working alliances." The process may occur quickly or it may take an entire session, even several. It involves both verbal and nonverbal techniques. Time spent establishing rapport is, however, seldom wasted. Lack of sufficient rapport is a major cause of failure in family therapy—and indeed in most endeavors that involve relationships with others.

b. Intervening in the family system. Having joined with the family, there are many ways the therapist may intervene in its transactional patterns. They may be divided into direct and indirect interventions.

A. Direct Interventions or Injunctions

Since family therapy aims to help families find new ways of functioning, a simple and straightforward approach is to offer the family suggestions, designed to help them make the changes that the assessment has shown to be needed in their way of functioning. The suggestions might be concerned with how family members could behave differently toward each other, or communicate more effectively, or alter their respective roles in the family—or whatever appears to be needed. They will also be related to the therapist's theory of change.

Direct injunctions should be more than the giving of common-sense advice, because they must be based on a careful assessment of the changes the family needs to make. Families presenting for therapy, while aware that they have problems, or that family members have symptoms, often do not know what changes are needed to achieve the objectives they desire. Indeed, when asked what they are seeking from therapy, many family members reply by saying that they want answers to "why" questions such as: "Why is my child stealing?" "Why won't my teenager daughter eat properly?" "Why have my husband and I drifted so far apart?"

"Why" questions are not unreasonable, but giving definitive answers to them is often difficult and frequently impossible. Who really knows the true motivation of anyone doing anything? It is generally better to focus on the changes that are desired by the participants, and how these may be achieved, than to spend time discussing the possible reasons why problems exist. The family members may be asked to describe, preferably in some detail, how things will be when treatment has come to a successful conclusion. (It is better to talk about *when*, not *if*, treatment has been successful; this is the process of "programming for success.") The desired state is sometimes referred to as the "outcome frame."

Once the outcome frame has been established the therapist, using the information that has been obtained during the assessment of the family, can then devise some interventions. Direct ones should probably be the first to be used, unless the history shows that they have been given a fair trial previously and have proved unsuccessful. Examples of direct interventions are:

• Rehearsing the family in communication techniques; these might aim to promote the direct, clear, and sufficient communication of information, opinions, and feelings between family members;
• Discussing the roles the various family members have been playing, and how these might be altered if it appears that alterations would be helpful;
• Proposing behavioral interventions to deal with undesired behaviors, or promote desired behaviors, on the part of the children;
• Suggesting, or modeling, more respectful ways for the family members to interact with each other;
• Helping family members to affirm and support each other, instead of the mutual criticism that is often encountered in families with problems.

Behavioral family therapy tends to use predominantly direct methods. The contingencies that appear to be controlling the behaviors that need to be changed are addressed directly.

Therapists of most schools are open to addressing dysfunctional patterns of interaction directly, and in some families this approach proves effective, especially when it is used in the context of a high degree of rapport. Unfortunately, especially in the more severely dysfunctional families, direct injunctions may be rejected or are not given an adequate trial even if lip service is paid to implementing them.

B. Indirect Interventions or Injunctions

The changes that may result from direct interventions, as outlined in the section above, tend to be what are often referred to as "first order change." This implies that although the behaviors of one or more family members have changed, there have not been the more fundamental changes in the family that may be needed and are implied by the term "second order change." Direct interventions may leave the functioning of the family system fundamentally unchanged, even though communication may be clearer, roles better defined, and so on.

The terms "strategic" and "systemic" are used for treatment approaches that aim to bring about more radical changes. These may involve alterations of perspective among the family members, so that some aspects of the way the family functions come to be viewed and understood in new ways. This is the process of "reframing"—the giving of different meaning to behavior, feelings or relationships. In "developmental reframing," for example, the antisocial behavior of an adolescent may be reframed as "immature," rather than "bad." "He's not really a bad kid, he's just having trouble growing up." Getting a family, including the young person who is displaying the troublesome behavior, to see the problem behaviors in this light represents second order change. The very process of developmental reframing may affect the young person's behavior. It may not be so acceptable to see oneself as immature, as opposed to being the strong, rebellious young person who does his or her own thing.

Many indirect interventions have been described. Here are brief descriptions of some of them:

• Reframing and positive connotation. Reframing— the giving of a different meaning to a behavior, or a pattern of behaviors—is the basic aim of most, if not all, indirect interventions. We have encountered one form—developmental reframing. Positive connotation is but a form of reframing, although it is an important one. For example, a parent's abusive behavior toward a child may be reframed (positively connoted) as a laudable attempt to correct the child's behavior. Therapy then can address the question of how the parent can develop better methods of achieving that goal. There are indeed few behaviors that cannot be positively connoted; what is required in doing so is the separation of the behavior from the motive behind it.

- Communication by metaphor. Metaphor is a long-established way of conveying messages indirectly and in a nonthreatening way. Situations may be reframed, new perspectives offered, and solutions to problems suggested without the issues being raised directly. Stories, anecdotes, other relationships, rituals, tasks, objects, and artistic productions may all carry meaning metaphorically.

- Paradoxical directives and related devices. When direct interventions have failed, it may be effective to suggest that, as "everything" has been tried, it may be better to leave things as they are. This effectively turns responsibility for change over to the family. Moreover, if they have, unconsciously, been trying to "defeat" the therapist, the only way they can now do so is by making the changes the therapist is advising against. Related to this are the declaring of therapeutic impotence and prescribing interminable therapy.

- Prescribing rituals and tasks. As we have seen, these may have metaphorical meaning, but they can also be used to interrupt repetitive, dysfunctional patterns of behavior. Examples are the "odd-days-even-days" routine, whereby parents take turns putting their children to bed; or the "same-sex parenting" plan, whereby the father is given responsibility for the boys in the family and the mother for the girls,

- Using humor. Helping family members to laugh at what they have been doing can, in the right situation, and in the context of profound *rapport,* be an effective change-promoting technique.

- Presenting alternative solutions or courses of action. This can be done by having the therapist admit to being uncertain about what is the best course of action and offering two or more; by having a "Greek chorus" observing though the one-way observation screen (a device widely used in family therapy) and sending in varying messages, or disagreeing with the therapist's ideas; or by staging a debate in the therapy room, the observers coming in to discuss possible solutions. Such strategies have several potential advantages. They make the point that there are choices to be made and that there is not necessarily only one possible solution to a problem; they invite families to take some responsibility for making changes; and they operate from the "one-down" position, that is, the therapist(s) are not presented as all-knowing experts seeking to impose their solutions on the family.

- Externalizing the problem. This is a process whereby a symptom is labeled or personified. "'Uncertainty' has taken over your life." "How can you win the battle with 'Mr. Anger'?" The family, or an individual, is then invited to consider ways of defeating or otherwise dealing with the externalized object.

The above are but examples of what are often called strategic therapy techniques. Others have been described and only the creativity of the therapist limits the possibilities. Such techniques are not used only in family therapy; they have application in individual therapy as well as in other fields of endeavor such as teaching and selling.

BIBLIOGRAPHY

Barker, P. (1992). *Basic family therapy* (3rd ed.). Oxford: Blackwell.

Barker, P. (1996). *Psychotherapeutic metaphors: A guide to theory and practice.* New York: Brunner/Mazel.

Duvall, E. M., & Miller, B. C. (1984). *Marriage and family development* (6th. ed.). New York: Harper & Row.

Epstein, N. B., Bishop, D. S., & Levin, S. (1978). The McMaster model of family functioning. *Journal of Marriage and Family Counselling, 4,* 19–31.

Imber-Black, E. (Ed.). (1993). *Secrets in families and family therapy.* New York: Norton.

Madanes, C. (1981). *Strategic family therapy.* San Francisco: Jossey-Bass.

Minuchin, S. (1974). *Families and family therapy.* Cambridge, MA: Harvard University Press.

Nichols, W. C. (1996). *Treating people in families: An integrative framework.* New York: Guilford.

Palazzoli, M. S., Boscolo, L., Cecchin, G., & Prata, G. (1978). *Paradox and counterparadox.* New York: Jason Aronson.

Steinhauer, P. D., Santa-Barbara, J., & Skinner, H. (1984). The process model of family functioning. *Canadian Journal of Psychiatry, 29,* 77–88.

Whitaker, C. A. (1976). The hindrance of theory in clinical work. In P. Guerin, (Ed.), *Family therapy: Theory and practice.* New York: Gardner.

Fathers

John Snarey

Emory University

Birth Fathers Men who are biologically generative through procreation and the initial care they provide for an infant.

Childrearing Fathers Men who are parentally generative through the care they provide to children and adolescents.

Father Involvement Level of a father's contribution to running a family, including involvement in childrearing and housework.

Generative Ethics An ethic of care; an ethical position that first considers effects on the next generation.

Generativity Psychologist Erik H. Erikson's term for the primary developmental task of the middle adulthood or seventh stage of the life cycle—caring for and contributing to the life of the next generation.

Generativity Chill The anxiety resulting from threats to an adult's generativity.

Negative Identity An imposed negative identification, which, in the context of fatherhood, presents fathers as absent, abusive, deadbeat, deficient, or unnecessary. Contrasts with a positive, generative identity.

Societal Fathers Men who are socioculturally generative by caring for the growth of younger adults or contributing to the well-being and continuity of the larger community.

Stages of Psychosocial Development Erik H. Erikson's life-span model of human development, which includes the following eight stages: (1) trust versus mistrust and (2) autonomy versus doubt, during the first 2 years of life; (3) initiative versus guilt, during early childhood; (4) industry versus inferiority, during later childhood; (5) identity versus identity confusion, during adolescence; and (6) intimacy versus isolation, during the early adult years; (7) generativity versus stagnation, during middle adulthood; and (8) the stage of integrity versus despair, during late adulthood.

FATHERS' contributions to their children's lives go well beyond that of traditional breadwinning. Today's couples, mental health workers, and social scientists are increasingly understanding that fathers are central, primary caregivers rather than secondary figures in childrearing or background variables in research. Most attempts to define the term *father* implicitly distinguish between (a) the biological progenitor of a child, (b) a male who performs the childrearing functions of a parent, and (c) a man who originates or takes responsibility for a larger social entity. Psychologist Erik H. Erikson's (1902–1994) concept of generativity—caring for and contributing to the life of the next generation—provides a developmental model that encompasses these three dimensions of fatherhood. Generativity provides the unifying theoretical framework for this article, just as it has begun to do for the field of fatherhood studies. Viewing fathers through the lens of generativity also helps delineate the practical contributions of fatherhood studies to mental health.

I. GENERATIVE FATHERING

Fathering is a primary psychosocial task of adulthood for most men. The concept of generative fathering brings psychological, sociological, and ethical perspectives to the experience of fathering.

A. Generativity and Care

According to Erikson, humans develop by journeying through a series of psychosocial tasks that intensify to a crisis or turning point in an ordered sequence of eight psychosocial stages across the life cycle (see Glossary). In middle adulthood, Stage 7, the challenge is to realize a favorable balance of generativity over stagnation or self-absorption. Generativity, broadly defined, includes any caring activity that promotes the development of others or otherwise contributes to the ongoing life of the generations.

The favorable resolution of each of the eight psychosocial tasks outlined by Erikson produces a particular personality strength or virtue. The successful realization of generativity gives rise to the ego strength of care—an inclusive concern for what love, necessity, and chance have generated. Generative care overcomes the ambivalence associated with irreversible obligations by being inclusively attentive to all that has been created. In contrast, the weakness that results from stagnation and self-absorption is rejectivity—an unwillingness to include particular persons or groups within the realm of one's generative care.

B. Three Types of Generative Fatherhood

Generativity is more complex and multifaceted than any other stage in the life cycle, in part because it spans more years than any of the other stages. Erikson, thus, implicitly distinguished among three types of generativity related to (1) biological procreation, (2) parenthood, and (3) societal productivity or creativity. Scholars of fatherhood have therefore distinguished between (a) birth fathers (biological generativity), (b) childrearing fathers (parental generativity),

and (c) societal fathers (sociocultural generativity). All three dimensions of fatherhood are interconnected because each potentially contributes to and renews the ongoing cycle of family life across generations. The work of fathers, therefore, is intertwined with the lives of others: the fathers' own fathers, their mothers and wives, daughters and sons, and others beyond the family sphere. These relations explain why there is an integral link between parenting and family mental health.

II. BIRTH FATHERHOOD

In early adulthood most men experience the first type of paternal generativity—becoming a birth father. More than 90% of all adult males in the United States eventually marry, and more than 90% of these married couples eventually have one or more children.

A. Becoming a Father

Birth fatherhood links intimacy, Erikson's sixth stage, to parental generativity. Becoming a father often makes a man intensely aware of the continuity of generations. Biological generativity calls upon a man and his partner to energetically expand their mutual interest to care for that which they have generated together. Becoming a parent may be the most complex and significant psychosocial milestone in the life of an adult. [*See* PARENTING.]

Biological generativity, according to John Kotre, also involves caring for an infant through its first year of life. An infant's physical viability is its parents' primary concern during the early months of the infant's life and, thus, biological generativity is incomplete without the initial care necessary to ensure the child's biological survival. Appropriate nurturing supports the infant's ability to develop a favorable ratio of trust over mistrust (Erikson's Stage 1).

B. Coping with New Fatherhood

Most new fathers, like mothers, typically feel a sense of achievement in biologically linking the generations. Most infants also captivate and engross their fathers, just as they do their mothers. The typical immediacy of a father's feelings suggests that he had become bonded with his child before its physical arrival. During the 21-month transition to becoming a father—the combined periods of expectant fatherhood (their wife's pregnancy) and new fatherhood (their child's first year of life)—many men also feel that they become more of an adult and more connected to their own fathers.

The afterbirth of fatherhood includes several initial stresses. Martin Greenberg and others have observed that new fathers experience an increased sense of economic responsibility and personal accountability. Stress is also associated with the realization that one must now care for a generation whom one cannot expect to outlive. New fathers today also may wonder about their adequacy to be fathers, given society's heightened expectations of men in dual-career families. In reaction to these and other stressors, couples sometimes experience an initial decline in marital happiness. Alan Hawkins and David Dollahite note that a new father must create a balanced identity between two extreme social expectations: the view that fathers are deficient or unnecessary, which leads to an imposed negative identity, and the exaggerated expectation of being a perfect father. This dilemma apparently prompts some new fathers to reflect on the meaning of life, which may be why many new parents show a renewed interest in spirituality and membership in a religious congregation. [*See* STRESS.]

Jay Belsky suggested that new fathers be informed of the everyday physical, psychological, and social strains of becoming a father and caring for an infant. By understanding that they can expect some difficulties, new fathers can anticipate and minimize stress. Perhaps mercifully, the sharp edges of these initial stressors are forgotten as the children grow. A related stress that is typically never forgotten by men who have experienced it, however, is the unexpected fear of possibly never having the experience of caring for a child.

C. Generativity Chill

With notable exceptions, most couples are better able to produce biological children in the period from the late teens to the early thirties. This biological foundation places time limits on biological procreation and promotes social expectations for having children "on schedule." The opposite of biological generativity is infertility. The current national primary infertility rate is 15% among all couples of childbearing age. This percentage has remained remarkably constant across historical and social contexts.

The experience of infertility may be the first time a man encounters generativity chill—an Eriksonian term coined by John Snarey to refer to the anxious awareness of the self as finite, arising from the threatened loss of one's child or potential child. Publications by Ross Parke, Alan Hawkins, and David Dollahite also suggest that the experience of generativity chill may be associated with late-time fatherhood and single fatherhood. Infertility is, therefore, a specific instance of biological generativity chill. It directly threatens a man's biological generativity, indirectly threatens his parental generativity, and can weaken his preparation for societal fatherhood or sociocultural generativity. [*See* INFERTILITY.]

Although it is often assumed that women experience a higher level of psychosocial stress associated with infertility than men, research suggests that this is inaccurate. Men may be more likely to minimize the personal impact of infertility because of social expectations. Close examination of men's psychological reaction to thwarted procreation often reveals experiences of high levels of anxiety, awareness of substantial loss (loss of status or prestige, loss of self-confidence, loss of hope), and depression. A husband may further feel guilty for depriving his wife of a child or feel resentful of his wife for depriving him of a child. Fortunately, 50% of infertile couples eventually achieve a pregnancy and, with the added option of adoption, the great majority of husbands and wives become childrearing parents.

III. CHILDREARING FATHERHOOD

Childrearing fathers exhibit their parental generativity by caring for their children's needs and supporting their children's physical, social-emotional, and intellectual development. Fathers vary considerably, however, in the manner and quantity of care they provide their children. A number of different approaches have been used to assess these variations.

A. Availability and Responsibility

The earliest and simplest approach used to study fathers is to classify them as absent or present. The results of this extensive line of research are usually interpreted as showing that fathers' absence predicts children's antisocial behavior, cognitive immaturity, poor academic achievement, sex-identity conflict, and low self-esteem. These findings are complex, however, and should be interpreted cautiously. Recent research on the consequences of a father's absence, for instance, has also shown that social support systems can moderate the impact of father absence. Furthermore, of course, father-absence research generally tells us little about the varieties of important ways fathers are present with their children. [See SOCIAL SUPPORT.]

Another group of studies has focused on how many hours a week fathers contribute to the total time couples devote to running a family, including both childcare and housework. National time-use data from the 1960s showed that fathers generally contributed about one-fifth of the total hours. This large difference reflected the allocation of time in the daily schedules of full-time housewives versus "breadwinning" fathers. National time-use data from the mid-1980s showed that men's average share rose to one-third of the total. During the current decade this time differential between fathers' and mothers' childcare is being further reduced although, as Rasmussen and colleagues have noted, men's responsibility for housework has not increased substantially.

Researchers have also asked how often fathers assume full responsibility for their children. Having the sole responsibility for a child's care during some portion of a day is far more demanding than sharing or being available to help with childcare. A caretaker with full responsibility, for instance, must be cognizant of all aspects of a child's needs and development—physical, intellectual, and emotional. The amount of time that fathers' have full responsibility for childcare is notably lower than mothers' but, again, the time differential is decreasing. One study from the early 1970s, for instance, estimated that fathers spent an average of only 1 hour per week taking sole responsibility, compared with mothers who reported that they had the sole responsibility an average of 40 hours per week. A 1987 U.S. Census Bureau survey, in contrast, showed that fathers in two-parent families were providing the primary care for 25% of preschool-age children and 11% of school-age children whose mothers work part time. Gallup Polls of both mothers and fathers conducted during the 1990s have shown that fathers are also increasingly assuming full responsi-

bility for childcare when their children are sick and home from school. Joseph Pleck and Michael Lamb, who have conducted the most detailed reviews of paternal involvement surveys to date, conclude that there have been clear increases in men's assumption of responsibility for childcare over the past three decades even though fathers still have a long way to go before they achieve parity with mothers.

B. Time Spent in Specific Childcare Tasks

The amount of time fathers typically spend in specific childcare tasks varies according to particular criteria and historical periods. Three decades ago, most reports estimated that fathers typically spent about 2 hours per week on childcare tasks (e.g., feeding, changing clothing). In contrast, more recent estimates that are also based on somewhat more diverse childcare activities (feeding, bathing, reading to, taking on trips) report that fathers average close to 2 hours of childcare per day rather than the similar figure noted above per week. Overall, comparisons of national surveys conducted between the mid-1960s and the early 1990s in the United States indicate that the time fathers spend in specific childcare tasks is gradually, but steadily, increasing.

An especially interesting version of the specific-task approach has been to ask how much time fathers spend playing with their children. This activity was, for some time, overlooked or mistakenly distinguished from childcare because much research on parenting focused on mothers. This limitation predisposed many researchers to discount the importance of the time men spend in play or athletic activities with their children, even though fathers invest the greatest proportion of the time they spend with their children in such activities. This line of research, which began with the fathers of infants, has shown that paternal care differs from maternal care: it consists of more limb movement, active arousal, initiative, and is generally more rough-and-tumble. Mothers' play, in contrast, involves more visual attention and perhaps more verbal interaction. Fathers do not restrict their preferences for stimulating and exciting physical-athletic childcare activities to young infants. Fathers of school children often participate in organized activities beyond the family sphere, such as Little League and scouting, that are also physically oriented. Fathers also use more verbal joking and rough physical play in their interactions with their older children. Similarly, fathers of adolescents spend more of the time they are with their children in activities that promote assertiveness rather than politeness. From birth through adolescence, a working-hard-at-playing quality tends to distinguish paternal from maternal childcare.

C. Generative Childcare

Global measures of time spent in childcare, while helpful, are not fully adequate because they can mask important differences between various types of childrearing involvement and usually lack a developmental perspective. This makes it difficult to consider that different types of fathers' childcare might vary in their relevance to different aspects of children's development during different age periods. Approaching men's parental generativity in developmentally sensitive ways also can increase our ability to understand fathers, including the origins and impact of variations in fathers' childcare practices.

A generative childcare approach was used by Snarey to analyze the childrearing careers of 240 fathers in the Glueck Longitudinal Sample, a study of working- and middle-class men who were born in Boston, Massachusetts, during the 1920s and 1930s. The concept of parental generativity was measured by examining all instances of constructive care for a child's personal course of development that were recorded in the interviews with the men that took place over four decades. Each instance of each man's actual childrearing activities was classified according to three areas of child development and two eras of childrearing. This method thus assessed six types of paternal support:

(1) social–emotional development in childhood;
(2) intellectual–academic development in childhood;
(3) physical–athletic development in childhood;
(4) social–emotional development in adolescence;
(5) intellectual–academic development in adolescence;
(6) physical–athletic development in adolescence.

The study found that many fathers promoted their children's maturity in the following ways:

• Social–emotional development was often supported through father–child companion activities. One father, for instance, took his son to the ocean shoreline to take a quiet walk up the beach and talk with him about his girlfriend problems. Another father, who had taken his daughter to a baseball game, took advantage of a quiet inning to talk about her concerns.

• Intellectual–academic competence was often promoted through intellectual-skill lessons and cognitive activities. One father, for instance, taught his son to identify star constellations and bird species. Another father taught his daughter how to calculate baseball statistics.

• Physical–athletic development was often supported through action-skill lessons and medical care activities. When one father challenged his son to a 50-yard dash and another father taught his daughter how to pitch horseshoes, they cared for their children's physical-athletic competence.

Among the men in the Glueck Longitudinal Sample, fathers who gave especially strong childrearing support in one area during childhood were not necessarily more inclined to offer support in other areas during childhood. But if a father had actively supported a particular area in the childhood decade, he tended to actively support that same area in the adolescent decade as well, suggesting some stability in childrearing style. During adolescence, however, fathers who were highly active in one area of childrearing during the adolescent decade tended to be notably active in the two other areas as well, suggesting that fathers may pursue an integrated approach to promoting their children's adolescent development. Overall, combining all three types of care, 24% of the fathers were very highly involved in childcare, 40% were significantly involved in childcare, and 36% were generally uninvolved in childcare. In other words, two out of three fathers were clearly involved in the actual day-to-day activities of rearing their children.

IV. PRECURSORS OF FATHERS' CHILDREARING

Research has revealed many boyhood precursors of men's active, positive involvement in childcare. By far the best predictor of adulthood parental generativity is the fathering that men themselves received in their family of origin. Scholars have offered two primary hypotheses to explain the intergenerational reproduction of good fathering: (a) modeling, in which a man replicates the strengths of the fathering he received, and (b) reworking, in which a man rectifies the limitations of the fathering he received.

A. Research on Modeling

The modeling hypothesis claims that fathers who are accessible, nurturing, and authoritative will serve as the most influential models for their sons. These sons, by a process of identifying with or modeling themselves after their fathers, will replicate the fathering they received as they raise their own children.

Empirical evidence in support of the modeling hypothesis comes from several studies that report that men who, as boys, experienced high levels of involvement with their fathers were significantly more likely to become highly involved with their own children. Henry Biller and others, for instance, have observed that fathers who provided nurturing, encouraging, attentive behavior toward their children served as a model for their sons who, in turn, were significantly more likely to identify with the male parenting role (e.g., to assume the role of the father doll in a doll-play activity and to score high on measures of masculinity).

The link between boyhood and adulthood was more directly addressed by the Berkeley Longitudinal Study. Boys who became the most well-adjusted men were significantly more likely to have had fathers who had shared responsibility for, and been highly involved in, their childrearing. Findings from the 4-decade Glueck Longitudinal Study also suggested that the boys in the study, as adults, built upon or employed their own fathers' strengths:

- Boys whose fathers had been relatively better educated tended as adults to provide significantly more support for their own children's social-emotional development in childhood.
- Boys whose fathers had been employed in relatively better or more complex blue-collar jobs tended as adults to provide significantly more support for their own children's social-emotional development in adolescence.
- Boys who grew up in a home where their father and mother worked together well to provide their children with a cohesive home atmosphere tended as fathers themselves to provide significantly more care and support for their own children's social-emotional development in adolescence. This pattern reminds us that a genuinely cohesive home

requires the active cooperation of both parents and, as Bill Peterson and Eva Klohnen have documented, generative women also are invested in the parenting process and provide models for boys' future behavior.

B. Research on Reworking

The reworking hypothesis, in contrast, claims that some sons of comparatively distant, nonnurturant, or powerless fathers will make extra efforts to be good fathers themselves in order to redress their fathers' shortcomings and to provide their own children with better fathering.

A considerable body of evidence supports this hypothesis. Several reviews of fatherhood studies have all concluded that men who experienced unsatisfyingly low levels of paternal involvement as boys were likely to adapt to, or compensate for, their negative role model by choosing to spend more time with their children. The ability of men to compensate for poor fathering is also consistent with Kohlberg and colleagues' review of longitudinal studies that showed that the long-term effects of boyhood emotional problems upon subsequent adult adjustment are usually slight.

The 4-decade Glueck Longitudinal Study of how fathers care provided three specific examples of how men rework and counterbalance their own fathers' shortcomings:

- Men whose relationships with their fathers had been distant or nonnurturant tended as adults to provide significantly above-average levels of care for their adolescent children's social–emotional development.
- Men whose fathers had inconsistently or inadequately supervised their physical well-being tended to provide significantly higher levels of support for their children's physical–athletic development in childhood.
- Men whose fathers had used physical punishment or threats of physical punishment, which instilled fear in them as boys, tended to provide significantly higher levels of positive care for their children's physical–athletic development in childhood.

Overall, the research suggests that the fathering men receive as boys does not necessarily place a straightjacket on their ability to be good fathers with their own children.

C. Beyond Modeling versus Reworking

It is often assumed that the modeling and reworking hypotheses are mutually exclusive, but the research may be more reasonably interpreted as showing that fathers' childcare may function as a positive model to be emulated and as a negative example to be learned from and reworked. Erik Erikson's case studies of adult development anticipated this perspective by showing the importance of positive social models in the development of psychosocial generativity and revealing the individual's power to transform prior negative experiences by a process of generative growth. All fathers, no doubt, provide their children with some mixture of experiences to be replicated and difficulties to be reworked.

These findings have practical implications. Men would do well to consciously observe the joint processes of modeling and reworking. When a childrearing situation or dilemma triggers a positive memory of one's own father, it is usually a good idea to try modeling one's own childcare after that of one's father, but when a childrearing situation triggers a negative childhood memory, it is important to seize the opportunity to rework one's own father's example and find a better way to handle the situation.

V. CONDITIONS OF FATHERS' CHILDREARING

The second broad category of paternal childcare predictors includes the current conditions or contemporary characteristics of men's wives, children, and themselves.

A. Wives' Characteristics

Wives' employment, educational level, and attitudes toward the father role are important factors in predicting fathers' total quantity of general parental generativity.

Mother's employment outside the home is one of the strongest predictors of her husband's heightened level of overall childcare. Wives increased breadwinning responsibility, that is, predicts increased childrearing responsibility by husbands. At all ages, including adolescence, children spend more time alone with their fathers when their mothers work outside the home. Ann Crouter and her colleagues, for instance,

have shown that the amount of time that fathers have the sole responsibility for children in dual-earner families is more than double that found in single-earner families. Fathers' childcare time is especially likely to increase when their wives work part time rather than full time because couples are more able to use a shift-work system when mothers work part time, but they often need a more highly structured system of outside care when mother and father both work full time.

The Glueck Longitudinal Study confirmed that wives' employment provides an immediate motivation for fathers to increase their level of childcare but the study also revealed that, once this is set in motion, the fathers' boyhood relationship with their own fathers still best predicts the specific areas of their children's development on which they will focus. This may be possible because, compared with mothers, fathers experience more cultural freedom regarding how they fulfill their role.

Education is also important. The Glueck Longitudinal Study showed that wives' educational level helped predict the fathers' total quantity of childcare beyond that accounted for by wives' employment. Fathers who were highly involved in childrearing were more likely to have wives with relatively *more* years of education than wives of less-involved fathers. Fathers with *less* educated mothers were also more likely to be involved in childrearing.

Attitudes of wives also help to predict their husbands' fathering behavior. A study by Rand Conger and colleagues showed that fathers were more likely to engage in constructive parenting when they and their wives believed that fathers' involvement would benefit their children's developing maturity. Research on dual-earner families has shown that, when a wife's attitude is liberal, her husband is more involved in parenting but, when her attitude is traditional, her husband does less. Husbands also participated more in childcare when their wives' fathers had been positively, but not highly, available; this may reflect a wife's desire to establish a less frustrating father experience for her children.

B. Children's Characteristics

The children's demographic characteristics represent another set of concurrent predictors considered in prior research. Below we will summarize the findings regarding age, gender, and generativity chill.

Age of children also helps to predict men's childcare because effective fathering, in part, is an interactional process of adjusting to children's different levels of competence and experience. During infancy, for instance, father–infant interaction is between two people of drastically disparate amount of experience and capabilities. As this balance gradually shifts during childhood and adolescence, fathers must reorient their fathering behavior accordingly.

The most frequent cross-sectional research finding regarding age is that men usually spend more time with younger children. When one examines different types of paternal generativity longitudinally, however, the findings become more complex. Among the fathers in the Glueck Longitudinal Study, the age of their children predicted their overall level of childcare, including the degree to which they cared for their children's social–emotional, intellectual–academic, or physical–athletic development. On average, fathers provided more childcare during the childhood decade than during the adolescent decade. During both decades, fathers supported their children's social–emotional development more than other types of childcare. They encouraged physical–athletic development in childhood, but this support declined in adolescence. In contrast, fathers' support for intellectual–academic development (the least frequent type of care provided in childhood) increased during adolescence. Interestingly, fathers who were highly supportive of their offspring's physical–athletic development in childhood tended to shift gears and encourage intellectual–academic development during adolescence. This suggests that fathers invest in different areas of development according to their awareness of their children's changing capacities and developmental tasks.

The gender of a child has been extensively investigated as a predictor of fathers' childrearing work, but the results are inconsistent. The age of the children involved in these investigations, Snarey has shown, partially explains the different findings. Studies of fathers of infants often indicate that fathers show more interest in sons than in daughters but, in contrast, studies of fathers of children and adolescents report few significant associations between fathers' childrearing and children's gender. Other background and cultural variables also have been found to moderate the impact of children's gender on fathers' childcare. Research by Crouter and colleagues, for instance, has suggested that fathers in single-breadwinner families spend more time in one-on-one activities with their sons than with their daughters, but that fathers in two-breadwinner families spend equivalent amounts of time with their sons and daughters.

Generativity chill, as discussed earlier, refers to the anxiety resulting from threats to an adult's generativity. Men most typically experience generativity chill when their child suffers a significant illness. Other forms of a potential loss of attachment to one's child, such as a custody suit, may possibly function in an equivalent manner. Generativity chill was investigated in the Glueck Longitudinal Study. The results showed that generativity chill significantly increased the total quantity of a father's childrearing activity. Generativity chill also predicted that fathers will provide high levels in three specific areas: physical–athletic support during both the childhood and the adolescent decades, social–emotional support during adolescence, and intellectual–academic support during adolescence. Fathers who experienced generativity chill commented that it taught them that children should never be taken for granted and that fatherhood should never take a permanent back seat to careers.

Underneath these specific findings, the generative encounters between father and child vividly illustrated the synchronization of life cycles. Children provided opportunities for fathers to exercise their own developmental need to be generative and, through their generativity, fathers promoted their child's development.

C. Fathers' Personal Characteristics

Many of men's personal characteristics and circumstances are associated with their level of childcare. Intelligence, employment status, and marital affinity are discussed below.

Intelligence, as indicated by IQ scores, has been shown to be higher among childrearing fathers. Intelligence predicts higher levels of both general childcare and specific care for children's intellectual-academic development. It is noteworthy that these involved fathers, as previously noted, also tended to be married to wives with higher than average levels of education, although their mothers had relatively low levels of education. This pattern suggests that men who are academically capable tend to compensate for their mothers' lack of education by marrying women with more education and then supporting the development of their children's academic abilities.

Employment status and work conditions have a major influence on fathering behavior. The detrimental impact of unemployment has been extensively documented by Glen Elder, Rand Conger, and their colleagues. Unemployment and the associated financial strain and loss of work status predict that fathers will experience marital tension, a deterioration of their relationship with their children, and a loss of influence over their children. Father–child relations are strained because unemployed fathers become less patient, more irritable, more controlling, and because their sons and daughters have to restrict their aspirations due to diminished financial resources. These combined stresses, in turn, often predict that their children will develop behavior and emotional problems, including depression, hostility, and aggression. [See UNEMPLOYMENT AND MENTAL HEALTH.]

Even gainfully employed fathers, of course, experience some degree of tension between childrearing and breadwinning obligations. This tension has produced the expectation of mutually negative tradeoffs between men's work and family life. Some cross-sectional studies do report negative correlations between measures of socioeconomic success and childcare involvement. Long-term studies, however, have shown that childrearing and occupational success are positively and reciprocally related over time, although these relations are not usually strong. Just as unemployment negatively influences father–child relations, for instance, occupational mobility may positively influence father–child relations, in part, because it increases economic security and provides greater self-esteem to counterbalance possible increases in stress. The 4-decade Glueck Longitudinal Study, for instance, showed that being highly involved or active fathers did not harm the men's long-term work success. By midlife, the men who gave priority to childrearing were actually somewhat more upwardly mobile in their occupations compared with men who had only focused on their work.

Marital affinity is another important concurrent predictor. It refers to a husband's ability to remain clearly committed to his wife despite the inevitable ups and downs in any family. Numerous studies have found that the quality of the marital relationship is a strong and consistently significant concurrent predictor of fathers' parental generativity. Among fathers of preschool children, for instance, the esteem their wives' held for them as husbands and the praise the men gave to their children are correlated. Among fathers of older children and adolescents, high levels of husband–wife conflict are associated with the use of punishment rather than reasoning as a disciplinary style. In a short-term longitudinal study of couples, Belsky and colleagues assessed marital affinity (defined as a low level of divorce contemplation) at four points during the first child's first 3 years of life. Husbands whose commitment to their wives decreased and misgivings about the durability of their marriage increased, interacted with their children in more negative and intrusive styles than did other fathers. In contrast, husbands whose marital relationship showed no such declines were significantly more likely to communicate positive emotions toward their sons and daughters and to interact with them in a responsive, encouraging style. In other research, marital affinity has also been found to predict fathers' care for their children's social-emotional development during both the childhood and adolescent childrearing decades, and to predict the total quantity of men's parental generativity.

Although the findings show that highly involved fathers are more likely to be men with strong marital affinity, a complicating factor is the likely possibility that marital affinity and fathering behavior are reciprocally related across the adult years. Improved parental practices and father–child relations could promote an improved marital relationship, just as improved husband–wife relations could also improve father–child relations. Nevertheless, the quality of the marital relationship is still probably a crucial, positive influence on the way that fathers parent because the marital relationship functions as the primary social support system available to the fathers and, as such, it exerts a direct influence upon fathers' parental generativity. [See MARITAL HEALTH.]

VI. CONSEQUENCES OF FATHERS' CHILDREARING

The quality of care fathers provide their children has consequences for their daughters' and sons' life outcomes. Paternal childcare usually predicts more of the variance in children's behavior than maternal childcare because fathers display greater individual variation in their childcare than do mothers. What is most noteworthy is that some types of paternal childcare

are of much greater benefit to daughters while other types are of more benefit to sons. This section will summarize research findings on the impact of fathers' childcare provided during the childhood and adolescent childrearing decades on the subsequent educational and occupational success of their daughters and sons by early adulthood.

A. Raising Daughters for Success

The importance of fathers' support of their daughters' physical–athletic development during childhood is an emerging theme in recent research. Biller and colleagues suggest that fathers make an important contribution to promoting their children's physical fitness and athletic abilities and that, in turn, fathers who encourage their daughters to participate in athletics help alleviate sex bias and promote sex role flexibility. Research by Parke and others supports this idea; they found that daughters exposed to higher levels of paternal physical play were more popular and assertive with their peers. Others have theorized that rough-and-tumble, challenging paternal behavior may promote the development of social independence in girls and make it less likely that they will passively accept their environment.

The Glueck Longitudinal Study found that daughters whose fathers promoted their physical-athletic competence during childhood were, as young adults, the most educationally successful. These daughters appeared to have experienced their fathers as challenging and as affirming of their ability to function autonomously and vigorously. In contrast, the consequences of fathers' social–emotional nurturance during the childhood decade are less clear. Norma Radin has suggested that unusually high levels of fathers' nurturing behavior during their daughters' childhood years may inhibit their daughter's cognitive development and sex-role flexibility. Retrospective studies of childhood have also reported that high achieving college women recalled that their fathers were challenging, but not smothering or overpowering, during childhood. Longitudinal evidence comes from the Glueck Longitudinal Study, which revealed that daughters' educational mobility was negatively predicted by only one type of paternal care: high levels of childhood support for social-emotional development. Girls who received high levels of support for social-emotional development from their fathers during their first decade

of life, that is, attained relatively lower levels of education in early adulthood than those who did not receive such support.

The father–daughter relationship is also very important during adolescence. The early father-absent research, for instance, showed that the apparent negative effects of father absence on daughters (e.g., difficulty maintaining relationships; low self-esteem; delinquency) did not become marked until girls reached adolescence. In contrast, retrospective studies of unusually competent women (e.g., doctoral students, managers, leaders) report that they often recalled their fathers as men who involved themselves in joint endeavors with their adolescent daughters. The fathers' styles were often recalled as active and encouraging, playful and exciting, but may also include a significant degree of father–daughter conflict. In addition, short-term longitudinal studies of adolescents have found that a strong father–daughter relationship that took place within the family context of a strong marital and parenting relationship predicted daughters' later academic and career success.

Douglas Heath's study of the wives of the men in the Haverford Longitudinal Study found that the women who succeeded in their work recalled their fathers as being steady, but not tender, in their social–emotional style. These same successful women also recalled fathers who prized their daughters' intellectual growth and actively urged their academic achievement. Heath also reported that fathers who urged daughters to participate in athletics significantly contributed to their daughters' subsequent adult success.

Daughters of the men in the Glueck Longitudinal Study who had experienced a high level of one-to-one involvement with their fathers during the adolescent decade, especially physical–athletic and social-emotional support, were significantly more upwardly mobile in educational and occupational levels by early adulthood. The ability of fathers' physical–athletic care to predict daughters who will go on to become high achievers suggests that their fathers contributed to their ability to compete with men beyond the family sphere. The importance of physical–athletic care during both decades again suggests that the nature of the father–daughter friendship was more vigorously challenging, affirming the daughters' ability to function autonomously and to transcend culturally determined gender roles. Girls raised by traditional fathers, in contrast, may remain at a competitive disadvantage.

B. Raising Sons for Success

Several cross-sectional and correlational studies of fathers' childrearing practices and sons' personal characteristics found that fathers' social–emotional nurturance positively predicts boys' academic skills, school grades, level of cognitive development, IQ scores, and other standardized test scores. Fathers' marital affinity has also been shown to be correlated with boys' intellectual functioning. In contrast, fathers' restrictiveness is negatively associated with these outcomes.

Heath's Haverford Longitudinal Study found that the men who had succeeded in their work during early adulthood or who were the most mentally healthy were also significantly more likely than the other men in the study to have recalled their boyhood fathers as men who were available, accessible, affectionate; helped them with their homework; and encouraged their physical–athletic growth. For the sons of the men in the Glueck Longitudinal Study, educational mobility was significantly forecasted by their fathers' care for their childhood intellectual–academic development and social–emotional development. Their occupational mobility was predicted by their fathers' care for their physical-athletic development. Thus, all three types of fathers' care during the childhood decade made a significant contribution to some form of their sons' social mobility.

The types of fathering that promote maturity in adolescent sons are also different from the fathering that promotes maturity among adolescent daughters. Cross-sectional and retrospective evidence show that fathers' involvement with their adolescent sons is positively associated with adulthood work success or occupational competency. One of the few longitudinal studies has been reported by Bell, who recorded the degree to which fathers, other adults, and siblings served as role models for boys when they were freshmen in high school and again when they had been out of high school for 7 years. At the latter time, Bell also measured six aspects of their vocational adjustments and behavior. Of all the occupational role models that subjects reported at the first period, only fathers' role-modeling was associated with their sons' vocational behavior a decade later. Fathers who were the most positive role models were more likely to have sons who attained their occupational goals and showed clear job satisfaction. Interestingly, fathers had ceased

to be the most important role models for these subjects during early adulthood. They were replaced by teachers, employers, other adults, and peers.

Among the fathers of adolescent sons in the Glueck Longitudinal Study, fathers who stayed involved with their son's intellectual growth significantly contributed to their sons' mobility. The care that fathers provided for their sons' social–emotional and physical–athletic development during adolescence, while positive, did not make a measurable contribution to their educational or occupational mobility.

C. Interpretations and Recommendations

These findings fit well with Eriksonian theory and suggest why highly generative fathers appear to engage their sons and daughters differently during the childhood and adolescent decades.

During childhood, both sons and daughters need their fathers to help them negotiate the first four of Erikson's psychosocial tasks. But the types of fathering that promote sons' and daughters' growth are not always identical. For boys, the early portion of the childhood decade requires them to separate from the mother and identify with the father, the same-sex parent, as part of the boy's gender identity development. Fathers' warm, close, guiding support of their sons' physical–athletic, intellectual, and social–emotional development promotes this transition. In contrast, daughters' primary identification remained with their mother. Fathers' friendly, but not overly warm or tender, childcare is an important support that does not draw them away from their primary identification. Fathers' exciting and rigorous physical–athletic interaction also appears to help their daughters to avoid an extremely traditional sex-role identification.

During adolescence, both sons and daughters are striving to establish their independence and distinctive identities. The type of fathering that will help adolescents fulfill these tasks again differs for sons and daughters. For adolescent sons, their psychosocial task includes achieving a significant degree of separation from their fathers. Their fathers' support from the sidelines, for instance, promotes their ability to achieve such a significant degree of separation from them while also providing them with an ongoing bridge back to the family. Thus, it is not surprising that fathering during adolescence has a weaker impact on sons. For adolescent daughters, in contrast, fathers' active, energetic involvement can promote their ability to achieve a significant degree of separation from their mothers. During a child's adolescence, a father's care can support his daughter in establishing an autonomous identity and providing her with opportunities for constructive, assertive interactions with males.

Fathers who continuously support their children's physical, emotional, and intellectual development (free of smothering involvement), help them to become capable, effective, well-rounded adults. Fathers need to understand, therefore, that almost any activity their children enjoy can be turned into an opportunity to promote their offspring's social, intellectual, and athletic maturity.

VII. SOCIETAL FATHERHOOD

By the time fathers reach midlife, most will have contributed to their children's care for more than 2 decades. Parenthood may function as a catalyst and model for generative care beyond the family sphere.

A. Societal Generativity

During intensive parenting, fathers develop important competencies for care. And, while parenting continues in some sense throughout the adult life cycle, young adult children are usually eventually launched from the nest. Concurrently, the larger society needs mature adults who are prepared to help establish the next generation of adults and ideas. Erikson suggested that realizing societal generativity may be easier for adults who have had the prior experience of parenting children. He was careful to acknowledge in a discussion of parenting, however, that there are people who, for a variety of reasons, channel their generativity through other benevolent concerns than parenting children. Parental generativity promotes societal generativity but living without children may not necessarily prevent societal generativity.

Societal generativity principally involves caring for other younger adults by serving as a mentor, providing leadership, and generally contributing to the strength and continuity of subsequent generations. Midlife men who are societally generative take on a sustained responsibility for the growth, well-being, and leadership of other adults (e.g., serving as a master in a master–apprentice work role, a labor union

leader, an athletic coach, a school board member, or an administrator at work). Societal generativity, therefore, is more broadly socially inclusive than the other types of generativity. Stagnation, in contrast, characterizes the failure to become societally generative. The widespread absence of generative care may threaten the future of a society's corporate life, Erikson suggests, because generativity is the link between the life cycle and the generational cycle.

B. Longitudinal Research Findings

Cross-sectional research suggests that adults who are effective, responsive parents are also more likely to score well on measures of psychosocial maturity. More authoritative, however, are the findings from longitudinal studies of the same men over decades.

The Haverford Longitudinal Study, conducted by Douglas Heath, followed a group of men from their entrance into college through their entrance to midlife. One of Heath's many aims was to test the Eriksonian idea that parenting contributes to societal generativity by investigating the impact of fathering versus other experiences on the way the men felt they had changed since leaving college. Heath found that the composite assessment of being a competent father was significantly related to almost a quarter of the assessed characteristics of the men's adult personalities and to a composite index of general competence in different roles. Fatherhood apparently promoted men's abilities to understand themselves, to sympathetically understand others, and to integrate their feelings. Heath also found that the men who had enjoyed being fathers were also more likely to serve in a community leadership position. As Heath concluded, the experience of being a father promotes an other-centered, generous character.

The Grant Longitudinal Study, directed by George Vaillant, also found that parental adaptation was related to later forms of psychosocial adaptation beyond the family sphere. More specifically, Vaillant investigated the level of men's personal, family, and career adjustment and related it to the men's psychosocial outcomes. Only 13% of the men who were found to have the highest degree of social adjustment reported greater psychological distance from their children than they wanted, while 50% of the men with the lowest social adjustment scores reported such distance. Similarly, men who had mastered the prior developmental task of intimacy, in the sense of having maintained a stable first marriage, had become more societally generative. In particular, they were more likely to evidence clear responsibility for the care and development of other adults at the workplace. In contrast, a high proportion of the men who received the lowest overall adjustment ratings had little work responsibility beyond themselves and had generally failed to show evidence of being societally generative.

The Glueck Longitudinal Study of how fathers care, conducted by John Snarey, specifically addressed the impact of childrearing fatherhood on later societal generativity. Each of the 240 men was rated for evidence of societal generativity, based on their age-47 interviews; the raters were blinded to their childrearing careers. The results showed that men who eventually became fathers also became more societally generative at midlife than the men who remained childless. And fathers who participated more in childrearing were also more likely to become societally generative at midlife. Fathers' care for their children's social-emotional development and for their adolescents' social-emotional and intellectual–academic development, in particular, were strong predictors of the men's societal generativity beyond the family sphere.

Finally, in the Nurturing Fathers Longitudinal Study, Kyle Pruett investigated 17 fathers who were highly involved in childrearing and their families. The study was conducted over a period of 8 years after the fathers became the primary childcare provider. Pruett did not find any association between occupational class and good fathering; rather, all of the men studied were quite able to perform the role of primary childcare provider. He did observe that the work of fatherhood empowered men to work through any lingering distress from their relationship with their own fathers. They became the active caring fathers with their own children that they wished their own fathers had been with them. Pruett also observed that fathering promoted the men's generative self-confidence—that they were generous and competent men who were capable of being responsible for the welfare and development of another human being. Their identity as fathers had become central to their lives.

The combined longitudinal findings are consistent with the Eriksonian thesis that the experiences of parenting or parentlike activities serve as a foundation, although not as a sufficient condition, for the later attainment of societal generativity at midlife.

C. Fatherwork

At different times in history people have had different levels of interest in different stages of life. For instance, men who came of age and entered the major professions before the value revisions of the feminist movement and in a time that provided few rewards for men's childrearing work were more likely to regard their occupation as more important than fatherhood for their personal generativity. In contrast, others have noted the emergence of a new cohort of fathers—postfeminist-era fathers who may express their generativity equally via parenting. These historical contrasts underscore the importance of societal supports for the work of fathers.

Fathers, today, are faced with numerous practical dilemmas because they cannot do all of the things they "ought" to do. Most employers, Pleck has observed, still assume that a father's involvement in childrearing and family life will not take precedence over their paid work, but that a mother's family roles will assume priority over her paid work. Most common conflicts derive from workplace policies that are insensitive to family life. The special significance of the workplace is simply because the majority of fathers and mothers work outside of the home and, thus, the principle non-home setting in which most fathers and mothers live their lives is the workplace.

New policies, according to Nancy Crowell and Ethel Leeper, can make society more friendly for men who are fathers. If both husbands and wives are given more control over their work schedules and work environments, for instance, they can create a better balance between work and family life. Paid infant-care leave for fathers as well as for mothers has the potential to significantly add to the quality of father–child relations. A gender-inclusive parental leave policy provides the flexibility needed to allow fathers as well as mothers to form early, firm bonds with their newborn or newly adopted infants, and to allow infants to become equally bonded with both of their parents. Alternate work schedules are even more essential. Fathers can join mothers in achieving a high level of childrearing involvement if both parents are able to make the adjustments in their work schedules necessary to allow some degree of shift work. Family support services also should be added to the workplace to counterbalance workplace structures that make it difficult for men and women to bring their childrearing concerns, let alone their children, to the workplace.

Generative policies and programs are needed to build an ethic of parental generativity into the structure of the workplace.

Fathering, like most aspects of family mental health, is multiply determined and has multiple consequences. Yet, the general pattern is quite simple: Children are psychologically highly significant to fathers and their psychosocial development, and, in turn, the impact of fathers' childcare work is positive and significant for their sons and daughters, their families, and the larger society. As Hawkins and Dollahite have emphasized, generative fathering is about the work men do to build connections across generations. Generative fathering, in fact, may be men's most important line of work.

BIBLIOGRAPHY

Belsky, J. (1995). *The transition to parenthood.* New York: Dell.

Biller, H. B. (1993). *Fathers and families.* Westport, CN: Auburn House.

Crowell, N. A., & Leeper, E. M. (Eds.). (1994). *America's fathers and public policy.* Washington, DC: National Research Council of the National Academy of Sciences.

Erikson, E. H. (1982). *The life cycle completed.* New York: Norton.

Hawkins, A. J., & Dollahite, D. C. (1997). *Generative fathering.* Newbury Park, CA: Sage Publications.

Lamb, M. (1997). *The role of the father in child development* (3rd ed.). New York: Wiley.

McAdams, D. P., & de St. Aubin, E. (1997). *Generativity and adult development: Psychosocial perspectives on caring for and contributing to the next generation.* Washington, DC: APA Press.

Parke, R. D. (1996). *Fatherhood.* Cambridge, MA: Harvard University Press.

Peterson, B. E., & Kohnen, E. C. (1995). Realization of generativity in two samples of women at midlife. *Psychology and Aging, 10*(1), 20–29.

Pruett, K. D. (1988). *The nurturing father.* New York: Warner Books.

Rasmussen, K. S., Hawkins, A. J., & Schwab, K. P. (1996). Increasing husbands' involvement in domestic labor: Issues for therapists. *Contemporary Family Therapy, 18*(2), 209–223.

Shapiro, J. L., Diamond, M. J., and Greenberg, M. (Eds.). (1995). *Becoming a father.* New York: Springer.

Snarey, J. (1993). *How fathers care for the next generation: A four-decade study.* Cambridge, MA: Harvard University Press.

Food, Nutrition, and Mental Health

Bonnie J. Kaplan

University of Calgary

Adverse Reaction A term used to describe an apparent negative response to a substance, but which does not presume any particular biologic mechanism.

Allergy A state of hypersensitivity that involves an antibody and an antigen.

Antibody An immunoglobulin molecule (such as IgE) that interacts with a specific antigen, resulting in an allergic response.

Antigen A substance such as a toxin or a bacterium that provokes the body to produce an antibody.

Attention Deficit Hyperactivity Disorder (ADHD) The diagnostic label currently used to describe the constellation of symptoms that includes hyperactivity, inattention, and impulsivity.

IgE Immunoglobulin E, a protein that functions as an antibody in allergic-type reactions.

FOOD and food substances affect mental health in the broadest sense inasmuch as the development and function of the human brain is dependent on the ingestion of appropriate nutrients. This article focuses more specifically on suspected adverse reactions to nutrients and food additives. Hyperactivity in children and depression in adults have often been reported to be examples of such reactions. Clinical anecdotes, the mass media, and publications for laypeople have reported many other examples of presumed food–mental health interactions. The focus here is limited to the areas for which scientific data are most readily available. A theoretical model of food–behavior interactions is also reviewed.

I. INTRODUCTION

This article demonstrates that far more is unknown about food–mental health relationships than is known. Although the clinical literature is replete with case reports dating back decades, and even though every bookstore sells monographs that claim to help people improve their mental health through better nutrition, the scientific studies lag far behind. It is essential to acknowledge that the evaluation of food–mental health interactions in humans is extraordinarily difficult, far more so than in many other areas of mental health. There are several reasons for this. First, expectancy effects are enormous. Everyone has strong feelings and beliefs about what they eat. People who would never venture a guess as to the neurologic implications of taking a certain medication are more than willing to make assumptions about the mood or behavioral effect of a certain food. Humans are all guilty of this, even scientists. Yet the truism "we are what we eat" surely reveals the paradoxical nature of this inconsistency: the ingestion of nutrients can influence brain function in the same manner as the ingestion of drugs.

A second reason for the extraordinary difficulty in assessing the mental health effects of food is that it is hard to control for long periods of time what people eat or the environmental stimuli to which they are exposed. Even in a person known to be somewhat sensitive to a particular ingredient, it is possible that the adverse reaction is not obvious unless exposure occurs for awhile and the behavior is monitored consistently over that time period. During that time, other events may occur in people's lives that also influence the outcome variables being studied. For instance, an evaluation of the impact of an additive on depression would ideally be carried out for a time period of sufficient length to observe the full range of moods normally occurring in that person, but with no life events occurring that might impinge on the subject's mood. Isolation of individuals for weeks at a time is hard to accomplish.

There are other reasons that scientists have found it arduous to study these relationships in humans: questions about dosage or exposure, uncertainty about length of exposure required, problems in obtaining ratings of behavior that are entirely blind with respect to exposure, and so on. Factors such as these mean that much research remains to be done before a comprehensive summary can be written that concludes just how important nutrition is for the mental health of the general public.

II. MALNUTRITION AND BRAIN DEVELOPMENT

Certainly, this area of nutrition research is the oldest, and also the best supported by animal studies. In hundreds of investigations over the past several decades, nutritional deprivation has been shown to influence negatively brain growth and learning skills in rodents and other mammals. In humans, the most extreme forms of protein-calorie malnutrition (marasmus and kwashiorkor) have an acute effect on mental functioning; mental apathy is a characteristic of both. [*See* PRENATAL STRESS AND LIFE SPAN DEVELOPMENT.]

War has provided a "natural" experiment on the mental effects of malnutrition. Studies from World Wars I and II have demonstrated high prematurity rates and low birth weights in the affected populations. Economic class has also been demonstrated to be a significant consideration, even in times of peace. Relatively poorer women generally have less nutritious diets and give birth to smaller babies; their

children are also at risk for more congenital anomalies, most of which affect the central nervous system (anencephaly, hydrocephaly, spina bifida, etc.). The causal nature of these associations has been demonstrated by nutritional intervention studies in economically disadvantaged populations, showing that dietary supplements consistently reduce the risk for these adverse outcomes.

The inescapable conclusion from this body of research is that intrauterine nutrition is very important for reducing the risk of prematurity and low birth weight, and also for ensuring adequate brain development. Many years ago, autopsies demonstrated convincingly that babies who died of malnutrition had significantly fewer neurons and lower overall brain weight. The insult appears to have been general, at least in these extreme cases: there was no localized effect detectable in any particular area of the brain.

Of great importance is the question of whether the human brain can ever fully recover from a period of malnutrition. The answer seems to be contingent on two variables: how early the nutritional deprivation occurred, and how long it lasted. Brain growth is not continuous throughout childhood. The fetal period and the first 2 years of life (when cell division is still occurring rapidly) appear to be the most significant, and studies have shown better recoveries from malnutrition when the deprivation occurs later rather than earlier. Recovery is also influenced by the background upon which the malnutrition has occurred. For instance, the children born during the Dutch blockade in World War II were born to women who had previously been well nourished; termination of the blockade resulted in dramatically improved nutrition. Long-term studies of prenatal exposure to famine in this population showed no effects on cognitive performance at age 19 years. These results are not generalizable to children in chronically deprived populations who suffer a period of severe malnutrition and who do experience concurrent depression of cognitive performance scores.

III. WHAT IS AN ADDITIVE?

In the 1970s in North America, the term "additive" became pejorative. Yet in previous decades, as food science developed to the point of being able to change food during the manufacturing process, additive had a far more positive connotation. Before that time, food staples such as bread and milk products had to be eaten within a day or so. Preservatives (a type of additive) changed all that. In addition, year-round accessibility became possible for fruits and vegetables that had previously been available only during summer months.

What, exactly, is an additive? Although at first glance this may seem obvious, consider the following examples. When whey powder, a "natural" ingredient, is used in another food as a thickener, it becomes an "additive"—is that necessarily negative? When ascorbic acid (vitamin C) is added to frozen vegetables to prevent browning, should we avoid it because it is an additive? To take a more extreme example, soy lecithin is often used as a filler and thickener. Not only is it a natural ingredient when viewed on its own, it is also a phytochemical, which current research suggests is beneficial to human health.

It is not only the word *additive* that is confusing; even the word *food* can be ambiguous. Consider substances such as herbs. When people drink chamomile tea to assist them in falling asleep, are they ingesting a food or taking a medicine?

Finally, it should be noted here that additives are not the only category of food substances that have been labeled as culprits in research on food–mental health interactions. There is probably just as much literature published on the adverse effects of naturally occurring substances (sugar, wheat, dairy products) as there is on additives put into food during the production process (artificial flavors and colors, preservatives).

IV. WHAT IS A FOOD–MENTAL HEALTH INTERACTION?

Obviously, certain basic nutrients are necessary for sufficient growth and development. Yet for many years the health literature seemed to assume that within the general guidelines of basic nutrition (e.g., the Recommended Daily Allowance of the U.S. Department of Health) there was no variation that would account for feelings of well-being (or, in contrast, mental distress). Likewise, adverse emotional/behavioral reactions to foods or food additives were generally assumed to be rare or of no clinical consequence. Early reports of the hallucinatory effects of wheat in

schizophrenia were never well accepted in the general medical/mental health literature. Until the 1970s, after Dr. Benjamin Feingold claimed that post-World War II use of food additives were directly contributing to childhood hyperactivity, there was little well-controlled mental health research on the effects of food substances. Because of the intriguing results reported in the last 20 years, this research is likely to increase in the future.

In its broadest and most accurate sense, a food–mental health reaction should encompass feelings of well-being elicited by the ingestion of food substances as well as adverse mental or emotional reactions triggered by such ingestion. In reality, adverse reactions have been studied the most, and public concerns about potential harm caused by what we eat have stimulated the majority of the research. In only one area do we know a bit about possibly beneficial effects of our diet on mental health: the research on selected populations "self-medicating" by eating carbohydrates, which will be reviewed in this context.

V. EFFECT OF ADDITIVES

Most of the world's population does not have the luxury of worrying about the ingredients of its food supply. In westernized, industrialized society, and especially in North America, an intensive concern has developed since World War II about the so-called additives in the population's food (as well as in water and air). These concerns have ranged across a wide variety of topics: the use of aluminum cooking pots, the application of irradiation to foods, genetically engineered vegetables, pesticides in agricultural products, hormones in beef, lead paint and leaded gasoline, and so on. Coupled with the North American public's general suspicion that an increasingly polluted environment is affecting our health (viz., sick building syndrome) was the feeling, apparent in the 1970s, that something was increasingly wrong with our children. A natural reaction was the connection of the two, which explains the fertile ground into which Dr. Benjamin Feingold planted his theory that food additives were causing hyperactivity (now referred to as Attention Deficit Hyperactivity Disorder, ADHD. [*See* ATTENTION DEFICIT HYPERACTIVITY DISORDER (ADHD).]

Just as subsequent research has shown that lead

does, in fact, affect intellectual ability, there is also support from careful studies that some people are influenced by food additives. In some ways, however, the analogy is better made with sick building syndrome: whereas environmental exposure to lead seems to put everyone at risk for impaired cognitive development, much of the research on food additives suggests idiosyncratic reactions. The public health implications of idiosyncratic reactions are far more difficult to evaluate. Because leaded gasoline was shown to be a danger to all humans (especially children), it was not difficult (once the danger from lead was clearly documented) to mobilize the public will necessary to change the regulations regarding acceptable levels of lead in gasoline. But when something in the environment (e.g., food substances) are shown to affect only a minority of people, social change is less likely to happen.

The Feingold Hypothesis, presented in the 1970s, was that artificial colors, artificial flavors, and naturally occurring salicylates were causing hyperactivity. On the basis of his clinical experience, Dr. Feingold claimed that the removal of these substances cured two thirds of the children that he treated. His concepts were presented on the floor of the U.S. Congress in support of a bill requesting that a new symbol be adopted by the food industry to clearly label each manufactured product that was additive-free. The bill did not pass, but the subsequent publicity resulted in huge interest from the public, and pressure for scientists to provide data.

With the public clamoring for scientific data, several scientists quickly conducted studies using a "challenge" paradigm. With this method, children were presented with cookies or drinks that had either artificial or natural colors. The emphasis was on colors for a practical reason: the Food and Drug Administration was able to provide clear data on the average amount ingested by each person per year. The results of the challenge studies have not changed over the last decades: each study has found a small number of children whose behavior worsened with the additive challenge, but the majority of children were unaffected. The public's response to these results was to dismiss the relevance of all food additives, but this was an overreaction for several reasons. First, in every challenge study conducted, at least a few children experienced an adverse reaction to the bolus of artificial colors. In some cases, these children were dropped from

the study, particularly if the adverse reaction included a somatic component such as a stomachache. Second, the challenge studies did not evaluate all food additives, nor salicylates. These studies evaluated a group of artificial colors, and so hindsight reveals that the proper interpretation would have been that this group of food colors adversely affects the behavior of a small minority of hyperactive children.

There have also been several studies that used a different method, namely, "elimination diets." This method is much more difficult in that it restricts the food intake of the children being studied and then has periods of time in which additive-laced foods are incorporated into the diet. Whereas the challenge paradigm usually ignores the background food intake of the children, the elimination diet approach actually replaces and controls the entire food intake. For these elimination studies, in general, it seems that the broader the net (i.e., the greater the number of items eliminated from the diet), the larger the capture rate (the greater the number of children exhibiting improved behavior). This is a logical result if one considers the proposition that each food–behavior interaction is specific to an individual. Thus, the combination of these two types of studies seems to provide a compelling argument that additive–behavior interactions in children with ADHD exist but are highly idiosyncratic.

By the 1980s, it became clear that idiosyncratic reactions of the type that concerned Dr. Feingold might not be limited to additives. A series of European cases demonstrated that some people become more hyperactive and emotional when exposed to certain natural foods, not necessarily those with salicylates. Although categories of foods such as dairy products, chocolate, wheat, and eggs appeared to be the most typical provocateurs, there is hardly a food substance on earth that has not been suspected of causing an adverse reaction in at least one person.

From a therapeutic perspective, the research on additive–behavior interactions in children with ADHD has been disappointing. It is certainly clear that the Feingold claim of a two-thirds cure rate for ADHD was highly inflated. Particularly in comparisons with stimulant medication, it has become obvious that elimination diets do not have nearly the beneficial impact that pharmacology has. In addition, elimination diets such as the one proposed by Feingold are extremely difficult for some families to follow, and they sometimes impose undue stress on already burdened families. The result is that long-term compliance can be problematic.

It would not be an exaggeration to say that research on additives and behavior has been more useful from a scientific perspective than it has been for the treatment of any mental health problem. Scientifically, Feingold's efforts, the media interest, and the early studies stimulated interest in food–behavior relationships beyond the specific focus of ADHD. As discussed later, one of the results of this broadened interest has been the development of some interesting models of food–mental health interactions.

VI. EFFECT OF SUGAR

A. Hyperactivity

No discussion of food–mental health interactions in children with ADHD is complete without a review of the impact of sugar. Even though the North American public has forgotten much of what Feingold initially hypothesized, it still believes that sugar makes children hyperactive. Understanding the source of such an entrenched (and unsupported) belief is a challenge.

Attempts have been made to evaluate the impact of sugar by challenging children with ADHD with either sucrose or a placebo (often aspartame). Interestingly, although increased motor activity has been shown in Sprague-Dawley rats fed sugar water, this effect has been hard to document in children. In contrast, sugar has consistently been shown to cause sleepiness in adults. If the variables studied in children with ADHD had emphasized the attentional problems, this apparent difference would be easy to reconcile: one could hypothesize that the soporific effect of sugar ingestion was resulting in degraded attention. But when people claim that sugar is adversely affecting their children with ADHD, they are generally referring to the motoric and emotional aspects, and there is no convincing evidence that sugar has a causal effect on these variables. The only research supportive of a sugar–hyperactivity link is correlational; a few studies have shown that the children with ADHD who eat more sugar are the ones who are more hyperactive. With correlational data such as this, however, it is essential to keep in mind that the direction of causation (if, indeed, causation is relevant) could be either way.

One of the most interesting aspects of the research on sugar–hyperactivity interactions in children with ADHD is that it has been totally parent driven. From the beginning, the scientific literature did not support such a link. Sugar is a carbohydrate. For many years it has been known that a carbohydrate-rich meal results in increased availability of tryptophan, increased brain serotonin, and sleepiness or at least impaired alertness. The pathway for this phenomenon has been defined in animal studies. Serotonin, a monoamine neurotransmitter, is synthesized in the brain. One factor that significantly influences how much serotonin is synthesized is the availability in the diet of tryptophan, the amino acid precursor of serotonin. Humans cannot synthesize tryptophan; we have to obtain it from the protein we ingest. Paradoxically, eating a high carbohydrate (not protein) meal is the most effective way to increase brain availability of tryptophan. The paradox occurs because of the ratio of tryptophan in protein and the competitive system that exists for the carrier molecules that cross the blood–brain barrier. In summary, the most effective way to elevate brain serotonin is by eating a high carbohydrate, low protein meal. Ingesting carbohydrates reliably *decreases* activity and alertness in humans. Several studies have confirmed that children who are given sucrose or fructose (two sugars that are carbohydrates) exhibit decreased motor activity.

There are several simple possibilities that might explain why the sugar–hyperactivity belief has become entrenched in our society. In the modern nutrient-conscious parent, the one situation in which children are still almost universally permitted to indulge in sweets and treats is a party, holiday, or other festive occasion. The social environment at such events is likely sufficient to provoke hyperactivity, impulsivity, and emotionality in children. Another perspective worth considering is that children rarely eat pure sucrose in isolation from additives. If a child is believed to be reacting adversely to a sweet food, it is possible that the reaction is being triggered by the other ingredients and is an example of an idiosyncratic reaction to an additive, as discussed earlier.

A more interesting finding is the clinical research that suggests that certain groups selectively crave carbohydrates and perhaps use them to self-medicate. For many years it has been known that some people with clinically diagnosed depression have a low level of 5-HIAA (5-hydroxyindoleacetic acid) in their cerebrospinal fluid. This chemical is a metabolite of serotonin and is an indirect measure of serotonin levels in the central nervous system. It is also known that the administration of some of the precursors of serotonin can result in elevated levels of 5-HIAA and improved mood. Clinical researchers report that craving for carbohydrates is commonly reported in some people with depression, and that the ingestion of carbohydrates can reduce their depression. Finally, in one study of nondepressed young men who were deprived of tryptophan, self-reported mood became more depressed. Thus, it appears that chemicals or foods that increase serotonin function are associated with mood elevation; serotonin depletion is associated with depressed mood, even in people not suffering from clinical depression. This pathway may explain why some people crave carbohydrates such as sugar: they may be unconsciously self-medicating in order to elevate their mood. [*See* DEPRESSION.]

B. Delinquency

What hyperactivity was to the 1970s, delinquency/criminal behavior seems to have been to the 1980s. Because of the great concern about increased juvenile delinquency, an association with their diet was hypothesized. Some studies seemed to indicate a correlation, which has even lead some correctional facilities to alter their institutional diets. In the last 5 years, more thorough studies of insulin secretion in response to sugar ingestion, as well as inquiries into the nutritional status of juvenile offenders, have not supported a general problem of sucrose tolerance. As with ADHD, it is possible that there are idiosyncratic reactions. The good single cases or small series of cases that would be necessary to determine whether this is true have not been done with this population. Consequently, at the present time, it is difficult to conclude that excessive sugar intake has a unique or reliable effect on criminal behavior. [*See* CRIMINAL BEHAVIOR.]

VII. MODELS OF FOOD–MENTAL HEALTH INTERACTIONS

One of the consistent findings in the literature is that many of the populations hypothesized to have adverse reactions to foods are also prone to an unusual number of allergies (especially IgE-mediated hay fever, asthma, eczema, etc.). This association has been reported in children with ADHD and in adults with clinical depression. One theorist has developed a model of food–mental health interactions that takes into account this alleged association with allergies.

Marshall's model of nutrient–mood interactions involves an imbalance between adrenergic and cholinergic activity in the autonomic (ANS) and central (CNS) nervous systems. For the ANS, physiological responsivity to cholinergic agonists of people with IgE-based allergies, asthma, and so on, is greater than in control nonallergic subjects. Marshall argues that there is reason to hypothesize that children with ADHD exhibit excessive cholinergic activity. Admittedly based on evidence from the ANS rather than from the brain, the theory is that many children with ADHD experience allergic reactions that induce cholinergic hyperresponsiveness. The excessive cholinergic activity is thus believed to be caused by allergic reactions and is believed to be responsible for poor regulation of arousal in ADHD. It is also hypothesized that cholinergic hyperresponsiveness induced by allergies would cause rebound effects that would ultimately lead to excessive adrenergic activity.

A similar model has been proposed to account for another observed association with IgE-mediated reactions: depression. Marshall has recently reviewed a large amount of research on depression, its association with allergy, and the possible mechanisms that could account for that association. His neurochemical threshold model interprets endogenous depression as being caused in part by allergy-induced supersensitivity of the cholinergic system of the CNS, as well as beta-adrenergic subsensitivity. His model integrates many well supported facts about CNS effects of allergy while still providing roles for genetic predisposition and the impact of acute or chronic stress. [*See* GENETIC CONTRIBUTORS TO MENTAL HEALTH; PSYCHONEUROIMMUNOLOGY; STRESS.]

BIBLIOGRAPHY

Christensen, L. (1996). *Diet–behavior relationships: Focus on depression.* Washington, DC: American Psychological Association.
Egger, J., Carter, C. M., Graham, P. J., Gumley, D., & Soothill, J. F. (1985). Controlled trial of oligoantigenic treatment in the hyperkinetic syndrome. *Lancet, 1,* 540–545.

Kaplan, B. J. (1988). The relevance of food for children's cognitive and behavioural health. *Canadian Journal of Behavioural Science, 20,* 359–373.

Marshall, P. (1989). Attention deficit disorder and allergy: A neurochemical model of the relation between the illnesses. *Psychological Bulletin, 106*(3), 434–446.

Marshall, P. S. (1993). Allergy and depression: A neurochemical threshold model of the relation between the illnesses. *Psychological Bulletin, 113*(1), 23–43.

Spring, B., Chiodo, J., & Bowen, D. J. (1987). Carbohydrates, tryptophan, and behavior: A methodological review. *Psychological Bulletin, 102*(2), 234–256.

Stein, Z., Susser, M., Saenger, G., & Marolla, F. (1975). *Famine and human development: The Dutch hunger winter of 1944–45.* New York: Oxford University Press.

Wachs, T. C. (1995). Relation of mild-to-moderate malnutrition to human development: Correlational studies. *Journal of Nutrition, 125*(Suppl.), 2245S–2254S.

G

Gambling

Douglas Carroll and Frank F. Eves

University of Birmingham

Arousal A state of activation or excitement manifest by heightened affect and increased physiological activity.

Cognitive Bias A term used to describe the biases in thinking that individuals may display.

Gambling Wagering money or goods on a game or sport in which the outcome is uncertain.

Pathological Gambling An impulsive disorder manifest by an addiction to gambling.

Personality The stable attributes and dispositions that characterize an individual.

Prevalence A measure of the rate of a particular phenomenon, such as pathological gambling, within a population at a particular time.

Reinforcement Schedule The pattern of outcomes associated with an individual's responses or actions.

GAMBLING is a strikingly ubiquitous human activity. For most people it constitutes a fairly casual pastime, amid a varied matrix of social and leisure pursuits. For some, however, gambling is anything but a casual activity: for the pathological gambler, gambling is preoccupying, consuming substantial time and money. The American Psychiatric Association regards pathological gambling as an impulsive disorder manifest as an addiction to gambling akin to alcohol

or drug addiction. This entry briefly describes the salient characteristics of the pathological gambler and indicates the current prevalence of the disorder. Explanations for pathological gambling are reviewed along with comments on treatment and intervention.

I. GAMBLING

Gambling, in some form or another, is legally sanctioned in more than 90 countries worldwide and in 48 of the 50 states of the United States. In 1988, it was estimated that Americans legally wagered some $210 billion; by 1991, the estimated expenditure on gambling had soared by 50% to $304 billion. The proliferation of video lottery terminals and the establishment of casinos on Native American lands, consequent on passage of the federal Indian Gaming Regulation Act in 1988, are just the most recent manifestations of the progressive loosening of legislative restrictions on gambling. In this context, it is worth noting that in 1974, the total of legal wagers in the United States was $17 billion, a mere 5% of the most recent expenditure estimates.

Other countries have increasingly adopted similarly supportive legislative postures and have shown similar expenditure trajectories. For example, government revenue from gambling in Australia rose from $168 million (Australian dollars) in 1972–1973 to $2.02 billion in 1992–1993. Indeed, some countries began relaxing strictures against gambling much earlier than the United States. Although the United Kingdom was slow to appreciate the fiscal possibilities of lottery gambling, the Gaming Act, which legalized gaming for profit, became law in 1968. Among other things, it allowed licences to be granted for slot machine installations in cafes, leisure centers, or dedicated slot machine arcades, with access policed only by a voluntary code of conduct, devised by the British Amusement and Catering Trade Association (BACTA). The BACTA code prohibits those under 16 years of age from entering slot machine arcades. However, the code does not apply to seaside arcades, does not bind owners who are not members of the association, and does not apply to nonarcade sites. Thus, while other European countries, Australia, and the states of the United States set the legal minimum age of access to slot machines at 18 or 21 years, the United Kingdom, in effect, exerts no legal restriction.

Not surprisingly, the legislative arrangements that govern gambling have implications for behavior. For example, whereas other countries are not without problems related to slot machine gambling, it would appear that the heavy involvement of young people is a particularly British phenomenon. In the United Kingdom, organizations such as Gamblers Anonymous (GA) report an increasingly large number of under-18 youths seeking help for excessive or uncontrolled slot machine use. In 1964, the typical British GA member was a 40- to 50-year-old horse race gambler; by 1986, approximately 50% of new members were slot machine players, half of these being adolescents.

Legislative relaxation in the United States has not only seen a massive increase in expenditure on gambling, it has also been associated with a substantial increase in participation. In 1974 in the United States, about 60% of the adult population were estimated to have participated in some form of gambling. By 1990, the figure had risen to just over 80%, and the most recent estimates, based on sampled states, suggest that the current lifetime participation rates may be even higher.

These figures are cited only as illustration. Nevertheless, they are broadly representative. With increasing legislative laissez-faire has come increased access and participation rates, as well as massively increased expenditure on gambling, not to mention, in many cases, vast increases in government revenues. In addition, where legislation and cultural values permit, gambling appears to be a prevalent activity among the young. For example, surveys show that between 3%

and 14% of British high school students are regular slot machine players. The figures for occasional use are more dramatic, with two thirds of British adolescents reporting use of gaming machines in arcades.

II. PATHOLOGICAL GAMBLING

While for most people gambling represents an occasional distraction, for the pathological gambler it is anything but. In contrast to the occasional or recreational gambler, the pathological gambler has lost control over his or her gambling behavior. Gambling has, for such an individual, reached the point of disrupting not only his or her life, but also the lives of close family members and friends. In 1980, the American Psychiatric Association (APA) formally recognized pathological gambling as a disorder of impulse control, similar in many ways to other addictions. Save for "chasing" losses, the criteria used for defining gambling as pathological were very much modeled on those used to define alcohol and drug abuse. Like the substance addict, the pathological gambler is consumed by gambling, and will beg, borrow, cheat, and steal to support their addiction. Like the substance addict, the pathological gambler often shows tolerance, needing to increase the size or the frequency of the bet to achieve the desired excitement or "high." Similarly, withdrawal symptoms of disturbed mood and behavior are evident when gambling is curtailed. With regard to withdrawal, one study interrogated 222 pathological gamblers. Sixty-five percent reported at least one of the following: insomnia, headaches, upset stomach, loss of appetite, physical weakness, heart racing, muscle aches, breathing difficulties, sweating, and chills. Indeed, the pathological gamblers reported, if anything, more withdrawal symptoms than did substance-addicted control subjects. Finally, there are many instances of cross-addictions among pathological gamblers. Some studies have observed that as many as 50% of pathological gamblers had abused alcohol or drugs at some point in their lives. [See IMPULSE CONTROL.]

The following criteria are currently recommended by the APA as being characteristic. A diagnosis of pathological gambling is registered if an individual meets five or more of these criteria, with the proviso that the behavior is not better accounted for by a manic episode. A person may meet the criteria if he or she

1. Is preoccupied with gambling (e.g., preoccupied with reliving past gambling experiences, handicapping or planning the next venture, or thinking of ways to get money with which to gamble)
2. Needs to gamble with increasing amounts of money in order to achieve the desired excitement
3. Has repeated unsuccessful efforts to control, cut back, or stop gambling
4. Is restless or irritable when attempting to cut down or stop gambling
5. Gambles as a way of escaping from problems or of relieving a dysphoric mood (e.g., feelings of helplessness, guilt, anxiety, depression)
6. After losing money gambling, often returns another day to get even ("chasing" one's losses)
7. Lies to family members, therapist, or others to conceal the extent of involvement with gambling
8. Has committed illegal acts such as forgery, fraud, theft, or embezzlement to finance gambling
9. Has jeopardized or lost a significant relationship, job, or educational or career opportunity because of gambling
10. Relies on others to provide money to relieve a desperate financial situation caused by gambling

III. PREVALENCE

Prevalence is the measure of the rate of a given phenomenon, such as pathological gambling, in a given population at a given time. Accordingly, the examples of prevalence rates cited here will necessarily be parochial. Although there are reasons for suspecting that the rates have increased in recent years, the data are circumstantial. As yet, there are no published reports of repeat prevalence surveys conducted on the same population. Nevertheless, there are clear trends apparent in research findings. Consider, for example, surveys of slot machine gambling among British high school students; in general, higher rates of pathological gambling appear in more recent surveys. Similarly, an escalation in pathological gambling can be inferred from the increase in treatment-seeking behavior. Consider the example of Holland and its alcohol and drug treatment centers. The number of individuals seeking treatment for gambling-related problems at these centers has increased strikingly over time. While only 10 individuals sought information or treatment in 1985, 400 did so in 1986, 1200 in 1987, and 3883 in 1991.

The only national survey in the United States was conducted in 1974. The authors concluded that 1.1 million Americans were probable pathological gamblers. More recently, researchers have relied for data on state-based prevalence surveys. Those carried out since 1990 report prevalence rates ranging from 1.4 to 2.8%. Surveys of gambling behaviors in Canadian provinces yield, if anything, slightly lower prevalence rates, but much depends on the definition of what constitutes pathological. One of the problems with the survey research is variation in the criteria used to define pathological gambling. For example, if one adheres to a strict definition of pathological gambling, the Canadian provincial rates range from 0.8 to 1.7%. However, if one relaxes the definition to include problem gamblers who possess almost, but not quite, a sufficient number of the defining characteristics to qualify as pathological gamblers, the prevalence rates range from 2.7% in Saskatchewan to 8.6% in Ontario. Other countries are gradually beginning to survey their populations. Rates of pathological gambling in regions of Spain currently run at about 1.7%. In Australia, a partial national survey revealed pathological gambling rates of 1.2%, an identical figure to that which emerged from the recent national survey in New Zealand. Some appreciation of what these figures mean in social problem terms can be obtained by extrapolating from the case of New Zealand. A prevalence rate of 1.2% implies that there are approximately 27,500 pathological gamblers in New Zealand. If we assume an overall current prevalence rate of 2% in the United States, a reasonable assumption given recent individual state estimates, and an age structure similar to New Zealand, we can calculate that there are more than 3 million pathological gamblers in the United States.

There are reasons for suspecting, however, that the prevalence rates revealed by many of these surveys are, if anything, underestimates. We have already alluded to the matter of the criteria used to identify pathological gambling; someone may have severe problems with gambling, yet fall just short of pathological status. Secondly, most of the prevalence surveys have relied on telephone data collection techniques. Such an approach has obvious pitfalls. Pathological gamblers may be underrepresented as they are more likely to have their telephones cut off periodically for nonpayment of bills, or to be too poor to possess telephones. Furthermore, telephone surveys have notoriously high nonresponse and refusal rates; pathological gamblers are less likely to be at home to telephone enquiries and, if they are, more likely to be reticent in the face of enquiries about gambling. This would again lead to pathological gamblers being undersampled. Problems also arise from unsampled groups, such as those in institutional care. Studies of patients in alcohol and drug treatment centers reveal prevalence rates of pathological gambling of 9 to 15%. The exclusion of such individuals from surveys of pathological gambling will consequently lead to underestimates of prevalence. There is also emerging evidence of relatively high rates of pathological gambling among adolescents. For example, recent surveys among high school age individuals in Canada registered pathological gambling prevalence rates of about 3%. Most general telephone surveys necessarily exclude adolescents and are, as a result, likely to yield prevalence estimates lower than the true figure.

Finally, individual surveys in the United States usually show that pathological gambling prevalence rates are higher among those with low levels of education, as well as being higher among males, young adults, and nonwhites. It is worth noting that young adults and nonwhites tend to be underrepresented in treatment programs. Thus, treatment may not be reaching many of those who need it most.

IV. EXPLANATIONS

Early attempts to account for pathological gambling relied either on psychodynamic metaphor or on a strict application of reinforcement theory. From a psychodynamic perspective, gambling was regarded as an attempt to resolve conflicts with parental figures through symbolic contests with a surrogate. Pathological gambling reflected an unconscious desire to lose such contests, thus appeasing the parental figures. Reinforcement theory regarded gambling as a learned response to intermittent schedules of financial reinforcement. Pathological gambling, from this perspective, was the result of repeated exposure to these pow-

erful schedules. Neither provide a satisfactory answer. While psychodynamic explanations are couched in a manner that renders empirical examination extremely difficult, strict reinforcement theory, with its emphasis on purely financial contingencies, gives improper regard to other motivating agencies and to intraindividual factors.

Other, recent theoretical models of pathological gambling are much more multifactorial in character, and, although retaining variable financial reinforcement schedules as part of the explanatory matrix, have incorporated a range of other factors. Most prominent among these are cognitive bias, personal disposition, and arousal.

A. Cognitive Bias

One of the most influential contributions to a cognitive psychology of gambling has been the work of Ellen Langer on the illusion of control. The illusion of control is defined as an expectancy of personal success inappropriately higher than the objective probability would warrant. In an elegant series of laboratory studies, Langer demonstrated that subjects' appropriate orientations toward chance events could be altered by a range of manipulations. For example, subjects who cut cards against a nervous competitor bet more than when playing against a confident competitor. Subjects would pitch the sale price of a lottery ticket that they had chosen themselves at a higher price than they would a ticket chosen for them. Subjects given the opportunity to practice a novel game of chance would bet more than those denied such an opportunity. Finally, subjects led to believe that they were particularly successful during the early trials of a cointossing task rated themselves as significantly better predictors of outcomes than subjects led to believe they performed poorly in the early stages of the task.

In summary, if devices conventionally characteristic of skill situations are introduced into chance situations, individuals will inappropriately shift their expectations of success to levels better than chance. For example, provision of "feature" buttons which control aspects of slot machine behavior may enhance beliefs that skill is relevant to this form of gambling. Studies of gamblers in naturalistic settings yield confirmatory data. Regular gamblers frequently deny the importance of chance factors in their chosen pursuit, erroneously believing that they have devised a winning system. They display flexible attributions in that success is attributed to their own skill, whereas external factors such as bad luck or fluke circumstances are invoked to account for losses.

It is also clear that individuals vary in the degree to which they generally attribute outcomes to internal factors, such as skill, or to external factors, such as luck. Thus, some individuals may be more likely to adopt a skill or control perspective in essentially chance situations. There is certainly evidence from studies of slot machine players that an internal locus of control may be particularly characteristic of young pathological slot machine gamblers. [See MENTAL CONTROL ACROSS THE LIFESPAN.]

B. Personality

Aside from orientations regarding the locus of control, other personality factors have been implicated as predisposing a person to pathological gambling. Given the variety of personality questionnaires that have been deployed and the variations in the populations studied, it is perhaps hardly surprising that not all studies point in the same direction. Nevertheless, some consistent themes can be discerned. Sensation-seeking, impulsivity, and lack of concern for others emerge as characteristic of pathological gamblers in a number of studies. [See PERSONALITY.]

Results from studies that have measured a disposition toward sensation-seeking have yielded equivocal results. However, perhaps sensation-seeking is best regarded in the context of prevailing levels of stimulation. Evidence seems to indicate that pathological gamblers, apart from their gambling, endure a lifestyle noticeably low in stimulation, and many report relief from boredom as a major motivating force. Accordingly, to the extent that sensation-seeking is implicated in pathological gambling, it is perhaps less as a personality trait, and more as a response to characteristically low levels of stimulation and arousal.

While caution is appropriate, given the bias toward male subjects in research, impulsivity and a lack of concern for others emerge from a number of studies of pathological gamblers. Pathological gamblers score high on a range of questionnaires devised to measure disregard for others, lack of empathy, inability to form and sustain relationships, attraction to risk and danger, and preference for immediate stimulation regardless of the consequences. Further evidence on im-

pulsivity emerges from electroencephalographic studies. Drawing on the theory that brain hemispheric dysregulation is related to poor impulse control, hemispheric activation was measured in response to simple verbal versus nonverbal tasks. Pathological gamblers showed a pattern of activation dissimilar to normal control subjects, but similar in many ways to children with attention deficit disorder. Probably the major behavioral characteristic of such children is impulsivity. It has been speculated that at the neurochemical level, poor control of impulses may reflect a deficit in a particular brain neurotransmitting substance, serotonin. There is some recent evidence in line with this speculation. A serotonergic probe was used to measure the degree of activity of the serotonin system in pathological gamblers and matched control subjects. The pathological gamblers showed hypoactivity relative to the controls. It would appear that pathological gambling may share common neurochemical features with other behavioral disturbances characterized by poor impulse control.

C. Arousal

A number of recent theories propose an important role for arousal in pathological gambling theories. Such theories add arousal, as a reinforcer on a fixed-interval schedule, to the more commonly hypothesized variable financial schedule to explain what sustains pathological gambling. Indeed, it has been argued that arousal as a reinforcer may be the most important determinant of loss of control. From this perspective, then, arousal in combination with irregular financial schedules is regarded as the driving force behind pathological gambling.

Early laboratory investigations of heart rate as an index of arousal suggested that gambling was not particularly provocative. However, the ecological validity of these studies has been questioned. Tellingly, a key study found only modest increases in heart rate among students and regular gamblers in the context of a laboratory casino. For the regular gamblers in a real casino, however, substantial increases in heart rate accompanied gambling. Furthermore, the magnitude of the increase was related to the size of the wager. In subsequent studies, reliable increases in cardiovascular activity has been observed during slot machine play and horse race gambling.

Nevertheless, there is still no strong evidence that

individual variation in arousal underlies pathological gambling; that is, there is no evidence that pathological gamblers are any more aroused by gambling than recreational gamblers. Furthermore, a recent study comparing pathological and recreational slot machine gamblers suggested that it might be baseline levels of arousal that are discriminating, and not the magnitude of the increase provoked by gambling; pathological slot machine gamblers tended to register low baseline arousal levels.

V. TREATMENT

A variety of treatments have been applied to pathological gambling, but have not, on the whole, been subject to systematic and controlled evaluation. Because, for many, GA is the main or only recourse available, it is unfortunate that its mixture of disclosure and social support has received so little formal evaluation. In a study of 232 GA attenders in Scotland, 8% were abstinent at the 1-year follow-up; by the 2-year follow-up, 7% remained abstinent. The addition of behavior therapy to the usual GA provisions seemed to produce better results; in one study in the United States that used this combination, 54% reported gambling less than they did before treatment. This latter study raises an, as yet, unresolved issue: the appropriate outcome measure. Whereas earlier studies championed complete abstinence, there has been a shift toward moderated gambling as the preferred treatment outcome. Moderated gambling is not necessarily, as critics claim, associated with an increased probability of a return to pathological gambling. There is even evidence that intermittent relapses from complete abstinence can occur without gambling returning to pathological proportions. [See BEHAVIOR THERAPY.]

A number of earlier studies applied behavioral techniques to the treatment of pathological gambling. The underlying assumption of the behavioral approach is that pathological gambling constitutes a learned response to schedules of intermittent reinforcement by money and arousal. The most common treatment procedures have been aversive conditioning and covert sensitization. In the former, unpleasant, but not painful, electric shocks are administered while individuals engage in gambling behavior. In the latter, aversive imagery is substituted for the electric shocks; the gambler is guided through a sequence of imagined gambling scenes characterized by unpleasant physical (e.g., nausea) or social (e.g., discovered gambling by spouse) consequences.

The application of both of these techniques has produced encouraging outcomes, with up to 40 to 50% of pathological gamblers reporting either complete abstinence or that gambling is under control at follow-up. Nevertheless, caution is warranted. None of the behavioral treatment studies to date has included proper control conditions, many have treated very small numbers of gamblers, and the follow-up period has often been of limited and insufficient duration.

More recently, cognitive therapies have been tried. These are based on the assumption that faulty and erroneous cognitions are important determinants of pathological gambling. The aim of therapy is to replace dysfunctional cognitions with adaptive and rationale thinking. While there are fewer data available, cognitive therapies would seem to produce outcomes not wholly dissimilar to more purely behavioral approaches; that is, about 40 to 50% of pathological gamblers derive benefit from the therapy. [See COGNITIVE THERAPY.]

Of the various behavioral and cognitive approaches that have been applied, currently the most promising is imaginal desensitization. In contrast to covert sensitization described earlier, imaginal desensitization promotes images in which the gambler is no longer excited by gambling and no longer thinks of it as a way of dealing with tension, stress, and boredom. Participants practice relaxation along with imaging four scheduled scenes. In the one published controlled treatment outcome study, imaginal desensitization was compared with aversive therapy. Whereas only 2 out of 10 of aversive therapy participants reported that they were abstinent from gambling at 1-year follow-up, 7 out of the 10 imaginal desensitization participants did so.

As gambling has become more accessible, so the casualties have increased. While the development of effective treatment is very much in the early stages, the need is pressing. It is clear that our general understanding of pathological gambling is improving, and, accordingly, more recent therapeutic initiatives are being informed by more sophisticated theory. However, in this context, we would do well to pay more heed to the models of behavior change being deployed elsewhere. Most relevant are the therapeutic models being applied to changing unhealthy behaviors, such as cigarette smoking and poor dietary habits. In particular, the stages-of-change model, described first in 1984 by Prochaska and Di Clemente, is worth close consideration.

The stages-of-change model has, as its starting point, a keen appreciation that people differ in their willingness to consider or to adopt behavioral changes. Furthermore, the process of change contains a series of stages through which individuals progress, reflecting the temporal dimension in which behavior change occurs. A stages-of-change model may be particularly applicable to changing gambling behavior in that it describes both the nature of change and the strategies most likely to facilitate change. Five stages of change are identified. The first stage is known as precontemplation. Here, no or only occasional thought is given to changing behavior. The next stage is known as contemplation, in which the individual begins to consider changing his or her behavior. However, contemplation does not guarantee action, and individuals can still slip back to the precontemplation stage. Nevertheless, contemplation may lead to active consideration, which is the necessary launching pad for behavioral change. These stages of active consideration and achievement of behavioral change are the planning and action stages. The final stage is one of consolidation and maintenance of behavioral change. From this perspective, intervention is about moving individuals from one stage to the next, from precontemplation to contemplation, from contemplation to active consideration, and so on. Thus, it is important that the therapist appreciates what stage the individual is at and also that different sorts of intervention are called for, dependent on stage. A number of researchers have identified phases in the career of a pathological gambler. At the very least, it has been argued, it is important to distinguish between acquisition and maintenance. Nevertheless, there has been, as yet, no systematic attempt to exploit a stages model in treating pathological gamblers.

Preventive strategies have received limited attention, although there are encouraging preliminary results from a high school-based program in Quebec. However, given the evidence implicating early initiation into gambling in the development of pathological gambling and the high prevalence rates of pathological gambling among adolescents in many countries,

substantially greater energies should be devoted to developing and evaluating preventive strategies.

VI. CONCLUSIONS

It is clear that relaxation of legislative strictures and easing of access are associated with increased gambling. This is evident both in the numbers gambling and the monies wagered. It is almost certain that such changes have consequences for the numbers who gamble pathologically.

While substantial progress has been made, the study of gambling has still to yield a definitive account of the mechanisms that lead some individuals to pathological gambling. A variety of factors are undoubtedly involved. It is also likely that these various factors assume a different importance during progression from acquisition to maintenance, that is, from induction to addiction. For example, at the induction stage, positive cultural attitudes toward gambling, legislative laissez-faire, and early age of initiation all undoubtedly increase risk. Subsequently, compelling schedules of monetary reinforcement, the consistently arousing nature of gambling in the context of an otherwise unfulfilling and unstimulating lifestyle, a tendency to presume control when it is chance that operates, and a personality high on impulsivity and low on social concern, are all likely to be significant factors. Nevertheless, this is merely the bare bones of a theory, and, aside from the proposed role of hemispheric dysregulation and serotonergic deficits in impulsivity, we are without any account of the mechanisms operating at a neurobiological level. Given that pathological gambling may not be phenomenally distinct from other addictive behaviors, it is perhaps to the neurobiology of other, more fully studied addictions that gambling researchers should look for clues.

Both behavior and cognitive treatment techniques have been applied to pathological gamblers with some success. However, there is a dearth of properly controlled therapeutic trials. In addition, the treatment of pathological gambling could well benefit from adopting the therapeutic models that have been used successfully in other areas of behavior change. In particular, much could be gained from adopting a model that appreciates stages of change. Furthermore, more attention needs to be paid to preventive strategies. Given the prevalence rates of pathology gambling in young people, it is imperative that effective school-based preventive programs are developed. Finally, there may be a need to consider selective legislative intervention. Many of the substantial numbers of young people in the United Kingdom who fall afoul of slot machines could be helped by effective treatment regimes. However, simple legislative reform, restricting access to those 18 years or older, would undoubtedly yield more immediate and cost-effective dividends.

BIBLIOGRAPHY

Blaszczynski, A., & Silove, D. (1995). Cognitive and behavioral therapies for pathological gambling. *Journal of Gambling Studies, 11*, 195–219.

Carroll, D., & Huxley, J. A. A. (1994). Cognitive, dispositional and psychophysiological correlates of dependent slot machine gambling in young people. *Journal of Applied Social Psychology, 24*, 1070–1083.

Galski, T. (Ed.). (1987). *The handbook of pathological gambling.* Springfield, IL: Charles C. Thomas.

Langer, E. J. (1983). *The psychology of control.* Beverley Hills, CA: Sage.

Lesieur, H. R. (1994). Epidemiological surveys of pathological gambling: Critique and suggestions for modification. *Journal of Gambling Studies, 10*, 385–398.

Lesieur, H. R., & Rosenthal, R. J. (1991). Pathological gambling: A review of the literature. *Journal of Gambling Studies, 7*, 5–39.

Prochaska, J. O., & Di Clemente, C. C. (1984). *The transtheoretical approach: Crossing traditional foundations of change.* Homewood, IL: Don Jones, Irwin.

Rosenthal, R. J. (1992). Pathological gambling. *Psychiatric Annals, 22*, 72–78.

Shaffer, H. J., Stein, S. A., Gambino, B., & Cummings, T. N. (Eds.). (1989). *Compulsive gambling: Theory, research, and practice.* Lexington, MA: Lexington Books.

Volberg, R. A. (1996). Prevalence studies of problem gambling in the United States. *Journal of Gambling Studies, 12*, 111–128.

Walker, M. B. (1992). *The psychology of gambling.* Oxford, UK: Pergamon Press.

Gender Differences in Mental Health

Esther R. Greenglass

York University

Coping The process of changing behavior and thoughts to manage the situation involving stressors.
Gender Role A set of socially significant activities associated with men or women.
Gender Stereotypes Beliefs about characteristics associated with or activities appropriate to men or women.
Panic Attack An anxiety disorder in which intense fear occurs without a fear-provoking situation.
Social Support Receipt of emotional, material, practical, or informational resources from friends and family.

In this article, discussion will center around the diagnosis of mental illness and how it varies with **GENDER**. Gender ratios in various indices of mental illness will be examined, along with the relationship between social roles, gender and mental health. Gender-role socialization predisposes each sex to different kinds of mental illness. In the discussion that follows, sociocultural and psychosocial models are applied to an understanding of the etiology of mental disorders in men and women. In addition, patterns of mental health as related to stress are compared in women and men. How people cope with their stress is important for mental health and in fact differs according to gender. Social support is related positively to mental health; gender effects in this relationship are examined. The process of psychotherapy is reviewed and traditional versus feminist therapies are compared. Drug therapy is also described.

I. DIAGNOSIS, MENTAL ILLNESS, AND GENDER

Men and women often receive different diagnoses for mental illness. Diagnosis according to a system of classification is a necessary part of treatment. In North America, the *Diagnostic and Statistical Manual of Mental Disorders* (*DSM*) of the American Psychiatric Association has become the standard used by mental health professionals in making a diagnosis. Currently, the fourth edition of the *DSM* is in use. Using this system clinicians match the patient's symptoms against a description and make diagnoses on each of five axes. The first three axes provide the diagnosis and the other two axes provide an evaluation of stressors and overall functioning. The manual consists of more than 200 different diagnoses with descriptions of symptoms that characterize the disorders. Women's higher rate of treatment and the gender differences observed in some categories have led some to argue that there is a gender bias in the *DSM*, especially in the personality disorder diagnoses that appear on Axis II. Some personality disorders are more common in women, whereas others are more common in men. Since the descriptions of these disorders seem like exaggerations or stereotypes of the male or female gender roles, the *DSM* classification system has been labelled as biased. [*See* DSM-IV.]

While the *DSM-III-R* was being revised, feminist therapists realized that several new categories were being considered for inclusion that had negative implications for women. Two of these were the "premenstrual dysphoric disorder" (now called the Late Luteal Phase Dysphoric Disorder) and "self-defeating personality." These correspond to what is popularly known as the premenstrual syndrome and the masochistic personality, respectively. This has the effect of labeling female experience and stereotypic feminine traits as mental illness symptoms. Despite widespread opposition, they are now included in the *DSM*. [*See* PREMENSTRUAL SYNDROME (PMS); PREMENSTRUAL SYNDROME TREATMENT INTERVENTIONS.]

Opposition to these kinds of labels is due to the observation that personality traits are enduring patterns of behavior or thinking about oneself. An example would be masochism, which, for many, is thought of as a trait. However, research has shown that many of the behaviors associated with this category decrease when the victimized person is removed from the abusive context. Such a quick response to a change in the environment would be evidence *against* underlying pathology and *for* a situational explanation for the behavior where the stimuli eliciting the behavior are present in the person's immediate environment. The "masochism" label obscures the role of the psychosocial and cultural environment in determining behavior but rather blames the woman for her problems. Gender bias in the *DSM* is not limited to women. Some of the *DSM* diagnostic categories seem to draw from certain dimensions of the masculine gender role. For example, one personality disorder, "antisocial personality disorder," appears to be an exaggeration of the traditional masculine gender role. It is described as a pattern of disregard for, and violation of the rights of others. And, as expected, men receive this diagnosis more often than women. In other research there is evidence that stereotypes regarding men influence behavior in that therapists have been found to urge men who have nontraditional life-styles to consider a change to more traditional masculine behavior.

Arguments that stereotypes have been applied to diagnosis go beyond the *DSM* and in fact affect the diagnosis of mental illness according to most systems. Much of the criticism that has been voiced refers to the bias against women and the labeling of feminine stereotypes as mental disorders. One of the earliest studies of gender stereotypes and their relationship to diagnoses is that of Inge Broverman and her colleagues conducted in the early 1970s. In this study, the standards of mental health for women and men were examined in mental health professionals including psychologists, psychiatrists, and social workers. Results were that clinicians held different ideals for mentally healthy functioning adult males and females. For example, they described the ideal healthy woman as being more submissive, less independent and adventurous, more easily influenced, less aggressive and competitive, more easily excitable in minor crises, more easily hurt, more emotional, less objective, and less interested in math and science than the ideal healthy man. Also, their ideal of the healthy man was similar to that of a healthy mature adult (gender unspecified), but their ideal of a healthy woman was quite different from both. One conclusion from the study was that women were caught in a double bind. If they met the standards for a healthy adult, they were defined as unfeminine and thus poorly adjusted. If they met the mental health standards for their gender, they were inadequate compared to the ideal for healthy adults. The study also demonstrated that clinicians shared with others popular beliefs about appropriate characteristics of men and women.

Today, while therapists no longer list different characteristics as desirable for mentally healthy women and men, studies find that in practice, clinicians' judgments about their clients are influenced by stereotypes about gender roles. And, naturalistic studies of therapists and their clients suggest that gender bias is still rampant. Thus, the evidence indicates that the practice of psychotherapy tends to work toward preserving traditional gender roles in both women and men.

II. MENTAL ILLNESS AND GENDER RATIOS

Women and men differ in the diagnoses they receive. There appears to be agreement among clinicians that three categories of mental illness are more likely to be found on average in women than in men. These are depression, anorexia, and agoraphobia. According to statistics, 20 to 26% of women will experience diagnosable depression at some time in their lives compared with 8 to 12% of men. Further, it is estimated that among individuals given some treatment for depression, the ratio of women to men is 2 to 1. Depressed individuals describe their emotional state in negative terms; they are sad; they may experience insomnia, fatigue, loss of appetite, slow speech, indecisiveness, hopelessness, and feelings of inadequacy. [*See* DEPRESSION.]

Reasons for depression can be found in both medical and social models. According to the medical model, women are biologically more vulnerable to certain disorders, especially depression. Women are seen as being at risk during periods of hormonal change such as menstruation, following childbirth, and at menopause. Three syndromes have been identified as being associated with various stages of women's reproductive cycle. These are the premenstrual syndrome or PMS, postpartum depression, and the menopausal syndrome. However, reproductively related symptoms are poorly defined, often lacking medical consensus for diagnosis and medical treatment. In fact, feminist theorists have charged that biological determinist causes of women's behavior are often used to ignore the social and political context of women's reproductive experiences. And, according to Rhoda Unger and Mary Crawford, the existence of so-called reproductive syndromes help to justify beliefs in the biological inferiority of women.

Research supports the idea that depression often has social roots. It has been argued that women suffer more from depression because of social roles, lack of reinforcement, helplessness, violence, and poverty. It is documented that an increasing number of those living below the poverty line are women and their children, a phenomenon known as the feminization of poverty. This, in turn, is related to factors such as the increased proportion of single-parent households headed by women, inadequacy of child support payments following divorce, and lack of affordable childcare and housing. Evidence shows a link between poverty and mental health problems. Therefore, higher poverty rates among women significantly contribute to their higher rates of depression. For example, studies have found that depression is high among women living in poverty with young children. Victims of sexual and physical abuse are also highly vulnerable to depression.

Others argue that the feminine gender role makes women susceptible to depression by encouraging them to feel helpless by teaching them to respond to stress in powerless ways. Martin Seligman's learned helplessness theory as a cause of depression may help explain women's depression. According to him, depressives have a history of learning that they are incapable of successful mastery and control over their lives. In short, they have learned to regard themselves as helpless. The sense of helplessness and lack of control he talks about sound very much like the powerlessness that is characteristic of many women. If women in our society lack power, this may contribute to a sense of helplessness and thus to depression. The sense of helplessness, that one's behaviors do not affect outcomes, can generalize to new situations. Thus, the individual learns that his or her behaviors will be ineffectual in dealing with stressful situations, thus leading to an increased susceptibility to depression. At the same time, when men are depressed, they engage in activities that tend to distract them from their feelings. Men are socialized to be active and to ignore their feelings of weakness. While men may be taught to be independent and not seek help for depression, expectations associated with the feminine gender role may stress the importance of the woman paying attention to her moods and seeking help.

Anorexia nervosa is an eating disorder characterized by overcontrol of eating for weight reduction. This disorder is present mainly in women, 90% of anorexics are females, and a majority of them are adolescents. This disorder has been estimated to affect 1 in 250 adolescent girls. A major symptom is loss of 20% or more of body weight. The anorexic's body image is distorted so that she believes herself to be fat even though she may be emaciated. Another eating disorder found disproportionately in females is bulimia, where the person binges on food and then purges the body of the calories by vomiting and/or using laxatives. Research on college populations indicate that as many as 13 to 20% of the women have engaged in bulimic behaviors. [*See* ANOREXIA NERVOSA AND BULIMIA NERVOSA.]

Several factors have been identified as contributing to eating disorders. A major factor is media-related. A generation ago, female models weighed 8% less than the average woman and today they weigh 23% less. Moreover, the average woman portrayed in the media today weighs less and looks thinner than 95% of the female population. The role models in the media, pressures for thinness ubiquitous in our society, along with strong desire for peer group acceptance and popularity combine to make the adolescent female highly vulnerable to eating disorders. Other predisposing factors include disturbed familial relationships, loss of a boyfriend, and disturbed cognitions such as a distorted body image. Once excessive dieting begins to occur, secondary gains include attention and positive reinforcement for weight loss. [See DIETING.]

Agoraphobia, in which there is anxiety about being in places or situations from which escape might be difficult or in which help may not be available in the event of having a panic attack, is more likely to occur in women. Such feelings of anxiety often result in the person avoiding situations that might elicit such feelings. Agoraphobia is an anxiety disorder and is considered to be the most common phobic reaction seen by psychotherapists. Agoraphobic individuals label themselves as anxious rather than angry or sad. They also see themselves as fearful of criticism, disapproval, and rejection. Individuals with this disorder are often passive and dependent, indecisive, and lack the ability to express their feelings. Explanations for the etiology of agoraphobia tend to be gender-role based, drawing on the differing expectations for coping with fear incorporated into feminine and masculine roles. For example, girls are reinforced not for mastery, but for expressing their fears and remaining helpless and dependent, whereas socialization of males encourages them to master their fears. It has been suggested that agoraphobia may be elicited when an individual who was socialized to be dependent becomes pressured to be independent. Agoraphobic women exhibit extreme forms of personal attributes associated with the feminine gender role, including helplessness, overdependency, and passivity. Lack of instrumentality, the capability of self-assertion and competence, the key aspect of traditional masculinity, also characterize agoraphobics. Women lower in instrumentality, mastery, and perceived control are also more likely to have helplessness expectancies and negative outcome expectancies combining to create hopelessness, which leads to a variety of mental illnesses. Existing evidence suggests that mental health outcomes are better understood using gender-based models. [See PHOBIAS.]

Men outnumber women in the substance-abuse disorders, particularly those involving alcohol and illegal drugs. In order to receive a diagnosis of one of the types of substance abuse, the individual must not only use the drug but must also exhibit a strong desire to use the substance and experience problems in social or occupational functioning due to drug use. The ratio of men problem drinkers to women is about 3 to 1, however, the number of women who drink alcohol has increased. Among younger age groups, 21 to 29 years old, a much higher rate of heavy drinking for women was found than in women of the same age group in previous generations. Research suggests that among younger women, those who are employed are more likely than housewives to be problem drinkers. It is hypothesized that alcoholism rates for males and females are getting closer in part because of the change in gender roles, making drinking more acceptable in women. Nevertheless, female drunkenness is viewed less tolerantly than male drunkenness. Alcoholism is judged more harshly in women. Illegal drug use is higher in men than in women, with men's use of drugs such as heroin, amphetamines, cocaine, and marijuana paralleling their use of alcohol. Some have suggested that men are more likely than women to use illegal drugs and alcohol to mask their depression rather than admit to feelings of weakness. [See ALCOHOL PROBLEMS; SUBSTANCE ABUSE.]

Some *DSM* categories of mental illness seem to be exaggerations of the traditional masculine gender role. Two of these are applied more often to men than women. For example, schizoid personality disorder is characterized by "detachment from social relationships and a restricted range of expression of emotions in interpersonal settings." And, antisocial personality disorder appears as a "pervasive pattern of disregard for, and violation of, the rights of others." These disorders also reflect the masculine gender role in that it stresses independence, separation, and strength. The strict prohibition against emotional expressiveness in men (except perhaps anger) is one of the most powerful masculine mental mandates influencing men and their behavior. Male inexpressiveness is the result of gender role socialization that begins early in childhood. Men are taught that emotional expressiveness is a feminine trait and they learn to distance themselves from femininity. At the same time, masculine socialization contributes to and encourages aggressive behavior in men. Men are more involved than women in violent crime, including armed robbery, spouse and child abuse, and rape. While aggression in the sports and military context is socially approved and rewarded, the social program associated with masculinity also includes competitiveness and aggression that are socially sanctioned as masculine coping styles. [*See* AGGRESSION; CRIMINAL BEHAVIOR.]

While women more often express distress in internalized and depressive symptomatology, men often cope with their feelings differently in that they are more likely to externalize their feelings such as becoming physically aggressive or by distracting themselves from their feelings by engaging in a variety of activities. The violence committed by men against women in its many forms is in part an outcome of a society that is dominated by men who see themselves as controlling women in many different contexts. Research suggests that power, sexual control, and aggression are amplified in men in a patriarchal society such as ours. The mental health costs of male violence justify reexamination of the prescriptions of the masculine gender role. The idea that gender-role socialization of men and women predisposes each sex to different kinds of mental illness may be viewed as an application of sociocultural and psychosocial models to the etiology of mental illness. This necessitates examining as well the relationship between social roles and mental illness.

III. SOCIAL ROLES, GENDER, AND MENTAL HEALTH

The notion that socially prescribed roles influence mental health is evident when examining research findings relating marital status to mental health, findings which at times differ according to gender. Early research indicated an interaction between gender and marital status regarding mental illness—married men had lower rates of mental illness than married women, but unmarried men had higher rates of mental disorders than unmarried women. Overall, more married than single women have been reported to be passive, phobic, and depressed. More married women than married men have been found to experience psychological and physical anxiety as well as immobilization. However, more recent research indicates that while married women do exhibit higher rates of distress than married men, sex differences in distress in the unmarried are either nonexistent or in the same dir-

ection, with women having higher rates of distress than men. And, psychological research evidence indicates that marriage may benefit mental health in both women and men.

Empirical research provides evidence that certain sets of multiple roles are beneficial for mental health. Involvement in multiple roles expands potential resources and rewards including alternative sources of self-esteem and social support, all of which can enhance mental health. The employment role provides financial, psychological, and social resources for women and men. Employed married women have lower rates of psychological distress than their unemployed female counterparts. And for both men and women, work provides an important link to social support providers. [*See* SELF-ESTEEM; SOCIAL SUPPORT.]

But, increasingly, research is suggesting that the quality of a person's experiences within and across roles and not merely role occupancy per se, are critical to understanding mental health outcomes. Women are more likely than men to experience high levels of demands with low control over those demands in the workplace. Having low-quality roles such as those with time constraints, irregular schedules, and low control may jeopardize mental health, whereas having high-quality roles may help maintain or enhance it. Positive mental health outcomes are associated with the degree of control a woman exerts over the demands in her environment. Research supports the idea that psychological well-being in women is related to greater equity in the marital relationship and greater decision making by women.

The consequences of multiple role occupancy are not uniformly positive, especially for women. Women in the labor force also perform most of the domestic work and on average spend more hours in housework and childcare than do men. Wives are still responsible for two-thirds of the housework and childcare and are doing from 13 to 17 hours more of work within the home than men. Employed married women still manifest higher rates of distress than employed married men. And, employed married women with young children experience higher rates of psychological distress than their childless counterparts or comparable men. Given the demands on women when combining employment and familial roles, many women experience interrole conflict and/or role overload. For women, familial obligations are expected to take precedence over those associated with employment. Compared with fathers, mothers are far more likely to fit their employment around their families' needs. Women's roles are inherently stressful in that they obligate them to respond to others, including the very young as well as the elderly. Informal care for elderly parents and relatives is generally provided primarily by women. These demands are a significant source of stress, thus playing an important role in women's mental health. Elements of the feminine gender role endanger women's mental health in that the provision of care for their families and friends can be and often is emotionally and physically draining, particularly given the relative lack of fathers' participation in work at home. [See PARENTING.]

Further research findings suggest that increased involvement in the fathering role can have positive mental health effects in men. In a review of research on paternal involvement, findings are that fathers who increased their involvement with their children experienced self-confidence in their parenting abilities, in satisfaction with their fathering role, and an increase in their overall self-esteem. Redefining the masculine gender role to include a nurturing dimension will not only place men in equivalent dual roles as women, but will also contribute to positive mental health outcomes in men. [See FATHERS.]

IV. STRESS, MENTAL HEALTH, AND GENDER

Research indicates that women not only experience stress more than men, they also have more symptomatology than men. Women are exposed to more stressful life events than are men and, as a result, they have higher rates of psychological distress. Women experience anxiety and mood disorders at a greater rate than men. Women may appear to be more distressed than men as a result of the kind of outcome measures that are typically used in research in this area. These studies tend to employ self-report measures of symptomatology. It is generally assumed that if an individual is coping reasonably well, she/he is free from anxiety and depression. This conceptualization of effective coping leads to a bias in research findings given that women, more than men, often express distress. Some argue that women appear more distressed because they are more likely than men to

report symptoms of all kinds. Gender-role factors contribute to the degree to which individuals report symptoms and seek help. Traditional masculine and feminine gender roles differ in the amount of vulnerability and permissibility in seeking help from others. Traditionally, men are seen as strong and invulnerable, thus restraining men from showing symptoms of mental illness or seeking help. The traditional feminine gender role allows and even encourages vulnerability to problems, thus resulting in the greater reporting of illness symptomatology. [See COPING WITH STRESS; STRESS.]

Notwithstanding women's greater "openness" regarding their psychological symptomatology, research indicates many reasons for women's greater distress. Despite their greater employment, women still tend to be concentrated in "female" occupational spheres including education, health care, clerical, domestic, and service industries. Women have less promotional opportunities, make less money, and often do not have access to membership in the "old boys' network," all of which restricts their advancement on the job. Women professionals and managers are subject to negative stereotyped attitudes that portray women as doing a poor job fitting into the male work world. Sex discrimination and harassment remain endemic in the workplace. Such attitudes not only harm salary and promotion prospects for women, they are also detrimental to their mental health.

Reproductive life events including menstruation, pregnancy, childbirth, and menopause are stressful for women, and fluctuations in women's hormones do not explain responses to them. Research shows that neuroendocrine responses are altered by social roles and other sociocultural variables. Personal and social coping resources affect how women respond to these changes, which necessitates placing reproductive life events within a broader psychosocial framework in order to understand their effects on women.

V. STRESS, COPING, AND GENDER

Gender affects the way people cope with stress. For many there is the stereotyped idea of men as problem-focused and women as emotion-focused in their coping efforts. For example, men have been reported to be more likely than women to engage in coping that alters a stressful situation. Some assert that men more often possess psychological attributes, that is, self-esteem and mastery, that influence their coping. However, as has been pointed out by others, gender differences in mastery or a related characteristic, self-efficacy, are likely to be linked to differences in social experiences. A consistently unresponsive or negative environment has been found to affect a person's sense of self-efficacy, which in turn leads to anxiety and depression. Studies of gender differences in psychological characteristics have pointed out that models of stress and coping were developed primarily on men without consideration of women's roles and experiences and may not encompass other aspects of coping, including relationship-focused coping techniques.

Research shows that when education, occupation, and/or position are controlled for, few gender differences are found in coping strategies. The type of coping an individual employs when dealing with stress is often related to the status, resources, and power associated with one's position. Many more women than men hold lower level jobs with less scope for use of problem solving and direct action strategies. Women are also more likely than men to experience high levels of demands with low control over those demands in the workplace.

In a similar vein, coping research tends to narrowly focus on individual behavior as the unit of analysis and sees autonomous, agentic, and independent behavior as synonymous with effective coping. But, research shows that coping is highly specific to both the individual and the context. It is important to investigate a wide range of situations before concluding that we have a general theory of coping. The social milieu in which a particular stressor is experienced should be incorporated into research paradigms that inquire into the relationship between gender and coping. Women may behave in a more passive way in groups with men, where stereotyped roles and social norms may be more strictly enforced. But, these women may appear different when acting alone or in a same sex group.

VI. SOCIAL SUPPORT AND GENDER: IMPLICATIONS FOR COPING

There is evidence that social support has a positive effect on one's mental health. And, research suggests that social relationships with women are more health promoting than those with men. Wives are better providers of both instrumental and emotional support than husbands. Wives function more often than husbands as an important part of their spouses' support system. Men tend to benefit from relationships with women; women generally benefit from relationships with their friends, mainly those of the same sex.

Close relationships can help a person cope with psychological distress. In such relationships people can disclose and discuss problems, share concerns, and receive advice that is keyed to their psychological needs. These relationships can also provide useful information, practical advice, and morale boosting, all of which can assist an individual in dealing with their stressors and lessen psychological distress. Research shows that the connection between social support and coping is stronger in women. Women employ more coping forms involving interpersonal relationships. Other research findings suggest that women use support from others through talking with one another. Women are able to make more effective use of their support networks since they talk more as a way of coping with stress. Women are also more emotionally involved in others' lives and tend to serve a nurturing role for a wider network of people. The extent to which women's roles obligate them to respond to others' needs and the psychological costs to women of this kind of caring are important factors in women's mental health.

VII. PSYCHOTHERAPY AND GENDER

Psychotherapy is often sought when individuals are experiencing mental or emotional distress. In psychotherapy, people receive help in coping with their problems. Women are more likely than men to consult a therapist. Some argue that traditional psychotherapy is a form of social control. This is due to the observation that therapy, like marriage, can put a woman into a dependency relationship with an authority figure, in this case, the psychotherapist. And, just as diagnosis of mental illness can be biased, psychotherapy and therapists themselves can reflect sexist beliefs. There are reports of sexist attitudes toward women patients, of psychotherapists fostering traditional gender roles, and not being aware of women's experience of social situations. Another problem with traditional psychotherapy is that rather than focusing on the social context, a psychotherapist, particularly one who adheres to psychodynamic theory, is more likely to blame the individual for her problems. Often, when individuals have problems, they are seen as the source of their distress. Therapy is directed toward changing her and helping her adapt to the situation rather than focusing on changing an intolerable social situation, which may be the source of the woman's problems. Sexism in traditional therapy resides in the belief system that promotes "cures" for women's distress through individual personal change while at the same time ignoring the status quo.

Awareness of the problems in traditional therapy, particularly with respect to gender roles, has given rise to an alternative, namely feminist therapy. Feminist therapy discards traditional gender stereotypic assumptions about behavior. Feminist therapy incorporates the view that the differential roles and statuses prescribed for women and men are potentially harmful to both sexes, especially to women. One of the basic assumptions of feminist therapy is that "the personal is political." That is, an individual woman's problems are a reflection of the social and political structure of the society. Instead of focusing only on individual difficulties, this approach encourages the client to see his or her problem in its social/political context. In therapy the client learns to understand how society plays a role in shaping an individual's behavior. At the same time, she learns to validate her own experiences and explore her own values. In feminist therapy the client is empowered, the distance between therapist and client is decreased, and the therapeutic process is thereby demystified. Men may also be clients in feminist therapy, but men are less often in therapy of any kind than women. Their reluctance to seek therapy for their problems is a reflection of the masculine gender role and its emphasis on independence and invulnerability.

VIII. DRUG THERAPY

In addition to psychotherapy, drugs may be prescribed for individuals with emotional or mental distress. Often, psychoactive (or mood-altering) drugs are prescribed for psychological problems. These include antidepressants, sedatives, and tranquilizers, and findings indicate that these are far more likely to be pre-scribed for women than for men. Drug advertisements are a major influence in differential patterns of drug prescriptions for women and men. Images they use support stereotypes of women patients who are depicted more often as complaining of diffuse anxiety, depression, stress, and tension. [See PSYCHOPHARMACOLOGY.]

IX. CONCLUSIONS

Gender-role socialization predisposes women and men to different kinds of diagnoses and mental illness. Often stereotypic male or female traits are labeled as mental illness symptoms. Gender bias is very much a part of the diagnosis of mental illness. The effect of gender roles is to make certain types of disorders more likely in one sex or the other. The feminine gender role encourages women to focus more on their feelings and amplify them, the masculine gender role encourages males to distract themselves from their feelings. It has been argued that women are considered less psychologically healthy than men because men constitute the standard for what is mentally healthy. Increasingly, it is recognized that socially prescribed roles influence mental health, findings that at times differ according to gender. Just as the diagnosis of mental illness has been found to be sexist, traditional psychotherapy may also be biased. By blaming the patient for her problems, traditional therapy seeks a "cure" through changing individual behavior rather than focusing on the social context. While in the past, explanations of mental illness and mental health relied primarily on biogenic mediating factors, increasingly psychological research points to the importance of the social context, expectations and socialization in the understanding of human behavior.

BIBLIOGRAPHY

Brannon, L. (1996). *Gender: Psychological perspectives.* Needham Hts., MA: Allyn and Bacon.
Greenglass, E. R. (1991). Burnout and gender: Theoretical and organizational implications. *Canadian Psychology, 32,* 562–572.
Greenglass, E. R. (1995). Gender, work stress, and coping. Special Issue on gender in the workplace (Ed.) J. Struthers, *Journal of Social Behaviour and Personality, 10,* 121–134.
Lips, H. M. (1993). *Sex and gender: An introduction* (2nd ed.). Mountain View, CA: Mayfield.

Phares, V. (1996). Conducting nonsexist research, prevention, and treatment with fathers and mothers: A call for a change. *Psychology of Women Quarterly, 20,* 55–77.

Russo, N. F. & Green, B. (1993). Women and mental health. In F. L. Denmark and M. A. Paludi (Eds.), *Psychology of women: A handbook of issues and theories* (pp. 379–436). Westport, CT: Greenwood Press.

Unger, R., & Crawford, M. (1992). *Women and gender: A feminist psychology.* New York: McGraw-Hill.

Waldron, I. (1991). Effects of labour force participation on sex differences in mortality and morbidity. In M. Frankenhaeuser, U. Lundberg & M. Chesney (Eds.), *Women, work and health: Stress and opportunities* (pp. 17–38). New York: Plenum Press.

Gender Identity

Beverly Fagot and Carie Rodgers

University of Oregon and Oregon Social Learning Center

Gender The dimensions of masculinity and femininity; the culturally defined characteristics that are correlated with sex.

Gender labeling The ability of the child to give defining verbal labels to males and females.

Gender role The behaviors, traits, and attitudes defined by the culture as belonging to one sex or the other.

Gender segregation The tendency for males and females to cluster in same–sex groups.

Sex The dichotomous classification of people as male or female based upon biological characteristics.

The importance of **GENDER IDENTITY** for adjustment and psychopathology in childhood, adolescence, and adulthood has been an area in which there are far more traditional notions or unsupported theories than empirical data. Recent epidemiological studies confirm some of the traditional notions concerning gender differences in different types of psychopathology, but age, social class, and ethnic background also influence rates of adjustment and interact with gender. In this article, we will first review theories of gender development and normative gender develop-

ment. Second, we will discuss differences in competencies of boys and girls and men and women. Third, we will discuss differences in diagnoses and other measures of adjustment by gender. In the final section, we will speculate about how differential socialization and different cultural expectations influence rates of adjustment among males and females.

First, a word about sex and gender: We see these terms as neither completely interchangeable nor completely distinct. For the most part, we will use sex to refer to the dichotomous classification of people as male or female, and sex typing and sex roles in talking about what is assigned to people on the basis of their biological sex. We will use gender where the dimensions of masculinity and femininity come into play. This is not to say that masculinity and femininity are excluded from sex roles and typing, but that these dimensions are always present in our usage, with their implications of social and cultural baggage, whenever gender is mentioned.

I. THEORIES

Modern theories of parenting have their roots in Freud's description of the family. Freud articulated very clearly the family roles that mirrored the upper-middle-class European family structure during the late 1800s, with the mother providing love and warmth and the father providing rules and discipline. This has had a profound effect on our thinking about parenting, about the roles of the mother and father within the family, and about the gender role identification of boys and girls. Freud's influence on modern thinking should not be underrated. We cannot really understand the theoretical and empirical literature on parenting since the turn of the century without understanding how Freud's views have permeated our thinking. With Freud's emphasis on the satisfaction of drives came a clearer articulation that the quality of early care affects later development. Our emphasis on providing a sensitive caregiving environment during early childhood, as well as our articulations of family roles, are influenced, either directly by or in opposition to, Freudian thinking.

Freud viewed sex role development as a function of the biological sex of the child rather than in terms of socialization differences. He proposed two types of identification. The first is called *anaclitic* (basically, *leaning upon)*, which is somewhat parallel to what is today called attachment, although Freud believed it occurred because the caregiver satisfied the infant's basic needs. This type of identification, usually with the mother or some substitute female caregiver, was not differentiated for boys and girls. The second type of identification occurred during the *phallic* period, at around 4 years of age. During this time the child comes to have active sexual desires directed toward the opposite-sex parent. However, it soon becomes clear to the child that the same-sex parent, whom they view as their competitor for the sexual attention of the opposite-sex parent, is more powerful and that this situation must be resolved.

The resolution of this conflict and its outcome are very different for boys and girls. The terms *Oedipal* and *Electra complex* have become almost "pop psychology," but the far-reaching implications of the differential resolutions of boys' and girls' conflicts cannot be overstated. The boy—from fear of the father (whom he fears as the aggressor) and through his own fear of castration—resolves his conflict by identifying with the aggressor, and by doing so internalizes the attitudes, behaviors, and moral standards of the male parent. In this way the boy develops a strong superego and a complete identification with all that is male. For the girl, who has already identified with her mother through anaclitic attachment, the situation is somewhat different. Her phallic identification, which Freud claimed is less complete than that of the boy, takes place through fear of loss of love of the mother. To Freud, girls never internalize the female role as completely as boys do the male role, because the paralyz-

ing fear of castration, said to be felt by all small boys, was never present. In Freud's view, many male and female differences come from the differences in resolution of the identification process. From this theory we see the picture of the girl as incomplete, because she has not gone through the male identification process. This scenario has had a profound influence on psychological thinking about males and females, far beyond the amount of scientific support available for the theory.

During the past 40 years, the two major positions within the field have been social learning and cognitive development. There are many viewpoints within each broad area and the two approaches have come closer together in the 1980s and 1990s, but research in psychology since 1960 has been shaped primarily by these two theories. Social learning theorists have focused upon how the environment shapes boys' and girls' development. Studies have confirmed that boys and girls receive different information from both home and school environments. Cognitive developmentalists, such as Kohlberg in 1966, have emphasized the regularities in the child's understanding of gender and developed a stage theory of gender role development, focusing on the unfolding maturational process by which gender role development takes place. Kohlberg emphasized the sequence of identifying one's own sex (*gender identity*), of understanding that sex remained stable over time (*gender stability*), and of understanding that sex remained constant despite perceptual changes (*gender constancy*). Early work within the Kohlbergian framework tested, and for the most part confirmed, that there is a consistent sequence to children's understanding. While social learning theory emphasizes the role of the environment, and cognitive development theory emphasizes the role of maturational changes, both portray the child as essentially passive in the development of gender role.

Beginning with Martin and Halverson's article in 1981, research started to show that children actively contribute to their own gender role development. This view emphasized the normative nature of cognitive development, with gender presented as a special case. Martin and Halverson adopted the term *schema* to describe the outcome of the developmental process; a schema is an organized knowledge structure, and a gender schema is a knowledge structure organized around gender or sex. Researchers began to study how children's understanding of gender influenced their memories and information processing as well as their choice of toys and activities. As they try to understand all they see and hear, children begin to form categories that help organize the flood of information that inundates them. The distinction between female and male, feminine and masculine, provides a readily available organizing principle that is relevant to the child.

During the 1980s there were several attempts to bring together views from cognitive development and social learning theories as applied to children's gender role development. Because children live in a sex-typed world, they develop gender schemas that guide the choice of "sex-appropriate" behaviors and the knowledge of the action patterns necessary for carrying them out. Gender role adoption is expected to occur as the self-concept is assimilated to the gender schema and as children adopt standards of sex appropriateness in accordance with the information to which they are exposed. Schema formation undoubtedly depends upon the child's own mental effort and developmental status, but the information being processed must reflect the degree and importance of gender typing in the child's surroundings. Thus, schema theory offers a framework for describing and integrating the development of gender understanding with environmental information and values.

II. GENDER IDENTITY DEVELOPMENT

Gender identity development includes the socialization of sex-typed values, behaviors, and attitudes by families, peers, and schools, as well as children's characteristics and cognitive capacities as they affect use of information provided by the environment. Our convictions that environmental influences are often more subtle and more powerful than has been asserted, and children's gender understanding more complex and less concrete, have both shaped and been shaped by the work we will discuss here.

Gender is the ultimate real-world category system. Every ordinary human being must deal with it in many ways, on many levels. Physiology defines the most fundamental level, designating people as male or female on the basis of their sexual anatomy, but every known society surrounds the basic facts of sexual form and function with a system of social rules

concerning what males and females are supposed to be and do. As children internalize and master this system, they learn to discriminate and label themselves and others on the basis of sex, to recognize attributes, attitudes, and behaviors that are typical of or considered appropriate for each sex, and to learn how to do what is seen as appropriate and to avoid what is not. What is more, the gender category system is infused with affect to an extent few other knowledge bases can match, making it the most universally salient parameter of social categorization available to the young child.

The raw materials of sex role acquisition are the child's physical makeup and inherent capacity to learn, and the information and consequences provided by the environment. What the child contributes and what the environment provides cannot be independent of one another. They interact, and interact dynamically. That is, each affects the other so that as the child grows neither child nor environment remain static. We agree with current cognitive-developmental theory that children construct their own understanding of the world as they go along, but we insist that the building blocks used in this construction include the information and consequences socializing agents and cultural practices provide.

The external powers of sex typing can be blatant, as are television commercials, and forceful, even cruel, as peer reaction to boys who try out cross-gender behaviors. More often they are ubiquitous and fairly subtle. To illustrate, in our laboratory we have found mothers more likely than fathers to use directions and instructions as they interact with their children. The disparity in parental verbalization emerges and is greatest when children are about 18 months old and are not yet showing many behavioral sex differences. Not only are mothers more inclined to use and model this kind of instructive interaction, girls receive more of it than boys do. In addition, boys and girls in play groups receive different types of attention from teachers. In our laboratory we observed children from 12 to 16 months of age in infant play groups who were engaged in either assertive behaviors or attempts to communicate with adults. There were no sex differences in the rate at which children showed these behaviors. However, girls were given more positive responses for their attempts to communicate with the teachers, and their interactions with teachers lasted longer. At the same time, boys received more adult attention for negative or acting-out behavior, whereas such behavior in girls tended to be ignored. When the same group of children were observed in play groups 12 months later, we found sex differences in aggression and in the amount of time boys and girls engaged in communication with the teachers. In other words, precursors to aggressive behavior tend to be strengthened in boys but extinguished in girls, while girls are learning how to communicate effectively with adults. By the time children are ready to enter school, adults respond to the type of behavior rather than the sex of the child, but by then boys show higher rates of aggression and girls are better prepared for the school role.

These examples from our work illustrate two of the ways in which environmental input and developmental status interact to facilitate the acquisition of gender roles. First, findings concerning family influences are very likely to be age- and behavior-specific. The latter part of the second year exemplifies a transition time in which it is particularly important to study the process of gender role socialization. Both children and parents are learning new skills and new ways of relating to each other. Children are starting to exert control of their environment as their developing capabilities allow them to do so, and parents feel a need to teach appropriate behaviors as the child begins to enter the larger world. We will argue that parental socialization of sex typing will be greatest at such times of transition and that once children have adopted traditionally sex-typed behaviors, many mechanisms in society maintain their choices. In addition, many differences in the treatment of boys and girls are small, subtle, and indirect, but even apparently minor differences in boys' and girls' environments at crucial times can have long-term consequences. We must not discount the power of these influences nor fail to investigate the ways in which they contribute to the "gendering" of the child.

However, there is also little doubt that children bring a good deal of organization to the gender identity process. One of the characteristics of infants is their ability to develop categories. Certainly, by a few months of age, infants show the ability to develop perceptually based categories. Infants in the second half of the first year, rather than focusing just on perceptual characteristics, show signs of incorporating functional and contextual information into the categorization process so that there is some indication that at least a basic conceptual understanding of objects has emerged. There is evidence that some 7-month-old infants categorize faces by gender, although it may be that they are using perceptual cues, and comparing as like/not like the exemplar. However, categorization does not appear to be related to family variables in the child's environment, nor does the age at which the child can categorize predict anything about the child's future gender role behaviors.

During the child's second year, language becomes increasingly important and gender categories now come to be labeled. In 1986, Leinbach and Fagot developed a gender-labeling task that consisted of 12 paired pictures of adults and 12 paired pictures of children. Children first learned the adult discrimination of either man or woman, or more usually of mommy and daddy, at about 20 months. The learning of gender labels for boys and girls came almost 8 months later at a mean age of 28 months. Unlike attainment of gender categories as measured by the habituation paradigm, the gender-labeling task appears to be related to a number of social behaviors.

In our laboratory we examined a sample of children, half of whom had passed the gender-labeling task and half of whom had not. The children were observed in ongoing play groups for 2 weeks after they had been given the gender-labeling task. Three different types of behavior (sex-typed toy choices, same-sex peer choice, and aggressive behaviors) were examined, as these are all behaviors that have shown gender typing in previous research. We did not find any effect of passing or failing the adult-labeling task, nor did we really expect to as we felt it was the ability to label self and others like self that would accelerate adoption of gender role behaviors. Children who showed knowledge concerning the boy-girl labels were more likely to play with same-sex peers. Finally, a rather unexpected finding was that girls who passed the boy-girl gender-labeling task showed much less aggression than those who failed the task. For boys there was no effect on aggressive behavior of learning gender labels. This was a cross-sectional study, and compared a group of rather mixed age children at a single point in time.

We have replicated these results with a group of children followed longitudinally from the time they were 18 months until they passed the boy-girl-labeling task. The age of passing ranged from 21 to 37 months. We had two goals: First, to determine if children who were early versus late labelers differed in their behaviors prior to labeling. Second, we were interested in seeing if the child's behavior changed between the term prior and the term after boy-girl gender labeling was obtained. Because we expected age related changes, we divided the children into two groups, one consisted of children who had passed gender labels by 28 months, the other consisted of children who passed later than that. We compared all of the children in their first term of play groups, when they were 18 to 21 months of age and had not passed the gender-labeling task. We used the same three sets of behaviors to compare the children: sex-typed toy play, play with same-sex peer, and aggression. We found no differences between the two groups who would become early versus late labelers on sex-typed toy play, but we did find the beginnings of sex-typed toy choices. Boys preferred playing with male-typed toys and avoided female-typed toys, whereas girls played more with female-typed toys but did not avoid male-typed toys. Neither boys nor girls nor early versus late labelers showed a significant preference for playing within their own-sex groups. There were no differences in aggression between boys and girls or between early and late labelers. Before any of them learned gender labels, the sex-typed toy play of children who would become early versus late labelers was very similar, but there were the beginnings of preferences in sex-typed toy play. [*See* PLAY.]

The next set of questions concerned changes in behavior as a function of gaining gender label understanding. We were interested in changes in children's behavior in the play groups as a function of change in labeling knowledge. We studied the children over 3 years. We used each child as his or her own control and compared their performance before and after learning gender labels. We continued to study the same variables: sex-typed toy play, play with same-sex peers, and level of aggression. The older the child, the more they played with same-sex toys and the less they played with opposite-sex toys. Children played more with same-sex peers after they learned gender labels than before learning labels. Girls showed a significant drop in aggression after learning gender labels. There was no such effect for boys. These longitudinal data support the earlier cross-sectional findings. Toy play does not appear to be guided by the child's knowing gender labels. There is undoubtedly so much available information from the environment about appropriate toys that children learn which toys are appropriate for them through association and reinforcement. However, for same-sex peer play, it appears that understanding that boys and girls carry different labels is related to a choice to play with peers of the same sex. For girls, the avoidance of aggression appears strongly tied to the development of gender labeling.

We see then that the developing capacities of the child and the information provided by the environment combine to produce strong gender schema in both boys and girls. One of the clear consequences of knowledge that gender exists and applies to oneself is the acceptance of stereotypes about gender learned from the environment. So in young preschool children we see play with same-sex toys, avoidance of the opposite sex, and less aggression in girls. Gender for these young children is still very much a matter of appearance and the adoption of what is for boys and what is for girls is often quite rigid.

As children grow they come to recognize the stability of gender, and they recognize that appearances alone do not dictate one's sex. We can then say that they have obtained gender constancy. There is some evidence to suggest that once children have obtained a better cognitive understanding of gender they are more flexible in their attitudes; however, behavioral manifestations of this flexibility are not very apparent. Another difference that occurs as children go beyond a simple perceptual understanding of gender is that individual differences in preferences for sex-typed behaviors can be studied.

III. DIFFERENT COMPETENCIES OF MALES AND FEMALES

If you read the current popular literature, you might conclude that all males care about are sex and aggression, and all females care about are intimate relationships. How true is this perception, and how much is simply a reiteration of well entrenched gender stereotypes? If you look at actual behavior, attitudes, and values, you find that the overlap between males and females is tremendous and that the differences are quite small. In 1974, Eleanor Maccoby and Carol Jacklin wrote a massive volume on sex differences and in their summary included a summary of unfounded beliefs. This summary indicated that the sexes did not differ on sociability, suggestibility, self-esteem, types of cognitive functioning, achievement motivation, or use of the senses. Since that time, no consistent findings in the research literature have been found to contradict these conclusions. That is certainly not the picture presented from the popular literature in which females' self-esteem is simply assumed to be lower, and males are assumed to be more analytic, and so on. Most often these stereotypic ideas are used to promote some particular point of view about males and females. Reader, beware. If a black-and-white picture of research findings is presented, they are misrepresented. Check the primary sources of the research.

This is not to say that males and females are exactly the same. Clearly, sex of a person determines many experiences, and those experiences in turn reflect the outcome of that person's life. When we say experiences, we are including the biological differences of a male and female body as well as the social consequences of being in those bodies. From a very early age children across many cultures see females as soft and males as rough. Young children will often pantomime the physical nature of their perceptions, such as a young boy, when asked if a sandpaper starfish is like a man or woman, feeling his own cheek and saying, "Feels like daddy." Many early descriptors that differ by sex appear to have their roots in physical differences, but of course these also become psychological descriptors.

By the time they are 3 years old, boys and girls around the world participate in different activities and show different behavioral styles, play more with same-sex peers, and avoid opposite-sex peers. Children are often taught their social roles through guided participation in ongoing family social groups or in either informal or formal peer groups. One point that has been noted by most researchers is the tendency for girls and boys of this age to group themselves or separate themselves by gender. This phenomena has been called gender segregation, and it appears across cultures and across age groups. This means that even though the process by which boys and girls define their gender is similar, the worlds in which they live may be very different. Boys' groups and boys' friendships appear to be based more on shared activities, and this is also true for men. Girls' groups and girls' friendships seem to be based more on a sharing of secrets or intimacy, and this difference also appears to be true for women. Another consequence of gender segregation, and it does appear to be a consequence not a cause, is that

boys and girls participate in very different activities. Peer groups are also organized differently, with boys' groups being more hierarchical, larger, and more openly competitive. Girls' groups are smaller, organized around friendships and later around intimacy, and are not as openly competitive. One learns different coping mechanisms in these groups, and some researchers suggest that the long-term success of men in terms of employment is directly related to the way they learn to interact with other boys in their peer groups. Girls never seem quite as tied into the peer group as boys, in part because there is more pressure from their families to remain in the family sphere. They therefore learn to see the family as their main sphere of competence. Mean differences between males and females in these types of peer interactions are reported consistently in the literature, but it should also be noted that the differences are relatively small and that there is a great deal of overlap in the worlds of boys and girls, at least in the Western cultures.

The history from two very different areas of research might be used to explore how sex differences may appear to be established and in fact are almost translated into stereotypes, but after several years of later empirical research such differences are not consistently found. The first is the area of achievement motivation, which in the 1960s was often cited as an area where large gender differences were present. However, once better methodology was used, males and females proved to be very similar in achievement motivation, although context differences did make it appear that a gender difference in the trait was present. An area of considerable controversy is that of moral development, wherein early reports suggested males showed higher levels of moral reasoning than females. Once comparable tasks and samples were compared, however, this difference was not replicated.

Even in areas in which sex differences seem well established there is evidence that contextual factors may play a role in maintaining such differences. For instance, girls appear to have somewhat higher verbal ability and boys somewhat better mathematical ability in the United States, but these differences do not seem to be true of children in Asia. The one difference that does seem to hold up across many cultures is that boys are somewhat more aggressive than girls in the same culture. However, the intensity and frequency of aggression varies by culture, so that girls in one culture may be far more aggressive than boys in many other cultures. It is often very difficult to untangle cultural maintenance of gender differences from differences that might result from biological sex differences. That is because most cultures work to maintain and perhaps widen differences between the sexes. [*See* Aggression.]

IV. SEX DIFFERENCES IN PATTERNS OF ADJUSTMENT

The title of Carolyn Zahn-Waxler's 1993 paper, "Warriors and Worriers," sums up the popular stereotypes concerning patterns of adjustment in males and females. The questions are: How true are these stereotypes? Do they hold across ages? And do they have anything to do with gender socialization? These are not easy to answer for the epidemiological studies and clinical rates of diagnoses differ considerably in some categories. There is a 75% to 25% male-to-female diagnosis rate for conduct disorders, which is close to the epidemiological rate of 77% to 23% for impulsive aggressive behaviors. However, the case of attention deficit disorder is more disturbing. Clinic rates run about 9 to 1, male to female, whereas rates in community samples suggest a rate closer to 3 to 1. This could be due to misdiagnoses of one or the other sex for a particular disorder, or it could be that certain sets of symptoms are more troublesome for males than females. [*See* Attention Deficit Hyperactivity Disorder (ADHD); Conduct Disorders.]

There appears to be a sex difference in prevalence and patterns of psychological adjustment during the early years after infancy. In a large epidemiological study in Australia, boys from 5 to 8 years old were reported by the teacher as having more problems on almost every measure, even on anxiety-fearfulness. In addition, the paths to problem behaviors for boys seems more rooted in temperamental factors than do those for girls.

There may well be different developmental paths toward disorders for boys and girls. One difficulty with much of the work examining paths to psychopathology is that most of the work has been done on clinical cases (i.e., with individuals who have been diagnosed with the disorder). Several studies have found that depression may be manifested differently in boys and girls. In a factor analysis of depression scores,

there appeared to be some support that, among depressed individuals, girls are more dissatisfied with their appearance and have feelings of low self-worth whereas boys are more likely to act out (e.g., fighting or having difficulty in school) and report having less positive affect and more problems with relationships. Depression also seems to be more related to loneliness for boys than it is for girls. In addition, depressive disorders in childhood and adolescence for boys appear to be related to other types of problems such as conduct disorders, although this does not seem to be true for girls. After adolescence, depressive disorders in both sexes appear more similar to adult patterns with associations with anxiety disorders, eating disorders, and substance-related disorders. It seems that females are more often diagnosed with internalizing problems, and these sex differences in diagnoses also appear among nonclinical cases. Interestingly enough, in normative samples, males and females do not report different levels of self-esteem. [*See* Anxiety; Depression; Substance Abuse.]

We see that when we investigate the relation of gender and adjustment the time in the life span makes a difference. In 1987 Nolen-Hoeksema documented a greater incidence of depression in women than in men. Most studies report that approximately twice as many women suffer from depression as men. This difference is apparent in people who present themselves for treatment of depression and meet the criteria for clinical depressioin, as well as in studies of community populations, wherein many of the subjects have not tried to obtain treatment but still meet the criteria for clinical depression. The female–male difference is also present for people with depressive symptoms who do not meet the criteria for clinical depression. However, this high ratio of females to males for depression is not consistent across the life span. The incidence of depression is the same for boys and girls until adolescence, when it becomes more prevalent in young women. There is also evidence that in elderly populations, men and women are equally likely to be depressed.

The evidence that the disparity in the incidence of depression in women and men occurs between adolescence and old age and not across the life span may indicate that social factors play a large role in the cause of depression for women. While there are hypotheses that attribute the differences in prevalence rates to hormonal changes across the life span, many researchers dispute these theories. There is some evidence that women seem to be most depressed in their twenties, long after hormonal changes have begun, but at the very time when pressures to start a family as well as a career are highest. Genetic hypotheses have also been presented, but evidence supporting them seems to be inconclusive at best. It is, therefore, important to investigate other changes that are taking place for young women at puberty and that are enduring until late in life.

Perhaps some of the most powerful forces that females encounter at adolescence are changing social demands. Until this time girls have more flexible social roles than boys. They are able to play with masculine sex-typed toys and participate in masculine sex-typed games with little stigma. At adolescence this changes. Young women are increasingly expected to conform to feminine social roles, limiting their range of activities considerably and, in fact, actually denying them access to activities they may have once enjoyed. Girls who try to resist these social demands may find that they do not receive support from their peers, which is extremely important during adolescence. There is also evidence that girls at this age become aware of pressure to curb their own assertiveness and hide their opinions and intelligence. The link between this pressure and depression is consistent with findings of a positive correlation between depression and intelligence in young women. Boys, from early childhood, experience much less flexible social roles and, as a result, do not have to adjust their behavior to conform to so many new expectations at adolescence. Therefore, the change in social expectations at puberty may be more extreme for young women and may account for some of the increase in depression for young women at this time.

Although some of these reasons remain present in women's lives as they move past adolescence they are not adequate to explain the difference in incidence of depression between women and men, which remains until late in life. It has been suggested that a large portion of the 2 to 1 ratio of women to men in depression can be attributed to married women aged 25 to 45 years with children. This, once again, certainly implicates different societal expectations for women and men. While many women work outside of the home, either by choice or necessity, in many families they are still expected to do most of the work in the home and most of the parenting. They are also pulled in different directions at work. The stereotypical feminine role calls for women to be demure and primarily con-cerned with the needs of others, but these attributes are not much valued in the working world and will not result in advancment. The demands society places on women in this situation may place them at greater risk for depression.

Although it can be established that the different incidence of depression for women and men between adolescence and old age can be attributed, at least in part, to social variables, how can equal incidence later in life be accounted for? Are women finally free of societal pressures that increase their risk for depression? Unfortunately, this does not appear to be true. Nolen-Hoeksema reports that the decrease in the ratio of women to men who become depressed is due to an increase in depression in men, not a decrease in depression in women. Perhaps because many cultures do not value the contributions of the elderly, men at this age experience a loss of prestige and power. They are expected to conform to a passive and powerless role, which may be similar to the loss of freedom that young women experience at adolescence when more stringent adherence to gender roles is expected.

Possible differences in the development of psychopathology between the sexes has been examined in the literature on the prevalence and manifestation of conduct disorder in boys and girls as well. As stated above, there is clearly a difference in the number of boys and girls who meet the criteria for this disorder. There also appear to be differences in the expression of the disorder by males and females. Girls with conduct disorder, while more aggressive than their female peers without conduct disorder, are less aggressive and less confrontational than boys with conduct disorder. They are not arrested as frequently as boys with conduct disorder, and when they are arrested it is usually for less violent offenses. In addition, in girls, somatic complaints seem to be linked with conduct disorder, but this pattern is not apparent in boys. [See GENDER DIFFERENCES IN MENTAL HEALTH.]

Prevalence rates for conduct disorder also seem to be related to life span. While it appears that more males than females are diagnosed with conduct disorder across all ages, onset in childhood is much more frequent in males and the ratio of males to females diminishes somewhat from preadolescence to adolescence as more girls are diagnosed. When adult disorders are examined in people who had conduct problems as children and adolescents, more men have externalizing disorders (antisocial personality disorder and substance abuse) and more women have nonexternalizing disorders (somatization, anxiety disorders, affective disorders, schizophrenia). In fact, somatization disorder is as likely to be an adult outcome for women with conduct problems as antisocial personality disorder, but is rarely seen in men. However, conduct problems in childhood and adolescence predict externalizing disorders equally well for both sexes while predicting nonexternalizing disorders slightly better for women.

There is some discussion in the literature on conduct disorder about the reason for the disproportionate number of boys compared with girls who are diagnosed with conduct disorder. Is the ratio of boys to girls an accurate reflection of the prevalence of conduct disorder between the sexes, or is it possible that as many girls as boys have the same underlying psychopathology, but girls express their problems differently than boys, and the current criteria are more focused on the behaviors of boys? Evidence of the effects of gender socialization are reflected in both scenarios. As Zahn-Waxler points out, gender differences in aggression are clear, and girls receive very different messages from an early age about appropriate ways to handle anger. Female infants receive more negative response than males when they express anger. Female toddlers are more actively discouraged from aggressive actions than boys of the same age. Caregivers are also more likely to use physical punishment with boys, perhaps modeling more aggressive behaviors. In addition, girls are better at interpreting the emotional cues of others and are more empathic than are boys, which may lead to a tendency to be less aggressive.

The constraints of social roles of girls may prevent them from having the opportunities to engage in more aggressive behaviors that would meet criteria for conduct disorder. As mentioned in the section on gender differences, the subcultures of boys and girls are highly segregated, and the differences between these subcultures may shed light on the development of conduct problems. Boys are more likely to engage in rough-and-tumble active play, are more likely to play in large groups, and are more likely to establish dominance by physical means. Girls are more likely to play in small groups, are much less likely to engage in rough-and-tumble play, and are more likely to establish dominance verbally rather than physically. Girls may also be more likely to be supervised by an adult in their play, making opportunities for aggression rare, especially in light of the discussion above. These differences in the everyday worlds of girls and boys

help explain the differences in the prevalence rates of conduct disorders for the sexes.

Perhaps the disorders with the largest sex difference are the eating disorders. Most estimates of the ratio of males to females for these disorders range from 1 to 10 to 1 to 20. When males do have eating disorders, however, the symptoms and course are very similar to those seen in females. Both suffer from weight loss, emaciation, and symptoms related to starvation as well as displaying fear of being fat and a refusal to maintain a normal body weight. Differences in the male to female ratio over the life span have been pointed out, the ratio of males to females being smaller in preadolescence, with around 20% to 30% of children in clinic samples of eating disorders being male. Gender may be less important in the development of eating disorders in preadolescent children than in adolescents and adults.

Gender and gender role expectations do seem to play a central role in eating disorders. The fact that eating disorders are a phenomena in Western cultures indicates that there is something specific about the socialization of these cultures that is a risk factor for these disorders. Certainly expectations about ideal body type for women, which begin to concern girls at adolescence, are important. Western cultures place value on being thin. In cultures that regard large women as beautiful, eating disorders that are characterized by starvation are rare.

There has also been some discussion in the literature about the gender role orientation of women who have eating disorders. While clinical lore has described women with eating disorders as very stereotypically feminine, almost to the extreme, empirical studies do not appear to provide evidence to support this theory. In fact, some have found women at higher risk for eating disorders to be more masculinely sextyped. It may be that eating disorders are not linked to feminine gender orientation, but to social pressure placed on all women to be thin. If men are placed under as much pressure to be thin, the ratio of men to women with eating disorders may grow smaller. [See ANOREXIA NERVOSA AND BULIMIA NERVOSA.]

V. GENDER IDENTITY DISORDER

The disorder that is most related to gender identity is the syndrome first identified formally in *DSM III* or *II* as gender identity disorder. This syndrome in both children and adults has had a controversial history and in fact continues to generate controversy. Most of the early work with children was done with feminine boys, and the assumption was that it was this pool of children who would be transsexual and homosexual as adults. Controversy concerning early treatment of the disorder resulted from the punitive, female-denigrating nature of the process and in some cases from the underlying assumption that homosexuality was an evil that needed to be addressed. A prospective study following up a large group of feminine boys found that the probability of a homosexual orientation increased, but transsexualism is such a rare disorder that it was not possible to examine increases over base rates. The argument in favor of treatment is that these children are extremely unhappy and confused, rejected by peers, and have other major problems. Certainly this appears to be true in the case of boys, but this argument is more suspect for girls except at very extreme levels. One of the difficulties of diagnosis is that cross-sex behavior is quite normative for girls so that a girl has to display more to be referred, whereas cross-sex behavior is very much frowned upon for boys so that boys are referred at much higher rates. The causality of gender identity disorder is not at all understood, although there have been many attempts to examine both biological and psychosexual factors. [*See* HOMOSEXUALITY.]

VI. THE RELATION OF ADJUSTMENT TO GENDER IDENTITY AND STEREOTYPING

The question of what is the optimal amount of gender stereotyping, if any, has been studied both theoretically and empirically over most of this century. Early theoretical work emphasized the importance of conforming to gender stereotypes, with the assumption that obviously the best-adjusted individuals did so. However, that notion was challenged quite early in the history of this type of research as it was clear that better educated, more successful individuals of both sexes, were less, not more stereotyped. Prior to 1974, only masculinity and femininity scores were available,

and often one was simply the obverse of the other. Sandra Bem proposed the androgyny model, in which the healthy individual has components of both masculinity and femininity. She proposed, and to some extent demonstrated, that androgynous individuals functioned better in a variety of sex-typed paradigms and in effect were more capable.

Probably no construct has generated more criticism and more empirical work than that of androgyny. Despite many problems of measurement and interpretation, the general idea that androgynous individuals do seem to be somewhat more capable and somewhat better adjusted is now more accepted than the original masculinity–femininity models. What the finding seems to imply is that rigid adoption of either the masculine or feminine stereotype does not allow for flexibility of responses to adjust in today's world. While there are certainly groups within Western society who wish the return to male dominance and female submission, at this point in time, the person who can function without their self-identity defined absolutely by sex stereotypes appears to have a better chance of achieving success in whatever domain they decide to practice.

BIBLIOGRAPHY

Bem, S. L. (1974). The measurement of psychological androgyny. *Journal of Consulting and Clinical Psychology, 42,* 155–162.

Fagot, B. I. (1995). Parenting boys and girls. In M. H. Bornstein (Ed.), *Handbook of parenting* (Vol. 1, pp., 163–183). New York: Erlbaum.

Fagot, B. I., & Leinbach, M. D. (1993). Gender-role development in young children: From discrimination to labeling. *Developmental Review, 13,* 205–224.

Green, R. (1987). *The "sissy boy syndrome" and the development of homosexuality.* New Haven, CT: Yale University Press.

Maccoby, E. E., & Jacklin, C. N. (1974). *The psychology of sex differences.* Stanford, CA: Stanford Press.

Nolen-Hoeksema, S. (1987). Sex differences in unipolar depression: Evidence and theory. *Psychological Bulletin, 10,* 405–422.

Zahn-Waxler, C. (1993). Warriors and worriers: Gender and psychopathology. *Development and Psychopathology, 5,* 79–90.

Zucker, K. J., & Bradley, S. J. (1995). *Gender identity disorder and psychosexual problems in children and adolescents.* New York: Guilford.

Genetic Contributors to Mental Health

David L. DiLalla

Southern Illinois University at Carbondale

Behavioral Genetics A field of study devoted to explaining the etiology of individual differences in behavior.

Environmentality Proportion of individual differences for a phenotype that is the result of environmental influences operating on a population of individuals.

Genotype The genes that are related to the expression of a particular behavior or characteristic.

Heritability Proportion of individual differences for a phenotype that is the result of genetic variation within a population of individuals.

Nonshared Environment Environmental influences that are unique to an individual, or that are uniquely perceived by the individual.

Phenotype A measurable, observable characteristic of an individual.

Shared Environment Environmental influences that are shared by two or more individuals (for example, influences that might be shared by siblings within the same family).

Research findings on the **GENETIC CONTRIBUTORS TO MENTAL HEALTH** are summarized in this article.

One of the major research goals of clinical psychologists, psychiatrists, and experimental psychopathologists has been the identification of factors that give rise to psychological disorder and distress. However, some researchers and practitioners have noted that this approach focuses too much attention on what goes wrong and it does not illuminate the "etiology" of healthy psychological development. Consistently, research findings have shown that genetic and environmental factors are related to the development of a variety of mental disorders including schizophrenia, bipolar affective disorder (manic depression), depression, and anxiety disorders. It is the goal of this chapter to summarize research findings that relate to potential genetic influences on mental health.

I. HOW MIGHT GENES INFLUENCE MENTAL HEALTH?

A. Evolutionary Psychology: A Broad Perspective on Genetic Influences

When thinking about evolution, what comes to mind initially is the development of physical, physiological, and biological systems. The field of evolutionary psychology, on the other hand, suggests that the same evolutionary pressures that shaped the physical development of our species also influenced the development of basic psychological characteristics of humans. Such an influence is predicated on the notion that basic human personality characteristics are influenced, at least in part, by genetic factors, a position strongly supported by a large body of research in modern behavioral genetics. To the degree that a particular behavioral or psychological characteristic proved to offer a reproductive advantage to individuals who possessed it (i.e., the characteristic makes it more likely that the individual successfully reproduces and passes on his or her genes), this characteristic would become increasingly prevalent among the population of individuals who experience similar evolutionary "pressure."

A number of potential examples of such behavioral systems come to mind. Perhaps the best known is John Bowlby's Attachment Theory. Bowlby posited that attachment bonds between infants and their primary caregivers (usually mothers) are found in all humans because such bonds offered survival advantage to human infants in the environment in which humans evolved (what Bowlby referred to as the "environment of evolutionary adaptedness"). For example, separation anxiety (emotional upset that occurs when separated from a caregiver) is a major component of the attachment system, according to Bowlby and others. For individuals who lived as hunter-gatherers, there was obvious danger to infants from predatory animals. As a result, infants who "signal" the caregiver by protesting when the caregiver moves beyond a certain distance away had clear survival advantage over infants who did not experience such distress upon separation. [*See* ATTACHMENT.]

It should be noted, of course, that evolutionary processes are generally thought of as related to the development of species-universal characteristics and not as explanations for current individual differences in those characteristics, although some recent hypotheses have been forwarded to explain individual differences in terms of evolutionary processes. With respect to the example of Attachment Bonds noted above, all individuals are assumed to be predisposed to form an attachment bond with a primary caregiver (because such a bond initially had evolutionary adaptiveness), but the quality of the attachment bonds observed at the present time (i.e., individual differences in attachment) are expected according to attachment theorists to be influenced by patterns of parent–child interaction during the first 6 months of life. It was this aspect of attachment theory that has been explicated by Dr. Mary Ainsworth and her colleagues over the past three decades.

B. Factors Influencing Individual Differences in Adjustment

This article is less concerned with broad evolutionary—genetic influences on species-specific character-

istics—and more with explanations for individual differences in psychological adjustment and well-being. In particular, what are we to make of individuals who might be considered at risk for developing psychopathology (either by way of familial risk or exposure to severe environmental challenges) but who do not exhibit maladjustment? Researchers have been extremely interested in studying such "resilient" individuals to gain potential insight into how mental illness might be successfully prevented. Although the bulk of this research has focused on protective factors that are environmental in nature, I will focus here on potential genetic influences on adaptation and resilience.

For example, it has been well documented that there is a moderate genetic influence on liability toward schizophrenia. Although lifetime risk for schizophrenia in the general population is approximately 1% (1 person in 100 is expected to be diagnosed with schizophrenia over his or her lifetime), risk to a first-degree relative of an individual diagnosed with schizophrenia—a parent, for example—is closer to 10%. Among children of individuals diagnosed with schizophrenia, what factors influence whether or not the illness will be expressed? Clearly, part of the answer lies in the degree to which children share the risk-relevant genes for schizophrenia. However, consider a theoretical situation in which two siblings could be determined to equally share the genes that confer risk for developing schizophrenia. What determines whether illness will or will not occur in this case? Again, it seems clear that environmental influences play a critical role, but it is also possible that other genetic factors function in a "protective" or buffering role. [*See* SCHIZOPHRENIA.]

Although the above example involves genes as buffering factors against a genetic liability toward mental illness, the same basic principle applies to buffering against environmental stressors. Much research has been conducted on individuals who, by virtue of their circumstances, might be expected to be at high risk for developing psychological problems, but who are mentally healthy. How do we understand the factors that produced such "resilient" individuals? Again, genetic factors might operate, either directly (for example by conferring a general "hardiness"), or more indirectly by way of mediating what might initially appear to be an "environmental" influence (for example, a strong positive relationship with a caregiver.

It is the goal of this review to summarize research findings and theorizing about the issues described above. The discussion will begin with a brief overview of the literature on resilience and adaptation. Subsequently, this literature will be evaluated in terms of potential genetic influences on adaptation. Such influences may be of at least five types. First, general intellectual ability has been shown to be a protective factor in terms of mental health. Second, temperamental characteristics may be related to a general resistance to stressful events. Third, personality traits may exert a direct influence on wellness and mental health. Fourth, positive mental attitude and a general sense of optimism have been linked to positive outcome. Finally, social support has been shown to play a crucial role in protecting individuals from psychological distress; it will be argued that some instances of "environmental" buffering of stressors can be reconceptualized, at least in part, in terms of what have been called Gene–Environment correlations (associations between an individual's genetic makeup and his or her environment. Each of the above influences on mental health will be discussed in turn. [*See* PROTECTIVE FACTORS IN DEVELOPMENT OF PSYCHOPATHOLOGY.]

Before embarking on this discussion, however, it is important to review some basic concepts in behavioral genetics, the branch of behavioral science involved with investigation of genetic and environmental influences on behavior. This will include a broad discussion of the mechanisms by which genes influence behavior, a discussion of the meaning of "heritability," one of the major statistics used by researchers in behavioral genetics, and a brief review of the basic methods in behavioral genetics. [*See* BEHAVIORAL GENETICS.]

II. HOW DO GENETIC EFFECTS ON BEHAVIOR OPERATE?

Throughout this discussion, it is important to keep in mind that genes do not "code" directly for behavior; there is not a one-to-one correspondence between genes and the behaviors of interest. Rather, genes provide the blueprint for the body to create amino acids, building blocks for proteins that have important roles in other physiological or hormonal processes (for example, the synthesis of neurotransmitters). For all of the behaviors and characteristics to be discussed here, the role of environmental factors is also extremely important, even though the precise pathways of environmental influence are still unclear. Many researchers describe the relationship between genetic and environmental factors in terms of a "probabilistic" or

"diathesis-stress" model. This means that genetic factors may confer some likelihood for development of a particular behavior pattern, but that environmental factors (which could be either protective or destructive) strongly influence whether or not the risk for the behavior pattern is actually expressed. It should be kept in mind that environment in this context is a broad term that includes prenatal influences and intrauterine biochemical and hormonal conditions, as well as postnatal social and nutritional influences.

III. WHY HAS HERITABILITY BEEN CONTROVERSIAL?

Given the historical influence of Behaviorism within psychology, investigation of genetic influences on human behavior has sporadically sparked controversy. At times, there have been concerns about the "deterministic" leanings of behavioral geneticists, coupled with fear that genetic findings might be used for eugenic purposes. It should be noted at the outset that one should not equate genetic determinism with the findings that have been reported in human behavioral genetics. Rather, researchers have discovered that even for disorders such as schizophrenia, which have been shown to have a strong genetic etiological component, the causal role of environmental factors is extremely strong. This is highlighted by the fact that among twins reared together, the average concordance rate for schizophrenia is roughly 50% among genetically identical twins where one member of the pair has been diagnosed with the disorder. To the degree that specific environmental triggering (or protective) factors can be identified, such findings hold out the possibility of environmentally-based preventive interventions for individuals who have some genetic risk of developing schizophrenia (for example, offspring or other first-degree family members of individuals with schizophrenia.

Another controversy surrounding behavioral genetic research is mistaken attempts to interpret the heritability statistic as a means for explaining differences *between* groups of people on a psychological characteristic. Heritability is defined as the proportion of individual differences on some characteristic within a given population that can be attributed to the effects of genetic variation within the population. Thus, heritability provides an estimate of the effects of genes on variability *within* a group, but it cannot be invoked to explain observed variability *between* two or more groups.

A brief classroom example will illustrate this distinction. Assume that we have two genetically heterogeneous groups of plants for which heritability for height has been shown to be equal. If the seeds from one group are planted in enriched soil and the seeds from the other group are sown in soil that was deficient with respect to nutrients, we will see a clear height advantage at maturity in favor of the plants placed in the enriched environment. Although we know that individual differences in height are influenced by genetic factors for both populations of plants, it would be *incorrect* for us to conclude that the height difference observed between the enriched and deficient soil groups is the result of genetic differences. In terms of human behavioral genetics, the methods described below *only* provide information about factors that influence differences among individuals *within* the population under study. Such studies should not be interpreted as providing an explanation for observed differences between groups of individuals.

IV. METHODS IN BEHAVIORAL GENETICS

A. Family Studies

Research in human behavioral genetics usually employs one of several basic research strategies. In family (or "pedigree") studies, the prevalence of a particular disorder or characteristic by which individuals may be classified is assessed among relatives of an identified individual who has the characteristic of interest (the "proband"). Of particular interest is the likelihood among biological relatives of possessing the target characteristic as a function of varying genetic relatedness. Similarly, family members may be compared to each other with respect to their similarity on some behavioral or emotional characteristic that is noncategorical (for example, a personality trait score). By assessing similarities and differences among family members who differ with respect to their degree of genetic relatedness, estimates of the importance of genetic and environmental influences on behavior can be made. Such studies generally must include large numbers of multigenerational families in order to estimate the relative contributions of genetic and environmental factors on the trait being studied.

B. Twin Studies

A mainstay in behavioral genetics is the twin method. The simplest method of twin analysis consists of a direct comparison of concordance rates (percentage of pairs where both twins are affected with the disorder under study) for monozygotic/identical (MZ) and dizygotic/fraternal (DZ) twin pairs, realizing that on average, DZ twins share half their genes, whereas MZ twins are genetically identical. The basic premise is that any difference between MZ twins must be due to environmental effects. Similarly, to the extent that genetic factors are important in the development of the disorder under study, MZ twins will more often be "concordant" for the disorder than will DZ twins.

As was the case for family studies, twin studies can also shed light on genetic and environmental influences on continuously distributed characteristics of people. Here, to the degree that MZ twins tend to be more similar to each than DZ twins are to each other—and assuming that MZ and DZ twin pairs generally experience the same environmental factors that are relevant to development of the target trait or disorder—the greater MZ similarity reflects the influence of genetic factors. A broad estimate of the degree of heritability (usually denoted h^2) can be obtained by doubling the difference between the MZ and DZ correlations for a given measure. As noted previously, heritability gives an indication of the percentage of variability among individuals that is the result of genetic factors. Analogously, the percentage of variance caused by environmental factors is sometimes referred to as environmentality and can be broadly derived as $1 - h^2$. Additional information about the heritability statistic can be found in Plomin and colleagues' book, *Behavioral Genetics*.

C. Adoption Studies

Another often-used technique in behavioral genetic research is the study of adoptees and their biological and adoptive relatives. This method has at its core the natural "experiment" wherein children leave the care of their biological parents early in life and are reared by persons to whom they are genetically unrelated. Genetic predisposition and influence of the rearing environment are thus separated. Similarities between adopted children and their adoptive parents are due to environmental effects or cultural transmission, whereas similarities between adopted children and their nonrearing biological parents represent the effect of shared genes or prenatal environmental influences. This assumes "random" placement of children into adoptive homes so that adoptive parents are uncorrelated with biological parents. To the extent that adoptive parents are systematically chosen so that they are similar to their adopted children's biological parents, selective placement has occurred. Such potentially biasing effects can be evaluated statistically to determine whether selective placement variables such as race, social status, or correlates of these affect the observed similarity among adoptive relatives.

Most of the research summarized in this article was conducted using either twin or adoption methodology, or in the case of studies of twins reared apart, an amalgam of the two methods. Although the methods are described above in terms of simple correlations between individuals on a single trait, modern multivariate statistical methods have been developed for evaluating the degree to which the observed variance in characteristics observed in twin and adoption studies is the result of genetic or environmental factors, or interactions between the two effects. Although the details of these methods are beyond the scope of this article, the book *Genes, Culture & Personality* by L. Eaves and colleagues provides an excellent review of the methods and their application.

D. Reliability and Validity of Measures

Studies in behavioral genetics typically report estimates of genetic and environmental influence on a phenotype (the measured characteristic or behavior of interest). In many studies, the phenotype is measured by some sort of rating scale, questionnaire, or behavioral checklist. Reliable and valid measurement of the phenotype is a crucial matter to researchers as well as consumers of research. A measure is reliable to the degree that it generates consistent, stable, reproducible estimates of the target characteristic. However, reliability is not sufficient; measurement devices must also be valid—that is, it must be shown that they truly tap into the construct that they were designed to measure. It should be recognized that most of the tests and questionnaires used in psychological studies are not perfect indicators of the traits they are designed to measure, even when the validity of the test has been well established. Thus, there is a varying degree of measurement error that must be taken into account. Critical evaluation of the measures employed in the

study will inform the confidence one places in the results of the research project.

V. FACTORS INFLUENCING ADAPTATION AND RESILIENCE

Researchers in psychology and psychiatry have clearly documented the influence of risk factors (both biological and environmental) on the development and course of psychopathology. At the same time, a compelling aspect of these findings has been the large proportion of individuals (often a majority) who are at risk but do not develop symptoms of psychological disorder or distress. A number of factors have been shown to be related to such positive outcomes in at-risk individuals including the following: (1) intellectual and cognitive abilities; (2) temperamental characteristics of the individual such as sociability and activity level; (3) personality characteristics such as extraversion, sense of well-being, and internal locus of control; (4) possession of a global sense of optimism or positive mental attitude; and (5) the buffering effects of social support from others, and in particular, the protective nature of "one good relationship" with another person. Evidence regarding the degree to which each of these protective factors may be influenced by genetic factors will be reviewed below.

A. Intellectual Ability

Research on twins, twins reared apart, and adoptees has implicated the influence of both genetic and environmental factors on IQ. It should be noted that there has been debate in the literature regarding the degree to which standard tests of IQ validly measure "intelligence," or whether such tests offer too narrow a view of human intellectual ability. Still, given the abundant research on the utility of IQ scores as predictors of outcomes such as academic achievement and employment success, it seems clear that IQ scores tap into skills and abilities that are associated with success in Western cultures. Moreover, many of the recent studies of heritability of intellectual ability employ multiple measures of ability that are then aggregated into a combined measure of general cognitive skill.

To summarize findings in this area, it has generally been found that roughly 50 to 60% of observed individual differences in IQ can be attributed to genetic variation among individuals. Some studies have reported heritability for IQ as low as 30% while other researchers have reported heritability as high at 70% for IQ. With respect to twin studies, the average identical twin correlation (summarized across over 4600 twin pairs) for IQ is .86 while the average correlation for fraternal twins (over 5500 pairs) is .60. It is noteworthy that the IQ correlation for identical twins reared apart (approximately 150 pairs) has been found to be roughly .74, not appreciably lower than the correlation for twins reared together. For purpose of comparison, studies of nontwin biological siblings reared in the same home have shown an average correlation of .47 and genetically unrelated children living together (adoptive siblings) have an average correlation about .32 for IQ. The average IQ correlation for children and their biological parents (by whom they are being reared) is .42 whereas the average correlation between children and their adoptive parents is .19. A summary of the findings to date in terms of genetic and environmental influences on IQ is presented in Fig. 1.

How, then, should these findings be interpreted? The results clearly indicate that genetic factors play a significant role in the expression of intellectual ability as measured by IQ. This effect appears to be polygenic (the result of the combined influence of multiple genes) rather than the result of a single "IQ gene." At the same time that genes are important, the results clearly highlight the crucial role of environmental influences on IQ. Genetically identical twins, though highly similar, are not identical with respect to IQ, and genetically unrelated individuals living in the same household are more similar to each other with respect to IQ than would be expected of unrelated individuals in general. Similarly, researchers have documented malleability of IQ in studies of individuals who are adopted from impoverished environments into families of higher socioeconomic status.

Many researchers in this area interpret these results in terms of genetic factors providing some upper and lower limits with respect to IQ, with actual IQ depending on environmental influences on the developing individual. There are some indications that this "reaction range" may be broader for individuals from lower socioeconomic samples than for those of higher socioeconomic status. Simply put, this would be reflected in *lower* heritability of IQ in low SES samples than in higher SES samples, indicating the more "potent" effect of environmental influences on developing IQ. In sum, the results of a large number of well-designed and well-executed studies indicate moderate genetic influences and environmental influences on measured IQ. [*See* INTELLIGENCE AND MENTAL HEALTH.]

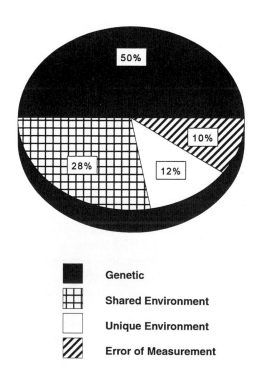

Genetic

Shared Environment

Unique Environment

Error of Measurement

Figure 1 Summary of genetic and environmental influences on IQ from family, adoption, and twin studies conducted through 1992 [Data summarized from Plomin, DeFries, McClearn, & Rutter (1997). *Behavioral Genetics*. New York: W. H. Freeman & Company.]

B. Temperament

In discussions about the roots of adaptation, temperamental characteristics are often suggested to directly contribute to psychological wellness, or indirectly promote adjustment by way of buffering the individual against the effects of stressors. Research on links between temperament and mental health has been hampered, however, by a lack of consensus among researchers regarding the definition, scope, and measurement of temperament. In very general terms, temperament can be understood as a group of characteristics that reflect the basic behavioral style of an individual. There is some consensus that temperament has biological underpinnings, particularly to the extent that reliable individual differences in temperamental characteristics have been documented within the first hours after birth. Most, although not all, researchers in this area focus on infancy and early childhood, given the assumption that associations between temperamental traits and actual behavior become more difficult to disentangle as the individual accrues life experience. There is also substantial blurring between definitions of temperament and personality, although there is some consensus that personality represents an outgrowth or development of basic temperamental traits.

Despite such definitional ambiguities, substantial research has demonstrated associations between individual differences in temperamental characteristics and psychological adjustment, coping with stressful events, and resilience. In particular, temperamental attributes such as activity level, emotional stability versus reactivity, cognitive-intellectual abilities (see discussion of IQ), the ability to reflect on one's behavior, and the degree to which one is socially responsive to others have been shown to function as protective factors in individuals at risk for developing psychological disorders.

Behavioral genetic studies of temperamental traits such as activity, sociability, behavioral inhibition, mood quality, and approach-withdrawal have generally found a moderate degree of genetic influence (heritability in the range of .3–.6), although the literature on this topic is relatively small. Most of these studies were conducted in the United States or in Western countries, although at least one major study of temperament in twins was undertaken in China with similar findings. Consistent with the results from the personalty literature, the effects of shared environmental influences on temperament appear to be fairly small.

Findings of significant heritability are not universal, however. In one twin study of neonatal (first 24 hours after birth) temperament there was no appreciable genetic effect on any of the temperament measures. Rather, unique environmental influences, including birth and neonatal complications, were the principal determinant of individual differences on temperament ratings. With respect to continuity of temperamental characteristics during infancy, maintenance of temperamental traits has generally been found to be related to genetic influences, whereas change over time is the result of uniquely experienced environmental effects.

C. Personality Traits

As early as 1935 researchers had begun comparative analysis of personality characteristics of identical (MZ) and fraternal (DZ) twin pairs and by the late 1950s there was a fairly steady stream of reports in the psychological literature on genetic influences on normal personality traits. These reports were received with great skepticism and, occasionally, some hostility from the psychological establishment of the time, which was strongly influenced by the behavioral tradition and which viewed the roots of important human behaviors as lying squarely in the environmental domain. The prevailing view, in its strongest form, could be summarized in terms of John Watson's description of the human infant as a blank slate (Tabula Rasa) upon which the environment writes its effects.

Although the early twin studies can be faulted on a number of grounds, including relatively small sample sizes and "uneven" measurement of personality traits, the results from these studies is remarkably consistent with the more methodologically sophisticated research that came later. Specifically, a meta-analytic summary of these findings reported by Lyndon Eaves and his colleagues indicated that heritability (percentage of variability in a sample that is the result of genetic influences) ranged from .29 to .38 for the "Big 3" personality traits of Neuroticism, Extraversion, and Psychoticism. Since that time, a number of well-conceived and well-executed twin, family, and adoption studies have converged on the conclusion that a wide range of normal personality traits, including the "Big 5" traits of Neuroticism, Extraversion, Openness/Intellect, Agreeableness, and Conscientiousness, are influenced, to a moderate degree, by the effects of genes. Judy Dunn and Robert Plomin summarized recent findings as pictured in Fig. 2.

Figure 2 indicates that, on average, 40% of variability in normal personality traits has been shown to be caused by genetic influences; 35% of the variation is accounted for by environmental influences unique to a particular individual; 5% of variation is the result of environmental influences that are shared (for example, by siblings within the same family); and 20% of variation can be explained by error of measurement of the personality traits under study.

A common question about results such as these has been how it is possible for the effects of shared family environment to be so small in terms of inducing similarity among individuals within the same family. The best explanation for this rather counterintuitive finding appears to be that environmental effects that we might initially assume to be shared by individuals within the same family (for example, parental disci-

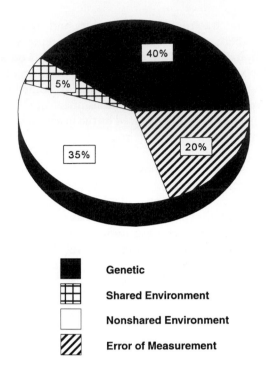

Figure 2 Percentage of variance in personality traits accounted for by genetic, shared environmental, and unique environmental influences, and by measurement error. [Summarized after J. Dunn & R. Plomin, 1990. *Separate Lives: Why Siblings Are So Different.* New York: Basic Books.]

Table I Genetic and Environmental Variance Components for Personality Traits in Twins Reared Together and Apart

Personality trait	Genetic effect	Shared environment	Unique environment
Well-being	.48	.13	.40
Social potency	.54	.10	.36
Achievement	.39	.11	.51
Social closeness	.40	.19	.41
Stress reaction	.53	.00	.47
Alienation	.45	.11	.44
Aggression	.44	.00	.56
Control	.44	.00	.56
Harm avoidance	.55	.00	.45
Traditionalism	.45	.12	.43
Absorption	.50	.03	.43
Positive emotionality	.40	.22	.38
Negative emotionality	.55	.02	.43
Constraint	.58	.00	.43

Summarized after Tellegen, A., Lykken, D. T., Bouchard, T. J., Wilcox, K. J., & Rich, S. (1988). Personality similarity in twins reared apart and together. *Journal of Personality and Social Psychology, 54,* 1031–1039.

pline style) are, in actuality, uniquely experienced by individuals (unique environmental effects) so that their effect tends to promote individual differentiation rather than similarity with respect to personality traits.

It is instructive to review in slightly more detail a combined study of normal personality similarity among identical and fraternal twins reared together and apart. The study, conducted by Auke Tellegen and his colleagues used the Multidimensional Personality Questionnaire (MPQ) as an index of normal personality characteristics. The MPQ measures a broad range of normal personality traits, many of which are related to personal and interpersonal adaptation. The main findings of this study are summarized in Table I.

The last three personality traits in Table I (Positive Emotionality, Negative Emotionality, Constraint) are similar in content to the broad personality traits of Extraversion, Neuroticism, and Psychoticism (in the reversed direction), respectively. Positive Emotionality is a composite of the traits of Well-Being, Social Potency, Achievement, and Social Closeness. Hence, it is related

to the broad experience of positive emotional states in an "individual" as well as "interpersonal" context. Well-Being, in particular, is related to a sense of optimism and hope about one's future, an attribute shown to function as a protective factor when faced with stressors that could place an individual at risk for emotional distress or disorder. Similarly, Social Closeness and Social Potency relate to the desire for and success at negotiating interpersonal associations with others. These characteristics, too, have been shown to function as "buffers" for individuals who are under stress. Hence, we see a moderate degree of genetic influence on personality characteristics that may play a role in promoting or maintaining mental health, as well as moderate unique environmental influence and a smaller but significant shared environmental influence on these traits.

Negative Emotionality (a composite of Stress Reaction, Alienation and Aggression) has been proposed as a general risk factor for emotional distress and disorder. Table I indicates moderate genetic and unique environmental influences on this group of traits, with little effect for shared environmental events. Although we can infer some genetic influence on risk for psychological disorder from this finding, it is important to recall that the genetic influence on the trait is not "all or nothing." Rather, the genetic effect on a personality trait is presumed to be an additive one; when one has "more" of the relevant genes, one is more likely to exhibit higher levels of the trait. By inverting the logic of this general approach, we also conclude that lower levels of Negative Emotionality will confer lower risk for development of psychological disorder. That is, a low score is just as influenced by genetic factors as a high score would be. Hence, genetic influences operate on the full continuum of scores from low to high.

Finally, if one considers the higher order trait of Constraint in Table I, it will again be seen that there is both significant genetic and environmental influence (principally of the unique sort) on the characteristics comprising the constraint factor (principally defined by Traditionalism, Harm Avoidance and Control). To the degree that conservatism, impulsiveness, and a thrill-seeking mentality are related to the likelihood that one might place the self in psychologically or physically risky situations, genetic influences on these traits also can be thought of being related to prevention (or risk) of psychological distress and disorder. [*See* PERSONALITY.]

D. Positive Mental Attitude/Optimism

Although we might consider optimism and the expression of a positive mental attitude as a personality characteristic, it seems reasonable to discuss separately the findings in this area given the importance accorded to these constructs in the literature on stress, coping, and resilience. Writers and researchers in this area have generally approached the topic from a purely "environmental" perspective, arguing that our expectations about the world (generalized to encompass a broad sense of optimism or pessimism) are essentially learned as a result of the history of our daily interchanges with people and things. This basic etiological model is reflected in the title of Martin Seligman's influential book, *Learned Optimism.*

However, a recent study by Robert Plomin and colleagues of twins reared together and apart, the first study of its kind, investigated the potential contributing role of genetic factors to the development of optimism and to the link between self-reported optimism and mental health outcome. Consistent with other

findings in the personality literature, this study indicated significant, but modest, heritability for optimism; roughly 25% of individual differences in self-reported optimism were attributed to the effects of genetic factors. Interestingly, and rather uniquely in the personality literature, the effect of shared environment on the development of optimism was also significant, accounting for approximately 13% of individual differences in the trait. This is evidenced by the fact that identical twins who were reared together in the same household were more similar with respect to optimism than were identical twins reared apart (who were still significantly more similar than fraternal twins reared together). In general, the results highlight the importance of both genetic, shared environmental, and unique environmental influences on the development of optimism.

Consistent with other research in the resilience literature, Plomin's study also indicated that optimism was a significant predictor of life satisfaction and (absence of) depression. In addition, however, the researchers also demonstrated that the observed association between optimism and mental health could be explained, at least in part, by a shared genetic effect. That is, the same genetic factors may influence both optimism and mental health status. [*See* OPTIMISM, MOTIVATION, AND MENTAL HEALTH.]

E. Social Support

The literature on stress and coping has shown conclusively that individuals who are able to draw on the emotional, physical, and material support of others are more resistant to the negative effects of stressful events. Such individuals, as a result of social environmental influences, are viewed as more psychologically healthy than their risk-inducing environments might predict that they would be. Although it might appear to be counterintuitive, recent work in behavioral genetics has shown that effects that have been historically viewed as purely environmental are, in fact, influenced in part by genetic factors. That is, it appears to oversimplify the real state of affairs to conceive of genes and environments as independent of each other and it suggests that thinking in terms of "nature vs. nurture" may be misguided. [*See* SOCIAL SUPPORT.]

The mechanism responsible for this shift in the way we might normally consider the effects of genes and environmental events has been referred to as the

"Gene–Environment Correlation" and was described in detail in the early 1980s by Scarr and McCartney. Essentially, the concept suggests that environmental events are not independent of genotype (the genetic make-up of the individual) because of links of various kinds between the genes an individual has and the environmental stimuli he or she experiences.

The links between genes and environments are of three basic types. In a Passive G–E Correlation, the association between genes and environment occurs without any direct involvement of the affected individual. This is best illustrated by the observation that biological parents provide *both* genes and environment for their offspring. For example, parents who are highly sociable and outgoing pass along to their children genes related to the expression of sociable behavior (to the degree that extraverted behavior is moderately heritable, as we have seen) and may be expected also to provide a home environment to their children that complements tendencies toward sociable behavior. Thus, the environment is indirectly related to the child's genotype.

The second type of Gene–Environment Correlation is called "Reactive." In this situation, we assume that an individual has particular characteristics that are influenced, at least in part, by genetic factors. To the degree that the environment that the individual is exposed to "reacts" to such characteristics, again, there is an association between the environment and the genotype. An example of this kind of effect is a school teacher providing an enriched learning environment to a student who shows high levels of intellectual ability, or a peer responding positively to an individual's positive social behavior. In this way, we might reconceptualize some of the reported protective, health-promoting effects of social support as being mediated, at least in part, by genetic influences by way of an individual's personal characteristics "evoking" a positive effect from the environment.

Some initial research consistent with this model has been reported by Robert Plomin and his colleagues in the area of adaptation to aging. In that particular study, genetic influences were shown to account for a significant portion of the observed association between psychological well-being and individuals' perceptions about the adequacy of their social support networks.

The concept of reactive Gene-Environment Correlation can also be offered as a partial explanation for the findings reported consistently by Michael Rutter, Norman Garmezy, and others that the experience of at least one strong interpersonal relationship with another person has salutary effects in terms of promoting psychological health and well-being among individuals at risk for developing psychological disorders. This idea has also been proposed as being potentially related to the finding that secure attachment to caregivers is associated with positive psychological outcome. That is, the personal, temperamental characteristics of individuals (which may be in part genetically influenced) can play a role in evoking positive responses from significant others and thus contribute to the development of a secure attachment relationship. This is, in part, an extension of the reasoning, long accepted by developmental psychologists, that there are "reciprocal" effects in parent–child interaction with the characteristics of each individual contributing to the development of the relationship.

Finally, an Active Gene–Environment Correlation reflects the notion that individuals may actively seek out environmental "niches" that are consonant with their personal styles and that foster positive development and adaptation. In terms of the examples already cited, this might entail an intellectually bright individual creating an environment that will further support development of cognitive skills, for example, by choosing intellectually stimulating peers or life situations. Similarly, in the emotional domain an optimistic individual may seek out situations and individuals that support an optimistic worldview and that contribute to positive outcome. As above, to the degree that intellectual ability or optimism, in this case, are influenced by genetic factors, we see that genes and environments are not independent of each other.

VI. CONCLUSION

In this article I set out to shed additional light on the question "What causes individuals to be psychologically well adjusted?" The research that has been summarized indicates that psychological adaptation and well-being may be directly promoted, or that psychological maladjustment may be avoided, by some basic characteristics of people and of situations, and that these characteristics and situations may be, in part, influenced by genetic factors. It should be noted that the magnitude of the genetic influences described here is moderate, usually accounting for roughly 30 to 60% of individual differences among individuals. The flip side of such heritability estimates is that between 40 and 70% of individual differences on these wellness-related characteristics is accounted for by environmental influences, usually of the sort that are uniquely experienced by individuals.

More interesting, perhaps, than the finding that there are genetic influences on characteristics related to psychological adjustment, is the observation that even those predictors of psychological health that we have assumed to be purely environmental in the past may, in fact, be mediated in part by genetic influences (see Gene–Environment Correlation). This underscores the immense complexity of human behavior and challenges simplistic assumptions about the world. We have seen that the question is not whether nature *or* nurture is the most important predictor of mental health, but how genetic and environmental factors act together to influence an individual's development.

VII. WHAT DOES THE FUTURE HOLD?

The findings summarized here suggest a number of interesting directions that future research on mental health might take. From an academic standpoint, it will be interesting to pursue recent findings that hint at the possibility that shared genes are responsible for the association between personality traits such as optimism and psychological health. This parallels recent research in psychopathology that has suggested that shared genes may influence both the expression of disorders such as depression and personality traits such as negative emotionality (suggesting continuity between normal personality traits and psychopathology).

It will also be intriguing to learn more about the precise mechanism by which genetic influences operate. As we have seen, it seems clear that single gene

effects are not operating with respect to basic psychological characteristics and that multiple genes combine in a generally additive fashion to produce their effects. A better understanding of the biological mechanisms of these genetic effects on mental health may begin to offer some glimpses into how individuals with psychopathology might better be treated (for example, with newly developed psychopharmacological interventions).

Most important from a pragmatic perspective, it is crucial to conduct research that uncovers the precise ways in which specific environmental factors combine with particular personal characteristics to produce a healthy outcome. Does a particular socially oriented intervention work well with some individuals but not with others? Are some interventions universally relevant? Such research will be difficult to undertake, but it is essential so that we may better understand the complex, multidimensional nature of psychological adjustment.

BIBLIOGRAPHY

Bouchard, T. J., Lykken, D. T., McGue, M., Segal, N. L., & Tellegen, A. (1990). Sources of human psychological differences: The Minnesota study of twins reared apart. *Science, 250,* 223–228.

Buss, A. H., & Plomin, R. (1984). *Temperament: Early developing personality traits.* Hillsdale, NJ: Erlbaum.

Dunn, J., & Plomin, R. (1990). *Separate lives: Why siblings are so different.* New York: Basic Books.

Eaves, L. J., Eysenck, H. J., & Martin, N. G. (1989). *Genes, culture and personality: An empirical approach.* New York: Academic Press.

Plomin, R., DeFries, J. C., McClearn, G. E., & Rutter, M. (1997). *Behavioral genetics.* New York: W. H. Freeman, Co.

Rolf, J., Masten, A. S., Cicchetti, D., Nuechterlein, K. H., & Weintraub, S. (Eds.). (1990). *Risk and protective factors in the development of psychopathology.* Cambridge: Cambridge University Press.

Seligman, M. E. P. (1991). *Learned optimism.* New York: Knopf.

Grief and Loss

Kathrin Boerner and Camille B. Wortman

State University of New York, Stony Brook

Bereavement   Objective situation of a person who has suffered the loss of someone significant.

Grief   Emotional response/experience of a number of psychological, behavioral, social, and physical reactions to one's loss.

Loss   The term loss can refer to a physical loss (loss of a person), and/or to a psychosocial loss (loss of a certain role in life, loss of hopes or expectations for the future).

Mourning   Actions expressive of grief, which are shaped by social and cultural mourning practices and expectations.

This article discusses **GRIEF AND LOSS**: its symptomatology, reaction to grief, and how the grief response can be mediated.

I. INTRODUCTION

Our goal in this article is to help clarify why different individuals react to a major loss in such different ways. There is a striking variability in response to the loss of a loved one: One person may experience intense initial distress, but return to normal functioning rather quickly. Another person may continue to suffer from deep agony and despair for several years. A third person may not be affected much, or may even feel relief as a result of the loss. Why do people react in such diverse ways?

To understand these patterns of responses, it is important to recognize that each bereaved person may experience a unique set of losses. For example, a widow may have lost an intimate friend, a child-rearing partner, a protector, and a sexual partner. Bereaved parents may experience their child's death as the loss of a central part of themselves, and of all their wishes, hopes, and expectations for the child's future. Bereaved siblings may have lost a confidant and a companion, and may also feel neglected because their parents are so absorbed by their own grief. People who lose a spouse or child in a traumatic incident such as a drunk-driving crash must endure the loss itself as well as the shattering of their basic assumptions about the world (safety, security, justice).

These examples point to the importance of understanding who and what is lost when a loved one dies. However, this still does not explain why even in the case of a similar loss, such as the anticipated death of a spouse, responses often differ enormously from person to person. Some investigators maintain that the extent of grief depends mainly on the quality of the relationship with the deceased. Others claim that personality differences are primarily responsible for the variability. What are the most important determinants of reaction to loss and how do they influence adjustment following the loss? A major goal of this article is to address these questions.

We begin by describing the range of symptoms that may occur as a consequence of a loss. Next, we review the theoretical perspectives that have been most influential in the bereavement literature, and consider whether they provide an explanation for the variety of grief reactions. We then describe and evaluate some new theoretical developments that challenge traditional ways of thinking about grief. Next, we discuss several factors that may mediate the grief response. We focus primarily on two areas that we feel are most essential in their impact on the grieving process: The nature of the lost relationship, and the circumstances surrounding the death. We then provide a discussion of different treatment options for bereaved individuals who seek professional help. In the concluding section, we review the current understanding of the grieving process and identify new research directions for the future.

II. SYMPTOMATOLOGY

Grief is regarded as a set of psychological, behavioral, social, and physical responses that can impact a bereaved person's life in a variety of ways.

Psychological responses comprise three different dimensions: emotions (e.g., depression, anxiety, yearning, helplessness, anger, guilt, and sometimes relief); cognitions (e.g., disbelief, confusion, and thoughts about how the loved one died); and perceptions (e.g., feelings of unreality, visual or auditory hallucinations, sense of the deceased person's presence). Behavioral responses include searching for the deceased, clinging, crying, avoidance of reminders, and restless hyperactivity or decreased energy and initiative. Social responses include lack of interest in others, social withdrawal, feelings of alienation, an overcritical or hostile attitude toward others, and heightened dependency. Common physical responses are symptoms that are indicative of depression such as loss of appetite, fatigue, and physical exhaustion, of anxiety such as trembling, heart palpitations, and hypervigilance, or of both such as sleep disturbances.

As noted above, the pattern of symptoms and the course of the grieving process depend on many factors (for instance, the type/mode of death, aspects of the bereaved person's personality and of the relationship to the deceased, and circumstances surrounding the loss). Most researchers consider a grief reaction problematic if the bereaved either does not show any of the aforementioned symptoms, or if they are manifested in an extreme or prolonged form. There is evidence that full-blown clinical complications (mainly major depression and anxiety disorders) occur in about 20% of bereaved persons.

III. THEORETICAL PERSPECTIVES

Several different theoretical statements have made important contributions to the current state of knowledge about loss and grief. An early paper that is generally referred to as a classic in the field of bereavement is Freud's paper, "Mourning and Melancholia." According to Freud, the psychological function of grief is to withdraw emotional energy (cathexis) and become detached from the loved one (decathexis). The underlying idea of this formulation is that people have a limited amount of energy at their disposal. Consequently, only by freeing up bounded energy will the person be able to reinvest in new relationships and activities. Freud believed that the mourner has to work through the grief by carefully reviewing thoughts and memories of the deceased (hypercathexis). He maintained that although the process of working through causes intense distress, it is necessary in order to achieve detachment from the loved one.

Another highly influential theoretical contribution has been advanced by John Bowlby. In his attachment model of grief, Bowlby integrated ideas from psychoanalysis, ethology, and from the literature on human development. Fundamental to his view is the similarity between children's reaction to early separation from their mother and the mourning behavior of adults and primates. He considers grief to be a form of separation distress that triggers attachment behavior such as angry protest, crying, and searching for the lost person. The aim of these behaviors is maintenance of the attachment or reunion, rather than withdrawal. However, in the case of a permanent loss the biological function of assuring proximity with attachment figures becomes dysfunctional. Consequently, the bereaved person struggles between the opposing impulses of activated attachment behavior and the need to survive without the loved one. Bowlby believed that in order to deal with these opposing forces, the mourner must go through four stages of grief: initial numbness, disbelief, or shock; yearning or searching for the lost person, accompanied by anger and protest; despair and disorganization as the bereaved gives up the search, accompanied by feelings of depression and lethargy; and reorganization or recovery as the loss is accepted, and an active life is resumed. Emphasizing the survival value of attachment behavior, Bowlby was the first to give a plausible explanation for responses such as searching or anger in grief.

In addition to Bowlby, a number of theorists have proposed that bereaved individuals go through certain stages or phases in coming to terms with the loss. One important model based on stages is Mardi Horowitz's stress response model. In this formulation, Horowitz asserts that a person reacts to the initial news about the death with extreme shock, responding with a sense of "No, that can't be true," termed "outcry." Then, the bereaved enters a stage that is characterized by denial. It is assumed that in this phase most individuals are overwhelmed by what has happened, and consequently avoid confronting thoughts and feelings about the loss in order to regain some equilibrium. After a while, however, the reality of the loss will break through, in the form of intrusive thoughts and memories. Because the intrusions are too painful to bear, the bereaved person is expected to engage in denial again. For some time, an oscillation takes place between these two states of mind. Horowitz maintained that this allows the individual to face the reality of the loss in low doses, and integrate it slowly with his or her general life conceptions.

One stage theory that has received a great deal of attention is Kubler-Ross's model, which addresses people's reaction to their own impending death. Individuals are assumed to go through stages of denial, anger, bargaining, depression, and ultimately acceptance. It was Kubler-Ross's model that popularized stage theories of bereavement. For the past several years, stage models such as Kubler-Ross's have been taught in medical, nursing, and social work schools. These models also have appeared in articles in newspapers and magazines written for bereaved persons and their families. As a result, stage models have strongly influenced the common understanding of grief in our society. There is evidence that health care professionals tend to use the stages as a yardstick to assess the appropriateness of a person's grieving. A negative consequence of this is that people who do not follow the expected stages may be labeled as responding deviantly or pathologically. For example, a person who does not reach a state of resolution after a certain time may be accused of "wallowing in grief." Also, legitimate feelings such as being angry because one's spouse died as a result of receiving the wrong medication may be discounted as "just a stage." Such a rigid application of stage models has the potential to cause harm to bereaved persons. For these reasons, the Institute of Medicine has warned against the use of "stages" in a review on bereavement. In that report, it was argued that the rigid use of stages may lead people to expect a bereaved person to progress through the grieving process in a more orderly manner than typically occurs.

Because of the widespread use and acceptance of stage models, in 1989 Wortman and Silver systematically examined all empirical studies that appeared to provide relevant data on the topic. What they found was that the available evidence did not support and in some cases even contradicted the stage approach. The research findings showed that few people pass through stages in the expected order, and that certain stages are sometimes skipped altogether. According to this evidence, the specific kinds of emotions experienced following a loss, the intensity of emotional responses, and the sequence of reactions are extremely variable. For example, in some of the reviewed studies, feelings of depression appeared to precede feelings of anger, which is the opposite of what is predicted by stage theories of grief. In other studies, it was reported that feelings of anger were not followed by depression. In fact, there were some studies in which anger was found to increase over time, contrary to what the stage models would predict. Furthermore, feelings of anxiety appeared to be as prevalent as feelings of depression, a pattern that is not predicted by the majority of stage models. Taken together, available evidence suggests that the reaction to loss varies considerably from person to person. The main weakness of stage models is that they cannot account for this variability in grief responses. [See ANGER; DEPRESSION.]

Recently, a different theoretical framework, the so-called stress and coping approach, has been applied to the topic of loss and grief. Stress and coping theorists maintain that life changes become distressing if a person experiences a discrepancy between the demands of a situation and the resources available to cope with them. According to this view, an individual's grief response is not determined by the mere exposure to a loss. Rather, it depends on the extent to which the demands created by the loss exceed the available coping resources. To explain why a given loss has more impact on one person than on another, stress and coping researchers have focused on the identification of potential risk factors (e.g., personality) that may make some individuals more vulnerable to developing complicated grief. They also have considered protective factors (e.g., social support) that may be strengthening, and, thereby, facilitate the coping process. A strength of the stress and coping approach is that it can account for variability in response to a major loss. [*See* COPING WITH STRESS.]

IV. CURRENT UNDERSTANDING OF GRIEF

As a result of the evidence reviewed above, most researchers to date conceive of the grieving process as a series of flexible, fluent phases, instead of a set of discrete stages. A model that represents this view has recently been advanced by Rando, who suggested that bereaved individuals typically go through three basic phases: avoidance, confrontation, and accommodation. She believes that an initial struggle to acknowledge and understand what happened is a common response to all losses. This phase is called "avoidance" because, initially, people are expected to avoid the reality of the death. Whether acknowledgment of the loss is avoided depends on such factors as how the death occurred. For example, an individual may find it particularly difficult to accept the reality of a loss if the death was sudden and traumatic—for example, if a young child playing on the sidewalk is struck and killed by a drunk driver. Once the reality of the loss is acknowledged, a person is expected to enter the confrontation phase, where grief is experienced and expressed. Rando maintains that during this phase, the relationship to the deceased must be remembered and reexperienced realistically, and the old attachment must be relinquished. Finally, in the accommodation phase, the symptoms of grief decline, and the mourner begins to accept the loss and its implications.

The loss is accommodated once the bereaved has developed a new relationship to the deceased, and a new way of being in the world without the loved one. The new relationship is usually based largely on recollection and past experience. It may involve celebrations for the deceased, commemorative activities, reviewing mementos, acting on the deceased's values and concerns, and appreciating the ways one has benefitted from having loved or been influenced by him or her. Regarding the development of a new way of being in the world without the deceased, it is important that over time, the bereaved undertake new roles, skills and relationships to deal with the absence of the loved one. It is important to reinvest in new activities that, unlike the deceased, can provide gratification to the bereaved. A person may choose to reinvest in new people (e.g., now that one is a single parent, forming friendships with other single parents); new activities (e.g., pursing activities that the bereaved has an interest in that the deceased did not share, such as tennis, sailing, or art), or new goals (e.g., going back to school to become a teacher).

In what way does Rando's phase model differ from the stage models described in the last section? What does this model add? First, Rando has taken into consideration the available knowledge about possible risk factors that may complicate the grief reaction. For each phase, she provides a detailed discussion about the influence of factors such as the mode of death, or the relationship to the deceased. Second, in contrast to many other stage theorists, Rando does not propose a final state of resolution. Most researchers believe that a state of resolution is reached when a bereaved person can accept the loss intellectually and emotionally. This means that the bereaved should have made sense of, or found some meaning in the death, and he or she can recall the deceased without intense distress. In contrast, Rando maintains that many bereaved individuals never fully resolve their grief. This view is supported by research studies investigating the long-term effects of loss. For example, in a study focusing on the loss of a spouse or child in a motor vehicle accident, a majority of respondents could not make sense of, or find any meaning in the loss, and continued to be intensely distressed when recalling their spouse or child, even 4 to 7 years later. Similarly, Rando claims that many bereaved individuals never completely recover, which means that they do not return to their previous state of functioning. Evidence shows that this is particularly likely to be the case if the loss was sudden and traumatic. According to these findings, many people struggle with the ramifications of their loved one's death for the rest of their lives.

Another interesting aspect of Rando's model is her focus on the importance of developing a new relationship to the deceased. Many theorists maintain that bereaved individuals must break the tie to their loved ones in order to recover from the loss. Some even consider this disengagement from the deceased as the major task a mourner has to accomplish. However, Rando believes that developing a new relationship to the deceased is an essential part of the accommodation process. The few available findings on this topic suggest that many bereaved persons remain attached to their loved one, and that this continuing relationship with the deceased not only can be adaptive but can also serve as a strengthening resource that helps the individual to cope with day-to-day life. In an example of this, one study found that a majority of widows endorsed items indicating a continuing relationship with their spouses (e.g., asking their spouse for advice regarding how to handle a problem) initially following the loss, and even 13 months postloss. Another study reported that a majority of elementary school children who lost a parent developed memories, feelings, and behaviors that kept them connected to the lost parent. A relinquishment of the tie did not seem to occur. Most of the children seemed to perceive their connection with their deceased parent as comforting and helpful. When they were asked what they would advise another bereaved child to do, they gave answers such as "just think of him (her) as often as you can."

An intriguing issue that has not been addressed in any of the models described previously, including Rando's, concerns those individuals who fail to become intensely distressed following a loss. Because the majority of people who experience a major loss go through a period of intense distress, it is believed that the failure to experience intense distress is not normal, and probably indicative of emotional shallowness or the inability to form close relationships. Furthermore, those who do not show intense grief are expected to develop some kind of delayed grief or subsequent health problems. However, a review of the available controlled studies has shown that a substantial minority of bereaved individuals do not go through an initial period of intense distress following the death of a loved one. Moreover, these people do not seem to develop a delayed grief reaction over time. On the contrary, those who do not show intense distress early in the grieving process often appear to be coping most successfully later. Conversely, those who are most distressed initially are more likely to experience a prolonged grief reaction. At this point, no controlled studies have examined the hypothesis that lack of distress after a loss is a sign of one's emotional shallowness or inability to form close relationships.

V. FACTORS MEDIATING THE GRIEF RESPONSE

At present, there is considerable interest in identifying factors that may influence why some people appear to be hit harder by the loss of a loved one than other people are. Different issues that have been addressed are the role of sociocultural factors (e.g., age, gender, social class, ethnic group), individual factors (e.g., personality, religiosity, health, means of coping), situational factors (e.g., negative life events prior to loss, mode of death, social support), and factors concerning the nature of the lost relationship (e.g., loss of a spouse or a child, loss of a highly conflictual or a harmonious relationship). Because a detailed review of these factors is beyond the scope of this article, we discuss those factors that we believe to be most critical in understanding reaction to loss, but that have generally received insufficient attention in the literature: the nature of the relationship to the deceased, and the circumstances that may surround the death. [*See* AGING AND MENTAL HEALTH; ETHNICITY AND MENTAL HEALTH; GENDER DIFFERENCES IN MENTAL HEALTH; INDIVIDUAL DIFFERENCES IN MENTAL HEALTH; RELIGION AND MENTAL HEALTH; SOCIOECONOMIC STATUS.]

A. Nature of the Lost Relationship

To explain the consequences of a particular loss, it is important to consider the nature of the lost relationship. Only by understanding what the loved one meant to a bereaved individual can we understand the impact of the loss. What place did the deceased have in the bereaved person's life? What roles did the loved one play? Has the deceased been a main source of emotional gratification and support? Was the relationship overly conflictual in nature? To elucidate the unique characteristics of different losses, we will discuss the loss of a spouse, a child and a parent.

1. Loss of a Spouse
Most studies in the field of bereavement have investigated the consequences of losing a spouse. Research findings show that the loss of a spouse is associated

with health problems and an elevated risk of mortality. A spouse may fill many roles in a person's life. This means that a bereaved individual may have to cope with a whole set of losses, such as loss of a lover, friend, protector, and financial or status provider. The fact that each bereaved person has to deal with a different set of losses may account for a considerable part of the variability in reaction to a loss. One person may have lost an intimate friend, a sexual partner, and a child-rearing partner. Another person may not have been so strongly connected to the spouse, but may still experience the loss of someone who helped with certain household responsibilities. For a third person, the loss may signify the end of a conflictual marriage, or the intense strain of caregiving for an ill spouse. It seems plausible to expect that these three individuals will show different grief reactions, even though they all experienced the loss of a spouse. These examples demonstrate that certain characteristics of the marital relationship may shape the grief response.

One factor that has consistently been found to influence the grieving process is heightened dependence on the spouse. There is clear evidence that a high level of dependency on the spouse enhances the risk for excessive yearning and complicated grief. Attachment theorists have suggested that emotional dependency signals insecurity, a lack of confidence, and a tendency to cling. These features may make it more difficult for a person to meet the challenges of a life without the spouse.

Another factor that has generated considerable research and interest is the impact of a conflictual marriage on grief. Unfortunately, the evidence on marital conflict is much less clear than the data on dependency. Clinical lore suggests that those involved in a troubled marriage are most likely to experience problems following the loss. This view is supported by some researchers who found that a highly conflictual relationship is predictive of long-term difficulties in the grieving process. However, other investigators have found that the happier the marriage was, the more intense and prolonged the grief.

A new way of conceptualizing marital difficulties, and their impact on the grieving process, has recently been developed by Blair Wheaton. He argues that the reaction to a partner's death is determined to a considerable extent by the amount of stress that is experienced in the marital role. He found that when widowhood signified the end of chronic role stress (e.g.,

a conflictual marriage or burdensome caregiving responsibilities), the usually detrimental effects of such a loss were moderated or eliminated. His data suggest that the mental health of a surviving spouse can actually improve after such a loss. Of course, these findings do not resolve the inconsistencies in the literature on how marital conflict impacts a bereaved person's grief. But they do challenge the traditional view that is held by most researchers and clinicians, and thereby provide a new perspective that may help to clarify the impact of marital conflict on bereavement in subsequent research.

2. Loss of a Child

There is consistent evidence that the loss of a child causes particularly intense and prolonged grief. In one study, parents who lost a child in a motor vehicle crash showed higher mortality, more depression, and were more likely to seek and obtain a divorce than control respondents. The enormous distress of losing a child may be due to the unique nature of the child–parent attachment. Because one's child is an extension of one's self, bereaved parents may feel that they lost a central part of themselves. The death of a child may also trigger a loss of purpose in life. Hopes and expectations about the future may be shattered. Also, core assumptions, such as the expectation that parents protect their children, or that children outlive their parents, may be violated.

For some types of child loss, parents' distress may be exacerbated by the fact that the significance of these losses is not recognized by society. Losses due to miscarriage or stillbirth may fall into this category. Not realizing to what extent a bond can be developed in advance of birth, people may show very little sympathy in such cases. For instance, they may make comments like "You can always have another child," or "It is much worse to lose a child one knows."

3. Loss of a Parent

Most studies that have investigated the loss of a parent have focused on young bereaved children. There is general consensus that the death of a parent is a stressful experience for pre- and grade school children. Researchers have reported that the loss of a parent during childhood is typically followed by depression and behavioral problems, such as acting out, sleep problems, bedwetting, and a tendency to cling to the surviving parent. Children may also develop somatic symptoms such as headaches, stomach aches or diarrhea in response to the loss. The risk of developing emotional and behavioral problems is minimized in cases where the surviving parent can be emotionally available to the child and can maintain family routines.

B. Circumstances Surrounding the Death

Next, we discuss the impact of the circumstances surrounding the death. In recent years, researchers have come to recognize that the circumstances under which a death occurs play a major role in shaping response to a loss. Below, we discuss the implications of sudden, traumatic deaths, deaths after a lengthy illness, stigmatized deaths, and deaths where the bereaved must cope with the loss without adequate social support.

I. Sudden, Traumatic Death

Research evidence demonstrates that a sudden, unexpected death typically results in more physical and mental health problems for a bereaved individual than an anticipated death. The likelihood of intense and prolonged grief is particularly enhanced if the loss was untimely, or traumatic, involving elements of maliciousness, negligence, or violence. Rando pointed out that, due to technological advances in society, the number of natural deaths had decreased, whereas sudden traumatic deaths are occurring with greater frequency. To date, accidental deaths are the leading, and homicide the second leading, cause of death for people under age 40.

The debilitating effect of a sudden, traumatic death is exacerbated if the death was violent or mutilating, if it was witnessed by the bereaved, or if the bereaved's life was threatened. Survivors of sudden traumatic deaths often not only suffer from intensified and prolonged grief but also experience massive anxiety, intrusive thoughts, and nightmares. Frequently, the symptomatology following such a loss resembles the typical picture of Posttraumatic Stress Disorder. Additionally, the mourner may have to contend with the shattering of basic assumptions about safety, security, and justice in the world. Moreover, if the death was caused intentionally, the bereaved person is confronted with the human potential for destruction and cruelty. If the death was a result of somebody else's negligence, the bereaved individual may struggle with the fact that the loss was unnecessary and preventable. [*See* POSTTRAUMATIC STRESS.]

2. Death after a Lengthy Illness

Research findings suggest that death caused by lengthy illness may also increase the bereaved person's risk of subsequent difficulties. At first glance, this notion appears to be inconsistent with evidence that clearly identifies a sudden, unexpected death as a risk factor for poor outcome. Especially if the bereaved individual was the primary caregiver, the benefits of having time to prepare for the death may be outweighed by the costs of a long period of emotional and physical strain. Caregivers often set aside their own needs and health concerns to cope with the day-to-day demands of caring. The exposure to the loved one's prolonged pain and physical deterioration may cause additional stress. In some cases, the person involved in caregiving may feel that the loved one does not appreciate the many sacrifices that are being made. After the death, they may not permit themselves to express any resentments, and feelings of anger, hostility, and relief may evoke feelings of guilt. Bereaved individuals who have devoted a significant part of their time to this task may have difficulties finding a new purpose in life. Furthermore, particularly in the case of the elderly, emotional and physical resources may have been so exhausted by the strain of the loved one's illness that survivors may have difficulty returning to their previous level of functioning.

3. Stigmatized Death

Deaths that are associated with a stigma put an enormous strain on the survivor because of the shame that surrounds the loss. Two causes of death that are often stigmatized in our society are suicide and AIDS. Research findings suggest that suicide is a precipitant for intense and prolonged grief. There is evidence that bereaved individuals who have lost a loved one through suicide show higher levels of depression and anxiety, and are more prone to commit suicide themselves, than other bereaved persons. Being blamed by others for not preventing the suicide or for having caused it may evoke feelings of anger or guilt. It is also common to feel rejected because the loved one has chosen death over a life with the bereaved. Additionally, the suicide may often be perceived as a sort of betrayal, and the loved one may be accused of abandoning the survivor: "How could he be so selfish?" "How could she do this to me?" Such thoughts may exacerbate already existing feelings of guilt, and nourish self-reproach. [*See* SUICIDE.]

Death from AIDS is probably the most stigmatized loss in our society. Despite efforts at education, AIDS is still stereotyped as a gay or an IV-drug user disease. As a result of the widely held notion that AIDS "punishes sinners," individuals who have acquired the disease, as well as their family or friends, often receive very little sympathy from others. Yet, they seem to have a special need for support. In fact, it has been suggested that individuals who experience a loss caused by AIDS are at risk for prolonged and intensified grief, if they have not received adequate help during the loved one's illness, and subsequently after the death. Certain characteristics of the disease and its implications may exacerbate the grief reaction. A lengthy period of physical deterioration may amplify the impact of the ultimate loss. This is true in part because the course of the disease is usually harsh and unpredictable, and observing the loved one's pain and physical deterioration can be very distressing. Moreover, watching a loved one die from AIDS may also elicit an agonizing fear of one's own vulnerability. Furthermore, survivors are often confronted with the death of multiple friends. In this case, it may be difficult to grieve adequately for a particular loss. The detrimental impact of each loss subsequently may be cumulative. [See HIV/AIDS.]

4. Lack of Perceived Support

Different factors that may ameliorate the impact of loss have been discussed in the literature. One of these is social support. The perception that social support is available appears to affect the grieving process after a major loss. Research findings suggest that following bereavement, the outcome is not predicted by the number of support providers, but rather by qualitative aspects of the received support (e.g., feeling loved and accepted, feeling free to express emotions).

In several studies, bereaved persons reported that what they perceived as most helpful was an opportunity to talk about their grief. At this point, research on social support suggests that the bereaved face a dilemma in obtaining adequate support. On one hand, there is consistent evidence that bereaved individuals value being allowed to express their feelings in nonjudgmental surroundings. Also, clinicians usually consider the expression of grief to be healthy and, therefore, encourage bereaved individuals to discuss their feelings. On the other hand, many findings indicate that revealing intense distress frequently evokes negative social responses. It has been reported that bereaved individuals frequently feel misunderstood, avoided,

and even blamed by others when expressing their grief. Evidence shows that, in many cases, other's responses add to their distress, and may lead the bereaved not to express their feelings anymore, or even to withdraw from social contact altogether. Some studies suggest that failure to express feelings may result in subsequent health problems.

Research findings indicate that although people make an effort to provide support to the bereaved, their efforts are often not perceived as helpful. Common statements made to bereaved individuals include, "You still have another child," "I know how you feel," "You should get out and meet people," "Think of the future," and so on. Even if motivated by good will, these comments may minimize the loss, put the bereaved under pressure to recover quickly, and discourage the expression of feelings. There is evidence suggesting that because these types of "condolences" serve to inhibit the display of grief, they are not helpful. Interestingly, these inappropriate responses are just as likely to come from family members or close friends as they are from casual acquaintances. Because those people are most affected by the bereaved person's anguish, and they have the greatest stake in his or her recovery.

Why do people often fail to provide adequate support? As was discussed above, our society holds certain assumptions about the typical duration and severity of grief that, according to recent research, seem to be incorrect. Thus, potential supporters may lack accurate information about what is normative and, therefore, may place inappropriate expectations on the mourner. In addition, contact with the bereaved also seems to evoke feelings of helplessness and vulnerability in the support provider, particularly if the bereaved person conveys intense distress. Helplessness may occur because there is so little one can to ameliorate the bereaved individual's agony. Facing the reality of death can also be anxiety provoking and high levels of arousal may interfere with providing effective support. Especially in the case of a traumatic death (e.g., by homicide), the confrontation with such a tragic event may threaten the helper's need for security and safety. Rando suggests that others blame, derogate, and avoid survivors of traumatic death in order to help maintain the illusion of personal safety and the belief in the avoidability of such events.

Negative responses such as avoidance are commonly experienced by bereaved parents. In our society, the loss of a child represents the worst of all possible fears. The idea of losing a child is so threatening that most people are extremely reluctant to be confronted with the possibility that such a tragedy could happen to them. This may cause them to either avoid the topic in conversations with bereaved parents, or to avoid bereaved parents entirely.

It seems ironic that what is considered most beneficial for a bereaved person—the expression of painful feelings—may be difficult for others to tolerate and may impede them from providing effective support. This raises the question of whether bereaved individuals should be instructed about how to minimize negative feelings in others. Some researchers have suggested encouraging alternative ways of expressing feelings (e.g., keeping a diary). It should be noted, however, that the failure to express grief verbally may contribute to false societal norms. For example, if a certain percentage of bereaved people inhibit the emotional expression of grief soon after the loss, the assumption that one can recover in a relatively short time will be maintained. As a result, it will be even more difficult for bereaved individuals to get the support they need. Considering the benefits and the difficulties of providing support for bereaved individuals, it may prove helpful to educate lay persons not only about the nature of grief, but also about specific strategies that are generally perceived as unhelpful and helpful. Avoidant responses, such as pretending you do not see the bereaved in the grocery store, are extremely hurtful, as are responses that impart blame (e.g., "If your son was wearing a seat belt, he probably would have lived."). Other unhelpful responses include asking inappropriate questions (e.g., "Did he leave a lot of insurance money?"), giving advice (e.g., "Isn't it time to take down the pictures of the bereaved?) presence ("just being there"), expressing concern, and providing appropriate tangible support (e.g., shoveling out an elderly widow's driveway). It is also helpful to provide the opportunity for the bereaved to express their feelings about the loss if they wish. Above all else, the support provider should try to listen nonjudgmentally, and thus help the bereaved person to feel understood. [*See* SOCIAL SUPPORT.]

VI. INTERVENTION

The evidence reviewed above shows that most bereaved individuals go through a period of enormous distress, and that many of them value the opportunity to talk about the loss and to disclose their feelings. This raises the issue of whether bereaved people could benefit from professional support, and what kind of intervention may be helpful. It should be noted that bereaved individuals rarely seek professional help in dealing with their grief. Approximately 5 to 10% turn to their clergy or their physician; a smaller percentage attends support groups, and even fewer see a psychotherapist. If many bereaved individuals have the need to express and share their feelings, why do so few seek out professional help? A reluctance to seek therapy may stem from a fear of not being understood, or from being overwhelmed by one's own emotions. Bereaved people may also think that they should be able to handle their grief, and that the failure to cope with it on one's own is a sign of weakness. This barrier toward help seeking may be eliminated if more information about different treatment options were available to lay persons. Options include different kinds of individual psychotherapy, group or family therapy, peer support groups, and medication.

There is some consensus that intervention should facilitate the expression of feelings, and provide reassurance that a certain intensity and duration of grief is normal. Professionals should assist a bereaved person in learning how to tolerate and modulate painful feelings, in reviewing positive and negative aspects of the lost relationship, and in reestablishing goals, interests and relationships that facilitate moving on with life. In addition to these goals, therapy provides an opportunity to monitor the risk of suicide, and the possible need for medication.

One important question that must be addressed is the following: under what conditions should an individual seek professional help in dealing with the death of a loved one? In our judgment, the bereaved are at heightened risk for a poor outcome, and hence likely to benefit from treatment, if they possess one or more of the risk factors discussed earlier. These include losing a spouse on whom one was highly dependent; experiencing the loss under traumatic circumstances (e.g., a loss that was sudden, untimely, violent, or mutilating); presence of concomitant stressors (e.g., chronic illness, job loss); and absence of social support. Available evidence also suggests that if the bereaved person experiences an extremely intense reaction to the death involving painful yearning and longing for the deceased, there is greater likelihood of a poor outcome, and it would be wise to consider treatment. Other symptoms that predict subsequent difficulties if they are marked and persist for at least two months include: feeling shocked or numb; attempting to avoid reminders of the loss; feeling that life is empty or meaningless; difficulty believing the death has occurred; feeling that part of oneself has died; feeling excessive irritability, bitterness, or anger related to the death; feeling a lost sense of security, trust, or control; and difficulty imagining a fulfilling life without the deceased.

Once a decision is made to seek treatment, the bereaved individual must consider the advantages and disadvantages of the many treatments that are available. The research evidence provides clear support for the efficacy of individual psychotherapy. Specific studies have focused on a variety of different treatments. Cognitive interventions have proved to be helpful in reducing a person's distress by gradual exposure to memories and reminders of the deceased. For survivors of traumatic loss, a combination of exposure and anxiety management (e.g., relaxation) seems to work best. Cognitive behavioral therapists have also focused on improving cognitions of helplessness, guilt, and low self-esteem. Brief focused psychodynamic therapy has also been successful in helping bereaved people, especially when symptoms such as avoidance or denial are prevalent.

Because many people lack the resources to afford individual therapy, there has been increasing interest in more economical treatments such as peer support groups. Support groups or one-on-one peer support can also serve as an important adjunct to psychotherapy. Listening to the stories of survivors who have experienced a similar loss can be uniquely empowering. Contact with others in similar circumstances can reassure the bereaved that their thoughts and feelings are normal and understandable. Groups can also provide a forum for the exchange of information about grief, PTSD, and community resources.

A handful of studies has examined the impact of peer support groups. In some studies no outcome differences were found between bereaved persons who attended such a group and those who did not. However, other studies have shown that participants benefitted a great deal from attending a support group. Why do support groups work for some people, and not for others? There is some evidence that peer support is most beneficial for bereaved individuals with an outgoing nature, good social skills, but insufficient coping strategies. Those with poor social skills may not benefit as much because they may find it difficult to become freely involved with the group.

Over the years, the use of medication (mainly antidepressants and antianxiety drugs) in the treatment of grief has been controversial. Some clinicians believe that drugs can interfere with the process of remembering and reexperiencing the loss—a process they maintain is essential to healing. However, as evidence has mounted that many of the symptoms of grief, such as depression and PTSD, have biological underpinnings, there has been enhanced interest in the use of medication. Although there are few carefully controlled studies addressing this issue, available evidence supports the judicious use of antidepressant and antianxiety drugs in the treatment of grief. In the acute stages of grief, evidence supports the use of drugs that decrease autonomic arousal, such as benzodiazepines. These drugs typically reduce nightmares and intrusive thoughts and promote sleep. By stabilizing clients, such medications can often free them to work through their painful feelings without becoming overwhelmed. However, it should be kept in mind that because such drugs have addictive properties, and because withdrawal can be difficult, the use of these drugs should be monitored carefully. Tricyclic antidepressants and selective serotonin reuptake inhibitors (SSRIs) have also been shown to be effective in alleviating depression and PTSD symptomatology. Since different drugs affect different symptoms for different people, the clinician may wish to try a second drug if response to the first medication is minimal or partial. [See [PSYCHOPHARMACOLOGY.]

There is general agreement that such medications should not be used routinely to manage grief, but are appropriate in cases where grief is unusually intense or prolonged, or where the client is at risk for a poor outcome. When medication is warranted, most practitioners feel that it should be prescribed in conjunction with psychological intervention.

Considering the variability in response to bereavement, it makes sense to assume that different interventions are more or less appropriate for different individuals. There is evidence that individual therapy is indicated if the level of distress is extremely high or if the possible necessity of prescribing medication needs to be monitored. If the loss was sudden and traumatic, and the bereaved person is suffering from PTSD symptoms like intrusive thoughts and nightmares, these symptoms may need to be treated before the process of grieving can take place. A therapist who is experienced in treating grief and trauma would be the best choice. For people with lower levels of distress, or people who are unwilling to consider individual therapy (or who cannot afford it), peer support groups are a good option. They may be helpful in providing reassurance about the normality of emotions, or in serving as a forum for the exchange of information and experiences. If possible, the bereaved person should select a support group comprised of mourners who have experienced a similar loss (e.g., perinatal loss, death of a young child, loss following a lengthy illness, suicide, etc.).

In sum, the evidence is clear in suggesting that professional interventions are effective in helping bereaved individuals who are judged to be at high risk for developing complications. Therefore, it is recommended that bereaved individuals who possess some or all of the risk factors discussed earlier, and/or who show an intense and extremely painful grief reaction that does not abate somewhat after a few months, give serious consideration to obtaining professional treatment. Without such treatment, symptoms like depression, painful intrusive thoughts, and the inability to concentrate can become entrenched, lasting for months or years.

VII. CONCLUSION

The loss of a loved one typically has a major impact on the future course and direction of a person's life. As the reviewed research shows, a permanent loss can seriously threaten and impair one's health, well-being and productivity. It may also challenge people's fundamental assumptions about themselves and their world, and shatter their hopes and expectations for the future. However, some bereaved individuals succeed in recovering from their grief to a certain degree, some seem to remain permanently damaged, and others appear not to be much affected by the loss. Our main goal in this article was to highlight and clarify this striking variability in response to loss. A related goal was to show that certain commonly held beliefs—for example, that the failure to experience intense grief following a loss is necessarily indicative of pathology; that a bereaved person needs to break down the attachment to the deceased in order to recover from the loss; and that people typically return to normal functioning after a relatively short time—are generally not supported, and in a few cases even contradicted, by empirical evidence. We urged readers to be more aware of the particularly devastating effect of certain losses such as sudden traumatic or stigmatized losses. Grief responses to these losses can be quite different from reactions to the timely deaths from natural causes that everybody encounters as an inescapable part of the life course.

Considering the great variety in grief reactions, why is the idea of universal stages, including the above-discussed assumptions about recovery and resolution, still so popular among workers in the field and among lay persons? Why are stage models of grief often applied in such a rigid way, probably more rigidly than they were ever meant to be used? It seems essential to understand this discrepancy between research evidence and practice. Direct contact with someone in the throes of grief can be demanding for the social network as well as for health care professionals. Relying on a framework or model may often help to interpret the bereaved person's behavior, or provide an idea of what to expect next. Because it can be very distressing to be confronted with another's persistent display of grief, believing in a state of complete resolution (as suggested in most of the models) may sometimes help to carry on, especially if the bereaved does not seem to improve despite efforts to help. The notion of a final stage of recovery seems to express the wish/hope that, in the end, "everything will turn out fine," rather than to represent a realistic normative goal.

If the idea of stages has a supportive function in coping with the intense grief of a bereaved person, what could serve as a substitute for this function? What can be done to ease the pain of bereaved individuals as well as the emotional strain for support providers? Findings show that bereaved people generally value a nonjudgmental attitude, and that disapproving reactions from others can intensify their already existing distress. However, as we have outlined above, it is often difficult for outsiders to remain nonjudgmental, even if they have the best intentions to do so. What may enable bereaved individuals and those in their social network to communicate in a way that is helpful and rewarding for both sides? These intriguing questions can only be answered by research that explores the transaction between bereaved individuals and support providers.

Also, much remains to be learned about other factors that may promote or inhibit healing. In our opinion, a number of topics have not received sufficient research attention to date: In what way do worldviews and prior aversive life events influence the grieving process? Clinical experience suggests that the more a person's fundamental views about the world are shattered by a loss, the more likely it is that subsequent difficulties will occur. Similarly, prior losses may influence coping with a current loss in that they shape people's expectations and beliefs about their lives. The current loss may also stir up distressing memories about the former event.

Another issue that seems important to us is the role of dependency versus autonomy. If high dependency is a risk factor for poor outcome, is high autonomy a protective factor? A related topic is the question whether the coping process is facilitated if a person had many different sources of gratification (e.g., different interests, people to confide in) prior to the loss.

However, retrospective ratings of mediating factors such as one's health or the quality of one's marriage are likely to be affected by the loss. Therefore, prospective designs with pre- and postloss assessments are required to identify risk and protective factors, and to assess their impact on the grieving process. In the framework of prospective designs, we need to complement self-report methodology with measures of physiological change in order to examine the long-term effects of bereavement on health. In so doing, we may be able to answer important questions such as whether the failure to express emotional distress following a loss results in subsequent health problems.

When thinking about processes that inhibit recovery, we may also want to consider the possibility that bereaved individuals process information about the world differently from those who did not experience a loss. For example, somebody who lost a loved one by homicide may be particularly sensitive to the presence of violence almost anywhere (e.g., in the news, in movies, or in newspapers), and this may interfere with the recovery process.

To complete the picture of how a major loss may influence a person's life, we need to measure personal growth in more bereavement studies. It is widely believed that the experience of distressing life events can promote personal growth. However, this has rarely been substantiated by research. There are some studies suggesting that as a result of coping with the death of their husband, women typically report becoming stronger, more self-confident and more independent.

In this section, we have raised more questions than we could answer. In so doing, we intended to show that there is still much to be learned and understood about how people cope with a major loss, and that those who suffer from the death of a loved one need and deserve an open-minded attitude toward their plight.

BIBLIOGRAPHY

Jacobs, S. (1993). *Pathological grief: Maladaption to loss.* Washington, DC: American Psychiatric Press.

Klass, D., Silverman, P. R., & Nickman, S. L. (1996). *Continuing bonds: New understanding of grief.* Bristol, PA: Taylor & Francis.

Parkes, C. M., & Weiss, R. S. (1983). *Recovery from bereavement.* New York: Basic Books.

Rando, T. A. (1993). *Treatment of complicated mourning.* Champaign, IL: Research Press.

Stroebe, W., & Stroebe, M. S. (1993). *Handbook of bereavement: Theory, research, and intervention.* Cambridge: Cambridge University Press.

Walker, C. L. (1993). Sibling Bereavement and Grief Response. *Journal of Pediatric Nursing, 8*(5), 325–334.

Wortman, C. B., & Silver, R. C. (1989). The myths of coping with loss. *Journal of Consulting and Clinical Psychology, 57,* 349–357.

Wortman, C. B., Silver, R. C., & Kessler, R. C. (1993). The meaning of loss and adjustment to bereavement. In M. S. Stroebe, W. Stroebe & R. O. Hansson (Eds.), *Bereavement: sourcebook of research and interventions* (pp. 349–366). London: Cambridge University Press.

Guilt

Donald L. Mosher

University of Connecticut

Affect Primary innate biological motivating system, consisting of nine primary affects, each defined by a discrete pattern of facial, vocal, breathing, neural, and endocrine responses to innate or learned activators.

Central Assembly All functionally joined units of the minding system during a quantum of time, including the transmuting mechanism which renders conscious a report selected from the larger set of messages.

Moral Ideology Module of moral rules, within a world view, that define which aspects of human conduct are to be celebrated as virtues or sanctioned as vices.

Scene Unit of analysis of the stream of life, defined as a happening with a beginning and an end, forming an organized pattern that includes affects, objects, times, places, events, actions, psychological functions, props, and outcomes.

Script Unit of analysis of personality, defined as a psychologically magnified set of rules for ordering information in a family of connected scenes to predict, control, defend, and evaluate variants and analogs of the family of scenes. *Sex* is to scene as *sexuality* is to script.

GUILT can be defined as the feeling of remorse for violating a moral rule. Within the script theory of Silvan Tomkins, guilt is the affect of shame when centrally assembled with a moral judgment that the self is blame-worthy. Such moral barriers interrupt ongoing excitement and enjoyment to trigger guilt. Shyness, shame, and guilt are identical as an innate affect, but as moral shame, guilt amplifies an evaluation that the self is responsible for violating a moral rule. Although free-floating guilt may not be assembled with perceptions of specific causes and consequences in consciousness, whenever moral self-blame is so assembled, a specific moral urgency is manifested. Guilt is the primary human motivator that prevents, inhibits, avoids, escapes, modifies, amends, or defends against possible or actual immoral fantasies or conduct. "Guilt" refers primarily to the affective–cognitive report of anticipatory, coincident, or consequent moral remorse and secondarily to the motivational disposition to minimize guilt.

I. A SCRIPT THEORY OF SEXUAL GUILT

The human infant is born into a world in which she quickly learns to continue or repeat good scenes and to escape or avoid bad scenes. Inevitably, the human being comes to want to maximize the discrete positive affects of interest–excitement and enjoyment–joy and to minimize the discrete negative affects of fear–terror, distress–anguish, anger–rage, shame, disgust, and dissmell (an auxiliary to olfaction, like disgust is to gustation). Disgust and dissmell are innate defensive responses that are auxiliary to the hunger, thirst, and oxygen drives and which generalize to learned sources. Shame is an affect auxiliary response that specifically inhibits interest and enjoyment whenever a temporary barrier interrupts those activated positive affects. Examples of temporary barriers include all sources of shyness, discouragement, exposure, and guilt. Surprise–startle resets the central assembly, commanding an immediate response to its activator regardless of the nature of the ongoing scene. [*See* ANGER; ANXIETY.]

Positive affects are experienced as rewarding and inherently acceptable from birth; just as the negative affects, in addition to their distinct qualia, are invariably experienced as punishing and inherently unacceptable. Just as pleasure and pain require no learning and are distinctive in their qualia, so too are innate affects unlearned and distinct in experience. Affects are innate biological entities, encoded in subcortical centers and activated by gradients of neural stimulation that match distinct innate programs. Learned activators of affect must match or mimic these gradients. Whether activated by innate or learned sources, each discrete affect conforms to its innate profile of activation. Tomkins's theory and empirical research on affect stimulated Paul Ekman's and Carrol Izard's independent demonstrations of the universal recognition of facial affect. Ekman's research continued to identify neural and physiological correlates of discrete affects; Izard's research demonstrated the unlearned appearance of affect in children.

The experience of affect is primarily the experience of patterned changes in the facial skin and secondarily in breathing and vocalization which may or may not be associated with perception, analysis, or memory in the central assembly. When in consciousness, however, the nine discrete affects acquire their nuance and meaning from the information that is centrally assembled and transmuted into a report. Affect is activated by only three classes—nonoptimally intense, accelerating, or decelerating gradients—of neural firing. Consciousness is biased toward the inclusion of affect because the governing principle for filling the limited channel of consciousness selects messages to report with the most dense neural firing from the larger set of messages until the limited channel is filled.

The human infant quickly learns to repeat, create, and evaluate whatever scene is the source or target of excitement and joy; just as she learns to predict, defend against, and evaluate whatever object poses a barrier to such excitement and joy (thereby, activating shame or guilt) or whatever activates fear, distress, anger, disgust, or dissmell.

Discrete affects motivate through their capacity to amplify by analogy any ongoing or recruited responses; such responses are correlated with their sources, both sharing a distinct affective qualia and a similarity to the innate profile of activation of the discrete affect. So, the activation of excitement from a sexual partner touching the sexual skin amplifies both the source (being touched) and target (the sexual partner) of that affect, giving both an excited qualia with a moderately accelerating profile as the specific gradient that triggers interest–excitement.

Any temporary barrier or interruption of ongoing sexual excitement or sexual enjoyment innately activates shame. Guilt is the variant of shame in which moral cognitions regard the source, the target, or sexual affect itself as violating a moral rule within an ideology of what sexuality means and how it is to be celebrated or sanctioned. The moral ideology of parents and other significant socializers affects their style of socialization of guilt, including their tolerance of sexual affect and how they link moral cognitions to sexual scenes.

Experience in sexual scenes or in vicarious sexual scenes that involve moral rules can be connected as sharing a family resemblance, including the interruption by guilt of sensory pleasure, excitement, and enjoyment. Whenever a good scene turns bad, it becomes a candidate for psychological magnification. Psychological magnification increases the urgency of rules concerned with interpreting and understanding, with predicting and managing, with creating and defending, and with evaluating and justifying a connected set of scenes that have been so amplified by affect that they have become urgent to understand and manage. The individual attempts to order the information from the family of scenes by sets of rules: psychological principles that govern psychological functions.

Like their rules, scripts are selective in the scenes they govern; incomplete, requiring auxiliary information as the scenes unfold; often conditional upon variables as alternatively specifying response, tactic, or strategy; variously accurate and inaccurate in their interpretation and management of the scene; and continually changing with disconfirmation or as new scenes are added to the family.

Fresh affect is activated during the process of ordering information in the family of scenes, thereby reamplifying the already once amplified scenes *and* their rules. The principal script factor is repeated dense change in the polarity of affect within the set of scenes.

Thus, the good sexual scene turned bad—sexual guilt interrupting sexual excitement and enjoyment—becomes the primary source of the sex-guilt script.

Scripts are modular, capable of combination, recombination, and partitioning. Sexual scripts are composed of modules of rules ordering information from several families of scenes, including affect socialization scenes, moral scenes, interpersonal scenes, sexual scenes, and gender scenes. For example, gender, interpersonal, and moral rules are learned respectively in scenes concerned with the socialization of gender, of interpersonal relations, or of morality. Later, these modules become connected with developing sexual scripts within the encompassing family of scenes relevant to sexuality.

The broadest classification of sexual scripts would order them based upon the overall ratio of positive to negative affect within the plot of a life, including sexual scenes: (a) affluent, (b) damage–reparative, (c) limitation–remediation, (d) contamination–decontamination, and (e) toxic–detoxification. Given its stable equilibrium of positive over negative affect, an affluent sexual script provides flexible and alternative paths to deepening sexual involvement. In damage–reparative sexual scripts, perceived damage activates shame–guilt that may be temporary when it is repaired by seeking forgiveness, avoiding specific sexual objects or sexual linkages, or by making amends for harming the partner. In limitation–remediation sexual scripts, some lifelong limit in the nature of the self (e.g., gender dysphoria) or sexuality (e.g., sin) or world (e.g., homophobia) requires remediation by continuing effort to remedy it (e.g., by a sex-change, or chastity, or coming-out). In contamination–decontamination sexual scripts, sexuality is replete with plurivalent conflict, impurity, and ambiguity—often creating nuclear scripts that constellate more and more scenes to the family—that require continual but failing efforts to decontaminate the multiple deep disgusts that a sexual scene activates. In the toxic–detoxification sexual script, which has a stable equilibrium of negative affects over positive, a lust-murderer, for example, must recast the scene in which he trembled in terror by venting his rage against a dissmelling oppressor (mother) or her analog (prostitute).

The sexual guilt script is a modular component of sexual scripts. It functions as an affect control script, in which guilt (in contrast to distress, fear, disgust, anger, or dissmell) controls sexual excitement and enjoyment. An affect control script regulates the density, display, vocalization, consciousness, communication, conditionality, and consequences of affect.

Sexual scenes and sexual guilt can be either rewardingly or punitively socialized. Ideology includes a world view about the nature of sexuality and affect that varies from left-winged humanist ideology, identifying with the oppressed and social change, to right-winged normative ideology, identifying with the dominant authority and the status quo. For the humanist, children and their playful affects, like human nature, are to be celebrated as exciting sources of enjoyment. For the normative, children must be taught to adhere to the norms, and, thus, positive affect should only occur when a norm is met. So, for the normative, the only good sex should be marital, monogamous, passionless sex in the missionary position to procreate. A rewarding socialization of sexuality contrasts with a punitive socialization in which sexual excitement and enjoyment must be interrupted or further controlled (as contaminating or toxic) by socializers who activate negative affect in an attempt to offset sexual affects. Thus, the punitive versus rewarding socialization of sexual affects, often joined with specifically stated moral rules that are either normatively inviolate or humanistically contextual, respectively, create either intolerance or tolerance of the density, display, vocalization, consciousness, communication, conditionality, and consequences of sexual excitement and enjoyment. Thus, a psychologically magnified sexual guilt script often produces a damage–reparative sexual script in which the conditionality of sex is inhibited and limited by invariant moral rules, the density of sexual affect is interrupted or diminished by guilt, the display and vocalization of sexual interest–excitement and enjoyment–joy are attenuated or suppressed, the consciousness of sex as perception and fantasy is selective and reduced, the communication of sexual interest and information is decreased or stopped, and the consequences of sexuality are often feared as sexual and moral failure or, still worse, as disgusting and dangerous. Shame–guilt is not a highly toxic affect; in contrast, the more strongly that sexuality is psychological magnified by more toxic disgust or still more toxic terror, rage, and dissmell, the more problematic the sexual script becomes. In the punitive socialization of sexual affects, these affects are both suppressed and conceptually linked to sexual sin (guilt) and dirt (disgust) and danger (fear) by the Normative socializer. The sexual sinner is perceived either as contaminated (disgusting) and as requiring decontamination or as so evil and perverse (dissmelling) as to be toxic and beyond redemption, activating righteous rage.

Whenever the punitive socialization of sexual affects has been predominantly associated with the use of disgust to minimize sexual affects, then a contamination–decontamination script becomes likely as the major sexual affect control script. Whenever the punitively socialization of sexual affects produces an affect control script based upon the socializer's rage and dissmell to sanction sexual affects, producing terror and dissmell and hidden rage in the child, then a toxic–antitoxic sexual script may be the outcome. Although such anti-sexual ideological scripts are intolerant of communicating about sex, the same inflexible, anti-sexual, moral rules may have been offered by the parent or inferred by the child as a rationale for their cruel behavior; the less toxic but still moderately punitive parent may use this same anti-sexual ideology when inducing shame–guilt. The rewarding socializers of sexual affect communicate conditional rules for sexual guilt that are flexibly tied to issues of caring and responsibility in interpersonal relations rather than to fixed and exceptionless rules (e.g., no masturbation or premarital sex or oral–genital sex *ever*). A rewarding socialization of sexuality celebrates sexual interest–excitement and enjoyment–joy as rewarding affects to be maximized in life; sexual scenes are good scenes, rewarding and valued.

II. THE MEASUREMENT OF GUILT

By the mid-1960s, Donald Mosher had developed sentence completion, true–false, and forced–choice inventories to measure the personality disposition of guilt. The items included (a) admissions of feeling guilty, sinful, ashamed, disgusted, or revolted by sexual, aggressive, or other immoral acts, intentions, or fantasies; (b) moralizing attitudes that characterized sexuality or aggression as abnormal, self-destructive, or detrimental to society; and (c) self-reports that judged the self to be blameworthy, even as evil and unworthy of forgiveness, as desiring punishment, as practicing ascetic denial, or as engaging in acts of confession, contrition, and restitution. Nonguilty items

included: (a) denials of shame or guilty feelings over immoral acts, intentions, or fantasies; (b) nonmoralizing attitudes toward sexuality and aggression as normal, expected, or pleasurable; and (c) self-reports of self-acceptance following sexual or aggressive behavior, plans to avoid detection, or to enjoy transgressions brazenly.

The construct of guilt is given meaning by a script theory that specifies the processes by which it effects scenes and scripts; *guilt* is given meaning by the rules for its use in the scientific context. As a script (or personality variable), guilt is a disposition to activate the affect of guilt and guilty responses that minimize guilt in a moral–conflict scene. An inventory of guilt should include psychometric referents faithful to the theory that reliably orders individuals' dispositions to guilty affect and responses. Construct validation requires using the measure of guilt to test theoretically generated hypotheses. Favorable empirical outcomes both corroborate the theoretical hypotheses and provide evidence of the construct validity of the inventory.

Influenced by the classic papers of Cronbach and Meehl on construct validity and Fiske and Campbell on the multitrait–multimethod matrix, Mosher, in a classic paper, demonstrated that his measure of three aspects of guilt (sex guilt, hostility guilt, and morality conscience) converged appropriately within subscales and discriminated guilt from social desirability and anxiety. However, these promising multimethod matrices used multiple psychometric measures of the same trait—guilt, not maximally dissimilar measures. Thus, they demonstrated the reliability more than the validity of the three aspects of guilt. These measures of guilt represented the state of the art in personality scale development in the mid-1960s, leading to 300 empirical studies.

Later, a factor analysis of the Forced-Choice Guilt Inventory demonstrated that the internal structure of each subscale was similar for males and females and that the factor structure was complex within each subscale. The four-factor structure for sex guilt was: (a) *childhood sexual experiences*, (b) *sexual relations before marriage*, (c) *feelings about adultery*, and (d) *sociosexual guilt*. Another study of the concept of item bias in item-response theory used a pool of 72 sex-guilt items; the authors concluded that, within items, the relationships of items to guilt were the same for men and women, but, across items, the relationships of items to guilt were different for men and women. Men had higher thresholds than women for feeling guilty over prostitution, adultery, childhood sexual play, sexual desires, and petting; men and women had about equal thresholds for guilt over obscene literature, unusual sex practices, sex relations before marriage, masturbation, and dirty jokes; and men had lower thresholds than women for guilt over homosexuality. Only 2 of the 72 items yielded poor item responses. Several studies had demonstrated that women usually scored lower on sexual guilt than men. These item-response results indicated that this is a function of differences to particular stems which appear to reflect differences in socialization and, consequently, in the gender and sexual scripts of men and women; the pattern of the data generated no real surprises, since men were known to be more homophobic than women and more accepting of heterosexual contacts outside of courtship or marriage.

To measure the affect of guilt, six adjective prompts (guilty, remorseful, repentant, sinful, blameworthy, and conscience stricken), usually embedded within Izard's Differential Emotions Scale, proved reliable and useful in many studies.

In 1975, Paul Abramson and Mosher developed an Inventory of Negative Attitudes toward Masturbation as a measure of masturbation guilt. Three factors were (a) *positive attitudes toward masturbation* ("Masturbation can provide harmless relief from sexual tensions"), (b) *false beliefs about harm* ("Masturbation can lead to homosexuality"), and (c) *negative affect over masturbation* ("When I masturbate, I am disgusted with myself.").

After 20 years, the means of sex guilt had fallen, the Revised Mosher Guilt Inventory (Mosher, 1988) was developed by using the old items with contemporary samples. The response format was altered to a limited-comparison format, which is like a forced-choice format in pairing stems, but uses a Likert rating scale on each item. This strategy of renewing the item pool, using contemporary internal consistency analyses from both sexes, permitted the retention of past evidence of construct validity while improving the predictive power of the inventory.

In 1988, Mosher and James Sullivan developed the Sexual Polarity Scale to measure sexual ideology (also included were items from Tomkins's Polarity Scale of Normatives and Humanists). *Sexual ideology*: (a) consists of a more or less organized set of ideas about

sexuality that orders information about norms and vices within a sexual world view; (b) polarizes individuals into communities that believe and share either a left-winged naturalist or a right-winged Jehovanist view of the sexual world; and (c) serves as an ideological script that interprets, manages, defends, evaluates, and criticizes ongoing, remembered, and imagined sexual scenes.

III. A SUMMARY OF RESEARCH ON SEX GUILT

A. Double-Entendre Words

The earliest research on sexual guilt examined reports of recognition and word association in a double-entendre (e.g., screw, rubber, prick, balls, snatch) paradigm. Across several studies, high-sex guilt men and women delayed recognition of sexual words and gave fewer sexual associates, although sexual associations were elicited from them by repetition of the list or by instruction. Frequency of sexual associations also were influenced by sexual arousal or priming by pin-ups, expectations of the experimenter's response, and the "approachability" and sex of the experimenter.

In a series of studies, Gary Galbraith succeeded in reconciling the initial failures to find the expected, delayed reaction times to double-entendre words by high-sex-guilt participants. By an instruction requiring either a sexual or a nonsexual association to a color-coded stimulus word, sexual responses produced longer latencies than nonsexual associations and high-sex-guilt men and women had longer response latencies to sexual responses but not to asexual responses.

B. Premarital Sexual Behavior and Moral Decisions

Several studies demonstrated that the personality disposition of guilt is negatively correlated with delinquent and criminal status and behavior. Among felons, their undetected and unreported totals of crimes were correlated in the .60s with sex guilt for sex crimes; hostility guilt for violent crimes, and total crimes with both hostility guilt and morality conscience. Among college students, similar negative correlations were reported with self-reported drug-use and delinquencies. Not only did high-guilt men and women use marijuana, depressants, stimulants, and hallucinogens less, but when they did use these drugs they found the drug experience less pleasant and reported more "bad trips."

A frequently replicated result found sex guilt to be inversely related to the cumulative level of premarital sexual experience. Also, sex guilt was inversely related to sexual standards, virginity, age of first coitus, lifetime and last-year frequencies of coitus, number of coital partners, and orgasmic frequency across several samples of men and women. As predicted, high-sex-guilt men and women expected to feel guilty, giving moral reasons for not participating in premarital sex. High-sex-guilt men, who have affiliative needs, attempted fewer passes and used less exploitative tactics when dating; just as, high-sex-guilt women reported experiencing less aggressive sexual behavior.

Decision making about beginning premarital coitus was studied by combining an interest in sex guilt with Lawrence Kohlberg's approach to moral judgment. Delinquents scored low on guilt and moral judgment, yielding a positive correlation in a truncated range without any postconventional scores. Within samples of college women or of men and women, high-sex-guilt subjects scored highest on the law-and-order stage of morality. Whether a couple decided to have coitus was predicted best by male sex guilt, then by male moral judgment, and then by female sex guilt. Males, but not females, with a law-and-order orientation reported more standing decisions not to begin coitus; the lesser power of women and the traditional norm that women should accept male dominance may overcome high-sex-guilt women's sexual restraint. Although uncorrelated with sex guilt in men, the need for autonomy was inversely correlated with sex guilt in women.

Among noncollege women, low-sex-guilt women were more sexually aroused or orgasmic: to fantasy and erotica, sex-play, masturbation, and coitus. Anorgasmic women reported greater discomfort communicating about the need for clitoral stimulation, more masturbatory guilt, more belief in sex myths, and more sexual guilt.

Using an interpersonal pleasuring paradigm, modeled after the aggression machine, high-sex-guilt males administered less pleasure to women. When they anticipated meeting the woman, they gave still lower levels of pleasure to her. All of the men increased their level of interpersonal pleasuring across trials, suggest-ing that giving pleasure is a rewarding response, but a less acceptable one for high-guilt men.

C. Contraception, Abortion, and STDs

Several studies reported an inverse correlation between sex guilt and attitudes toward and the use of effective premarital contraception. Masturbation guilt appeared specifically to inhibit women's use of the diaphragm that requires, for them, a disgusting (when imagined or when inspecting) manipulation of the vulva for vaginal insertion. Also, high-masturbation-guilt women reported more distress from genital herpes, less sexual interest, and less willingness to tell partners; Abramson also found that high fear combined with high masturbation guilt led to more frequent outbreaks of genital herpes among infected women.

High-sex-guilt men and women not only disapproved of abortions but were reluctant to grant them, particularly when pregnancies resulted from casual sex. Yet, an abortion clinic reported their clients were higher on sex guilt than nonpregnant, sexually active women; high-sex-guilt women cannot plan to sin by seeking oral contraceptives. High-sex-guilt men know less about condoms and are reluctant to use them, even when they have a sexually transmitted disease.

Having found that high-sex-guilt women had coitus despite their reservations, failed to contracept or delayed the onset of contracepting, and had unwanted abortions, Meg Gerrard's research program sought answers. Noting that it was easier to prefer and recognize high levels of moral reasoning than to produce and articulate high levels of moral reasoning, Gerrard demonstrated that college women's level of endorsed moral reasons from a prepared list was higher than their ability to verbally articulate their own moral reasoning. The less sexually experienced, high-sex-guilt women had the largest gap between their preferences and their articulated moral reasoning. Gerrard concluded that the relationship between sex guilt and specifically sexual moral reasoning was strongly negative and was mediated by sexual experience. She argued that these women's maladaptive sexual behavior (coitus without contraception) resulted indirectly from their lack of sexual experience and, thus, their relative inexperience in coping with moral dilemmas. Pursuing this hypothesis, Gerrard and her associates studied the effects of sexual experience and sex guilt on the recall of sexual and nonsexual moral dilemmas. In particular, high-sex-guilt, sexually active women were compared to low-sex-guilt, sexually active women. Women whose sexual behavior violated their sexual norms had difficulty remembering sexual vignettes. What they did remember were the reasons *in favor of,* rather than against, participating in sexual activities, which the authors interpreted as an avoidant and repressive defense against guilt.

D. Sexual Fantasy and Pornography

High-sex-guilt women who read erotica were sexually aroused but felt guilty. While viewing sexually explicit films, high-sex-guilt men and women not only felt guilty but also rated the films as more pornographic, disgusting, and offensive; they considered oral-genital sex to be abnormal.

In general, men reported sexual arousal and positive affect to pornographic stimuli, whereas women reported a mix of sexual arousal and disgust. This reflects the bias in commercial pornography toward a male audience who reports more exposure to pornography. Nonetheless, high-sex-guilt men had less exposure to pornography in the past and looked less at *Playboy* while waiting for an experiment to begin. Viewing time of pornographic slides generally increased as a positive linear function of ratings as pornographic—highly arousing but disgusting images. But, unobtrusive timing during the viewing of sexually explicit slides revealed that high-sex-guilt men did not increase their exposure to more explicit slides, thereby minimizing their exposure to "forbidden" porn.

In a study of sex guilt and gender, "correct" choices in a discrimination task were followed by erotic slides, "incorrect" choices by nonerotic slides. Both females and high-sex-guilt subjects made fewer erotica-producing choices and also were less positive in their affective responses to the erotica. For individuals who experienced positive affect to the slides, they were experienced as rewarding; whereas for others, they were punishing.

When men and women viewed experimental films of a male or a female masturbating, the men were turned on by the female and turned off by the male masturbating; women were about equally responsive to both. Men and women high on either sex guilt or masturbation guilt reported more disgust, guilt, shame, and anger; men high on masturbation guilt reported the most disgust to the film of the male mastur-

bating. Women, but not men, wrote a more elaborate sexual fantasy to the same-sex film of masturbation. For both sexes, high masturbation guilt was associated with less positive affect about the fantasy or about orgasm.

Given this difference in the ability of women relative to men to identify positively with same-sex masturbation, another study tested two plausible hypotheses that such negative responses were due either to guilt over masturbation or to homosexual threat in men. Results indicated that men's adverse reactions to a film of a male masturbating were consistent with both masturbation guilt *and* homosexual threat.

Recent research demonstrated that women responded more positively to X-rated videos designed for and by women than to X-rated videos intended for a male audience; men were responsive to both. Ideological beliefs about the harms of pornography—moral corruption and incitement to violence—influenced subject's rating of harmful effect on others.

Like the studies of pornography, studies of guided imagery of sexual encounters continued to find that high sex guilt was associated with less sexual arousal and more negative affect during imagined sexual scenes across a variety of experimental conditions. A causal model was posited and supported across free fantasy, remembered interpersonal sex and masturbation, and guided imagery of a sexual scene. Derived from script theory, the model specified: (a) sex guilt and masturbation guilt have both direct and indirect effects on subjective sexual arousal, (b) positive affects amplify, whereas negative affects attenuate, sexual arousal, and (c) affects mediate the indirect effects of sex guilt and masturbation guilt.

Sexual guilt was associated with: fewer sexual fantasies during intercourse, more guilt over such "abnormal" and "immoral" fantasies, and more sexual dissatisfaction and dysfunction. Studies of sexual fantasy production found that high-sex-guilt men and women produced more restricted content and shorter fantasies and reported more embarrassment and less sexual arousal while writing them.

E. Guilt and Defensive Processes

Defensive processes are inferred from correlates rather than directly observed in action. Still, a number of studies have documented the potential role of the modulation of various responses from guilty motives. When watching erotic videotapes, high-sex-guilt women reported less subjective sexual arousal but had more vaginal engorgement according to vaginal photoplethysmography. Because women low in sexual arousability and sexual experience showed a similar pattern, Patricia Morokoff concluded that a history of inhibited sexual behavior facilitated increased responsiveness to "forbidden" stimuli. Although difficult to untangle, it appeared that sexual guilt mediated differential past exposure to sexual stimuli (a known outcome) or inhibited awareness of subjective sexual arousal despite physiological signs of arousal.

In a balanced placebo design (alcohol dosage crossed with expectancy), alcohol expectancy, but not alcohol itself, yielded greater penile tumescence and subjective sexual arousal to audiotapes of consenting intercourse, rape, and sadistic sexual aggression. High sex guilt (and hostility guilt) was inversely correlated with subjective sexual arousal for the consenting and rape tapes. Another investigation using a balanced placebo design had individuals watch sexual slides that were unobtrusively timed. The high-sex-guilt men reported less sexual and masturbatory experience and fewer orgasms; they rated the slides as more pornographic, had less experience with porn, and more negative attitudes toward it. Nonetheless, believing that they had imbibed alcohol permitted them to view the more pornographic material longer; thus, they now showed the same positive linear function of time with ratings of pornographic explicitness as the low-sex-guilt men.

A similar study with women had a less clear-cut outcome. More inhibited or less interested, women did not show a linear increase of viewing time with pornography ratings. It was only the low-sex-guilt women in both the placebo (expect alcohol/receive tonic) and antiplacebo (expect tonic/receive alcohol) who viewed the slides significantly longer than the control women (expect tonic/receive tonic). Thus, only the least inhibited women were responsive to either alcohol expectancy or alcohol dose. Although the high-sex-guilt women did not change their viewing behavior, they reported the highest level of subjective sexual arousal.

Using a balanced placebo design in an information processing context, high-sex-guilt men increased penile tumescence to both heterosexual and homosexual videos only in the placebo condition of falsely expecting to receive alcohol. From these studies, it appears that, although many men may use alcohol to minimize the affective inhibition of sexual affects, high-sex-guilt men need only to expect alcohol/receive placebo to reduce their personal responsibility and to permit them to respond sexually to "forbidden" sources.

In 1974, false heart rate feedback was shown to influence high-sex-guilt men's ratings of attractiveness of sexual slides. In 1978, Frederick Gibbons demonstrated increased consistency between pre-experimental attitudes toward erotica and laboratory response to erotica when men were self-focused, using a mirror to create self-focus. Women were more consistent in their rating as a function of self-focus, but high-sex-guilt women were less capable of enjoying erotica when self-focused.

Other investigators pointed out that less subjective sexual arousal in high-sex-guilt subjects might represent either suppression or denial of arousal in self-focused conditions. Supplying high-sex-guilt men with alternative attributions (either sexual arousal or undifferentiated arousal) produced denial, reports of decreased sexual arousal, and somewhat more undifferentiated arousal when viewing slides of nude women. Gibbons continued by examining motivational biases in causal attribution of arousal by introducing a placebo pill, asserted to create arousal. High-sex-guilt men and women who viewed an erotic video attributed their arousal to the drug rather than to the erotica. Attributing their arousal to a nonthreatening source reduced their guilt over transgressing a sexual standard that prohibits sexual arousal to erotica.

In self-awareness theory, self-focused attention increases consistency with standards of "correctness," whether such standards are internal or external. Gibbons asked what happens when a personal standard conflicts with external standards? Self-focused, high-sex-guilt women conformed more than others, supporting the *social* standards hypothesis. But, postexperimentally, they also had maintained their own personal standards. After modifying their responses in the liberal direction in response to conformity pressure, they reasserted their personal standards.

IV. IMPLICATIONS FOR THE SOCIALIZATION OF GUILT

The critical question in the socialization of sexual affect is whether the parent regards the sexuality of the child as positive or as an alien entity to be shaped to fit antisexual norms. If the parent can empathize with the child's sexual excitement and with the complexities of an emerging gender and sexual identity, then sexuality is neither an affront to the authority of the parent and society nor sinful, dirty, and dangerous. Instead, it is another aspect of interpersonal relationships. A humanist morality requires a rewarding socialization of sexual affect while helping the child tolerate the negative affect triggered by the inevitable shameful and guilty failures and distressing limitations that must be faced and tolerated before the young adult can be said to have mastered a moral sexuality. The parent will attempt to minimize shame and guilt and to remedy limitations, but will neither contaminate sexuality with disgust nor make it toxic by fear, rage, or dissmell. Sexual morality will be justified by reasoned argument from moral principles, rather than consisting of draconian threats of punishment for engaging in sexual scenes defined as either conditionally or forever taboo.

Sex guilt is associated with religiosity, generational differences, and a normative and Jehovanist ideology, creating a continual tension between the sexuality of youth and the "morality" of conservative adults. Yet, a moral view of sexuality requires the same moral rules that govern all human relationships; it does not require an ideology that sex equals dirt and danger nor an affect socialization that instills sexual disgust, fear, and dissmell. Sexual dissmell motivates hatreds that cannot be morally justified. Social acceptance of sexual diversity requires tolerance of sexual affect in children and adults. At its best, sexual guilt is only a temporary barrier, not a permanent wall forbidding sexuality. At its best, a critical morality fosters nonmalevolence and benevolence in sexual relationships, not a moralistic intolerance of sex and sexuality.

This article has been reprinted from the *Encyclopedia of Human Behavior, Volume 2.*

BIBLIOGRAPHY

Creighton, M. R. (1990). Revisiting shame and guilt cultures: A forty-year pilgrimage. *Ethos* **19**, 279–307.

Kelly, M. P., Strassberg, D. S., & Kircher, J. R. (1990). Attitudinal and experiential correlates of anorgasmia. *Arch. Sex. Behav.* **19**, 165–177.

Kugler, K., & Jones, W. H. (1992). On conceptualizing and assessing guilt. *J. Pers. Soc. Psychol.* **62**, 318–327.

Mosher, D. L. (1988). Revised Mosher Guilt Inventory. In "Sexuality-Related Measures: A Compendium" (C. M. Davis, W. L. Yarber, and S. L. Davis, Eds.). Graphic Press, Lake Mills, IA.

Mosher, D. L., & Sullivan, J. P. (1988). Sexual Polarity Scale. In "Sexuality-Related Measures: A Compendium" (C. M. Davis, W. L. Yarber, and S. L. Davis, Eds.), Graphic Press, Lake Mills, IA.

Mosher, D. L. (1994). Sexual guilt. In "Human Sexuality: An Encyclopedia" (V. L. Bullough and B. Bullough, Eds.). Garland Press, New York.

Scheff, T. J. (1988). Shame and conformity: The deference emotion system. *Am. Soc. Rev.* **53**, 395–406.

Tomkins, S. S. (1991). "Affect Imagery Consciousness: Anger and Fear," Vol. III. Springer, New York.

Happiness: Subjective Well-Being

Ed Diener

University of Illinois

Mary Beth Diener

University of Kentucky

Adaptation Organisms react more strongly to novel stimuli, but over time they habituate and react either weakly or not at all to those same stimuli. In the area of subjective well-being, adaptation refers to the fact that people react emotionally to new events, whether good or bad, but over time adapt to these events so that they have less impact on SWB.

Affect Feelings with a pleasant or unpleasant quality that include moods (usually longer term than emotions and with an unknown cause) and emotions (often short-term, frequently more intense than moods, and with a clear cause).

Context Theories Scientific explanations of subjective well-being that stress that events and circumstances do not have a uniform relation to subjective well-being across all people and life circumstances. Instead, the context in which an event occurs determines its effect on the person's SWB.

Happiness A term that conveys several different meanings, including momentary joy, satisfaction with life, and long-term enjoyment. The term is also used as a popular and short-hand way of speaking about subjective well-being.

On-Line Experience The experiences that are felt moment by moment over time. On-line subjective well-being refers to the positivity of one's experiences over a period of time. On-line experience is often contrasted with global reports that are made retrospectively for a defined period of time. The experience sampling method (ESM) is often used to record on-line affect over time.

Pleasant Affect Emotional experiences and moods that are pleasant and sought after, including joy, affection, and pride.

Social Comparison The belief that people compare themselves to others in order to gain information and evaluate their outcomes. In the realm of subjective well-being, the idea that how well off other people are in the domain compared to oneself influences whether one is satisfied with that domain. In *imposed social comparison* approaches, the focus is on comparisons thrust on the individual by virtue of the people who are in his or her vicinity.

Subjective well-being (SWB) A person's evaluation of his or her life, including ongoing affective reactions and conscious evaluations, reported either at the moment or globally for a longer time period.

Temperament Individual differences in psychological tendencies that are present early in life, are fairly stable, and have some genetic basis.

Unpleasant Affect Emotional experiences and moods that are unpleasant and are usually avoided, including sadness, guilt, anger, shame, and anxiety.

SUBJECTIVE WELL-BEING (SWB) is how a person evaluates his or her life, and varies from utter dissatisfaction and depression to complete satisfaction and enjoyment. This entry focuses on defining and measuring SWB, the correlates of SWB found in survey research, and the temperament and psychological processes that are likely to influence SWB.

I. DEFINING AND MEASURING SUBJECTIVE WELL-BEING

Subjective well-being (SWB) is synonymous with one meaning of the lay term "happiness." The term subjective well-being, however, is preferred because happiness has several different meanings in popular usage. It can mean a pleasant momentary mood ("I am happy on payday") or the cause of such moods (e.g., "Happiness is a 3-day weekend"). Happiness can refer to life satisfaction (e.g., "I am happy with my life"), to long-term pleasant affect (e.g., "I have been happy since I changed jobs last year"), or to a predisposition to pleasant affect (e.g., "She has a happy personality"). Because of these diverse meanings, researchers prefer the term subjective well-being to refer to the global state of evaluating one's life in a positive way.

The idea of subjective well-being or happiness has intrigued thinkers for millennia, although it is only in the last several decades that it has been defined and empirically measured in a systematic way. Subjective well-being is a person's evaluation of her or his life. This evaluation may occur in the form of cognitions when a person makes conscious evaluative judgments about his or her satisfaction with life as a whole, or evaluative judgments about specific aspects of his or life such as work or recreation. This evaluation may also occur in the affect system when people experience unpleasant or pleasant moods or emotions. Affect is a term that includes both moods and emotions, both of which can be described as pleasant or unpleasant.

People constantly evaluate what is happening to them so that they are usually able to offer judgments about their lives. Furthermore, people virtually always experience moods and emotions, which have an hedonic component that is pleasant, signalling a positive reaction, or unpleasant, signalling a negative reaction. Thus, SWB refers to a person's perceptions of his or her well-being that are based on both affective and cognitive appraisals. The cognitive and affective components of SWB are highly intertwined.

A. Hallmarks of Subjective Well-Being

There are several hallmarks of the study of SWB. First, the field covers the entire range of well-being, from agony to ecstasy. It does not focus only on undesirable states such as depression; instead, individual differences in levels of positive well-being are believed to be important. Second, SWB is defined in terms of the experience of the individual. An external frame of reference is not imposed when evaluating subjective well-being. Although many criteria of mental health are dictated from outside by researchers and practitioners (e.g., maturity, autonomy, realism), SWB is measured from the individual's own perspective.

A final hallmark of SWB is that it pertains to longer term states, not just momentary moods. Although a person's moods are likely to fluctuate with events, the SWB researcher is most interested in the person's average mood over time. Whereas the emotion theorist may be interested in affect that sometimes lasts only microseconds, researchers in the field of SWB focus on understanding satisfaction and levels of mood that persist for weeks, months, or years. Often, what leads to happiness at the moment may not be the same as what produces long-term SWB.

B. Is SWB Necessary and Sufficient for Mental Health?

Subjective well-being is not synonymous with mental health. A delusional person may be happy and satisfied with his or her life, and yet we would not say that he or she possesses consummate mental health. Thus, SWB is not a sufficient condition for psychological well-being. Carol Ryff outlines other characteristics beyond SWB (e.g., the ability to control one's environment) that are important to complete mental health.

Is SWB a necessary condition for mental health? It appears that some people function well in many aspects of their lives but are not particularly happy. Examples come to mind of individuals such as Elie Wiesel and Sylvia Plath who were frequently dysphoric, but who made significant contributions to society. Some might argue, however, that SWB is a necessary condition for mental health. The argument is that individuals such as Wiesel and Plath did not enjoy full mental health because they were so frequently in depressive mood states. We have not yet determined the level of SWB that is optimal for mental health and good functioning. [*See* DEPRESSION.]

Subjective well-being is only one aspect of psychological well-being. Nevertheless, the subjective frame of reference implicit in the concept of SWB has the strength of being based on the respondent's own internal perspective, and thus gives priority and respect to people's own views of their lives. Rather than a standard imposed by a mental health professional, SWB grants importance to the experience of people. Subjective well-being clearly represents what most people believe to be an extremely important aspect of life. At the same time, the focus on an internal perspective means that other criteria of well-being, recognized by the community, philosophers, or mental health professionals, may not be met in every individual who has high subjective well-being. Although we cannot say whether high SWB is absolutely necessary for mental health, we can say that most people consider it to be a desirable characteristic.

C. Components of SWB

There are three primary components of SWB: satisfaction, pleasant affect, and low levels of unpleasant affect. Subjective well-being is structured such that these three components form a global factor of interrelated variables. Each of the three major facets of SWB can in turn be broken into subdivisions. Global satisfaction can be divided into satisfaction with the various domains of life such as recreation, love, friendship, and so forth, and these domains can in turn be divided into facets. Pleasant affect can be divided into specific emotions such as joy, affection, and pride. Finally, unpleasant affect can be separated into specific emotions and moods such as shame, sadness, and anxiety. Each of the subdivisions of affect can also be subdivided even further. Subjective well-being can be assessed at the most global level or at progressively narrower levels, depending on one's purposes. The justification for studying more global levels (rather than just focusing on the most molecular concepts) is that the narrower levels tend to co-occur. In other words, there is a tendency for people to experience similar levels of well-being across different aspects of their lives.

One of the most important findings emerging from research on SWB is Bradburn's (1969) finding that pleasant and unpleasant affect are separable and are not exact opposites, as was once thought. At the individual level, this means that people who experience a specified level of pleasant affect may feel either high or low unpleasant affect. Not only are there individuals who are high in one type of affect and low in the other, but there are also individuals who experience low levels of pleasant *and* unpleasant affect, as well as individuals who experience high levels of both. In addition to the independence of the two types of affect, there are different correlates for each type of affect. For example, social contact and close relationships tend to correlate more strongly with pleasant affect than with low unpleasant affect, as do extraversion and positive events. On the other hand, neuroticism (the personality trait that is based on a reactive punishment system) and negative life events predict unpleasant affect more strongly than they predict the lack of pleasant affect. Thus, contrary to popular opinion, happiness should not be thought of as a unidimensional variable that varies from depression to elation. Instead, scientists must consider people's levels of both pleasant emotions and unpleasant moods in order to understand fully their affective well-being.

Affect forms two strong, separable factors. Within each factor, however, people who experience much of one type of affect also tend to experience more of other emotions of that same valence. For example, people who frequently experience high levels of sadness are also likely to experience frequent anger, anxiety, and guilt. Similarly, people who are often joyful are likely to experience affection and pride frequently. Although high life satisfaction tends to be experienced by people with a high hedonic balance (pleasant emotions strongly predominate over unpleasant emotions), life satisfaction and hedonic balance can diverge. For instance, some elderly people are very satisfied with their lives but they do not experience intense levels of joy. Some young adults report a positive hedonic balance, but low life satisfaction. Thus, to understand SWB, we must be able to measure and understand all three of its components—satisfaction, pleasant and unpleasant affect—and their causes.

II. COGNITION AND SUBJECTIVE WELL-BEING

An idea that has long captivated writers is that how we perceive and think about the world determines our SWB. In certain philosophical and religious traditions, advice and exercises on proper thought are offered that appear to be designed to guide one's moods and emotions. For example, mental detachment from the world is counseled in some religious traditions in order to dampen one's unpleasant emotions. Philosophical traditions such as stoicism also recommended specific thoughts in order to steel oneself against adversity. [*See* EMOTIONAL REGULATION.]

Cognitive theories of well-being and ill-being within the behavioral sciences were developed in the last decades. For example, the attributional theory of depression is well known. Depressed individuals are more likely to believe that negative events are caused by global and stable causes so that negative events are very likely to continue to happen to them. In the area of SWB, researchers find that one can dampen or amplify one's emotions by what one thinks, and thereby experience more or less intense emotions. Thus, the belief of the stoics, ascetics, and others that how "attached" or involved one becomes with goals and life circumstances can influence how intensely one reacts has been confirmed empirically. [*See* EMOTION AND COGNITION.]

Happy people experience more events that are considered desirable in the culture, but they also have a propensity to interpret ambiguous events as good. People with high SWB are also more likely to perceive "neutral" events as positive. Thus, people with high SWB may not only experience objectively more positive events, but they may also perceive the same events more positively than do people who are low in SWB.

Theories of coping are based on the idea that in order to cope with problems, happy people initiate thoughts and behaviors that are adaptive and helpful, whereas on average, unhappy people cope in more destructive ways. For example, happy people are more likely to see the bright side of affairs, pray, directly struggle with problems, and seek help from others, whereas unhappy people are more likely to engage in fantasy, blame others and themselves, and avoid working on problems. What is not yet known is whether these coping styles are the cause or effect of SWB. [*See* COPING WITH STRESS.]

Many suggestions have been offered about how people increase their SWB by control of their thoughts. For example, perhaps happiness can be increased by believing in a larger meaning or force in the universe. Support for this proposition comes from findings that, on average, religious people are happier than nonreligious people. Furthermore, SWB is higher if one concentrates on smaller goals rather than focus attention exclusively on distant, difficult goals. Finally, one can

heighten SWB by being optimistic about one's future. It is not known whether these cognitive factors correlate with SWB because of the influence of some third variable such as temperament, or whether the cognitions have an independent long-term influence on SWB. More research is needed on whether attempts to purposefully alter cognitions can lead to permanent increases in SWB. [*See* RELIGION AND MENTAL HEALTH.]

III. CROSS-CULTURAL FINDINGS

People in extremely poor nations show average SWB scores close to neutrality or slightly below it. Countries that are wealthier, have greater freedom and human rights, and emphasize individualism have citizens with higher SWB. Surprisingly, other factors such as the economic growth and the cultural homogeneity of a society do not correlate with average levels of SWB.

Reports of SWB are higher in individualistic nations, even when income is statistically controlled. The cultural dimension of individualism versus collectivism produces complex effects, however. Individualistic cultures are those that emphasize the individual in terms of autonomy, motives, and so forth. In contrast, in collectivist cultures, the group (e.g., the family) is believed to be more important than the individual. There is an emphasis on harmonious group functioning and the belief that the individual's motives and emotions should be secondary. In individualistic nations, reports of global well-being are high and satisfaction with domains such as marriage are extremely high. Nevertheless, suicide rates and divorce rates in these individualistic nations are also high. It may be that people in individualistic nations make more attributions for events internally to themselves, and therefore the effects are amplified when things go either well or badly. It might also be that individualists are more able to follow their own interests and desires, and therefore more often find self-fulfillment. At the same time, individualistic cultures may offer less social support during difficult times. Furthermore, individualists are more likely to opt out of marriage, or even out of life, if things do not go well. Thus, individualists may experience more extreme levels of SWB, whereas collectivists may have a safer structure that produces fewer people who are very happy but also fewer people who are isolated and depressed. Our data support this line of reasoning in that not only do individualistic nations have higher suicide and divorce rates, they also have higher reports of subjective well-being.

IV. TEMPERAMENT AND PERSONALITY

Temperament is a powerful influence on SWB. Studies of heritability, in which twins separated at birth are studied as adults, found that both pleasant and unpleasant affect have a genetic basis. In the case of pleasant affect, about one half of the variation between individuals appeared to be heritable in a western sample, and a small proportion of variance seemed to be due to common family environment. In the case of unpleasant affect, the heritability coefficient is even stronger, and little variation was due to shared family environment. Although heritability coefficients may be different in other environments, these data show convincingly that some proportion of SWB is due to genetic makeup. Further supporting the idea of an inborn influence on SWB, measures of heart rate in utero and of reactivity in young infants predict later fear responses. Thus, even before socialization and rearing, individuals react in a characteristic way to stimuli. Another piece of evidence supporting the importance of temperament to well-being is that people who undergo changes in marital status, employment status, or residence are not much less stable in SWB over the long-term than individuals who do not change status in these areas. [See GENETIC CONTRIBUTORS TO MENTAL HEALTH; PERSONALITY.]

In adults, optimism, self-esteem, a sense of personal control, and extraversion are several of the personality traits possessed by happy people. For example, informant reports of extraversion and sociability correlate with the amount of pleasant affect that nursing home residents display. Extraverts in a national probability sample who lived in a variety of different circumstances experienced higher subjective well-being than did introverts. It is useful, however, to differentiate the separate components of SWB. The two major forms of affect, pleasant and unpleasant, appear to be related to the separate personality factors of extraversion and neuroticism, respectively. Although extraverts experience more pleasant affect, they do not experience a predictable level of unpleasant affect. Neurotics are likely to experience high levels of un-

pleasant affect, but are less predictable when it comes to levels of pleasant affect. When measurement error is controlled, the relations between these two facets of affect and these two personality dimensions are very strong. [See OPTIMISM, MOTIVATION, AND MENTAL HEALTH; SELF-ESTEEM.]

Extraversion and neuroticism are two cardinal traits that are part of a system of personality labeled the Five Factor Model. Two more traits in this model, agreeableness and conscientiousness, are correlated moderately with SWB. Whereas extraversion and neuroticism might relate to SWB because they are rooted in biologic propensities in the basic biologic approach and avoidance systems, agreeableness and conscientiousness might relate to SWB because of environmental rewards. That is, in many or most environments, people who are agreeable and conscientious may receive more positive reinforcements from others, and therefore may experience higher SWB. For example, a conscientious person might receive better grades in school, better pay at work, and may even be more likely to have a good marriage. Thus, although conscientiousness might not directly produce greater SWB, it might result in receiving rewards that heighten one's SWB.

The fifth cardinal trait in the Five Factor Model, openness, may relate to emotional intensity (having both intense unpleasant and pleasant emotions) rather than to hedonic balance. Much more research is needed to understand the relation of the "Big Five" traits to SWB. For example, we do not know which facets of extraversion (e.g., warmth vs. surgency) most relate to pleasant affect, and we are uncertain about the causal direction between pleasant affect and extraversion.

Self-esteem correlates with SWB; this relation is strongest in individualistic societies, where the self is paramount. Not surprisingly, optimism is also related to subjective well-being. Agency, a trait that was formerly labeled as masculinity, also has an association with hedonic balance.

Although many personality predispositions have been related to SWB, most of this work has not yet been replicated across cultures. Without such cross-cultural replication, it is not known whether the relations uncovered between personality and SWB are due to environmental rewards or to universal biological systems. A fundamental question for mental health practitioners is whether teaching people to have the personality characteristics of happy people will increase their SWB.

V. CONTEXT THEORIES

Some theorists, such as Veenhoven, maintain that subjective well-being is caused by the satisfaction of basic, universal human needs. He maintains, for example, that people can only be happy if needs such as hunger, warmth, and thirst are fulfilled. Thus, like the temperament approach, the basic needs approach relies on a biological substrate for explanations of SWB. In the case of basic needs models, however, the biological substrate is universal across people, whereas in the temperament approach, the biological substrate of SWB is based on individual differences in people. In contrast, context theories emphasize that the factors that influence SWB are variable across both time and individuals, and how good or bad life events are perceived to be is based on the circumstances in which people live. The relevant context varies in different theories. In adaptation theory, for example, the relevant context is the person's past life. In social comparison models, the context is the social others of whom the target individual is aware. Other contexts that could influence SWB are a person's ideals and the imagining of counterfactual alternative situations. Finally, in the goal approach, the context is the person's conscious aims. In each of the context models, whether something is good or bad, and how good or bad it is, is thought to be based on changeable factors rather than on biological universals.

A. Adaptation

Demographic variables such as age, education, sex, and ethnicity have weak relations to subjective well-being. For example, across 16 nations, women and men, and people of different ages, on average hardly differed in SWB. The absence of large demographic differences in SWB led researchers to examine the process of habituation or adaptation to new conditions. The idea of adaptation is that people initially react strongly to new life events or circumstances, but over time they habituate and return to baseline. For example, a positive event such as winning the lottery is likely to boost a person's mood, but the person is likely, over time, to return to his or her original level or baseline. Parducci offers a mathematical formula-

tion of adaptation theory. The context for events in Parducci's theory is based on the range of events (from a person's best to worst events), as well as on the frequency distribution of events. The current range and frequency of a person's events in an area determines how a new event is evaluated. Thus, in context theories, events do not have an inherent value, but instead are evaluated against a backdrop of other factors.

Indirect support for the idea of adaptation comes from data that show that many demographic variables correlate only weakly with SWB. For example, income in the United States correlates only about .12 with SWB—almost no correlation at all. Furthermore, in one study, lottery winners were nonsignificantly happier than others. Physical attractiveness among young adults, like wealth, shows only a weak covariation with subjective well-being. Perhaps most surprising, objective health among the elderly is only faintly correlated with SWB. In another study, people with disabilities who were confined to wheelchairs were about as happy as a nondisabled comparison group. The presence of positive SWB in groups who suffer incapacities in daily living is indicative of adaptation to even severe conditions.

More direct evidence for adaptation comes from longitudinal studies in which significant events are greeted with strong emotions, but these emotions dampen over time. One dramatic study found that spinal cord-injured paraplegics and quadriplegics experienced, not surprisingly, a large amount of unpleasant affect after the accident that produced their paralysis. Within 8 weeks, however, the pleasant affect of these accident victims was stronger than their unpleasant affect. In another study, the average life events of students after college graduation (events such as getting married, obtaining a new job, being promoted at work) had an impact lasting 3 months or less. This did not mean that events never had a longer impact, but that most events produced a short impact on subjective well-being.

It appears that one's long-term baseline of well-being is strongly influenced by one's temperament, for example, by traits such as extraversion and neuroticism. Good and bad events cause a positive or negative deflection, respectively, from this baseline. Nevertheless, over time, the person drifts back to his or her baseline. In an Australian panel study spanning an 8-year period, it was found that the adaptation model provided a good description of the interaction of life events, personality, and SWB.

The idea of adaptation cannot be pushed to the extreme position that environment has absolutely no long-term influence on subjective well-being, because some circumstances do seem to influence it on a continual basis. For example, as reviewed earlier, there are substantial differences in SWB between nations. These differences relate to the income, human rights record, and democratic institutions in these societies. Nations with few human rights and dire poverty report levels of subjective well-being that are substantially lower than wealthier societies with a good record on human rights. These findings suggest that people may not adapt completely to all conditions, no matter how bad. For example, family caregivers of Alzheimer's patients do not appear to adapt to their burden. A nationally representative sample of people with disabling conditions did report lower life satisfaction on average, especially if they suffered from multiple disabilities. Thus, although adaptation is a powerful force that may dampen the impact of virtually all conditions, it may not be complete or may not occur in all circumstances. Research is needed to discover the limits of adaptation.

B. Social Comparison and SWB

In 1972, Easterlin proposed that nations do not differ in SWB because people within nations compare only to each other on attributes such as income. Therefore, according to Easterlin, although richer people within a nation are likely to be happier than poorer people in that country, *nations* should not differ in SWB. Furthermore, based on the imposed social comparisons approach, the average person in any nation ought to be neutral in subjective well-being because about half the people will be above average and about half will be below average. Research demonstrates, however, that most people have SWB above neutral. In the United States, for example, about 85% of people report a positive level of subjective well-being. In some domains, such as family life, even higher percentages report satisfaction. For global SWB, investigators have replicated the "most people are happy effect" using measures other than global self-reports (e.g., memory measures, experience sampling, and informant reports). More surprising is the fact that even disadvantaged persons, such as the disabled and chronically mentally ill, also report SWB above the neutral point. Representative surveys conducted in industrialized nations reveal the same pattern, with most societies falling in the slightly to moderately happy range. It is not yet known why most respondents report positive SWB—whether this is because most people live in generally positive life circumstances or whether most people have a biological set-point that returns them to pleasant affect. Nevertheless, these data seem to cast doubt on Easterlin's thesis. Another damaging piece of evidence is that nations do differ in predictable ways in SWB.

Other evidence also casts serious doubt on imposed social comparison approaches to subjective well-being. This evidence shows that people with similar characteristics who live around fortunate or unfortunate others do not differ as predicted by the idea of imposed social comparisons. For example, people with similar incomes who live either in wealthier or in poorer neighborhoods do not differ in the way predicted by the idea of imposed social comparisons. That is, people who have a moderate income were about equally happy whether they lived either in a poorer or wealthier geographic area. Social comparison does not automatically produce happiness when one is around others who are inferior on some characteristic. Instead, the data support a coping model of social comparison in which people selectively choose others with whom to compare. In some cases, people even imagine someone with whom to compare in order to achieve their objectives. The coping idea is that people can look to others to help motivate themselves, to boost their moods, and to gain specific knowledge. People can increase their SWB by attending to others who are either superior or inferior to themselves. Thus, the idea that people's SWB is usually influenced by whether they are better off than those who are immediately around them seems incorrect in most circumstances.

C. Values, Goals, and Meaning

Telic theories are those approaches that posit that SWB is dependent on people's goals. Different aspects of goals are related to different components of subjective well-being. For example, one study found that possessing important goals correlated with life satisfaction, success in achieving one's goals correlated with pleasant affect, and conflict between goals was related to the experience of unpleasant affect.

According to telic theories, to the extent that people have different goals, the causes of SWB ought to differ. There are now numerous studies that find variations between individuals and between groups in terms of what correlates with SWB. For example, the resources (e.g., money and social skills) that most strongly predict SWB for an individual are those that are required to gain his or her specific aims. If a person does not value athletic achievement and has no athletic goals, athletic ability is unlikely to be related to his or her subjective well-being. If a person desires to be a model, then physical attractiveness is more likely to be related to SWB. An individual's life tasks or goals are influenced by cultural goals and individual needs. The success of people in meeting their goals depends on their strategies and situational affordances. In the telic approach, SWB ought to follow from people using strategies that are successful in their environment in pursuing their goals. [*See* INTRINSIC MOTIVATION AND GOALS.]

Although the telic approaches treat a wide variety of goals as equivalent in desirability in terms of SWB, it is possible that the *content* of goals differs in terms of efficacy in producing SWB. In other words, some types of goals may be more beneficial than others. Veenhoven proposed that aims related to universal human needs are those that produce long-term SWB. According to this approach, people cannot be happy when experiencing chronic hunger, danger, or isolation. In this view, some goal strivings and successes may not produce SWB because they are based on superficial desires that are not based on human needs. In contrast, obtaining food and other biological needs is more likely predictive of subjective well-being, according to Veenhoven. A related approach states that some goals serve intrinsic needs, whereas other goals are extrinsic in nature (instrumental or substitutes for deeper needs). Goals that meet intrinsic needs such as autonomy, relatedness, and competence are hypothesized to predict SWB, whereas goals reflecting extrinsic needs are hypothesized to be negative predictors of well-being. Supportive data showed that needs for financial success, social recognition, and physical attractiveness were predicted by having cold, uninvolved parents, and were inversely correlated with SWB. In contrast, the intrinsically rewarding activities of personal growth, satisfying relationships, and community contributions were positively related to SWB. Thus, a worthwhile research agenda is to determine which human goals are most likely to produce subjective well-being.

It is in the area of goals and values that SWB transcends the boundaries of hedonism. One objection to using subjective well-being as a criterion for mental health, as discussed earlier, is that a person might live an immoral life and be happy. Thus, SWB does not seem to be a complete definition of the "good life," as was suggested by ethical hedonists such as Jeremy Bentham. When one finds, however, that subjective well-being is at least partially dependent on fulfilling one's goals, which in turn are related to one's values, SWB becomes defensible as an essential ingredient of the good life. If an individual's subjective well-being depends on engaging in activities that are congruent with her or his values, then SWB cannot be thought of as a simple form of hedonism that follows from bodily pleasures. Instead, SWB, especially life satisfaction, is likely to reflect the person's fulfillment of his or her values and goals. Thus, SWB becomes a broader measure of quality of life, because it reflects deeper values than physical pleasure.

A related point is that it is not desirable to have a happy society based on drugs or other interventions that circumvent values and goals. For example, few would support the idea of creating a euphoric nation by adding drugs to our drinking water supply. Similarly, few would advocate placing millions of human brains in laboratory jars and titrating hormones into the container to maintain the brains in ecstasy. We hold other important values besides subjective well-being, and a fear is that happiness could become such an important goal that these other values are forgotten. However, short of drug interventions, it appears that people's SWB is to some degree related to their fulfillment of their values. To the extent that this is true, value-based quality of life and SWB merge. The ideal society socializes its citizens to cherish certain values. In such a society, the citizens are likely to achieve SWB by working toward cultural values.

VI. ACTIVITY THEORY OF SUBJECTIVE WELL-BEING

An approach related to goal models is the hypothesis that SWB depends on being involved in interesting activities. The idea is that humans are constructed, because of their large brains and reliance on knowledge for survival, so that interest (vs. boredom) is a compelling motivation. Interesting activities are those in which there is a balance between challenge and skill, and which relate to the person's values and goals. Such activities are pleasant because they provide an optimal level of new information that is novel, yet not overwhelming. In activity theory, goals are related to SWB primarily to the extent that they provide involvement in interesting goal-striving activities.

Two important variables that can be interpreted in terms of activity theory are marriage and work. Married people of both sexes report more happiness than those who are never married, divorced, or separated. One benefit of marriage may be to provide interesting and supportive social interactions for the individual. Furthermore, there is evidence that happy people are more likely to marry in the first place, so the causal influence between SWB and marriage may travel in both directions. In the work arena, occupational satisfaction is a predictor of life satisfaction. Furthermore, unemployed people have lower SWB than do employed persons. Activity theory may once again provide a partial explanation for this outcome, although, of course, other factors such as income and societal status are also likely to be influential. Activity theory points to the fact that interesting activities can supplement the pleasures that are achieved through people's emotions and physical comforts.

VII. MEASURING SUBJECTIVE WELL-BEING

The usual method of measuring SWB is through self-report in which the respondent judges and reports his or her life satisfaction, the frequency of pleasant affect, or the frequency of unpleasant emotions. For example, Pavot and Diener review evidence using the Satisfaction With Life Scale (SWLS).

Using the 1–7 scale below, indicate your agreement with each item by placing the appropriate number on the line preceding that item. Please be open and honest in your responding.

> 7—*Strongly agree*
> 6—*Agree*
> 5—*Slightly agree*
> 4—*Neither agree nor disagree*
> 3—*Slightly disagree*
> 2—*Disagree*
> 1—*Strongly disagree*

_____ *In most ways my life is close to my ideal.*
_____ *The conditions of my life are excellent.*
_____ *I am satisfied with my life.*
_____ *So far I have gotten the important things I want in life.*
_____ *If I could live my life over, I would change almost nothing.*

The SWLS is in the public domain and is free to all users. Other questionnaires are available to measure pleasant and unpleasant affect. The assumption behind self-reports of SWB such as these is that the respondent is in a unique position to report on his or her experience of well-being. After all, only the respondent can experience her or his pleasures and pains and judge whether his or her life seems worthwhile based on internal experience.

Self-report questionnaires designed to measure SWB usually converge with each other, and with SWB assessed by other methods. A variety non-self-report alternative methods are available for measuring SWB. For example, people's frequency of smiling, their ability to recall positive versus negative events from their lives, and reports from the target respondent's family and friends are useful measures of SWB. In addition to standard questionnaires, alternative methods based on self-reports such as interviews and the experience sampling method (mood reports are collected at random moments over a period of weeks) can also be helpful. In addition, behavioral observations of affect expression in natural settings correlate with informant reports of emotion. Finally, electrophysiological measures such as electroencephalographic frontal laterality and electromyographic facial recordings also converge with self-reports of SWB. It is encouraging that measures based on diverse methodologies correlate and provide similar estimates of well-being, because the multimeasure approach helps rule out artifactual explanations of self-report data. There should also be recognition that other methodologies complement self-reports in their strengths, and that self-report scales are not the only method by which to assess experience.

Measures of SWB show moderate to high temporal reliability. For example, life satisfaction correlates .58 over a 4-year period, and this correlation remains strong (.52) when informant reports of life satisfaction are substituted at the second testing. In addition, pleasant affect and unpleasant affect have a degree of stability across a period of many years. These findings suggest that SWB does change, but that there is some constancy in it even over a prolonged period.

A. On-Line Versus Global SWB

Another intriguing area in conceptualizing SWB is the distinction between on-line measures of well-being at the moment and global reports of longer time periods that are based on memory. If we sample people's experiences over time, we can obtain a measure of their on-line levels of SWB. Are most of their moments pleasant or unpleasant? In contrast, we can also ask respondents for a retrospective, global evaluation. For example, "How happy have you been during the past year?" Or, "How frequently have you felt pleasant emotions during the past month?" For most animals, we assume that their on-line experience is equivalent to their subjective well-being. For a dog, high SWB is being happy during most moments. For humans, however, memory, symbolism, expectancies, and imagination are so important and so fundamental to functioning that global judgments are very meaningful. For a person who has no hippocampus and no memory, only the immediate moment matters. But for most people, the past and future are more important than the current instant in time. Thus, some incidents may be unpleasant as they are experienced moment by moment, but may be perceived in a positive manner when they are over. Therefore, global judgments and on-line feelings may both be quite important in humans.

The distinction between the two types of SWB is heightened because certain "biases" exist when momentary affect is translated into global reports. That is, on-line or momentary moods are not reflected in a straightforward way when global judgments are requested. For instance, in formulating global judgments, people heavily weight the peak moment during the episode, and also strongly attend to how the episode ended. Kahneman, Fredrickson, Schreiber, and Redelmeier (1993) call this the Peak/End Rule. They find that people show relative neglect for how long an episode lasted in evaluating how pleasant it was. Therefore, people tend to ignore the duration of the episode when they evaluate how pleasant it was. Kahneman and Fredrickson found, however, that people rely on the most intense moment in conjunction with how the event ended in giving their global report of how pleasant the episode was. An episode that ends well is more likely to be remembered positively, regardless of how pleasant or unpleasant it was earlier. Thus, we are beginning to develop an understanding of subjective well-being defined as a series of happy moments versus happiness defined as global judgments. Although on-line and global subjective well-being are related, they are not identical. The understanding of the causes of these two different modes of SWB is in its infancy, although this area does have applied implications. For example, clients reporting on their moods to their therapist are likely to weight heavily recent episodes, and might also give special significance to their most intense moods.

VIII. CONCLUSIONS

Subjective well-being is a rapidly growing research and applied domain in the mental health arena. Although assessment issues related to SWB are not completely resolved, the measures appear to have adequate validity to allow progress in the area. Subjective well-being is on average positive in industrialized nations, although people do differ in their levels of pleasant affect, unpleasant affect, and life satisfaction. Several potential causes of the individual differences in SWB have been explored, and temperament looms as an important influence. People's goals, cognitive styles, and activities are also likely influences of SWB. External circumstances seem less important to subjective well-being than is often believed, probably because people so readily adapt to them. Nevertheless, extreme situational differences, such as that between life in the wealthiest and poorest nations, do affect SWB. Values are related to positive subjective well-being in that people who are involved in goal activities that they believe are important are more likely to experience feelings of well-being.

BIBLIOGRAPHY

Argyle, M. (1987). *The psychology of happiness*. London: Methuen.

Bradburn, N. M. (1969). *The structure of psychological well-being*. Chicago: Aldine.

Campbell, A., Converse, P. E., & Rodgers, W. L. (1976). *The quality of American life*. New York: Russell Sage Foundation.

Diener, E. (1984). Subjective well-being. *Psychological Bulletin, 95*, 542–575.

Diener, E. (1994). Assessing subjective well-being: Progress and opportunities. *Social Indicators Research, 31*, 103–157.

Diener, E., & Larsen, R. J. (1993). The experience of emotional well-being. In M. Lewis & J. M. Haviland (Eds.), *Handbook of emotions* (pp. 405–415). New York: Guilford.

Kahneman, O., Fredrickson, B. L., Schreiber, C. A., & Redelmeier,

D. A. (1993). When more pain is preferred to less: Adding a better ending. *Psychological Science, 4,* 401–405.

Kozma, A., & Stones, M. J. (1980). The measurement of happiness: Development of the Memorial University of Newfoundland Scale of Happiness (MUNSCH). *Journal of Gerontology, 35,* 906–912.

Myers, D. G. (1992). *The pursuit of happiness: Who is happy—and why.* New York: William Morrow.

Myers, D. G., & Diener, E. (1995). Who is happy? *Psychological Sciences, 6,* 10–19.

Pavot, W., & Diener, E. (1993). Review of the Satisfaction With Life Scale. *Psychological Assessment, 5,* 164–172.

Watson, D., Clark, L. A., & Tellegen, A. (1988). Development and validation of a brief measure of positive and negative affect: The PANAS scales. *Journal of Personality and Social Psychology, 54,* 1063–1070.

Hardiness in Health and Effectiveness

Salvatore R. Maddi

University of California, Irvine

Existential Psychology The view that people construct the meaning in their lives by recognizing that (a) everything they do constitutes a decision, (b) decisions invariably involve pushing toward the unknown or shrinking into the familiar, and (c) choosing the unknown expands meaning, whereas choosing the familiar contracts it.

Hardiness A disposition formed of three interrelated beliefs concerning oneself in interaction with the world. The beliefs are *commitment* (the belief that being involved in whatever is going on provides the best chance of finding what is personally interesting and worthwhile), *control* (the belief that through struggle one can usually influence the outcome of ongoing events), and *challenge* (the belief that what is ultimately most fulfilling is to continue to grow in wisdom through what is learned from experiences).

Hardiness Training A procedure, usually done in small groups, by which the beliefs forming hardiness are learned through feedback from the process of using particular techniques (*situational reconstruction, focusing,* and *compensatory self-improvement*) to gain broadened perspective and deepened understanding of current stressful circumstances, the better to formulate and carry out action plans to transform these circumstances so as to be less debilitating and more advantageous.

Personal Views Survey-II (PVS-II) The most recent hardiness questionnaire, comprising 50 rating scale items, including positive and negative indicators, which yields part scores of *commitment, control,* and *challenge,* as well as a total *hardiness* score. Studies have shown adequate reliability and construct validity for this test, and the three moderately related part scores have been substantiated by factor analysis.

Strain The bodily mobilization (fight or flight reaction) resulting from the appraisal of circumstances as acutely or chronically stressful. If it is too intense or prolonged, this mobilization can lead to wellness breakdown.

Stress The characteristic of situations or circumstances that is perceived as dangerous and which can thereby provoke strain reactions. Acute stresses involve disruptive changes, whereas chronic stresses involve continuing mismatches between what one wants and what one gets.

Transformational Coping The way of dealing with stressful circumstances, whether acute or chronic, that decreases their stressfulness by putting them in a broader perspective, gaining a deeper understand-

Encyclopedia of Mental Health
Volume 2

ing, and carrying out the actions that solve the problems they represent. The opposite is regressive coping, or the attempt to deal with stressful circumstances through denial and avoidance.

Wellness Breakdown This possible end result of unrelieved stress and strain includes physical disorders (e.g., heart disease, cancer, stroke, obesity), mental disorders (e.g., burnout, anxiety, depression), and performance and conduct failures (e.g., disorganization, memory problems, violence).

HARDINESS is conceptualized as a personality disposition influencing how people interact with each other and the environment. Hardiness plays a role in decreasing the likelihood of stress-related illnesses and performance decrements, and is believed to be learned rather than inherited. As such, hardiness is an important factor in wellness. This entry examines (a) the status of hardiness as a disposition, (b) the relationship of this disposition to health and illness and performance effectiveness, (c) the mechanisms underlying this relationship, and (d) relevant training procedures.

I. ROLE OF HARDINESS IN TURBULENT TIMES

Because of its stress-buffering effects, hardiness would be valuable under virtually any circumstances. Its value is especially enhanced, however, in the current turbulent times, so characterized by megatrends beyond individual control. Think of the dramatic transition we are making from a traditional, industrial society to an information society, the values of which have yet to be determined. At the same time, there is the collapse of the Soviet Union and the U.S. defense industry along with it. For some time, we have been experiencing a worldwide increase in competition and redistribution of wealth as U.S. post-World War II supremacy declines. Furthermore, needed assaults on discrimination toward women and minorities has led these progressively less disadvantaged groups to demand equality at work and at home, sending shock waves throughout society. Less tangible but undoubtedly of increasing impact on living are global warming, overpopulation, and pollution.

The trickle-down effect of these megatrends, whether socially advantageous or disadvantageous,

is a dangerously high level of stressful circumstances in our daily lives. As shown in longitudinal and cross-sectional research, both the acute stress of disruptive changes and the chronic stress of continuing mismatches between what one wants and gets are on the rise. Many people are overwhelmed by all of the changes, feeling continually confused as to why their lives are so unsatisfying and chaotic. As shown in Figure 1, acute and chronic stresses are appraised as danger and responded to with a mobilization or strain response. Evolutionarily, this mobilization was intended to be brief and decisive, as indicated by its identification as the fight or flight response. But, as acute and chronic stresses mount, their accumulation produces ever more intense and prolonged strain reactions. This phenomenon is augmented by social propriety, which usually precludes literal fighting or running away with regard to stressful circumstances. This unfortunately intensified and prolonged mobilization is aptly called strain, because the ensuing depletion of bodily resources increases the likelihood of wellness breakdown. As shown in Figure 1, wellness breakdown may take the form of stress- and strain-related physical illnesses, mental illnesses, or performance/conduct decrements. [*See* COPING WITH STRESS; STRESS.]

In these turbulent times, there are signs of stress- and strain-related wellness breakdown everywhere. Most degenerative, or wear and tear diseases, such as cancer, diabetes, osteoporosis, and obesity, have been rising precipitously of late. And heart disease, after soaring in the recent past, has leveled off at a still unacceptably high rate. In mental illnesses, eating disorders continue to increase, as do depression and anxiety disorders, although the latter two are masked by effective mood-altering medications. [*See* ANOREXIA NERVOSA AND BULIMIA NERVOSA; ANXIETY; CANCER; DEPRESSION; OBESITY.]

Whether or not performance and conduct problems reach the status of mental illnesses, they are certainly on the rise. In the workplace, performance of U.S. employees lags behind that in many other countries, and there is an unacceptably high rate of job-related violence here. American employees seem bogged down in the negative emotions of job insecurity, disloyalty, internal competition, and generalized distrust and dissatisfaction. In private life, ever more people live alone and in single-parent homes, and a 50% divorce rate seems to persist. In our solitude, we seem to have lost

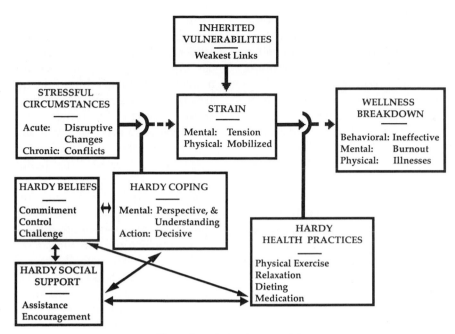

Figure I   The hardiness model.

the sense of cooperative sharing, and are certainly not happier for that. In recent years, the rate of substance abuse, violent crimes, homicides, and suicides has increased, especially among adolescents and children. In those younger age groups, accidents have also increased.

Although some bewildered people hope for the return of "the good old days," traditional values appear too outmoded to help. What is needed is a personality disposition that inclines one to address stressful circumstances by (a) accepting them as a natural, even developmentally important, aspect of life, (b) believing one can transform them into opportunities rather than letting them debilitate, and (c) proceeding to cope decisively with them. And that is precisely what dispositional hardiness does.

II. DERIVATION OF HARDINESS FROM EXISTENTIAL PSYCHOLOGY

Hardiness is the concretization of the concept of courage that appears in the optimistic theme of existential psychology. In existentialism, people are viewed as constructing meaning in their lives by recognizing that (a) everything they do constitutes a decision, (b) deci-

sions invariably involve pushing toward the future or shrinking into the past, and (c) choosing the future expands meaning, whereas choosing the past contracts it. Though positive in terms of meaning and possibilities, choosing the future raises anxiety over the unpredictable nature of things not yet experienced. To accept this so-called ontological anxiety and push ahead with choosing the future anyway requires courage, according to existentialists.

Substituting hardiness for courage lends precision to the existential formulation by emphasizing the three interrelated beliefs about one's interaction with the world: commitment, control, and challenge. People strong in the *commitment* component of hardiness believe that by involving themselves actively in whatever is going on, they have the best chance of finding what is interesting and worthwhile for them. They experience the opposite—being or feeling uninvolved or alienated—as wasteful. People strong in the *control* component believe that through struggle they can usually influence the outcome of events going on around them. They experience the opposite—being or feeling powerless—as wasteful. People strong in the *challenge* component believe that what is ultimately most fulfilling is to continue to grow in wisdom through what they learn from experience, whether positive or negative. They experience the opposite—the wish for easy comfort and security—as overly entitled. Conceptualized as positively interrelated, these three Cs combine additively to yield a hardiness disposition that is especially helpful in turbulent times.

As indicated in the lower portion of Figure 1, hardiness is assumed to decrease the likelihood of stress-related physical illnesses, mental illnesses, and performance/conduct decrements. Hardiness achieves this by motivating (a) transformational (active, decisive) rather than regressive (denial, avoidance) coping with stressful circumstances, (b) the search for activistic social support that assists transformational coping, and (c) beneficial rather than detrimental health practices (diet, exercise, relaxation). Through the mechanisms of coping and health practices, hardiness has a buffering effect on otherwise debilitating stressor levels. [See EXERCISE AND MENTAL HEALTH; FOOD, NUTRITION, AND MENTAL HEALTH; MEDITATION AND THE RELAXATION RESPONSE; OPTIMISM, MOTIVATION, AND MENTAL HEALTH; SOCIAL SUPPORT.]

III. DEVELOPMENT OF HARDINESS

Hardiness is conceived of as learned, rather than inherited. Parent–child interactions are the important natural context for learning hardiness. The child brings to these interactions a pattern of inherent needs and capabilities, as do the parents. But the parents have lived long enough to have views about themselves, the world, and child rearing, and these views influence the parent–child interactions.

In order to build the commitment component of hardiness, the majority of the parent–child interactions must help the child to feel accepted and encouraged. Children will attempt to satisfy their needs (e.g., for safety or love) and express their potentialities (e.g., mathematical or artistic ability) in many ways. When parents usually meet these efforts with approval and encouragement, the child feels supported enough to come to view the self and the world as interesting and worthwhile, and this view is the cornerstone of commitment. But if parents are regularly hostile, disapproving, or neglectful toward expressions of needs and potentialities, the child develops the view of self and world as empty and worthless, and this leads to alienation. [See PARENTING.]

As to the development of the control component of hardiness, it is important to recognize that, as children grow older, their maturing physical and mental capabilities lead them to try to accomplish things. In the developmental process, it is best for children when, in trying to accomplish things, the tasks they encounter are just a bit more difficult than what they can easily perform. If the task is too easy, then succeeding at it will not bring a sense of accomplishment or mastery. Conversely, if the task is too hard, the child is likely to fail and feel powerless. What builds a sense of control is for the child's interactions with the environment to be characterized by tasks that can be mastered regularly through effort. In order to bring this about, it behooves parents to ensure that the child's tasks are always just a bit more difficult than easily accomplished.

To build a sense of challenge, that third component of hardiness, the child's environment must include frequent changes construed as richness rather than chaos. In the construal of richness, it helps if (a) the changes are small (e.g., varying tasks around the home, contact with lots of people who talk and act in differing ways) rather than large (e.g., many changes in residence, divorces and remarriages), and (b) the parents themselves see changes as interesting rather than threatening and convey this to the child. If children are regularly encouraged to see changes as interesting possibilities, they will develop a sense of challenge. If, however, children are taught that changes are dire, disruptive losses, they will develop a sense of threat instead.

IV. MEASUREMENT OF HARDINESS

The first measure of hardiness combined already existing scales that seemed conceptually relevant, although they had originally been devised with other concepts in mind. Although all of the selected scales had adequate reliability, the resulting hardiness measure was a hodgepodge of true–false, forced-choice, and rating scale items. Even worse, although the commitment, control, and challenge subscales showed the expected positive intercorrelation in samples of working adults, challenge appeared unrelated to the other two in samples of undergraduates. The difficulty appears to have been the use of challenge items that signify socioeconomic security/insecurity for working adults, but political conservatism/liberalism for undergraduate students.

Faced with these results, some investigators suggested emphasizing either each hardiness component separately or discarding the challenge component altogether. But the hardiness conceptualization stemming from existential psychology highlights the dynamic interplay between all three components. Specifically, each component is seen as influencing and tempering the others. The cognitive flexibility associated with challenge should keep a person high in control from becoming too compulsive. Furthermore, the openness to experience and interest in new learning also associated with challenge should protect those high in commitment from becoming blindly dedicated to a single cause. Those high in commitment would be stopped from accepting the status quo through unquestioned involvements by also being high in control, with its implications of proaction and initiative in solving problems. Those high in control would be saved from the Type A behavior syndrome if also high in commitment, with its implications of enjoyment of ongoing activity, and challenge, with its implications of continuing to learn by experience rather than insisting on uniform perfection.

In short, those high on all three hardiness components would be trying out many roles in life, while at the same time remaining focused on fundamental sources of meaning and their accumulation into an overall direction. Their satisfaction would be based not only on being involved, being an initiator, or being in a continual learning process, but on all three together. Therefore, it is worth expending effort on developing a hardiness measure that adequately assesses all three components—commitment, control, and challenge. And however much some investigators may be interested in exploring the construct validity of the component scores, it is the total hardiness score that conveys the major conceptual uniqueness of this approach.

Fortunately, the current hardiness measure, the Personal Views Survey-II (PVS-II), appears to avoid the difficulties of previous measures. In developing the PVS-II, many rating scale items were composed or compiled to express specific aspects of commitment, control, or challenge beliefs. After considerable psychometric analysis, the surviving 50 items yielded commitment, control, and challenge scores that are internally consistent, moderately intercorrelated, and substantially correlated with the total hardiness score. In addition, the PVS-II correlates at .91 with the ear-

lier hardiness measure, and at .71 when only nonredundant items are used.

By now, studies have shown the PVS-II to have adequate internal consistency (.70 to .75 for commitment, .61 to .84 for control, .60 to .71 for challenge, and .80 to .88 for total hardiness) and stability (for total hardiness, .58 over 3 months, and .57 over 6 months). Factor analyses done with adults and adolescents have confirmed the postulated existence of three interrelated components of hardiness. Examples of PVS-II items are, for commitment, "I really look forward to my work" and "Ordinary work is just too boring to be worth doing"; for control, "What happens to me tomorrow depends on what I do today" and "Most of what happens in life is just meant to happen"; and for challenge, "It's exciting to learn something about myself" and "The tried and true ways are always the best." [1]

V. EARLY HARDINESS RESEARCH AT ILLINOIS BELL TELEPHONE

Through the early 1970s, the message concerning stressful circumstances was that they are debilitating forces best avoided. Expressive of this view was the emphasis on protecting oneself through relaxation, physical exercise, and nutrition if stressors could not be avoided. This seemed a limited view to our research team at the University of Chicago. First, it seemed unrealistic in these turbulent times to advocate avoidance of stressful circumstances. Second, we believed that people could take more initiative to decrease the stressfulness of circumstances through transformational coping than is implied by exclusive reliance on protecting the organism.

To test our views, we launched hardiness research with a longitudinal study of lower, middle, and upper level managers at Illinois Bell Telephone (IBT). This study began 6 years before and continued 6 years after the colossal upheavals in 1981 surrounding the AT&T federal deregulation and mandated divestiture. In the wake of the deregulation and divestiture,

---

[1] The PVS-II is self-administering and can be completed in about 10 minutes. A computer scoring diskette and associated manual (with adolescent and adult norms) is available, along with copies of the test, from The Hardiness Institute, Inc., 4425 Jamboree, Suite 140, Newport Beach, CA 92660, phone: 714-252-0580, fax: 714-252-8087.

IBT dramatically downsized and reorganized in order to become competitive in the new telecommunications industry. Not only did job descriptions change completely or terminate, so did all strategies, goals, and procedures of doing business. Consequently, every employee's work life changed radically, and this often had major ramifications in private life as well. In short, IBT during this peiod constituted a good model for understanding the stress effects of turbulent times.

In initiating our study in 1975, a demographically representative pool of lower, middle, and upper level managers was approached, with 75%, or 259 subjects, agreeing to participate on a volunteer basis for the duration of the research. Three years before the end of the study, the sample was enlarged to 430. Subjects were tested once a year, mostly by questionnaires. In some years, for some subjects, additional testing procedures, such as interviews and behavioral sampling sessions, were also used. In addition, subjects' yearly medical examination records were also available.

The measurement of hardiness and frequency of stresses and illnesses involved self-report. Self-report is methodologically the best approach in measuring hardiness, as it is the subjective perceptions of self and world that are conceptually relevant. Arguably, self-report is also sensible in measuring stressors, as their mere occurrence may not have much effect on any given person. Although self-report addresses the personal impact of stressors, it is possible that one person may perceive a stressful event to have occurred when another does not. This latter problem is especially likely when minor stresses, or "hassles," are involved. Thus, our approach was to provide subjects with a checklist of major or at least clear-cut stressors (e.g., job loss, new supervisor, residential move, divorce); frequency was determined by recording the dates of occurrence. Although methodological reliance on self-report of illnesses and symptoms also seems sensible, it is possible that certain persons may exaggerate while others are in denial. To avoid this latter difficulty, we validated the symptom and illness checklist used in our research program against physicians' conclusions in the IBT medical charts updated yearly on our sample.

On the basis of the initial testing, a subsample of managers high in stressors and high in illness severity was compared with another subsample also high in stressors but low in illness. Discriminant function analysis established that the self-perceptions we called hardiness were the most potent discriminators of whether a person had stayed healthy or became ill under stressors. Later, this buffering role of hardiness in the stress–illness relationship was demonstrated prospectively in an analysis of covariance study which measured stressors and hardiness first and illness a year later, with the added feature of a statistical control for initial illness level. Another study added to the mix of independent variables by demonstrating the increase in the likelihood of becoming ill under stress produced by inherited vulnerabilities, and the buffering role of hardiness on the effect of inherited vulnerabilities. Throughout these studies, hardiness was generally independent of education, age, managerial level, marital status, ethnicity, and religious conviction.

A later study in the series suggested a synergistic effect of multiple lifestyle factors in decreasing stress-related illness by focusing on physical exercise and social support along with hardiness. Table 1 shows that, in a subsample of managers, all of whom were selected because they were above the stress mean for the entire sample, a low level of all three buffers involved a 92.5% likelihood of at least one serious illness in that year. High levels of one, two, and all three buffers decreased illness likelihood to 71.8%, 57.7%, and 7.7%, respectively. The strongly accelerating drop-off of ill-

Table I Illness as a Function of Number of Resistance Resources among Subjects High in Stressful Life Events

Resistance resources, 1980	n		Mean illness		Illness probability[a]	
	1980	1981	1980[b]	1981[c]	1980[d]	1981[e]
All three high	13	13	357.04	601.46	7.69	23.11
Two high	26	22	2049.27	1702.13	57.69	50.00
One high	32	24	3336.18	2715.58	71.87	62.50
None high	14	11	6474.35	5635.91	92.85	81.80

Note. Reproduced from Kobasa, Maddi, Puccetti, and Zola, 1985, p. 529.

[a] Entries indicate the percentage of subjects in the various resistance resource categories falling above the illness median for all 71 subjects.

[b] For entries in this column, $F = 8.38$ $(p < .0001)$.

[c] For entries in this column, $F = 4.94$ $(p < .003)$.

[d] For entries in this column, Kendall's $\text{Tau}_C = 0.52$ $(p < .0001)$.

[e] For entries in this column, Kendall's $\text{Tau}_C = 0.39$ $(p < .001)$.

ness likelihood as buffers increased suggests a synergistic effect. A similar, although not quite as dramatic, pattern is still apparent 1 year later. Further scrutiny of the relative role of the three buffers showed that hardiness was almost twice as effective in decreasing illness likelihood as was either physical exercise or social support.

VI. SUBSEQUENT HARDINESS RESEARCH

As hardiness research at IBT became known, other investigators instituted relevant studies. In addition, members of the original hardiness research team have continued their work despite the end of the IBT project. By now, a lot of ground has been covered.

A. Methodological Concerns

With the earliest measure of hardiness, a methodological concern arose that questioned whether hardiness is indeed a composite of commitment, control, and challenge. In several studies of undergraduate samples, the challenge component appeared unrelated to the other two, although this problem did not apply to samples of working adults. The difficulty was the inclusion of items on the challenge component that represented socioeconomic security/insecurity for working adults, but political conservatism/liberalism for undergraduates. In any event, the current hardiness measure (PVS-II) has corrected that problem and yields intercorrelated commitment, control, and challenge components not only on adults, but on adolescents as well. Currently, there is no obstacle to regarding hardiness as a composite of those three components.

Another methodological concern that arose questioned whether the negative relationship between hardiness and self-reported illness severity was anything more than a negative affectivity or neuroticism confound. People strong in negative affectivity or neuroticism might well endorse items in such a way as to receive both low hardiness and high illness severity scores on questionnaires. Rebutting this criticism in 1994, Maddi and Khoshaba showed that the pattern of negative relationships between hardiness and the clinical scales on the Minnesota Multiphasic Personality Inventory (MMPI) persists despite statistical control for scores on an accepted measure of negative affectivity. At least one other study has also shown that

the relationship between hardiness and self-reported illness severity survives controlling for negative affectivity. Such results are all the more remarkable because typical measures of negative affectivity are rather indistinguishable from strain, a factor that conceptually should be inversely related to hardiness (see Figure 1). Regrettably, the conceptualization of negative affectivity or neuroticism has not improved to the point where it can be distinguished in measurement from strain. Until the time of such conceptual improvement, attempts to control for negative affectivity will severely jeapordize the legitimate explanatory domain of hardiness. Fortunately, there are also by now several demonstrations that hardiness is negatively related to illness measured objectively. It seems unlikely at this point that hardiness is nothing more than the opposite of negative affectivity.

Further evidence of discriminant validity continues to accumulate. As mentioned earlier, the IBT longitudinal project showed the independence of hardiness from various sociometric indices. In addition, there is now evidence that hardiness is unrelated to the social-desirability bias.

B. Hardiness in Health and Illness

By now, hardiness research has been done on many different groups experiencing characteristic stresses and in contexts that are particularly stressful. This expansion of hardiness research has gone beyond our study of business managers and undergraduates to military personnel of two countries, clergy of various religions, bus drivers, printers, nurses, lawyers, physicians, university employees, social workers, elementary and secondary school teachers, adolescents, the elderly, immigrants to the United States, American civilians working overseas, chronic illness sufferers, Japanese business persons, and athletes. Studies in progress include not only these groups and contexts, but also police officers, victims of job discrimination and harrassment, workers' compensation claimants, and patients with degenerative diseases.

The common denominator in these studies of various groups and contexts is to find out whether some persons weather the storm of stressful circumstances better than do others, and if so, how. Happily, gone is the old belief that stressors have a uniformly debilitating effect on those experiencing them. Now, we search for individual differences in reactions to stressful circumstances, highlighting those reactions that preserve and even enhance health. In this trend, hardiness has been a pivotal concept.

A particularly active research area has been hardiness in nurses. Several studies have shown that this personality disposition decreases the risk of burnout among nurses involved in a variety of caregiving settings. Also demonstrated is the effectiveness of nurses' hardiness in resisting debilitation by intense, prolonged noise in critical care units. Furthermore, hardy student nurses were found to appraise their first medical/surgical experience as positive compared with their nonhardy counterparts who found it a negative experience. [See BURNOUT.]

Another burgeoning research area concerns hardiness in particularly stressful military contexts, both in the United States and in other countries. Studies have focused on men and women undergoing the rigors of officer training school, seasoned military personnel on a dangerous training mission, army helpers providing support to survivors of a major military disaster, and navy personnel recovering from a wartime engagement. The results are similar in all of these extremely stressful contexts: hardiness preserves mental health, physical health, and performance adequacy.

In other research areas, where there are fewer relevant studies, the emerging picture is nonetheless quite similar. The higher their hardiness, transit workers remain freer of illness symptoms, elderly persons are more physically and mentally active, seriously ill people have better quality of life and health, undergraduates use alcohol and drugs less frequently, and both immigrants to this country and American citizens on peacetime work missions overseas adjust better despite culture shock and show fewer illness symptoms over time. It appears that in determining whether wellness will be preserved or undermined in the face of stressful circumstances, the personality disposition of hardiness is an important factor.

C. Hardiness in Performance

The beneficial effects of hardiness are apparently not limited to matters of health, but also concern performance effectiveness. Several of the studies already mentioned accumulated evidence that hardiness not only preserves health and minimizes illness, but also enhances performance. In particular, studies of com-

bat and officer training in the military have linked hardiness to successful graduation as well as to health preservation. Also, studies of the reactions to culture shock of immigrants and overseas workers indicate that hardiness enhances adjustment and task performance, not just health. In most of these studies, hardiness was measured before the performance criteria, suggesting the expected direction of causality.

There are additional studies that focus on the role of hardiness in performance rather than in health and illness. For example, in a study of high school varsity basketball players, hardiness levels in the summer predicted a variety of performance excellence indices (e.g., field goal average, rebounds, turnovers) throughout the season. The only performance index unrelated to hardiness was free-throw average, which is the one kind of shot taken in relative calm during the otherwise tumultous, split-second, stressful action of a basketball game. These findings have stimulated several ongoing studies of hardiness and sports around the world.

More studies of the link between hardiness and performance effectiveness are needed. Also, research should expand to include not only performance but also conduct, in the sense of ethical and legal, as opposed to deceitful and criminal, behavior. If results continue along present lines, it will become clear that hardiness is an essential ingredient of the good life.

D. Mechanisms of the Hardiness Effect

What are the mechanisms by which hardiness has its beneficial effects on health and performance? Available results concerning appraisal of and coping with stressful circumstances fit well into hardiness theory as summarized in Figure 1. As to appraisal, research shows that the greater the hardiness, the stronger the tendency to perceive events or circumstances as less stressful. It is theoretically understandable that persons who feel committed, in control, and positively challenged by life circumstances would see the stresses as manageable rather than overwhelming. Also fitting well with hardiness theory are findings that hardiness may encourage active or decisive coping efforts in stressful circumstances. Along with this are results that the frequency of alcohol and drug use is inversely related to hardiness. In hardiness theory, alcohol or drug reliance would constitute regressive or avoidant coping, that is, a means of dealing with stressful circumstances that may bring short-term relief but that is ineffective as a way of life.

At the physiological level, there is evidence that hardiness is positively related to the vigorousness of the immune response. This is understandable in light of the accumulating evidence that anxiety, depression, and other aspects of a prolonged fight or flight reaction can suppress immune system functioning. The courageous and effective quality of hardiness, as expressed by perceiving circumstances as manageable rather than overwhelming and by coping with them decisively rather than by avoidance, should minimize the magnitude and length of fight or flight reactions, thereby preserving vigorous immune functioning.

Research also shows that there is an interaction between hardiness and social support in buffering the otherwise debilitating effects of stressful circumstances. At IBT, subjects high in both social support and hardiness showed the lowest level of illness severity. But, subjects with the combination of high social support and low hardiness were the sickest in the sample. In this study, the stresses were typically in the rapidly changing workplace, and the social supports tended to involve family and nonwork friends. Perhaps, subjects high in hardiness asked for or accepted as social support assistance and encouragement in doing the hard work of decisive, active coping. In contrast, perhaps subjects low in hardiness asked for or accepted as social support overprotection or subtle competition, both of which would encourage avoidant and passive coping while undermining decisive and active coping. More research is needed to be sure of this interpretation.

A final mechanism involves such health practices as sound nutrition and exercise. There is evidence that the higher their hardiness level, the more subjects are conscientious in pursuing positive health practices. Thus, the attitudes of commitment, control, and challenge are apparently related to pursuing physical fitness through sound exercise and dietary programs.

VII. HARDINESS TRAINING

The longitudinal nature of the original IBT research program permitted a charting of stress and illness severity scores over a period of years. Figure 2 shows a

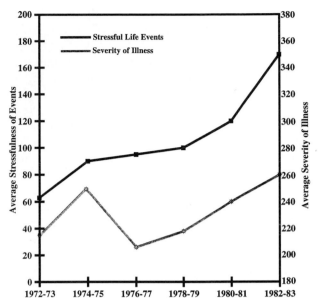

Figure 2   Stressful life events and illness over time.

precipitous rise in reported stressor severity, accompanied by a less dramatic but substantial rise in reported illness severity. Understandably, the rise in stressor severity is sharpest after the AT&T deregulation and divestiture in 1981. In the attempt to assist IBT with this employee problem, we instituted a hardiness training program for managers who wished help in remaining healthy and productive despite the mounting stresses.

We reasoned that for the commitment, control, and challenge self-perceptions of hardiness to increase in adulthood would require properly processed feedback from successful efforts to cope with stressful circumstances. In this process, trainees would increase their beliefs in commitment, control, and challenge by acting consistently with these beliefs in their coping efforts. Accordingly, transformational coping was emphasized in a process that began with each trainee: (a) identifying an ongoing stressful circumstance to be resolved, (b) applying one, two, or all three techniques we provided to stimulate their imagination, and (c) using the ensuing perspective and understanding to fashion an action plan for decreasing the stressfulness of the circumstance by turning it to advantage. The techniques provided are *Situational Reconstruction,* (using imagined better and worse alternatives to the stressful circumstance in fashioning solutions), *Focusing* (exploring feelings that may be obstructing solutions), and *Compensatory Self-Improvement* (regaining momentum when the stressful circumstance emerges as unchangeable). The second step in the transformational coping process is for the action plan to be carried out and for the trainee to remain alert to feedback (a) from observations of self, (b) from observations by others, and (c) about the effect of the actions on the targeted stressful circumstance. The third step is to learn to use the feedback from all three sources to deepen the sense of commitment, control, and challenge. The presumption is that hardiness will increase through this process and that when the training is over, the increased hardiness will motivate transformational coping efforts with future stressful circumstances. By now, there are detailed workbooks for this hardiness training that can be used for individuals or groups.

At IBT, the hardiness training was planned to take place in small groups for two reasons: so that each trainee could receive from fellow trainees (a) activistic social support in planning the difficult steps of the transformational coping process, and (b) feedback as the action plans were carried out. The training sessions were led by psychologists experienced in the hardiness approach and who were skilled at letting trainees follow their own imagination to resolve stressful circumstances.

Early results of this joint service and research effort indicated the effectiveness of the training and are reported in Table 2. An experimental group received hardiness training in the first wave, and a waiting list control group was trained later. The pattern of results for the first wave supports expectation. As a result of training, hardiness and job satisfaction increased, while such indices of strain as anxiety, depression, obsessiveness, interpersonal sensitivity, somatization, and blood pressure decreased. No pattern of this sort appeared in the subjects on the waiting list; but when the waiting list control group was subsequently trained, the same pattern emerged. The effects of training persisted over time, as there were no statistically significant declines in the posttraining scores during the 6-month follow-up period.

The effectiveness of the hardiness training was affirmed by trainee evaluations. When asked to estimate (on a 4-point scale, from "not valuable" to "of marked value") whether the training improved their understanding of stress problems, 90% of the trainees

Table II   Pre- and Posttraining Averages of IBT Managers

	First wave (N = 27)		Second wave (N = 19)		
Outcome variables	Pretraining	Posttraining	"Pretraining"	"Posttraining"	Posttraining
Personality hardiness	7.00	17.00[a]	8.52	9.41[b]	18.23[c]
Job satisfaction	135.54	147.04[a]	136.61	135.38[b]	144.05[a]
Mental strain					
Anxiety	4.54	2.19	4.00	4.30	2.02
Depression	8.31	3.62	7.46	6.92	3.15
Obsessiveness	7.27	3.38	7.61	5.85	1.75
Interpersonal sensitivity	6.38	2.42	6.46	5.50	2.33
Somatization	7.15	4.15	7.00	6.85	4.06
TOTAL	41.15	19.58[a]	40.65	35.00[b]	18.62[a]
Physical strain:					
Blood pressure	130/82	120/77[c]	128/84	129/83[b]	119/74[c]

Note. Reproduced from Maddi, 1987, p. 110.

[a] The comparison of this mean and the relevant one in the preceding column was significant beyond the .01 level by *t* test.

[b] The comparison of this mean and the relevant one in the preceding column was not significant by *t* test.

[c] The comparison of this mean and the relevant one in the preceding column was significant beyond the .05 level by *t* test.

found it of marked value. Similarly, 93% thought that they had "definitely improved" in managing stress and expected that these changes would "definitely last." Both of these ratings were the most positive of their 4-point scales.

When asked for qualitative comments on their course experience, trainees were also extremely positive. One male trainee said, "Your hardiness training has made an almost incredible difference in my life. Use of these skills is becoming second nature. Application of the mental exercises now brings a climax to what had become a scattering of thoughts." This manager lost 20 pounds during the course because he found it much easier to stay on his diet. Also, his outlook toward himself, work problems, relationships, and IBT in general became dramatically more positive.

A female trainee listed the following as specific changes in her view of herself: "I feel more in control. I feel I have more energy. I'm not depressed. I feel I can change." With regard to changes in her behavior, she said, "I'm tackling the computer (which I successfully avoided previously). I've improved my relationship with my fiance by discussing more problems with him. I'm attempting more work (different kinds) at work." In commenting on the course, she said, "I think it was great. I think most people would profit from this course if they want to self-reflect." This trainee's test scores also showed considerable improvement in hardiness and job satisfaction.

Another female trainee listed as specific personal changes that resulted from the course: "Becoming more assertive at the start of a problem instead of waiting to become more upset. Feeling more valuable as a person. Thinking more about ways to resolve a problem instead of just mentally or verbally complaining. Allowing me to put my problems in perspective." Her test scores also reflected the gains she mentioned.

Returning to a male trainee's view of the specific changes in himself: "I now approach all situations with the feeling that I have positive control. I try to eliminate worry as a result of fears of what *might* happen. I eliminate self-pity and reduce procrastination." And about the course: "I enjoyed it. There were a couple of times because of the press of business that I resented having to go, but every time I went I was glad I had attended." And finally, 6 months after the training was over, one female manager asserted: "Things have never been better. I went from being frightened for my son, who you remember wanted to start a rock

band, to supporting him—its his life, after all. . . ."

Although this study shows promising results, it needs to be supplemented in various ways. The number of trainees was small and there was only one trainer. A waiting list control is a step in the right direction, but it does not control for possible placebo or social support effects. Also, it would be helpful to compare the relative effectiveness of hardiness training with various other stress management techniques currently in use.

VIII. SOME RELATED CONCEPTS

Four concepts appear conceptually related to hardiness. The first is Antonovsky's sense of coherence, which combines meaningfulness, comprehensibility, and manageability. Like hardiness, coherence concerns conceptions of self-in-world that can influence behavior and organismic responsivity in a broad manner. Like hardiness, coherence is regarded as valuable for maintaining wellness, and has an existential flavor emphasizing meaning.

Despite these similarities, there are important differences as well. Antonovsky's concept grew out of sociology, conditioned by his immersion in Israeli culture, whereas hardiness reflects psychology and American culture. Where hardiness emphasizes taking the initiative, exerting influence, turning disruptive events to advantage, developing continually through change, and relying on oneself while maintaining relationships with others, coherence emphasizes understanding and accepting more than acting, relying on others and community, persisting in the face of adverse change, and remaining oneself. Although these differences were more apparent in Antonovsky's earlier work, they are still apparent now and help explain why hardiness work has combined research with application through training interventions and coherence work has remained more academic.

Another similar concept is the Type A behavior pattern, which might be regarded as the opposite of hardiness. Conceptually, Type A persons are impatient to the point of hostility, concerned with control issues, and feel as if they never have enough time. In hardiness, a sense of time urgency does suggest the opposite of challenge, and hostile impatience, the opposite of commitment. But the emphasis on control is similar in both concepts. This mixed picture translates into the hypothesis that measures of hardiness and Type A behavior should be negatively correlated at a moderate level, which is what research has found. Findings also show the predisposition to illness present in persons high in Type A behavior to be nullified if they are also high in hardiness. Perhaps hardiness adds to control the mellowing effects of commitment and challenge, making the critical difference in whether the predisposition is to health or illness.

Another relevant concept is optimism. The main similarity to hardiness lies in the contention that through optimism and optimism training, one can maintain and enhance wellness. Optimism is also part of a hardy outlook, but here a crucial difference emerges. The main source of optimism for hardy people is reliance on their mental and action capabilities for dealing effectively with whatever comes their way. But whatever comes their way could be exciting or devastating, and would need to be perceived clearly for what it is—the better to formulate effective solutions. In contrast, optimism theory emphasizes the generalized expectation of beneficial outcomes to stressful circumstances, without this being tied in any necessary way to one's own active coping efforts. Consequently, optimism is more likely than hardiness to include elements of denial, naivete, or complacency such as failure to recognize the seriousness of a stressor or the passive conviction that all will resolve itself automatically. Research appears to support the hardiness view, as hardiness in candidates in officer training school correlated both with graduating successfully and with experiencing the training as stressful. After all, officer training school is intended to be stressful. The candidates low in hardiness tended to describe the training as not stressful, and, in their optimism, they also failed the program. Failing to perceive a problem clearly may jeopardize coping with it effectively.

A final concept bearing some similarity to hardiness is resiliency. Resiliency refers to constructive rather than debilitating reactions to disadvantage of one sort or another and has been studied primarily in youngsters. Conceptually, hardiness is a personal disposition, rather than a reaction, involving attitudes that increase the likelihood of resiliency reactions. And just as there are other factors contributing to resiliency (e.g., social or family support), there are other, nonresiliency expressions of hardiness (e.g., reaching one's potential even when there are no dis-

advantageous circumstances with which to contend). The differences between the two concepts stem from the fact that resiliency refers to behavioral reactions and hardiness refers to a personal disposition.

IX. CONCLUSIONS AND APPLICATIONS

Hardiness emerges from research as a personal disposition, formed of attitudes about self-in-world regarding commitment, control, and challenge. The evidence suggests that hardiness protects physical and mental health, even as stressors mount. As to the mechanisms of this health-maintaining effect, it has been shown by comparison with others that hardy people perceive circumstances as less stressful, cope in decisive rather than avoidant ways, are less physiologically reactive, and engage in health practices more conscientiously. In addition, hardiness appears positively related to performance effectiveness. Hardiness studies have included both experimentally contrived and naturally occurring circumstances. Among the latter are a wide variety of occupationally and contextually stressful circumstances.

There is now a reliable and valid questionnaire for assessing hardiness level and a systematic hardiness training procedure. This opens the way for a variety of applications of the hardiness approach to health and performance enhancement. One arena is tertiary prevention or helping those already seriously ill to recover or at least to get no worse. Here, hardiness assessment and training can well serve as adjuncts to medical treatment in such disorders as heart disease, cancer, diabetes, morbid obesity, and psychopathologies. Evaluation of such applications can determine the role of hardiness in enhancing or preserving quality of life and in the physical course of the disease.

Another application is secondary prevention or the attempt to keep those at risk of serious illness and performance collapse from succumbing. People can be at risk either because their lives are very stressful (e.g., emigrating, being downsized, participating in wars, being on the spot for superlative performance) and/or because they are showing definite signs of strain reactions or disease and performance deficit precursors (e.g., hypertension, coronary artery blockage, excessive irritability, chronic gastrointestinal difficulty, anger erupting into behavior, concentration and memory problems, anxiety, depression, creeping obesity). Accordingly, contexts in which to apply hardiness assessment and training include, for occupations, the military, sports, and the corporate sector, and for social categories, the unemployed, the elderly, the uprooted, and the abused. To judge from available research, hardiness assessment and training should be extremely helpful to those at risk of wellness breakdown.

The third application is primary prevention or helping people develop skills for remaining free of debilitating levels of stress and strain throughout their lives. It is not at this time a feasible approach to control the environment in order to minimize stressors. As indicated earlier, there are megatrends at work that none of us can really control. Consequently, for individuals to build a life around stressor avoidance would mean to also give up opportunities by shrinking their lives to the size of a postage stamp. The more effective answer is to build hardiness in youth, with its emphasis on accurately perceiving stressors and coping with them effectively. Hardiness training can easily be adapted for the curriculum of secondary, and even primary, schools. The youngsters advantaged by this training may well, as they grow into adulthood, specialize in succeeding in turbulent times by turning what could be disasters into opportunities and capitalizing on them.

BIBLIOGRAPHY

Antonovsky, A. (1987). *Unraveling the mystery of health*. San Francisco: Jossey-Bass.

Funk, S. C. (1992). Hardiness: A review of theory and research. *Health Psychology, 11*, 335–345.

Kobasa, S. C., & Maddi, S. R. (1977). Existential personality theory. In R. Corsini (Ed.), *Current personality theories*. Itasca, IL: Peacock.

Kobasa, S. C., Maddi, S. R., Puccetti, M. C., & Zola, M. (1986). Relative effectiveness of hardiness, exercise, and social support as resources against illness. *Journal of Psychosomatic Research, 29*, 525–533.

Maddi, S. R. (1987). Hardiness training at Illinois Bell Telephone. In J. P. Opatz (Ed.), *Health promotion evaluation*. Stephens Point, WI: National Wellness Institute.

Maddi, S. R. (1988). On the problem of accepting facticity and pursuing possibility. In S. R. Messer, L. A. Sass, & R. L. Woolfolk (Eds.), *Hermeneutics and psychological theory: Interpretive perspectives on personality, psychotherapy, and psychopathology*. New Brunswick, NJ: Rutgers University Press.

Maddi, S. R. (1990). Issues and interventions in stress mastery. In H. S. Friedman (Ed.), *Personality and disease*. New York: Wiley.

Maddi, S. R. (1994). The Hardiness Enhancing Lifestyle Program (HELP) for improving physical, mental, and social wellness. In *Wellness Lecture Series*. Oakland, CA: University of California/HealthNet.

Maddi, S. R., & Khoshaba, D. M. (1994). Hardiness and mental health. *Journal of Personality Assessment, 63*, 265–274.

Maddi, S. R., & Kobasa, S. C. (1984). *The hardy executive: Health under stress*. Chicago, IL: Dorsey Press.

Orr, E., & Westman, M. (1990). Hardiness as a stress moderator: A review. In M. Rosenbaum (Ed.), *Learned resourcefulness: On coping skills, self-control, and adaptive behavior*. New York, NY: Springer.

Ouellette, S. C. (1993). Inquiries into hardiness. In L. Goldberger & S. Bresnitz (Eds.), *Handbook of stress: Theoretical and clinical aspects* (2nd ed.). New York: Free Press.

Tillich, P. (1952). *The courage to be*. New Haven, CT: Yale University Press.

Werner, E. E., & Smith, R. S. (1982). *Vulnerable but invincible: A study of resilient children*. New York: McGraw-Hill.

Westman, M. (1990). The relationship between stress and performance: The moderating effect of hardiness. *Human Performance, 3*, 141–155.

Headache

Glen D. Solomon

The Cleveland Clinic Foundation

Cluster Headache A syndrome of recurrent, short duration, excruciating, one-sided headaches. They occur around the eye and are associated with multiple signs and symptoms. These include eye redness and tearing, nasal congestion, runny nose, forehead sweating, and droopy, swollen eyelids on the side of the headache. Cluster headaches occur one to four times nightly during the 1- to 3-month cluster period and last from 20 minutes to 2 hours. Cluster headache periods typically occur every year or every other year.

Migraine A syndrome of intermittent, moderate to severe intensity headaches, lasting from 4 to 72 hours. The headaches are typically unilateral, throbbing in quality, and are associated with nausea or vomiting and sensitivity to light and/or noise. Aura, usually scintillating scotomata or fortification spectra, precede the headache in about 15% of patients.

Nociception Pain sensation. Pain is generally thought of as having two components: a fast, localized sensation carried by myelinated A-delta fibers, which respond to mechanical (i.e., sharp) or thermal stimulation, and a slower, more unpleasant and diffuse sensation carried by unmyelinated C-fibers.

Serotonin (5-hydroxytryptamine) A peptide found in blood platelets and brain that acts to constrict blood vessels and stimulate smooth muscle. Within the brain, it acts to modulate moods, pain, appetite, sleep, energy, and sex drive.

Tension-type Headache A bandlike pressure headache without associated symptoms.

Trigeminal Nerve Fifth cranial nerve. The sensory nerve of the head and face. It carries pain sensation from the blood vessels and pain-sensitive structures in and around the brain.

HEADACHE has been called the most common medical complaint of civilized people and is the seventh most common reason for outpatient medical visits in the United States. The problem of headache generates more than 18 million outpatient physician visits per year in the United States. Although usually not a life-threatening health concern, chronic headache is a major health problem because of its frequency in the population, its impact on the health-related quality of life of headache sufferers, and its cost to society in terms of medical expenses and decreased productivity. While headache is common and only infrequently associated with organic disease, headache may be the presenting symptom in catastrophic illnesses, such as cerebral hemorrhage, meningitis, or brain tumor. To ignore the symptom of headache may risk the life of the patient. Headache may be intense whether its source is benign or malignant.

Copyright © 1998 by Academic Press.
All rights of reproduction in any form reserved.

I. CLASSIFICATION OF HEADACHE

The classification of any disease is difficult, and the disorder "headache" poses particular hardship. The primary headache disorders constitute a group of syndromes of uncertain pathophysiology and a complete absence of laboratory or radiographic tests which could be used for diagnostic criteria. The headaches of a patient may change over their lifetime both in quantity and in quality. Patients may have multiple types of headache. Although "pure" forms of headache exist, many patients experience transitional forms of headache.

The most comprehensive classification scheme for headache was developed by the International Headache Society (IHS) and published in 1988. This provides an in-depth diagnostic classification of more than 100 types of headache divided into 13 groups. The IHS classification has become the standard for diagnosing patients for research purposes, and virtually all new headache research makes use of these diagnostic criteria. The clinical utility of the IHS criteria in medical practice has been questioned by both primary care and headache specialists. A more clinically useful classification scheme for headache was designed by Diamond and Dalessio. They divide headache into three groups: vascular, tension-type, and traction and inflammatory headaches.

Vascular headache includes migraine with aura (classic migraine) and without aura (common migraine), hemiplegic, basilar, and ophthalmoplegic migraine, cluster headache and the cluster headache variants (chronic paroxysmal hemicrania, idiopathic stabbing headache, exertional headache), toxic vascular headache, and hypertensive headache. Common to all of these headaches is the tendency for cerebral blood vessels to dilate (vasodilation). Whether the vasodilation causes the headache or is merely an epiphenomenon is unknown. Constriction of cerebral blood vessels may also occur and may be responsible for the painless sensory and motor auras that precede the migraine. Toxic vascular headache refers to a headache evoked by a systemic vasodilation produced by fever, alcohol ingestion, poisons, low levels of oxygen in the blood, high altitude, carbon monoxide poisoning, and medications that dilate blood vessels, such as nitroglycerin.

The tension-type or muscle contraction headache is the most common form of headache in Western populations. Tension-type headache is typically described as a bandlike pressure headache without associated symptoms. This headache most commonly occurs as an episodic discomfort that responds well to over-the-counter medications and rest and rarely requires medical intervention. When it occurs chronically, as it does in 3% of the population, it can markedly impair the sufferer's quality of life. Chronic tension-type headache can be a common physical manifestation of depression, and occurs frequently in patients with diseases such as fibromyalgia and chronic fatigue syndrome. [See DEPRESSION.]

When chronic tension-type headache occurs in patients with frequent migraine attacks, the terms "mixed headache syndrome," "chronic daily headache," or "transformed migraine" are often used. Because there is no evidence that migraine "transforms" into chronic tension-type headache, and because tension-type headache itself is often a chronic daily headache, the term mixed headache syndrome is used here.

Traction and inflammatory headache includes most of the dangerous or secondary causes of headache. These include headache evoked by organic diseases of the skull or its components, including the brain, meninges, arteries, veins, eyes, ears, teeth, nose, and paranasal sinuses. Traction headache describes the often nonspecific headache seen with mass lesions of the brain, including tumors, hematomas, abscesses, and brain swelling. Headaches from subarachnoid hemorrhage, meningitis, sinusitis, and disorders of the teeth and joints of the jaw and neck are included in the traction and inflammatory group.

The management of the traction and inflammatory headache generally involves specific treatment for the associated underlying disease. These patients may require extensive investigation, neuroimaging, and consultations with ophthalmologists, otolaryngologists, dentists, neurologists, or neurosurgeons.

A. Mechanism of Headache

Despite years of research, there is still a great deal that is not known about the pathogenesis of migraine. Early headache researchers proposed that migraine is a vascular disease initiated by spasm of cerebral blood vessels, while others have believed that migraine originates from nerve discharges within the brain. Recent theories have suggested that spreading neuronal depression may be the cause of migraine with aura.

Research on cerebral blood flow has convincingly shown that dilatation of intracranial and extracranial arteries is a prominent feature of migraine in the headache phase, in both patients with and without aura. In addition, medication-induced constriction of the dilated arteries relieves migraine headache.

Episodic tension-type headache may be caused by increased pain signals from strained muscles, as occurs with inadequate rest or poor posture, or increased muscle tension, as occurs with stress. Increased pain impulses may cause an increased sensitivity of nerves of the trigeminal tract and pain may then propagate itself to some extent. Recurrent bouts of tension-type headache may lower the threshold for new episodes by altering the myofascial tissues, potentiating nociceptive (pain) neurons, or by decreasing the activity of the brain system for fighting pain (antinociceptive system). It is probable that episodic tension-type headache is predominantly a disorder of nerves and muscles of the head and neck, while chronic tension-type headache reflects a central (brain) pain disturbance.

Chronic tension-type headache appears to be one of a group of disorders marked by low levels of the brain chemical serotonin. Patients with chronic tension-type headache commonly report symptoms of constant headache, generalized muscle aching, difficulty initiating and maintaining sleep, chronic fatigue, carbohydrate craving, decreased sex drive, irritability and mood swings, and disturbed memory and concentration. This disorder is similar to the disease depression; however, in chronic tension-type headache, anhedonia (inability to experience pleasure) is not present, the mood disturbance is less marked or may even be absent, and the primary symptom is headache pain.

Many patients with "mixed headache syndrome" have a history of migraine beginning in their teens or early twenties, with the development of daily, tension-type headaches between the ages of 35 and 45. It is less common for patients to present with both migraine and daily headaches beginning at the same time. Because many of these patients have had a long history of migraine, they are well-versed in the use of vasoconstrictor and analgesic medications. When their headache cease being intermittent and become daily, patients with this syndrome often resort to frequent or excessive analgesic or vasoconstrictor medication use. Use of excessive medication can lead to habituation and the problems of medication withdrawal or rebound headaches.

One theory of the pathophysiology of mixed headache syndrome is based on the concept of serotonin depletion. Serotonin depletion causes increased pain sensitivity and arousal. Symptoms common in patients with the proposed serotonin depletion syndrome include chronic daily headaches, sleep disturbances (initial and/or late insomnia), mood disorder (dysthymia and/or depression), carbohydrate craving, decreased sex drive, premenstrual syndrome (PMS) in women, and difficulties with memory and concentration. Other conditions associated with low levels of serotonin may include fibromyalgia, depression, alcoholism, and premenstrual syndrome.

This theory proposes that patients with mixed headache syndrome initially suffer migraine headaches. Migraine attacks are marked by acute decreases in brain and plasma serotonin levels. Between attacks, the serotonin levels return to normal. After a number of years, some migraine sufferers develop chronically low levels of serotonin. Over several years, the level of serotonin in the brain drops below a critical level and symptoms of serotonin depletion emerge. These patients develop chronic tension-type headaches as a manifestation of their chronically low serotonin levels, and continue to have migraine attacks caused by intermittent acute decreases in brain serotonin.

The likely anatomic locus of pathology for cluster headache is the superior pericarotid cavernous sinus. This hypothesis is based on the unique convergence of fibers from the ophthalmic trigeminal division, the maxillary division (a small branch of the orbitociliary nerve), the superior cervical ganglion controlling pupil and lid function, and the sphenopalatine ganglion.

B. Epidemiology of Headache

In spite of the enormous scope of the problem of headache, until recently, little had been known about the prevalence of this common disorder. Most data about headache sufferers came from specialized headache clinics, but little was known about the majority of headache sufferers—those who do not consult physicians about their headaches.

The advent of sophisticated epidemiologic methodology and the widespread acceptance of the IHS criteria for the diagnosis of headache disorders stimulated a new understanding of the epidemiology of headache in the early 1990s. Four key studies, each using a different methodology, definition of migraine, and population group, were performed in the late 1980s and early 1990s to detail the prevalence of headache disorders.

II. PREVALENCE OF HEADACHE

To determine the overall prevalence of headache in the general population, Rasmussen and colleagues examined 740 persons randomly chosen to constitute a representative sample of the population of Copenhagen, Denmark. The group was aged 25 to 64 years old and was representative of the Danish population in sex and age distribution and marital status. Subjects underwent a structured interview, examination by a neurologist, and laboratory evaluation. Headache disorders were classified according to the IHS criteria.

Rasmussen's group reported a lifetime prevalence of headache of 96%; prevalence was significantly higher among women (99%) than among men (93%). Only one case of cluster headache was found in this group. Men aged 55 to 64 had the lowest lifetime and last year prevalence of headache. Headache at the time of examination (point prevalence rate) was twice as common in women as in men.

The overall lifetime prevalence of migraine was 16%, 25% among women and 8% among men. A migraine occurring during the last month was reported by 4% of patients. The male:female ratio was about 1:3. There were no significant differences in migraine prevalence rates according to age. Of migraine sufferers, 15% had migraine 8 to 14 days per year and 9% had it more than 14 days per year, and 85% of migraine sufferers reported severe pain intensity.

The lifetime prevalence of tension-type headache was 78%, 88% among women and 69% among men, and 48% of subjects had a tension-type headache in the previous month. The male:female ratio was about 4:5. Men aged 55 to 64 had the lowest lifetime prevalence of tension-type headache. Among women, there was a significant decrease in prevalence of tension-type headache with increasing age.

Of tension-type headache sufferers, 23% had headache 8 to 14 days per year, and 36% had it several times per month. Chronic tension-type headache (i.e., tension-type headache occurring 180 or more days per year) was reported by 3% of the population. Only 1% of tension-type headache patients reported severe pain intensity, while moderate pain was noted by 58% and mild pain by 41%.

A. Headache Prevalence in Young Adults

To assess the prevalence of headache in young adults and their use of medical care, Linet and her associates performed a population-based telephone interview study of 10,169 young adults (ages 12 to 29 years) in Washington County, Maryland. This study evaluated a community population sample to obtain specific data on medical help and medication use. This methodology did not allow for the diagnosis of specific types of headache.

More than 90% of males and 95% of females had a history of headache during their lifetime; 57.1% of males and 76.5% of females reported that their most recent headache occurred within the previous 4 weeks. Only 9% of males and 5% of females had no headache during the previous year. Of the headache sufferers, 6.1% of males and 14% of females noted four or more headaches in the preceding month. Migraine headache, defined in this study as (a) headache with nausea or vomiting and a visual prodrome, (b) unilateral headache with a visual prodrome, or (c) unilateral headache with nausea or vomiting, was reported by 3% of males and 7.4% of females as having occurred within the previous month.

Headaches caused significant disability. Almost 8% of males and 14% of females reported missing work or school. Disability was greatest for women aged 24 to 29 years. In addition, women described headaches that were more severe and longer in duration than men.

In spite of the disabling nature of their headaches, 85% of male and 72% of female headache sufferers never consulted a physician for a headache-related problem. Family practitioners, internists, and ophthalmologists were the physicians most commonly consulted for headache problems. Neurologists were consulted by only 5% of headache sufferers.

The most common nonprescription drugs used for headache were acetaminophen (Tylenol, Tylenol Extra Strength), aspirin, ibuprofen (Advil), and aspirin with caffeine (Anacin). The most common prescription medications used for headache were acetaminophen with codeine (Tylenol with Codeine), butalbital with aspirin and caffeine (Fiorinal), butalbital with aspirin, caffeine, and codeine (Fiorinal with Codeine), and isometheptene muscate with acetaminophen and dichloralphenazone (Midrin).

B. Headache in the Elderly

Headache in the elderly (defined in these studies as age 65 or older) is less prevalent than in younger age groups. Cook and associates found 53% of women and 36% of men reported headache in the past year. Headaches occurring several times a month or more were reported by 17% of their elderly population. The overall prevalence of migraine was 12% among women and 7% among men. The prevalence of migraine fell with advancing age from 14% in women aged 65 to 69 to 6% in women over 90 years old. In men, the prevalence fell from 10% in those aged 65 to 69 to 0% in men over 90 years old. Solomon and Kunkel found that older headache sufferers attending a referral medical center had more tension-type headache (27 vs. 20%) and less migraine headache (15 vs. 31%), when compared with younger headache patients.

To describe the magnitude and distribution of the public health problem posed by migraine, Stewart and colleagues sent a self-administered questionnaire to 15,000 households representative of the U.S. population. Each household member with severe headache was asked to respond to detailed questions about his or her headaches. Responses were obtained from 20,468 subjects between 12 and 80 years old. The large sample allowed the authors to evaluate migraine prevalence, frequency, and disability by gender, age, race, household income, and geographic factors.

In this study, migraine was defined as at least one severe headache in the last 12 months, in patients not experiencing daily headaches, with one of the following sets of symptoms associated with their severe headaches: (a) unilateral or pulsatile pain and either nausea or vomiting or phonophobia with photophobia, or (b) visual or sensory aura before the headache. These criteria are consistent with the IHS criteria and are somewhat more broad than the criteria used by Linet.

Migraine prevalence was 5.7% of males and 17.6% of females. Black and white females had the same prevalence of migraine, but migraine was less common in black males than in white males (3.3% and 6.1%, respectively). Migraine prevalence was highest in both men and women between the ages of 35 and 45. Migraine prevalence was strongly associated with household income; prevalence in the lowest income group was more than 60% higher than in the two highest income groups.

Projecting this data onto the U.S. population, it is estimated that 8.7 million females and 2.6 million males suffer from migraine headache with moderate to severe disability. Of these, 3.4 million females and 1.1 million males experienced one or more attacks per month. Females between the ages of 30 and 49 from lower-income households were at especially high risk of having migraines and were more likely to use emergency care services for their treatment.

There are several theories to explain the higher prevalence of migraine in lower-income groups. Diet, stress, and other factors associated with poverty may have triggered migraine attacks. Alternatively, access to good health care by higher-income groups may have decreased the duration, and therefore the prevalence, of migraine. In some sufferers, the frequency of debilitating headaches may have led to loss of job or income, resulting in a downward drift of socioeconomic status. [See FOOD, NUTRITION, AND MENTAL HEALTH; SOCIOECONOMIC STATUS.]

III. IMPACT OF CHRONIC MIGRAINE

To determine recent trends in the prevalence of chronic migraine and the impact on disability and use of medical care, the National Health Interview Survey (NHIS) collected data through personal interviews with a representative sample of the U.S. population. Interviews were conducted from 1979 to 1989 from population samples of 60,000 to 125,000 persons. This study compared migraine prevalence for 1980 and 1989.

In the NHIS study, migraine was defined by answering yes to the question, During the past 12 months, did anyone in the family have (a) migraine headache?, or by reports of migraine headaches that restricted or limited activity or resulted in hospitalization. This definition of migraine was the most broad of the four studies reviewed here; however, its utility was limited by patient self-diagnosis.

In contrast to Linet, who showed that about three-quarters of headache sufferers did not seek medical care for their headaches, the NHIS study showed that more than 80% of female and 70% of male migraine sufferers had at least one physician contact per year because of migraine headaches. Of these, 8% of female and 7% of male migraine patients were hospitalized at least once per year for migraine. Long-term limitations in ability to function due to migraines were reported by 3% of females and 4% of males.

The NHIS reported the prevalence of migraine in the United States in 1989 (previous year prevalence) to be 41 out of 1000 persons (4.1%). This represented a 60% increase in prevalence from 10 years earlier (25.8 per 1000 in 1980). These figures are considerably lower than the 10% previous year prevalence reported by the Danish group. The difference in prevalence rate likely represents the method used to diagnose migraine rather than a difference in the populations studied. The NHIS study used self-diagnosis, while the Danish study used physician evaluation to diagnose migraine. Patients often misdiagnose themselves as having sinus headache or stress headache when migraine is the appropriate medical diagnosis.

The NHIS report found that most (71%) of the increase in migraine occurred among persons younger than 45 years of age. In each year of the study, the prevalence of migraine was greater in women than in men, and the rate of increase in migraine was greater in women than in men, 77% and 64%, respectively.

IV. CLUSTER HEADACHE

In contrast to migraine and tension-type headache, cluster headache is rare. At specialized headache clinics, its incidence has been reported as ranging from 2 to 16% of headache patients. The prevalence of cluster headache is approximately 1 cluster case per 1000 population, compared with a migraine frequency of 41 per 1000 (by NHIS).

Cluster headache is the only major headache that is more common in males. Studies suggest a male-to-female ratio of between 5 and 9 males to every 1 female cluster sufferer. The average age at onset for cluster is 26 years. Cluster headache in children is unusual, with only isolated cases reported. Although migraine is a hereditary disorder, familial cluster headache is unusual, reportedly occurring in only 3% of cluster patients. A family history of migraine is reported in 15 to 17% of cluster patients, a figure compatible with the frequency of migraine in the general population.

There is a significant association between cluster headache and cigarette smoking: 71% of patients with episodic cluster and 93% of patients with chronic cluster smoked cigarettes at the time of initial presentation. This contrasted with the American population, in which 25% were smokers. It has been reported that, with few exceptions, cluster patients were chronic, heavy cigarette smokers who began smoking during adolescence. Cigarette smoking may be etiologically related to cluster headache. There is a small percentage of cluster headache patients who have been lifelong nonsmokers.

V. ECONOMIC COST OF HEADACHE

The economic toll from headache is enormous. The expense of physician appointments, emergency room visits, laboratory and radiographic studies, and prescription and over-the-counter medications is staggering. In addition to the expense of treatment, the high cost of headache includes the cost to society in lost productivity.

In the United States, $1 billion are spent annually on over-the-counter medications for headache. In addition, the annual medical expense for migraine care, excluding medications and radiographic studies, averages $817 per migraine patient.

Estimated productivity losses attributable to migraine range from $6.5 to $17.2 billion per year in the United States. The lost productivity of females because of migraine was conservatively estimated at $4.3 to $4.7 billion in 1990. These figures address only labor costs related to lost workdays and lost productivity. Extrapolated to 1 year, the annual cost of lost labor from migraine was $2712 to $3072 per person ($256 per person per month). From the employer's perspective, incorporating benefits and wages, the annual cost of lost labor due to migraine was $4752 to $5112 per employee per year ($396 to $426 per employee per month). These costs did not include direct costs associated with treatment (physician visits, medications, increased insurance premiums, etc.).

VI. PATIENT HISTORY IN HEADACHE

The first step in evaluating any patient with headache is to obtain a thorough headache history. The history is the key to making the correct diagnosis. Because the physical and neurological examination, laboratory tests, and radiographic studies are usually normal, the headache history determines whether a headache is migraine, cluster, or tension-type, or whether it represents a symptom of underlying disease. Most often, a careful and complete history will provide a presumptive diagnosis, which can then be confirmed by physical examination and laboratory or radiographic studies.

Evaluating factors such as age of onset, temporal pattern, quality and location of pain, and settings that trigger headaches usually allow the physician to diagnose the headache problem and initiate therapy.

Most important at the beginning is the determination of how many types of headache does the patient experience. For each type of headache the patient describes (and many patients have two or more types), a detailed headache history should be obtained.

Duration of the headache problem, or age of onset, is often a key indicator as to probable underlying cause. Severe headache of sudden onset, especially if associated with abnormal neurological findings or changes in level of consciousness, suggests serious illness, such as hemorrhage or meningitis. Recurrent episodic headache dating back many years, on the other hand, more likely reflects a type of vascular headache—migraine or cluster. A long history of daily headaches without associated symptoms suggests chronic tension-type headache. The patient's initial migraine headache, unless preceded by a characteristic aura or warning, may be confused with serious neurological problems, such as meningitis or intracerebral hemorrhage.

Among the most difficult headaches to interpret are those developing over weeks or months. These may be benign or arise from conditions as diverse as sinusitis, eye disease, subdural hematoma, brain tumor, or—in the patient over age 60—giant cell arteritis.

After establishing the frequency and duration of the headache, the timing with respect to other physiological events can be crucial to correct diagnosis of the recurrent headache. Time of day the headache occurs, its relationship to puberty, menses, pregnancy, menopause, or the use of hormones are also significant for diagnosis.

Migraine often initially occurs during puberty and may resolve after menopause. It may occur irregularly for months to years, or it may follow a regular pattern of occurring with menses. An acute migraine attack can last from 4 to 72 hours, with headache-free intervals between attacks.

Episodic cluster headache follows a pattern of cyclic bouts of attacks, lasting from 2 weeks to several months, often in the spring and fall. These bouts are separated by headache-free periods lasting from months to years. During these bouts, severe headaches lasting from 15 minutes to 3 hours may occur from one to four times a day, often awakening the patient from sleep at night.

The duration of the cluster headache attack distinguishes it from trigeminal neuralgia, which presents with recurrent jabs of pain lasting less than a minute. Cluster variant headaches, such as chronic paroxysmal hemicrania, show a pain pattern similar to cluster headache, but attacks are more frequent and predominantly occur during the day.

Chronic tension-type headaches show no periodicity and have rare headache-free intervals: the patient typically describes a daily, unrelenting headache. The mixed headache syndrome is characterized by intermittent paroxysms of severe, throbbing, "sick" (migraine) headache superimposed on a constant daily headache.

Location of the head pain can sometimes aid in diagnosis, such as in cluster headache or trigeminal neuralgia, but also can be misleading. Although migraine is unilateral (one-sided) two-thirds of the time, it is bilateral one-third of the time. Chronic tension-type headache is usually bilateral, but may be unilateral. Cluster headache, trigeminal neuralgia, headache linked to local disease of the eye, nose, sinuses, or scalp is typically unilateral. Headaches arising from hemorrhage or brain tumor may begin unilaterally but usually become bilateral. Migraine usually alternates sides with different attacks, but may be predominantly unilateral throughout life. Cluster headache is invariably unilateral and affects only one side during a series of attacks.

The description of the quality of the pain can be valuable. Migraine is usually throbbing or pulsatile, whereas a constant ache suggests tension-type headache, and deep, boring intense pain points to cluster headache. Trigeminal neuralgia is marked by short, intense, shocklike jabs.

The intensity of pain in cluster headache and trigeminal neuralgia is invariably described as severe, so much so that the cluster headache patient usually cannot remain still. The migraine sufferer, by contrast, often tries to rest in a dark, quiet room.

If the patient tells of an aura or warning signs, this generally means migraine with aura (classic migraine), the only type of headache with a recognizable pro-drome. Visual or neurological symptoms commonly precede the headache by 10 to 60 minutes (usually 20 minutes). Premonitory symptoms, which can include euphoria, fatigue, yawning, and craving for sweets, may occur 12 to 24 hours before an attack.

Associated symptoms that may accompany migraine include light and/or sound sensitivity, loss of appetite, nausea, and vomiting. Seen with cluster headache are eye redness and tearing, nasal congestion, runny nose, forehead sweating, and droopy, swollen eyelids. Runny nose and nasal congestion are also common in sinusitis.

Neck stiffness or other signs of meningeal irritation can signal meningitis, encephalitis, or hemorrhage. A brain tumor, hydrocephalus, or encephalitis may be suggested by a decreased level of consciousness. Seizures can reflect brain irritation resulting from a tumor or vascular malformation. Fever and sweating suggest an infectious process.

There may also be precipitating factors. Fatigue, particularly loss of sleep, may trigger either migraine or tension-type headache. Stress may exacerbate tension-type headache, whereas migraine may occur after a period of stress, often occurring on weekends or vacations. Migraine sufferers may associate their headaches with menstrual periods, missing meals, or eating foods rich in the amino acid tyramine, such as found in red wine or aged cheese. Alcohol may trigger a cluster attack during a series, but will have no effect during a quiescent period. Weather changes can be associated with migraine or exacerbation of sinusitis. Commonly associated with chronic tension-type headache are symptoms of depression, such as sleep and appetite disturbances. [*See* STRESS.]

An assessment of possible exposure to occupational toxins, chemicals, or infectious agents should also be made. Carbon monoxide poisoning, for example, often manifests as headache. Certain chemicals such as nitrates induce withdrawal and reintroduction headache.

The patient's medical–surgical history and history of current and previous medications can aid in diagnosis. Head trauma, for instance, may suggest subdural hematoma or skull fracture. Certain medications can trigger the onset of headache or exacerbate headache in patients with an underlying headache disorder. Chronic use of some drugs, including narcotics, barbiturates, caffeine, and ergots, can lead to rebound or withdrawal headaches.

The final step in history taking includes assessment of psychological functioning. It is necessary to identify or rule out psychiatric disease or personality disorders. If these are present, concomitant psychological or psychiatric management must be considered. Second, the psychological reaction to pain should be recounted. The reaction to pain reflects the underlying personality or coping style. Third, general health behaviors are reviewed (i.e., exercise, alcohol use, recreational drug use, sleep and eating habits, smoking). These may reflect the patient's perceived locus of control for their health. Previous health behaviors, as well as the patient's reaction to the suggestion that they modify current health behaviors, can be important data in predicting success with nonpharmacologic therapy for headache.

VII. FAMILY HISTORY

Reviewing the patient's family history may prove rewarding. Migraine is a hereditary disorder, with a positive family history in two-thirds of cases. Seventy-five percent of patients will have a family history of migraine on the maternal side only, 20% on the paternal side only, and 6% on both the maternal and paternal sides. Based on a number of studies, there is approximately a 70% risk of migraine in offspring when both parents suffer from migraine, a 45% risk when only one parent is affected, and less than a 30% risk when both parents are unaffected. The risk for siblings of an affected child but with unaffected parents is estimated at 20%.

Cluster headache is familial in only about 3% of patients. In tension-type headache, a family history of depression or alcohol abuse is common. This may reflect a hereditary abnormality of serotonin neurotransmission, which has been associated with tension-type headache sufferers, depressed patients, and alcohol and physical abusers.

VIII. SCREENING AND EARLY INTERVENTION

The purpose of early detection of headache is to diagnose the organic etiologies of headache, initiate therapy, and reduce the morbidity caused from chronic headache disorders.

Because headache is often a disorder of otherwise healthy young adults, the practitioner often is able to use the headache evaluation to encourage a healthy life style. Patients are usually relieved when their headache evaluation shows no abnormalities, and this can open the door to a dialogue on maintaining health. This opportunity to reach young, health-conscious patients should not be overlooked.

One valuable intervention for the headache patient is smoking cessation. Cigarette smoking is associated with increased headache intensity. One-third of patients believe that smoking precipitates or aggravates their headache symptoms. The initial headache evaluation serves as an ideal time to initiate smoking cessation as part of the overall therapeutic plan.

The morbidity from chronic headache can be financial as well as physical: 55% of migraine sufferers missed 2 workdays per month and 88% worked 5.6 days per month with migraine symptoms that reduced their productivity. Migraine was more prevalent in the lowest income group. This was postulated to be due to downward socioeconomic drift caused by disruption of function at school or work related to recurrent migraines. Early intervention may stop the downward economic spiral caused by recurrent migraine headaches.

The value of early intervention is largely determined by the effectiveness of therapy. Some therapies appear to be more effective is used early in treatment. Biofeedback therapy for headaches is more effective in younger subjects who are not chronically habituated to pain medications. Patients older than 60 had a poor response to biofeedback and relaxation therapy, with only 18% noting clinical improvement. Therefore, if headache patients are identified at a young age and before they become habituated to pain medications, biofeedback therapy has a 60 to 65% likelihood of inducing improvement. The percentage of patients reporting continued significant improvement at 3 to 5 years posttreatment with biofeedback ranges from 30 to 80%.

Prophylactic drug therapy of migraine is effective in reducing headache frequency for about two-thirds of patients. Because the efficacy of drug therapy, like biofeedback, is reduced in patients taking large amounts of habituating pain medication, early intervention with appropriate prophylactic therapy is quite valuable. Because the efficacy of prophylactic therapy is reduced by excessive use of habituating medications, early intervention permits the selection of nonhabi-

tuating medications to treat acute headache attacks. Furthermore, early intervention may reduce the morbidity caused by frequent use of over-the-counter analgesics (peptic ulcer diseases, analgesic-induced kidney disease).

IX. DRUG HABITUATION IN HEADACHE

Because drug habituation is a common accompaniment of many chronic headache syndromes, this is an important issue in patient management. Medications that are known to cause habituation and rebound headaches include narcotics, barbiturates, ergotamine tartrate compounds, benzodiazepines, and caffeine preparations. There is no evidence that simple analgesics such as aspirin, acetaminophen, or nonsteroidal anti-inflammatory drugs cause rebound headaches with daily use.

Detoxification from habituating drugs is the initial step in the treatment of patients who are taking excessive pain medications (i.e., using daily or almost daily habituating pain medication, or taking ergotamine more than twice weekly). Preventive medication is ineffective in patients suffering from rebound or withdrawal headaches. Frequently patients will say that they "would stop taking pain medication if only the preventative medication prevented the headaches." Patients must be instructed that the "pain medication" is part of the cause of the headaches, and that headache therapy is futile until the rebound/habituation cycle is resolved.

X. TRIGGER FACTORS IN MIGRAINE

It is important to understand how trigger factors work in precipitating migraine. Most migraines are precipitated only when several triggers occur in close temporal proximity, usually in the 12 hours preceding the migraine onset. The simultaneous elimination of multiple headache triggers has an additive effect in decreasing the probability that the migraine threshold will be crossed. Migraines are rarely induced 100% of the time upon exposure to individual triggers. For example, alcohol exposure will precipitate migraine 60 to 80% of the time in headache-prone individuals. The triggers may vary from migraine attack to migraine attack in the same patient, although patients may have their own typical triggers. The combination of trigger elimination with medication management will improve headache control in more patients than either approach alone.

Identification and elimination of headache triggers has been found to be a highly effective and long-lasting migraine treatment. An English study reported a 50% reduction in migraine attacks in approximately 80% of previously intractable migraine patients by the elimination of multiple triggers. The key to treatment success was careful physician questioning and education about precipitating factors. Individuals were usually able to identify four to five trigger factors.

The most common migraine trigger factors are alcohol and four food substances: tyramine (found in aged cheese, fermented foods), aspartame (found in many diet soft drinks), monosodium glutamate (MSG, found in Chinese restaurant food, flavor enhancers), and phenylethylamine (found in chocolate). Additional common trigger factors are hormonal changes (menses, climacteric), alterations in sleep patterns (shift changes, jet lag, sleeping late on weekends), fasting, weather changes, and "let down" after stress (weekends, vacations).

XI. TREATMENT OF HEADACHE DISORDERS

A. Nonpharmacologic Therapy

Nonpharmacologic therapy has an important role in the management of chronic headache syndromes. The most commonly used techniques are biofeedback, acupuncture, and physical therapy.

Biofeedback can help patients to change vasomotor tone and to relax tight muscles. Biofeedback refers to a collection of techniques in which the physiologic activity of unconscious bodily functions is monitored and provided instantly by audio or visual instruments to enable the patient to gain control over these functions. The rationale underlying biofeedback assumes that the physiologic activity being monitored is causally related to a clinical problem, and that alteration of the physiologic activity can lead to resolution of that problem.

Biofeedback for tension-type headache primarily measures electromyographic (EMG) changes in the tension of the frontalis muscle or in the most tense muscle in the head or neck. The patient is instructed to use thoughts, feelings, or other strategies to reduce the muscle tension. Daily home practice of these skills is encouraged. Meta-analysis of this technique showed posttreatment improvement of 61% (compared with a placebo response of 35%). Relaxation training alone was statistically equivalent to biofeedback (59%), and the combination of relaxation training and EMG biofeedback was also equivalent (59%) in efficacy.

Biofeedback for migraine may also utilize EMG, but usually includes thermal biofeedback. Patients are taught to increase the surface temperature of their hands, causing a reduction in sympathetic tone. The technique of thermal biofeedback is similar to EMG biofeedback. Meta-analysis of frontalis EMG biofeedback with relaxation training in migraine subjects showed posttreatment improvement of 65%, relaxation therapy showed posttreatment improvement of 53%, and thermal biofeedback showed posttreatment improvement of 52%.

The appropriate role for biofeedback in headache remains uncertain. In its 1985 position paper on biofeedback for headaches, the American College of Physicians concluded that there is insufficient evidence of the efficacy of biofeedback to recommend it for the treatment of mixed headaches. It stated that biofeedback may be useful adjunctively in some patients with tension-type or migraine headaches to assist relaxation, or in patients whose headaches are refractory to other forms of therapy. They also concluded that biofeedback was no more effective than other relaxation techniques. A review of biofeedback for chronic headache concluded that biofeedback has a high degree of short-term efficacy, which has been maintained on long-term follow-up. Comparisons of biofeedback with relaxation have shown similar effectiveness. The review also concluded that there is little apparent benefit from repeating biofeedback for more than a maximum of 12 sessions. [See BIOFEEDBACK.]

Physical therapy is used to train patients to strengthen neck muscles, improve mobility, and correct poor posture. Physical therapy should not be limited to heat and massage. Although heat and massage provide short-term pain relief, only strengthening exercises provide long-term benefit.

Acupuncture has been shown to be effective for the treatment of migraine and tension-type headache in a number of controlled clinical studies. Pain reduction of 31% was reported in tension-type headache. No major side effects were reported with acupuncture.

B. Counseling and Compliance

In an effort to evaluate the nature of consumer expectations, barriers to care, and levels of satisfaction, researchers surveyed subjects attending an educational seminar on headache. Most subjects (86%) had seen physicians for headache, and 82% used prescription medications for headache. Subjects desired one or more helpful outcomes of their visits to physicians: pain relief, 90%; medication and related advice, 66%; explanation of the cause of the headache, 55%; opportunity to be listened to, 43%; and reassurance as to absence of serious disease, 40%.

Three out of four subjects indicated the presence of factors that made it difficult to see physicians for headache. These included attitudes and behaviors of physicians ("doctors won't listen") by 27% of subjects, and high cost or inconvenience by 18% of subjects.

A lack of satisfaction with treatments received from physicians for their headaches was indicated by 34% of subjects. The most frequently cited reasons for dissatisfaction were ineffectiveness of medications and physician behaviors. The most frequent suggestion made by subjects to improve medical care for headache was to change physician behavior or performance ("know more," "listen more," or "try harder").

It is estimated that nearly one half of all migraine sufferers have given up seeking help for their headaches from their physicians. Although patients sometimes find their headache medications to be ineffective, it is physician behavior toward the headache patient that discourages continuity of care. Counseling the patient on the mechanisms of headache, trigger factors, expected outcome of therapy ("control" of headaches and improvement in lifestyle without "cure" of disease), and reassurance of the absence of serious disease, should help to cement the therapeutic relationship. Further discussion on the wide varieties of medications available to aid the headache sufferer should encourage the patient to continue care if the initial therapy is ineffective or poorly tolerated.

When the patient and physician have bonded a relationship based on an understanding of the disease, the patient's response to her or his illness, and knowledge of the risks, benefits, and goals of therapy, compliance rarely is a problem. Limiting the dietary and lifestyle restrictions (reduction of trigger factors) to those that apply to a given patient will improve compliance. For example, a woman who gets migraines only with menses should not be asked to eliminate chocolate and cheese from her diet. Patients with cluster headache must eliminate alcohol during the cluster cycle, but abstinence between cycles will not influence the headache pattern. Smoking cessation, however, may benefit the headache problem.

The physician treating headache patients must be available to handle the episodic worsening of headache and the occasional headache that does not respond to usual medications. Additionally, the patient and physician must forge a long-term relationship to deal with the chronic nature of headaches. The management of chronic headache disorders requires close follow-up and frequent physician visits until therapy is successful with a minimum of adverse effects. Although this takes commitment on the part of both the practitioner and the patient, good results should be expected in the vast majority of cases.

C. Medications

A wide variety of medications have been used in the prevention of migraine, including methysergide (Sansert), beta blockers, calcium channel blockers, nonsteroidal anti-inflammatory drugs (NSAIDs), tricyclic antidepressants, divalproex (Depakote), and cyproheptadine (Periactin). Methysergide (Sansert) is less commonly used today for migraine prophylaxis because of the risk of serious complications. Cyproheptadine (Periactin) is generally used for migraine prophylaxis in children. Adults often find the side effects of fatigue and weight gain from this antihistamine/antiserotonin drug to be intolerable.

Beta blockers, calcium channel blockers, divalproex, and NSAIDs are considered first-line drugs for the prophylaxis of migraine. Several beta blockers have been shown to be effective in migraine prophylaxis. Among these are propranolol (Inderal) and timolol (Blockadren), the only beta blockers currently approved by the U.S. Food and Drug Administration (FDA) for migraine prophylaxis, nadolol (Corgard), metoprolol (Lopressor, Toprol), and atenolol (Tenormin). Beta blockers with intrinsic sympathomimetic activity, such as pindolol (Visken) and acebutolol (Sectral), have not been found useful in migraine prophylaxis.

Calcium channel blockers are useful in the prophylaxis of migraine and cluster headache. Several calcium channel blockers have been shown to be effective in migraine prophylaxis, including verapamil (Isoptin, Calan, Verelan, Covera), diltiazem (Cardizem), flunarizine, nimodipine (Nimotop), and nicardipine (Cardene). Nifedipine (Procardia, Adalat) is either weakly effective or ineffective for migraine prophylaxis, and can exacerbate migraine in some patients because of profound vasodilation. In the United States, verapamil is the calcium channel blocker of choice for migraine and cluster prophylaxis.

Divalproex (Depakote) is an anticonvulsant medication approved by the FDA for migraine prophylaxis. It is thought to work by modulation of GABA within the brain.

Nonsteroidal anti-inflammatory drugs (NSAIDs) are valuable in both the prophylaxis of migraine headache and as adjunctive therapy for tension-type headache. This dual effect on migraine and tension-type headache allows NSAIDs to be used as a single-drug therapy in some patients with the mixed headache syndrome.

Several NSAIDs have been reported to have prophylactic activity in migraine. Among these are aspirin, naproxen (Naprosyn), flurbiprofen (Ansaid), ketoprofen (Orudis), and fenoprofen (Nalfon).

For the patient who has failed conventional therapy, alternatives include the monoamine oxidase inhibitor phenelzine (Nardil) or methysergide (Sansert). Because of their potential for serious toxicity, these agents for headache should be prescribed only by physicians experienced in their use.

For the abortive (acute) treatment of migraine headaches, a NSAID or isometheptene compound (Midrin) is generally prescribed initially. The most effective NSAIDs to abort migraine attacks are naproxen sodium (Anaprox, Aleve), flurbiprofen (Ansaid), and meclofenamate (Meclomen).

When initial therapy is ineffective, or the migraine is associated with significant disability, serotonin agonist agents should be considered. Sumatriptan (Imitrex), a serotonin 1-D agonist, is effective in about 60% (with oral formulation) to 80% (with subcutaneous formulation) of migraine attacks. Limitations to its use include expense and the problem of recurrent headache in up to 40% of patients. Dihydroergotamine (DHE-45) can be given intramuscularly (1 mg), subcutaneously (1 mg), or intranasally (2 mg). Repetitive doses of intravenous dihydroergotamine (DHE-45) may be given to abort prolonged (status) migraine. Parenteral dihydroergotamine (DHE-45)

will usually induce nausea; pretreatment with an antiemetic is recommended. Several other serotonin agonist drugs are under development for the acute treatment of migraine.

Ergotamine tartrate (Wigraine, Cafergot) is often effective for the acute treatment of migraine. When ergotamine tartrate is prescribed, it should be given no more often than every four days to prevent rebound headaches. Vasoconstrictors, such as ergotamine preparations, sumatriptan, and isometheptene products, should be avoided in patients with coronary artery disease, peripheral vascular disease, or poorly controlled hypertension.

Antidepressants are the drugs of choice for chronic tension-type headache, and several of these agents are also effective in migraine prevention. Of the antidepressants, the tricyclic drugs and the newer serotonin reuptake inhibitors are usually the agents of first choice because of the lower incidence of side effects and less serious drug interactions compared with the monomine oxidase inhibitors (MAOIs).

The selection of a specific antidepressant drug should be based primarily on whether or not the patient has a sleep disturbance. Patients who initiate and maintain sleep easily generally tolerate nonsedating drugs better than sedating agents. Those patients who have difficulty initiating or maintaining sleep respond better to sedating drugs. Patients often will note improvement in headaches within 1 or 2 weeks after their sleep disturbance is corrected.

The second consideration, after effect on sleep, is whether the patient is likely to be intolerant of anticholinergic side effects. The common anticholinergic side effects with tricyclic antidepressants are urinary retention (primarily in men with prostatic hypertrophy), dry mouth, blurred vision, and constipation.

Treatment of the daily, tension-type headache with abortive medications is difficult. Muscle relaxants such as chlorzoxazone (Parafon forte), metaxalone (Skelaxin), and orphenadrine citrate (Norflex), either alone or in combinations with aspirin and caffeine (Norgesic Forte), are generally helpful. NSAIDs are also useful as analgesics for daily headache. The prescription of benzodiazepines, butalbital combinations (Fiorinal, Fioricet, Esgic, Axotal, Phrenelin), and opiates should be carefully controlled or avoided because of the risk of habituation and rebound headaches.

Prophylactic therapy of the mixed headache syndrome generally consists of treatment of both the daily tension-type headache and the migraine component. This often requires the use of more than one daily preventative medication. Treatment of acute headache attacks is a major challenge in patients with the mixed headache syndrome. Because headaches occur daily, with intermittent severe attacks, the patient may use abortive drugs quite frequently. Avoidance of habituating medications is critical.

Medications used in the prophylaxis of cluster headache include ergotamine, glucocorticoids, methysergide (Sansert), verapamil (Isoptin, Calan, Verelan), and lithium carbonate (Eskalith, Lithobid). Verapamil (Isoptin, Calan, Verelan) is useful in both episodic and chronic cluster headache, and is generally considered the drug of choice for cluster prophylaxis.

For the acute treatment of cluster headache, the drug of choice is oxygen, given at 8 to 10 liters per minute by mask for 10 minutes. Other useful abortive medications include ergotamine (Wigraine, Ergomar), dihydroergotamine (DHE-45), sumatriptan (Imitrex), and lidocaine (Xylocaine) nosedrops.

BIBLIOGRAPHY

Cook, N., Evans, D., Funkenstein, H., Scherr, P., Ostfeld, A., Taylor, J., & Hennekens, C. (1989). Correlates of headache in a population-based cohort of elderly. *Archives of Neurology, 46,* 1338–1344.

Diamond, S., Dalessio, D. J. (Eds.). (1992). *The practicing physician's approach to headache* (5th ed.). Baltimore: Williams and Wilkins.

Headache Classification Committee of the International Headache Society. (1988). Classification and diagnostic criteria for headache disorders, cranial neuralgias, and facial pain. *Cephalalgia, 8*(Suppl. 7), 1–96.

Linet, M., Stewart, W., Celentano, D., Ziegler, D., & Sprecher, M. (1989). An epidemiologic study of headache among adolescents and young adults. *Journal of the American Medical Association, 261,* 2211–2216.

Olesen, J., & Schoenen, J. (Eds.). (1993). *Tension-type headache: Classification, mechanisms, and treatment.* New York: Raven Press.

Olesen, J., Tfelt-Hansen, P., & Welch, K. M. A. (Eds.). (1993). *The headaches.* New York: Raven Press.

Rasmussen, B., Jensen, R., Schroll, M., & Olesen, J. (1991). Epidemiology of headache in a general population—A prevalence study. *Journal of Clinical Epidemiology, 44,* 1147–1157.

Solomon, G. D. (1990). Pharmacology and use of headache medications. *Cleveland Clinic Journal of Medicine, 57,* 627–635.

Solomon, G. D. (1991). Concomitant medical disease and headache. *Medical Clinics of North America, 75*(3), 631–639.

Solomon, G. D. (1995). The pharmacology of medications used in treating migraine. *Seminars in Pediatric Neurology, 2*(2), 165–177.

Stewart, W., Lipton, R., Celentano, D., & Reed, M. (1992). Prevalence of migraine headache in the United States. *Journal of the American Medical Association, 267,* 64–69.

Tollison, C. D., & Kunkel, R. S. (Eds.). (1993). *Headache diagnosis and treatment.* Baltimore: Williams and Wilkins.

Health Beliefs and Patient Adherence to Treatment

M. Robin DiMatteo

University of California, Riverside

Barriers to Adherence Circumstances that interfere with carrying out an intended health behavior.

Commitment A stated obligation or pledge.

Health Belief Acceptance as true of a health-related idea.

Health Professionals Individuals providing health care to patients, including physicians, nurses, nurse practitioners, physician assistants, physical and occupational therapists, chiropractors, psychologists, psychiatrists, therapists, and counselors.

Interpersonal Communication The unimpeded transmission or exchange of factual or emotional information from one individual to another through spoken, written, or nonverbal (gestural) means.

Patient Adherence (interchangeable with patient compliance) The accurate following by patients of health-related actions recommended by their health professionals (e.g., taking medication, following a special diet).

Patient Nonadherence (Noncompliance) The patient's failure to follow treatment recommendations correctly because of misunderstanding, ignoring, or forgetting what was recommended.

Rapport A harmonious, understanding relationship between people.

Treatment Regimen The course of health-related action recommended by a health professional.

PATIENT NONCOMPLIANCE OR NONADHERENCE refers to when patients ignore, forget, or misunderstand their health professionals' directives and proceed, instead, to engage in behaviors that are detrimental to their health. This problem is common in clinical practice. Patients may take their antibiotics with incorrect dosing or only until the symptoms abate but not long enough to eradicate their infections; patients may forget or refuse to take long-term medications, such as for diabetes or hypertension; or patients may persist in dangerous and unhealthy lifestyle activities, such as cigarette smoking and eating a high-fat, low-fiber diet. This article examines the causes and consequences of patient nonadherence and suggests ways that health professionals can work with their patients to enhance cooperation with treatment recommendations.

I. INTRODUCTION

Despite the potential of modern medicine to control or eradicate disease and improve patients' quality of life, two out of every five patients on average fail to take prescribed medication correctly. Up to as many as 75% fail to follow life-style modifications that are essential to their health.

Obtaining medical care requires the investment of time, expertise, and financial resources, and when patients do not adhere to the recommendations given, these resources may be completely wasted and medical care may become unnecessarily costly. Worse yet, as a result of failure to adhere, patients may become more and more seriously ill, appropriate therapy may be seriously delayed, treatment-resistant pathogens may develop, physicians may inappropriately alter patients' treatments (e.g., by increasing medication dosages), and physicians may be misled about the correct diagnosis. Furthermore, medical practitioners and patients may become frustrated and disillusioned with each other, or with a valuable pharmaceutical or pharmacotherapy in general, and as a result choose more invasive treatments such as surgery.

Nonadherence varies with the regimen. Patient noncompliance occurs in all sorts of medical practices, from the poorest county clinics to the plushest private offices, among uneducated and highly educated patients alike. The more difficult the regimen, the less likely all patients are to follow it. About 20% of patients fail to take correctly a 10-day course of antibiotics, whereas more than 50% fail to follow long-term therapy for a symptom-free condition like hypertension (high blood pressure). [*See* HYPERTENSION.]

Studies show that fewer doses of medication per day bring about greater adherence and that annoying side effects are likely to influence patients to be nonadherent. More than 75% of patients fail to adhere to lifestyle change recommendations they receive, such as limiting the consumption of alcohol and dietary fat, exercising, or ceasing the use of tobacco products.

II. ASSESSING ADHERENCE

Research demonstrates that medical providers rarely address or even concern themselves with adherence problems in their own patients. Instead, they tend to believe that patient noncompliance is a problem for other practitioners but not for them. It is relatively easy for medical practitioners to remain unaware of noncompliance; their patients tend to hide it. Partly because they want to be seen as "good patients," those patients with problems adhering to recommended regimens tend to hide those problems and few patients admit to having any difficulties at all. Patients rarely tell their providers that they have no intention of following the regimen.

Health professionals should always consider the possibility that a patient may be nonadherent, particularly if the patient has no response, or an inconsistent response, to treatment. Nonadherence may also be to blame when the patient's clinical picture is confusing.

III. JOINT DECISION MAKING WITH PATIENTS

Many patients misunderstand directions they are given or forget what has been told to them. Others question the value of the regimen or fear its effects. Patients typically do not speak up, however, about their confusions or their fears. Studies show that health professionals should be particularly sensitive to the possibility of noncompliance when patients appear passive, uninvolved, and unquestioningly obedient. Patients who appear to have no opinions of their own, and who defer to "physician authority," are more likely to be noncompliant than those who question recommendations, offer ideas and opinions, and even attempt to negotiate more acceptable regimens than what has been offered to them.

Why is this the case? Although they may not tell their providers, most patients make their own decisions about whether or not to adhere to what has been prescribed. Patients at all levels of education and social class consider any prescribed courses of action in light of their own health beliefs. These beliefs are typically based on various preconceived notions about health and health care, as well as on recommendations received from others (including sources of information far outside the health care field).

The beliefs that influence a patient's intention to adhere are usually about the disease and about the regimen. Patients are more likely to (at least *intend to*) adhere if they truly believe that the condition to be treated is serious and poses the possibility of danger to them. Adherence depends, too, on the patient's belief that the recommended treatment is worth the effort—that the benefits outweigh any costs (in time, trouble, money, embarrassment, etc.) and that the regimen is likely to be effective.

Patients are likely to be circumspect about their adherence difficulties if they anticipate any criticism, belittling, or negation of their beliefs or of their right to make self-determined choices about what they will and will not do for their health. The goal in questioning patients about their adherence should never be to "catch" and reprimand them or to assert provider authority. Instead, questions about adherence should focus on helping the patient to understand the regimen and its necessity, formulate and support beliefs that are consistent with the regimen, and make collaborative choices with his or her health professionals.

IV. COMMUNICATION AND PATIENT ADHERENCE

Health professionals' emotionally sensitive and supportive discussions with patients are absolutely necessary for determining the level of adherence and enhancing it. Through effective communication, health professionals can foster patient beliefs that support the regimen and help patients to overcome practical barriers to adherence.

It should be remembered that even highly educated patients may not understand the meaning of their conditions. Physicians sometimes find, for example, that hypertensive patients take their medication only when they feel "hyper" or "tense." They may not understand or believe in the efficacy of taking medication regularly, think it is dangerous, or feel embarrassment at being dependent on medication. Only when patients are intellectually and emotionally committed to the regimen will they try to incorporate it into their lives and tackle the inevitable barriers that interfere with adherence. Effective communication is essential to uncovering and dealing with these important aspects of patients' health beliefs.

Patients may abandon a regimen that is, in practical terms, too difficult for them to follow. When patients experience unpleasant side effects, for example, they may unilaterally, without telling their physician, stop taking a medication to which they initially made a commitment. Often, patients forget to take a medi-

cation, even one they believe in, because remembering several daily dosages in the midst of a busy lifestyle is too great a challenge.

V. COMMUNICATION AND PATIENT SELF-DETERMINATION

One of the primary causes of patient noncompliance is a poor provider–patient relationship in which trust and caring are not established. If health care providers behave in a controlling, paternalistic manner, patients have little opportunity to make their own personal commitment to the regimen. Effective communication is essential if potential barriers to patient adherence (such as the inability to afford costly medication, or a hectic and irregular daily schedule) are to be disclosed and discussed.

Noncompliance is sometimes a patient's way of resolving distress at a paternalistic health professional and the apparent inequality of decisional power in the provider–patient relationship. When patients cannot assert their preferences, even if these preferences are unrealistic and must be modified, they often privately make plans for their own medical well-being. Noncompliance may be an active coping strategy to restore a lost sense of control in the medical interaction and in response to illness.

VI. THE HEALTH CARE TEAM

Members of the health care team, working with each other and with the patient, play an important role in enhancing patient adherence. Adherence is fostered when health professionals encourage their patients to ask questions and to describe their personal expectations for treatment outcomes and when they choose regimens that are in concert with patients' expressed preferences for outcomes. Adherence is furthered when health professionals obtain feedback about patients' beliefs in the benefits and efficacy of treatment and patients' understanding and acceptance of risk. Health professionals must elicit patients' concerns, discuss with patients precisely how they intend to implement treatment, facilitate patient commitment, and build support for and reduce barriers to successful treatment implementation.

Patients typically encounter many providers in the

course of their care. Each one of these providers is important to patient adherence. Opportunities for building rapport exist from the first encounter with the patient by the receptionist and the billing clerk. Nurses can make it clear that they respect the patient's intelligence and autonomy and will convey concerns to the physician and function as patient advocates. Physicians can remain sensitive to input from their nurses regarding patient concerns or distress about the regimen. Appointment clerks should inform physicians and nurses about patient "no-shows" or repeated cancellations. Physicians should tell nurses when patients seem to need additional information or support beyond what the physicians have time to provide. Pharmacists might alert physicians to patients who fail to pick up their medication or to renew when appropriate. Physicians might ask pharmacists to follow up on patient experience with the medication. All of these actions require providers to work together as a health care team toward the goal of improved patient adherence.

VII. RESPECTING PATIENT AUTONOMY

Philosophers and ethicists are very clear about the admonition that patients have every right to make their own decisions about their medical care. In practice, respecting patient autonomy and interacting with patients in a collaborative relationship works best to achieve the best possible therapeutic outcomes. Adherence is highly dependent on patient involvement in making medical choices and treatment decisions. Patient responsibility for self-management and adherence require effective practitioner–patient communication and collaboration.

The cost of avoiding this collaboration is high for both patients and health professionals. When they avoid discussion and its inevitable *but manageable* conflicts regarding both expectations for and goals of treatment, providers and patients create paternalistic, one-sided relationships. On the other hand, physician–patient negotiation about the possible course and outcomes of treatment make both parties equal participants. When patients are fully informed and involved in their care, they take more responsibility for implementing the jointly decided on treatment plan, and nonadherence is avoided.

The most effective approach to adherence is recognizing and accepting that patients are autonomous and appropriately make their own personal choices to maximize their own quality of life *as they see it*. Adherence requires that patients be recognized as experts about their own values, preferences, and capabilities, just as providers are experts in the realms of medical diagnosis and treatment. The ideal provider–patient relationship is one in which the provider approaches the patient as a sensitive, supportive advocate, and not as an authoritarian adversary. This acknowledges that the patient has unique values and lifestyle, and a unique definition of what constitutes a high quality of life. This uniqueness must be incorporated into all medical treatment decisions.

VIII. ACHIEVING PATIENT COMMITMENT

The achievement of patients' commitment to adherence requires the simultaneous management of a number of elements of care. Effective, accurate communication of information to the patient is essential. Such communication is not standard, however, as nearly half of all patients leave their doctors' offices not knowing what they have been told. Physicians regularly use medical terms that patients do not understand, and patients tend to be unwilling or lack sufficient skill to articulate their questions. Although about 90% of patients highly value having as much information as possible and want to know about potential outcomes of and alternatives to treatment recommendations, this information is rarely provided to them; less than 5% of the medical visit is spent giving patients any information at all. Although they may not realize that they are doing so, physicians often discourage patients' voicing of their concerns and requests for information by exhibiting hurried behaviors such as by looking at their watches and interrupting patients. In response, patients ask few questions and provide little information beyond that which is directly requested. A patient's ability to participate in his or her own health care, and ultimately to adhere to an appropriate treatment regimen, depends on having information.

Effective communication requires empathy, an understanding of patients' feelings, and a building of interpersonal trust in the provider–patient relationship. If a provider attends only to the disease and ignores the patient as a person, he or she may fail to form a therapeutic relationship that can contribute to healing. Supportive interpersonal behavior by health care providers has been found to be associated with patients' recall of medical information provided and their subsequent adherence to prescribed regimens. Patient satisfaction with medical treatment is greater when patients trust their providers, and emotional support of patients enhances positive expectations for patient healing. Providers who are more sensitive to and emotionally expressive with nonverbal communication have more satisfied patients and have patients who are more adherent to recommended treatments. On the other hand, physicians who make their patients feel rushed or ignored, who devalue their views and fail to respect and listen to them, and who fail to understand patients' perspectives contribute to patient dissatisfaction and are even more likely to be sued for medical malpractice. [*See* NONVERBAL COMMUNICATION.]

Patient adherence depends on patient commitment to what may be a disruptive, difficult course of treatment. Patients' commitment depends on their clear understanding of and belief that the regimen is worth following—that it is likely to be effective and that the benefits outweigh the costs in time, money, embarrassment, and lifestyle adjustment. Such a commitment by the patient requires detailed discussion about the recommendation, including its value compared with other courses of action and any potential risks or problems that may be encountered. The time for discussion of any possibly problematic elements of a choice is *before* the choice is made, not after, when difficulties and challenges (such as side effects) have contributed to patient abandonment of the regimen.

Striving for patient adherence to a provider's unilateral goals will likely result in patient dissatisfaction, patient nonadherence, and poor health outcomes. The intent of treatment should not be to achieve the provider's own personal agenda for the patient. Instead, there needs to be an emphasis on the *patient's* agenda, and his or her own unique quality of life. There needs to be a clear recognition that the patient will always know more about himself or herself than the clinician ever will. Furthermore, it must always be remembered that the patient is the one who has to live with the results of medical treatment decisions. Providers and patients must explore together various ways to achieve the goals that they have jointly decided on, and consider together the chances of the patient achieving an outcome that allows the patient to live life as he or she would like to live it. Together, practitioner and patient must work to consider various alternative futures for the patient that may result from various types of treatment (including no treatment at all). Only under these circumstances, when the groundwork has been laid for patient commitment to the therapeutic regimen, can the patient begin to try to incorporate the regimen into his or her daily life.

IX. PRACTICAL REALITIES FOLLOWING COMMITMENT

After a patient has truly come to understand and believe in the value of the regimen, he or she is ready to state a commitment to fulfill its requirements. It is at this point of stated commitment that provider and patient can begin to work together to develop a plan for *precisely how* the recommended treatment will be incorporated into the patient's lifestyle. The health care team must strive to identify ways to overcome potential *practical* problems that may serve as barriers to adherence. For example, some patients have difficulty remembering to take their medication several times a day. Linking the taking of medication with other regular activities such a eating meals or brushing teeth can enhance adherence. At this stage of adherence advancement, it is essential for practitioner and patient to work together to determine precisely how the regimen can be implemented by the patient for maximum clinical effectiveness. It is important to develop with a patient various methods for follow-up and continued maintenance. These might include regular telephone contact with the health care team as well as office visits to check on progress and solve inevitable difficulties. Some health care teams may write out brief "contracts" with their patients, specifying what the patient will do (the details of the treatment regimen) and what the providers will do in return (e.g., regular telephone contact from the nurse for encouragement). The pharmacist may serve a particularly important role as well. He or she might help the patient to understand the regimen more fully, emphasize the importance of full adherence, review with the patient ideas for implementation, provide the patient with continued informational and emotional support, and recognize problems about which the physician and nurse should be alerted.

Many physicians may find it difficult or impossible to devote extended time to patient education, follow-up, and maintenance. Written materials may be useful, but only if they supplement what has been discussed with the patient in person. An office nurse, health educator, or health psychologist can provide valuable adjunctive care to patients. Many patients may need additional referrals, such as to a nutritionist for dietary modification and to an exercise counselor/personal trainer for fitness education and training. Many patients who have chronic diseases are helped by support groups from which they may learn ideas for coping and receive practical help from others with similar illness experience. [See CHRONIC ILLNESS; SUPPORT GROUPS.]

The practical problems that patients face can derail their best attempts to comply with their treatment. All effort should be made by both provider and patient to anticipate and prepare for these practical problems and to develop a repertoire of solutions. For example, any medication that is prescribed should be evaluated not only in terms of its effectiveness and cost, but also in terms of its adherence potential. A slightly more expensive medication may be a worthwhile choice if it is less problematic in terms of daily dosing and side effects. The cost of patient noncompliance can be very high, and it should be factored into all treatment decisions.

X. PHILOSOPHY OF ADHERENCE

Both patients and health professionals must recognize the inevitability and tremendous value of negotiation in their relationship. The mutual exploration of alternatives toward the goal of agreement on a course of action can help providers and patients to form realistic expectations of outcomes and to learn to work together despite their likely differing perspectives on the clinical situation.

Because patient involvement in the decision process has been demonstrated to lead to more satisfactory outcomes, providers should work with their patients to involve them actively in their care. Providers should work to unearth patients' objections in the process of negotiation and collaborative decision making. Constructive challenge leads provider and patient to examine their points of disagreement and avert patients' expressions of disagreement and dissatisfaction through noncompliance and malpractice litigation. The purpose of provider–patient negotiation is to help the patient to understand the provider's view of the problem and preferred solution, as well as to have the provider understand the patient's possibly different definition of the problem. Only through negotiation can provider and patient recognize that they might have different goals and a different idea of what methods are acceptable for achieving those goals. There needs to be recognition that the most effective interaction occurs when providers and patients fully understand each others' goals and preferences. Achieving patient adherence does not depend on provider authority or coercion, but rather on having all members of the health care team focus their full attention on the patient's decision-making autonomy and on quality of life as the patient defines it.

BIBLIOGRAPHY

Brody, H. (1992). *The healer's power.* New Haven: Yale University Press.

Cassell, E. J. (1985). *Talking with patients. The theory of doctor–patient communication* (Vol. 1). Cambridge, MA: MIT Press.

DiMatteo, M. R. (1991). *The psychology of health, illness, and medical care: An individual perspective.* Pacific Grove, CA: Brooks/Cole.

DiMatteo, M. R., & DiNicola, D. D. (1982). *Achieving patient compliance: The psychology of the medical practitioner's role.* New York: Pergamon Press.

Haug, M. R., & Lavin, B. (1983). *Consumerism in medicine: Challenging physician authority.* Beverly Hills, CA: Sage.

Kleinman, A. (1988). *The illness narratives: Suffering, healing, and the human condition.* New York: Basic Books.

Roter, D. L., & Hall, J. A. (1992). *Doctors talking with patients/patients talking with doctors.* Westport: Auburn House.

West, C. (1984). *Routine complications: Troubles with talk between doctors and patients.* Bloomington: Indiana University Press.

Healthy Environments

Hugh Freeman

Green College, Oxford

Ecology The relationship between a local territory and the people occupying it.
Incivilities Signs of physical deterioration of an area or of criminal activity.
Noise Unwanted and intrusive sound.

ENVIRONMENT refers to people's surroundings as expressed in their homes, districts, regions, and countries. It also includes the social groupings outside the immediate family, beginning at the level of a residential community or ethnic or occupational group and going on to higher levels of social organization.

I. INTRODUCTION

In this encyclopedia, a discussion of environments will clearly be from the point of view of mental health. However, it would be quite wrong to start from an assumption that physical aspects of the environment affect only physical health, while psychological and social aspects affect only mental health. The evidence is that no such sharp dichotomy exists: studies will be reviewed below that show that structural features of the environment have measurable effects on behavior, interpersonal relationships, and actual mental states. Similarly, social processes may have effects on bodily health. Although the title of this article is "Healthy Environments," scientific concern has in fact focused more on *unhealthy* situations, and this has been for several reasons. In the first place, it is easier to measure morbidity in a standardized way than it is to measure "mental health," and this relates to problems of definition whereby "mental health" has often been constructed in idealized and unrealistic terms. Second, there is obviously more social and political concern about bad than about good environments. Third, both research and remedial action—whether medical, architectural, or other—are focused primarily on unfavorable environments.

Freeman pointed out that in spite of the great amount of attention and concern that the subject of the environment has attracted in recent years, its relationship with mental health still lacks both adequate data and rigorously defined concepts. René Dubos, a great environmentalist, stated that, "The study of man as an integrated unit and of the ecosystems in which he functions is grossly neglected because it is not in the tradition which has dominated science since the seventeenth century." Therefore, those aspects of people's physical and social surroundings that would be likely to influence mental health still need to be examined in more systematic and scientific ways. Here, problems can arise at the interface between disciplines—particularly between psychiatry and sociology; for instance, how far is the sociological concept of "adjustment" equivalent to the medical concept of mental health? There may be some justice in the complaint that psychiatrists vaguely conglomerate family, neighborhood, community, and other social configurations into a single factor of "social environment," whereas for sociology, each of these represents a separate, highly structured element, with dynamics of its own.

Scientific study cannot examine something as broad as "the environment" (home, neighborhood, region, country, etc.) as if it was a unitary factor. To be studied, it must be disaggregated into elements that are homogeneous enough to be investigated on their own—so far as this is possible. Exactly the same is the case with "mental health"; this has only a limited (and often vague) meaning in itself, so that changes are difficult to identify. It needs to be split into diagnostic categories and into factors such as depression or anxiety, for which assessments and changes can be measured with reasonable validity and reliability. But if it were found that the number of people in a population reporting symptoms of depression or anxiety had reduced over a period of time, it would no doubt be reasonable to say that the overall mental health of that population had improved. If, during the same period, there had also been changes in that population's environment, then it is possible that these environmental changes could be connected with the improvement in mental health. But such a connection should not be assumed, without further evidence.

Practical considerations require a number of exclusions to be made from the topics covered in this article. First, the design of psychiatric hospitals and other therapeutic settings is a considerable subject in itself and one that is currently in a state of flux, as conventional hospitals are tending to be replaced by "community" units. It is not at all clear at present to what extent this change is a positive process for the mentally ill. Second, the immediate family environment, which is now widely believed to have significant effects in schizophrenia through "expressed emotion," and to be influential in other disorders, for example, through levels of support. Some of these processes are largely independent of the environment in a structural sense. Third, conceptual developments such as social network theory do not necessarily relate to any specific forms of physical environment and would enter too far into the specific territory of sociology. How-

ever, social support is strongly related to social networks and is also an important aspect of mental health. This illustrates the problem of disciplinary interfaces, mentioned above. [See COMMUNITY MENTAL HEALTH; SOCIAL NETWORKS.]

II. ENVIRONMENTAL TOXICITY

It is only possible here to refer briefly to this enormous and controversial subject; in the case of lead particularly, there is bitter disagreement not only as to what should be done, but as to what the scientific evidence means. Psychiatric texts make little reference to neurotoxicity, except for gross events such as overdoses, and the subtle dysfunction that can come from ambient poisons tends to be overlooked. These risks are likely to be maximal in industrial workplaces, although areas with heavy traffic pollution may also affect people adversely. Because of its unimaginable complexity and the large number of its specialized components, the central nervous system is particularly vulnerable to such toxicants. In the case of metals, manganese, mercury, and lead all have well-known neurotoxic effects; the latter is the most important of these toxins because of its presence in motor vehicle exhausts, although the exact amount of harm that is done in this way remains a matter of dispute. There can be little doubt that transport and fuel policies in most countries have taken less account of this risk than they should have. Pesticides also have neurotoxic effects and poisoning from the organophosphorous compounds is not uncommon; early signs of this may be relatively subtle, so that toxicity is difficult to identify.

Since the early 1980s, a new syndrome has been increasingly reported by those working in large, usually air-conditioned office buildings—the "sick building syndrome"—typically consisting of fatigue, dizziness, upper respiratory irritation, and eye irritation. Factors that may contribute to the emergence of this disorder include: inadequate ventilation, tobacco smoke, and vapors from building materials, furniture, and paint; artificial materials such as plastics may be particularly at fault here. Also, fungi, bacteria, and viruses may grow throughout air-conditioning systems, which themselves may be drawing in air pollution from vehicle exhaust fumes. However, no consistent difference has been found up to now in indoor air quality between "healthy" and "sick" buildings; possibly most of the symptoms are due to a complex interaction between physical, chemical, and psychosocial factors, although more systematic studies are needed. There are also a number of uncontrolled reports that people living in close proximity to electrical power lines suffer a higher rate of morbidity than the average, both for somatic and psychiatric disorders. On theoretical grounds, such an effect would not be impossible, but it remains very uncertain with present evidence.

III. HOUSING AND REDEVELOPMENT

Housing, no doubt, represents that part of the physical environment that is most important for any person's mental health and, since it usually contains the immediate family, it also relates to the most significant aspect of the social environment. Although people obviously prefer good accommodation to bad, when there is a choice, relatively little is known about the effects of any specific aspects of housing on morbidity. Much of the research undertaken in the field has actually focused on residential movement rather than residence, but this encompasses many factors in addition to the housing itself. For instance, a move to the suburbs is accompanied by changes that were the reason the move was made, and not its effects, for example, entering a different age-band.

Since World War II, in the United States, United Kingdom, and in other industrialized countries, there has been an enormous outward migration of people from the older, more central parts of all large cities. This move has been mainly to suburbs and peripheral housing developments, but also to expanded rural communities and (in the U.K.) to new towns. At the same time, the vacated inner-city accommodation has been reoccupied (where not demolished) mostly by minority races or groups with socially marginal characteristics, including those with chronic mental illness. In this process, the nature of inner urban communities was changed fundamentally, and in such a way as to produce a whole series of major social problems, particularly as it began to coincide with economic decline and deindustrialization. [See URBAN LIFE AND MENTAL WELL-BEING.]

Compared with previous forms of mass housing, suburbs have been profligate in their use of land: the built-up area of London doubled between 1919 and 1939, but with only a one-fifth increase in population. Landmarks tend to become submerged as the combination of large built-up areas with unrelieved uniformity of style and layout produces a peculiarly disorienting effect. In sociological terms, "control" mechanisms are not induced here by a web of kinship ties, but by accepted patterns of work and leisure and by a set of social expectations such as those on the role of women in the home.

The suburban problem was summed up by the architect Oscar Newman: "New suburban communities house few extended families and facilitate little contact with one's neighbours or between different ethnic and income groups. They are spread over too large areas and provide little incentive (for) residents in one group to seek out the community or institutions of another, when both are identical. Each . . . is intentionally designed to be self-contained, and because of the small size of its population, each can support only the most mundane of communal and commercial facilities." Suburban residential areas become fluid and transient, rather than developing firm social networks, while the immediate family takes on an increasingly important role and inward focus, replacing the traditional role of the community.

In England, "suburban neurosis" was first described just before World War II: the stresses that commonly occurred after removal from a central city area to a peripheral housing estate (higher expenses, social isolation, distance from work, loss of familiar surroundings) seemed to result in a higher incidence of neurotic disturbances, particularly in women. However, in 1965, a direct comparison was made between residents of a new housing estate and those of an older, central area of the town from which they had moved. There was no significant difference between the two, although in each case, mental ill health and physical ill health were strongly associated in those who were affected. It was concluded that every population contains a vulnerable group that is more prone than the rest to the development of illness, both mental and physical; this group will tend to complain about its surroundings, and such complaints may be mostly a projection of its poor health. At the same time, the process of moving, that is, rapid cultural change, may cause a temporary exacerbation of symptoms in those who are already neurotic.

This minimalist view of environmental influence

on mental health has not been generally accepted, though. The hope was expressed that since children growing up in the new housing areas seemed to have better physical health than their parents, they might also have better mental health when they grew up. There is no evidence that this has happened, however; in fact, drug-taking and unemployment—almost unknown in the early 1960s—have made things much worse in general.

Empirical studies of involuntary relocation have been few, but the most significant one was that of the West End of Boston, an area that had been occupied by successive waves of immigrants; at the time of its demolition (1958–1960), it had a mixed White ethnic population. Yet despite the physically poor quality of the buildings and the fact that most of the residents could easily have afforded to live elsewhere, the overwhelming majority said that they liked their old apartments. In 1963, Fried studied a sample of the residents in their new environments, finding that 46% of the women and 38% of the men had suffered "severe grief reactions." More than 2 years after the demolition, 26% of the women were still depressed. Not surprisingly, those residents who reported the highest levels of satisfaction with living in the West End before the demolition were the ones who showed the most severe grief reactions afterwards.

In the process of "slum clearance" the boundaries and spatial arrangements that different ethnic or social groups have established over time are wiped out, and with these, often their *modus vivendi* with society in general—having predictably adverse effects on the social order of cities. The demolition of a neighborhood is not just the destruction of buildings, but also that of a functioning social system, with a characteristic culture of its own and important social networks that could never be reproduced artificially. These networks provide not only social support, which is important in the maintenance of mental health, but mutual advice and assistance, sometimes extending over several generations.

The unhappiness and isolation that are likely to be experienced by a proportion of incoming residents to a new housing development might be reduced if vulnerable individuals could be identified by psychiatrists before the move, and support and counseling offered at an early stage. Yet any intervention of this kind would be extremely difficult in practical terms, unless the people concerned were already under medical care. Other mental health professionals—social workers, psychologists, and nurses—might be helpfully involved in this work, particularly if they were attached to primary medical care.

A further aspect of the housing question is the relative merits of houses versus apartments; the frequency of each of these depends mainly on two factors—national tradition and urban versus rural situation. In continental European and American cities, urban housing was primarily in apartments, whereas in Britain separate houses were the norm. On the other hand, in rural and suburban areas, separate houses have been almost universal. It is very likely that where there is no significant tradition of apartment living, as in Britain, difficulties in adjustment to this kind of living situation will be relatively frequent. In fact, a number of studies have suggested adverse effects on the mental health of residents, particularly young children and their mothers, although these effects have not been strong. Yet in high-rise buildings, people may well feel cut off from community life, with no real neighborly contacts, yet at the same time lacking privacy because of poor sound insulation, and so on. The elderly and physically handicapped particularly often find these situations hazardous and stressful because of their dependence on elevators and garbage chutes, which may fail to work, because of their physical isolation, and because they are often harassed by groups of adolescents who hang around public areas and are remote from any adult observation or control. The pollution of public areas by litter, vandalism, graffiti, urine, or feces is also a source of much distress to residents, not only because it is offensive, but also because it demonstrates a breakdown of the moral order of society.

For those whose social situation is initially unfavorable, living in a high-rise building with hundreds of other families is likely to exaggerate feelings of fear, suspicion, and isolation. The satisfactory use of multistory housing requires residents to show methodical habits, self-restraint, and social competence, which may not be possible for those who are below average in social assets. It is also much easier for those who can afford such compensations as the use of a car, holidays, or outdoor sports. If young children cannot be allowed out of apartments on their own—because there is no safe and supervised play space—the restriction of stimuli and personal interactions, together with those imposed outside by traffic dangers and urban sprawl, could well hinder children's social and perceptual development, which may now largely occur at second hand, through television. For school-age children, the high-rise environment is lacking in environmental interest, is deprived of the supervisory care of adults, and is more vulnerable to damage, compared with the traditional street. Because of this, play and sport facilities are particularly important, yet exist hardly anywhere to the extent that is needed.

The methodological problem in all research on residential environments is to separate the influence of housing itself from the matrix of individual and social factors in which it is embedded. These include: income, family structure, physical health, public safety, social networks, culture (e.g., of minority groups), civic facilities, transport, and so on. "Housing" has extensive meanings beyond those of mere living space, providing the essential basis for personal and family well-being. Because of this complexity, the influence of residential crowding on mental health, for instance, has remained very uncertain.

A study of working-class women in London found that those living in homes of poor environmental quality were more likely to be suffering from depression than those in better homes. While this may well indicate that the poor environment contributed to depression, it might also be the case that those women acquired worse homes because they were already vulnerable. In other words, the direction of causality must remain uncertain until subjects are examined before moving into one kind of home or another.

In a study of working-class housing schemes in New York, Newman found that the rates of crime, fear of crime, and instability of the resident population were related to four main factors. These were: the size of the building; its accessibility for unauthorized entry; a combined factor of low incomes and proportion of one-parent families; and the ratio of teenagers to adults. Residents' control of space outside their apartment ("defensible space") had an important influence on the rates of burglary, personal crime, and fear of crime. Another major factor that was related to both the volume and type of crime was the number of families using the same entrance to a block; the larger this number, the more difficult it is for people to identify the building as being theirs or to feel that they have any right to control the activities taking place in communal spaces, through an established code of behavior. A complex, anonymous environ-ment, poor maintenance, and social instability of the resident population will all tend to have adverse effects on the quality of life for people living in any development.

Halpern has emphasized the importance of an ability to control one's environment. "The negative impact of environmental stresses is greatly reduced when people feel that they have control over them. Similarly, the impact and quality of people's relationships with their neighbors is critically mediated by the extent to which they are able to regulate their interactions with them." However, environments that facilitate social contacts between neighbors will not necessarily lead to positive social relations, if residents are unable to regulate these contacts. Semipublic spaces, used by a restricted number of residents, are generally helpful in this respect. On the whole, people of similar background and income level tend to get on better with each other than those who are not, although the positive effect of such local homogeneity tends to become a negative one if extended over too large an area. Apartment blocks containing only older people without children generally function well, provided that the services and maintenance are reliable.

IV. NOISE

Noise, which is defined as "unwanted sound," is the kind of stressor that might be expected to have a harmful effect on mental health. It is generally believed that noise will cause annoyance to the individual, as well as disturbing communication and activities, thus leading to stress responses, symptoms, and possibly illness. [See STRESS.]

Industrial workers regularly exposed to high levels of noise tend to report a variety of symptoms, but the relationship of these to noise is uncertain because these workers often experience other stressors at the same time, for example, physical danger or heavy work demands. Also, there may be selective processes in the choice of personnel for jobs with a high exposure to noise—they might have poor health and have been unable to obtain a more desirable job, or might be unusually tough. Outside work settings, environmental noise is usually less intense, but may be more difficult to avoid, for example, from traffic, aircraft, or neighbors (particularly where sound insulation is poor).

Noise impairs several aspects of human functioning, particularly sleep; although these effects may habituate over time, they do not necessarily do so in all cases and deficits may persist for years. It also affects performance by increasing arousal and decreasing attention through distraction, and can impair social behavior, for example, through impairing communication or removing attention from important behavioral cues. All these processes could have potentially harmful effects on mental health. The most common subjective response to noise is annoyance, which includes mild anger, fear, and a feeling that one's personal privacy is being invaded. However, the meaning of a noise for any individual is important in determining whether or not that person will be annoyed by it, and the context in which the noise is heard may also be influential. Those who already have minor psychiatric disorder or who are most vulnerable to developing it are likely to experience the most annoyance from noise. Also, noise-sensitive people show slower physiological habituation to noise. The relationship between noise and actual symptoms seems to be very complex, though.

In spite of the intrusiveness of noise in modern society, particularly from vehicles and amplified sound, the evidence so far shows it to have only a limited effect on mental health, and then only on less severe disorders. In the case of traffic noise, people's negative feelings about it may be strongly influenced by concern about road safety and by annoyance from pollution. However, the subject remains to be investigated more thoroughly, traffic noise in particular needing systematic research.

V. ECOLOGY

In human studies, ecology refers to the relationship between a local territory and the people occupying it; these relationships are found to be influenced by the characteristics of that territory, such as whether it is urban or rural.

This principle was applied to the study of cities, which can be divided into zones, showing distinctive socioeconomic characteristics. Faris and Dunham plotted the home addresses of people admitted to mental hospitals with schizophrenia from the city of Chicago. They found that the highest rate was in the center, and that it became steadily less toward the outer suburbs. The central areas were characterized by a declining population, environmental deterioration, much casual employment, and a high rate of people living alone. It was concluded that these environmental conditions led to social isolation, which in turn promoted the development of schizophrenia. [*See* SCHIZOPHRENIA.]

However, when the study was repeated some years later and population movements were examined, an entirely different picture emerged. The overall high-rate areas, combining old and new cases, were still central, and the low-rate areas peripheral. But new cases of schizophrenia were randomly distributed throughout the city, in terms of their family homes. The central excess came from the migration of individuals who were becoming ill or had already been ill, and who had deteriorated in social performance. They had become unable to continue living in better residential districts. Thus, being resident in a poor environmental area was not an etiological factor in itself, but rather one associated with the adverse effects of developing schizophrenia.

This migration, which also applied to other socially marginal groups, such as Skid Row alcoholics, was described as "social drift." In schizophrenics, it also involves a general drift downward in the social class scale. In this way, the process tends to concentrate people who are less able and more impaired in less desirable areas. At the same time, healthier and more economically active people tend to move out to suburban areas.

Although prevalence rates of schizophrenia are generally higher in cities, the same excess can be found in some areas that have the opposite environmental characteristics. One notable example is the rural West of Ireland. There, it has been shown that the very high prevalence rate of total cases is not due to a higher-than-average incidence rate of new cases. This excess prevalence rate in Ireland seems to be related to a number of social processes, of which the overall decline in population, associated with migration, is probably the most important.

Ecological studies indicate that a number of adverse social factors related to psychiatric disorder show spatial variations and that these tend to cluster in either a positive or a negative direction. These factors include: poverty, mental or physical handicap, some forms of minority status, role disturbance (e.g., one-parent families), prolonged unemployment, and crime.

Where the clustering is negative, there is likely to be an association with higher levels of both psychiatric illness and of social pathology such as drug-taking, child abuse, delinquency, and attempted suicide. There is also likely to be more pollution in such areas. Completed suicide does not show the same association, but is maximal in areas which have the highest measures of social isolation.

A California study showed that air pollution had no direct effect on mental health, but that it did act as a vulnerability factor; the effects of pollution were only evident in the simultaneous presence of a stressful life event. The significance of this finding is that the cost to the individual of coping with such an undesirable polluted environment is a reduced ability to deal with new stresses. However, the methodological issues in such studies are extremely complex.

VI. URBAN–RURAL DIFFERENCES

It has long been believed that living in cities is unhealthy, because of presumed greater social stress in urban life, as well as the very real problems of hygiene and infection in earlier periods. More recently, psychological work has suggested that in cities, the volume of stimuli—both coming from other people and from the ambient level of signals and messages—could be too much for those with a vulnerable nervous system to process.

However, the evidence for this hypothesis remains uncertain, probably because the usual urban-rural dichotomy, which is used in studies, no longer represents a meaningful difference. In industrialized countries, a distinct rural culture has largely ceased to exist due to depopulation, increased mobility, and the universal influence of the mass media. Also, the term "urban" has been used for anything from a town of 20,000 people to a city of nearly 20 million; most existing data do not distinguish between the various orders of magnitude of urban populations. Cities certainly do contain concentrations of multiply disadvantaged people, many of whom have poor mental health along with other unfavorable attributes, but this picture should not be overgeneralized.

Blazer and colleagues showed that in North Carolina, major depression was much more common in the urban counties than in the rural ones. But it was concluded that place of residence now serves largely as a proxy for social processes that affect the risk of developing psychiatric disorder. In other words, that vulnerable people tend to live in certain kinds of places, rather than that the conditions of these places cause greater morbidity.

It may also be wrong to think of environmental stress as primarily an urban phenomenon. Rural people have always been vulnerable to such stresses as bad weather and social isolation. "Sociocultural disintegration"—a process most often thought of in connection with inner cities—also affects many rural areas, for example, the mountainous districts of Spain and Italy, which have been largely abandoned by their former peasant populations. It used to be widely believed that people in remote and unsophisticated situations suffer less emotional distress and fewer psychiatric disorders than those in industrialized societies. However, a survey of women in a Ugandan village found that they had the same levels of depressive illness as women in London, while women in two mountain villages of the Himalayas had even more anxiety and depressive disorders than a comparable sample in Europe.

VII. CROWDING AND DENSITY

The relationship of crowding and density to each other and to mental health remains far from clear. "Density" should be used to represent the number of people resident in a geographical unit of area—purely a mathematical ratio. "Crowding" describes the number of people in an area of dwelling; it varies mostly with local socioeconomic circumstances, whereas density does not. Thus, the two may not necessarily correspond at all: for instance, a high-rise block of expensive apartments may have a high density (per hectare), but a very low ratio of crowding.

What is regarded anywhere as "crowding" is strongly affected by culture, and is largely a psychological experience: people feel that their personal space has been invaded. Social interaction then becomes involuntary and unpredictable, resulting in high arousal of the central nervous system, and so of the endocrine and other bodily systems. There is also likely to be a higher rate of life events, which may have an adverse effect, particularly in precipitating depression. In the near presence of too many people, social support may break down. However, any stress associated with the experience of crowding probably derives more from disordered social relationships than from actual lack of physical space. It should not be forgotten that the opposite of crowding, that is, living alone, is also associated with stress and with insufficient social support. Also, most people welcome intense physical crowding at certain times, such as at a party.

In Western societies, cross-sectional analyses of population density—as opposed to crowding—have failed to show any significant relationship with psychiatric morbidity. One likely reason for this is that the range of densities found in industrialized countries is now fairly narrow, and another is that longitudinal studies over time are really needed, but these are extremely difficult to complete. On the other hand, in a study in Chicago, Gove and colleagues found that the number of persons per room correlated with rates of psychiatric symptoms and rates of nervous breakdown in the previous year. Many studies of crowding are confounded by such factors as low income, social class, and education but the Chicago effects remained positive after adjusting for gender, race, marital status, education, age, and family income.

The importance of culture can be seen in the fact that in parts of Asia, very low rates of household space per person do not seem to be associated—at least up to now—with the kinds of adverse results that have been described in European or American populations. This applies both to psychiatric disorder and to social pathology, and seems to result from different social norms on the sharing of space that have been incorporated into these cultures, particularly among people related by kinship. Individual privacy is felt to be less important than it is in Western populations, except among nonkin.

VIII. CHILDREN AND ADOLESCENTS

It has been pointed out that certain areas of cities show a connection between psychiatric disorder and high rates of social deviance; this is most marked in the case of children. There is also an excess of both among inner-city children, compared with those living in more rural situations. Rutter and colleagues compared 10-year-old children in inner London with others living in the Isle of Wight. Both psychiatric morbidity and delayed reading were twice as common in the city children. The correlates of this morbidity—family disturbance, parental deviance, social disadvantage, and school difficulties—were also much more common in London. Environmental effects seemed to be mediated through families and schools to the children, who may have been more susceptible than adults to these effects because they had less control over resources and fewer coping abilities. However, the exact nature of this inner-city effect on children's psychiatric morbidity has not yet been identified; it was not poverty alone.

Yet even in a deprived neighborhood, many children show no evidence themselves of delinquency or other antisocial behavior. There is considerable individual variation, probably of genetic origin in the main, in response to environmental stress, and so it may be useful to focus help on the most vulnerable. Investigation of risk factors for psychiatric disorder in children has shown that a single one does not increase the likelihood of disorder, but that when two or more factors are present together, the risk of disorder increases greatly, due to interaction effects. [See CHILD-HOOD STRESS.]

Children and adolescents have suffered particularly from the consequences of contemporary environmental changes in many cities—destruction of established neighborhoods, high-rise housing, urban highways, loss of public transport, and so on. They can no longer play spontaneously in their street or go by bicycle to school. These urban environments are unfriendly and fail to provide opportunities for the kind of social interactions and physical activity that children and adolescents need. In these circumstances, vandalism, drug-taking, and the defacement of every accessible surface with graffiti are likely to occur on a massive scale, compared with more human environments. Such "incivilities" are especially frightening to older people, leading to a deterioration in the community's morale and so to poorer mental health.

Jane Jacobs first pointed out that established neighborhoods are largely self-policing, in that outside their homes, children are constantly seen by passing neighbors or relatives, as well as being observed by "the eyes in the street"—people who watch the passing scene from their homes. Contact with many adults then provides a variety of role models for the process of socialization into the society's mores. However, in many redeveloped areas, particularly with high-rise buildings, this informal supervision can no longer take place—there is no passing scene from the 14th floor.

Young people also tend to remain completely separate from adults in these environments, for example, in the gang territory of empty spaces.

IX. UNDERLYING MECHANISMS

Two concepts have been mainly used in investigating the relationship between environmental factors on the one hand and the characteristics of individuals or communities on the other.

The first of these is social support, which is related to the theory of social networks. The relationship between social support and psychiatric disorder may operate in both directions (e.g., support reduced by the personal withdrawal of schizophrenia), but social support does seem to be an important factor in depression, in many neurotic disorders, and in buffering the effects of stress. The structure of the environment can have a strong influence on the degree to which human interactions occur, from which support may be derived. Features such as cafes, pubs, or pedestrian streets (particularly for the "paseo" of Mediterranean countries) provide sources of support that are part of local culture. In more dispersed, motorized societies, though, such informal, unplanned social support becomes less and less possible. The endless spread of housing around large cities requires more and more car travel for any activity. Out-of-town shopping centers are so large and draw on such a huge catchment area that the likelihood of meeting anyone familiar is considerably less than in a local shopping street. Yet the possibility of chance meetings and face-to-face encounters is a fundamental part of human life and social support. A vibrant, diverse, and fairly densely populated environment is one that fosters these interactions in the best way. [*See* SOCIAL SUPPORT.]

The effects on mental health of commuting have been little studied, but there are reasonable grounds for proposing that this is often harmful—to the commuter, the family, and to society in general. The consequence is that residential areas become dormitories, which are largely devoid of activity during weekdays, while the business or industrial districts are deserted in the evenings and on weekends; in both cases, social support is absent for much of the time. The intermediate areas also suffer because of the volumes of traffic that pass through them.

The second conceptual model used in analyzing these relationships with environmental factors is that of stress. This is a poorly defined concept, but there seems to be no alternative to using it. Psychiatry has a long tradition of regarding external stress as a causal factor in mental disorder, and the regime of psychiatric hospitals can be seen partly as a protection from environmental stress. However, hardly any direct relationships have been found between particular forms of environmental stress and specific psychiatric disorders. An important exception is the posttraumatic stress disorder that follows environmental disasters— whether natural, such as Australian bush fires, or man-made, such as Chernobyl. The Athens earthquake of 1981 was found to have been associated with a measurable epidemic of heart attacks, a few days later, providing a remarkable natural experiment of the pathogenic effects of environmental stress.

X. CRIME AND FEAR OF CRIME

A factor of increasing importance in cities, particularly large cities, is that they contain more crime and social pathology of all kinds than less densely populated areas. Therefore, both fear of crime—seen as chronic anxiety disorder—and the consequences of crime—such as posttraumatic stress disorder—must be present at a higher rate in cities than elsewhere. Such an excess must make a significant contribution to mental ill health in city residents; fear of crime also causes social withdrawal, which undermines supportive social networks.

"Incivilities" such as environmental degradation (litter, graffiti, etc.) and frightening behavior are symbols of danger and environmental decline that raise anxiety levels and discourage people from using public areas. Their avoidance then increases the level of danger because fewer people are about and isolated individuals are more vulnerable. People who have been victims of crime are more disturbed by environmental incivilities than are those who have not been victimized. There is evidence that control of such low-level infringements of public order helps to militate against more serious crime, and thus improves the mental health of a population.

Rates of crime can also be influenced by architectural policies. Newman's work on "defensible space" showed that structural changes to public housing developments can promote that informal control by residents that is the strongest deterrent to crime. The presence of "confused space," for which no one is responsible, has been shown to increase the local rate of offenses. An environment concerned with the promotion of mental health would pay attention to these questions.

XI. CONCLUSION

There is very little reliable information in the scientific literature as to whether the mental health of a population can actually be enhanced by improving the environment; hardly any have been studied before and after such a change. However, Halpern took a random population sample from a public housing area in Britain that the city was proposing to improve comprehensively. This sample was given a questionnaire to estimate levels of anxiety and depression—both of which were present to a surprisingly large extent. There was also a generally high level of social distrust and withdrawal. After the environmental improvements, both symptoms were significantly reduced, but anxiety more than depression; social withdrawal was also reduced. Halpern proposed that mental improvement was not just due to the structural changes, but also to the consultation process with the residents that preceded them. These data provide some encouragement to the view that mental health can in fact be improved by environmental changes.

Currently, enormous environmental changes are going on throughout the world. In the United States, with the growing phenomenon of "edge cities," unrelated to any central focus, it may often be difficult to decide where a city begins or ends. In developing countries, cities have already reached sizes never previously known in human history; but in scientific terms, practically nothing is known about their populations. The task of psychiatry—so far as it can—is to draw attention to environmental factors that have been shown to be harmful to mental health, and to suggest ways in which these might be modified, primarily by political action.

BIBLIOGRAPHY

Blazer, D. *et al.* (1985). Psychiatric disorders: a rural/urban comparison. *Archives of General Psychiatry, 42,* 651–656.

Dubos, R. (1972). *A God within.* London: Scribners.

Faris, R. E., & Dunham, H. W. (1939). *Mental disorders in urban areas.* Chicago: Hafner.

Freeman, H. L. (1984). *Mental health and the environment.* London: Churchill Livingstone.

Fried, M. (1963). Grieving for a lost home. In L. J. Duhl (Ed.), *The urban condition.* New York: Basic Books.

Gove, W. R., Hughes, M., & Galle, O. R. (1979). Overcrowding in the home—An empirical investigation of its possible pathological consequences. *American Sociological Review, 44,* 59–80.

Halpern, D. (1995). Mental health and the built environment. London: Taylor & Francis.

Jacobs, J. (1961). *The death and life of great American cities.* New York: Random House.

Newman, O. (1980). *Community of interest.* New York: Anchor.

Rutter, M., Yule, B., Quinton, D., Rowlands, O., Yule, W., & Berger, M. (1975). Attainment and adjustment in two geographical areas, II. *British Journal of Psychiatry, 126,* 520–533.

Heart Disease: Psychological Predictors

Howard S. Friedman

University of California, Riverside

Coronary Heart Disease Blockage and hardening of the coronary arteries which supply the heart, due to build-up of fatty plaques on the artery wall.

Fight or Flight Response The body's physiological response to significant challenge, involving activation of the sympathetic nervous system and the release of stress hormones.

Self-Healing Personality A psychosocial reaction pattern that leads to good physical health, characterized by an enthusiastic, positive emotional style, an alert, energetic motivation, and secure, constructive interpersonal relations.

Social Support Emotional, informational, or tangible resources provided by family or friends.

Type A Behavior Pattern An emotional and behavioral style characterized by a chronic, aggressive struggle to accomplish more and more in the shortest possible time period.

There is substantial evidence that psychological factors predict **HEART DISEASE** and premature mortality. What is less clear are the causal pathways and causal mechanisms. Many people assume that stressful pat-terns of psychological reaction and associated unhealthy habits can increase the likelihood of heart disease—a blockage (occlusion) of a coronary artery or an irregular heartbeat (arrhythmia). There is relatively little surprise among observers when a heart attack victim is a hard-working 50-year-old obese businessman who is known for chain-smoking cigarettes and compulsively devouring doughnuts while screaming into two telephones that he wants that shipment "YESTERDAY." The scientific difficulty comes in separating fact from stereotype—that is, in discerning which if any behavioral patterns are solid predictors of increased likelihood of heart disease.

There are three basic kinds of relations between psychology and heart disease. First, psychological factors can play a direct causal role in increasing the likelihood of disease. That is, physiological stress reactions and unhealthy habits can dramatically increase one's risk. Second, underlying (third) variables like genetic abnormalities can produce both distinctive psychological profiles and elevated disease risk. In such cases, psychological patterns are associated with disease but interventions to affect the psychological factors may or may not have any effect on the likelihood of disease; the relation may be spurious. Third, psychological correlates of disease may be the result of the disease process. For example, depression may follow a heart attack. In such cases, psychological interventions obviously will not affect health risk unless the factors are also tied through other pathways. All of these three sorts of ties between psychological factors and heart disease have been shown to exist, thus making simple explanation and simple amelioration problematic. Nevertheless, much is known about healthier and unhealthier psychosocial living patterns.

I. HISTORICAL PERSPECTIVE

Psychological predictors of heart disease have been noted since ancient times. There are biblical proverbs on this matter, such as "Gladness of the heart is the life of a man, and the joy of a man prolongs his days" (Apoc. 30:22). The ancient Greeks were especially keen observers of the relations between psychological factors and illness. They were good at describing nature, but not so good at causal mechanisms. Their idea of essential bodily fluids or "humors" was intriguing but of course erroneous. The four bodily humors—black bile (or melancholy), blood, yellow bile (or choler), and phlegm—were said to lead to proneness to depression and degenerative disease, or to a sanguine and ruddy disposition, or an angry (choleric), bitter and unhealthy persona, or to a phlegmatic, cold, apathy. As this humoral explanation of physiology was found to be incorrect, it was gradually discarded over the centuries. Unfortunately, so too was the scheme of the four emotional aspects of personality that so influenced medical practice for 2000 years. Hostility, cheerfulness, depression, and apathy are indeed useful patterns for understanding psychology and health. The ancient Greeks had correctly observed psychosocial correlates of disease but their causal mechanisms were wrong.

In the first half of the 20th century, there was again considerable interest in the psychological predictors of heart disease. The influential medical educator Sir William Osler proposed a link between high-pressure activity and coronary heart disease; and the well-known psychiatrists Karl and William Menninger asserted that heart disease is related to repressed aggression. Psychosomatic theorists developed and applied the psychoanalytic notions of Sigmund Freud to their patients, looking for repressed conflict as a cause of chest pain and heart disease. Psychological treatments often proved helpful. These physicians were all trying to account for the dramatic rise in coronary heart disease that was occurring in the 20th century. Since the 20th century was also a time of rapid social and technological change, it made sense to look for explanations in the pressure and demands of modern-day

life. However, most of this work was clinical and speculative. It was not until the 1950s that the idea of a Type A person was proposed and led to substantial controlled empirical research.

The Type A behavior pattern was proposed by two cardiologists—Ray Rosenman and Meyer Friedman—who noticed that their patients possessed a distinctive constellation of psychological characteristics. Since traditional risk factors like high blood pressure hardly did a complete job in accounting for heart disease risk, the cardiologists began a systematic search for psychosocial and behavioral predictors of heart disease. These efforts led to three decades of intensive research, upon which our current understanding rests. [See TYPE A–TYPE B PERSONALITIES.]

Current research indicates that certain people are psychologically vulnerable or resilient due to a combination of temperament and early socialization. When vulnerable people encounter psychosocial environments that are a poor match for their needs, chronic negative emotional patterns often result. These reactions are accompanied by physiological disturbance—high levels of sympathetic activation and cortisol, and possibly other hormones. And, unhealthy behaviors such as substance abuse may also occur. Finally, these disturbances interact with disease-proneness caused by heredity (e.g., proneness to the build-up of plaque in the coronary arteries) and environment (e.g., high fat diets). The resulting increased risk of illness is comparable in size to that of many other commonly noted health risks.

II. DISEASE-PRONE PERSONALITIES

There is strong reason to believe that stress, chronic negative emotions, and poor social relations can play a role in the development or triggering of cardiovascular disease and heart attacks, and in impairing postsurgical recovery. The evidence is as strong as or stronger than the findings usually trumpeted about concerning the effects of diet, environmental pollution, body weight, exercise, and similar health factors. Unfortunately, this psychosocial evidence often goes mostly unnoticed by a biomedically oriented health care system. For an acute, life-threatening illness like a heart attack, doctors in their super-high-tech medical centers often work miracles. Yet there is a hefty percentage of the population heading for expensive and dangerous coronary bypass operations (or the newest high-tech equivalent), while psychosocial preventive measures are sometimes ignored.

Originally (in the 1960s and 1970s), research on the Type A behavior pattern focused on individuals who are aggressively involved in chronic struggle to quickly achieve more and more in less and less time. But many active, expressive people often tend to work hard and hurry around like Type A people but are not at all coronary-prone; on the contrary, they are especially healthy! In addition, many so-called "Type B" people (supposedly stress-free) are not really calm and healthy, even though they look superficially like Type B's; rather their emotional conflicts are repressed. The Type A concept has therefore been deemed inadequate to capture the richness of individual differences in emotional response. It often is too imprecise to predict heart disease. Rather than being "wrong," the Type A construct has inspired research that has led to its being surpassed and encompassed. Subsequent research suggests that hurrying around or working hard is not necessarily unhealthy. Rather, hostility and aggressive or cynical struggle seem predictive of disease.

Use of the statistical technique called meta-analysis (which is a sophisticated kind of statistical average, across different studies) has allowed investigators to address the broad issue of psychological predictors of heart disease and to help us look at how big an effect is; it also points us toward specific patterns of findings, rather than just vague general impressions. The degree of consistency in the overall findings is remarkable. Results consistently indicate significant relations between chronic emotional disturbance—namely, hostility and depression—and coronary heart disease. These associations are similar in size to those of other risk factors such as diet and lack of exercise.

III. SOCIAL INTEGRATION

A variety of sociological and epidemiological investigations indicate that people who are well-integrated into a stable community are less likely to develop heart disease or die prematurely. It appears that when faced with life change and the stress experienced as a result of it, the support of family and friends can significantly aid one's coping. (Social support comes from the friendly ties an individual has with family, associates, neighbors, and the community.) Conversely, the sudden loss of social ties seems to have a dramatically negative effect. Community studies have consistently shown effects of social ties on cardiovascular health—people with fewer community ties are more likely to become ill and die. [*See* COPING WITH STRESS; SOCIAL SUPPORT.]

How does social support work? First of all, social support can sometimes influence an individual's coping by affecting how stressful events are appraised. For example, if one knows other people who have gone through the same challenging experience, the experience may be seen as less stressful. More importantly, social support may help one deal with the emotional consequences of stress. (Not surprisingly, this is termed emotional social support.) Social support can also help the stressed individual develop new coping strategies by providing information about how to deal with the stress. This informational support often goes hand in hand with emotional support, but sometimes it comes alone in the form of written materials about how to deal with the challenge. Finally, social support may also operate by providing tangible resources. This is called instrumental support. Instrumental support might sometimes be harmful if it makes the recipient feel inadequate, indebted, or unduly manipulated. Social support is especially important when a person faces a severe challenge such as the challenge of chronic cardiovascular illness.

Social integration may also protect against heart disease by providing an opportunity for self-disclosure. Scattered lines of evidence suggest that it is healthy to be able to discuss one's feelings and self-image with at least one intimate friend or companion. The degree of importance and the generality of this phenomenon are not yet known.

Hostile and cynical people are likely to have interpersonal disputes, due to their suspicious, competitive, irritating style. This may lead to poor health in three ways: by interfering with social support, by exacerbating any tendencies toward physiological hyperreactivity, and by placing the individual into more stressful situations—an onslaught of major and minor hassles. In short, although there is good evidence that people who live in stable families and in stable communities are more protected from heart disease, it is not yet well understood how these factors are related to the other relevant psychosocial influences on health.

IV. CAUSAL MECHANISMS

Efforts to identify a coronary-prone personality or a coronary-prone behavior pattern focus on two sorts of mechanisms or pathways through which psychological factors can help bring about disease. These are nervous system and hormonal mechanisms, and behavioral mechanisms.

A. Psychophysiological Mechanisms (Nervous System and Hormonal)

Most often implicated are physiological disturbances involving high sympathetic (and sometimes parasympathetic) activation. This activation is commonly summarized as the "fight or flight" response—the immediate internal bodily response to danger. However, some people are quite frequently in this state of agitation. The links to sudden death via autonomic nervous system-induced arrhythmias of the heart are documented: when psychological stress, such as seeing a shocking scene of mutilation, or when physical stress such as shoveling heavy snow becomes too great, the heart may beat uncontrollably and irregularly and soon fail. But such fatal events are relatively rare, especially as compared to chronic but slow artery obstruction. It is also the case that such irregular, fatal heartbeats are much more probable when there is partial pre-existing heart disease.

The links to atherosclerotic disease—the major type of heart disease in which fatty plaques build up on the arteries that supply the heart with blood—are necessarily more problematic. Sympathetic nervous system arousal has numerous effects, including increased physical stress on the arteries and changes in lipid (fat) metabolism. It appears that both the physical stress of high blood pressure and the metabolic effects on blood lipids (fats) promote plaque formation.

Experimental studies demonstrate that social stress promotes atherosclerosis among monkeys straining to maintain a position of social dominance. When the composition of monkey groups is changed by the experimenter, those monkeys struggling for dominance face ill health. Further, those animals with the greatest heart-rate reactivity show the most coronary artery

damage and act more aggressively, again suggesting the relevance of the "fight or flight" physiological response. These experiments confirm clinical studies of humans regarding aggressiveness and struggle. Since this artery damage in monkeys can be prevented by a beta-blocker (Propanolol), the evidence again points to harmful effects of excessive activation of the sympathetic nervous system, by social struggle. Everything else being equal, the modulation of sympathetic arousal is likely to promote physical health, in both monkeys and people.

Less well understood are hormonal effects. Both nervous system arousal and other forms of psychophysiological imbalance such as depression alter the usual complement of bodily hormones. For example, stress, helplessness, and depression are linked to high cortisol levels; and stress, anger, and frustration are linked to high levels of catecholamines (such as of norepinephrine). Increasing attention is turning to the possible links between such matters and heart disease. Other stress-related or stress-influenced hormones such as thyroxin, testosterone, and other hormones have also been shown to play a significant role in stress-related homeostasis and physical health. No study has yet followed the whole process, showing for example that hostile people develop certain psychophysiological disturbances that impair metabolism and thereby bring on heart disease. [*See* PSYCHONEUROIMMUNOLOGY.]

There is weak but accumulating evidence that the repression of thoughts or feelings, partly genetically based, is a form of stress that is accompanied by detrimental psychophysiological arousal similar to that of the other disease-prone states. Speculation has centered on chronic autonomic arousal. Ongoing research will shed light on the complex issues of emotional self-regulation; it is unlikely that a simple hydraulic model of "bottling-up" versus emotional "discharge" will prove relevant. Indeed, the issue of whether to repress or express negative emotion may be somewhat of a red herring; the problem seems to arise from having the chronic imbalance in the first place.

B. Behavioral Mechanisms

Personality-based behavioral patterns likely have an independent effect as well as interacting with stress-related psychophysiological influences on cardiac health. For example, a major problem in medical care is the patient's failure to cooperate with treatment. A host of individual and psychosocial characteristics affect whether a patient will take medication, follow a low-fat diet, return for follow-up, and so on. The patient's sense of self-efficacy and confidence that success is achievable is one dimension often found to relate to healthy behavior. Relatedly, failure to take prophylactic measures may be associated with sensation-seeking, low conscientiousness, hostility, low self-esteem, or other traits. Tendencies toward denial or excessive optimism may result in a deadly delay in seeking treatment. [See SELF-EFFICACY; SELF-ESTEEM.]

Regarding substance abuse, there is evidence that hostile and neurotic people are more likely to smoke, drink to excess, and/or use drugs, thereby increasing their risk of heart disease. There is also evidence that people low in ego strength, that is, low on conscientiousness, are similarly at risk. Surprisingly, there is very little prospective study of such potentially important relations of personality, unhealthy behavior patterns, and subsequent health. [See SUBSTANCE ABUSE.]

Depression (and possibly repression) is clearly associated with a whole host of behavioral risk factors for disease including disturbances in eating and sleeping, impaired social relations, as well as substance abuses. Here again, however, little is known of the causal pathways. Prospective clinical studies of depression and of substance abuse could prove especially informative if they also included psychophysiological measurement, general assessment of health behaviors, and heart disease outcomes. [See DEPRESSION.]

V. NONCAUSAL EFFECTS

Some of the association between psychological variables and heart disease is due to noncausal pathways. The development of heart disease can produce dramatic psychological and social changes in the patient's life. Heart attack victims (who survive) may become angry at the world for their plight. Or they may become depressed about the new limitations on their activities. They may lose their job or may be treated differently by their employers or their colleagues. Sexual relations with one's partner may change, as fear, fatigue, or resentment enters the relationship. In all of these cases, psychological and behavioral patterns are a result rather than a cause or predictor of heart disease. (Nevertheless, these factors or patterns may

then predict or contribute to further deterioration, through the causal mechanisms described above.) Interestingly, some disease predictors may act differently following a heart attack. For example, anxiety that contributes to the development of disease may prove helpful after the attack if it leads the patient to cooperate more fully with medical treatment. We should not expect the same factors to predict disease and recovery from disease, although this error of inference is often made.

Spurious relations between psychological variables and heart disease may result from underlying third variables that produce both the psychological characteristics and the disease. For example, men are less likely to be nurturant than are women, and men are more likely to die prematurely from heart disease; but it is not likely that nurturance is a key causal factor. Similarly, various genetic patterns affect both personality and health, but interventions to change these aspects of personality would not necessarily lead to improvements in health.

A final type of noncausal association between psychological variables and heart disease results from methodological artifacts. A common artifact here is a selection artifact or bias. For example, consider the case of neuroticism, angina, and angiography. Neurotics are more likely (than nonneurotics) to persistently seek out medical care, even when there is little or no discernible organic disease. When such patients are referred by their cardiologists for angiography (a picture of their coronary arteries), an interesting relation emerges. Neuroticism is found to be inversely related to arterial blockage, since only the neurotics (with clean arteries) and nonneurotics (with true blockage-caused pain) are in the sample. This artifact might obscure a true causal relation between neuroticism and the development of disease, and so such artifact-laden studies should not be undertaken. Analogously and more simply, a high percentage of cardiology patients may be found to be neurotic; the explanation is a selection artifact.

VI. SELF-HEALING PERSONALITIES

In the field of medicine, it is too often assumed that health is simply the absence of disease. In medicine, a negative test result is good news—it means the disease is not there. But little attention is paid to the positive, proactive elements of good health. In fact the word "health" itself is often corrupted. To speak about people who stay healthy and resist disease, the awkward term "wellness" must be used. However, despite a few polite nods toward behavioral science, most medical students do not take serious courses on wellness after their pathology course. This problem is not the fault of individual health care providers, but rather is a systemic flaw. That is, the medical care system is designed mostly to fix illness problems, not to prevent health problems. What is a healthy psychological pattern?

Briefly stated, a good way to characterize the self-healing personality is in terms of enthusiasm. The word enthusiasm literally means "having a godly spirit within." Enthusiastic people are alert, responsive, and energetic although they may also be calm and self-assured. They are curious, secure, and constructive. There are several good clues that indicate emotional balance and an inherent resilience. Enthusiastic, sanguine people tend to infect others with their exuberance. They are not ecstatic but rather are generally responsive and content. They are people one likes to be around. They are not downcast or shifty-eyed. They smile naturally—the eyes, eyebrows, and mouth are synchronized and unforced; there is usually no holding back of expression of pleasant feelings. Such enthusiastic people have smooth gestures, that tend to move away from the body; they are less likely to pick, scratch, and touch their bodies. They are not apt to make aggressive gestures with their hands. Emotionally balanced individuals not only walk smoothly, they talk smoothly. They are inclined to show fewer speech disturbances such as saying "ah," and their speech is modulated rather than full of sudden loud words. Their voices are less likely to change their tone under stress. Obviously, there are exceptions to these rules: A single nonverbal gesture does not tell us much. Still, lab research has shown how valid information can be gathered about a person's healthy emotional style from just a few episodes of social interaction.

A sense of continual growth and resilience is also relevant. Dr. Walter Cannon, who developed the ideas of homeostasis upon which modern notions of self-healing are built, emphasized that the body has developed a margin of safety. By this Cannon meant that the body has allowance for contingencies, that we may count on in times of stress. The lungs, the blood,

and the muscles have much greater capacity than is ordinarily needed. In other words, the body naturally prepares itself for the rare "extra" challenge, and self-healing people do what they can to increase these margins of safety. William James, who anticipated much of our modern scientific understanding of emotional responses, summed up this idea succinctly when he advised, "Keep the faculty of effort alive in you by a little gratuitous exercise every day. That is, be systematically ascetic or heroic in little unnecessary points, do every day or two something for no other reason than that you would rather not do it, so that when the hour of dire need draws nigh, it may find you not unnerved and untrained to stand the test" (*Principles of Psychology*, 1890, Chapt. 4).

Self-healing personalities have often been described by existential and humanistic psychologists, although they usually thought they were describing only mental health, not physical health. For example, Abraham Maslow pointed out that healthy people first need to achieve balance in their basic biological needs, and then affection and self-respect. But he emphasized what he called self-actualization—the realization of personal growth and fulfillment. People with this growth orientation are spontaneous and creative, are good problem-solvers, have close relationships to others, and have a playful sense of humor. They become more concerned with issues of beauty, justice, and understanding. They develop a sense of humor that is philosophical rather than hostile. They become more ethical and more concerned with the harmony among members of the human race. These characteristics of the self-healing personality are not merely the opposite of such disease-prone characteristics as suspiciousness, bitter cynicism, despair and depression, or repressed conflicts, but are positive, meaningful motives in their own right. Similarly, Viktor Frankl, the existential philosopher and therapist who developed his theories of a healing personality as an inmate in a Nazi concentration camp, noted that survival was more likely for those who tried living in a meaningful way, even in dire straits.

Like much of social and behavioral science, psychosocial prescriptions for good cardiovascular health often sound like "common sense," until the matter is examined more closely. In actual fact, it is very difficult to walk the fine line between narrow-minded biomedical views of the nature of health that exclude psychosocial factors, and the unscientific touchy-feely health gurus who proclaim oversimplified and overgeneralized prescriptions for good health.

VII. INTERVENTIONS

In the practice of medicine, and to a lesser extent in the practice of public health, the relevant question that always jumps to the forefront is "What psychosocial interventions can be made to reverse, prevent, or stop the progression of heart disease?" Given that cardiovascular disease is by far the greatest cause of premature mortality, and given that the social and economic costs of heart disease are overwhelming for both families and society, what can be done? Unfortunately, various sorts of unsubstantiated advice are often given based on scanty evidence. Since the various elements of a self-healing (or a disease-prone) personality are usually intercorrelated, teasing out the causal pathways is a major challenge, one that has been given relatively little research attention or funding.

There is good evidence that lifestyle changes affect the incidence of heart disease. Most of this evidence is epidemiological and anthropological, showing that when people move from one country or one cultural group to another, their heart disease rate can change dramatically. There is also some experimental evidence indicating that dramatic lifestyle changes can improve aspects or correlates of cardiovascular health. A serious problem with this work is that little is known about which components of the healthy, self-healing lifestyle are the necessary causal elements.

For example, consider Japanese immigrants entering America. They leave a close-knit, well-ordered society with an Asian diet and Asian recreation patterns, and they (or their children) enter an individualistic, heterogenous American society with very different social and recreational patterns and a hamburger stand on every corner. If heart disease rates rise, what is to blame? We simply do not know. Nutritionists may point to fish oils or fat intake; religionists may point to meditation patterns; sociologists may point to family structure; psychologists may point to stress reactions. There is evidence that some or all of these points may be valid.

What about specific recommendations that are of-ten heard regarding individuals at risk for an initial or recurrent heart attack? For example, is it really healthy to retire and get away from the stresses of the workplace? In fact, retiring may be very stressful and unhealthy, or it may be helpful. It all depends upon the particular individual and the particular situation. Retiring has been shown to be unhealthy if it results in a diminution of social ties, inadequate financial resources, and psychological states of uselessness or boredom. On the other hand, retirement may be healthy if it reduces the psychosocial stress of the workplace and increases opportunities for healthy habits. In addition, changing societal reactions to retirement can be extremely important—in terms of social security programs, health insurance, laws that prohibit age discrimination, opportunities for educational and social activities, and so on.

Can heart disease be reversed by meditation? Meditation is now being used in several popular programs, in combination with diet and exercise to reduce stress. This is sometimes even covered by medical insurance. Is stress a risk factor for heart disease? Yes. Has it been shown through controlled study that increasing the incidence of meditation is key to reducing the incidence of heart disease? No. Meditation is wonderful for some people, but others may find it stressful or silly. And, there is no good evidence that meditation is superior to other forms of systematic relaxation.

Is it healthy to be optimistic and look on the bright side? Although it seems to be the case that a sense of willpower and positive hopes for the future can help us through difficulty, it is also the case that optimism can lead us to be shocked by reality or to avoid taking necessary prophylactic measures. It makes sense, as has been found, that for a heart disease surgical patient, optimism is helpful. It does not, however, make sense to assume that optimism will prove helpful to a chain smoker or an ice cream addict. The emphasis on optimism without sufficient regard to context is an example of the search for the psychosocial equivalent of a "miracle drug" that can cure all disease.

Are societal pressures encouraging jogging the key to protecting one's heart? It is very clear that a cigarette-smoking obese person who cannot walk up a flight of stairs is at markedly increased risk of heart disease; and this often has led to the incorrect belief that being in shape means the ability to run 6 miles each morning. In actual fact, the benefits of aerobic exercise rapidly reach an asymptote. A brisk walk or swim for 30 minutes every other day seems to do it. People struggling miserably each morning to get "in shape" may be harming their health.

Is it unhealthy to work long hours? In actual fact there is no evidence at all that it is unhealthy to be a "workaholic" if all the other elements of self-healing are in place. That is, hard work and long hours themselves have never been shown to be a risk factor. On the contrary for example, many powerful or influential executives, leaders, artists, and scientists work exceedingly long hours and live long and healthy lives. This is an illustration of where an overgeneralized stereotype of Type A behavior leads to an inaccurate conclusion about behavior and health.

Is all this information common sense? Do physicians and others commonly accept that psychoemotional reactions can affect cardiovascular health and recovery? Not at all. There are regularly major reports published which break the "news" that some medical researchers are now urging that psychological and emotional reactions of patients be taken into account. Such considerations generally still lie outside the traditional medical model of disease that focuses primarily on pharmaceuticals and surgery.

VIII. CONCLUSION

Contrary to some common conceptions, most of the past increase in adult life expectancy in the developed countries has come not from high technology medicine but rather from infection control techniques, low-cost inoculations, improved sanitation, nutrition, and other public health improvements. Antibiotics have also made a significant difference, but visits to super-specialized cardiologists at university hospitals produce limited impact overall when the big picture is considered. This is not to say that a heart disease patient would not be wise to seek out such a specialist, but only that the overall public health benefit of such high-cost cardiology care is relatively small. However,

there is reason to suspect that dramatic (and low-cost) improvements can be realized if we put our knowledge of self-healing to good use. Societal and lifestyle changes may be the psychosocial equivalents of improved sanitation, nutrition, and infection control.

The scientific evidence for self-healing—prevention of and recovery from heart disease—is much stronger than many skeptical doctors imagine, but different from what many health gurus proclaim. Individuals who learn their own psychosocial needs and develop appropriate techniques of self-regulation can maximize their potential for good health. And these psychological styles can be significantly complemented by societal structures that promote healthy reaction patterns and behaviors.

This article has been reprinted from the *Encyclopedia of Human Behavior, Volume 3,* "Psychological Predictors of Heart Disease."

BIBLIOGRAPHY

Friedman, H. S. (Ed.) (1990). "Personality and Disease." Wiley, New York.

Friedman, H. S. (1991). "The Self-Healing Personality: Why Some People Achieve Health and Others Succumb to Illness." Henry Holt, New York.

Friedman, H. S. (Ed.) (1992). "Hostility, Coping & Health." American Psychological Association, Washington, DC.

Houston, B. K., and Snyder, C. R. (Eds.) (1988). "Type A Behavior Pattern: Research, Theory, and Intervention." Wiley, New York.

Matthews, K. A., *et al.* (Eds.) (1986). "Handbook of Stress, Reactivity, and Cardiovascular Disease." Wiley, New York.

Miller, T. Q., Turner, C. W., Tindale, R. S., Posavac, E. J., and Dugoni, B. L. (1991). Reasons for the trend toward null findings in research on Type A behavior. *Psychol. Bull.* **110**(3), 469–485.

Sarason, B. R., Sarason, I. G., and Pierce, G. R. (Eds.) (1990). "Social Support: An Interactional View." Wiley, New York.

Schneiderman, N., McCabe, P., and Baum, A. (Eds.) (1992). "Stress and Disease Processes." Erlbaum, Hillsdale, NJ.

Schneiderman, N., Weiss, S. M., and Kaufmann, P. G. (Eds.) (1989). "Handbook of Research Methods in Cardiovascular Behavioral Medicine." Plenum, New York.

Siegler, I. C., Peterson, B. L., Barefoot, J. C., and Williams, R. B. (1992). Hostility during late adolescence predicts coronary risk factors at mid-life. *Am. J. Epidemiol.* **136**(2), 146–154.

HIV/AIDS

Lydia R. Temoshok

Division of Mental Health, World Health Organization

AIDS The abbreviation for the Acquired Immuno-deficiency Syndrome, refers to the late stages of infection with the human immunodeficiency virus (HIV), when a person's severely deteriorated immune system can no longer fight off various opportunistic infections and cancers. In 1981, the first cases of AIDS were recognized in New York and California among homosexual men, where it spread rapidly within this population. In the first decade of the U.S. AIDS epidemic, the main AIDS-defining clinical conditions were the opportunistic infection *Pneumocystis carinii* pneumonia (PCP, a protozoan organism normally well contained in the body), Kaposi's Sarcoma (a skin cancer that forms large bluish or brownish discolored blotches on the skin, frequently on the legs, but also on other parts of the body, including the lungs and internal digestive organs), and lymphomas (cancers that affect lymphoid tissue, found mostly in the lymph nodes and spleen, but that can affect other organs such as the brain). Another important indicator condition for AIDS diagnosis is HIV encephalopathy or "AIDS dementia," involving disabling cognitive and/or motor dysfunction that interferes with work or activities of daily living. Effective in 1993, the U.S. Centers for

Disease Control and Prevention (CDC) expanded the definition of AIDS to include pulmonary tuberculosis (TB), recurrent pneumonia, invasive cervical cancer, and an HIV-infected person with a very low count of helper (CD4+) T-lymphocytes. In other parts of the world, particularly countries in sub-Saharan Africa, TB is the most common AIDS-related condition. Particularly in developing countries, AIDS is characterized by various combinations of symptoms and diseases such as diarrhea, fever, wasting ("slim disease"), and failure to thrive among children.

Asymptomatic HIV Infection After initial ("acute") infection with HIV, which is characterized by a syndrome much like the flu or mononucleosis and lasts 3 to 14 days, the virus retreats from the blood into the immune cells. During this stage of HIV infection, which is sometimes called the "incubation period," the person appears healthy and feels well, but is infectious and can still transmit the virus to others. This stage can last up to 10 years or longer, and gradually ends with the development of HIV-related symptoms, such as herpes zoster ("shingles," a localized blistering rash caused by the chicken-pox virus), candidiasis ("thrush," a fungal infection of the mouth causing white plaque to form), or persistent generalized adenopathy (PGL, or enlarged lymph nodes in the armpits, neck, groin, or collar-bone area).

Helper (CD4+) T-lymphocyte This important regulatory immune cell directs both antibody and cell-mediated immune responses, much like a conductor leading a symphony orchestra. The helper T-cell is the primary target for HIV infection, which partly explains how HIV can cause such massive dysregulation of the immune system. The virus has an affinity for the CD4 surface marker or receptor site, which allows the virus to attach to, and enter the cell. The CD4+ T-lymphocyte coordinates a number of important immunologic functions. Loss of these functions results in progressive impairment of the body's immune response and disease-fighting capacities. As the number of these lymphocytes decreases, the risk and severity of opportunistic illnesses increase.

HIV Human immunodeficiency virus was first isolated and identified as the causal agent of AIDS in 1983. There are two main types of the virus, HIV-1 which is the most common, and HIV-2, found especially in West Africa, but also in Angola and Mozambique. Although both types are transmitted by the same means (sexually, perinatally, and parenterally), the likelihood of transmission of HIV-1 through heterosexual intercourse appears to be about 3 times higher per exposure than for HIV-2. In addition, perinatal transmission rates of HIV-2 are significantly lower: less than 4% for HIV-2 compared with 25 to 35% for HIV-1. The development of symptoms and progression to AIDS is much slower in people infected with HIV-2. There exist at least 10 genetic subtypes of HIV-1, but their biological and epidemiological significance is currently not well understood.

HIV Testing Serologic (blood) tests for HIV have been commercially available since 1985. The most commonly used test is the ELISA (enzyme-linked immunosorbent assay), which does not detect the actual presence of HIV, but rather antibodies produced by the immune system in reaction to HIV exposure. When these antibodies are detectable, the person is said to have "seroconverted." Although the ELISA is relatively sensitive as an initial screening test (i.e., it fails to identify very few of those with antibodies to HIV), it is not very specific. To reduce the false positive rate (which is higher in populations with low HIV prevalence), positive ELISA tests require confirmation by another method, usually the Western blot test. Because it takes from 4 to 12 weeks for HIV antibodies to form after exposure to the virus, people in this "window period" may test negative on the ELISA, even though they are infected with HIV. To be reasonably sure that a person is free of the virus, a second serologic test must be negative following a 6-month period of abstinence from sexual or drug use behaviors where exposure to HIV could occur. In 1995, home access rapid HIV testing, as an alternative to conventional testing in anonymous testing sites or medical laboratories, was approved by the U.S. Food and Drug Administration.

IDU Injection drug use, the use of needles and syringes to inject drugs intravenously or subcutaneously, is the main route for parenteral transmission of HIV. "IDU" also refers to "injection drug user."

Perinatal Transmission The "vertical" transmission of HIV from an infected woman to her fetus or newborn child can occur during the perinatal period—before, during or shortly after the time of birth.

PLWHA Persons Living With HIV or AIDS, include people who are HIV-infected ("HIV seropositive," "HIV-positive," or "HIV+"), whether they are asymptomatic, symptomatic, or have developed AIDS-related conditions. This term is considered preferable to other possible designations such as "AIDS patients," "sufferers," or "victims."

Sexual Transmission There is a great deal of epidemiological and clinical evidence that sexual transmission of HIV can occur most efficiently through insertive penile-anal sex; that is, from an infected man inserting his penis in the anus or rectum of an uninfected sexual partner, whether male or female. There is also risk of sexual transmission, albeit substantially lower, when the infected man is the recipient of anal sex. It has been estimated that the probability of HIV transmission during penile–vaginal sex is significantly greater when the man rather than the woman is the infected partner. The likelihood of a women infecting a man during penile–vaginal sex is increased when either partner has another STD, particularly syphilis or genital ulcer disease (which disrupts the mucosal integrity). Studies of serodiscordant couples (where one person is HIV-infected and the other is not) have shown that correct and consistent use of condoms during sexual intercourse can greatly reduce the risk of transmission. Condoms are more likely to tear, slip, or break during anal sex (because there is no natural lubrication), particularly for the inexperienced user. Therefore, the best way to protect against the high risk of transmission during anal sex is to engage in nonpenetrative practices only (e.g., manual sex or masturbation), or to reduce risk by always using condoms for penile–vaginal sex. Transmission risk for orogenital sex (stimulating the genitals with the mouth or tongue) between two women appears to be negligible. There is, however, some degree of risk for transmitting HIV during orogenital sex when this involves an infected man who ejaculates into the mouth of an uninfected partner. Recent studies suggest that the risk of orogenital sex has been underestimated (i.e., it cannot be considered "safe"); however, it is still substantially less risky than penile–anal or penile–vaginal sex.

STD Sexually transmitted disease refers to all infections that are transmitted mainly through sexual contact, during unprotected vaginal or anal intercourse. STDs include HIV/AIDS, gonorrhea ("clap" or "drip"), syphilis, Chlamydia, hepatitis B, genital herpes, trichomoniasis ("Trich"), and chancroid.

The impact of the **HIV/AIDS** pandemic has been demographic, economic, social, and political, as well as medical, and presents daunting challenges to public health, biomedical, and behavioral sciences. It can be argued that effective methods of HIV prevention and intervention can best be developed and implemented from a biopsychosocial perspective that takes into account the complex interactions across biological, psychological, and social dimensions or levels.

I. EPIDEMIOLOGY

Epidemiology is the science of the natural history of diseases, including the frequency of a disease in a given population ("prevalence"), its geographic distribution, and the characteristics of the individual, the population, or the environment that affect its course and the number of new infections within a given time period ("incidence"). Epidemiologists try to determine whether there has been an increase or a decrease of a disease over the years; whether the frequency of a disease in one geographical area is higher than that in another, and whether various characteristics (e.g., sociodemographic factors, age, gender, or behaviors) of persons with a particular disease distinguish them from others who do not have that disease.

The worldwide epidemiological dimensions of HIV/AIDS defy the imagination: the World Health Organization (WHO) and the United Nations Joint Program on AIDS (UNAIDS, the U.N. agency responsible for coordinating international action against HIV/AIDS) estimate that in 1997, there are over 30 million people worldwide currently living with HIV, including 1.1 million children. Ninety percent of these people live in developing countries. The cumulative number of cases of HIV infection in the world since the beginning of the pandemic (worldwide epidemic) is estimated to be 29.4 million, including 15.5 million men, 11.3 million women, and 2.6 million children. It is estimated that around 8500 new HIV infections occur every day. By the year 2000, up to 40 million people are expected to be infected.

There are vast geographic differences in the worldwide epidemiology of HIV/AIDS. It is believed that the epidemic has been developing longest in the sub-Saharan Africa, where the general population prevalence is 5.6% but is much higher in urban areas, and in certain countries. According to UNAIDS, an estimated 17% of the adult population in Zimbabwe and Zambia, and 13% in Malawi are thought to be HIV-infected. Because the principal mode of infection in Africa is heterosexual, women and men have been infected in about equal numbers. Due to inadequate HIV antibody testing of blood donations in most countries in the region, blood transfusions continue to play a role in the spread of HIV to those most likely to receive transfusions: women of reproductive age and children.

By 1995, more than half of all new infections of HIV worldwide were in Southeast Asia. South and Southeast Asia now have an estimated million adults living with HIV/AIDS (prevalence 0.6%, or more than half a percent of the region's population). Another seriously affected region is the Caribbean (prevalence 1.7%), where the principal mode of infection is also heterosexual.

In contrast, a much lower HIV prevalence of 0.3% is found in North America, Australia, New Zealand, Northern and Western Europe, as well as in parts of South America (prevalence 0.6%), where the main mode of transmission has been through male–male sexual relations and injection drug use (IDU), and then to the heterosexual partners of IDU. Information on HIV infection in North Africa and the Middle East, where the virus was introduced more recently, is sparse. For example, IDU in Djibouti has contributed to relatively high levels of HIV infection there, but for the region, overall, prevalence is estimated to be 0.1%.

The epidemic continues to evolve and change in various parts of the world. The epidemic in Thailand is among the best documented in the world. Nationally, HIV prevalence among IDU rose quickly in 1988 to approximately 35%. HIV among brothel-based sex workers rose from 3.5% in 1989 to 33% by late 1994. Current (1997) figures suggest that the epidemic has reached its peak and is beginning to level off, or even reverse in some population groups such as young men conscripted into the military. However, HIV prevalence in women attending antenatal clinics has continued to rise, along with the numbers of infected infants.

Countries in the world which are experiencing a very rapid increase in numbers of new cases include India (especially Bombay), Cambodia, Vietnam, Myanmar, China, and some Eastern European countries that were former Soviet republics, including Ukraine, Russia, Belarus, and Moldava. Ukraine, for example, which used to be among the countries with the lowest level of AIDS, now has 16,500 HIV+ persons officially registered. These cases probably represent only the tip of the iceberg, perhaps only one-tenth the actual number of cases. The rapid increase of AIDS incidence in Ukraine, as well as in the two Western European countries of Portugal and Spain, is associated with IDU. Based on the explosive increase in several former Soviet republics in the incidence of syphilis and other STDs that typically precede increased HIV incidence, experts predict one million PLWHA in Russia alone by the year 2000.

The prevalence of HIV infection and AIDS also varies considerably within countries. The U.S. cities with the highest prevalence of AIDS cases in 1996, as reported by the Centers for Disease Control and Prevention (CDC), were New York, Miami, Jersey City, N.J., and San Francisco. In the United States, deaths from AIDS began to decline in 1996 for the first time, according to the CDC. AIDS deaths in the United States fell 26% in 1996; and the disease was no longer the leading cause of death for Americans between the ages of 25 and 44, as it had been the previous two years. Every region of the United States, as well as every racial/ethnic group, experienced a significant drop in mortality. Although some experts have attributed this decline to new and improved ways to manage the disease, the drop in mortality occurred before widespread use of the new and effective treatments in the last months of 1996. (see Section III). The changes are more likely attributable to "dynamics of the epidemic"; that is, differences in the introduction and spread of HIV within different segments of the population. This is one explanation for the finding that the

number of AIDS deaths among U.S. women actually rose by 3% between early 1995 and early 1996, while the number of AIDS deaths among men fell sharply: Men who had sex with men tended to be infected early in the epidemic, and thus progressed to AIDS and died sooner than did women, who tended to be infected later in the course of the epidemic through sex partners who were IDU. Early epicenters of the disease were San Francisco, Los Angeles, and New York; it then spread throughout the East Coast, where it began to level off in 1996. Therefore, it is likely that the southeastern U.S. will experience a later peak in AIDS cases and subsequent mortality rates. Other factors, such as differential socioeconomic status and access to health care may also play a role in affecting mortality statistics: the CDC estimates that the rate of progression from HIV infection to AIDS is seven times higher for African Americans and three times higher for Latinos, than it is for Whites.

II. RELATED CONDITIONS

A. Tuberculosis

Because the immune suppression associated with HIV infection increases susceptibility to a large number of diseases, it is not possible to separate completely the impact of HIV from that of these other opportunistic infections. Probably the most significant disease of this nature is tuberculosis (TB). The AIDS and TB epidemics are locked in a vicious spiral of mutual reinforcement: millions of carriers who would otherwise have escaped active TB are now developing the disease because their immune systems are weakened from HIV. There are an estimated 8 million new cases of TB, and 3 million deaths per year, mostly in resource-poor countries. About 9% of global TB cases are attributable to HIV infection; this figure is projected to increase to about 15% by the year 2000. Many countries in South and Southeast Asia, sub-Saharan Africa, and Eastern Europe are reporting annual increases in TB cases in excess of 10%. TB is endemic in sub-Saharan Africa, and for most countries in this region, the majority of adults who have been infected with HIV will harbor latent TB. When HIV-infected persons experience a decline in cell-mediated immunity, their latent TB is reactivated. Many countries have experienced a resurgence of TB, complicated by an increase in the proportion of patients with multidrug-resistant strains. Death rates among HIV+ persons newly infected with drug-resistant TB range from 91 to 100%, with most dying less than 16 weeks after infection. A WHO study released in 1996 reported that TB caused 30% of all deaths among HIV+ persons, worldwide. Because of the lethality of active TB for HIV+ persons, and the potential for rapid spread to others, WHO has strongly advocated a treatment strategy known as Direct Observed Treatment Short-course (DOTS) in which patients are given a full course of drugs under the strict supervision of health workers. The high effectiveness of the DOTS method has suggested that it would be useful to implement such programs in conjunction with TB and HIV testing programs, particularly in countries experiencing great increases in both TB and HIV, so that infected individuals can receive prompt and life-saving therapy, and preventive therapy can be initiated.

1. Implications for Biopsychosocial Interventions

A fundamental issue is the rapid and correct diagnosis of TB in HIV-infected persons. This implies the need for people to be able to recognize the early symptoms of TB, and to seek preventive and therapeutic care. Because of TB's high infectivity, the possibility of infected family members, and levels of TB infection in the community should also be considered. Because a critical failure of many programs has been nonadherence to therapy (which leads to treatment failure, continued TB transmission, and development of lethal, drug-resistant strains), interventions that facilitate adherence would have considerable impact on TB treatment and prevention.

B. Other Sexually Transmitted Diseases (STD)

A major cause of the rapid spread of HIV in poorer countries, particularly in sub-Saharan Africa, are other STD, which facilitate HIV transmission through genital sores and ulcers. UNAIDS estimates that more than 330 million people, worldwide, contract a curable but nevertheless dangerous STD every year. In addition to their impact on HIV, STD have serious health and social consequences themselves, particularly for women and infants, including pelvic inflammatory disease, infertility, ectopic pregnancy, fetal

abnormality and childhood mortality. Failure to diagnose and treat gonorrhoea, chlamydia, and syphilis can cause serious complications of pregnancy such as miscarriage, prematurity, congenital and neonatal infections, and blindness. Unusual courses of syphilis have been reported in HIV-infected individuals, including more frequent ulcerating secondary syphilis. Moreover, syphilis in HIV+ persons progresses much more rapidly to advanced stages, may not respond to conventional treatment, and may progress prematurely to neurosyphilis. A number of studies have documented the negative impact of HIV-related immunodeficiency on the course of genital ulcer disease, on HPV-mediated cervical abnormalities, and cervical cancer. Sexual transmission of Hepatitis C virus (HCV) appears to be enhanced in patients with concomitant HIV infection. Among the most alarming aspects of HCV are its high rate of persistence and its ability to induce chronic liver disease. Coinfection with HCV and HIV may hasten the onset of cirrhosis or liver failure. Several studies have shown that herpes viruses directly activate HIV production, and contribute to HIV progression. Herpes virus (HPV)-associated genital lesions in HIV+ women are of particular concern because they are likely to progress to invasive cervical neoplasia.

1. Implications for Biopsychosocial Interventions

An issue of recent debate concerns the best strategy to treat STD in countries where such diseases are highly prevalent, such as in sub-Saharan Africa. Although mass treatment may have an initial impact, this strategy may lead to antibiotic resistance in the future, particularly if individuals fail to follow the full course of antibiotics. Another approach is syndromic treatment (treatment based on symptoms), which has been shown in randomized trials to reduce the incidence of HIV by about 40% (through reducing viral load in HIV+ persons and therefore reducing the rate of HIV transmission). Several other recent studies have shown that a program of STD treatment, combined with condom promotion, can have dramatic effects on reducing HIV incidence. As several experts have cogently noted, solutions to the STD/HIV problem do not lie exclusively or even largely in the development of biomedical treatments or vaccines; control requires a broad-based approach that goes beyond the medical model to address prevention, and low cost/

low technology approaches to diagnosis, treatment and care. For example, it would be important to assess the availability of simple, affordable, and noninvasive diagnostic and screen tests for STD. Equally critical is the availability of facilities for syndromic treatment and counseling, including adequate provision of condoms and encouragement of partner notification and treatment. An assessment of educational and informational needs would focus on awareness and recognition of STD symptoms for oneself, sexual partners, and family members, as well as on the importance of early identification and treatment of STDs.

C. Diarrhea and Other Constitutional Symptoms

For people with HIV infection, the first symptoms to appear are the "constitutional" symptoms that often accompany chronic illnesses, including weight loss, weakness, diarrhea, fever, and fatigue. Diarrhea, a common infective complication of HIV disease, causes emotional as well as physical distress, has profound negative effects on quality of life, and is responsible for significant morbidity and mortality, especially in developing countries. Malabsorption of carbohydrates, which has been described in HIV-infected persons in the absence of diarrhea, becomes more severe as the disease progresses, particularly in those with protozoal infections. In Zaire, mortality from diarrhea increased elevenfold among HIV-infected children, largely because of increased fatalities associated with persistent diarrhea. A number of studies have suggested that vitamin A supplementation appears to lower the risk for severe infection, reduces the incidence of severe diarrhea, and reduces mortality rates by 23% in children 6 months to 5 years of age.

D. Pain

Pain is a common and debilitating symptom of HIV disease which is gravely underestimated and undertreated. In a recent multicenter study in the United States, from 30% of outpatients to 62% of inpatients reported pain due to HIV disease. Opportunistic infection by cytomegalovirus (CMV) also causes painful neuropathy. Pain severity significantly decreases patients' quality of life. Undertreatment of pain in HIV disease is related to doctors both underestimating pain and underprescribing analgesics. [See PAIN.]

I. Implications for Biopsychosocial Interventions

WHO guidelines for cancer pain relief are useful for categorizing "worst" pain severity reported by patients. Part of the problem in a complex disease such as HIV infection is the subjectivity of pain, where somatic, visceral, and neuropathic pains are often associated with anxiety and depression. Pain assessment in persons with HIV may require development of multi-symptom assessment scales.

E. Psychological and Psychiatric Disturbances

Compared with research on HIV pathogenesis (how HIV causes disease), disease progression, and biomedical interventions, mental health has been a relatively neglected area in HIV research, with some important exceptions. Published studies on stress and psychological functioning in HIV+ persons have been limited (largely to homosexual men in the United States, Europe, and Australia), but have consistently shown the relationship between social support, stressful events, and coping on the one hand, and depressive symptomatology, distress, and poorer health on the other.

The prevalence of psychiatric disorders, other than substance use-related disorders, in PLWHA tends to vary with the population under study. In a recent U.S. study of depression in seropositive compared to seronegative homosexual men, there did not appear to be an overall increase in depressive symptoms in HIV+ men from the time of infection until prior to AIDS. HIV+ homosexual men did report specific depressive symptoms more often, including less hope, more fearfulness, more insomnia, and more anorexia. In community samples, the prevalence of current major depression among HIV+ persons has been estimated to be from 4 to 15%, whereas the prevalence is from 20 to 35% for any current substance use disorder, including chronic alcohol and drug use. Rates of psychiatric distress in inner-city adult HIV clinics in the United States are much higher (e.g., 52% scoring above the screening threshold on standardized self-report measures of global distress and depression) than in the general population or than in other outpatient medical clinics. A comorbid substance use condition was the most powerful and consistent predictor of psychiatric distress, probably reflecting the high lifetime prevalence of these disorders in uninfected homosexual and IDU in the United States or Europe. [*See* DEPRESSION.]

Although many people believe that suicidal behavior is more common in PLWHA, recent epidemiological reviews suggest that suicidal acts are not more frequent in PLWHA, compared with uninfected persons from the same subpopulation (for example, IDU or homosexual men). The prevalence of suicidal acts is higher in PLWHA only if they are compared to the general population. [*See* SUICIDE.]

I. Implications for Biopsychosocial Interventions

The term "HIV spectrum" was coined by the CDC to describe affected populations and the range of symptomatology involved in HIV infection as a pyramid model, with the tip representing those with AIDS—both the smallest population, and those with the most severe symptomatology. The "HIV mental health spectrum" is a parallel model that provides a framework for understanding the mental health consequences associated with the potential range of HIV-affected populations and with increasing HIV symptomatology. At the base of the pyramid are those non-infected individuals who are psychologically and socially affected by this disease, including the so-called "worried well," and those in particularly affected communities. Health care providers are at the next higher level in terms of how directly they are affected by HIV, followed by family members and significant others of PLWHA, and those caring for infected loved ones. At the next level, are the large numbers of individuals whose behaviors and/or situations put them "at risk" of becoming infected with HIV. Increasing degrees of symptomatology that accompany HIV progression describe the next levels, from asymptomatic infection, to those with early manifestations of HIV, and then significant symptoms. At the tip of the pyramid are those with severe AIDS-related infections or cancers, and those dying of AIDS. Each level of the mental health spectrum has different and specific needs for mental health services. Ideally, these services would be offered as part of a comprehensive set of health services, which would integrate biomedical and psychosocial interventions for PLWHA.

F. Neurocognitive Disorder

This refers to a disturbance in function resulting from the presence of a neurocognitive impairment. A neurocognitive (neuropsychological) impairment exists when there is a deficient performance in some area of neurocognitive functioning, including attention/speed of information processing, verbal/language skills, reaction time and other perceptual/motor skills, and memory functions, including learning and recall of information. Three levels of severity of neurocognitive disorder, generally associated with time course considerations, have been widely described in HIV-infected persons: (1) mild neurocognitive disorder; (2) HIV-associated dementia (disabling cognitive impairment, usually accompanied by motor dysfunction and behavioral change); and (3) delirium associated with HIV disease.

There are wide geographic variations in incidence and prevalence of various HIV-related neurological disorders. For example, the most common neurological disorder in asymptomatic HIV+ persons in Africa is isolated herpes zoster (5–10%). Guillain Barre syndrome, Konzo, and other neurological disorders are apparently much more prevalent in parts of Africa than in the United States or Europe. As a group, the major central nervous system (CNS) complications share some of the highest mortality rates among AIDS-defining diseases. Neurological disease adds considerably to the morbidity of HIV infection, interfering with the capacity of infected persons to lead independent and fruitful lives. Thus, the number of individuals worldwide with HIV dementia will continue to increase, posing enormous burdens on health care services, home care providers, and families and communities where individuals who normally provide food and compose the active workforce will be unable to function, or even to care for themselves in the late stages of infection.

There is wide agreement among neuropsychologists that the incidence of HIV-associated neuropsychological impairment increases as individuals progress from asymptomatic disease to symptomatic disease to AIDS. A WHO cross-cultural study, reporting on data from Munich, Sao Paulo, Kinshasa, Nairobi, and Bangkok, noted a prevalence of dementia, as defined by the International Classification of Diseases, ranging from 5.9 to 6.9% among symptomatic HIV+ persons. Current estimates are that from 15 to 20% of individuals with AIDS will develop frank dementia, while another 20 to 30% will manifest lesser degrees of cognitive and motor dysfunction. Most CNS diseases complicating HIV infection occur in its late or AIDS phase; however, uncommon encephalopathies resembling postinfectious autoimmune diseases can develop during the initial period of acute HIV infection and seroconversion, and a second type of presumed autoimmune brain disorder has been described in the "asymptomatic" or "middle" phase of systemic HIV infection. Autoimmunity also seems to be the cause of peripheral nervous system complications, such as demyelinating neuropathies that usually develop during the stage of clinical latency.

Although it is clear that HIV-1 can be detected in the central nervous system early in the course of disease, there is debate about whether this presence is related to neurobehavioral functioning, especially when individuals are medically asymptomatic. There is evidence across a number of recent studies for median rates of neurocognitive impairment in 35% of asymptomatic HIV+ individuals. Rates of impairment appear to be even higher in studies that included measurement of certain specific "subcortical" functions: reaction time, attention, and speeded information processing. To the extent that such functions are important, even critical, to certain occupations (e.g., piloting aircraft, driving trains and buses, operating dangerous equipment, as well as other highly technical jobs that depend upon these skills), it has been suggested that consideration should be given to periodic skills assessment of HIV+ persons in these and related occupations.

I. Implications for Biopsychosocial Interventions

There have been reports of a dramatic decline in the frequency of HIV dementia related to the earlier and more widespread use of antiretrovirals such as zidovudine (ZDV or "AZT"), but these are not widely available for 90% of the persons with HIV in the developing world. It has been suggested that the experience of neurological dysfunction is a key contributor to hopelessness in HIV-infected individuals and their loved ones and caretakers, and may accelerate an overall decline in health. Subjective cognitive complaints in asymptomatic individuals are significantly associated with depressive symptoms. Psychosocial interventions that reduce the effects of perceived stress can also help PLWHA to maintain a sense of autonomy, optimism, and control in their lives. Also important are interventions that help PLWHA obtain and maintain support in social relationships, including relationships with health care workers and employers, as well as significant others.

There is almost no research on occupational or employment-related functioning in relationship to neuropsychological impairment in HIV infection. There is also little research on psychological, psychiatric, and/or neurocognitive disorders in HIV-infected persons in developing countries. Moreover, these conditions are rarely taken into account in national plans or community responses to the epidemic. The emotional, cognitive, and behavioral reactions to perceived problems in neurocognitive functioning can complicate provision of care at home or in the clinical setting, and cause significant distress in PLWHA.

III. INTERVENTIONS AND TREATMENT ADVANCES

A. AZT and Preventing Disease Progression

This antiretroviral drug, formally known as zidovudine, was the first treatment shown, in 1987, to prolong survival in persons with AIDS. In 1989, two studies showed that AZT may delay progression to severe symptomatic states and AIDS in patients with earlier stages of HIV infection. In 1993, however, a large cooperative trial called the Concorde showed that there was no difference in survival over 3 years' average follow-up between those in whom treatment was started early and those in whom it was delayed until clinical symptoms had developed or CD4 lymphocyte count had fallen. Then, AZT-resistant strains of HIV began to appear. Three pivotal studies on treatment of people with AIDS marked 1996 as the end of the "AZT Era" of therapy. Use of the drug AZT alone ("AZT monotherapy") was clearly shown to be not as effective in treating AIDS as combinations of antiviral drugs, which could attack HIV strains that had become resistant to AZT.

B. Preventing Vertical Transmission

HIV can be transmitted from an infected woman to her fetus or newborn during pregnancy, during labor and delivery, and during the postpartum period through breastfeeding. Without treatment, an HIV-infected mother in the United States faces about a 25% risk of passing the virus to her child perinatally; in developing countries, this risk is significantly higher, about 40%. It is estimated that breastfeeding increases by about 25% the risk of passing HIV from HIV+ mothers to those infants who escape perinatal infection. In 1985, the U.S. CDC recommended that HIV-infected women forgo childbearing until more was known about the risks of perinatal transmission. Although the estimates of maternal–fetal transmission rates have improved, the prognosis for children with AIDS has not. Treatment during pregnancy and for 6 weeks after birth with AZT can reduce HIV transmission to newborns by 70%, and is recommended by most HIV specialists. Such treatment is, however (a) often financially out of reach for women in developing countries, and (b) dependent on identification of the mother as HIV+, and thus on the availability of routine HIV screening in maternity clinics in high prevalence areas. One of the simplest regimens, however, uses just two doses of a single drug, nevirapine—one dose to the mother when she comes to the hospital in labor, the other to the baby soon after birth. The cost of this treatment—about $2—is cheap enough for international health organizations to offer everywhere. Testing pregnant women in order to prevent transmission to the baby has raised concerns among AIDS activist groups about confidentiality for the mother. Recommendations for using AZT to prevent mother to child transmission were published in the United States in August 1994, but have not been adopted by most countries, or by any in the developing world. Although voluntary testing and counseling for pregnant women was strongly recommended in 1995 by the CDC as a means of identifying and treating HIV+ women to reduce perinatal transmission, hospitals in New York City first began widespread, mandatory HIV testing of all newborns in February 1997. This policy does not permit, however, testing and treatment of pregnant women, which has been shown to be critical for reducing infant infection. With the opportunity to reduce significantly the risk of vertical transmission with AZT, it is even more important to develop strategies to ensure that all pregnant women are offered HIV testing.

C. Combination Therapies

The year 1996 will probably be remembered as a landmark year in efforts to combat or even "cure" AIDS. The reason for this optimism is the success of the new "combination therapies," or "cocktails," which involve combinations of drugs, including AZT, 3TC (another drug that, like AZT, disrupts an early stage of viral replication), and one of a new class of drugs called "protease inhibitors" (protease is an enzyme necessary for viral replication). Clinical trials with combination therapies have shown dramatic results, in which the "viral load" (the amount of HIV that can be measured in blood and other tests) is reduced in some PLWHA to undetectable levels. If the virus cannot reproduce, theoretically it may eventually die out as the cells it has infected die. Clinically, these treatments are prolonging and transforming the lives of thousands of HIV+ persons who have begun to feel much better, look better, and to resume their work and former quality of life. For the first time, it appeared as if AIDS was treatable—and perhaps curable.

There are reasons to be less than fully optimistic about these remarkable medical developments. First, these treatments cost more than $15,000 per person per year, beyond the means of all but the wealthiest nations and their citizens. They are thus effectively out of reach for the 90% of PLWHA living in developing countries. Second, AIDS researchers are cautious in not saying that these treatments have cured patients by completely ridding their bodies of HIV after only a year. The virus may still be hiding in lymph tissue or elsewhere in the body, and may require taking these or progressively stronger drugs for a lifetime. Third, there is the problem of adherence—if a patient skips even a single dose of any one drug in the combination, HIV could press this small advantage to mutate into a strain that resists all current medications. Therefore, a critical question is how long the new combinations of anti-HIV drugs will work before resistant strains of the virus appear, as they quickly did with first-generation treatments such as AZT.

I. Implications for Biopsychosocial Interventions

Because of the effectiveness of these combination treatments and the importance of starting therapy as soon as possible, HIV experts are now strongly advocating early detection of HIV infection and initiation of these combination treatments among everyone infected with HIV, but particularly those with CD4 cell counts below a certain level (500 cells per cubic millimeter of blood). This suggests that it would be important for behavioral HIV scientists to develop messages and methods to encourage anyone who has any risk for being HIV-infected to be tested and then to enter treatment. This could involve new ways of helping people recognize the often vague or general flu-like symptoms associated with initial infection with HIV, as well as to evaluate more accurately their risk for exposure to HIV.

The importance of consistent adherence to a regimen of more than a dozen pills a day (for the combination treatments) in keeping drug resistance at bay poses a great challenge to behavioral scientists and clinicians, who need to work closely with physicians to understand—and to help patients understand—that strict adherence is the key to success of this regimen. Concomitantly, methods to increase adherence behavior as well as motivation, are important, not only for the individual patient, but to avoid creating a potentially disastrous public health risk through the spread of a multidrug-resistant virus. Taking the full course of prescribed medications and making doctors' appointments have long been recognized as problems for many PLWHA who are homeless, drug users, sex workers, or who otherwise lead marginalized lifestyles.

IV. PREVENTION

A. Ensuring Safe Blood Supplies

The most basic measure that a country can take against HIV—safeguarding the blood supply from infection—has still not been achieved in many developing countries. UNAIDS estimates that up to 10% of new HIV infections in developing countries, more than 15 years into the pandemic, are caused by infected blood transfusions. A large reason is cost: a single transfusion of blood from volunteer donors (donors who seek payment for their blood are often at high risk for being HIV-infected through their lifestyles), using safe and sterile equipment, and screened for HIV, costs an estimated $20 to $30. Although it is cheaper to ask donors questions about previous experiences that might have exposed them to HIV, it is much easier to get honest answers from volunteers than from paid donors. A recent study found, however, that a "measurable percentage" of U.S. voluntary blood donors do not report risk factors (such as IDU, sex with a prostitute, or recent blood transfusion) at the time of donation. Although all donated blood is tested for seven infectious diseases, only 8% of those who reported such risks were screened out by laboratory testing.

B. Education, Condoms, and Behavioral Prevention Strategies

Most HIV prevention efforts over the last 15 years have concentrated on advocating correct and consistent condom use for every act of sexual intercourse to prevent sexual transmission, and on advocating the use of clean needles and syringes and not sharing drug-using equipment to prevent parenteral transmission. There is evidence that some of these prevention programs are working. Between 1991 and 1995, young men in northern Thailand became less likely to have intercourse with commercial sex workers, and more likely to use condoms when they did so. During the same period, the rate of infection with HIV and the proportion of men with STD fell substantially. Although this was not a clinical trial, and thus, it could not be proven that the drop in HIV/STD infections was causally attributable to use of condoms with sex workers, there is a likely association. Further, the increased use of condoms by young Thai men does appear to be the result of the Thai government's aggressive "100 Percent Condom" campaign, which involved not only educating people about safer sexual practices, but providing condoms to commercial sex establishments, and enforcing condom use among clients of these establishments.

There are mixed results for the effects of HIV prevention in developed countries, particularly in the United States, Canada, and Europe. Transmission by men having sex with men (MSM) has slowed considerably in many developed countries, but it is difficult to establish that this is because of changes in dynamics of the epidemic (cf. section I), or because prevention has worked for this subpopulation. There is more compelling evidence, however, that HIV prevention can work well when strategies to control the spread of HIV are implemented early—as in certain cities (e.g., Glasgow, Lund, Sydney, Toronto, and Tacoma), which began early to make treatment for drug use and clean syringes available on demand, and consequently have a very low HIV prevalence among IDUs (<5%), compared to rates over 50% in cities without such early prevention efforts. Australia and New Zealand also implemented sound HIV prevention policies and practices early, slowing the spread of HIV among IDUs and heterosexuals, and decreasing the spread of new infection transmitted by MSM. None of the developed countries has experienced the kind of heterosexually transmitted epidemic typical of developing countries.

There have been no successful strategies to prevent the major route of heterosexual transmission in the United States, Canada, and Europe—from IDUs to their sexual partners.

In developing countries, heterosexual transmission accounts for almost 75% of HIV infections. Prevention strategies have had limited impact on the general spread of the epidemic. The most frequent prevention programs are national mass-awareness campaigns and interventions consisting of three interrelated strategies—reduction of number of partners, promotion of condom use, and control of STDs—targeted at populations at risk. There is a need to complement current prevention efforts that concentrate on influencing individual behavior, with approaches that take into consideration the social, economic, and structural determinants of risk that act as barriers to the adoption of preventive behavior. Many studies have shown that strategies that are effective for certain at-risk groups are not meeting the needs of those most vulnerable to infection—namely, women, youth, single-gender migrant groups, and other marginalized segments of the population, who live under economic and social deprivation. Unfortunately, theories of behavior change have become synonymous with HIV prevention, although these theories have limited application to, for example, monogamous wives at risk because of their husbands' extramarital relationships, or to populations who have no access to health services. Studies on sociocultural and programmatic barriers to seeking health care for HIV and other STD are necessary to make services more accessible and responsive to user's needs.

C. Other Prevention Methods

One problem for women who want to protect themselves against HIV is that they have little power to ensure that their husbands or partners wear condoms during sex. The female condom—a sheath that lines the vagina—appears to be a promising option to increase the options for women to protect themselves. It has been reported that women like it, use it, and often men do not even notice it. Currently, however, the female condom costs $3, which is impractical for most people in the world who need it. An agreement to make the female condom cheaper and more widely available would help and is being sought by UNAIDS.

UNAIDS has also been conducting tests on "chemical condoms," in the form of a vaginal microbicidal pill or gel, to be used by women. The question remains, however, whether the vaginal microbicide will actually protect people from HIV infection and if it can kill the virus.

D. HIV Vaccines

According to UNAIDS, probably the only solution for the 90% of people living with HIV/AIDS in developing countries, who have little access to health care and expensive anti-HIV medications, is prevention, particularly development of a vaccine. Early optimism about developing a vaccine against AIDS faded in the 1980s and early 1990s, but recent scientific developments have renewed hopes for the eventual deployment of an effective vaccine. Tests of the safety and immunogenicity (ability to stimulate immune responses thought to be salutogenic) of several potential vaccine products have been carried out or are underway in the United States, Europe, Thailand, Uganda, and Cuba. The question is how effective these will be in preventing infection in large-scale trials. One challenge to possible efficacy is the existence of different strains of HIV—and whether a vaccine which protects against the "B" strain found mainly in North America and Europe will protect about other strains (particularly "E" found in Thailand, or "A" in Uganda). Another challenge is whether a vaccine that protects IDUs, who are infected through the blood, will also provide "mucosal immunity," thought necessary to prevent heterosexual transmission.

1. Implications for Biopsychosocial Interventions

Behavioral science can contribute to the design, conduct, analysis, and interpretation of scientifically and ethically sound vaccine trials in various ways: by helping to understand incentives and disincentives to participate in trials, to help improve the consent process to ensure that consent is both truly "informed" and truly voluntary, and to assess behavioral risk for HIV exposure during a trial—which if not taken into account, could cloud interpretation of a study's results.

E. Populations for Which HIV Prevention Is Urgently Needed

1. Prisons

In the United States, the concentration of IDUs in correctional institutions is associated with a high prevalence of HIV infection among inmates. By December 1994, the prevalence of reported cases of AIDS in the prison population was 5.2 per 1000, or 6 times the total U.S. adult population rate of 0.9 per 1000. There is pressing need for HIV testing, prevention and education programs, counseling, provision of condoms, and medical care for STDs and HIV in jails, prisons, and youth correctional facilities. It is also important to develop and support discharge planning and supportive services in the community that assist ex-offenders in instituting and maintaining needed behavior changes.

2. HIV-Infected Individuals

Since the first AIDS cases were described in the medical literature in 1981, HIV prevention efforts in both developed and developing countries have continued to concentrate on preventing exposure and infection in vulnerable or at-risk individuals and populations. Little attention, however, has been devoted to the complementary perspective, preventing transmission by PLWHA, despite accumulating evidence that disturbing numbers and proportions of PLWHA continue to engage in behaviors that could infect others. Studies of the impact of HIV voluntary testing and counseling programs suggest that many individuals who learn they are HIV+ make appropriate behavioral changes, but that, in general, reductions in transmission risk behaviors are limited, even among those who are aware of their infection and who have been counseled about how to avoid transmitting the disease. Messages and methods need to be developed to encourage those at high risk of being infected to seek testing, and to motivate those who know they are infected to inform their sexual partners of their infection, as an important component of promoting sexual responsibility. It would be essential to develop specific interventions for PLWHA to enhance coping and relationship dimensions of quality of life that will have an impact, ultimately, on preventing transmission of the virus to loved ones and other sexual partners.

3. Military Populations

There is mounting evidence that a number of national militaries, particularly those in sub-Saharan Africa where the virus has been spreading longer, have estimated HIV prevalences as high as 50 to 60%, compared to less than 10 to 20% among civilian populations in the same countries. Even militaries with a low HIV prevalence, such as in the United States, appear to provide inadvertent opportunities for exposure to HIV during, for example, deployment or rest-and-recreation (R & R) leave to areas of the world where there is high HIV prevalence. Historically, soldiers, prostitutes, and the spread of STD have long been linked. Other factors thought to contribute to higher risk for HIV infection in military populations include: different cultural norms in military compared with civilian communities (e.g., higher risk-taking), the relative unavailability of women as steady sexual partners, being stationed far from the stabilizing influences of family and "hometown," and increased opportunities for casual sex during leave periods, overseas assignments, or deployments. Behavioral and infection surveillance systems must be established, not only in areas of high HIV prevalence, but in populations and subpopulations where new infections are likely to occur, and, as in many military populations, where high levels of risk behavior have created a "tinderbox" situation.

V. QUALITY OF LIFE

Since 1948, when the World Health Organization defined health as not merely the absence of disease and infirmity but also as physical, mental, and social well-being, quality-of-life issues have become increasingly important in health care research and practice. "Objective" health status and functioning in physical, psychological, and social domains are influenced by "subjective" perceptions, experiences, beliefs, and expectations to such a degree that two people with the same level of severity of the same disease could have markedly different perceptions of their quality of life. Moreover, there is much evidence to suggest that psychosocial dimensions of quality of life, particularly hope (or its converse, depression and hopelessness), perceived social support (or its converse, isolation and social inhibition), and fighting spirit (or its converse, resignation), can have striking effects on disease susceptibility as well as on biomedical issues such as recovery and survival time for persons with cancer and heart disease, as well as AIDS. In patients with most organic medical disorders, functional health status is strongly influenced by mood, coping skills, and social support; yet, it has been argued that the mental, emotional, and behavioral dimensions of illness are typically neglected by predominant medical approaches. By helping patients manage not just their disease but also common underlying needs for psychosocial support, coping skills, and sense of control, health outcomes as well as quality of life can be markedly improved, and at significantly lower costs than when medical interventions alone are used. [*See* COPING WITH STRESS; SOCIAL SUPPORT.]

All these considerations suggest that "quality of life" is a concept that is broader than health, and that necessarily extends beyond the limitations of the medical model, and physical or chemical interventions. Quality of life needs to be understood as a multidimensional construct incorporating the complex interrelationships among physical health, psychological state, coping, role functioning, social relationships, and cultural values, as well as personal goals, beliefs and concerns.

Although there are many commonalities between HIV/AIDS and other chronic and/or life-threatening conditions, HIV/AIDS presents a number of unique problems and challenges to quality of life. For example, cancer is usually characterized as a chronic condition, and indeed, many cancers are considered curable, particularly if diagnosed and treated early. Such is not the case for HIV/AIDS, which has been assumed to be inevitably fatal, at least until the recent announcement of the dramatic effects of retroviral drug combinations and protease inhibitors on slowing, even halting progression of disease (cf. section III). As many have commented, however, these treatments are not currently available nor are they likely to become so for the 90% of persons with HIV in the developing world.

Much more stigma is attached to having HIV/AIDS, in part, because the disease first appeared in stigmatized groups where it still has increased prevalence (homosexual and bisexual men in developed countries, sex workers in developing countries, injecting drug users in many cities around the world). Unfortunately, this is still true in most parts of the world, and ignorance of how the disease can and cannot be spread has resulted in the rejection and ostracization of PLWHA from their families and communities. To a far greater degree than for people with cancer, those with HIV/AIDS suffer discrimination in employment, housing, access to health care, travel, and other areas.

Unlike most cancers, HIV disease, particularly in the latter stages, involves mental, as well as physical symptoms and deterioration. Because HIV, unlike cancer, is an infectious disease, the burden of HIV is often exponential in families, as productive adult members become sequentially infected, and children are born with the disease. This results in substantial decreases in the general standard of living of the family due to cessation of productive work by the sick individual and expenses related to caring for the sick. Finally, PLWHA are more likely than those with cancer to be young and more critically needed in their roles as providing for and raising their families. This has devastating socioeconomic impact on families and communities, particularly in developing countries.

It is critical to understand the salient components, influences and determinants of quality of life that are affected as a result of HIV infection in various parts of the world. Such an understanding is essential in developing, evaluating, and improving biomedical as well as psychosocial interventions that aim to ameliorate quality of life for persons living with HIV/AIDS (PLWHA). At another level, studying quality of life in large populations of PLWHA can furnish information to help government and health policymakers allocate funds to those interventions shown to elicit the best quality of life outcomes.

VI. BIOPSYCHOSOCIAL ISSUES IN AFFECTED POPULATIONS

A. The Increased Vulnerability of Women, Youth, and Children

Women are the group most rapidly becoming infected with HIV. It is estimated that women may ultimately account for half of all AIDS cases in the United States, as they do globally. As the numbers of HIV-infected women increase, so do the numbers of HIV-infected infants. Of the 3 million HIV-infected infants born since the beginning of the pandemic (worldwide epidemic), more than 90% have been born in Africa. Many of these children typically develop AIDS and die within a few years. Although the most important route of transmission in children is through their HIV-infected mothers, a smaller number of children are infected through use of infected blood products (e.g., the chilling situation of children in Romanian orphanages infected through HIV-infected needles used inadvertently to administer various inoculations). Children of HIV+ mothers, even if they themselves are not affected, suffer social exclusion from the community.

A variety of gender-based problems affecting HIV-infected and at-risk women have been reported for developed and for developing countries. These problems are both causes and consequences of HIV infection, and thus, impossible to consider separately. Around the world are reports of young women and girls who are increasingly vulnerable to violence and sexual abuse, and concomitantly, infection with HIV/STD. During the 1994 genocide in Rwanda, HIV was used as a weapon of war, as HIV-infected soldiers deliberately raped women after killing male members of their families. Many of these women became HIV-infected, as well as pregnant, and as a result, have faced the compound traumas of having being raped, infected with HIV, and giving birth to a potentially unwanted and HIV-infected baby fathered by the perpetrator of this violence. The millions of youth who work as domestic laborers are often subject to sexual and physical abuse. Traditional healers in some African countries prescribe sexual intercourse with minors as a "cure for AIDS," which is probably responsible for the 100% increase in incidence in juvenile rape in these countries in recent years.

Many women with HIV in sub-Saharan Africa and in Asia were not infected through their own high-risk sexual activity, but rather through the high-risk behaviors of their husbands or partners. Infection rates as high as 25% have been reported among women with only one lifetime partner in Rwanda, for example. In Thailand, husbands bring home HIV acquired from sex workers, which are patronized by more than one in five Thai men. A study from Costa Rica found that most women with AIDS had been infected by their steady male partners or husbands, who did not inform the women of their high-risk sexual behaviors.

An unfortunately common situation in India is for a husband to become HIV-infected from an extramarital relationship with a sex worker, to subsequently infect his wife, and then to join his relatives in blaming the wife for infecting him. The HIV+ wife is then thrown out on the streets to fend for herself and her HIV+ children. UNAIDS has estimated that India will have between 5 and 8 million people with HIV in the year 2000, many having experienced this tragic scenario.

The needs of women living with HIV/AIDS in various countries are particularly acute. In Zimbabwe, reports indicate that 90% of the women faced discrimination in health, education, professional, and legal rights. Wife inheritance is a problem in some East African tribes. When a woman's husband dies, often of

AIDS, it is the tradition to marry the brother of her dead husband. If she refuses (or he will not marry her because she has become HIV-infected), she faces eviction, loss of her children, and disinheritance of property left behind by her husband. Without access to land and means of production, widows and children are often forced into petty theft or commercial sex work, where they continue the vicious cycle of poverty and concomitant vulnerability to HIV. In many countries, women have little control over sexual relations within marriage, which renders them economically and legally vulnerable. The dilemma for many married women is that in most cultures, women do not have the right to refuse sex with their husbands, even if they know or suspect that he is HIV-infected. Rural women appear to be at even higher risk for discrimination due to ignorance.

The social impact of HIV is differentially hardest on women, particularly in developing countries, even if women are survivors and not direct casualties of AIDS. Women are not only the main care providers, but also largely responsible for food production, agricultural labor, and the raising of children. When mothers are infected with HIV and subsequently die, the responsibility to feed, clothe, shelter, and educate these children falls on grandparents, extended families, and increasingly, women friends of women who die of AIDS.

B. "AIDS Orphans"

The estimated proportions of children under 15 who have lost their mothers to AIDS in various countries have been reported as: 2.9 to 4.6% in Zambia, 1.5 to 3.3% in Uganda, 1.3 to 1.8% in Tanzania, 1.2% to 1.7% in Ivory Coast, and 1.1% to 1.7% in Kenya (WHO and UNICEF, 1994). The number of children who will have been orphaned by HIV/AIDS by the year 2000 has been estimated to range from 5 to 10 million. Despite the variety of services and growing number of involved organizations, the needs of orphaned children are not being met. In some African countries such as Zimbabwe, grannies are increasingly assuming the role of parents for the growing population of AIDS orphans. Often ill or infirm themselves, usually poor, uneducated as well as unemployed, these grannies are not able to cope with a problem that grows more overwhelming by the day. In Africa, orphaned children have relatively few legal or customary rights to property or to decision making about their future, unless the father has made specific provisions for them. As a result, AIDS orphans are at risk for exploitation, deprivation of property rights, abuse, and neglect; girls are particularly vulnerable to sexual exploitation and consequently, to HIV infection.

C. Sex Workers

From Honduras to Ethiopia to Thailand, women who are sex workers are at high risk of becoming infected with HIV and other STD, and of suffering a lower quality of life than infected women who are not sex workers. Prevalence rates can be as high as 75% among female sex workers, up to 90% in urban centers, and incidence rates of 38% per year or even 10% per month have been reported in some African and Asian countries. Data from 1991 to 1993 for urban women sex workers in countries in sub-Saharan Africa show infection levels of greater than 30% for many countries, including Ivory Coast (86%), Kenya (85.5%), Ethiopia (65.6%), Mali (52.8%), Cameroon (45.3%), Tanzania (42.9%), Ghana (37.5%), The Gambia (35%), and Zaire (30%). HIV seroprevalence among women sex workers in Asia from 1986 to 1994 was highest in Madurai, India (54.7%), and above 30% in several other regions in India and Thailand. The sex industry in India, along with other Asian countries, displays often appalling conditions of forced prostitution and sexual exploitation.

In general, commercial sex work is a direct result of economic pressures, not choice. When sex workers rely on a client for money to pay for food, housing, or drugs, they are not in a position to be adamant about demanding that condoms be used. Once sex workers have contracted HIV, which is virtually inevitable in high-prevalence areas, survival for themselves and their children becomes an immediate and all-consuming problem.

Police commonly raid brothels in Mumbai (formerly Bombay), forcibly testing women for HIV and putting those found to be HIV+ in detention centers, where they are treated not as victims but as criminals. The sudden raids mean that women often leave behind money, belongings, and even children. TB is common in the detention centers, and HIV+ women easily contract the disease. Many of these women had been kidnapped from Nepal or otherwise forced into prostitution, and are unable to return home to obtain support from their families and communities.

These problems are exacerbated for very young girls who are often sold into prostitution by their families, and thus in a very real sense are sex slaves with no rights and no one to whom to appeal for help. Younger females are especially vulnerable to HIV infection because their greater susceptibility to tearing and immature cervical cells allow the virus easier access to the bloodstream. Fear of AIDS is primarily responsible for the spiraling demand for younger and younger children. There is a growing trade in child prostitution as a result of "sex tourism" in countries such as Cambodia and Thailand, where it has been estimated that as many as 50% of underage sex workers have the virus. Child prostitution is also gaining ground in Latin America and particularly in Eastern Europe, where HIV is rapidly spreading among intravenous drug users and homeless persons.

I. Implications for Biopsychosocial Interventions

Because of the illegality of prostitution, and women's consequent fear of loss of business or arrest by police, it is extremely difficult for sex workers to be reached through the usual health or social care system. Their access to medical care is minimal, and they rarely if ever go to public hospitals, so this route is usually effectively closed, as well. Another difficulty is that many sex workers are not citizens of the countries in which they work, so that their plight and even their numbers are not the concern of local health organizations. Outreach to nongovernmental organizations (NGOs), women's groups, and organizations offering health or legal services to women would be important. Needs assessments should be appropriate and applicable to the situation of sex workers. Such questions, for example, about perceptions of (a) special barriers to health care or housing, (b) violence and abuse, and (c) unfair or discriminatory treatment could also be applicable to other marginalized groups such as refugees (discussed below).

D. Pregnant Women and Parents

In every culture, having children and raising the next generation are highly valued and central to the definition of quality of life. These values and new lives are being threatened by the HIV pandemic. Although strategies to prevent transmission from mother to child, such as counseling women considering pregnancy, avoiding invasive procedures during labor, and administering HIV treatments (especially AZT) to

HIV-infected pregnant women, the number of infected children is still increasing. Many women are not aware that they are infected, and seek help only at a late stage of the disease. Frequently, the diagnosis of maternal HIV infection is made only after their children begin to manifest HIV symptoms.

HIV seroprevalence among pregnant women in urban areas in Thailand has increased to levels as high as 4% (1994) in the northern region. Figures for HIV seroprevalence among pregnant women in India were highest in Pune. In maternity clinics in Mumbai, 2.8% of women are HIV+. Recent HIV seroprevalence rates among pregnant women in other countries have been reported as follows: 33% in urban areas of Rwanda, 29% in Uganda, 23% in Malawi, and 33.6% in Zambia.

Infected women who would wish to terminate their pregnancy are confronted with societal and legal barriers: a 1992 survey on AIDS in the world showed that abortions were never or seldom offered in government facilities in over three-quarters of the developing countries surveyed. In more than one-half of the developing countries surveyed, abortion was illegal with no exception in the case of maternal HIV infection.

It is now well established that breast-feeding by HIV-infected women is a significant additional factor in the transmission of HIV from mother to newborn, especially in developing countries. The dilemma for mothers is that withholding breast-feeding will significantly increase the risk of diarrheal diseases, nutritional problems, and increased mortality in the newborn.

HIV-infected parents are faced with an array of stressors, including disclosure to children, disclosure to schools, guardianship, and additionally for women, issues of child care, meal preparation, and housework when feeling sick or otherwise weak. Disclosing HIV to children is a difficult and emotional task for parents. Poverty and its consequences force women to relinquish children to relatives or child welfare agencies. Losing custody heightens a sense of loss in infected women who feel they may not live long enough to see a child raised to adulthood.

I. Implications for Biopsychosocial Interventions

Theoretically, testing and counseling can assist women in assessing their current or future risk for infection and allow for referral to other HIV prevention services.

It is not clear to what extent these objectives are met in most developing countries. It would be important to assess whether knowing that they are infected allows women to obtain early diagnosis and treatment for their infants, make informed reproductive decisions, use methods to reduce the risk for perinatal transmission, receive information to prevent HIV transmission to others, and obtain referral for psychological and social services.

What are pregnant women's perceptions of the HIV test, and about various kinds of interventions to protect their future children from HIV? What interventions do they have knowledge about, and which would they accept? In terms of spiritual and cultural meaning, how does an HIV+ woman come to terms with her natural desires to give life and to see her life continue through her children, and the realistic fear that her children will die painfully and early from AIDS? HIV testing and counseling for women of childbearing age appear to offer important prevention opportunities for both uninfected and infected women and their infants, but what testing and counseling are available to women, and how is it perceived? Is confidentiality of test results indeed a concern that outweighs benefits of testing to mother and baby? If so, what could be done to decrease problems related to testing confidentiality? What information do HIV+ women have about decreasing the risk of transmitting HIV to their children?

E. Refugees and Displaced People

The United Nations Program on HIV/AIDS (UNAIDS) recently reported that there are around 40 million refugees and other displaced people in the world today; about 75% of all refugees are women and children. Forced from their homelands by war, civil strife, floods, or earthquakes, they often live in special refugee camps where they are at risk for an array of health problems and diseases, including HIV/AIDS. Because transfusions are often needed in large numbers in situations of war and other emergencies, there is a great danger of spreading HIV throughout refugee camps from the transfusion of infected blood. Sexual contact presents another risk for infection, particularly for women refugees. Living with HIV/AIDS in a foreign country is particularly distressing, because of unawareness of and/or ineligibility for health services in that country.

Although prevalence of HIV infection was not assessed directly in the recent Rwandan refugee crisis, more than 50% were infected with agents causing vaginitis, and the prevalence of active syphilis was 4%. STD case detection and management in such situations could be improved by training health workers to use the syndromic approach and through information campaigns encouraging attendance at clinics.

According to recent reports, many women refugees from Myanmar on the Thai border have been forced into prostitution to provide for their families. They face harassment by Thai authorities on the one hand, and by the Myanmaran military on the other, with the threat of HIV infection a constant but background threat. It is critical to understand the unique and salient issues affecting quality of life for refugees who are either already HIV-infected or in danger of becoming so, although it is obviously very difficult to conduct such assessments, upon which appropriate, multidimensional and timely interventions depend. UNAIDS has recommended that relief workers follow universal medical precautions in all medical procedures with refugee populations, that condoms should be made available early in an emergency, and that following the acute phase of an emergency, relief agencies should provide information on HIV risks and safer sex.

F. Home Care, "Burnout," and Grief

In sub-Saharan Africa, home care support services are the predominant organizational response to the need to provide care for PLWHA, but serious problems arise concerning the quality, coverage, cost, and sustainability of these programs. A major problem appears to be reliance on narrow health/medical care models, instead of a more sustainable, community-rooted approach that utilizes community centers, volunteers, local remedies, and traditional knowledge structures, and that empowers women who are the de facto primary caregivers.

I. Implications for Biopsychosocial Interventions

Home-based care models for supporting PLWHA in Thailand offer multidisciplinary support for the whole person (including spiritually) as well as for the family, who are provided informal education on HIV prevention, on the disease process, and how to care for their family member(s). In Mexico, as in many other coun-

tries, the family is primarily the main support for persons living with AIDS. In order to prevent burnout of the caregiver (usually wife, mother, daughter, or sister), it is important to strengthen community structures to respond to caregivers' emotional support needs. Informed families and communities are more accepting of PLWHA, making it easier for these individuals to come to terms with their HIV status and to have an acceptable quality of life within the context of a supportive community. [*See* BURNOUT.]

G. Death and Dying

In addition to the emotional exhaustion that is a frequent consequence of caring for family members with chronic/fatal diseases, especially when suffering is intense, there is also the experience of grief when those individuals die. In AIDS-saturated communities, there are cumulative losses of members of one's immediate and extended families, as well as friends. Issues concerning death and dying are often paramount for PLWHA, for themselves, as well as for their loved ones, for whom they are often caregivers. Fears about death are often overshadowed by fears about the process of dying. What seems to make the critical difference is quality of dying, for example, whether one can imagine or anticipate being "ready," in control, aware, surrounded by loved ones, comfortable, and not in pain. Other important aspects that have been reported to affect "quality of dying" experiences include: the experience of other losses, grief, and bereavement for others who have recently died or who are in the process of dying; whether the person feels resolved about or "can't get over" these deaths; whether death is accepted as "inevitable" or denied; belief in life after death; whether there is a "conspiracy of silence" among those closest to the person; and the personal or cultural significance of dying and/or being buried in a special place or with one's family and ancestors. [*See* DYING.]

I. Implications for Biopsychosocial Interventions

A number of studies have documented the negative health effects of grief and multiple loss, including effects in communities where many people have died from AIDS. There have been no published studies, however, concerning the impact on quality of life of anticipated death and quality of dying, or the impact of witnessing loved ones die from the same disease from which one is suffering. Perhaps more than any other HIV-related issue discussed above, it is necessary to understand the social and cultural context in which individuals' subjective views of death and dying are necessarily embedded.

VII. CONCLUDING COMMENTS

There can be no conclusion here, because the story of HIV and AIDS is still being written, and very rapidly, in many areas of this field—epidemiology, treatment, and prevention. Despite recent promising advances in treatment, the epidemic is not only far from over, but is a growing threat to certain population groups where it was previously less common—women, children, as well as to new populations in Eastern Europe and Asia. As is the case for other diseases, probably the only true hope lies in more than an once of prevention—in multidimensional and comprehensive prevention programs that are rooted in a biopsychosocial understanding of the dynamics and complexities of this pandemic disease.

BIBLIOGRAPHY

DiClemente, R. J., & Peterson, J. L. (1994). *Preventing AIDS: Theories and methods of behavioral intervention.* New York: Plenum.

Grant, I., & Martin, A. (Eds.). (1994). *Neuropsychology of HIV infection.* New York: Oxford University Press.

Kalichman, S. (1995). *Understanding AIDS: A guide for mental health professions.* Washington, DC: American Psychological Association.

Maj, M., Starace, F., & Sartorius, N. (Eds.). (1993). *Mental disorders in HIV-1 infection and AIDS.* WA: Hogrefe and Huber.

Mann, J. M., & Tarantola, D. (Eds.). (1996). *AIDS in the world II: Global dimensions, social roots, and responses.* Oxford: Oxford University Press.

O'Leary, A., & Jemmott, L. S. (Eds.). (1996). *Women and AIDS: Coping and care.* New York: Plenum.

Pizzo, P. A., & Wilfert, C. M. (Eds.). (1994). *Pediatric AIDS: The challenge of HIV infection in infants, children, and adolescents.* (2nd ed.). Baltimore, MD: Williams & Wilkins.

Temoshok, L., & Baum, A. (Eds.). (1990). *Psychosocial Perspectives on AIDS.* Hillsdale, NJ: Lawrence Erlbaum.

Wasserheit, J. N., Aral, S. O., & Holmes, K. K. (Eds.). (1991). *Research issues in human behavior and sexually transmitted disease in the AIDS era.* DC: American Society for Microbiology.

Wu, A. W., Mead, S. C. W., van Dam, F., & Temoshok, L. R. (Eds.). (1994). Quality of life and HIV: A symposium on quality of life methodology. *Psychol. & Health, 9,* (Number 1–2) 1–160.

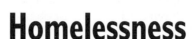

Homelessness

Marybeth Shinn and Beth C. Weitzman

New York University

Kim Hopper

Nathan Kline Institute

Literally Homeless   Those living in shelter, on the streets, or in other places not intended as normal dwelling units.

Period Prevalence   Number of cases over some specified period of time.

Point Prevalence   Number of cases at a particular point in time.

Precarious Housing   Substandard housing, seriously overcrowded conditions, or unstable doubled up arrangements that place people on the verge of homelessness.

Runaway Youths   Youths who leave home without parental permission.

Systems Youths   Youths who live in or leave foster care or institutional settings.

Throwaway Youths   Youths who are neglected, abused, or asked to leave by parents.

Although definitions of **HOMELESSNESS** vary, this article, like most research, focuses on the literally homeless: people living in shelter, on the streets, or in other places not intended as normal dwelling units. It examines different definitions, shows how definitions affect understanding of the scope of the problem, describes different groups of people who become homeless, and discusses solutions.

I. DEFINITIONS OF HOMELESSNESS

By the early 1980s, significant numbers of Americans found themselves unable to obtain, or maintain, a place of their own. Although skid row communities had existed in most cities throughout the decades, not since the Great Depression had this nation seen so many men, women, and children living on the streets and in shelters, or doubled and tripled up with family and friends. Occurring within years of the movement to deinstitutionalize the mentally ill, the phenomenon of homelessness was quickly linked with mental illness in the media and in the public debate. This link was further enforced by the visibility of "street people" suffering from unmistakable signs of severe mental illness. Yet, research and the experience of service providers have demonstrated that the relationship of homelessness and mental health is complex, and those who experience homelessness are heterogeneous in regard to their demographic characteristics, their pathways to homelessness, and their mental health status.

A firm and enduring definition of homelessness has proven elusive. Rather than two categories of people—one homeless and one housed—researchers, service providers, and policymakers are faced with a myriad of housing conditions, which can be loosely placed on a continuum of inadequate and atypical housing arrangements. There remains substantial debate concerning where on this continuum the line should be drawn between housed and homeless. At one end are those places never intended as homes, such as streets, public parks, subways, or cars. On any night, in virtually all of our nation's cities and towns, some people are living under these extreme conditions. At the other end of the continuum are stable doubled up situations in which people beyond a nuclear family share a dwelling unit, as well as residential and Single Room Occupancy hotels (SROs) and other forms of shared housing. Between these two points are shelters for the homeless, domestic violence shelters, institutional facilities (such as hospitals) where people are housed because other appropriate arrangements are unavailable, and more conventional but still precarious housing situations: physically inadequate housing where heat and running water, for example, are lacking for much of the time, badly overcrowded housing, and unstable doubled up arrangements.

In reality, people move among these different housing conditions, so that a temporary dwelling place should not be confused with a class of homeless people. For example, rather than living continuously on the streets where they might be dubbed a "street population," a substantial number of homeless individuals move frequently among the streets, short-stay hotels, doubled-up arrangements, and institutions, including prisons. Homelessness in this broader sense is best characterized by instability across a variety of impermanent and often inadequate living situations. The research on homeless people, however, has been more narrowly focused. Difficulties in identifying homeless people who are doubled-up, and in interviewing people in institutional facilities, have resulted in an operational definition of homelessness that is almost always limited to sheltered populations, users of related services (such as soup kitchens) who have no permanent address, or people visibly living on the streets or in encampments.

To no one's surprise, estimates of the number of "homeless people" in America have varied greatly, ranging from less than half a million to more than two million each year. Some estimates have been based on sophisticated sampling techniques, while others are at best educated guesses. The variations in the count, however, are not simply the result of variations in scientific rigor. Rather, differing definitions of what qualifies as homelessness (as discussed above) and differing time periods result in variations in the estimates. Epidemiologists draw a useful distinction between point prevalence, or the number of people in a given condition at a particular point in time, and period prevalence, or the number of people experiencing the condition at any time during some stipulated period. If some people experience a condition only briefly, period prevalence may be many times greater than point prevalence. Such is the case of homelessness; for some people homelessness proves to be cyclical, for others it involves an acute, single episode, and in other cases it is chronic.

Given these patterns, counts of homeless people that focus on a single point in time, for example, how many people are homeless on a given day, result in much lower estimates than measures of period prevalence, for example, how many people are homeless over the course of a year. As many as seven million Americans were literally homeless at some time during the later half of the 1980s. However, in any given week, approximately 350,000 were literally homeless.

In addition, if the characteristics of those who are only briefly homeless differ from the characteristics of those who remain homeless for extended periods—that is, if "exit" rates are not uniformly distributed among those who become homeless—a point-in-time estimate can yield a distorted picture of the whole. The longer the period of homelessness, the greater the likelihood of being "captured" by point-in-time methods. For example, when studies use point-in-time approaches, the composition of homeless populations includes higher proportions of single adults; this is because single adults are more likely than families to experience chronic or repeated homelessness. The same logic is applied to mental disabilities below.

It is generally agreed that the numbers of homeless people grew substantially throughout the 1980s, that the problem has continued into the 1990s, and that it is a problem of national (and, in fact, international) scope. Significantly, the growth in the numbers of homeless people has been concurrent with a dramatic growth in the number of Americans living in extreme poverty and a decline in the number of affordable housing units. As a national phenomenon, homelessness may best be understood as a structural problem, namely, increasing numbers of poor people chasing after declining numbers of low-cost rental units. The upshot is a musical chairs game where some portion of the population is, inevitably, left without a home. The losers, by default, are the most vulnerable among us; their vulnerability may be due to extreme poverty, youth, race, physical disability, mental illness, substance abuse, or badly frayed social networks.

II. RELATIONSHIP OF HOMELESSNESS TO MENTAL ILLNESS

Given this framework, it is not surprising to find that rates of mental illness tend to be higher among homeless populations than among those housed. But it is incorrect to take these elevated rates as clear evidence that mental illness causes homelessness. A number of serious methodological caveats stand in the way of this interpretation. The relationship between mental health and homelessness may be differently understood depending on the operational definition of homelessness chosen by the researcher. Where will homeless people be sought? Location may determine the nature and extent of the mental health problems uncovered; for example, studies done in shelters with strict restrictions on alcohol use are likely to result in undercounts of alcohol problems. Similarly, operational definitions of mental health and illness will influence the relationship detected. Does the study rely on service utilization, observer impression, or diagnostic instruments? [*See* ALCOHOL PROBLEMS.]

Static portraits of homeless people may further confuse the relationship between homelessness and mental illness for several reasons. As noted above, people move in and out of homelessness. Mental health problems, too, vary in intensity and duration. For many conditions, lifetime prevalence rates are significantly higher than point-in-time rates. The lifetime prevalence rates used in many studies overestimate the proportion of homeless people currently suffering from a particular disorder. [*See* EPIDEMIOLOGY: PSYCHIATRIC.]

Many studies "capture" people in the middle of an episode of homelessness. Given this methodology, it is difficult to discern whether mental problems are the cause, consequence, or, merely, a correlate of homelessness. In order for mental illness to be a cause of homelessness, several conditions must be demonstrated. First, homeless people must be found to have higher rates of such conditions than other poor people. Second, these elevated rates must precede homelessness. Third, some mechanism must be proposed that plausibly shows how such problems elevate risk of homelessness. Certain mental illnesses, such as schizophrenia, fulfill such criteria and may be argued to cause some people to become homeless. [*See* SCHIZOPHRENIA.]

Elevated rates of other mental health problems may be a consequence, rather than the cause, of homelessness. In such a situation, rates would also be higher among the homeless than the housed but the elevation in rates would begin only after entry to homelessness. That is, homeless and housed people would look the same prior to homelessness, but would be significantly different during or after becoming homeless. Certain types of depression follow this pattern. [*See* DEPRESSION.]

Finally, mental health problems may be neither cause nor consequence, but a correlate of homelessness that may contribute to people's inability to extricate themselves from the situation. In this case, rates of the problem would not necessarily be greater among those recently made homeless. Rather, those with the problem would be more likely than those without it to experience extended episodes of homelessness. If mentally ill people are more likely to be chronically homeless, they will be oversampled in cross-sectional studies. As a result, these studies may overestimate the extent of mental illness among people who become homeless.

Patterns of homelessness, and the demographic characteristics of those people who are homeless, are quite diverse. There are differences between urban and rural areas, across geographic regions (e.g., the Southwest and Northeast), and over time. There are differences between those who are in families and those who are on their own. For purposes of this discussion on the relationship between homelessness and mental health, four broad populations have been identified. They are: single men and women, parents in families, children in families, and adolescents on their own.

III. HOMELESS SINGLE ADULTS

Adults who are living separately from their families of origin and often from families of procreation, are the single largest group of literally homeless people. They make up a clear majority of all who become homeless, and an even larger proportion of those who are homeless at any point in time. During the surge of homelessness in the 1970s and 1980s, younger minority men replaced older White men as the predominant group of single adults in many cities, and were joined by increasing numbers of women. Most of what is known about homeless adults comes from studies of people living in shelter or on the street, sometimes using sophisticated sampling strategies to account for the fact that a single individual may move between various conditions and locations. Studies rarely include comparison groups of poor adults, because it is difficult to define and sample an appropriate group, but sometimes use comparison data from epidemiological studies.

In addition to the problems of definition and method already discussed, taking the measure of mental illness among homeless single adults presents distinctive problems of its own. The assessment of symptoms among the street-dwelling population is especially problematic. To begin with, troubling behavior that would usually be taken as a sign of psychiatric disorder may, in the case of people who are homeless, reflect the influence of an unusually stressful environment, lack of access to washrooms ("poor hygiene," "a disheveled appearance"), or strategic adaptations to the hazards of street life (certain bizarre behaviors may function as a defense against unwanted attention). The complex and varied contexts of homelessness present further difficulties. Without a thorough accounting of the places in which (even literally) homeless people can be found, the representativeness of the samples drawn, sites recruited from, and season of study cannot always be judged. Subpopulation differences complicate matters further. Substantial investments of time, innovative recompense, and flexible assessment strategies may be necessary if a study seeks a representative sample of people whose survival skills place a premium on avoiding detection.

For these and other reasons, reported rates for the prevalence of mental illness have varied wildly in the literature. As noted above, most studies report lifetime prevalence, from cross-sectional surveys, primarily of homeless single adults. Even so, prevalence rates for mental illness have ranged from 1 to 70%. More rigorous meta-analysis of published studies can cull for poorly designed research, inadequately defined samples, and vague diagnostic procedures, while restricting mental illness to present-day conditions that are both severe and persisting. Under such strictures, the range of reported prevalence rates for single homeless adults shrinks significantly to 13 to 26%. Applying similar restraints to the assessment of drug and alcohol dependence produces ranges from 26 to 67% and 11 to 58%, respectively. The range for co-

occurring disorders (severe mental illness and substance use) is from 12 to 26%, although ethnographic studies of street-dwelling populations tend to report higher figures. Doubtless methodological differences explain some of the reported variance. But real differences in the causes of homelessness from place to place in all likelihood make for different compositions of local homeless populations. If so, there should be no charmed generic figure for the prevalence of mental illness among single homeless adults.

Comparisons with housed populations generally show that severe mental illness is many times more common among the literally homeless, while rates for drug use, although higher, are less strikingly so. Gender differences—homeless men are less like than homeless women without children to show evidence of severe mental illness—probably reflect the operation of several factors. First, doubling up with others is often an alternative to, and last stop before, literal homelessness. Because the cultural threshold of tolerance for dependence and for disruptive behavior seems to be set higher for women than for men, women may be permitted to stay with family and friends in circumstances where men would be ejected. If so, women who exceed the threshold may be expected to show substantially more severe disorders than their ejected male counterparts. Also, the forms of mental illness most common among women are less often associated with threats or violent behavior than those common among men. Further, as discussed later, the population of single homeless women may include a fair number of mothers who have lost custody of their children due to mental illness. [See GENDER DIFFERENCES IN MENTAL HEALTH.]

Although there is little question that rates of mental illness are elevated among single homeless populations, the interpretation of that fact has occasioned much dispute. Research has discredited the two extreme positions: either, that preexisting mental illness so disables its casualties that they are unable to hold on to housing of their own; or, that homeless people are "just like you and me," except for the damage sustained after they lost their housing. It is clear today that severe mental illness generally predates first episodes of homelessness; it is also clear that the strains of street and shelter life (lack of sleep, the threat of danger, self-medication with drugs or alcohol) can disrupt treatment regimens, exacerbate symptoms, feed depression, and fuel disorganization.

Careful documentation of histories of residential instability holds the potential to elucidate the dynamics of homelessness in particular lives, but such histories are difficult to reconstruct reliably. Ironically, first person accounts can overplay the role of disability, ignoring the fact that such conditions had long been present in one's life without causing homelessness. The negotiation of life transitions (either expected or unexpected) can be especially tricky, and their difficulties are compounded when mental illness intrudes. The few longitudinal studies available show that although many people with severe mental illness manage to leave the streets and shelters, such unassisted "exits" tend to be short-lived, shallow, and unstable, such that returns to homelessness are common.

Conceptual difficulties compound the practical ones. Once crude notions of causation have been replaced by the more flexible epidemiological constructs of risk and vulnerability, researchers can begin to pinpoint those factors that, singly and in combination, appear to raise the likelihood of homelessness. Studies consistently find poverty, major mental illnesses, substance abuse, and disruptive childhood experiences to be risk factors for later homelessness. Mental illness and substance abuse are widely distributed across the socioeconomic spectrum, whereas homeless people with such problems come largely from low-income backgrounds. Substance abuse co-occurring with mental illness appears to be a particularly destabilizing combination. [*See* SUBSTANCE ABUSE.]

Homeless mentally ill persons also have fewer supportive relationships and more troubled kinship ties than their non-mentally ill counterparts. Closer examination of the histories of homeless individuals has begun to refine pictures of long-standing vulnerability. Foster care placements figure much more commonly (11 to 39%) in their childhoods (and even more so in those with severe mental illness); so, apparently, do episodes of abuse (physical and sexual), although comparative figures are difficult to come by. How such early events exert their destabilizing effect over time—whether, for example, foster care signifies developmental damage to coping abilities, the loss of kinbased support later in life, or the sudden cessation of public support at an age when few are prepared to be self-sufficient—remains open to interpretation.

Remarkably, apart from their treatment histories, the biographies of mentally ill and non-mentally ill homeless single adults do not show marked differences. This finding further confirms that illness, even severe psychiatric disorder, is not the sole factor in predisposing people to homelessness. It also suggests that a shared complex of early deprivation and/or harm may help explain both later homelessness and accompanying mental illness and substance abuse.

A different approach to the overrepresentation of severe mental illness in single homeless populations shifts attention from the traits of individuals to the structure of the system designed for their care. Traditional, highly centralized mental health systems have been dismantled. The achievements and coverage of community-based approaches have been mixed. Budget cutbacks have further limited the role of local psychiatric resources. Significant gaps in systems of coordinated treatment remain. Under such circumstances institutions not usually considered part of the psychiatric establishment have effectively been pressed into service to provide extended supervised care, permanent housing, temporary lodging, or discharge planning. To the degree that psychiatric hospitals today discharge individuals to nominally "homeless" facilities instead of halfway houses or other parts of the "mental health" system, the presence of individuals with psychiatric symptoms in shelters and other places serving the homeless poor becomes a foregone conclusion. Formerly, disreputable sections of inner-city neighborhoods (the tenderloins, skid rows, and rooming-house districts) had served as habitats of last resort for those who found it difficult to fit in elsewhere. With the loss of such places (and the destruction of cheap residential hotels in the 1970s), shelters increasingly assumed that role by default.

For most unattached homeless adults, the crisis of homelessness appears to be a passing one, limited to a brief stay or two in a shelter. Longer term homeless men and women may make use of shelters or drop-in centers, patronize soup kitchens, and avail themselves for the services of street outreach teams. But they still must contend with the elements, fend off the advances of passersby who approach them for sex or treat them as cruel sport, and maintain vigilance for safety's sake. Not only are they are burdened with the usual diseases of poverty, especially functional disabilities and chronic disorders, but such ailments are worsened by the stresses and isolation of street and shelter life. More recently, resurgent old afflictions (like tuberculosis), lethal new ones (like HIV-related illnesses), and infectious agents that have mutated into more deadly forms (like drug-resistant TB strains) have made their appearance. [*See* HIV/AIDS.]

The rigors of homelessness add their own toll, from the demoralization long documented among shelter residents, to the deterioration in mental state observed in street-dwellers over time, to the difficulties of getting appropriate care in supportive settings, to the pervasive loss of civil rights on the street. Not surprisingly, the quality of life of homeless adults with severe mental illness has been found to be much poorer than that of their housed counterparts. But close documentation of the daily lives of long-term homeless adults has identified relatively few differences in the subsistence circumstances of those with severe psychiatric disorders versus those without, a fact attributed to the "leveling" effects of homelessness itself. Those most severely hampered in meeting basic subsistence needs proved to be people suffering from both severe mental illness and substance abuse problems.

All the same, the ingenuity, resiliency, and resourcefulness often shown by people accustomed to long periods of homelessness should not go unremarked. Ethnographic studies have been especially revealing about the sheer effort it takes to survive from one day to the next on the street or in shelters, ostensibly established to help homeless people. It demands not only perseverance and a thick skin, but tolerance for bureaucratic stupidities and a sometimes surprising ability to connect with others in like circumstances.

During the 1980s, substantial progress was made in engaging and rehousing homeless people suffering from severe mental illness. The demands of such work proved formidable and the trust-building involved can be time-consuming. But given patience and consistency, attention to expressed preferences, a discerning sense of boundaries and possibilities, and a secure stock of back-up resources—drop-in centers or other safe havens, medications, clinical personnel, affordable housing, willing landlords—many former street-dwellers have been coaxed inside by skilled outreach workers. Such skills can be taught, and formerly homeless persons have proven adept practitioners of the trade. Two difficulties arise: how to transfer the hard-won trust between outreach worker and homeless client to local service providers, who have often proven indifferent to the special needs and circumstances of the homeless poor; and how to compensate for the "eventfulness" of street-living foregone once a settled (and sometimes tediously "straight") life has been resumed.

Supportive housing couples an affordable place to live with needed services. It has been shown to be a flexible enough model to handle even traditionally "difficult" clientele, although substantial investment is needed to expand alternatives for those with both mental illness and substance abuse problems. Follow-up studies have shown most of these supportive housing placements to be remarkably stable, although continuing substance abuse markedly increases the risk of recurring homelessness. Noteworthy innovations include the delivery of appropriate services with adjustable levels of intensity; the development of "mixed" housing, where people with and without disabilities live side-by-side and sources of rent are more diversified; and contrived communities of formerly homeless persons living in self-governing settings. Additional resources are needed to replicate proven models and further innovation is needed to rectify the shortcomings of existing designs. Single-room-occupancy living, for example, raises awkward questions about the architecture of privacy and security when housing the elderly, mobility-restricted, or HIV-infected.

IV. PARENTS IN HOMELESS FAMILIES

About 40% of those who become homeless do so as parts of families, but families are a smaller proportion of those homeless at any given point in time. Most homeless families use shelters, both because shelters are more available to families than to other groups and because even poor shelters may be better environments for children than life on the streets. Thus, much that is known about homelessness among families comes from studies of families in shelter, sometimes with comparison groups drawn from the public assistance rolls or other sources. Patterns of shelter use reflect shelter policies and the other resources available to families, resources that are frequently not available to single individuals.

Before becoming homeless, many families have never had a house or apartment of their own; the vast majority have doubled up with others or moved frequently before turning to shelter. They have often lived in overcrowded or substandard housing. Families who have never had their own home, or who have lost one, frequently do not have the resources to secure a place on their own (including rent, security deposit, furniture, and other costs of moving in), and so stay in or move between shelter and the homes of families and friends. However, when given access to subsidized housing and income support, usually welfare, the vast majority of families who have experienced homelessness are able to stay out of shelter. These facts suggest that housing and economic conditions play a central role in family homelessness.

Although homeless families are diverse, some generalizations are possible. Parents tend to be young, with most studies finding an average age between 25 and 30. They tend to receive public assistance or be eligible for it, and have incomes well below the poverty line; many are from ethnic minority groups. Most are women and many are single mothers, both because single parenthood is associated with poverty and because welfare and shelter policies often separate fathers from their families. (The men then enter the population of "single" adults.) Homeless mothers' education and work histories are poor, but not appreciably different from those of mothers on public assistance. Family sizes are typically small, averaging two to three children. Bouts of homelessness are generally shorter than for homeless single adults, in part because more resources are offered to families.

As a rule, homeless parents have many fewer mental health problems than homeless single adults. Parents in shelter often report high levels of distress, but psychotic disorders are rare, and rates of clinical depression do not appear to be elevated before families become homeless. Levels of substance abuse are higher than among other poor families before families enter shelter, and are exacerbated while families are in shelter, but remain substantially lower than in studies of homeless single adults. Rates of hospitalization for psychiatric problems, although higher than among poor families generally, range from 4 to 12%—far lower than among homeless single adults.

Studies differ in whether they find parents in families that are homeless to have smaller or less helpful social networks than parents in other poor families. Certainly most families get material support, often a place to stay, before entering shelter. It is possible that differences in social networks arise only after families lose their homes. Many homeless mothers are victims of domestic violence, which is sometimes a precipitating factor in loss of a dwelling. Homeless parents are more likely than other poor parents, but less likely than homeless single adults, to have been abused as children or separated from their families of origin. [*See* SOCIAL NETWORKS.]

A large proportion of homeless parents (estimates range across studies from a fifth to a majority) also become separated from their own children, in a process that is not well understood. A majority of the children are with relatives, suggesting voluntary placement, at the initiative of parents or the request of family members, but substantial numbers of children are in foster care. According to model child welfare guidelines, homelessness is not by itself a reason for removing children from a family, yet one study found that nearly one-fifth of children in foster care in one state were there only because their families had no place to live. Shelters sometimes exclude older children or male children as well as fathers forcing families to make difficult choices between shelter and family integrity. Although risk factors such as maternal substance abuse and domestic violence predict separation of children from both housed and homeless families, homeless families are far more likely than housed families to lose children at every level of risk. Many single homeless adults are in fact parents who have become separated from all of their children. To the extent that separations from all children are more common for parents, especially mothers, with serious substance abuse or mental health problems, this may further explain why single homeless women have more troubled mental health profiles than homeless mothers with children.

Solutions to the problem of homelessness for families are primarily economic. Targeted efforts to provide emergency aid to keep families housed and transitional funds to move families into apartments of their own have shown promise in preventing homelessness. Although families who leave shelter on their own often return to doubled up situations that do not last, families who obtain access to subsidized housing and income supports typically manage to stay out of shelter. An exception may be the minority of homeless families with parents who abuse substances, who are more likely than others to have a repeated bout of homelessness even after obtaining sustainable housing. There is a clear need for programs that permit parents who abuse substances to undergo treatment while remaining with their children. While they are homeless, families need access to shelters that will house the entire family unit, without arbitrary limits on length of stay that often require families to move from place to place.

To emphasize the importance of housing is not to deny that many homeless families, like other poor families, would benefit from other services to enhance their mental health and quality of life. Housing, by itself, does not cure mental health problems, although it at least prevents homelessness from exacerbating problems or impeding their treatment. Similarly, mental health services, by themselves, do not cure homelessness. Housing programs for homeless families are often accompanied by case management services, but rigorous research is needed to demonstrate whether these specialized services result in greater stability or better mental health than do community-based services that are not associated with shelter or housing programs. Homeless families, unlike many homeless individuals with mental health problems, do not appear to require a lengthy process of engagement and building trust before services can be rendered.

V. CHILDREN IN HOMELESS FAMILIES

Virtually nothing is known about the mental health or development of children who are separated from homeless families and placed with relatives or in foster care, although the fact that separation from the family of origin in childhood is consistently associated with later homelessness may mean that these children are at special risk. Much more is known about the health, emotional, developmental, and educational status of children who are with their families in homeless shelters. Because children's problems only rarely put families at risk of homelessness, most problems children experience can be seen as consequences of poverty and homelessness, although some may also be due to characteristics of families. Most children in homeless families are fairly young, so that there are many more studies of preschool and elementary school children than of adolescents, but findings are reasonably consistent across age levels.

In a number of studies, children who are homeless have more health problems than other poor children, with differences more pronounced when medical records or doctors' reports rather than parental reports are the source of data. Infant mortality rates are higher for children born in shelter, and homeless children are more likely to be hospitalized, to have elevated levels of lead in the blood, and to experience delays in immunizations. Studies without comparison groups find high levels of a number of other chronic and acute health problems.

Children in shelters are also somewhat more likely than housed poor children to experience mental health and emotional problems—particularly depression and anxiety—as well as behavioral problems, including aggression, but both groups have elevated levels of problems relative to general population samples. This pattern has been described as a continuum of risk, with homeless children at greater risk than other poor children, who are in turn at greater risk than are middle-class children. Differences between adjacent groups on the continuum are not always large. In some studies, differences due to residential status (homeless versus housed) are not as great as differences due to the experience of maternal distress or recent stressful life events.

A similar pattern is evident for children's development. Again, many but not all studies find that young children surveyed while in shelter are delayed in social and motor development and language relative to other poor children, who in turn are delayed relative to children who are not poor. Early childhood education is protective for both housed and homeless children, but homelessness may impede access to such programs.

Homeless children of school age suffer educational impairments relative to housed poor children or general population samples. They have poorer school attendance and more often repeat grades. Homeless children also score lower on reading and on tests of educational achievement, and have lower expectations for future educational and occupational attainment. Even normative school transitions are times of stress for children, and frequent residential and school moves put housed children at risk for mental health and academic problems. The non-normative transitions associated with homelessness are likely to lead to greater risk. In addition, schools often fail homeless children, delaying enrollments or denying them special services, from remedial education to gifted programs, for which they are eligible. Homeless children are frequently stigmatized by peers and sometimes teachers.

Little is known about whether the problems of homeless children persist after they and their families leave shelter for more permanent housing, although several studies are underway. Research reported to date concerns children in shelter in the midst of an episode of homelessness, when both they and their parents are under a great deal of stress, and it is possible that emotional or behavioral problems demonstrated under such circumstances are transient. To the extent that families are homeless for relatively brief periods, and children are resilient, the effects of homelessness may not be enduring. However, some problems documented for homeless children may have long-term consequences. Elevated serum lead levels can have permanent neurological effects and absenteeism or poor performance in school can affect later class placement and eligibility for educational opportunities. For children who are separated from homeless families, the separations may also have long-term legacies for mental health.

Solutions to the problem of homelessness for children, as for their families, must include permanent housing. In addition, because stability is important to children's development, programs for homeless families should be arranged so as to minimize disruptions in living situations and schooling. Frequent forced moves, which are required when shelter programs place limits on the time that families can stay, are likely to be detrimental to children, particularly when residential changes lead to school moves as well. Federal law (the McKinney Act and its amendments) mandates that homeless children receive comparable school services to those provided to housed children, and that the child be permitted to remain in the school of origin or transfer to a school serving the new area, whichever is in the child's best interests. Full enforcement of the provisions of the law would help to minimize the effects of homelessness for children. Small investments of resources for transportation that permits continuity in schooling and for school supplies can also make a major difference for children of school age. Developmentally appropriate child care has major benefits for preschoolers.

VI. YOUTHS ON THEIR OWN

Youths who are homeless on their own are the least studied group of homeless people. They represent a distinct population with different problems and needs from youths who are homeless as part of family units. Researchers describe at least three categories of homeless children: runaways who have left home without parental consent; "throwaways" whose parents have asked them to leave or who subjected them to serious abuse or neglect; and "systems youths" who have been living in foster homes or institutional settings. The categories are frequently blurred, with many runaway youths reporting parental neglect and abuse or prior foster care or institutional placements. The reported numbers and characteristics of homeless youths, like those of other homeless groups, often vary from study to study, depending in part on how homelessness is defined and on how youths are sampled. For example, many adolescents—about 130,000 in 1988—run away from home for a night or two, but fewer stay away for long periods, or run away repeatedly and take up more permanent residence on the street. Youths sampled in shelters are approximately evenly divided by sex, but boys predominate among youths sampled on the street. Adolescents are more likely than other homeless groups to mirror the ethnic composition of their communities.

The poverty and shortage of affordable housing that play a large role in homelessness among adults and families play at most an indirect role in homelessness among American youths on their own. Welfare, or Aid to Families with Dependent Children, provides some income to families with minor children so that children in the United States rarely leave home for subsistence reasons; it remains to be seen whether new limits on the length of time families can receive welfare change this dynamic. Children who become separated from homeless families are most often placed with relatives or in foster care. It is not known whether any large number of these children later become homeless on their own.

Youths who are homeless on their own often cite abuse or family conflict as their reason for leaving, and indeed many come from families with various degrees of dysfunction. Across studies, about one- to two-fifths of children have experienced physical or sexual abuse and about two-fifths have been in foster care, often due to parental abuse or neglect. A Government Accounting Office study suggested that a sixth of homeless children left home because of substance abuse by a parental figure. Family conflicts can also occur over youths' behavior, including school problems, substance abuse, and sexual activity. Homeless gay and lesbian youths often report family rejection over their sexual orientation.

By the time they are recruited into studies, youths who are homeless on their own have a variety of mental health and behavioral problems; in one study a quarter reported one or more stays in a psychiatric hospital, and in two studies, half or more had been in juvenile detention. Few attend school. Unlike the case of adolescents who are homeless with their families, rates of mental illness in youths who are homeless on their own greatly exceed that in the general population, although the precise rates vary greatly from study to study, depending on both the sample and the diagnostic methods employed. Rates of depression, alcohol and substance abuse, posttraumatic stress disorder, and especially conduct disorder are all high, although the last diagnosis may follow from its definition: running away from home and skipping school are considered symptoms of conduct disorder, and subsistence on the streets may require other behaviors (e.g., stealing) that also qualify. Across several studies, a fifth to a half of homeless youths have attempted suicide. [See SUICIDE.]

Life on the streets is extremely dangerous for children, and hardly conducive to healthy development. There are few legitimate ways for youths with little education and few skills to earn money, and many engage in subsistence crime or subsistence prostitution—trading sex for food, shelter, drugs, or protection. Unprotected sex and intravenous drug use put youths at risk of HIV infection, so that it is not surprising that infection rates are far higher than in the general population, ranging up to 6% among older youths in epicenters of the AIDS epidemic. Many youths live in shelters, but an unknown proportion live in public places or "squat" in abandoned buildings, without proper sanitation or protection from exposure. Many are poorly nourished. Youths outside of shelters often form social groups that look after and protect one another.

Homeless youths on their own face even more formidable barriers to accessing services than do single homeless adults. Many have been victimized or exploited by adults, and mistrust service providers, so that engaging youths and building trust can be difficult. As legal minors, they may fear loss of control over their fate, being returned to a family where relationships are at best strained, or loss of confidentiality. Medical care is particularly problematic. Depending on their age and state laws, youths may not be able to give consent for their own medical treatment.

Despite the difficulties, a number of programs have succeeded in engaging homeless youths. Successful programs typically provide flexible, comprehensive, and coordinated services including outreach and drop-in centers that allow youths control over their contacts with service providers, residential options, educational and vocational opportunities, access to counseling or mental health and substance abuse services, advocacy, AIDS education and prevention. They work to promote independent living or reunification with parents or other members of the extended family, as appropriate.

BIBLIOGRAPHY

Baumohl, J. (Ed.) (1996). *Homelessness in America*. Phoenix: Oryx.

Center for Mental Health Services. (1994). *Making a difference: Interim status report of the McKinney demonstration program for homeless adults with serious mental illness*. Rockville, MD, Center for Mental Health Services Administration, US Department of Health and Human Services. DHHS Publication No (SMA) 94-3014.

Groth, P. (1994). *Living downtown*. Berkeley: University of California Press.

Jones, J. M., Levine, I. S., & Rosenberg, A. A. (Eds). (1991). Special Issue: Homelessness. *American Psychologist, 46*(11).

Lehman, A. F., & Cordray, D. S. (1994). Prevalence of alcohol, drug, and mental disorders among the homeless: One more time. *Contemporary Drug Problems, 20*(3), 355–381.

Liebow, E. (1994). *Tell them who I am*. New York: Free Press.

Robertson, M. J., & Greenblatt, M. (Eds.). (1992). *Homelessness: A national perspective*. New York: Plenum.

Shinn, M., & Weitzman, B. C. (Eds.). (1990). Urban homelessness (Special issue). *Journal of Social Issues, 46*(4).

Snow, D. A., & Bradford, M. G. (Eds.). (1994). Broadening perspectives on homelessness (Special Issue). *American Behavioral Scientist, 37*(4).

Homosexuality

Scott L. Hershberger

University of Kansas

Androgen   A family of hormones, of which the principle member is the sex steroid testosterone.

Anthropometric   The measurement of somatic characteristics such as height and weight.

Dizygotic Twins   Twins who share, on the average, 50% of their genes by descent.

Heritability   The proportion of observed variation in a trait that is due to genetic variation.

Lateral Preference   A preference for the right or left version of symmetrically appearing structures (e.g., hands, feet).

Lordosis   Female-typical sexual behavior in which the back is arched.

Monozygotic Twins   Twins who share 100% of their genes.

Probands   Target cases in a study.

Sexually Dimorphic   Traits that differ between men and women.

Twin Concordance   The degree to which two twins are identical on a trait.

HOMOSEXUALITY is sexual attraction to someone of the same anatomical sex. Closely allied to sexual attraction is fantasy: If someone has sexual fantasies about others of the same sex, then the fantasies are homosexual in content. If the person's sexual attractions and fantasies are primarily homosexual in content, then that person may be labeled a homosexual. Attraction/fantasy are not the only dimensions that could be used to define a person as homosexual but they are typically the most reliable. Physiological responses to erotic stimuli are one alternative but men and women respond differently to stimuli of different sensory modalities. Same-sex sexual behavior could serve as another criterion of homosexuality but personal and environmental constraints on sexual activity restrict its usefulness. Asking individuals whether they would self-identify as homosexual is another possibility, but this has the limitation that responses to this question are often based on social and political aspects of homosexuality and not sexual desire. Nonetheless, attraction/fantasy, physiological responses, behavior, and self-identity are significantly and positively correlated.

I. PREVALENCE

Magnus Hirschfeld in 1903 conducted what was probably the first survey of male homosexuality by mailing a questionnaire to 3000 college students in Berlin and 5000 metal workers. About 1 to 2% of the respondents indicated an exclusive sexual attraction to men. From 1938 to 1963, The Kinsey Institute for Research in Sex, Gender, and Reproduction conducted extensive interviews with more than 17,000 men and women. If sexual behavior is used as the criterion, the Kinsey study indicates that about 4% of men and 1% of women are exclusively homosexual throughout their lives. A 1994 British study of 19,000 men and

Copyright © 1998 by Academic Press.
All rights of reproduction in any form reserved.

women found that 1% of the men and 0.5% of the women were sexually attracted "mostly" or "only" to persons of the same sex or had sexual relations with someone of the same sex in the previous 5 years. A 1992 National Opinion Research Center survey conducted in the United States found that about 3% of the men and 1% of the women identified as homosexual. Other studies conducted in the United States and Europe find highly similar results: The prevalence of homosexuality, no matter how defined, is below 5% for men and women, and the rate is somewhat lower in women.

II. ORIGIN OF TERM

The term "homosexual" was first used in a letter by the German writer Karl Maria Kertbeny in 1868. He defined "homosexual" as referring to erotic acts performed by men with men and women with women. In this same letter, Kertbeny coined the term "heterosexual" to refer to erotic acts between men and women. The first public use of the term "homosexual" was by Kertbeny in a 1869 political tract. The first public use of the term "heterosexual" occurred in a 1880 book published in Germany by a zoologist, *The Discovery of the Soul*. "Homosexuality" was first publicly defined in the 1909 edition of Merriam-Webster's *New International Dictionary* as a medical term meaning "morbid sexual passion for one of the same sex." Although several well-known sexologists, including Richard Von Krafft-Ebing and Havelock Ellis had previously used "heterosexual" to refer rather neutrally to love between the sexes, the 1923 edition of the *New International Dictionary* first defined "heterosexual" as a medical term meaning "morbid sexual passion for one of the opposite sex." However, by the 1934 edition, both "homosexuality" and "heterosexuality" were given their contemporary definitions. "Heterosexuality" was defined as a "manifestation of sexual passion for one of the opposite sex; normal sexuality," and "homosexuality" was defined as "eroticism for one of the same sex." Most terms used to describe homosexuals have biblical, legal, or clinical origins, and are derogatory in meaning and intent; for example, "sodomite," "pederast," and "invert." One of the few exceptions was suggested by Karl Heinrich Ulrichs in the mid-nineteenth century. Ulrichs coined the Greek-

derived terms "urning" for male homosexuals and "urningin" for female homosexuals (and "dionings" for male and female heterosexuals). These terms never became very popular and eventually disappeared from use. The contemporary, nonclinical terms for homosexual men is "gay" and for homosexual women, "lesbian." The origins of "gay" and "lesbian" are rather unclear. Some have written that "gaie" (the feminine form of "gay") was used in sixteenth-century France to describe homosexual men, and first made its appearance in homosexual circles in the United States around World War I. Common use of "gay" started after World War II. The origins of "lesbian" are more obvious, inspired by the seventh century B.C. Greek female poet Sappho, who was born on the island of Lesbos. Sappho's poems frequently contained declarations of love for other women.

III. PUBLIC ATTITUDES

It would be fair to say that throughout a large part of modern history public attitudes toward homosexual behavior were negative, if not violent. Certainly in Europe and the United States, biblical injunctions against homosexual behavior influenced the creation of laws in which such behavior was dealt with severely. Nonetheless, it is true that within the last two decades, the general public's comfort with homosexuals as a group has increased. For example, a Gallup poll asking respondents for the acceptability of homosexuals in various professions has been conducted intermittently since 1977. In 1977, 68% endorsed the idea of lesbians and gays as salespersons, 51% endorsed the idea of lesbians and gays serving in the military, 44%, the idea of a lesbian or gay person entering the medical profession, 36%, the idea of a lesbian or gay cleric, and 27% endorsed lesbians and gays as teachers. By 1992, these percentages had risen to 82% (an increase of 14%, 57% (an increase of 6%), 53% (an increase of 9%), 43% (an increase of 7%), and 41% (an increase of 14%), respectively. However, comfort with a lesbian or gay person performing in a particular occupation is not the same as comfort with the idea of homosexuality itself. A 1973 National Opinion Research survey found that 73% of the respondents responded "always wrong" to the question: "Are adult homosexual relations wrong?" as opposed to only 19%, who responded that such relations were "never" wrong. By 1989, these percentages had barely changed: The "always wrong" response was given by 74% of the respondents (an increase of 1%) and the "never wrong" response was given by 22% of the respondents (an increase of 3%). Ideas concerning the malleability and etiology of homosexuality are not academic issues, but are important in determining how positive attitudes are toward homosexuality. A *New York Times*/CBS News poll conducted in 1993 asked respondents whether homosexuality could be changed and whether homosexuality is morally wrong. Among the respondents who endorsed the view that homosexuality is chosen, 78% indicated that homosexuality was morally wrong; among respondents endorsing the view that homosexuality cannot be changed, only 30% indicated homosexuality was morally wrong. Similarly, a Gallup poll in 1994 asked respondents to indicate whether people are born homosexual, homosexuality develops, or people prefer (choose) homosexuality. Respondents were also queried about various legal rights for gays. The most striking group differences were found for the item, "Are gay rights coming too quickly?": 28% of the respondents who indicated that people are born homosexual responded affirmatively; this number increased to 58% and 59% for the "homosexuality develops" and "people prefer homosexuality" endorsers, respectively. Obviously, people who believe homosexuality is biologically determined hold more positive views about homosexuals and homosexuality.

IV. PHYSICAL AND MENTAL HEALTH ISSUES

Several physical and mental health issues are of particular relevance for gays and lesbians.

A. Breast Cancer

There is a perception that the incidence of breast cancer among homosexual women is significantly higher than that of the general population. To date, no large prospective studies have been conducted to confirm this perception. In support of the likelihood that breast cancer is more prevalent among lesbians is the greater prevalence of risk factors associated with breast cancer in this group: Nonmaternity, late age of first preg-

nancy, above-average height and weight, high-fat diet, and high consumption of alcohol.

B. Sexually Transmitted Diseases (STDs)

STDs include syphilis, gonorrhea, nongonococcal urethritis, vaginitis, herpes, venereal warts, chlamydial infections, and yeast infections. Acquired immune deficiency syndrome (AIDS) can also be classified as an STD. The risk for acquiring an STD increases with the number of one's sexual partners. Gay men tend to have more sex partners than either lesbians or heterosexuals, and are thus at a greater risk for STDs. Just prior to the advent of the AIDS epidemic, the prevalence of STDs within the gay male community reached an all-time high. In the early years of the AIDS epidemic, as gay men became more conscious of the risks of sexual behavior, the incidence of STDs decreased. Although the reason for it are unclear, recent years have seen a renewed increase in the incidence of STDs. One popular reason given for this increase is the false sense of complacency among gay men based on recent advances in fighting AIDS. Whatever the reason, gay men should be aware that condoms, although extremely effective in preventing HIV transmission, are much less so in preventing STDs. [*See* HIV/AIDS.]

C. Weight

Evidence exists that lesbians may be more prone to obesity than heterosexual women. This evidence has come from studies directly comparing the weights of these two groups, as well large national surveys of lesbian health. For example, the National Lesbian Health Care Survey, completed by 2000 lesbians, found that being overweight was the most frequently reported health problem: More than one-third reported being overweight. If lesbians are more prone to obesity than others, the cause could lie in the stress and anxiety that comes with being a lesbian in this society. The cause could also lie in biological factors: The same biological factors that lead to female homosexuality might also affect weight. On the other hand, gay males have a tendency to be less heavy than heterosexual men. A significant weight difference between homosexual and heterosexual men is one of the most reliable group differences found in research comparing these two groups. As for women, the reason for the weight difference may lie with either socioenvironmental or biological factors. On the environmental side, evidence exists that gay men are more self-conscious about their bodies and hold themselves to higher standards of physical attractiveness than do heterosexual men. Biologically, the weight difference could simply be a result of the reliable height difference that exists between homosexual and heterosexual men: Several studies have found gay men to be shorter than heterosexual men.

D. Alcohol and Drug Abuse

Substance abuse is far more common among lesbians and gay men than among heterosexuals. Numerous studies have found more illicit drug use and alcohol use in the homosexual population. Alcohol consumption among gays and lesbians differs from the rest of the population in at least three respects. One, alcohol consumption is about equal for lesbians and gay men, whereas in the general population men consume more alcohol than women. Two, alcohol consumption does not decrease with age among homosexuals as it does for heterosexuals. Three, the higher rate of alcohol consumption among gays and lesbians is due primarily to an elevated rate of moderate drinkers; the prevalence of heavy drinking is the same for homosexuals and heterosexuals. Several reasons can be proposed as to why lesbians and gays take more illicit drugs and drink more alcohol. First, bars are an important meeting place within the homosexual community. Second, the challenge of a homosexual identity in a heterosexually dominated culture contributes to stress, which could find an outlet in substance abuse. Third, marriage and parenthood are two life events that are associated with a decrease in substance abuse, both of which are not available to most lesbians and gays. Fourth, drugs and alcohol could be used to overcome inhibitions or ambivalence about engaging in same-sex sexual intercourse. Obviously, programs designed to treat alcohol and drug abuse will have to be specially tailored to the needs of lesbians and gay men. [See ALCOHOL PROBLEMS; SUBSTANCE ABUSE.]

E. Domestic Violence

Domestic violence is not confined to heterosexual relationships: Some homosexual males abuse their partners, and some homosexual females abuse their partners. Unlike domestic violence in heterosexual relationships, abuse in homosexual relationships is largely hidden from society. A common emotion expressed by victims of domestic violence is shame; this shame is compounded when it occurs in the context of same-sex relationship. Shame over the abuse prevents the victim from informing the proper authorities; the fear that the victim's homosexuality may be revealed also serves to inhibit the victim from seeking help. The homosexual victim, whether rightly or wrongly, may also believe that the sympathy of others will be muted. After all, the victim muses, people can understand how a man can physically abuse a women, but how can one man physically abuse another, or a woman physically abuse another woman? Further discouraging the victim from coming forward are laws in many states that exclude domestic violence between same-sex couples. [See DOMESTIC VIOLENCE INTERVENTION.]

F. Victimization

The victimization of lesbians and gay men, through either verbal harassment or varying degrees of physical assault, is the most common kind of bias-related violence. More than half of the lesbian and gay male adult population have encountered some form of verbal harassment or violence in their lives. The physical and psychological well-being of many lesbians and gay men is compromised by this victimization. Adverse consequences include: Physical injury, behavioral and somatic reactions, interference in interpersonal relationships, self-blame, heightened internalized homophobia, disruptions of the coming-out process and diminished feelings of trust, security, and self-worth. Lesbian and gay youth are particularly vulnerable to the deleterious consequences of victimization. The prevalence of violence against gay youth is perhaps greater than for adults; in addition, there are additional stressors in the lives of these youth. Most prominent among these is fear of disclosing one's sexual orientation to family members. The victimization event is not shared with the family, and thus, the victim is denied emotional support from the family. Further, violence from the family against homosexual youth who do disclose their sexual orientation is not uncommon. This violence takes many forms; emotional rejection, verbal and physical abuse, and banishment from the home. Fortunately, more and more community services are being developed to assist these youths. In addition, laws concerned with bias-related crimes have been broadened in many states to include violence against homosexuals.

G. Suicidality among Homosexual Youth

Suicide is the third leading cause of adolescent mortality in the United States, accounting for nearly 5000 (13.3%) of the 37,000 annual deaths in the 15- through 25-year-old age category. Among adolescents, lesbian and gay youth have been identified as being at particular risk for suicide. Although it is difficult to assess to what degree sexual orientation plays a part in completed suicides, lesbian and gay youth report a high rate of suicide attempts. The prevalence of suicide attempts varies depending on the study (e.g., from 21 to 42% of the youth reporting at least one attempt) but every study finds a rate significantly elevated compared to the general adolescent population (estimates here range from 8 to 13%). Risks factors for homosexual youth include: low self-esteem, psychiatric symptomatology, difficulties in romantic relationships, family discord, difficulties with acceptance of one's sexual orientation, rejection by family and friends due to sexual orientation, physical and verbal victimization provoked by sexual orientation, and gender atypicality. These last four risk factors are probably largely responsible for the elevated rate of attempted suicides by lesbian and gay youth. [*See* SUICIDE.]

H. Mental Health

In 1973, homosexuality was officially deleted as a mental disorder by the American Psychiatric Association (APA) from its *Diagnostic and Statistical Manual of Mental Disorders (DSM-III)*. In its place, the APA created a diagnosis of "ego-dystonic homosexuality" to refer to those homosexuals who were unhappy about their sexual orientation. Ego-dystonic homosexuality was itself removed from the *DSM-IV* in 1987. Following the APA decision in 1973, other organizations, including the American Psychological Association, the American Medical Association, and the American Psychoanalytic Association, also decided that homosexuality should not be considered a mental illness. Most contemporary medical and psychological opinion views homosexuality as another normal

dimension of individual differences, with homosexuals capable of leading emotionally and medically healthy lives no different from that of heterosexuals. The beginnings of this change in attitude can be traced to at least two events. The first was the publication in 1948 of the Kinsey Report on sexual behavior in men. The high prevalence of homosexual behavior reported by Kinsey—and the rather liberal attitude of Kinsey toward homosexual behavior—did much to undermine the idea that homosexuality was a form of psychopathology. The second event occurred in the 1950s, with Evelyn Hooker's findings that the mental health status of an individual (as measured by the Rorschach inkblot test) was not associated with sexual orientation. Concurrent to these and other events was the rise of the gay movement within the United States. The political and social influence of lesbians and gays grew throughout the 1960s. In 1968, gay groups organized to initiate a campaign to pressure the APA to remove homosexuality as a disorder from the *DSM*, a campaign, as noted above, that was eventually successful. The success of the gay movement in removing the *DSM* is not meant to imply that all psychiatrists and psychologists changed their opinions concerning homosexuality. Most prominent among these individuals have been psychoanalysts Irving Bieber, Charles Socarides, and Joseph Nicolosi. In addition to equating homosexuality with mental illness, Bieber, Socarides, and Nicolosi have claimed success in being able to "cure" homosexuality. Most of the psychological community doubts the validity of the small amount of data presented by these psychoanalysts in support of their claims. The contemporary view held by most psychological workers is that a homosexual individual cannot be genuinely converted to a heterosexual individual, and legitimate reasons for wanting to do so are very limited in number. So-called "reparative therapy" does not work. As a result, the American Psychological Association in 1997 issued a resolution condemning the practice of reparative therapy. [*See* DSM-IV.]

V. BIOLOGICAL ETIOLOGY

Researchers have employed two broad, independent approaches to the biological etiology of homosexuality: neurohormonal and genetic. In one way or another, all biological approaches can be traced to either one of these views. The neurohormonal approach is motivated by the hypothesis that sexual orientation depends on the early sexual differentiation of hypothalamic brain structures. According to this view, homosexual men and heterosexual women have neural sexual orientation centers that are similar to each other and different from those of heterosexual men and homosexual women. Furthermore, the differentiation of these structures depends on prenatal androgen action. More generally, the neurohormonal approach suggests that male homosexuality may best be understood from the perspective of somatic feminization, and female homosexuality, from the perspective of somatic masculinization. Masculinization of brain structures in heterosexual men and homosexual women occurs because of relatively high levels of androgens, whereas feminization of brain structures occurs in the absence of sufficient levels of androgen. Androgens influence the development of the organizational structure of the nervous system. Thus, during adulthood, the neurohormonal view does not predict that homosexuals and heterosexuals will have different levels of circulating hormones. Rather, the theory predicts that comparable levels of the same hormones will have different activational affects based on different prenatally organized neural structures. The second, genetic approach has primarily involved the application of techniques from human behavioral genetics (a branch of population genetics), such as family, twin, and adoption studies, to investigate the degree of genetic influence on individual differences in sexual orientation. Recently, techniques from molecular genetics have supplemented the behavioral genetic approach.

A. Neurohormonal-Based Theories

Evidence consistent with the neurohormonal theory of sexual orientation has been obtained from nine areas of research: (1) the manipulation of the sexual behavior of nonhuman animals; (2) the examination of humans subjected to atypical patterns of prenatal hormone exposure; (3) the detection of neuroanatomical differences in the neural structures of homosexuals and heterosexuals; (4) the identification of cognitive and (5) anthropometric traits that differentiate homosexuals and heterosexuals that are also thought to be sexually dimorphic; (6) differences in lateral preference between homosexuals and heterosexuals;

(7) differences in birth order between homosexuals and heterosexuals; (8) gender identity atypicality of homosexuals in childhood; and (9) sibling sex ratio differences.

1. Sexual Behavior of Nonhuman Animals

Numerous studies exist examining the effects of prenatal patterns of sex steroid secretion on the development of sexually dimorphic behaviors in nonhuman animals. Nearly all of these studies support the idea that the prenatal hormonal environment influences predispositions toward certain sexually dimorphic behavioral patterns. The basic paradigm of most of these animal studies is to manipulate or change the prenatal hormonal environment so that it is more consistent with the hormonal environment of the other sex. Animals exposed to such hormonal changes frequently exhibit postnatal behaviors of the opposite sex. For example, male rats who have experienced prenatal androgen deficient hormonal environments exhibit lordosis, unusual levels of nonaggressiveness, and atypical play behavior. On the other hand, female rats who have experienced unusually high levels of androgen exhibit mounting behavior, increased levels of aggressiveness, and an avoidance of maternal rearing behaviors.

2. Humans Exposed to Atypical Patterns of Prenatal Hormone Exposure

The importance of prenatal sex hormones in nonhuman animals has encouraged researchers to examine their effects in humans. Leaving aside the complicated issue of whether animal sexual behavior provides a valid model of human sexual behavior, there remains the problem of how the prenatal hormonal environments of humans can be ethically manipulated. Researchers rely on experiments of nature, individuals whose prenatal sex steroid environment has been atypical due to some disorder. Congenital adrenal hyperplasia (CAH) has undoubtedly been the most studied. CAH is an inherited, autosomal recessive disorder of adrenal steroidogenesis, and effects about 1 in every 5000 to 15,000 births. CAH causes an excessive production of adrenal androgens; in females this results in full or partially masculinized external genitalia at birth. It is possible to treat CAH so that the excessive androgen production ceases and to surgically repair the genitalia. The question remains, though, whether

CAH females exhibit masculinized postnatal behavior due to the prenatal effects of atypical androgen levels. The consensus of a number of studies is that behavioral masculinization does occur in several areas. These include "masculine" toy preferences, high rates of a masculine gender identity, elevated rates of homosexual fantasy and behavior, and low rates of marriage. Thus the consequences of an unusual prenatal hormonal environment on the sexually dimorphic behavior of humans is consistent with that found in nonhuman animals.

3. Neuroanatomical Differences

Neuroanatomical differences between men and women in the hypothalamic region have suggested the possibility that such differences could exist between homosexuals and heterosexuals. In 1985 Swaab and Fliers reported that the sexually dimorphic nucleus (SDN) within the preoptic area (POA) of the hypothalamus was 2.5 times larger in men as in women and contained 2.2 times as many cells. In a later study, Swaab and Hofman found no difference in the volume or cell number within the SDN in homosexual and heterosexual men but did find a difference in the suprachiasmatic nucleus (SCN) of the hypothalamus: the SCN was 1.7 times larger in homosexuals as in heterosexuals and contained 2.1 times as many cells. In this case, an initially discovered sex difference did not generalize to sexual orientation differences. In 1989 Allen and colleagues studied sex differences in four cell groups within the preoptic-anterior hypothalamic area (PO-AHA): each was named the interstitial nuclei of the anterior hypothalamus (INAH) and numbered from INAH-1 to INAH-4. INAH-1 corresponded to the area Swaab and Fliers had named the SDN-POA. No sex differences were found in the volumes of INAH-1 (SDN-POA) and INAH-4 but sex differences were found in the volumes of INAH-2 and INAH-3: Both were significantly larger in males. LeVay attempted to generalize this sex difference in the INAH to homosexual and heterosexual men: In his 1991 study, INAH-1, INAH-2, and INAH-4 did not differ between the two groups but INAH-3 was significantly larger in heterosexual men. Thus, the INAH-3 appears significantly larger in heterosexual men compared to heterosexual women and homosexual men. Sex and sexual orientation differences have also been found in the anterior commissure (AC) of the brain. The AC is larger in heterosexual women and homosexual men than in heterosexual men. In addition, the volume of the central subdivision of the bed nucleus of the stria terminalis (BSTc) of the hypothalamus, a brain area known for its importance in sexual behavior, has been found to be larger in men than in women and male-to-female transsexuals; however its volume was unrelated to sexual orientation.

4. Cognitive Ability Differences

Findings that homosexual and heterosexual men differ on a number of cognitive abilities that also show differences between men and women supports a neurohormonal explanation of sexual orientation. A neurohormonal explanation would predict that homosexual men would show a pattern of performance closer to that of heterosexual women, and that homosexual women would show a pattern of performance closer to that of heterosexual men. Sex differences are well established for certain cognitive abilities, in particular the spatial abilities of mental rotation and spatial perception (with men performing better typically) and verbal fluency (with women performing better typically). Strong evidence also suggests that spatial ability and verbal ability are highly influenced by prenatal androgenization affects on brain lateralization. Table I summarizes the information obtained from 29 studies examining cognitive ability and sexual orientation in men, and Table II summarizes the information for women. On seven factors of cognitive ability, homosexual men performed better than heterosexual men: general intelligence, verbal intelligence, performance intelligence, vocabulary, logical reasoning, openness to experience, and perceptual motor speed. On four factors, heterosexual males performed better than homosexual males: verbal memory, mental rotation, spatial perception, and psychomotor skill. Most of these differences are consistent with predictions derived from sexually dimorphic abilities. For women, sexual orientation differences were found in favor of homosexuals for general intelligence, verbal intelligence, performance, logical reasoning, judgment, and perceptual motor speed. No differences were found in favor of heterosexual women. The differences found for the women are more difficult to interpret, in part probably due to the smaller number of studies examining women. They are certainly less consistent with a neurohormonal explanation; for

Table I Differences in Cognitive Ability between Homosexual and Heterosexual Men

Factor/Specific tests	Studies	N	Weighted effect size[a]
General intelligence/	1,2,12,15,16,20,25,26	745	.26*
Wechsler Adult Full Scale IQ	2,15,20,25	336	.78
General Technical and Aptitude Test	1	24	−.13
Peabody Picture Vocabulary Test	26	54	−.69
Raven's Progressive Matrices	16	141	.47
California Capacity Questionnaire	12	190	−.48
Verbal intelligence/			
Wechsler Adult Verbal Scale IQ	2,15,20,25	336	.92***
Performance intelligence/			
Wechsler Adult Performance Scale IQ	2,15,20,25	336	.47***
Verbal memory/	4,5,23,25	810	−.26***
Wechsler Adult Digit Span	4,5,25	752	−.30
Wechsler Memory Scale Story Passages	4	26	.60
Fargo Map Test	23	32	.16
Visual memory/			
Wechsler Memory Scale Visual Designs	4	26	.81
Vocabulary/	2,4,10,22,25,28	703	.29*
Wechsler Adult Vocabulary	2,4,22,25,28	453	.51
Quick Word Vocabulary Test	10	250	−.11
Logical reasoning	10,25,28	646	.20*
Wechsler Adult Similarities	25,28	196	.64
Wechsler Adult Picture Arrangement	25	100	.03
Wechsler Adult Picture Completion	25	100	.49
Alternate Uses Test	10	250	−.05
Judgment/	10,25	350	.09
Wechsler Adult Comprehension	25	100	.67
Wechsler Adult Consequences	10	250	−.14
Openness to experience/	7,8,9,10,11,13,18,19,21,27	1288	.45***
16PF Intelligence Scale	8,9,11,13,18,19,21,27	838	.25
Openness to Experience Inquiry	10	250	−.47
Openness to Experience Factor	7	200	.34
Verbal fluency/	4,5,6,10,14,23	1053	.71*
Animal Naming Test	4,14	102	.35
Controlled Oral Word Associates Test	4,5,23	684	.50
Remote Associates Test	10	250	−.02
Associational Test	6	17	−.03

Table I *Continued*

Factor/Specific tests	Studies	N	Weighted effect size[a]
Mental rotation/	14,22,23,26,28,29	478	−.67***
Primary Mental Abilities Spatial Rotation	14,28	172	−.41
Vandenburg and Kuse Mental Rotation	22,23,26,29	274	−.82
Everyday Spatial Abilities Test	23	32	−.76
Spatial perception/			
Piagetian water level task	14,17,22,23,26,29	434	−.28***
Spatial visualization/	3,4,6,14,17,25,28	531	.16
Differential Aptitude- Spatial Relations	14	76	−.25
Wechsler Adult Block Design	3,4,6,25,28	296	.34
Vincent Mechanical Diagrams	17	42	−.28
Wechsler Adult Object Assembly	25	100	−.05
Wisconsin Card Sort Test	6	17	−.03
Psychomotor skill/	24	124	−1.40***
Throw task	24	62	−2.08
Purdue Pegboard	24	62	−.72
Perceptual motor speed/			
Wechsler Adult Digit Symbol	2,3,4,14,25,28	438	.22*
General knowledge/			
Wechsler Adult Information	22,25,28	344	.25
Numerical ability/			
Wechsler Adult Arithmetic	25,28	196	.22

[a] Effect size $= \dfrac{\overline{X}_{Homosexual} - \overline{X}_{Heterosexual}}{\sigma}$.

*p < .05. **p < .01. ***p < .001. Significance tests reported only for factors.

Studies: 1=Druss (1967); 2=Evans (1992); 3=Robertson *et al.* (1993); 4=Saykin *et al.* (1988); 5=Selnes *et al.* (1991); 6=Zmachinski (1991); 7=Bernard (1982); 8=Bernard & Epstein (1978); 9=Cattell & Morony (1962); 10=Domino (1977); 11=Evans (1970); 12=Houston (1965); 13=Langevin *et al.* (1978); 14=McCormick & Witelson (1991); 15=Mohr *et al.* (1964); 16=Rabach & Ši'pova' (1974); 17=Sanders & Rossfield (1986); 18=Turner *et al.* (1974); 19=Visser (1971); 20=Willmont & Brierley (1984); 21=Duckin & du Toit (1990); 22=Gladue & Bailey (1995); 23=Gladue & Beatty (1990); 24=Hall & Kimura (1993); 25=Liddicoat (1961); 26=Tkachuck & Zucker (1991); 27=Tuite & Luiten (1986); 28=Tuttle & Pillard (1991); 29=Wegesin (1996).

example, a difference in mental rotation in favor of homosexual women would be expected but is not found.

5. Anthropometric and Related Physical Differences

Sexually dimorphic anthropometric and related physical differences are well established; these differences also appear to generalize to sexual orientation status. Table III summarizes the relevant information for men and Table IV summarizes the relevant information for women. The most striking and consistent results from Table III are: the earlier puberty of gay men, the greater leanness of gay men, and their shorter stature. Gay men also tend to have wider hips and narrower shoulders. Conversely, for women, Table IV indicates that

Table II Differences in Cognitive Ability between Homosexual and Heterosexual Women

Factor/Specific tests	Studies	N	Weighted effect size[a]
General intelligence/	25,26	147	.40*
Wechsler Adult Full Scale IQ	25	100	.75
Peabody Picture Vocabulary Test	26	47	−.35
Verbal intelligence/			
Wechsler Adult Verbal Scale IQ	25	100	.72***
Performance intelligence/			
Wechsler Adult Performance Scale IQ	25	100	.61***
Verbal memory/	23,25	130	−.22
Wechsler Adult Digit Span	25	100	.25
Wechsler Memory Scale Story Passages	23	30	−1.79
Vocabulary/			
Wechsler Adult Vocabulary	22,25,28	305	.30
Logical reasoning	25,28	364	.39***
Wechsler Adult Similarities	25,28	164	.33
Wechsler Adult Picture Arrangement	25	100	.44
Wechsler Adult Picture Completion	25	100	.55
Judgment/			
Wechsler Adult Comprehension	25	100	1.02***
Openness to experience/			
16PF Intelligence Scale	21,27	97	.08
Verbal fluency/			
Controlled Oral Word Associates Test	23	30	.03
Mental rotation/	22,23,26,28,29	352	−.11
Primary Mental Abilities Spatial Rotation	28	64	−.03
Vandenburg and Kuse Mental Rotation	22,23,26,29	258	−.02
Everyday Spatial Abilities Test	23	30	−1.11
Spatial perception/			
Piagetian water level task	22,23,26,29	258	−.08
Spatial visualization/	25,28	264	.17
Wechsler Adult Block Design	25,28	164	.39
Wechsler Adult Object Assembly	25	100	.06
Psychomotor skill/	24	32	.90
Throw task	24	16	1.17
Purdue Pegboard	24	16	−.27
Perceptual motor speed/			
Wechsler Adult Digit Symbol	25,28	164	.46***
General knowledge/			
Wechsler Adult Information	22,25	241	.11

Table II Continued

Factor/Specific tests	Studies	N	Weighted effect size[a]
Numerical ability/			
Wechsler Adult Arithmetic	25,28	164	.15

[a] Effect size $= \dfrac{\overline{X}_{\text{Homosexual}} - \overline{X}_{\text{Heterosexual}}}{\sigma}$.

$*p < .05.$ $**p < .01.$ $***p < .001.$ Significance tests reported only for factors.

Studies: 1=Druss (1967); 2=Evans (1992); 3=Robertson *et al.* (1993); 4=Saykin *et al.* (1988); 5=Selnes *et al.* (1991); 6=Zmachinski (1991); 7=Bernard (1982); 8=Bernard & Epstein (1978); 9=Cattell & Morony (1962); 10=Domino (1977); 11=Evans (1970); 12=Houston (1965); 13=Langevin *et al.* (1978); 14=McCormick & Witelson (1991); 15=Mohr *et al.* (1964); 16=Rabach & Ši'pova' (1974); 17=Sanders & Rossfield (1986); 18=Turner *et al.* (1974); 19=Visser (1971); 20=Willmont & Brierley (1984); 21=Duckin & du Toit (1990); 22=Gladue & Bailey (1995); 23=Gladue & Beatty (1990); 24=Hall & Kimura (1993); 25=Liddicoat (1961); 26=Tkachuck & Zucker (1991); 27=Tuite & Luiten (1986); 28=Tuttle & Pillard (1991); 29=Wegesin (1996).

Table III Anthropometric and Other Physical Differences between Homosexual and Heterosexual Men

Variable	Effect size[a] (Study #)
Age of first ejaculation	−.27 (1)
	−.40 (2)
Age of first masturbation	−.42 (1)
Age of puberty	−.24 (1)
Age of pubic hair development	−.09 (10)
Age of sudden growth onset	−.00 (10)
Age of height completion	.10 (10)
Age of voice change	.05 (10)
Biacranial diameter	−.39 (3)
	−.30 (4)
	−.58 (5)
Bi-iliac diameter	−.31 (3)
	−.08 (5)
Ratio of biacranial to bi-iliac:	−.68 (3)
((3 × biacranial) − (bi-iliac))	−.50 (6)
	−.58 (5)
Body mass (weight/height²)	.30 (7)
Fatness	−.18 (3)
	−.39 (6)
Height	−.07 (1)
	−.37 (8)
	−.01 (3)
	.28 (6)
	−.17 (5)
Ectomorphy (height/³√weight)	.74 (6)

Table III Continued

Variable	Effect size[a] (Study #)
Hand grip	−1.14 (6)
Muscularity	−.59 (6)
Penis length (erect)	.79 (4)
	.67 (5)
Penis length (flaccid)	.32 (5)
Penis width (erect)	.56 (4)
	.08 (5)
Foreskin coverage of penis	.14 (10)
Phimosis	.13 (10)
Meatus location	.10 (10)
Longest continuous erection	.23 (10)
Frequency of morning erections	.40 (10)
Amount of pre-ejaculatory mucus	.14 (10)
Weight	−.25 (1)
	−.64 (8)
	.13 (3)
	−.76 (6)
	−.06 (4)
	−.40 (9)
	−.28 (5)

[a] Effect size $= \dfrac{\overline{X}_{\text{Homosexual}} - \overline{X}_{\text{Heterosexual}}}{\sigma}$.

Study: 1 = Blanchard & Bogaert (1996a); 2 = Stephan (1973); 3 = Coppen (1959); 4 = Freund (1963); 5 = Mellan et al. (1969); 6 = Evans (1972); 7 = Siever (1994); 8 = Blanchard et al. (1996); 9 = Gettelman & Thompson (1993); 10 = Hershberger (1997b). Studies 1 and 10 were based on reanalyses of Kinsey et al. (1948).

Table IV Anthropometric and Other Physical Differences between Homosexual and Heterosexual Women

Variable	Effect size[a] (Study #)
Age of breast development initiation	.05 (4)
Age of growth completion	.07 (4)
Age of sudden growth onset	−.01 (4)
Age of pubic hair development	.05 (4)
Age of first menses	.06 (4)
Age of puberty	.04 (4)
Use of tampons for menstrual flow	.09 (4)
Amount of vaginal lubrication when aroused sexually	.26 (4)
When most arousable in menstrual cycle	.18 (4)
Regularity of menstrual cycle	.03 (4)
Length of menstrual cycle	.12 (4)
Age of menopause onset	−.01 (4)
Age of menopause completion	.01 (4)
Arm girth	1.37 (1)
Biacranial diameter	−.07 (1)
Bi-iliac diameter	−1.10 (1)
Ratio of biacranial to bi-iliac: ((3 × biacranial) − (bi-iliac))	.33 (1)
Body mass (weight/height²)	.53 (2)
Fatness	.06 (1)
Height:	.15 (1)
	.07 (4)
Leg girth	.20 (1)
Ectomorphy (height/³√weight)	−1.2 (1)
Muscularity	1.20 (1)
Weight	.57 (3)
	.12 (4)

[a] Effect size $= \dfrac{\overline{X}_{Homosexual} - \overline{X}_{Heterosexual}}{\sigma}$.

Studies: 1 = Perkins (1981); 2 = Siever (1994); 3 = Gettelman & Thompson (1993); 4 = Hershberger (1997b). Study 4 is based on a reanalysis of Kinsey *et al.* (1952).

lesbians enter puberty later and that lesbians are heavier, less lean, and taller.

6. Lateral Preference Differences

Lateral preference is another sexually dimorphic characteristic that is believed to be related to cerebral lateralization. In general, men are more lateralized and exhibit higher rates of left-handedness than women.

The primary model used to explain brain lateralization was developed by Geschwind and Galaburda. In this model, high levels of prenatal testosterone slow the development of the normally dominant left hemisphere. This allows the right hemisphere to become predominant, thus causing left-handedness. This is why more men than women are left-handed. The model predicts that homosexual women should also show elevated rates of left-handedness, based on the alleged prenatal presence of atypically high testosterone levels. On the other hand, the prediction for homosexual men is less straightforward. Elevated rates of left-handedness are also predicted for homosexual men due to the timing and amount of the testosterone production. It is hypothesized that initially gay men experience atypically high levels of testosterone (during the phase of fetal development in which cerebral lateralization occurs) and then later experience atypically low levels of testosterone (during the phase of fetal development in which sexual orientation is determined). Atypically high levels of prenatal testosterone are supposedly experienced because of maternal stress, a conjecture which has received mixed support. Handedness is not the only measure of lateral preference found to be related to sexual orientation. For example, Hall and Kimura report a bias toward leftward asymmetry in dermal ridges in gay men.

7. Birth Order Differences

A birth order difference between homosexual and heterosexual men is perhaps the most consistent and strongest research finding related to sexual orientation. In every study that has examined the issue, gay men are born later than members of the general population. A close examination of the data also suggests that the later birth of gay men depends only on the number of older brothers and not on the number of older sisters. A birth order difference has not been found between heterosexual and homosexual women. One hormonal explanation for the later birth of gay men implicates a maternal immune response to testosterone developed over the previous male pregnancies, compromising the sexual differentiation of the fetal brain, but this conjecture remains controversial. Psychosocial explanations for the birth order effect could be advanced as well; for example, fathers have less time to spend with later born male children when there are older male children present.

8. Gender Identity Atypicality during Childhood

Along with the birth order effect, the greater gender identity atypicality of gay men during childhood is the most robust finding in sexual orientation research. If hormones influence the development of sexually dimorphic behavior and sexual orientation, an atypical gender identity would be expected among homosexuals. Retrospective and prospective studies have shown that male homosexuality is strongly associated with childhood gender identity atypicality, including decreased aggression, decreased sports participation, the desire to be female, and being perceived as a "sissy" by others. Retrospective studies of lesbians produce similar results, with lesbians being perceived as being "tomboys" in childhood. However, the effect is significantly smaller for women. [*See* GENDER IDENTITY.]

9. Sibling Sex Ratio

In the 1930s, before the availability of techniques for karotyping the sex chromosomes, it was mistakenly suggested that homosexual males were genetic females. A prediction that followed from this hypothesis was that homosexual males would have more brothers than heterosexual males. Given the slight imbalance in the birth of males compared to females (106 males to every 100 females), a "genetic female" would be more likely to have brothers than a genetic male. Thus, the sibling sex ratio among homosexual men should significantly exceed the 106:100 ratio. Table V reports the results of studies which have calculated sibling sex ratios among homosexual men. Early studies found sibling sex ratios that significantly exceeded the population norm but later, more rigorously conducted studies using "normal" homosexual probands failed to find a difference between the ratios of homosexual and heterosexual men. Two contemporary studies which do find an excess of brothers among homosexuals; Blanchard and Sheridan and Blanchard and colleague sampled gender-dysphoric gay men.

B. Genetic-Based Theories

Genetic differences could also trigger differences in sexual orientation, perhaps by inducing differences in prenatal androgen levels or sensitivity to androgen. The evidence for genetic influences on sexual orientation is reviewed from (1) twin studies, (2) family studies, and (3) molecular genetic studies.

Table V Sibling Sex Ratio (SSR)

Study	Number of probands	Number of brothers	Number of sisters	SSR[a]	Number of controls	Number of brothers	Number of sisters	SRR
Jensch (1941)	2072	3794	3333	114/100	—	—	—	—
Darke (1948)	100	178	168	106/100	—	—	—	—
Kallmann (1952)	112	263	208	126/100	—	—	—	—
Lang (1960)	1777	2878	2287	126/100	—	—	—	—
Blanchard & Sheridan (1992)	193	353	270	131/100	273	337	288	117/100
Blanchard & Zucker (1994)	575	583	561	104/100	284	283	269	105/100
Zucker & Blanchard (1994)	106	86	88	98/100	100	83	67	124/100
Blanchard & Bogaert (1996a)	844	1027	927	111/100	4104	4669	4486	104/100
Blanchard & Bogaert (1996b)	302	376	359	105/100	434	496	481	103/100
Blanchard et al. (1996)	83	141	105	134/100	53	88	78	113/100

[a] Ratios are number of brothers:number of sisters.

Table VI Concordances for Twin Studies of Male and Female Homosexuality

Study	MZ		DZ		Ascertainment method
	N^a	%	N	%	
		Males			
Kallamann, 1952a,b	37/37	100.0	4/26	15.4	Word of mouth
Heston & Shields, 1968	2/4	50.0	1/7	14.3	Serial admission
Buhrich et al., 1991	8/17	47.1	0/3	0.0	Twin registry
Bailey & Pillard, 1991	29/56	51.8	12/54	22.2	Advertisement
King & McDonald, 1992	2/16	12.5	2/16	12.5	Advertisement
Whitam et al., 1993	22/34	64.7	4/14	28.6	Advertisement
Bailey et al., 1996	30/150	20.0	6/0	0.0	Twin registry
Hershberger, 1997a	4/16	25.0	2/8	25.0	Twin registry
		Females			
Bailey et al., 1993	34/71	47.9	6/37	16.2	Advertisement
Bailey et al., 1996	25/104	24.0	19/181	10.5	Twin registry
Hershberger, 1997a	6/11	54.5	2/8	25.0	Twin registry

^{a} The number of probands/the number of proband co-twins concordant for homosexuality.

1. Twin Studies

Table VI summarizes the twin concordance rates for homosexuality found in large sample male and female twin studies. In the case of males, with two exceptions (Hershberger; King & McDonald) the MZ (monozygotic twin) concordances are higher than the DZ (dizygotic twin) concordances. However, the concordances and implied heritabilities vary dramatically among studies. For example, Kallmann's results imply a heritability of 1.0, whereas King and McDonald's imply a heritability of 0.0. Thus, although the studies generally support a genetic contribution to male sexual orientation, the magnitude of the potential contribution varies widely. For females, all three studies imply significant heritability but again of varying magnitude. One possible source of variation among these studies is the method for recruiting subjects. It has been argued, for instance, that advertising for twins will more likely result in the participation of twins who are more alike than twins who are sample from a population-based twin registry.

2. Family Studies

Although less conclusive concerning the role of genes than studying the concordance of twins, sibling studies at least confirm whether a trait runs in families. Table VII summarizes the sibling concordances from a number of sibling studies of sexual orientation. Two findings are readily apparent in this table. First, ho-mosexual probands tend to have more homosexual siblings than heterosexual probands. Second, male homosexual probands are more likely to have male homosexual siblings than female homosexual probands, and to a lesser extent, female homosexual probands are more likely to have female homosexual siblings than male homosexual probands. In other words, male or female homosexuality may run in families, but usually not both. Two other studies have examined parental influence on offspring homosexuality. Bailey and colleagues found that the heterosexual and homosexual adult sons of gay fathers did not differ in the length of time they had lived with their fathers, the amount of contact they had with their fathers, how much they accepted their fathers' homosexuality, and the quality of the relationship with their fathers. These results argue against a psychosocial explanation for the development of a homosexual orientation. A second study, Golombok and Tasker, examined longitudinally the development of the children of lesbian and heterosexual mothers. No significant difference was found between the children of lesbian and heterosexual mothers in the proportion identifying as lesbian or gay as an adult.

3. Molecular Genetic Studies

The first molecular genetic study to address the location for specific genes for homosexuality was conducted by Hamer and colleagues in 1993. A linkage

Table VII Sibling Concordance for Sexual Orientation

Study		Heterosexual(HT) probands		Homosexual (HS) probands	
		HT siblings	HS siblings	HT siblings	HS siblings
		Male probands			
Henry (1940)	Brothers	——	——	93.3%	6.7%
	Sisters	——	——	93.8%	6.2%
Pillard *et al.* (1982)	Brothers	92.5%	7.5%	71.9%	28.1%
	Sisters	95.2%	4.8%	93.5%	6.5%
Pillard & Weinrich (1986)	Brothers	96.4%	4.6%	77.9%	22.1%
	Sisters	91.0%	9.0%	91.7%	8.3%
Bailey (1989)	Brothers	100.0%	0.0%	79.0%	21.0%
	Sisters	100.0%	0.0%	90.2%	9.8%
Bailey & Pillard (1991)	Brothers	——	——	90.1%	9.2%
Bailey & Bell (1993)	Brothers	95.8%	4.2%	91.0%	9.0%
	Sisters	99.1%	0.9%	97.1%	2.9%
Hamer *et al.* (1993)	Brothers	——	——	86.5%	13.5%
Hershberger (1997a)	Brothers	97.4%	2.6%	75.3%	24.7%
	Sisters	98.1%	1.9%	93.3%	6.67%
		Female probands			
Henry (1940)	Brothers	——	——	85.0%	15.0%
	Sisters	——	——	90.7%	9.3%
Pattatucci & Hamer (1995)	Brothers	97.9%	2.1%	93.2%	6.8%
	Sisters	98.8%	1.2%	89.9%	10.1%
Hershberger (1997a)	Brothers	98.7%	1.3%	83.8%	16.2%
	Sisters	99.1%	0.9%	58.8%	41.18%

between the distal portion of Xq28, the subtelometric region of the long term of the X chromosome, and a male homosexual orientation was discovered. In 1995, Hu and colleagues replicated the Hamer results for men—but with a lower effect size—and failed to find a relation with the Xq28 region and female homosexuality.

VI. PSYCHOSOCIAL ETIOLOGY

Two broad psychosocial approaches to the etiology of homosexuality are described: The psychoanalytic view and the learning theory view.

A. Psychoanalytic View

Freud's writings indicate a belief in two separate routes to male homosexuality. The first route begins during the phallic phase of development where the libido's attention is focused on the child's own body. Following the phallic phase, the libido's attention is admiringly redirected toward the genitalia of other males. Most male children leave this "homosexual phase" of development by turning their libido toward persons of the opposite sex. Adult homosexuals, however, are individuals who have never progressed beyond the homosexual phase of development. As Freud wrote in 1911, "Persons who are manifest homosexuals in later life have, it may be presumed, never emancipated themselves from the binding condition that the object of their choice must possess genitals like their own . . ." The second route to homosexuality suggested by Freud is better known. Having its origins during the Oedipal phase of development, adult homosexuals are individuals who never redirect their libido to females other than their mothers (in other words, resolve the Oedipal complex). As the future homosexual enters puberty, identification with the mother is retained by choosing as sex objects other individuals who resemble himself during the Oedipal phase (other males). Castration anxiety, provoked in childhood by paternal hostility or excessive maternal intimacy, is an additional important factor. Subsequent to this theory, Freud proposed in *Some Neurotic Mechanisms in Jealousy, Paranoia, and Homosexuality* (1922) a variant of the Oedipal theory of homosexuality. In the later theory, the future homosexual is still fixated upon his mother but now that person has a brother who becomes a rival for his mother's love. The future homosexual cannot harm his brother, so he represses and transforms his hostility in sexual attraction to the brother. Freud gave much less attention to the etiology of female homosexuality, most of which is contained in *The Psychogenesis of a Case of Homosexuality in a Woman* (1920). In this case study, Freud attributed a young woman's homosexuality to her wish to have her father's child. Instead, the mother (a rival for her father's affections) bore a child, instilling within the young woman a bitterness that lead to the rejection of all men. It is important to point out that Freud believed that homosexuals could not be "cured" (e.g., converted to heterosexuality). This was because homosexuality was not a neurosis but a perversion. Whereas a neurosis involves a repression and rechanneling of the libido (and thus susceptible to later, appropriate redirection), a perversion was an inhibition of sexual development. Psychoanalysis could only work with what the individual already had, not create something that never developed. The idea of homosexuality being a neurosis or a perversion is important because later, some American psychoanalysts relabeled homosexuality as a neurosis and thus "curable." This view is no longer held by a majority of psychoanalysts. Alternative theories in the psychoanalytic tradition have been developed. For example, Richard Isay has suggested that in the Oedipal phase, the prehomosexual boy does not develop sexual feelings toward the mother but toward the father. Knowing that the father is heterosexual, the boy cultivates feminine attributes to make himself an attractive sex object. Rather than succeeding in this, the boy's gender nonconformity evokes hostility in the father, often leading to rejection. It is this paternal rejection, Isay argues, that is at the basis of the poor self-esteem of many gay men. Isay does admit that the predisposition to be attracted to the father and the gender nonconformity may be inborn. Contemporary lesbian psychoanalysts have done much to remedy the relative neglect of lesbians in the psychoanalytic literature. For example, Leslie Deutsch has suggested that prehomo-sexual women fall in love with their mothers during the Oedipal phase, only to be rejected by their mothers for their seductive efforts. Adult homosexual behavior is viewed as an attempt to regain maternal affection. [*See* PSYCHOANALYSIS.]

B. Learning Theory View

Almost all learning theories have their origins in behaviorism; that is, behavior is determined by the schedule of reinforcements associated with it. Wainright Churchill was the first to propose that sexual orientation was determined by the pleasurable/unpleasurable events surrounding early sexual encounters. If early sexual encounters with individuals of the opposite sex were pleasurable, a heterosexual identity would be formed. Conversely, if early opposite sex sexual encounters were not pleasurable and/or same-sex sexual encounters were pleasurable, then a homosexual identity would be formed. A more sophisticated version of this theory was proposed by McGuire, Carlisle, and Young. It was not the early sexual encounter(s) themselves which provided the reinforcement that influenced sexual orientation but rather memories of these encounters during masturbation. McGuire and colleagues suggested that if masturbation provided the reinforcement that influences sexual orientation, then a homosexual orientation can be changed to a heterosexual one by substituting heterosexual fantasies. This suggestion initiated a number of conditioning paradigms to cure homosexuals: these included aversion therapy, covert sensitization, and in its most extreme form, electroshock treatment to disrupt the cognitive engrams developed by earlier conditioning. Studies examining the effectiveness of these conditioning paradigms for converting homosexuals to heterosexuals reach a uniform conclusion: No permanent change in sexual orientation ever results.

BIBLIOGRAPHY

Alexander, C. J. (Ed.). (1996). *Gay and lesbian mental health: A sourcebook for practitioners*. New York: Haworth Press.

Allen, L. S., Hines, M., Shryne, J. E., & Gorski, R. A. (1989). Two sexually dimorphic cell groups in the human brain. *Journal of Neuroscience, 9*, 497–506.

Bailey, J. M., Bobrow, D., Wolfe, M. & Mikach, S. (1995). Sexual orientation of adult sons of gay fathers. *Developmental Psychology, 31*, 124–129.

Blanchard, R., & Bogaert, A. F. (1996a). Biodemographic comparisons of homosexual and heterosexual men in the Kinsey interview data. *Archives of Sexual Behavior, 25,* 551–579.

Blanchard, R., & Bogaert, A. F. (1996b). Homosexuality in men and number of older brothers. *American Journal of Psychiatry, 153,* 27–31.

Blanchard, R., et al. (1996). Birth order and sibling sex ratio in two samples of Dutch gender-dysphoric homosexual males. *Archives of Sexual Behavior, 25,* 495–514.

Blanchard, R., & Sheridan, P. M. (1992). Sibship size, sibling sex ratio, birth order, and parental age in homosexual and nonhomosexual gender dysphorics. *Journal of Nervous and Mental Disease, 180,* 40–47.

Blanchard, R., & Zucker, K. J. (1994). Reanalysis of Bell, Weinberg, and Hammersmith's data on birth order, sibling sex ratio, and parental age in homosexual men. *American Journal of Psychiatry, 151,* 1375–1376.

D'Augelli, A. R., & Patterson, C. J. (Eds.). (1995). *Lesbian, gay, and bisexual identities over the lifespan.* New York: Oxford University Press.

Golombok, S., & Tasker, F. (1996). Do parents influence the sexual orientation of their children? Findings from a longitudinal study of lesbian families. *Developmental Psychology, 32,* 3–11.

Hall, J. A. Y., & Kimura, D. (1994). Dermatoglyphic asymmetry and sexual orientation in men. *Behavioral Neuroscience, 108,* 1203–1206.

Hamer, D., & Copeland, P. (1994). *The science of desire: The search for the gay gene and the biology of behavior.* New York: Simon & Schuster.

Hershberger, S. L. (1997). A twin registry study of male and female sexual orientation. *Journal of Sex Research, 34,* 212–222.

Hu, S., et al. (1995). Linkage between sexual orientation and chromosome Xq28 in males but not in females. *Nature Genetics, 11,* 248–256.

Isay, R. A. (1989). *Being homosexual: Gay men and their development.* New York: Farrar Straus Giroux.

King, M., & McDonald, E. (1992). Homosexuals who are twins. A study of 46 probands. *British Journal of Psychiatry, 160,* 407–409.

LeVay, S. (1993). *The sexual brain.* Cambridge, MA: MIT Press.

McGuire, R. J., Carlisle, J. M., & Young, B. G. (1965). Sexual deviations as conditioned behavior: A hypothesis. *Behavior Research and Therapy, 2,* 185–190.

Zucker, K. J., & Blanchard, R. (1994). Re-analysis of Bieber et al.'s 1962 data on sibling sex ratio and birth order in male homosexuals. *Journal of Nervous and Mental Disease, 182,* 528–530.

Hope

C. R. Snyder

University of Kansas, Lawrence

Agency The perceived capability to initiate and sustain movement toward a desired goal.

Appraisal A cognitive analysis of an imagined event.

Coping Attempts at lessening the physical or psychological pain that is associated with stressors.

Dispositional Pertaining to enduring characteristics that individuals display across times and in differing situations.

Expectancy A cognitive evaluation of the probability of attaining a goal.

Goal Any object, event, or outcome that is cognitively represented and desired by an individual.

Pathways A cognitive sense of being able to generate routes to an envisioned goal or goals.

Reliability Refers to the internal consistency of a measurement instrument, or the stability of scores on an instrument taken after a time interval.

State Pertaining to how one is thinking at a particular moment in time and in a given situation.

Stressor An event that is perceived as being the cause of physical or psychological pain.

Validity The extent to which a scale measures what it purports to measure.

HOPE reflects a positive cognitive set that people have about their future outcomes in life. Hopelessness, on the other hand, reflects a negative, often catastrophizing perspective about what is to subsequently transpire.

I. HISTORY

The history of attitudes related to hope has been mixed. Consider the most famous story about hope. According to mythology, hope was the only force remaining in Pandora's dowry chest after envy, spite, and revenge had been unleashed on the world. Unfortunately, the historical interpretation of this well-known tale is ambiguous. Was hope to be the antidote for these various evils, or was it just an illusion that would prolong human suffering? To this question, the Judeo-Christian tradition weighs in on the virtues of hope (the triumvirate is faith, hope, and charity).

In contrast to this positive view, other views have been quite damning. Such noted thinkers as Sophocles and Nietsche saw hope as a vehicle for stretching out human suffering. Plato called it a "foolish counselor," and Euripedes said it was a "curse upon humanity"; moreover, Francis Bacon served his doubts in a culinary analogy, "Hope is a good breakfast, but a bad supper." Indeed, for many writers, hope could not be discussed without labeling it as "false hope." Such views portray hope as whimsical and lacking in thoughtful analysis. Finally, hope has been criticized because of its definitional vagueness and difficulty in measuring.

Contrary to the negative historical perspectives, researchers in the last three decades have offered more positive views of hope. These models present clear definitions and cognitive bases for hope. Additionally, the research runs counter to the historical "false hope" view and suggests that hope offers several advantages.

II. DEFINITIONS AND MEASUREMENTS

A common dictionary definition of hope is that it is a "perception that something desired may happen." Although recent researchers probably would agree that these words can be applied to hope, there are varying perspectives regarding the exact nature of the construct. Generally, however, the writers about this topic suggest that hope rests on positive expectancies about future events. Conversely, hopelessness reflects the construal of the future in more threatening, negative terms. Various approaches to the conceptualization of hope, along with the corresponding measurement techniques, are described next.

A. Averill and Colleagues

Averill and his colleagues have used a questionnaire approach to ascertain the circumstances under which hope is appropriate. Their conclusion is that hope is a "relatively short-term response tendency, usually initiated and terminated by specific environmental conditions." In this regard, the persons surveyed indicated that hope is appropriate when a goal has some degree of perceived control, about a 50% probability of attainment, some significance, and socially and morally acceptable bases.

This constructivist approach is explicitly tied to an understanding of the rules that people espouse for using hope. As such, it necessitates knowing what people think about when and where it is appropriate to hope. In turn, measurement must reflect careful questioning about the appropriate circumstances in which hope can occur.

B. Stotland

Based on goal-related behaviors, expectancies, and social-psychological theory related to cognitive schemas, Stotland posited that the essence of hope was "an expectation greater than zero of achieving a goal." Within this perspective, hope reflects one's perceived probability of goal attainment. Similar to Averill and colleagues, Stotland held that the goal needs to have some importance ascribed to it before hope and the

subsequent potential for action become applicable.

For Stotland, hope helps to elucidate how antecedent events lead to a subsequent outcome. One means of measuring hope is to ask the person directly about his or her expectations of goal achievement. Because this is not always possible, hope typically reflects an inference made about another person's thinking in a given set of circumstances. More specifically, a higher level of hope is inferred by an observer in the degree to which the outcome is obtained in response to a set of antecedent events.

C. Snyder and Colleagues

Snyder and colleagues have theorized that goal-directed expectancies are made up of two separable, additive cognitive components. First, there is agency, which reflects a person's perceived capability to initiate and sustain movement toward a goal. Second, there is pathways, or the person's perceived capability to produce workable routes to reach goals. In more specific terms, Snyder et al. have defined hope as "a cognitive set that is based on a reciprocally derived sense of successful (a) agency (goal-directed determination) and (b) pathways (planning of ways to meet goals)." For goal-directed movement to occur, both the sense of agency and pathways are necessary.

With this two-component model of hope, a dispositional Hope Scale containing four agency, four pathways, and four distracter items has been developed (respondents indicate the applicability of each item on an 8-point continuum, see Table I). By summing the four agency and four pathways items, a total hope score is derived. The Hope Scale meets the requisite psychometric standards for self-report scales regarding internal reliability, and scores are relatively stable when retaken after intervals of several weeks. Additionally, the concurrent validity of the Hope Scale is demonstrated in several studies where it has correlated in predicted directions with other related self-report indices.

D. Overview of Additional Approaches

There are many other conceptualizations of hope that have appeared in the last three decades. For purposes of brevity, these approaches merely will be listed, along with a short definition of the premise that underlies each.

Table I The Dispositional Hope Scale[a]

Directions: Read each item carefully. Using the scale shown below, please select the number that best describes YOU and put that number in the blank provided.

$$1 = \text{Definitely False}$$
$$2 = \text{Mostly False}$$
$$3 = \text{Somewhat False}$$
$$4 = \text{Slightly False}$$
$$5 = \text{Slightly True}$$
$$6 = \text{Somewhat True}$$
$$7 = \text{Mostly True}$$
$$8 = \text{Definitely True}$$

_____ 1. I can think of many ways to get out of a jam. (Pathways)
_____ 2. I energetically pursue my goals. (Agency)
_____ 3. I feel tired most of the time. (Distracter)
_____ 4. There are lots of ways around any problem. (Pathways)
_____ 5. I am easily downed in an argument. (Distracter)
_____ 6. I can think of many ways to get the things in life that are most important to me. (Pathways)
_____ 7. I worry about my health. (Distracter)
_____ 8. Even when others get discouraged, I know I can find a way to solve the problem. (Pathways)
_____ 9. My past experiences have prepared me well for my future. (Agency)
_____ 10. I've been pretty successful in life. (Agency)
_____ 11. I usually find myself worrying about something. (Distracter)
_____ 12. I meet the goals that I set for myself. (Agency)

Note. From C. R. Snyder, C. Harris et al., *The Journal of Personality and Social Psychology,* © 1991, Vol. 60, p. 585. Reprinted with permission of the American Psychological Association and the author.

[a] When administering, the information in parentheses following each item is deleted, and the scale is labeled the Future Scale. The total Hope Scale score is derived by summing the four agency and the four pathways items.

Erickson and colleagues developed the Hope Scale as a 30-item index that taps a person's future goal orientation. In a modification of the Erickson et al. approach, Stoner developed a 20-item Hope Scale to tap more of the relational aspects of future expectancies. Obayuwana and colleagues introduced the Hope Index Scale as a 60-item measure of five themes (religion, education, perceived family support, ego strength, and economic assets) that supposedly reflect hopefulness. Miller developed a 40-item scale reflecting content about the continuation of a present positive state, improvement of that state, or the release from an aversive circumstance. Staats introduced a 16-item measure combining what a person wants and the associated expectations of attaining these desired goals. Nowotny posited that hope is activated when encountering stressful events, and, as such, the related 29-item scale taps the respondent's inner readiness, active involvement, spiritual beliefs, relations to others, perceived future possibilities, and confidence in desired outcomes. Herth reasoned that hope involves the realistic perception of upcoming positive outcomes, a feeling of confidence about one's plans to achieve goals, and the recognition of the importance of the interaction between self, others, and spiritual matters. Herth used this definition to develop a 30-item scale.

In contrast to the preceding approaches to the measurement of hope, Gottschalk developed a scale for analyzing hope based on samples of talk. Defining hope as the sense that favorable outcomes are forthcoming in one's activities, a rater makes judgments about the degree to which this motive is inherent in the speaker's words.

E. Beck and Colleagues

Beck and his colleagues developed the Hopelessness Scale as a brief (20-item) self-report index of the negative expectations that people hold toward their present and future. More specifically, hopelessness taps a lack of enthusiasm, a motivational propensity to not try (and, to give up if one does try), and a general lack of positive expectancies toward the future. This scale provides a reversed image of hope in that it is slanted toward the measurement of negative rather than positive expectancies. It is not the case, however, that hope and hopelessness are exact mirror images of each other. On this point, the magnitudes of the negative correlations between scores on the Hopelessness Scale and scores on hope indices generally run in the −.40 to −.50 range. The Hopelessness Scale has received considerable supporting research with regard to its internal reliability, stability over time, and validity.

F. Temporally Specific Approaches

Hope may operate as either a disposition or a state. Dispositional hope reflects thoughts that the person experiences over periods of time and varied situations; relatedly, dispositional hope is less malleable because of changes in time or life events. Contrary to this dispositional perspective, state hope refers to the thoughts that the individual experiences at a particular time and in a given situation; moreover, such state hope may change over time and should do so as a result of impactive interventions or life events. The approaches described previously typically have assumed that hope is a disposition.

Stotland theorized that hope occurs in particular situational contexts, and he was a proponent of conceptualizing hope as state expectancies that vary according to a given time and circumstance: however, he also allowed for the dispositional possibility, in that certain individuals may have higher or lower levels of hope across situations.

Using hope theory, Snyder and his colleagues have posited that there should be a dispositional hope that transcends times and situations (this is the basis of the Hope Scale; see Table I), and that there should be a state hope that reflects a given point in time and a particular situation. In this latter regard, they have developed and validated a brief six-item (three agency and three pathways) index of state hope in order to tap goal-directed cognitions at a given point in time. This scale (see Table II) meets the psychometric standards regarding internal reliability, and it has received construct validation support as the scores increase or decrease depending on perceived situational success in the pursuit of goals.

G. Age-Specific Approaches

In addition to the emphasis on the conceptualization and measurement of hope as applied to persons in their adult years, researchers also have given some attention to samples of people who are either quite young (i.e., children) or old (i.e., elderly persons).

To measure negative expectancies about one's self and future, Kazdin and colleagues developed the Hopelessness Scale for Children. The resulting 17-item self-report scale, for use with children 7 years of age or older, was patterned after the Beck Hopelessness Scale. This dispositional Hopelessness Scale for Children has received considerable research support with regard to internal reliability and construct validity.

Using hope theory as a basis, Snyder and his colleagues have developed and validated a brief, six-item (three tapping agentic beliefs and three tapping pathways thoughts) self-report dispositional measure called the Children's Hope Scale. This measure is applicable for children ages 8 through 16. The Chil-

Table II The State Hope Scale[a]

Directions: Read each item carefully. Using the scale shown below, please select the number that best describes *how you think about yourself right now* and put that number in the blank provided. *Please take a few moments to focus on yourself and what is going on in your life at this moment. Once you have this "here and now" set,* go ahead and answer each item according to the following scale:

> 1 = Definitely False
> 2 = Mostly False
> 3 = Somewhat False
> 4 = Slightly False
> 5 = Slightly True
> 6 = Somewhat True
> 7 = Mostly True
> 8 = Definitely True

_____ 1. If I should find myself in a jam, I could think of many ways to get out of it. (Pathways)
_____ 2. At the present time, I am energetically pursuing my goals. (Agency)
_____ 3. There are lots of ways around any problem that I am facing now. (Pathways)
_____ 4. Right now I see myself as being pretty successful. (Agency)
_____ 5. I can think of many ways to reach my current goals. (Pathways)
_____ 6. At this time, I am meeting the goals that I have set for myself. (Agency)

Note. From C. R. Snyder, S. C. Sympson et al., *The Journal of Personality and Social Psychology,* © 1996, Vol. 70, p. 335. Reprinted with permission of the American Psychological Association and the author.

[a] When administering, the information in parentheses following each item is deleted, and the scale is labeled the Goals Scale. Subscale scores for agency or pathways are derived by adding, respectively, the three even- and three odd-numbered items, and the total State Hope Scale score is the sum of all six items.

dren's Hope Scale has met the psychometric standards regarding internal reliability, temporal stability over time, and construct validity.

Hinds and Gattuso have designed and tested a 24-item index for use with adolescents. This Hopefulness Scale for Adolescents asks respondents open-ended questions about what is hoped; in turn, these responses (or goals) are rated subjectively by the researcher for the probability of actual attainment.

Turning to the other end of the age spectrum, Fry developed the Geriatric Hopelessness Scale on the premise that elderly persons often may perceive some pessimism and futility in projecting themselves into the future. This instrument contains 30 items covering topics such as diminished abilities, lost interpersonal worth, difficulty in recovering spiritual faith, and skepticism about being respected and remembered.

H. Gender Differences

The research generally has not addressed possible gender differences in hope, with one reported exception. This has been the work by Snyder and colleagues in which no differences have appeared between female and male adults as measured by dispositional and state indices of hope. Similarly, no gender differences have appeared with the Children's Hope Scale. These results, reflecting the scale responses of more than 10,000 adults and 1000 children, run counter to the stereotype that men are more likely than women to think in terms of acting independently and accomplishing goals.

III. RELATIONSHIPS WITH OTHER MARKERS

The relationships of individual differences in hope to other markers can be summarized in four areas: perceptions about one's life, coping, performance, and survival.

A. Perceptions of Self and Life Experiences

Many of the previously described models of hope implicitly assume that the ongoing experiences related to goal-directed activity should have an impact on one's emotions. More specifically, by experiencing positive movement toward a goal, positive emotions should follow; on the other hand, when experiencing difficulties or blockages related to the attainment of a desired goal, negative emotions should result. Research examining the emotional states of people under varying degrees of success in their goal-directed activities supports these speculations. Such research illustrates the pivotal role of the ongoing cognitive appraisal process in the pursuit of goals. In this regard, it should be noted that an important factor pertains to whether the probability of goal attainment is perceived as increasing or decreasing. Consider the individual with an initial 50% perceived probability of goal attainment.

When such a person perceives that the changes of goal attainment are increasing, this sense of gain produces positive emotions; conversely, when the chances of goal attainment are perceived as decreasing, the sense of loss results in negative emotions.

In contrast to the situationally induced changes in hope, it is also possible to examine the goal appraisal processes of people who are dispositionally low or high in hope. High- as compared to low-hope people appraise their goals as potential successes rather than as failures waiting to happen; not surprisingly, they also have a high perceived probability of goal attainment. More generally, these high-hope people are more likely to experience positive emotions than low-hope people.

B. Coping

The benefit of hopeful thinking is that people appraise their goals positively in normal daily goal pursuits, and this advantage is amplified when stressors are encountered. On this latter point, higher-hope people are not overwhelmed by situational stressors, and they expect that blockages sometimes will be encountered on their way to goals. Part of the superior coping of higher-hope persons may relate to their capabilities in producing alternative pathways to their goals.

Other coping strategies of higher-hope people include a propensity to look outward and problem solve, to call upon helpful social support networks, to laugh at themselves and their circumstances when they get stuck, to exercise, and to take care of themselves physically. There is evidence that higher- as compared to lower-hope persons also experience less burnout in a stressful job and have recovered better from spinal cord injuries. [*See* Burnout; Coping with Stress.]

C. Performance

Research on dispositional and state measures of hope consistently reveals that higher levels of this cognitive set relate to successful outcomes. For example, college students who score higher in hope achieve better grades, and this relationship holds even when the influences of previous school achievement are statistically removed. It should be emphasized that hope scale scores of adults and children have displayed only small positive correlations with measures of intelligence.

Other research has shown that dispositional hope

as measured by the Hope Scale can significantly predict athletic performance (female college track and field events), and this predictive relationship remains even when the natural athletic ability (as measured by coaches' estimates) is statistically removed.

From these results, it can be said that dispositional hope is not synonymous with intellectual capability, previous history of academic achievement, or athletic ability. Nevertheless, elevated hope is positively related to markers of academic and athletic success.

D. Survival

Although hope yields the benefits described previously, it may be surprising that it relates to the very survival of people. When hope dies, so, literally, do people. For an excellent description of the process of giving up hope and dying shortly thereafter, Victor Frankl's classic, *Man's Search for Meaning*, gives vivid and horrific examples. Based on his years in Nazi concentration camps, Frankl describes a recurrent pattern in which a prisoner who finally loses all hope would give up and die.

Research conducted with adults and children corroborates the link between hope and death. In particular, greater hopelessness, as measured by the Hopelessness Scale, has been related to the intention for and completion of suicides. Furthermore, although hopelessness and depression are positively correlated, hopelessness more strongly predicts suicidal intent. Similar findings have emerged with children, where children with higher scores on the Hopelessness Scale for Children have exhibited increased ideation about and attempts at suicide. Likewise, although the hopelessness in children relates to elevated depression, it is hopelessness that tends to be more robust in predicting suicidal tendencies.

IV. DEVELOPMENTAL PROCESSES

Having examined the individual differences in hope and the repercussions of those individual differences on various outcomes in life, we now turn to the issue of how the normal developmental processes can contribute to hopeful thinking. In order to build the case of how hope develops, we move from the infant/toddler through the adolescence stages and review those

events that can undermine the normal development of hopeful thought.

A. Infant to Toddler Years

The newborn is often portrayed as being quite helpless, and to some extent this is true. It is also the case, however, that the newborn is exquisitely equipped to acquire the essential components of hopeful thought. From birth, infants are using their senses to form images of shapes. Raw sensation is quickly supplanted by perception when a particular input is recognized in the infant's mind. This process of learned "What's out there" forms the basis for later selection of certain objects in the world as being more desired than others. For example, the mother's face is recognized very early; this can be conceptualized as the emergence of goals in the sense that the infant is desirous of perceiving and interacting with mom.

Infants also learn to link events temporally in their early months. That is to say, the infant learns that one thing seems to be followed by another, and, as such, events co-occur. By the end of their first year, babies can anticipate events and engage in intentional acts. Among such actions, babies begin to point at recognized objects in their environment (e.g., a toy, food, dad). Babies must learn "what goes with what" as a matter of survival; they attend to those persons and things in their environments that will fulfill their biological (food) and psychological (nurturance/interaction) needs. It is instructive, in this regard, to examine the utterances of toddlers. Their talk is full of statements about what they want and what they can do. By age 2 to 3, therefore, the child has been socialized by caregivers to articulate his or her expectations about desired outcomes or objects. In short, the toddler has received instruction by those in the surrounding environment about how to hope for future outcomes. Indeed, the foundation of hopeful thinking has been laid by toddlerhood.

Additional lessons related to hopeful thinking in toddlerhood relate to giving the child encouragement and instruction about how to overcome the obstacles that she or he may encounter. Likewise, the baby in the first 2 years typically establishes a secure attachment to a caregiver. Such positive attachments provide a context of empowerment so that the child learns how to work to meet goals and how to do this in concert with other people so that expectations can be fulfilled.

B. Preschool Years

From ages 3 through 6, the basic lessons in hopeful thinking are solidified. Although the brain grows from 50 to 90% of its adult weight, it is instructive to examine how the thoughts in these young minds also are growing. During this period, the child's use of language increases from a vocabulary of approximately 50 words to 10,000 words. Because language provides the structure for describing reality and communicating with others about this reality, it is the very medium through which hopeful thinking operates. In other words, language provides the vehicle for describing what the child wants, and it is used to help the child achieve his or her goals in the social context.

A second major developmental stage during the preschool years is the transition away from the totally egocentric perspective of the toddler. More specifically, the preschool child learns to understand and take the perspective of other people. By understanding the viewpoints of others, hopeful thinking is facilitated because the child's personal desires must be considered in the context of those other important people in the preschooler's environment.

C. Middle Years

From ages 7 through 12, children are expanding in both physical size and breadth of activities. In underpinning this newly acquired independence, hopeful thinking progresses on two major fronts. First, during the middle years, a variety of mental boosters become operative. For example, the child expands his or her storehouse of knowledge, which can be used for goal pursuit activities. Through actual physical exploration, or through reading, the child's knowledge base grows. In this latter regard, contrary to the preschool years during which the child is learning to read, in the middle years, the child is reading to learn. Additionally, the child's memory capacity expands during these middle years.

A second set of hope-related lessons that burgeon during the middle years involves the fact that the child continues to learn how to balance his or her desires within the social context. Expanding on the lessons that begin in the preschool years, the child in the middle years builds interpersonal skills related to communication, conflict resolution, reciprocity, and so on. These latter hope-related processes trade on the notion that hopeful expectancies often must be negotiated in the context of important other people in the child's environment.

D. Adolescent Years

During the adolescent years, ages 13 through 18, there are two sets of hope-related issues that are tackled. First, the adolescent gains a more sophisticated understanding and set of experiences related to relationships and sexual expression. In fact, the garnering of relationships and sexual expression become goals that will extend well into the subsequent adult years. Part of the high-hope perspective, and one that is born out by research, is the establishment of effective interpersonal relationships (both those with and without a sexual component).

The second hope-related process during adolescence is the solidifying of personal identity. Although the younger child may often act differently from situation to situation, the adolescent begins to resolve this personal sense of contradiction and moves toward a sense of coherence about who and what she or he is. It is difficult, for example, to engage in consistent goal-directed thought when one is ambiguous about one's values and desires. To establish a firm sense of self, however, enables the adolescent to have a platform from which to launch goal-directed, hopeful thinking.

E. Factors Undermining Hopeful Thinking

There are several factors that appear to negate or lessen the instillation of hopeful thinking as described. These hope-negating events can occur at any time in the developmental sequence, but generally the effects are more damaging when encountered earlier in the child's life and when these forces continue over longer periods of time.

If the child has experienced a caregiving environment that is neglectful or abusive, the bases of hopeful thinking are not established in the early infant/toddler period; moreover neglect or abuse occurring later in the developmental sequence may serve to squelch whatever hopeful thinking may have been established.

The loss of one's parents can also diminish hopeful thinking. This can come either through the death of a parent or a divorce that results in separation from one caregiver. What can happen in such losses is that the child not only loses the nurturance of a caregiver who can model hopeful thinking, but that child also is left with questions about the viability of interpersonal relationships.

Another set of hope-reducing forces pertains to caregiving environments where there are no consistent boundaries or any consistency in applying the rules. Likewise, the learning of goal-pursuit thinking can be undercut by caregivers who do not give support and reinforcement to the child's efforts.

V. MEANS OF INCREASING HOPE

In this section, the various approaches for nurturing hope are explored. For purposes of clarity, these interventions will be examined separately for children and adults, with a closing section on how hope is the process that is common to all psychotherapy techniques.

A. In Children

To explore the means by which the hope of children can be increased, it is helpful to break down the overall hope process into the components of goal thinking, agentic thought, and pathways cognitions. This section gives suggestions for improving a child's hope in the context of each of these three components.

First, for goal-related thinking, whatever a caregiver can do to aid the baby in identifying and naming objects in the surrounding environment helps to set the stage for goal thinking. Pertinent to this issue, it has been suggested that helping the young child to use specific words to pinpoint a desired object is useful. This by necessity means that the caregiver must carefully attend to the child so as to be sensitive to his or her desires. Relatedly, it is helpful if the caregiver shows an interest in the child's goals and talks with him or her about these goals. If a child appears to too quickly settle on one desired goal, the caregiver may want to teach the child how to consider several goals first before settling on one. Furthermore, because high-hope children appear to prefer goals that are difficult

but not impossible to attain, the caregiver should try to have children seek out stretch goals that necessitate some effort. In this process, a sense of ownership is produced if the children make their own decisions about desired goals. Finally, goal-making thought should be reinforced by praise from the caregivers.

Second, agentic thinking about the child's capacity to initiate and sustain action toward a desired goal can be facilitated in several ways. One way to encourage agentic thoughts is to remind children that they are responsible for making something positive happen. Likewise, praise for the child when showing determination to reach his or her goals is beneficial. The caregiver can teach children to accentuate their strengths and to minimize weaknesses. Likewise, the teaching of positive self-talk has been advocated, along with lessons about how roadblocks are a normal part of life and are not something that needs to be demoralizing. In this latter regard, caregivers can tell stories from their own lives about how they maintained their determination in the face of adversity; similarly, stories can be read to or read by the child to bring to life how other children have kept energized. Even more impactive may be when the child is reminded of previous difficult circumstances in which he or she remained motivated for a desired goal. Because higher-hope children view barriers as challenges rather than as defeats, this lesson also may be worth imparting. Also, showing a child how to have a good laugh, especially when she or he is stuck, can improve mental willpower. And, because agentic thinking may be drained for physical reasons, it is important to make certain that children have the proper dietary nourishment, exercise, and rest.

Third, pathways thinking toward desired goals can be promoted by varying means. For babies and toddlers, it is important to show them how causality works and to use nearby objects (e.g., blocks, drums, pull toys) in order to vivify these lessons. As these lessons in causality are being taught to toddlers, have them verbalize in their own words what is happening. Songs and stories, including nursery rhymes, offer excellent examples of how words go in a sequence and how one thing leads to another. As children tell or read stories, attend to how they are conceptualizing causality and talk with them about this process. Because pathways thinking may be related to actual skills, it is important to build a child's skill bases in athletics, scholastics, and social matters. To help children cope with the various situations they are to encounter, teach them mental scripts about what they are to do in given situations. Another approach that may be helpful is to instruct the child about how to break a long route to a desired goal into smaller steps that are more easily understood and achieved. Borrowing from a technique that high-hope children appear to use, teach them that those instances when they do not attain their goals are related to the fact that they used an ineffective strategy; this has the added advantage of disabusing the child of any incorrect attributions that she or he may be making about lacking the requisite talent or ability. Finally, throughout the developmental sequence, it may be helpful if caregivers talk with their children about their plans for attaining specific goals.

Although the means for producing increases in hope have previously been broken down into goal-related cognitions, agentic thinking, and pathways thoughts, there are three processes that cut across these components. The first is the forming and continuation of a firm attachment by the child to a caregiver. This means that at least one caregiver should spend large amounts of time with and attend to the child. The hopeful child needs to feel connected and able to communicate with an adult. A second common process that facilities all aspects of hopeful thinking is discipline. Forming a firm attachment also means being a consistent and dependable source of guidance for the child. Boundaries of acceptable behavior are important, and yet this should be done in a loving atmosphere. Finally, the caregiver serves as a model for hopeful thinking. Children watch and learn from their caregivers, and therefore parents need to let their children observe them as they pursue their adult goals. Part of this may be a joint project where the child and adult work together for a goal. In summary, forming an attachment, providing consistent boundaries, and modeling are common processes that adult caregivers need to provide to children in order to foster hopeful thinking.

B. In Adults

As was the case for the previous section dealing with the means of increasing hope in children, in this section the processes for raising hope are examined as they pertain to goal-related thoughts, agentic cognitions, and pathways thoughts.

First, on the topic of improving the goal-related thinking of adults, it is helpful to make certain that the person is setting a goal because it is something he or she wants, rather than what others want for this person. Likewise, anything that can be done to sensitize the person to the fact that he or she is constantly making decisions about important goals serves to bring this process more into awareness. Goal-setting thoughts sometimes are so automatic that people do not process them with the care that is warranted. Given that high-hope adults have goals in the differing arenas in their lives, it is often helpful to facilitate the person's production of an array of goals. It is also hope-inducing to set goals at levels that stretch one's talents, and therefore the person may want to set new goals at a somewhat higher level than previous ones in the same arena. Furthermore, teaching the person to prioritize goals from the least to the most important serves to clarify where his or her efforts should be spent. Along with this lesson, the person needs to specify his or her important goals in terms of concrete markers and do whatever is necessary to focus a majority of time on the important goals. Assuming that the person has made the aforementioned changes in goal-setting, a pivotal lesson is to make certain that sufficient time is allotted to spend on the important goals. This may mean that the person must set up his or her schedule so as not to be interrupted by outside demands that distract attention from the important goals. [*See* INTRINSIC MOTIVATION AND GOALS.]

Second, to enhance the agentic thinking of adults, one approach is to promote positive self-talk that can be used during normal times and especially during difficult times. In this latter regard, by anticipating that one will run into blockages in goal pursuit activities, the person may be better prepared to remain determined when actual adversity hits. Borrowing from the thought patterns of high-hope persons, it often may be uplifting to think of problems as challenges. Furthermore, because people sometimes forget what they have endured during previous difficult periods, remembering such previous experiences may provide a lift to persevere in the present situation. Cultivating the ability to laugh at one's circumstances, especially when one is experiencing a blockage of some sort, can be energizing. Learning to enjoy the process of moving toward one's goals, and not just focusing solely on goal attainment, also can be uplifting. Another tip from high-hope people is that a sense of agency can be renewed when one switches from a truly blocked goal to a new or substitute goal that is more reachable. Furthermore, monitoring and controlling one's eating and drinking patterns, particularly the avoidance of caffeine-, nicotine-, and alcohol-laden products, can provide a boost. Likewise, eating properly, resting, and exercising are effective means of improving one's sense of goal-directed energy. Finally, given the advances that have been made in producing antidepressant medications, seeing a physician about an appropriate prescription drug may provide another means of raising one's sense of agency. [See FOOD, NUTRITION, AND MENTAL HEALTH.]

Third, there are many approaches for enhancing one's pathways thinking. One such technique is to break a long-range goal down into smaller, more workable subgoals and to begin working on the first, most easily reached subgoal. In this regard, high-hope persons use a mental road map for detailing the step-by-step route to an end goal. Sometimes, it is useful to plan for alternative routes to get where one wants to go before setting out to attain the goal. In this way, the person may be better prepared should one of the routes prove to be impassable. By using mental rehearsals, the person may practice how to move toward desired goals, and in doing such mental rehearsals, the person can use the technique of anticipating blockages. When persons find that a given route to a goal does not work, they need to make attributions that they did not use the best strategy, rather than blame themselves and their lack of talent. This latter technique makes it more likely that a person may adaptively begin to search for another route, rather than give up. As was the case for children, if an adult can profit by learning a particular skill that will facilitate a desired goal pursuit, that person should try to acquire the necessary skill. On a similar theme, the person should realize that it is acceptable to ask for directions or aid in reaching a desired goal. Sometimes self-reliance can stifle the full search for pathways to goals. Finally, because high-hope people report that friendships are a powerful source of guidance for reaching goals, whatever can be done to enhance the adult's propensity to make and sustain friendships is advisable. Friendships offer the additional advantages

of helping the person to form appropriate goals and to remain energized in the pursuit of those goals.

C. In Psychotherapy

Survey results reveal that Americans view hope as being linked to action toward goals through organized, effortful thought and subsequent follow-through. Indeed, as noted previously, elevated hope appears to be related to enhanced performances. Laboratory and applied research also indicates that changes toward enhanced hope result in more favorable outcomes in a variety of settings, including psychotherapy. In fact, it has been argued that the positive effects of psychotherapy are basically mediated by increases in hope. For example, persons who are judged to have improved as compared with those who have not improved in psychotherapy, have increased their sense of positive goal-related expectancies. Whatever the techniques and interventions associated with a given psychotherapeutic approach may be, therefore, all may share a common theme in that they enhance the hope of clients. For the reader who is interested in the specific psychotherapy techniques that induce hope, most any book or manual by the proponents of the particular approaches will give detailed descriptions.

VI. CONCLUSIONS

The emerging viewpoint among researchers is that hope is not a vague, philosophical notion that is impossible to measure. Indeed, several psychometrically sound and valid self-report measures of hope are available.

Contrary to historical doubts about the usefulness of hope, relevant recent research suggests that higher hope is related to greater satisfaction in life, enhanced coping, and positive performance outcomes; conversely, hopelessness is related to ideations about and completions of suicide.

The inculcation of hopeful thinking is inherent in the developmental sequence of learning to master one's environment; moreover, although there are exceptions related to neglect, abuse, loss of parent, and inconsistency in caregiving, hopeful thinking typically is established by toddlerhood and reinforced throughout the subsequent years of childhood.

With regard to goal cognitions, as well as to the agentic and pathways thinking that are related to those goals, there are specific suggestions about how each of these components can be instilled to improve the overall hope in both children and adults. Finally, it can be argued that hopeful thinking underlies the effectiveness of psychotherapeutic approaches that may vary in technique.

BIBLIOGRAPHY

Averill, J. R., Catlin, G., & Chon, K. K. (1990). *Rules of hope.* New York: Springer-Verlag.

Beck, A. T., Brown, G., Berchick, R. J., Stewart, B. L., & Steer, R. A. (1990). Relationship between hopelessness and ultimate suicide: A replication with psychiatric outpatients. *American Journal of Psychiatry, 147,* 190–195.

Beck, A. T., Weissman, A., Lester, D., & Trexler, L. (1974). The measurement of pessimism: The Hopelessness Scale. *Journal of Consulting and Clinical Psychology, 42,* 861–865.

Dweck, C. S. (1986). Motivational processes affecting learning. *American Psychologist, 41,* 1040–1048.

Erickson, E., Post, R., & Paige, A. (1975). Hope as a psychiatric variable. *Journal of Clinical Psychology, 31,* 324–330.

Farran, C. J., Herth, K. A., & Popovich, J. M. (1995). *Hope and hopelessness: Critical clinical constructs.* Newbury Park, CA: Sage.

Frank, J. D., & Frank, J. B. (1991). *Persuasion and healing.* Baltimore, MD: Johns Hopkins University Press.

Frankl, V. E. (1992). *Man's search for meaning: An introduction to logotherapy* (4th ed.). Boston: Beacon.

Fry, P. (1984). Development of a geriatric scale of hopelessness: Implications for counseling and intervention with the depressed elderly. *Journal of Counseling Psychology, 31,* 322–331.

Goleman, D. (1995). *Emotional intelligence.* New York: Bantam.

Gottschalk, L. (1974). A hope scale applicable to verbal samples. *Archives of General Psychiatry, 30,* 779–785.

Herth, K. A. (1991). Development and refinement of an instrument to measure hope. *Scholarly Inquiry for Nursing Practice, 5,* 39–51.

Hinds, P., & Gattuso, J. (1991). Measuring hopefulness in adolescents. *Journal of Pediatric Oncology Nursing, 8,* 92–94.

Ilardi, S. S., & Craighead, W. E. (1994). The role of nonspecific factors in cognitive-behavior therapy for depression. *Clinical Psychology: Science and Practice, 1,* 138–156.

Kazdin, A. E., French, N. H., Unis, A. S., Esveldt-Dawson, K., & Sherick, R. B. (1983). Hopelessness, depression, and suicidal intent among psychiatrically disturbed children. *Journal of Consulting and Clinical Psychology, 51,* 504–510.

Kirsch, I. (1990). *Changing expectations: A key to effective psychotherapy.* Pacific Grove, CA: Brooks/Cole.

Miller, J. F., & Powers, M. (1988). Development of an instrument to measure hope. *Nursing Research, 37,* 6–10.

Nowotny, M. (1989). Assessment of hope in patients with cancer: Development of an instrument. *Oncology Nursing Forum, 16,* 75–79.

Obayuwana, A., Collings, J., Carter, A., Rao, M., Mathura, C., & Wilson, S. (1982). Hope Index Scale: An instrument for objective measurement of hope. *Journal of the National Medical Association, 74,* 761–765.

Schulman, M. (1991). *The passionate mind.* New York: Free Press.

Snyder, C. R. (1994). *The psychology of hope: You can get there from here.* New York: Free Press.

Snyder, C. R., Harris, C., Anderson, J. R., Holleran, S. A., Irving, L. M., Sigmon, Yoshinobu, L., Gibb, J., Langelle, C., & Harney, P. (1991). The will and the ways: Development and validation of an individual-differences measure of hope. *Journal of Personality and Social Psychology, 60,* 570–585.

Snyder, C. R., Irving, M. M., & Anderson, J. R. (1991). Hope and health. In C. R. Snyder & D. R. Forsyth (Eds.), *Handbook of social and clinical psychology: The health perspective* (pp. 285–305). Elmsford, NY: Pergamon Press.

Snyder, C. R., Hoza, B., Pelham, W. E., Rapoff, M., Ware, L., Danovsky, M., Highberger, L., Rubinstein, H., & Stahl, K. (1997). The development and validation of the Children's Hope Scale. *Journal of Pediatric Psychology, 22* (3), 399–421.

Snyder, C. R., Sympson, S. C., Ybasco, F. C., Borders, T. F., Babyak, M. A., & Higgins, R. L. (1996). Development and validation of the State Hope Scale. *Journal of Personality and Social Psychology, 70,* 321–335.

Staats, S. (1989). Hope: A comparison of two self-report measures for adults. *Journal of Personality Assessment, 53,* 366–375.

Stoner, M. (1988). Measuring hope. In M. Stromborg (Ed.), *Instruments for clinical nursing practice* (pp. 133–140). Norwalk, CT: Appleton & Lange.

Stotland, E. (1969). *The psychology of hope.* San Francisco: Jossey-Bass.

Human–Computer Interaction

Miriam W. Schustack

California State University, San Marcos

Cognitive Ergonomics A branch of the discipline of ergonomics that focuses on accommodating the ways in which workers deal with information.

Ergonomics The science of adapting work and working conditions to suit the worker.

Human Factors Psychology An applied subfield of psychology that addresses how machinery and workplace environments can be tailored to suit the cognitive skills and limitations of the workers. It differs from ergonomics in its exclusive focus on psychological aspects of human performance.

Phobia An anxiety disorder, characterized by fear of some particular situation or entity that is irrational, excessive, and persistent, and that disrupts the normal functioning of the individual.

Technophobia An irrational fear of technological devices, especially computers.

User Interface The part of a computer system that the user actually sees, hears, and touches, such as the screen images, warning sounds, and the input devices.

HUMAN–COMPUTER INTERACTION encompasses all the ways in which people use and are influenced by computers. The pervasive and ever-increasing presence of computers in people's lives makes this an important topic for psychologists with a variety of in-

terests. This article summarizes how people respond to computers, how behavior is influenced by computer usage, and how good computer design can accommodate the different strengths and weaknesses of people and computers.

I. THE PERVASIVE PRESENCE OF COMPUTERS

Not too many years ago, professionals who studied how people used computers were part of an esoteric field of study called "man–machine interaction," a subfield of the discipline of ergonomics. That old term reflected not only an outdated worldview of masculine dominance of the workplace, but also carried with it the assumptions that the domain of computer use was limited to the workplace, and that the issues of importance in using computers were largely overlapping with the issues entailed in using other machinery, especially industrial equipment.

Those assumptions seem obsolete now, with computerized equipment of many sorts (including video games and VCRs) in almost all homes in the United States. Home computers are commonplace in the homes of middle-class Americans, used for a wide variety of functions that were difficult to foresee even as the computer industry was blossoming—in 1977, the founder and head of a major computer manufacturer (Digital Equipment Corporation) was quoted as saying, "There is no reason anyone would want a computer in their home." That was just incorrect: People have many reasons for wanting and using computers at home, and computers have become an almost inescapable part of daily life in activities like shopping, traveling, banking, getting medical care, or engaging in transactions with government. The use of computers is no longer limited to a small and exclusive group of people with intensive special training—in fact, that was true for only a very short era early in the development and dissemination of computer technology. As computers have entered the lives of ever larger numbers of people, the issues that arise in their use have become more important because of the magnitude of the consequences.

By definition, a computer is "an entity that computes"—the term has a long history prior to the electronic revolution. During World War II, there were many people employed by the military in a job category called "computer," to do the mathematical calculations necessary for determination of settings for optimal bomb trajectories. Mechanical adding machines (of varying levels of complexity) were also often referred to as computers long before the era of the microchip. Since about the 1960s, though, the term "computer" has normally been used to refer to digital electronic machines that are capable of complex symbolic computation.

Currently, there are many other machines in common use (in addition to computers per se) that use computer technology. Many of the psychological consequences of interacting with computers hold true for these other devices as well, to varying degrees. To use a concrete and very common example, there are probably millions of people who have VCRs in their homes that have never had their time set—leaving the ubiquitous blinking 12:00. The devices can be so unintuitive to program (and the manuals so incomprehensible) that people find other ways within their technological competence to achieve their goals— many people do not know how to program their VCR in advance to record a show that will be on later, so they set an alarm clock instead to remind them to start recording, or ask someone else to record it for them. One way of describing this situation is that many people have devices in their possession that they do not know how to use properly. This description places the blame on the users for being insufficiently sophisticated to master their equipment. Another description that better captures this mismatch between the device and the user is that the designers of the device have failed to understand the needs, attitudes, and skills of their intended users—under this description,

the user interface of the device is at fault rather than the user. This more psychological perspective is the appropriate one for discussing how people interact with computers (and other sophisticated electronic devices).

The characteristics of the user that can influence how the device is used constitute what are called the human factors aspects of the person–machine dyad. In explaining the reasons underlying unsuccessful (or suboptimal) human–computer interactions, there are two important threads that are separable but not completely independent. One is the role of negative attitudes among users toward computer-mediated tasks ("computer phobia" or "computer aversion"), and the other is inappropriate interface design. Although these are discussed below in separate sections, they are interrelated, each reinforcing the negative consequences of the other.

II. COMPUTER PHOBIAS

One of the most striking characteristics of human interaction with computers (and related electronic devices) is the extent to which such interactions can provoke fear and avoidance in some users (or potential users)—often to the point that the person's response can reasonably be characterized as a phobia. Certainly, there are many situations where people seek to avoid interacting with computers for reasons other than fear—the person may be uninterested, inexperienced, or may not think a computer will help them reach any of their goals. A substantial number of people, though, do appear to be excessively anxious in their attitudes toward computer use—that is, they have an irrationally high level of fear associated with computers. Sometimes the terms "technophobia," "cyberphobia," "computer anxiety," or "computerphobia" are used to describe this phenomenon, although there is no consistent and systematic distinction among these terms. While there is no single definition of this phenomenon that is used across all research on this issue, there is general agreement that computer phobia includes components of fear and anxiety about interactions with computers, lack of confidence in one's ability to use computers, dislike of computers, and negative attitudes about computers. Studies that have attempted to measure the prevalence of computer phobia employ a variety of measurement instruments that define and assess people's attitudes and behaviors somewhat differently, so that the absolute numbers are not always directly comparable across different sets of data. But the general trends in the prevalence of computer phobia emerge across these studies, despite their minor variations. [*See* ANXIETY; PHOBIAS.]

In general, there is only limited evidence for a consistent or substantial effect of age: In only some of the studies is a larger proportion of older people than younger people found to be computer phobic (and in virtually every study many young people are excessively fearful as well). This general age trend appears to be interpretable in terms of computer experience. Because of the historical pattern of when computers became prevalent in different environments over the past decades, younger people, as a group, are much more likely to have been exposed to computer use in a variety of contexts. There is one further issue about older people and computer phobias: The surveys show that there is a large subgroup of older people (many retired) who are very active and accomplished computer users, many of whom had their first exposure to computers quite late in life.

But the phenomenon of excessive fear of computers is not restricted to older people by any means. We need to temper our culturally prevalent image of the teenaged hacker who is fanatically computer involved and enormously computer literate with the images of a sizable proportion of teens and young adults who are phobic or avoidant around computers. According to recent research, the young technophobes include a sizable representation of university students in many nations (in addition to those in the United States): One large-scale study across 23 countries showed high rates of technophobia, with one-third or more of the sampled university students in some countries classified as technophobic. It is important to keep the magnitude of this phenomenon in mind—if one-third or more of university students are technophobic, and better-educated people are disproportionately involved with computers, our society has a major task to perform in accommodating people to the tools with which they need to work. The study showed that there was some influence of experience: In countries where the students typically had greater exposure to computers, there were lower rates of computer phobia. But the effects of exposure may require extensive computer use, not just a few episodes: Many of the stu-

dents who were classified as technophobic also reported that they had previously used a computer to do schoolwork.

Many studies have addressed the question of whether there are differential rates of computer phobia in males and females. The results of these are mixed, with some studies showing higher rates of phobia among women and others showing no sex difference. Differences in computer usage between male and female children are consistently found, though: Boys participate in computer activities of many types to a greater extent than do girls. Measurement of both the proportions of each group who have had each type of computer experience, and the number of hours per month they spend engaged in computer-based activity shows that boys consistently do more computer-based activities than girls. These include use at school, playing video games at home and at commercial arcades, attending computer-oriented programs after school and at summer camp. For some of these activities highly skewed gender ratios are found (greater than 3-to-1 in some cases). In addition to disparity in computer usage among male and female children, there is also evidence that children perceive computers as more appropriate for boys than for girls. This disparity in overall computer use (that is, the technological "gender gap") probably reflects many factors that are relevant to the differential socialization of boys versus girls, but lower in-school computer usage is probably a consequence of the same pressures that lead to decreases in girls' math and science achievement by early adolescence. If these pressures can be reduced in the school environment so that access is more equal, however, the evidence suggests that the female students, when they later reach college, will achieve gender equity in their college computing performance.

One explanation for higher levels of computer phobia on the part of older adults is lack of exposure to computer technology, or perhaps to their intimidating exposure to early computer-based technologies that were very forbidding to novice users. Other explanations will be required to account for computer phobia on the part of children, teenagers, and young adults, however. One possible influence is negative and/or fearful attitudes toward computers that are learned from teachers in school. While there is some computer presence in virtually all elementary and secondary schools in the United States, the use of these machines is often quite limited. Unfortunately, schoolchildren often get their first exposure to computers from a teacher who is somewhat computer phobic, and may convey negative expectations to the children. A study published in 1995 reported on the attitudes and behaviors of 600 school teachers, among whom over one-third reported not using computer technology personally or with their pupils due to discomfort, lack of confidence, and a fear of the equipment. It is understandable that children whose computer experience is designed and overseen by such teachers often pick up on the teacher's negative attitudes.

The ways in which computers are made available in schools may compound the problem. Sometimes, there are one or two computers in each classroom, so that a child working at the computer is not engaged in whatever activity most of the other children are doing. It becomes difficult to integrate computer use with other classroom activities under this setup, even if the teacher is motivated to do so. The computer remains a peripheral activity unconnected with the main body of classwork. The separate computer laboratory gets around this problem—when the whole class is in the computer lab, everyone is focused on the same task. The downside of this approach, though, is that computer use under these circumstances tends not to be connected to other classroom activity. Think about how "physical education" is usually presented in school—the class goes (together) to a special place where this one activity occurs, there might be a different, specialized teacher who does only this one activity with the students, and the activity has virtually nothing to do with the rest of the school day. In many schools, unfortunately, the computer lab has these same features. The extent and nature of computer usage in school (to be described in the section on Computer-Assisted Learning) may be a major influence on the attitudes and skills that the children develop.

The likely importance of early and sustained interaction with computers has the potential to intensify and increase social-class polarization over the long term. Home computers are much less common in households at the lower end of the socioeconomic spectrum. Children in these homes do not get the benefit of computer exposure (and they may have less school-based computer exposure as well, in their less-well-equipped schools). In addition, there is some evidence that among non-Whites, children's attitudes (and teen attitudes to an even greater extent) discour-

age computer use. In one study, for example, high school students who were members of ethnic minority groups (Hispanic and African American) had less favorable attitudes toward computers and made fewer favorable attributions to computers than their White classmates.

There is a clear negative correlation between having a computer at home and computer phobia—people with computers at home (children as well as adults) are less likely to be computer phobic. Of course, this correlation alone cannot illuminate the causal structure of the effect. People who are computer phobic are certainly much less likely than others to purchase a computer for home use. For the children, the direction of influence is also unclear: maybe the children with computers at home become less computer phobic due to exposure, or maybe children who have positive attitudes toward computer use influence their families to purchase a computer.

III. PSYCHOLOGICAL ISSUES IN ERGONOMICS

Traditionally, the field of ergonomics has included both physical and psychological issues of how job tasks and equipment are adapted to the worker. With the prominence of computers in the workplace, both these classes of issues remain important. Most workers who make extensive use of computers are not found in the kinds of industrial environments that can endanger life and limb. Nonetheless, there are common physical risks as well as psychological ones in computer use in the workplace.

The physical risks involve conditions that can interfere with the productivity of the worker, and even disable the worker for extended periods of time. Examples of these risks are poor design or poor positioning of the input devices, such as keyboards, keypads, touchpads, and so on, which can cause so-called repetitive strain injuries to the hands and arms. These are injuries that are caused by motions that would be harmless if they were done once in a while, in the context of a variety of other motions, but are damaging when they are done hundreds and thousands of times in close succession without other motions intermixed. In addition, many work environments do not provide appropriate seating, lighting, and/or screen positioning for the user, leading to higher rates of headache, eyestrain, and back and neck pain.

While many of these physical risks can be remedied in a straightforward fashion, the psychological risks are less visible and often less amenable to change. Primary among these is stress. It is common for workers to feel that they are under pressure in their job performance—they feel that they are being asked to do more than they can reasonably do (in terms of quantity, quality, and speed of work), with tools that they may feel uncomfortable using. Job-related stress has been on the increase, according to the National Institute for Occupational Safety and Health (which is the government agency responsible for monitoring workplace conditions). While there are surely many causes for this increased level of worker's compensation claims associated with job stress, some of the increase seems attributable to the increased use of computers in the workplace. Psychological stress leads to a wider variety of types of ailments than the direct physical stressors—and each individual may react with a unique mixture of physical and psychological symptoms. Workers whose behavior is being directly monitored on a moment-to-moment basis seem to be especially vulnerable. Unfortunately, as technology improves, it becomes ever easier to keep tabs on workers, with techniques such as keystroke recording and covert surveillance of telephone conversations. [*See* STRESS.]

Computerized work environments have the capacity, in theory, to be better workplaces along many dimensions: For example, routinized tasks can be handed off to machines, and tools can be easily customized for each worker. The opposite alternative, though, is also possible: Computerized workplaces can be more inflexible, allow less independence on the part of workers, and isolate workers more from one another. Although computerization can be a powerful force in changing the world of work, the scope of the possible changes includes both helpful and harmful effects.

A. Cognitive Ergonomics and User-Centered Design

There are many sets of principles of computer system design that have been put forward as appropriate for the development of an effective system. In many cases,

these principles do not include concern for the intended users of the system. Admittedly, the tasks of system design and programming are very complex and difficult for computer systems of even moderate complexity. But if the ultimate goals of such a system include any criteria that concern ease of learning and/or ease of use by the intended users, then the design process must give major emphasis to the users. That is, the nature of the users and the nature of the tasks they will perform with the system must be a focus early on and continuously during the design and implementation processes.

Until recently, there were many within the computer community whose position could be characterized as "the peanut butter theory of usability"—concern for the users is something spread on at the end of system development, after all (or most) of the major decisions have been made. In this view, taking users' skills and goals into account is part of a fine-tuning process that might affect the packaging of the system long after its content and operation has been set. This approach, of course, severely limits the impact that the user issues can have on the system, because change is so difficult, expensive and time-consuming at that point.

Commonly, software developers did not view the user interface as a domain that needed any special expertise relevant to the human factors issues. Many software companies did not even have a formal process of incorporating the perspective of the user in the design of the system. In assembling a technical team to develop a product, the programmers and other technical specialists would use their own intuitions about the intended users as a basis for designing and implementing the product. These intuitions often provided an unrealistic and inappropriate set of expectations—the programmers may have had little knowledge about the intended users and how those users were likely to approach the task. Formal evaluation of potential designs in terms of their usability for the target population (called usability evaluation) was rarely done.

There has been some increased attention paid to the needs and responses of potential users—by the early 1990s, human—computer interaction had come to be considered one of the nine "core areas" of the discipline of computer science by a major professional society in the field of computer science (the Association of Computing Machinery), and was recommended as a requirement for all college-level computer science programs. Methodologies have been developed and adapted that facilitate greater responsiveness to user needs within the design process. For example, sometimes members of the intended user community are included on the design team; in other situations, there is careful observation of users interacting with prototypes of a product in the lab or in the "natural habitat" of the work settings where the software is intended to be used.

We are not yet a point, though, where the needs of the user have been given adequate weight in designing computer systems. Insensitivity to the needs of the user still shows up in many features of software—this is often quite obvious just from looking at the system's documentation (both manuals and on-line help). When a user cannot easily figure out how to do some task or operation that the user knows or expects the software to be able to perform, the user turns to the documentation—and often has great difficulty in finding the relevant information in a comprehensible form. The documentation is often organized and written in accordance with how the system developers conceptualized the functions of the software: This may bear little resemblance to how the actual users think about the task that they are performing. This mismatch in task perspectives limits the usefulness of the documentation that is provided, and ultimately the usefulness of the software itself.

By contrast, under the perspective of cognitive ergonomics, system design is centered on the user: Understanding the user and the user's perspective on the task is seen as central to the design of an effective human interface. As software becomes more sophisticated and powerful, the importance of understanding the user becomes even more important. Powerful tools have the potential to confuse or intimidate their users—but, appropriately designed, they can be "user-friendly" instead. This appropriate fit to the user can come about from multiple sources. First, the designers must develop an understanding of the model(s) the users have of the task—how the users think about the objects and operations involved. With this understanding, the developers can then exploit the users' preexisting expectations about how the software would work, and can avoid contradicting those expectations—both of which should make the software work better for the users. In addition, the

developers can develop an understanding of how the software will be used in actual work settings, with their complex social interactions and power relationships, and with additional tools available.

IV. COMPUTER-ASSISTED LEARNING

The popular media as well as some professional literature in education often herald the coming revolution in education that will occur as computers pervade the classroom. This is not the first time that machines have been promised to bring an educational revolution, and it remains to be seen if the PC/Internet revolution will have any deeper effects than the revolution brought about by the introduction of B. F. Skinner's "teaching machines" and "programmed instruction" in the years just after World War II. That older "revolution" (which passed with hardly a trace) focused on applying behaviorist principles of reinforcement to learning in school. The material to be learned was organized into logical sequences of small bits of the subject matter, with each bit contributing to clearly identified, concrete objectives for what was to be learned. The student progressed step-by-step through small lessons, self-paced, with immediate reinforcement provided for each correct response. The actual instruction was done by presenting the lessons on rudimentary machines that were programmed with the correct responses. The "teaching machine" approach had a brief stay in the limelight, but mainstream educational practice in the ensuing 40 years was hardly changed by it.

As multimedia and electronic communications technologies continue to improve, educational opportunities are created. Some schools have well-equipped computer labs (although many schools only have older, less powerful machines). More and more schools are being connected to the Internet, which can be used for a variety of educationally appropriate activities. As costs have fallen for both the machines and the mass storage media (such as optical videodisks and compact disks), opportunities are created for a variety of instructional activities. Children can be supplied with CD-ROM encyclopedias, which have much better search and cross-referencing capability than paper encyclopedias. With Internet capability, the children can seek out up-to-date information from sources worldwide, and can pursue electronic communication with others who share their interests, in either structured or informal ways. In addition, commercial educational software can be used in the classroom to support the children's learning of basic skills with computer-based practice in a game format.

A. Computers in Primary and Secondary Schools

How much change these technologies will bring in day-to-day classroom practice at the primary and secondary school level remains to be seen. Perhaps it would be more appropriate to view the changes as evolutionary rather than revolutionary. The computer use (as mentioned earlier in the section on computer phobias) tends not to be well integrated with the rest of the classroom activity, which continues in conventional format.

B. Computer Usage as a Factor in College Instruction

The same limited impact holds true at the college level. The computer "revolution" has, to some extent, arrived. College students communicate with their professors via e-mail and class mailing lists, they use computerized searches to find library materials, they use computers in the classroom and for homework in the sciences, the arts, the humanities. But the sorts of deep structural changes that many have prophesied—the death of the university as we know it—have been slow in coming. There surely are new, technology-dependent initiatives and programs: distance education via interactive video, self-paced video lecture courses, computer-based exercises, and the like. But, as of yet, these have not had much impact on most aspects of university life.

C. Computer-Based Instruction

For many years, a variety of computer-based techniques and technologies have been developed for education, many tracing back to Skinner's programmed instruction approaches. Because of the possibilities afforded by advanced computers, new approaches (or improved versions of older approaches) can become feasible. In the early years of computer-based instruction, most materials were limited to drill-and-practice approaches reminiscent of Skinner's teaching ma-

chine. The most important feature of the computer, for this approach, was that it never gets impatient or bored—but what can be learned via drill and practice is very limited in scope. The same complaint is often applied to commercial educational software: that flat drill and practice is not a very valuable exercise, no matter how flashy the sounds and graphics that accompany it. But computers make sophisticated and subtle approaches possible as well. For example, in military and industrial training, extensive use is made of large-scale computer simulations. In addition to learning about some complex task through traditional descriptive material, the student can get hands-on experience in performing the task, without the risks entailed in live training—fighter pilot trainees get to crash a simulator many times before they handle the controls of a plane in the air, and a sailor can damage or blow up a simulation of a ship's steam propulsion system before going out to sea.

V. TECHNOLOGICALLY MEDIATED COMMUNICATION

With the refinement of many forms of computer-mediated communication, we have many alternatives to live, face-to-face encounters. In our changing worlds of work and recreation, probably the biggest changes in communication have been relatively low-tech, from our current perspective: the use of computers for the exchange of written messages. Electronic mail (e-mail) has become a very heavily used communication mode in many environments.

A. Choosing Mediated Interaction over Direct Interaction

In many situations, we find people choosing an electronically mediated conversation even when a face-to-face conversation is possible. This is not a new phenomenon of the computer age—it used to occur when people would choose to make a telephone call rather than walk down the hall to a coworker's office. The reasons behind such a choice may apply to the use of electronic mail as well—people may perceive such communication to be more efficient in achieving their task goals. After all, if you walk down the hall you may find your coworker not at her desk, or on the phone, or talking to someone else. Using the phone does not protect you from initiating contact at a time that turns out to be inconvenient—but it minimizes the effort you expended to make the contact. E-mail can be viewed similarly—not necessarily an avoidance of personal contact, but a more efficient way to get the message across. In all cases, the less direct the contact, the more that is lost of the interpersonal contact—the social greeting, the "small-talk," the nuances of voice tone and visual nonverbal cues (gesture, posture, facial expression). Some of these cues are lost or degraded in telephone conversation, and are even less available when the medium shifts to e-mail.

Psycholinguistic research over many years has explored the differences between spoken and written communication. Until recently, the computer was not part of this focus—the comparisons were between what we say and what we write down on paper, along many dimensions. Those findings, very succinctly, are that changing the medium has powerful and broad effects on many aspects of a message—the wording, the tone, the way in which errors are corrected, the formality of the language used, the structure of the communication, the ways in which reference is made, and many other features. As the computer became a common mode of communication for many people, the research focused on how using electronic mail as the communication channel influences communication. Early findings (e.g., by Sara Kiesler and her colleagues) were that the use of electronic communication systems tended to reduce the inequalities among participants of differing status levels. Much was made of the notion of the computer network as a leveler of status and a reducer of social distance. More recent work, though, fails to show that communication is any more egalitarian in e-mail than elsewhere: As people have become more comfortable with the medium of electronic communication, they have become adept at picking up on the same sorts of social status cues (gender, race, age, education) that commonly influence interactions in other communications media. Of course, they must get the social-status information via slightly different means, but it appears to be used in similar ways regardless of the medium.

One major concern about computer-mediated communication is how it will change the ways in which people interact. In fact, it does have important differences from other forms of communication, and these have some negative consequences—but also some positive ones. For example, many people who use

voice-mail systems report that they can go through a series of several telephone interchanges with a colleague or client without ever talking to the person "live." They may get all their business done without ever having an interaction in real time. Typically, such interchanges tend to be more task-focused and less sociable than comparable real-time telephone conversations. Whether this should be viewed as a negative or a positive difference, though, clearly depends on the perspective of the evaluator. Objectively, it is probably positive in the short term, with people getting their business done more efficiently via voice mail than in repeated rounds of trying to reach one another live via "telephone tag," or leaving written messages via dictation to a third party. In the longer term, though, employers need to be concerned that the reduction in off-task socializing might result in a less cohesive workforce, poorer employee morale, poorer information distribution within the organization, and poorer relationships with clients.

B. Automated Administration of Test Instruments

In the computerized administration of psychological tests, respondents interact with a computer to provide information that is as valid and reliable as it is when they respond to the same test items administered in person by an examiner, without technological assistance. Computer-assisted psychological assessment is actually preferred in some situations by the test-takers, who may feel more comfortable in disclosing sensitive information when there is no human interviewer to face. This benefit is in addition to the more practical advantage of efficiency in the use of the practitioner's time, uniformity in the presentation of the questions, and a reduction in potential bias and error that the practitioner can introduce.

C. Online "Chatting" as a Mode of Communication

One use of technologically mediated communication that has blossomed in recent years is the "online chat." In this mode of communication, an interactive conversation is carried on among a varied number of people who (metaphorically) enter a room to take part in a conversation about a given topic, while they each sit at their personal computers, networked from anywhere in the world. People who "meet" via a chat room can choose to continue their conversation privately (leaving the metaphorical common room for a private room). How these interactions are generally perceived provides interesting information about how our society views social interaction and friendship. In many instances, two people "meet" in a chat room and begin a relationship that may go on for weeks or months of intensive on-line communication. Despite the fact that these conversations may have entailed enormous amounts of information exchanged (about backgrounds, beliefs, daily activities, etc.), many people view such relationships as not being "real" because the parties have not seen one another in the flesh. The parties involved are warned about the dangers of a face-to-face meeting, reflecting the belief that a potential partner found in a singles bar is for some reason less likely to be a creep or a pervert than one found on-line. People tend to feel confident in their greater ability to detect deception in person—but unfortunately that confidence is misplaced.

D. Computer-Oriented Addictive Behavior

In fact, there are potential dangers even if the user remains in cyberspace—Internet addiction. While this is not yet a disorder recognized by the *Diagnostic and Statistical Manual of Mental Disorders,* many clinicians see a syndrome of addiction to on-line computing, analogous to pathological gambling (including features of preoccupation, lack of control, risk to relationship or career, and withdrawal symptoms). While the availability of on-line access cannot be blamed for creating this addictive behavior (just as the availability of food cannot be blamed for creating eating disorders), we need to become sensitive to the signs of this maladaptive behavior.

E. The Emergence of Technological Support for Shared Work

Over the last several years, tools have been developed to support multiple people jointly participating in a task. Often termed "computer-supported cooperative work" or "computer-supported collaborative work," this area of research and development has worked to create computer-based tools that facilitate the completion of collaborations. There are many different

sorts of tools, with different goals: some tools support shared work on documents (allowing multiple authors to edit and comment on a jointly produced document), others are targeted for the support of productive teleconferencing, joint scheduling, workflow management, concurrent engineering, and other types of tasks.

F. Societal Polarization Effects

The rising usage of technologically mediated communication has the potential to further separate the information elite from others in society, especially those who are poor and/or members of linguistic and ethnic minority groups—to isolate the information haves from the have-nots. Current trends seem to point to increasing polarization, as the wealthier and more technologically literate segments of society adopt a variety of computer-mediated techniques—not only e-mail, but on-line typed conversation, interactive audio (basically using the computer as a substitute for a telephone), and two-way interactive video, with live video of each participant being captured by a camera. (Ironically, it seems as though the "picture-phone" that the telephone industry has been promising since the 1960s is finally available to many people—but not as a telephone-based technology!)

G. Societal Inclusiveness Effects

On the other hand, in many respects computer-mediated communication has the potential to provide opportunities for greater inclusion as well. Poor people living in rural areas can get access via their telephone lines to tremendous resources, equivalent to the resources available on-line in major metropolitan areas. Distance learning via computer can enable everyone to get equal access to educational activities at any level (from the elementary grades and vocational training through graduate work). Minority groups that are geographically dispersed can build a "community center" in cyberspace for the support of their language and culture, and for the coordination of their activities. This potential for benefit, though, will not necessarily be realized, unless various economic and cultural barriers are lowered. If minority-group members, poor people, rural people, and other marginalized constituencies do not get past the first few steps of getting access to the technology and becoming comfortable with it, their ultimate representation in "cyberculture" will be minimal.

H. Benefits for People with Disabilities

Electronic communication can be useful to people in the political, geographic, and ability mainstream, but it can be even more useful to those who are not. People in physically remote areas or those who are confined to their homes by illness or disability can interact with friends or colleagues via e-mail. The deaf can communicate with deaf and hearing others, and those who cannot speak intelligibly can substitute a keyboard. Communication opportunities for the disabled are only a small part of the impact of computer technology on the disabled community—many disabled people who would otherwise be unable to work are able to hold jobs with the help of sophisticated computer-based assistive devices of many sorts, ranging from "talking computers" that replace the words that normally would appear on the computer screen with synthesized speech (for the visually impaired), and voice-recognition systems that allow the user to talk to the computer instead of typing (for users unable to use a keyboard).

VI. IMPLICATIONS FOR THE FUTURE

A. Changes in the Workplace

The importance of the computer as part of the work environment interacts with other emerging changes in working patterns. The trend toward telecommuting makes workers more dependent on their computer technology and their technologically mediated communication to accomplish their jobs. Patterns of employment are changing in several ways that have relevance to human—computer interaction. For example, more and more workers are expected to change careers multiple times, and will need to learn new skills with each career change. As people remain in the workforce until later in life (a pattern that is expected to accelerate), we will have to deal with the changes in the demographic mix of workers. As immigrant and ethnic minority populations grow, we will have to find ways to accommodate cultural and educational differences in interactional styles and technological attitudes.

B. Changes in Leisure and Recreation

Recreational computer use seems to be on the increase, and there is always some new technology just around the corner that promises to keep people glued to their tubes. In the future, the distinctions among media will probably lessen, as your computer communicates over the cable television lines and you get live TV over the Internet. But in terms of human interface issues, we may see an intensification of the poor interfaces that characterized VCRs (and many other computerized products) until recently, magnified by the complexity of the new devices.

C. Changes in Interpersonal and Societal Structures

We know that many aspects of our society are being deeply changed by the pervasive presence of computers across the recreational, educational, and workplace domains. For example, people sometimes feel they need to use a phrase like "real reality" to mark that the term "reality" is not referring to the concept of "virtual reality." Or they will feel the need to qualify the phase, "I sent her mail" by specifying U.S. mail (or "snail-mail"). From a psycholinguistic perspective, such an adaptation means that the core meaning of the word is no longer restricted to its original value—the more recently introduced usage of these terms has changed the meanings that the words have when standing alone.

Our world has changed, and it continues to change as technology perfuses ever more of our daily lives and our society at large. A better understanding of the psychological factors that underlie how people adapt to those changes will enable us to make more intelligent decisions about where and how that technology should be used.

BIBLIOGRAPHY

Baecker, R. M. (1995). *Readings in human-computer interaction: Toward the year 2000.* (2nd Ed.). San Francisco: Morgan Kaufman.

Carroll, J. M. (1997). Human computer interaction: Psychology as a science of design. *Annual Review of Psychology, 48,* 61–83.

Collis, B. A., Knezek, G. A., Lia, K.-W., Miyashita, K. T., Pelgrum, W. J., Plomp, T., & Sakamoto, T. (1996). *Children and computers in schools.* Hillsdale NJ: Erlbaum.

Coordinating Committee for the Human Capital Initiative (1993). *Report of the committee on the changing nature of work*. Washington, DC: American Psychological Society.

Eberts, R. E. (1994). *User interface design*. Englewood Cliffs, NJ: Prentice-Hall.

Edwards, A. D. N. (1995). *Extra-ordinary human-computer interaction: Interfaces for users with disabilities*. Cambridge & New York: Cambridge University Press.

Helander, M. (1988). *Handbook of human—computer interaction*. Amsterdam: North Holland.

Hoc, J.-M., Cacciabue, P. C., & Hollnagel, E. (Eds.). (1994). *Expertise and technology: Cognition and human—computer cooperation*. Hillsdale NJ: Erlbaum.

Norman, D. A. (1990). *The design of everyday things*. New York: Doubleday.

Pfleger, S., Goncalves, J., & Varghese, K. (Eds.). (1995). *Advances in human-computer interaction: Human comfort and security*. Berlin and New York: Springer.

Schneiderman, B. (1992). *Designing the user interface: Strategies for effective human-computer interaction (2nd Edition)*. Reading, MA: Addison-Wesley.

Schofield, J. W. (1995). *Computers and classroom culture*. Cambridge: Cambridge University Press.

Thomas, P. J. (Ed.). (1994). *The social and interactional dimensions of human—computer interfaces*. New York: Cambridge University Press.

Humor and Mental Health

Nicholas A. Kuiper and L. Joan Olinger

University of Western Ontario

Change of Perspective A means of distancing oneself from the negative effects of a stressful event by generating different viewpoints that also incorporate humorous elements.

Cognitive Appraisals An evaluation of the positive or negative implications of an event for the self. Potential stressors can be viewed as positive challenges to overcome, or as a threat to self and well-being.

Laughter A reflex-like behavioral and physiological response, most often to humorous material, that includes guttural vocalizations, the baring of teeth, and increased heart rate, blood pressure, and respiration, combined with spastic head, body, and arm movements.

Positive Enhancement Effects The beneficial aspects of humor that add a degree of richness and fullness to the enjoyment of life experiences, including the expression of more positive emotions and a more positive self-concept.

Sense of Humor A multidimensional set of individual difference characteristics that describe core aspects of humor, including the ability to appreciate humor, produce humor, respond with laughter, and use humor to cope effectively with stressful life experiences.

Stress-buffering Effects The proposal that a good sense of humor provides an effective defense against the detrimental impact of stressful events, thus reducing both physical and mental health problems.

HUMOR and laughter have often been tied to mental health issues. Numerous writers have suggested that a good sense of humor can facilitate social interactions and buffer the negative effects of stress. The research findings reviewed here provide reasonable support for both of these mental health-related functions of humor. Humor and laughter have also been incorporated into a wide variety of programs and clinical approaches that seek to promote or restore mental health. Often this is done by teaching individuals to use humor or laughter as a coping strategy that provides effective distancing from a stressor, or by using the social facilitation aspects of humor and laughter to enhance interpersonal relationships, either in a clinical or social context. Although these mental health applications have demonstrated some degree of success in improving quality of life and subjective well-being, it is clear that major limitations remain. In particular, additional research findings are reviewed that indicate that humor and laughter may not always be beneficial to mental health, and may even prove detrimental. This major issue is addressed by first clarifying the basic concepts associated with humor, laughter, and mental health. A detailed examination of the empirical and theoretical links between humor, laughter, and mental health is provided. In addition to describing traditional theoretical models of laughter and humor as they relate to mental health, more recent refinements in theoretical constructs and models are also presented. This latter work integrates concepts and findings from several domains of psychology, including the stress and coping literature, personality theory, and quality of life.

I. HUMOR AND ITS LINKS TO MENTAL HEALTH

A. Descriptive Aspects of Humor

Humor is a pervasive and powerful force in our everyday lives. Reflecting the ubiquitous nature of this phenomenon, there has been a centuries-long interest in describing the various facets of humor and how these may relate to mental health. The past two decades, in particular, have witnessed a resurgence of empirically based research on this topic. At a basic descriptive level, this work has shown that humor and laughter occurs most often in social encounters. In recording more than 1200 public social interactions, for example, one study found that laughter was expressed in fully 99% of these episodes, and appears to function as a primary facilitator of these interactions. Other research has investigated what people report as humorous and funny in everyday life, with the majority of remembered incidents focusing on the foolishness of someone, and not necessarily on sexual or aggressive humor themes. A large number of research studies have investigated different aspects of humor as they may relate to jokes, cartoons, bloopers, and television advertisements. This work has provided evidence for a wide variety of categories of humorous material, including word play, nonsense or silly humor, slapstick humor, aggressive humor, sexual humor, sick humor, comic humor, disparaging jokes, put-downs, dry wit, and good-natured play. In addition, some of this work has also focused on determining which types of individuals may prefer which types of humor.

Of particular interest from a mental health perspective is personality-based research, which examines how individuals may differ in terms of their sense of humor. This research has adopted a trait approach that considers sense of humor to be a stable personality characteristic, with reliable and valid distinctions being evident across individuals. A number of self-report measures have been developed to assess these individual differences for various components of sense of humor, including laughter responsiveness, humor appreciation, humor production, coping humor, social humor, and degree of wittiness. Subsequent research has investigated various parameters associated with these individual differences. Expected life span distinctions emerge, for example, with younger children showing greater difficulties with humor appreciation and comprehension. Similarly, an observational study of naturalistic humor production and appreciation in children with either autism or Down's syndrome showed the expected reduction in both these humor components when compared with matched controls. Other research examining the correlates of higher levels of humor has often revealed patterns that are consistent with the proposal that enhanced humor may benefit mental health. Across a number of studies, individuals with higher levels of humor also report lower levels of depression and perceived stress, lower levels of loneliness, higher levels of intimacy and self-esteem, and higher levels of optimism, internal locus of control, and extraversion. As one specific example, a detailed study of more than 120 gifted adolescents revealed that those with higher levels of humor were also more creative, extraverted, and lower in need for social approval than those with low humor scores.

B. Functional Aspects of Humor

In addition to descriptive research, there has also been long-standing interest in the functions or roles that humor might serve. Congruent with repeated observations that humor is highly prevalent in social interactions, and is also linked to higher levels of personal sociability and extraversion, it has often been proposed that laughter and humor function to facilitate effective social interactions, smooth over interaction difficulties, and help maintain positive relationships with others. These proposed social interaction functions of humor have been highlighted by a number of humor theorists and have been empirically documented in several recent studies. As one illustration, a detailed analysis of more than 400 everyday social interactions revealed that the increased display of humor positively facilitated these encounters. In a second study, almost 600 individuals described the strategies they used to maintain various relationships with others (e.g., lovers, friends, relatives), with humor being one of the ten most beneficial strategies (along with positivity and openness in relationships). Using the naturalistic setting of a photography shop, a field study found humor to be a particularly effective tool for dealing with interpersonal conflicts and difficulties often associated with face-to-face bargaining. Finally, the "lubricating" value of humor has been acknowledged in a set of interviews with 10 successful mediators, with humor benefits being reduced tension and threat, increased security, and a broadening of perspectives. Taken together, these findings support the proposal that one of the functions of humor is to facilitate interpersonal communication and enhance social interactions, while simultaneously diffusing conflict and tension. From a mental health perspective, these social interaction functions of humor are extremely important, as they may help promote a more positive social environment that reduces interpersonal distress and contributes to greater psychological well-being.

A second mental health-related function of humor that has been repeatedly recognized throughout the ages is that a good sense of humor is an effective defense against stress. As described by a number of philosophers and psychologists, this stress-buffering function of humor is purported to reduce both mental and physical health concerns. Earlier in this century, Freud wrote that a good sense of humor is a rare and precious gift that functions as one of the highest ego defense mechanisms. This theme is also evident in contemporary approaches in the personality and psychopathology domains, with both characterizing a good sense of humor as one of the most mature, adaptive, and highly developed defense mechanisms available. In detailing the various characteristics that help protect a child from stressors, a good sense of humor is rated as one of the more prominent factors, along with good problem-solving abilities and a positive sense of self-worth. Also consistent with this proposal, research has found higher rates of humor use and creativity in gifted women, and lower rates in individuals with borderline personality disorders. Finally, and as described previously, several studies have shown that higher levels of humor are associated with lower levels of perceived stress and depression. [*See* COPING WITH STRESS; DEPRESSION; STRESS.]

Other lines of evidence converge on the proposal

that humor may be used as a defense mechanism or coping strategy for dealing with stressful life events. When faced with extraordinary circumstances, for example, humor was one of the strategies used by nurses when responding to victims of hurricane Hugo. Humor was also one of the documented coping techniques used by the victims of this natural disaster when discussing their plight. Similarly, in adapting to the hardships and rigors of a war zone, hospital ship personnel deployed in Operation Desert Storm were found to use a variety of psychological defenses, including humor. The use of humor has also been reported in a number of studies describing how professionals deal with violent deaths or the terminally ill. In discussing their responses to traffic deaths, homicides, and suicides, police officers indicate the use of humor as one effective form of release. Humor has also been used as a coping strategy by therapists working with terminally ill patients, helping to provide perspective and balance for both client and therapist. Further examples of the use of humor in a medical context are also evident. In dealing with cataract operations, for example, humor was among the most common defense mechanisms used by 100 elderly persons over the age of 70. The greater acceptance and use of humor has also been found to be a significant predictor of lower psychological distress in a sample of more than 50 patients coping with the effects of breast cancer.

In addition to extraordinary events, further research has documented that humor is often used as a coping strategy to handle the more routine daily stresses, strains, and conflicts encountered in everyday life. In this regard, humor has been used by married couples as one technique to deal effectively with job stress that may bear negatively on their relationships. Humor has also been used by teachers to cope with the demands of the classroom, and by students when faced with academic stressors, such as upcoming examinations and evaluations.

C. Using Humor to Promote Mental Health

There have been a number of programs developed that incorporate humor as an active component to promote better psychological adjustment in nonclinical populations spanning a considerable age range. These programs vary tremendously in terms of their specific aims. A common theme, however, is the use of humor to promote a more positive quality of life by dealing more effectively with stress. In the case of students, for example, this has included teaching stress management programs that use humor as one technique to cope with academic, interpersonal, and environmental concerns that may otherwise impede their academic progress. One specific illustration is grief programs for students who have lost a parent. Humor and laughter are used in these groups to help cope with the unpleasant reality of death, to gain control over fears, and to provide a safe counterpoint to grief and loss. For elderly populations, programs have been developed that use imagery techniques to enhance humor production by allowing these individuals to see potential problems from a different, more humorous perspective. This change in perspective results in greater distancing from the potential stressor, which contributes to an overall reduction in stress levels for these individuals. Humor has also been used in a year-long program in a nursing home to improve quality of life for the elderly residents. Follow-up results from this study indicated that humor was beneficial and resulted in more effective social interactions.

Several other programs have also used humor to improve social interactions and relations. As one example, humor was used extensively in a telephone support group for visually impaired elderly persons, resulting in a positive impact on mental health, especially for those persons living alone. As a second illustration, rehabilitation programs have been used with physically disabled individuals to add humor to their repertoire of interpersonal skills. Congruent with the social lubricating function of humor, these skills helped reduce feelings of interpersonal anxiety during social interactions, and this reduced tension resulted in smoother interactions.

Humor has also been used in several programs that address quality of life issues in the medical domain. With respect to cancer, for example, laughter therapy has systematically used humorous books and films to help alleviate suffering in these patients. Although it is clearly recognized that this therapy is not curative, psychological benefits include more positive emotions, increased social communication, and a degree of enhancement in quality of life. Laughter and humor are prominent in some group programs for helping individuals deal with AIDS-related deaths. One "last

rights" group, for example, specified a set of rights for dying people that included being in control, being able to laugh, feeling connected to a family, and using imagery experiences to share humor with others. Although stemming from physical health concerns, these programs clearly have a mental health focus in terms of preparing individuals to cope as effectively as possible with the psychological sequelae associated with suffering and terminal illnesses.

D. Using Humor to Restore Mental Health

In a clinical context, much has been written about the use of humor in psychotherapy to help restore an individual's mental health. Clinicians from a wide variety of therapeutic approaches, including both psychoanalytic and cognitive perspectives, have proposed that humor can be used to enhance and manage the client–therapist relationship for a variety of clients, including children, adolescents, and adults. In accord with the social interaction function of humor, it has been suggested that humor can alleviate tension and anxiety in the therapeutic setting, thus facilitating client–therapist communication. This increased rapport and strengthening of the patient–therapist bond provides a helpful adjunct to therapy by fostering a more positive therapeutic atmosphere. As one specific example, some research has shown that clients may engage in greater laughter and humor when disclosing more sensitive personal information about themselves. At a more general level, further benefits may accrue in terms of heightened client motivation, reduced feelings of inferiority, an increased degree of client insight and self-directedness, and greater social interest.

A second theme in the treatment literature follows directly from the proposed stress-reducing function of humor. It has been suggested by a number of clinicians that humor and laughter can be taught as viable coping techniques during therapy to assist clients in resolving personal conflicts and alleviating stress. In both cognitive therapy and rational emotive therapy, for example, clients are taught to dispute their irrational beliefs and interpretations by generating a series of alternative perspectives. Humor is one means of accomplishing this change of perspective that challenges these irrational thoughts. In other words, humor can provide a new way of thinking about formerly stressful situations or events that may allow clients to escape from formerly ingrained and automatic dysfunctional interpretations.

E. Limitations in the Effectiveness of Humor

Despite widespread acceptance of proposals that increased levels of humor can facilitate social interactions and alleviate stress, it should be pointed out that evidence can also be marshaled against both these propositions. The expression of laughter, for example, may sometimes be an indicator of pathology rather than of pleasure or social facilitation. Research findings indicate that patients with lesions or strokes often show emotionalism (i.e., inappropriate laughter and crying) that has very little to do with the positive functions of humor. Uncontrollable bouts of inappropriate laughter have also been observed in a number of other conditions, including epilepsy, multiple sclerosis, kuru, Alzheimer's disease, manic-depressive disorder, metabolic defects, drug use, and certain forms of schizophrenia. Rather than a social lubricant, laughter in these cases may be abrasive and serve as a further source of social impediment and emotional distress for these individuals. Although etiological factors are complex and not yet clearly understood, behavioral management programs have been used with some degree of success to curb the inappropriate laughter expressed by certain patients in clinical settings.

Other lines of evidence converge on the notion that the use of humor in social situations may not always be facilitative. In studying children's patterns of social interactions, for example, researchers have shown how humor may be used as an aggressive teasing response to promote conformity within groups, allowing bullies to dominate less assertive children. Instead of promoting social interactions, this ridiculing use of humor can lead to increased hostility and social withdrawal. Inappropriate humor on the part of adults can also have a negative social impact on the child. One observational study examined the ways in which parent–child interactions may subsequently hinder the child's ability to interact successfully with peers. Prominent negative factors included parental intrusiveness, low engagement, and the use of derisive humor. Similarly, in the classroom, the teacher's use of hostile humor can create a negative learning climate

that is perceived as low in social support. Finally, the effects of humor that may be socially facilitative in one culture may be detrimental in another. In dealing with embarrassing situations and social predicaments, North Americans rely much more extensively on humor and laughter as coping responses than do persons from Japan. The latter are much more likely to apologize, viewing humor and laughter as inappropriate social responses in these situations.

The proposal that humor may alleviate or buffer stress has also been challenged by some research findings. For nurses faced with a variety of stressors, including heavy workloads and the emotional demands of terminally ill patients and their families, one field study found that the use of humor in the work setting did not contribute significantly to reduced levels of stress. Further work has demonstrated, by inclusion of appropriate comparison conditions, that humor's beneficial effects may sometimes be less substantive than originally envisioned. One study, for example, found that laughter therapy, when compared directly with standard relaxation training, was less effective in reducing the physiological components of stress. Other research has shown that watching humorous films provided the expected increase in tolerance for physical stressors, but watching tragic films before the stressor test also provided the same increase. Finally, and in contrast to the findings reviewed earlier, several studies have reported that higher levels of humor are not always significantly associated with lower levels of depression, higher levels of verbal ability and creativity, greater happiness in childhood, or better overall mental or physical health. In fact, one study using longitudinal data across a 20-year time span found that the personality construct of "cheerfulness" (consisting of an amalgamation of optimism and sense of humor) was actually inversely related to longevity.

With regard to therapeutic applications, there is a need to clearly distinguish between humor that enhances therapeutic effectiveness and humor that detracts. In particular, humor should not be used to avoid uncomfortable aspects of the client–therapist relationship or to serve only the needs of the therapist. Some clinicians feel that the inappropriate use of humor in psychotherapy can have a number of detrimental effects. These include creating an imbalance in the client–therapist relationship, blocking effective communication, and generating negative feelings among clients. Therapists should also be aware that individual differences in both client and therapist may sometimes contraindicate the use of humor in therapy, or otherwise limit the type of humor that is used and for what purpose. In describing these limitations, it should be noted that relatively little well-controlled clinical research has been conducted on the therapeutic effectiveness of humor. An urgent need to conduct this research is therefore one of the major recommendations of a recent 20-year retrospective report on the role of humor in psychotherapy.

F. Summary

Thus far, we have highlighted the pervasive nature of humor and its possible benefits for mental health, including both social facilitation and stress reduction. Research supporting both of these functions of humor was presented, indicating how both functions are evident in a variety of humor-related programs and therapeutic approaches focusing on the promotion and restoration of mental health. Other research findings and clinical comments, however, have indicated that certain limits may be evident and humor may not always exert a beneficial effect on mental health.

Overall, then, sufficient evidence exists to support the general proposal that humor does play a role in mental health. What is much less clear, however, are the precise conditions or circumstances under which humor might either facilitate or impede an individual's mental health. This important issue is addressed in detail in the remainder of this entry.

II. CLARIFYING BASIC CONCEPTS OF MENTAL HEALTH, LAUGHTER, AND HUMOR

Traditional approaches to mental health have often defined this construct solely in terms of the presence or absence of psychopathology. Thus, individuals scoring high on measures of depression or anxiety, for example, would be considered mentally unhealthy, whereas those scoring low on these negative affect measures would be viewed as mentally healthy. Although this approach certainly captures one aspect of mental health, it generally ignores positive features that are also important.

A broader orientation is evident in contemporary approaches in both the subjective well-being and qual-

ity of life domains, which have clearly acknowledged that mental health is much more than just the absence of psychopathology. In accord with the personality theories espoused by Erikson, Maslow, and Rogers, these domains view personal growth and positive life enhancement as integral components of mental health. Thus, in addition to incorporating traditional measures of negative affect, these domains also include a focus on problem-solving abilities and coping skills that contribute to increased levels of positive self-esteem, greater life satisfaction, and more positive affect. This integrative approach to mental health further stresses the importance of everyday social interactions and personal resources in contributing to mental and physical well-being. Social support networks and personality characteristics, such as levels of optimism and hardiness, are viewed as essential factors underlying a healthier life style, greater life satisfaction, and enhanced emotional well-being. In adopting this broader approach to mental health, we conceptualize humor and laughter as important personal resources that not only affect the quality of an individual's social relationships, but also contribute significantly to subsequent perceptions and interpretations of a wide range of life events and experiences. [See HARDINESS IN HEALTH AND EFFECTIVENESS; OPTIMISM, MOTIVATION, AND MENTAL HEALTH; SOCIAL SUPPORT.]

Considering the concept of humor in more detail, there is a general recognition in the research literature that humor should be treated as a multidimensional rather than a singular construct. The most basic distinction is between laughter and humor, with the latter category divided into further components. Although both laughter and humor have been described as universal phenomena, they are differentiated on a number of features. Humor is a complicated higher order perceptual-cognitive-emotional process, whereas laughter is a more reflex-like physiological-behavioral response. Prominent behavioral aspects of laughter include guttural vocalizations, the baring of teeth, and pronounced facial grimaces and contortions. Skeletal muscles are exercised with the head often thrown back and spastic body movements accompanied by the flailing of arms. Laughter provides physiological stimulation in the form of increased heart rate, blood pressure, and respiration. Skin temperatures also rise and endocrine flow is stimulated, and overall immune system effectiveness is enhanced.

Research findings have confirmed that laughter appears early in life, before the more complex cognitive processes associated with humor become evident. By the age of 1, various parameters associated with infant laughter, such as rate of laughter, duration, and reciprocity, already show a high degree of stability. Individual differences in frequency of laughter are also evident at this age. Congruent with the social facilitative effects of laughter, research with adult samples has demonstrated the contagious nature of laughter, with laughter itself being a sufficient stimulus for more smiles and laughter. In adult samples, pronounced individual differences in the frequency of laughter are revealed by both behavioral observations and a variety of self-report scales. Perhaps the most widely used scale is the Situational Humor Response Questionnaire (SHRQ), which provides a psychometrically sound assessment of individual differences in laughter responsiveness across various life situations. A typical SHRQ item describes the following situation: "You are eating in a restaurant with some friends and the waiter accidentally spills a drink on you." For each item, respondents indicate the degree to which they would smile or laugh in that situation by endorsing one of five response choices ranging from "I wouldn't have found it particularly amusing" to "I would have laughed heartily." The SHRQ has been translated into at least 10 different languages and administered to a wide range of age groups and cultures. A recent overview by one of the original developers of this scale (Martin, in press) indicates a high degree of empirical support for the construct of laughter responsiveness and its clear separation from other self-report measures that focus on different components of humor, such as coping humor or humor appreciation.

The multidimensional aspects of sense of humor have been tapped by a number of published self-report scales. These measures assess such components as humor production and creative ability, playfulness, the ability to use humor to achieve social goals, humor appreciation, the value of humor in one's life, and the use of humor to cope with stressful situations. Across a number of research studies, the patterns of intercorrelations among these measures have typically been in the moderate range (i.e., $r = .25$ to $.55$), supporting the proposal that each scale assesses a somewhat different component of sense of humor. The Coping Humor Scale (CHS) is one of the more prominent measures here, both in terms of accumulated research

findings and in its most direct relevance to mental health concerns. The CHS was developed by the same researchers responsible for the SHRQ, but in contrast to mirth and laughter responsiveness, it was designed to assess the degree to which individuals report that they actively use humor as a means of coping with stress in their lives. An example item from the CHS is "I have often found that my problems have been greatly reduced when I tried to find something funny in them." Overall coping humor scores are obtained by summing an individual's level of agreement across the several items on this scale. As is the case with the SHRQ, the CHS is psychometrically sound and has been translated into several different languages for use in humor research around the globe.

III. LAUGHTER AND MENTAL HEALTH

In describing research findings and associated theory pertaining to the role of laughter in mental health, two themes are apparent. First, individual differences in laughter responsiveness, particularly as assessed by the SHRQ, are often related to the degree to which laughter may have a beneficial impact on stress reduction. Second, the theoretical models used to explain an association between laughter and mental health provide a useful general starting point but appear to lack specificity in terms of accounting for the more precise conditions under which laughter may or may not alleviate stress. We elaborate on each of these themes below.

In laboratory settings, two recent studies have linked the presentation of humorous stimuli and greater laughter responsiveness to heightened tolerance levels for stress. The first study assessed participants' thresholds for discomfort when administered transcutaneous end nerve stimulation. Individuals watching a humorous videotape showed higher thresh-olds than participants watching a nonhumorous tape, but this effect was qualified by individual differences in laughter responsiveness. In particular, when not provided with the humorous videotape, individuals with a low level of laughter responsiveness showed a much larger drop in their stress tolerance than individuals with higher laughter scores. A similar pattern was obtained in the second study, which monitored individuals while they waited several minutes ostensibly for a painful electric shock. Those individuals listening to a humorous tape showed lower levels of anxiety on physiological and self-report indices than those individuals listening to a nonhumorous tape. Again, however, this effect was qualified by individual differences, with those participants lower in laughter responsiveness showing the highest anxiety levels when not listening to a humorous tape. In contrast, individuals scoring higher on the SHRQ showed much lower anxiety levels, regardless of the presence or absence of a humorous tape. Taken together, these findings are congruent with the proposal that individuals with higher levels of laughter responsiveness can more effectively use this personal resource to cope with stress in a wide variety of life circumstances, especially situations that do not necessarily incorporate humor as an explicit element.

Other research has documented the relationship between increased laughter and enhanced immune system functioning. In the health psychology literature, immune competence is a key mechanism linking certain psychological variables to an individual's level of susceptibility to infectious disease. Laughter responsiveness appears to be one such variable, as research indicates that individuals reporting higher levels of mirth also indicate lower levels of physical illness. Of particular interest here are studies that have directly assessed activity of the immune system, including salivary immunoglobin A concentrations (S-IgA). These concentrations are important in the body's defense against upper respiratory infections, and in several studies they have been found to increase after presentation of humorous material. Furthermore, these studies have noted even higher levels of S-IgA concentrations for those individuals scoring high on the SHRQ, once again supporting the importance of this individual difference factor. Finally, with a different type of longitudinal design, other research has shown that laughter responsiveness can moderate the relationship between the daily hassles experienced by an individual and their subsequent level of S-IgA. Hassles refer to everyday irritating, frustrating, or stressful events, such as misplacing things, having too much to do, or various interpersonal conflicts. For individuals low on laughter responsiveness, a higher frequency of hassles was significantly related to lower levels of S-IgA concentrations 6 weeks later. In contrast, a high level of hassles did not lead to lower S-IgA concentrations for individuals with higher scores on the SHRQ. In other words, increased laughter responsiveness served to buffer these individuals from the immune suppressive effects of daily hassles that were quite evident for individuals with low levels of mirth.

Theoretical accounts of the positive relationship between laughter and increased mental and physical health have generally emphasized the physiologic benefits, with laughter often hailed as being "good for the body." These accounts suggest that laughter stimulates the muscular and cardiovascular systems, facilitates digestion, oxygenates the blood, and massages the vital organs. In addition, the activity of the immune system is enhanced and levels of stress-related chemicals in the body are reduced. When combined, these physiological and behavioral effects produce a general sense of well-being that contributes positively to the maintenance of health and survival. As described earlier, some research evidence supports this basic physiologic model, with higher immune competence being related to greater laughter. In addition, other research has found that the presentation of humorous stimuli results in increased laughter and heart rate and a subsequent decrease in negative affect. Finally, an evolutionary theoretical perspective stressing the metacommunicative signaling function of laughter in social interactions has been advanced by some writers. This perspective is in accord with the social facilitative effects of laughter and points specifically to the adaptive aspects of laughter that reward individuals for continuing with positive social interactions. Indirect evidence supporting this position includes findings that individuals significantly prefer speakers that elicit laughter from their audience.

Both of these theoretical perspectives, namely, the physiologic benefits and social adaptive views of laughter, are quite compatible with general arousal or tension-reduction theories of laughter. In 1860, Herbert Spencer proposed that one of the functions of laughter is to reduce arousal stemming from a buildup of tension and energy. From a mental health perspective, stress can be viewed as an undesirable increase in tension or arousal. Thus, social interactions marked by embarrassment or conflict, for example, may have heightened levels of tension that are reduced by the effects of laughter. Similarly, in describing the physiologic benefits of laughter, some theorists have proposed that laughter takes the place of negative emotions that may have further untoward effects. Thus, the energy related to these negative emotions is dissipated in a more positive manner. Freud's theory proposes a similar notion by suggesting that jokes may sometimes provide socially appropriate means of expressing unconscious aggressive or sexual impulses that would normally be repressed. This release of inhibitory energy is expressed in the form of laughter that is both pleasurable and tension-releasing for the individual.

Overall, then, these theoretical perspectives provide some useful insights regarding the possible conceptual underpinnings between greater laughter and enhanced mental and physical health. These theories are less successful, however, in terms of explaining instances when laughter does not have a facilitative effect on well-being, or may even prove detrimental. In other words, these theories seem to lack precision in terms of predicting the exact conditions under which laughter's effects on mental health may be benign, or even harmful, rather than facilitative.

IV. SENSE OF HUMOR AND MENTAL HEALTH

A. Stress Buffering Effects

The important role of individual differences in determining the more precise relationship between humor and mental health has been demonstrated in a series of studies examining the stress buffering effects of sense of humor. In the personality domain, it has been a long established finding that various personality characteristics, such as locus of control or hardiness, can moderate the negative effects of stressful life events on an individual. Drawing from this literature, the developers of the CHS hypothesized that individuals scoring higher on this measure may be more resistant to the negative impact of stressful life events than individuals displaying less coping humor. In particular, it was thought that individuals with higher levels of coping humor could deal more effectively with adverse life situations by generating a more humorous perspective on their problems. In turn, this alternative perspective would help these individuals distance themselves more fully from their stressors, taking them less seriously, and thus reducing their negative personal impact. Typical findings from this research provide reasonable support for this notion, as individuals with a higher sense of coping humor showed little or no increase in negative affect with a reported increase

in stressful life events. In contrast, a greater number of negative life events did result in more depressive affect for those individuals scoring low on the CHS. Similar stress-buffering effects for higher levels of coping humor have also been found when the level of S-IgA is the outcome measure. Again, for all individuals reporting higher levels of negative daily events, it was only those scoring low on the CHS who showed a significant decrease in S-IgA levels. In other words, high coping-humor individuals did not show a reduction in immune system effectiveness when faced with a large number of stressful events. [*See* PSYCHONEUROIMMUNOLOGY.]

At a theoretical level, the stress-moderating effects just described have been attributed to humor-related cognitive changes in perspective that allow for more effective distancing from the immediate threat of a prospective stressor. This notion is consistent with the often-described theme that a good sense of humor fosters and encourages mental flexibility, including changes in perspective and divergent thinking. This notion is also consistent with incongruity theories of humor that view the essence of humor as the unexpected and surprising joining together of two normally separate ideas or concepts. Incongruity theories propose that this type of cognitive activity, which is also evident in scientific discoveries and artistic creativity, is one of the hallmarks of humor. Applied to a mental health perspective, this greater cognitive flexibility allows more humorous individuals to generate alternative perspectives for a given scenario rapidly, ultimately contributing to healthier responses to a variety of challenging life circumstances.

Although the change of perspective notion provides a certain degree of theoretical explanation for the documented stress-buffering effects of humor, there are limitations. At an empirical level, at least one study has failed to demonstrate this stress-moderating effect. In this research, a large sample of undergraduates completed measures of sense of humor (including the CHS), negative life events, and depressive and physical symptomatology. Contrary to predictions, a greater sense of humor did not produce lower levels of depression or physical illness for those individuals experiencing a large number of stressful events. Conceptually, this failure suggests that the cognitive processes presumed to underlie the stress-buffering effect of humor still require further empirical and theoretical clarification.

In further accord with this suggestion, it should be noted that the stress-buffering studies have not provided any direct empirical assessment of change of perspective. As this cognitive variable is presumed to play a critical role in stress reduction, subsequent work has overcome this limitation by focusing directly on this measure. In this research, participants described negative stressful events that occurred to them in the previous month. In support of incongruity theories of humor and the stress-buffering interpretations described earlier, individuals with higher levels of coping humor reported that they were able to see these stressful events from a different perspective more frequently than those with lower levels of humor. High CHS scorers also indicated that this change in perspective resulted in more positive perceptions of these events and that they made more of a conscious effort to view their problems from an alternative perspective. These findings are important, as they appear to offer the first direct test of the change of perspective notion that has been repeatedly espoused by humor theorists as one of the keystones of humor-related stress reduction.

Other cognitive variables and processes that may contribute to the stress-reducing impact of sense of humor have also been examined more directly in recent research. Both the quality of life and stress and coping literatures have suggested that the degree of upset experienced by an individual in response to a potential stressor may, in large part, be determined by the way the individual appraises that event. These cognitive appraisals can be positive in orientation, such as viewing the potential stressor as a challenge to overcome, or negative, such as viewing the event as a threat to self and well-being. In the humor literature, it has been proposed that a shift in cognitive perspective may reduce the adverse effects of stress in at least two ways. First, individuals who generally respond to life in a humorous manner may be less likely to appraise their environment as threatening, and therefore may experience less stress overall. Second, individuals with a greater sense of humor may be able to cope more effectively in stressful situations by making more facilitative cognitive reappraisals. Evidence consistent with both of these proposals was found in a recent study in which university students with high scores on the CHS appraised an upcoming examination as more of a positive challenge than did individuals scoring low on this humor scale. In further accord with these appraisals, high-humor individuals also reported lower

levels of perceived stress and greater use of distancing as a coping strategy for academic evaluations when compared with low-humor individuals. Finally, when actual examination performance proved discrepant from initial expectations, it was only the high-humor individuals who readjusted their positive challenge appraisals in a healthier direction for the next examination.

B. Positive Enhancement Effects

In addition to alleviating stress, a good sense of humor may also add a degree of richness and fullness to one's life. As written about in the humor literature, these beneficial aspects of humor include enhanced enjoyment of positive life experiences, greater positive emotions, a more positive orientation toward self, and greater psychological well-being. This theme has a long tradition, with a number of personality theorists, including Rollo May and Sigmund Freud, describing humor as a positive, life-affirming approach to both the world and one's self. This positive orientation is a healthy way of preserving one's sense of self by facilitating psychic integration and insight.

Various research findings provide some initial indirect empirical support for the positive enhancement effects of humor. Factor analytic work, for example, has noted separate positive affect components, such as exhilaration, in several existing measures of humor appreciation. At a descriptive level, children in the sixth grade already see humor as a positive aspect of caring that serves to enhance growth and development. Similarly, in a large sample of 14- to 15-year-old adolescents in the Netherlands, their views on work and leisure linked higher levels of humor and relaxation to a greater quality of life. Finally, a series of in-depth interviews with 24 individuals spanning a wide age range found that humor was a positive life force that boosts self-esteem and other aspects of well-being.

The enhancement of quality of life in a positive direction is an important aspect of mental health, with greater subjective well-being including more life satisfaction and heightened positive affect. In the humor domain, several studies provide evidence that both of these positive mental health components are associated with a greater sense of humor. In assessing long-term marriages, data gathered from 100 older couples married at least 45 years identified sense of humor as being quite important to higher satisfaction with and success in marriage. The proposal that sense of humor is a positive element of marriage that leads to increased happiness has also been advanced by marital therapists, several of whom suggest that a healthy sense of humor can increase the number of positive experiences a couple shares, strengthening their relationship. Increased satisfaction is also evident in other domains, for example, older patients are more satisfied with their family doctors if shared humor and laughter form part of their relationship. Finally, a broad-based study of social role evaluations found that higher levels of sense of humor were significantly associated with greater satisfaction and pleasantness ratings for the most important life roles for each individual.

In a somewhat different vein, the social roles study also found that as the number of positive life events increased, it was only the more humorous individuals, as assessed by the CHS, who showed an increase in their positive affect levels. Low-humor individuals did not experience this heightened positive affect for more positive life events. This study further showed that high-humor individuals were much better able to maintain their positive affect in the face of increasingly negative life events, whereas low humor individuals showed a significant drop. Overall, this pattern supports a positive affect enhancement effect for sense of humor and was corroborated in another research study conducted in a laboratory setting. Here, it was found that more humorous individuals provided higher positive challenge appraisals for a drawing task and also displayed increased personal motivation levels for this task, and greater positive affect after task completion, when compared with those scoring low on the CHS. These laboratory-based findings again support a more positive orientation on the part of humorous individuals toward life activities, with higher humor levels associated with more positive challenge appraisals and greater enthusiasm and enjoyment for task engagement and completion.

Although humor theorists have often proposed that a good sense of humor contributes to a more positive self-concept, they have rarely specified any operational measures of this construct. This limitation has been addressed in a recent empirical study that used operational indicators of a healthy self-concept borrowed from the clinical and social psychology domains. Over the past 30 years, work in these two domains has

shown that smaller discrepancies between an individual's actual and ideal self-concept perceptions are associated with increased levels of self-esteem and a reduction in adjustment concerns. Accordingly, the degree of self-concept actual–ideal congruence, along with measures of self-esteem, perceived stress, and sense of humor, were assessed in a large sample of undergraduate students. Replicating earlier work, this study found that larger discrepancies between actual and ideal self-ratings on a set of 60 personality characteristics were highly correlated with reduced levels of self-esteem and heightened levels of stress. Sense of humor played a fundamental role in these relationships, with further analyses revealing that the lowest discrepancies between actual and ideal self-concept perceptions were obtained for those individuals scoring highest on the CHS. In addition, more humorous individuals also endorsed the most realistic standards for self-evaluation on a measure of self-worth contingencies. Taken together, this pattern provides some basic empirical support for the often proposed link between higher levels of sense of humor and a more positive and healthier self-concept.

V. NEGATIVE IMPACT OF LAUGHTER AND HUMOR ON MENTAL HEALTH

In detailing links to mental health, we have focused primarily on the facilitative and productive aspects of nonhostile laughter and humor. It is clear, however, that laughter and humor can also incorporate negative elements that can be destructive rather than constructive. Recent empirical work has documented several of these less desirable aspects of laughter and humor, especially as they may pertain to broader mental health issues associated with quality of life and subjective well-being. In a teaching context, for example, inappropriate humor can detract from effective learning, be it directly in the classroom or through educational television. Similarly, the inappropriate use of humor can be detrimental for effective mediation in industrial organizational settings. With regard to individual differences, research has found that higher levels of laughter responsiveness are also marked by an increased preference for sick humor (e.g., dead baby jokes) and a self-reported increase in alcohol consumption. Moreover, a survey of more than 100 alcoholic clients receiving outpatient treatment revealed that these individuals described themselves as laughing often and that their drinking increases their sense of humor.

The association between humor and aggression has frequently been commented on; disinhibiting effects revealed in a study in which participants instructed to use humor in a creative task also generated more aggressive responses. The merger of these two elements has been demonstrated in gifted humorous children, their spontaneous witty remarks also incorporated components of attention seeking, verbal aggression, and dominance. Teasing, disparaging remarks, and degrading put-down humor are all forms of interpersonal communication that synthesize aspects of ridicule, aggression, and humor. Research evidence indicates that as early as fourth grade, children begin to use humor to deliver antisocial messages. Negative consequences are quite apparent, with recipients of teasing viewing these actions as painful and hostile. Disparaging humor, in which an individual or group is belittled or insulted, can also result in negative outcomes. One study, for example, found that freely telling disparaging jokes about a given group resulted in the development of less favorable attitudes toward that group. Finally, another study found that the greater use of disparaging or put-down humor is associated with increased physical health problems and illness. This is in direct contrast to additional findings from the same study which revealed that nonhostile forms of humor, such as good-natured play and fantasy, are related to increased levels of well-being. [*See* AGGRESSION.]

The notion that laughter and humor may sometimes reflect the base, ugly, and aggressive elements of humanity is certainly not new. Superiority or disparagement theories of humor, which date back to Plato and Aristotle, have strongly emphasized negative laughter and humor at the expense of others. As suggested by Hobbes, laughter is the "sudden glory" experienced when we celebrate our own eminence and triumph over the weak, infirm, and foolish. The downgrading of more unfortunate others may be therapeutic to the extent that it enhances one's self-esteem and perceptions of mastery. The additional social costs, however, may ultimately outweigh these benefits. Ridicule and contempt form the root of superiority or disparagement theories. As such, they provide little room for the expression of caring and facilitative social interactions that mark more positive approaches to psychological well-being.

VI. CONCLUSIONS AND FURTHER CONSIDERATIONS

Over the centuries, there have been long-standing presumptions that a greater sense of humor functions to moderate the effects of stress as well as enhance the enjoyment of positive life experiences. Both of these themes can be traced back to ancient philosophers and biblical writings and have reemerged in a number of guises over the past 2400 years. In more recent times, for example, Norman Cousins published an account of his recovery from a serious disease through the use of humor and laughter. Although an anecdotal single-case report, Cousin's 1979 book was extremely influential in spurring a renewed interest in exploring the role of humor and laughter in contributing to both mental and physical well-being. As described here, there has been a flurry of research activity in this domain over the past two decades, with some of this work continuing at the anecdotal or descriptive level. Noteworthy, however, is the increased emphasis on providing more scientifically rigorous and controlled tests of hypotheses relating humor and laughter to mental health concerns.

When taken together, the research findings reviewed in this article form a reasonable empirical foundation for arguing that humor and laughter, under certain conditions, are both beneficial to psychological well-being. It is also apparent, however, that exceptions exist, and that laughter and humor may sometimes prove counterproductive to an enhanced quality of life. Accordingly, there is a clear need to develop more precise theoretical models that specify the exact conditions under which humor and laughter may or may not benefit mental health. Of special promise in this regard is the work that has begun to articulate more fully the cognitive processes and structures that may be involved in these relationships, including cognitive appraisals, change of perspective, and standards for self-evaluations. In keeping with the broader definition of mental health, this recent work has also focused more directly on the positive impact of sense of humor on subjective well-being and life satisfaction measures.

In providing further theoretical elaboration and clarification of the possible links between humor, laughter, and mental health, several concerns might be kept in mind. First, the relationships between the multidimensional aspects of sense of humor and other personality constructs, including extraversion, locus of control, sensation seeking, conservatism, optimism, and neuroticism, should be more fully documented and researched. This is of particular importance in determining which of these constructs takes on a primary explanatory role in predicting mental health outcomes. Second, there is a need to clarify possible gender differences in the links between humor, laughter, and mental health. Current findings provide little closure, with some studies finding no gender differences and others revealing quite distinct gender-related humor preferences and outcomes. Consistency is minimal, with gender findings reversing across studies or showing substantial changes across the life span. To date, gender-related work on humor and laughter has been largely atheoretical and may thus benefit from the development of theoretical formulations that also acknowledge life span changes. Finally, there is a need to clarify possible cross-cultural distinctions in the associations between humor, laughter, and mental health. Some basic research has documented culture-specific humor findings, with the value and nature of humor varying from one culture to the next. Again, however, other research findings suggest underlying commonalities that may serve to moderate the degree to which cross-cultural distinctions may affect the relationships between humor, laughter, and mental health.

BIBLIOGRAPHY

Cousins, N. (1979). *Anatomy of an illness.* New York: Norton.

Dixon, N. F. (1980). Humor: A cognitive alternative to stress? In I. G. Sarason & C. D. Spielberger (Eds.), *Stress and anxiety* (Vol. 7, pp. 281–289). Washington, DC: Hemisphere.

Fry, W. (1994). The biology of humor. *Humor: International Journal of Humor Research, 7,* 111–126.

Keith-Spiegal, P. (1972). Early conceptions of humor: Varieties and issues. In J. H. Goldstein & P. E. McGhee (Eds.), *The psychology of humor: Theoretical perspectives and empirical issues* (pp. 3–39). New York: Academic Press.

Kuiper, N. A., McKenzie, S. D., & Belanger, K. A. (1995). Cognitive appraisals and individual differences in sense of humor: Motivational and affective implications. *Personality and Individual Differences, 19,* 359–372.

Lefcourt, H. M., & Martin, R. A. (1986). *Humor and life stress: Antidote to adversity.* New York: Springer-Verlag.

Martin, R. A. (in press). The Situational Humor Response Questionnaire (SHRQ) and Coping Humor Scale (CHS): A decade of research findings. *Humor: International Journal of Humor Research.*

Martin, R. A., Kuiper, N. A., Olinger, L. J., & Dance, K. A. (1993). Humor, coping with stress, self-concept, and psychological well-being. *Humor: International Journal of Humor Research, 6,* 89–104.

Morreall, J. (1991). Humor and work. *Humor: International Journal of Humor Research, 4,* 359–373.

Shaughnessey, M. F., & Wadsworth, T-M. (1992). Humor in counseling and psychotherapy: A 20-year retrospective. *Psychological Reports, 70,* 755–762.

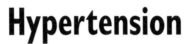

Hypertension

Barbara S. McCann

University of Washington School of Medicine

I. Hypertension Detection and Prevalence
II. Consequences of High Blood Pressure
III. Behavioral Factors in Hypertension Etiology
IV. Behavioral Treatment of Hypertension
V. Conclusion

Adherence Adherence (often termed "compliance") refers to the extent to which a patient follows the advice of his or her health care provider. The advice followed may be the taking of medications, or following any other recommendations (such as exercise, diet, and smoking cessation).

Biofeedback Biofeedback, literally, is feedback on a bioelectrical response. The term refers to a treatment modality in which some aspect of the patient's physiology (such as heart rate, skin temperature, or skeletal muscle activity) is recorded with instrumentation that converts the signal into an electrical response, such as a tone or light. This enables the patient to modify the response, often to achieve a relaxed state.

Personality Personality refers to stable predispositions of the individual that determine how the individual will behave in a variety of situations.

Reactivity Reactivity refers to acute physiological responses (for example, changes in heart rate, blood pressure, epinephrine concentrations) to a stimulus.

Stress The term "stress" has multiple meanings. Stress can refer to the body's physiological responses to a stimulus. The term stress is also used to refer to stimuli that elicit reports of fear, anger, or other negative affect from the individual.

HYPERTENSION, or elevated arterial blood pressure, occurs in more than 60 million people in the United States and is a leading cause of heart disease and stroke. Treatment of hypertension includes management with medications, diet, and exercise. In this article, behavioral approaches to improving patient adherence to these treatments will be reviewed. This article will also discuss behavioral factors in the development of high blood pressure, including environmental stress and personality, and behavioral approaches to the treatment of hypertension, including relaxation and biofeedback.

I. HYPERTENSION DETECTION AND PREVALENCE

A. The Detection of Hypertension

It is estimated that more than one-third of hypertensive individuals in the United States are not aware of their elevated blood pressure. However, detection of high blood pressure is inexpensive and straightforward. Blood pressure is measured using a sphygmomanometer, which is an inflatable cuff that is wrapped around the upper arm. The cuff is attached to a mercury column, and the column rises as pressure in the cuff increases. As the cuff is deflated, the examiner listens to arterial sounds using a stethoscope. The examiner records the point at which sounds are heard, and the point at which sounds disappear. Blood pressure is expressed in two numbers: systolic blood pressure (SBP), or the pressure in the arteries when the heart contracts (the appearance of sound), and diastolic blood pressure (DBP), or the pressure in the arteries when the heart relaxes between beats (disappearance of sound). These two numbers are expressed in millimeters of mercury (mmHg).

Normal blood pressure, among adults age 18 and older, is a systolic reading below 130 mmHg and a diastolic reading below 85 mmHg. In 1993, the Joint National Committee on Detection, Evaluation, and Treatment of High Blood Pressure established criteria for classifying high blood pressure, as shown in Table I. This classification of hypertension in stages replaces an earlier classification system that designated hypertension as mild, moderate, or severe. However, these terms are still in use today.

Increased efforts to screen individuals for elevated blood pressure have undoubtedly saved lives through enhanced detection of hypertension. However, blood pressure measured in the doctor's office is frequently higher than blood pressure assessed throughout the day. Elevated blood pressure that is detectable in the office but not at home or work is often referred to as "white coat" hypertension. This observation has led to the development of techniques to measure blood pressure repeatedly, throughout the day, while a person suspected of being hypertensive engages in his or her regular activities. Referred to as ambulatory blood pressure monitoring, this diagnostic procedure has aided in differentiating those who are truly hypertensive from individuals who only exhibit "white coat" hypertension. In addition to its use as a diagnostic tool, ambulatory blood pressure is useful for monitoring patient response to treatment. However, widespread use of ambulatory monitoring to evaluate high blood pressure is not currently routine, due to the cost and inconvenience of this method. Aside from treatment considerations, ambulatory blood pressure monitoring has served as a useful research tool for exploring relationships between blood pressure and events throughout the day.

B. Causes of Hypertension

A number of physical conditions can lead to elevated blood pressure. These include pheochromocytoma, Cushing syndrome, renal artery stenosis, aldosteronism, and coarctation of the aorta. Oral contraceptive use is also associated with elevated blood pressure. Hypertension that is attributable to a physical condition or medication is called secondary hypertension.

In most cases (as much as 95%), the cause of high blood pressure is unknown. This hypertension of unknown cause is referred to as idiopathic, primary, or essential hypertension. It is this form of hypertension that is the focus of this article. The cause of essential hypertension is likely to be a combination of genetic and environmental influences, and is still under extensive study. Stressful environments, or a predisposition to experience events as stressful, may be of etiologic significance in hypertension.

C. Hypertension Prevalence

Approximately one in four adults in the United States has high blood pressure. Hypertension disproportionately affects ethnic minorities, particularly African Americans. It is estimated that 15 million African Americans are hypertensive, accounting for more than one-quarter of all patients in the United States with high blood pressure. African Americans are more often affected by the physical sequelae of hypertension compared to Whites: 50% more likely to develop stroke, 50% more likely to develop kidney disease, and 30% more likely to develop heart disease.

In addition to race, other common demographic factors are also relevant. Young and middle-aged men have a higher prevalence of hypertension than do women, but among older adults, high blood pressure is more common in women. Elevated blood pressure is also more common in individuals with lower educational attainment and income levels. Blood pressure

Table I Guidelines for Defining Hypertension

Category	Systolic blood pressure (mmHg)	Diastolic blood pressure (mmHg)
Normal	<130	<85
Borderline	130–139	85–89
Stage 1	140–159	90–99
Stage 2	160–179	100–109
Stage 3	180–209	110–119
Stage 4	≥210	≥120

Source: The Fifth Report of the Joint National Committee on Detection, Evaluation, and Treatment of High Blood Pressure, National Institutes of Health; National Heart, Lung, and Blood Institute, NIH Publication No. 93-1088, January, 1993.

levels increase with age. While only 11% of people aged from 30 to 39 years are hypertensive, 54% of people between the ages of 60 and 69 are hypertensive. The demographic composition of the United States is changing: the population as a whole is getting older. Thus, the prevalence of hypertension in the United States is expected to continue to rise.

II. CONSEQUENCES OF HIGH BLOOD PRESSURE

Cardiovascular disease—notably, coronary heart disease (CHD) and cerebrovascular disease—is the leading cause of death and disability in the United States. The primary manifestation of CHD is myocardial infarction (MI), commonly referred to as heart attack. Factors that put people at risk for the development of CHD include smoking, high blood cholesterol, physical inactivity, and hypertension.

Stroke is the primary cerebrovascular disease related to hypertension. Risks of stroke are highest in individuals who smoke, in people with heart disease, and in people who experience transient ischemic attacks (brief reductions in blood flow within the brain). High red blood cell counts, older age, family history of stroke, and diabetes are also risk factors for stroke. However, hypertension is the single most important factor contributing to stroke, and control of blood pressure significantly reduces the risk of stroke.

Although heart disease and stroke are the most common consequences of high blood pressure, other debilitating diseases may result from uncontrolled high blood pressure, including congestive heart failure, renal insufficiency, retinopathy, and peripheral vascular disease.

A. Cognitive Effects

In some studies, individuals with hypertension show subtle neurological deficits. These deficits include impairment in perceptual, cognitive, psychomotor, and memory functions. However, these deficits are only evident during careful testing, and do not appear to affect day-to-day activities at home and work. In addition, the deficits seen during testing do not appear to worsen over time, and the underlying pathophysiology is unknown. Treatment with antihypertensive medications may improve neuropsychological functioning, but this is a question requiring further study.

III. BEHAVIORAL FACTORS IN HYPERTENSION ETIOLOGY

A. Stress

Psychologists Richard Lazarus and Susan Folkman have proposed that individuals differ in how they interpret environmental events, and that such differences in appraisal can determine whether such events are regarded as positive, negative, or neutral. Psychologists generally regard negative events as stressors, keeping in mind that situations that are stressful for some may not be regarded as stressful by others. Events that threaten control, self-esteem, and general well-being are generally regarded as stressful. [See STRESS.]

Exposure to psychological stress generally leads to an abrupt and transient increase in blood pressure. Elevated blood pressure when faced with stress is part of a constellation of physiological changes during challenge; others include increased heart rate, sweating, increased rate of respiration, muscle tightness, and hypervigilance. Under normal circumstances, these bodily changes during stress are adaptive, and are typical of the "fight or flight" response. However, it has long been hypothesized that inappropriately exaggerated responses to stress lead to the development of disease. Thus, the observation that blood pressure increases during exposure to stress has led researchers to hypothesize that prolonged exposure to stress, or inappropriately large blood pressure increases in response to stress, leads to sustained elevation in blood pressure, namely, hypertension.

Studies in controlled laboratory situations support the hypothesis that hypertension may develop due to exposure to stress. Two theories to explain this association between stress and hypertension have been proposed. One, the autoregulation theory, holds that increased cardiac output (due in part to increased heart rate) during stress leads to overperfusion of tissues with oxygenated blood, resulting in a compensatory (autoregulation) response of increased peripheral resistance. The persistence of this resistance constitutes essential hypertension. Another theory, that of structural adaptation, holds that elevations in blood pressure lead to changes in the heart and blood vessels that make them more susceptible to higher blood pressure during stress. The structural adaptation theory also holds that there may be genetic susceptibility to these changes.

The reactivity hypothesis is supported by numerous laboratory studies. One consistent finding is that many patients with borderline hypertension have higher circulating norepinephrine levels than people with normal blood pressure, indicative of greater sympathetic nervous system activity. Such individuals also show greater blood pressure and heart rate responses to stress. Another finding is that offspring of hypertensives show greater blood pressure and heart rate responses to stress than do offspring of normotensives.

B. Environmental Contributions

A number of studies have shown that people exposed to stressful work environments show higher blood pressure levels than people in relatively low-stress work environments. In particular, jobs that are high in demands—that is, jobs that are difficult, include many deadlines, or entail unpleasant interpersonal interactions—and jobs low in decision latitude, or the ability to control one's work, contribute to high levels of job strain. Job strain has been linked to higher blood pressure levels at work. Other studies have compared the jobs of hypertensive individuals with the jobs of people with normal blood pressure, and have found that hypertensives are more likely to be in high strain jobs. Finally, individuals living in crowded environments are more susceptible to the development of high blood pressure.

C. Personality

There has long been speculation that a "hypertensive personality" exists. The hypothesis that emotional factors contribute to the development of hypertension dates to at least 1939, when Franz Alexander proposed that the suppression of anger, hostility, and frustration contributes to high blood pressure. Recently, data from the Normative Aging Study based in Boston provided evidence for the existence of a hypertensive personality. The Normative Aging Study began in 1961, when more than 6000 men were recruited and received periodic medical examinations for an average of 17 years. A personality questionnaire was administered at one of the earlier visits. Men

who were more emotionally stable had a 13% lower risk of developing hypertension.

Anger expression and hostility are important personality characteristics that may influence the development of hypertension. Some studies have associated the tendency to "bottle up" feelings of anger with greater likelihood of exhibiting large blood pressure increases in response to laboratory stressors. However, anger, rather than mode of anger expression per se, may be related to an increased risk for developing hypertension. In the Israeli Ischemic Heart Disease Study, men who reported that they brood and harbor feelings of retaliation against supervisors were more likely to develop hypertension than their less hostile co-workers. [See ANGER.]

Another personality factor related to hypertension is John Henryism. John Henryism is a construct developed by Dr. Sherman James and his colleagues at the University of Michigan to explain the high prevalence of hypertension in African Americans. John Henryism refers to the belief that determination and hard work can be used to overcome any obstacle. The term derives from the legend of John Henry, a black steel-driver who challenged a steel driving machine. In his battle against the machine, John Henry won, but died from the tremendous effort. Because African Americans continually face obstacles due to discrimination and economic circumstances, they may be particularly susceptible to the effects of John Henryism, which include chronic excessive arousal with high blood pressure as a result. [See RACISM AND MENTAL HEALTH.]

Finally, a repressive style of coping, defined as high defensiveness and low levels of anxiety, has been associated with hypertension, and with greater blood pressure responses to stress in the laboratory. [See COPING WITH STRESS.]

IV. BEHAVIORAL TREATMENT OF HYPERTENSION

A. Stress Management

Based on the notion that high blood pressure is due, at least in part, to the effects of stress, a number of stress management techniques have been employed to lower blood pressure in hypertensive individuals. It is assumed that sustained elevations in blood pressure are due, at least in part, to increased arousal of the sympathetic nervous system. Some stress management techniques are aimed at controlling the nervous system's response to stress through general relaxation. These strategies include progressive muscle relaxation, meditation, autogenic training, and biofeedback. It should be noted that while stress management may be useful for some people with hypertension, such as individuals facing extreme and prolonged stress, stress reduction techniques are not currently recommended in the treatment of high blood pressure.

Progressive muscle relaxation (PMR) was developed by Edmund Jacobson in the 1930s. Two basic forms of PMR are in use today; one form, based on the original technique developed by Jacobson, entails careful, systematic tensing and relaxing of specific skeletal muscles in order to heighten the patient's awareness of muscle tension, thereby increasing his or her ability to "switch off" muscle tension when it is noticed throughout the day. The other, more popular technique, calls for tensing and relaxing of larger groupings of muscles, under the assumption that the relaxation phase of this sequence produces greater overall arousal reduction than does simply relaxing the muscles without the tensing sequence. Both approaches are similar because they focus on skeletal muscle arousal, and patients are advised to set aside at least a half hour per day to engage in the exercises.

Meditation to induce a state of relaxation has its roots in yoga and other Eastern practices that have been adapted and popularized by Westerners. Most forms of meditation require the participant to focus attention on a single stimulus, which can be a tangible object, breathing, or a repeated sound or mantra. Psychophysiological studies have shown that meditation is accompanied by reduced arousal. [See MEDITATION AND THE RELAXATION RESPONSE.]

Autogenic relaxation strategies encompass a wide range of mental imagery techniques to induce relaxation. Patients are encouraged to turn their thoughts inward, and visualize a number of changes in physical sensations, including increased warmth, comfort, relaxation, and a sense of inner calm. Autogenic training is often combined with another form of relaxation training that utilizes biofeedback.

B. Biofeedback

The term biofeedback, literally, means feedback on a biological response. As a treatment modality, biofeedback was developed in the 1960s as a means of teaching people how to exercise voluntary control over autonomic functions, such as heart rate and sweating. Sophisticated machines that can detect subtle changes in skin temperature, muscle changes, sweating, and other bodily functions are used to provide the patient with information through the use of auditory or visual signals that vary in tandem with these changes. As a general relaxation strategy, patients can use biofeedback to learn how to relax. [See BIOFEEDBACK.]

Several different biofeedback modalities have been used in the treatment of essential hypertension. Temperature biofeedback promotes general relaxation. Increased finger temperature reflects increased blood flow to the hands, indicative of vasodilation. By monitoring finger temperature, patients learn to recognize a state of relaxation, and become capable of voluntarily producing this state. Electromyography (EMG) biofeedback reflects tension in the muscles. As with temperature biofeedback, EMG biofeedback promotes general relaxation. Skin conductance biofeedback, also referred to as the galvanic skin response (GSR) or the electrodermal response, reflects sweating in the hands. GSR biofeedback promotes general relaxation.

Blood pressure biofeedback gives the hypertensive patient direct information about blood pressure, which can facilitate blood pressure lowering. However, feedback on actual blood pressure is difficult to produce with current technology. Consequently, this treatment modality has not seen widespread use.

In addition to these techniques that promote general relaxation, other stress management strategies are sometimes used that help individuals decrease the amount of stress they face in their day-to-day lives. These include time management, cognitive behavioral therapy, and assertiveness training. The rationale for the use of these approaches is that they promote blood pressure lowering by reducing the stressfulness of interactions. In contrast, the rationale for the aforementioned relaxation procedures is they reduce the physiological arousal that often accompanies exposure to stressful situations, thereby lowering blood pressure.

C. Antihypertensive Medication

There are several different types of drugs used to control hypertension. The most common of these antihypertensive agents are the diuretics, which lower blood pressure through increased water and sodium excretion. Beta blockers, another common class of medications used to treat high blood pressure, slow the heart rate, which in turn lowers blood pressure. Sympathetic nerve inhibitors reduce blood pressure by inhibiting nerves that cause constriction of blood vessels. Angiotensin converting enzyme (A.C.E.) inhibitors interfere with an enzyme that causes vasoconstriction and subsequent water and sodium retention. The calcium antagonists (also known as calcium channel blockers) reduce the heart rate and cause the blood vessels to relax, thereby reducing blood pressure.

A number of randomized, controlled clinical trials have shown that these medications are effective in controlling blood pressure, and they reduce the risks of heart attack and stroke. Studies evaluating pharmacological agents in the treatment of mild hypertension have generally found that lowering DBP by from 5 to 6 mmHg results in a 42% reduction in stroke incidence and a 14% reduction in CHD incidence.

Despite the success of medications for controlling blood pressure, compliance with antihypertensive drug therapy is problematic. It is estimated that from 20 to 50% of hypertensive patients discontinue their medication after 1 year. Overall, the adherence rate among people with hypertension is approximately 65%. Poor compliance may be due in part to the side effects often associated with these medications, including weakness and fatigue, dizziness, headaches, drowsiness, elevations in blood cholesterol levels, and sexual dysfunction. Other explanations for poor compliance include inadequate instructions to patients regarding medication use, patients' personal beliefs regarding the efficacy of medications, and an environment that is not conducive to medication adherence (for example, difficulties in getting prescriptions filled due to financial limitations or inadequate transportation).

Health psychologists, nurse practitioners, and other health professionals are often called upon to assist with medication compliance among people with high blood pressure and other chronic illnesses. Although empirical research on the efficacy of these interventions is sparse, a number of behavioral management strategies are promising. Self-monitoring is a useful tool in enhancing medication compliance. By recording medication use, and by self-monitoring blood pressure at home, patients can improve adherence to dosing schedules. Contracting with the health care provider is another effective technique for improving patient compliance at the outset of treatment. Cuing, or the provision of reminders to patients, serves as another useful intervention for addressing adherence.

These may take the form of written or telephoned reminders to patients, initiated by the health care provider.

D. Diet and Exercise

In 1993, the National High Blood Pressure Education Program Working Group recommended that the U.S. population could prevent the development of hypertension by losing weight, reducing sodium intake, reducing alcohol consumption, and increasing physical activity. Dietary changes and increased physical activity may also facilitate high blood pressure control in people who are hypertensive. Some individuals are salt-sensitive and can lower their blood pressure by reducing the sodium in their diet by avoiding salty foods. It is estimated that nearly half of hypertensive patients are salt sensitive and will respond to reductions in sodium intake with decreased blood pressure. This is particularly true of African Americans and the elderly. Some people find that excessive alcohol intake raises their blood pressure; consequently, alcohol intake should be restricted. Finally, obesity contributes to high blood pressure. Weight loss often results in lower blood pressure, particularly in individuals who are markedly overweight. Recent studies have shown that weight loss through caloric restriction, often in combination with sodium reductions and reductions in alcohol use, can produce beneficial changes in blood pressure among hypertensives, and can decrease their need for antihypertensive medication. In addition, dietary changes among people with established hypertension are effective in reducing left ventricular mass, one of the changes in heart size that accompanies sustained blood pressure elevations.

Although controlling hypertension through dietary changes and increased physical activity has considerable appeal, maintenance of these life-style changes is difficult, even in highly motivated individuals. Nutritional education forms the cornerstone of dietary change; patients require a careful explanation of the changes they need to make. Behavioral scientists have developed a number of approaches to assist patients with changes in life-style, and these have been shown to be effective in nutritional interventions.

One important component of behavioral interventions to change diet is the setting of appropriate and specific dietary goals with the patient. Goals that are too broad and nonspecific leave patients feeling frustrated and uncertain of the health care provider's expectations. In contrast, clear and specific goals make life-style changes seem much more manageable, and they are more likely to be met, thereby promoting a sense of accomplishment. A related component of behavioral interventions is self-monitoring. Patients who are trying to make dietary changes often find it useful to record certain aspects of their diet on a daily basis, such as the amount of sodium consumed (in grams). Frequently, the act of self-monitoring itself contributes to improvement in the monitored behavior. In addition, self-monitoring serves as an index of progress, and is a more immediate yardstick of improvement than is the occasional blood pressure measurement in the doctor's office.

Stimulus control training is another behavioral strategy that is relevant to dietary changes. Many dietary habits are dictated by the environment. For example, patients often report that certain sights and smells will trigger hunger, and may affect the food choices they will make. In addition, the ready availability of high sodium foods (such as potato chips left on the kitchen countertop) acts as a cue to eat foods the hypertensive patient should avoid. Thus, patients are often advised to limit their exposure to such stimuli in their environment, enabling them to exert greater control over their diet.

A similar concept to enhance dietary compliance is to encourage patients to engage in problem solving around dietary changes. People are often able to predict when they will be in situations that will make it difficult to maintain a healthy diet. One important part of behavioral intervention is to help the patient anticipate these situations and develop plans for minimizing the effects of such situations on their diet.

Relapse prevention training was developed by G. Alan Marlatt at the University of Washington to address the problem of relapse among people who have stopped using addictive substances such as alcohol, illicit drugs, and tobacco. Relapse prevention training has also been used in behaviorally oriented dietary programs to help patients deal effectively with the inevitable slip-ups they experience when trying to modify their eating behavior. According to Marlatt, patients who deviate from a successful pattern of behavioral changes—by eating a bag of salty potato chips, for example—experience an Abstinence Violation Effective (AVE). The AVE leaves the patient feeling as though he or she is a failure, lacks self-control, and cannot face situations that challenge habit control. Relapse prevention training addresses the AVE by encouraging patients to regard such slips, or relapses, as isolated incidents, rather than harbingers of failure. Patients are also encouraged to learn from these inevitable slips, which ties in with the aforementioned principles of problem solving.

A number of observational studies have found that physical activity is inversely related to blood pressure. In addition, several studies have shown that average blood pressure reductions of from 6 to 7 mmHg can result from interventions that promote increased physical activity. Low to moderate physical activity is sufficient to produce these gains. Based on these observations, increased physical activity is often recommended for people with mild hypertension. When dietary changes are recommended, particularly for weight loss, increased physical activity is generally recommended as well, as it promotes initial weight loss and maintenance of weight loss. As with dietary changes, however, maintenance of a program of regular exercise is often difficult. Many of the behavioral strategies outlined in this article, particularly goal setting and self-monitoring, are used to achieve better exercise compliance. [See EXERCISE AND MENTAL HEALTH; FOOD, NUTRITION, AND MENTAL HEALTH.]

Although the various strategies for blood pressure reduction have been described separately, probably the best way to achieve blood pressure reductions is through a combination of antihypertensive medication and changes in life-style. A recent clinical trial that combined dietary changes, exercise, and medication to reduce blood pressure in mildly hypertensive individuals is the Treatment of Mild Hypertension Study (TOMHS). The life-style intervention, which used many of the behavioral strategies outlined in this chapter, included dietary changes and increased physical activity. Participants achieved an average weight loss of 10.5 pounds at the end of 1 year, and by 4 years maintained a weight loss of 5.7 pounds. Leisure activity also showed substantial increases. Participants who received the life-style intervention, but did not receive an active antihypertensive medication, achieved average blood pressure reductions of 10.6/8.1 mmHg (SBP/DBP). The TOMHS experience attests to the value of life-style changes in achieving blood pressure control.

V. CONCLUSION

Although this article has outlined many of the behavioral and life-style factors that can be modified to lower blood pressure, several factors that affect blood pressure cannot be changed. These factors include age, genetic factors, and race. As people age, they are more likely to develop high blood pressure. People whose parents are hypertensive have an increased likelihood of developing high blood pressure. Finally, certain racial and ethnic groups, notably African Americans, are more likely to develop high blood pressure than are Whites. Nonetheless, there is considerable evidence for the role of personality and environmental factors in the development of high blood pressure, and the behavioral strategies discussed in this chapter are useful in the primary prevention and treatment of hypertension.

BIBLIOGRAPHY

Blanchard, E. B., Martin, J. E., & Dubbert, P. M. (1988). *Non-drug treatments for essential hypertension.* New York: Pergamon.

Dunbar-Jacob, J., Dwyer, K., & Dunning, E. J. (1991). Compliance with antihypertensive regimens: A review of research in the 1980's. *Annals of Behavioral Medicine, 13,* 32–39.

The Fifth Report of the Joint National Committee on Detection, Evaluation, and Treatment of High Blood Pressure. (1993). *Archives of Internal Medicine, 153,* 154–183.

Fray, J. C. S., & Douglas, J. G. (1993). *Pathophysiology of hypertension in blacks.* New York: Oxford University Press.

Krakoff, L. R. (1995). *Management of the hypertensive patient.* New York: Churchill Livingstone.

Langford, H., Levine, B., & Ellenbogen, E. (1990). *Nutritional factors in hypertension.* New York: Alan R. Liss.

National High Blood Pressure Education Program. (1993). Working Group Report on Primary Prevention of Hypertension. U.S. Department of Health and Human Services, NIH Publication No. 93-2669.

Turner, J. R. (1994). *Cardiovascular reactivity and stress.* New York: Plenum Press.

Hypnosis and the Psychological Unconscious

John F. Kihlstrom

University of California, Berkeley

Automatic Processes Perceptual–cognitive processes that are initiated involuntarily, executed outside phenomenal awareness, and consume no attentional resources.

Data-Driven Processes Perceptual–cognitive processes that are based on the perceptual structure of a stimulus.

Episodic Memory Memory for personal experiences, each associated with a unique spatiotemporal context (see contrasting *Semantic Memory*).

Explicit Memory Conscious recollection, as manifested in a person's ability to recall or recognize some past event (see contrasting *Implicit Memory*).

Factor Analysis A statistical technique that provides a concise summary of the correlations among a large number of variables.

Hypnotizability Individual differences in response to hypnosis, as measured by standardized psychological tests such as the Stanford Hypnotic Susceptibility Scales.

Implicit Memory Any effect on task performance that is attributable to a past event, independent of conscious recollection of that event (see contrasting *Explicit Memory*).

Preattentive Processing The perceptual–cognitive processing that occurs before attention has been paid to a stimulus.

Priming The facilitation of perceptual–cognitive processing of a stimulus (known as a target) by presentation of a prior stimulus (known as a prime). In repetition priming, prime and target are identical (e.g., water–water); in semantic priming, prime and target are related in terms of meaning (e.g., ocean–water).

Semantic Memory Context-free memory for factual information (see contrasting *Episodic Memory*).

HYPNOSIS is a social interaction in which one person (the subject) responds to suggestions given by another person (the hypnotist) for imaginative experiences involving alterations in perception, memory, and the voluntary control of action. In the classic case, these responses are associated with a degree of subjective conviction bordering on delusion and an experience of involuntariness bordering on compulsion. The psychological unconscious refers to the proposition that mental states—cognitions, emotions, and motives—can influence ongoing experience, thought, and action outside of phenomenal awareness and voluntary control.

I. HISTORY OF HYPNOSIS

The origins of hypnosis extend back to the ancient temples of Aesculapius, the Greek god of medicine, where advice and reassurance uttered by priests to sleeping patients was interpreted by the patients as the gods speaking to them in their dreams. Its more recent history, however, begins with Franz Anton Mesmer (1734–1815), who theorized that disease was caused by imbalances of a physical force, called animal magnetism, affecting various parts of the body. Accordingly, Mesmer thought that cures could be achieved by redistributing this magnetic fluid—a procedure that typically resulted in pseudoepileptic seizures known as "crises." In 1784, a French royal commission chaired by Benjamin Franklin and including Lavoisier and Guillotin among its members concluded that the effects of mesmerism, while genuine in many cases, were achieved by means of imagination and not any physical force. In the course of their proceedings, the commissioners conducted what may well be the first controlled psychological experiments.

Mesmer's theory was discredited, but his practices lived on. A major transition occurred when one of Mesmer's followers, the Marquis de Puysegur, magnetized Victor Race, a young shepherd on his estate. Instead of undergoing a magnetic crisis, Victor fell into a somnambulistic state in which he was responsive to instructions, and from which he awoke with an amnesia for what he had done. Later in the nineteenth century, John Elliotson and James Esdaile, among others, reported the successful use of mesmeric somnambulism as an anesthetic for surgery (although ether and chloroform soon proved to be more reliably effective). James Braid, another British physician, speculated that somnambulism was caused by the paralysis of nerve centers induced by ocular fixation; in order to eliminate the taint of mesmerism, he renamed the state "neurhypnotism" (nervous sleep), a term later shortened to hypnosis. Later, Braid concluded that hypnosis resulted from the subject's concentration on a single thought (monoideism) rather than from physiological fatigue.

Interest in hypnosis was revived in France in the late 1880s by Jean Martin Charcot, who thought hypnosis was a form of hysteria. Charcot believed that both hypnosis and hysteria reflected a disorder of the central nervous system. In opposition to Charcot's neurological theories, A. A. Liebeault and Hippolyte Bernheim, two other French physicians, emphasized the role of suggestibility in producing hypnotic effects. Pierre Janet and Sigmund Freud also studied with Charcot, and Freud began to develop his psychogenic theories of mental illness after observing the suggestibility of hysterical patients when they were hypnotized.

In America, William James and other early psychologists became interested in hypnosis because it seemed to involve alterations in conscious awareness. The first systematic experimental work on hypnosis was reported by P. C. Young in a doctoral dissertation completed at Harvard in 1923, and by Clark Hull in an extensive series of experiments initiated at the University of Wisconsin in the 1920s and continued at Yale into the 1930s. Also at Wisconsin during Hull's time was Milton Erickson, whose provocative clinical and experimental studies stimulated interest in hypnosis among psychotherapists (Hull knew Erickson at Wisconsin, but the immediate source of Hull's interest in hypnosis was Joseph Jastrow, who was Hull's mentor). In England, Hans Eysenck studied hypnosis and suggestibility as part of his classic explorations of personality structure.

After World War II, interest in hypnosis rose rapidly. Ernest Hilgard, together with Josephine Hilgard and Andre Weitzenhoffer, established a laboratory for hypnosis research at Stanford University. Hilgard's status as one of the world's most distinguished psychologists helped establish hypnosis as a legitimate subject of scientific inquiry. Also important in this revival were Theodore Sarbin, Martin Orne, Theodore Barber, and Erika Fromm. Hypnosis is now a thriving topic for both scientific inquiry and clinical application, and is represented by such professional organizations as the Society for Clinical and Experimental Hypnosis, the American Society of Clinical Hypnosis, and other affiliates of the International Society of Hypnosis. The *International Journal of Clinical and Experimental Hypnosis,* the *American Journal of Clinical Hypnosis,* the *Australian Journal of Clinical and Experimental Hypnosis,* and *Contemporary Hypnosis* (formerly the *British Journal of Experimental and Clinical Hypnosis*) are among the leading journals publishing hypnosis research.

II. INDIVIDUAL DIFFERENCES

The Abbe Faria, another follower of Mesmer, recognized individual differences in response to animal magnetism as early as 1819, and there are large individual differences in response to hypnosis as well. Hypnosis has little to do with the hypnotist's technique and very much to do with the subject's capacity, or talent, for experiencing hypnosis. Hypnotizability is measured by standardized psychological tests such as the Stanford Hypnotic Susceptibility Scale or the Harvard Group Scale of Hypnotic Susceptibility. These instruments are work samples, analogous to other performance tests. They begin with a hypnotic induction in which the subjects are asked to focus their eyes on a fixation point, relax, and concentrate on the voice of the hypnotist (although suggestions for relaxation are generally part of the hypnotic induction procedure, people can respond positively to hypnotic suggestions while engaged in vigorous physical activity). The hypnotist then gives suggestions for further relaxation, focused attention, and eye closure. After the subjects close their eyes, they receive further suggestions for various imaginative experiences. For example, they may be told to extend their arms and imagine a heavy object pushing their hands and arms down, or that a voice is asking them questions over a loudspeaker, or that when they open their eyes they will not be able to see an object placed in front of them. Posthypnotic suggestions may also be given for responses to be executed after hypnosis has been terminated, including posthypnotic amnesia, the inability to remember events and experiences which transpired during hypnosis. Response to each of these suggestions is scored in terms of objective behavioral criteria—do the subjects' arms drop a specified distance over a period of time, do they answer questions realistically, do they deny seeing the object, and so on.

Hypnotizability, so measured, yields a roughly normal (i.e., bell-shaped) distribution of scores. Most people are at least moderately responsive to hypnotic suggestions, while relatively few people are refractory to hypnosis and relatively few (so-called hypnotic virtuosos) fall within the highest level of responsiveness. Cross-sectional studies of different age groups show a developmental curve, with very young children relatively unresponsive to hypnosis and hypnotizability reaching a peak at about the onset of adolescence; scores drop off among middle-aged and elderly individuals. Hypnotizability assessed in college students remains about as stable as IQ over a period of 25 years.

Although hypnotizability is generally assessed in terms of a single-sum score, factor-analytic studies reveal a degree of multidimensionality. Hypnotic suggestions can be classified roughly as ideomotor (involving the facilitation of motor responses), challenge (involving the inhibition of motor responses), and cognitive (involving alterations in perception and memory). These factors are themselves intercorrelated, so that a general dimension of hypnotizability emerges at a higher level, much like Thurstone's solution to the structure of intelligence in terms of primary mental abilities and a superordinate general intelligence.

Even though hypnosis is a product of suggestion, it is a mistake to identify hypnotizability with suggestibility. In fact, suggestibility itself is also factorially complex. Eysenck distinguished among primary (e.g., direct suggestions for the facilitation and inhibition of motor activity), secondary (implied suggestions for sensory–perceptual changes), and tertiary (e.g., attitude changes resulting from persuasive communications) forms of suggestibility; a further form of suggestibility is the placebo response. Hypnotizability is correlated only with primary suggestibility, and this is carried mostly by the relation between primary suggestibility and the ideomotor and challenge components of hypnotizability.

There is some controversy over whether hypnotizability can be modified. Some clinical practitioners, influenced by the theories of Milton Erickson, believe that virtually everyone can be hypnotized, if only the hypnotist takes the right approach, but there is little evidence favoring this point of view. Similarly, some researchers believe that hypnotizability can be enhanced by developing positive attitudes, motivations, and expectancies concerning hypnosis, but there is also evidence that such enhancements are heavily laced with compliance. As with any other skilled performance, hypnotic response is probably a matter of both aptitude and attitude: negative attitudes, motivations, and expectancies can interfere with performance, but positive ones are not by themselves sufficient to create hypnotic virtuosity.

The role of individual differences makes it clear that

in an important sense, all hypnosis is self-hypnosis. The hypnotist does not hypnotize the subject. Rather, the hypnotist serves as a sort of coach, or tutor, whose job is to help the subject become hypnotized. Although it takes considerable training and expertise to use hypnosis appropriately in clinical practice, it takes very little skill to be a hypnotist. Beyond the hypnotist's ability to develop rapport with the subject, the most important factor determining hypnotic response is the hypnotizability of the individual subject.

III. CORRELATES

Hypnotizability is not substantially correlated with most other individual differences in ability or personality, such as intelligence or adjustment. Interestingly, it does not appear to be correlated with individual differences in conformity, persuasibility, or response to other forms of social influence. However, in the early 1960s, Ronald Shor, Arvid Ås, and others found that hypnotizability was correlated with subjects' tendency to have hypnosis-like experiences outside of formal hypnotic settings, and an extensive interview study by Josephine Hilgard showed that hypnotizable subjects displayed a high level of imaginative involvement in domains such as reading and drama. In 1974, Auke Tellegen and Gilbert Atkinson developed a scale of absorption to measure the disposition to have subjective experiences characterized by the full engagement of attention (narrowed or expanded) and blurred boundaries between self and object. Absorption is the most reliable correlate of hypnotizability (by contrast, vividness of mental imagery is essentially uncorrelated with hypnosis), although the statistical relation is too weak to permit confident prediction of an individual's actual response to hypnotic suggestion. So far as the measurement of hypnotizability is concerned, there is no substitute for performance-based measures such as the Stanford and Harvard scales.

Absorption seems to be a heretofore unappreciated aspect of individual differences. The scales of the Minnesota Multiphasic Personality Inventory, California Psychological Inventory, and other such instruments do not contain items related to absorption, which may explain their failure to correlate with hypnotizability. However, absorption is not wholly unrelated to other individual differences in personality. Recent multivariate research has settled on five major di-

mensions—the Big Five—which provide a convenient summary of personality structure: neuroticism (emotional stability), extraversion, agreeableness, conscientiousness, and a fifth factor often called openness to experience. Absorption is correlated with openness. [*See* PERSONALITY.]

Actually, the definition of the fifth factor as openness is somewhat controversial, with some theorists arguing for alternative interpretations in terms of intellectance (i.e., the appearance of being intelligent) or culturedness. Openness itself proves to be heterogeneous: some facets (richness of fantasy life, aesthetic sensitivity, and awareness of inner feelings) resemble absorption, while others (need for variety in actions, interest in ideas, and liberal value systems) relate to sociopolitical liberalism. In fact, hypnotizability is correlated with the absorption component of openness, but not with liberalism or intellectance. This pattern of differential correlates indicates that intellectance, absorption, and liberalism are different dimensions of personality and should not be lumped together. In stimulating the discovery of absorption, and in clarifying the nature of the fifth factor in the Big Five structure, research on individual differences in hypnotizability has contributed to understanding in the broader domain of personality.

Researchers have been interested in biological correlates of hypnotizability as well as in those which can be measured by paper-and-pencil tests. Although hypnosis is commonly induced with suggestions for relaxation and even sleep, the brain activity in hypnosis more closely resembles that of a person who is awake. The discovery of hemispheric specialization, with the left hemisphere geared to analytic and the right hemisphere to nonanalytic tasks, led to the speculation that hypnotic response is somehow mediated by right-hemisphere activity. Studies that used both behavioral and electrophysiological paradigms have been interpreted as indicating increased activation of the right hemisphere among highly hypnotizable individuals, but positive results have proved difficult to replicate and interpretation of these findings remains controversial.

It should be noted that hypnosis is mediated by verbal suggestions, which must be interpreted by the subject in the course of responding. Thus, the role of the left hemisphere should not be minimized. One interesting proposal is that hypnotizable individuals show greater flexibility in deploying the left and right hemispheres in a task-appropriate manner, especially when they are actually hypnotized. Because involuntariness is so central to the experience of hypnosis, it has also been suggested that the frontal lobes (which organize intentional action) may play a special role. A better understanding of the neural substrates of hypnosis awaits studies of neurological patients with focalized brain lesions, as well as brain-imaging studies (e.g., positron-emission tomography, magnetic resonance imaging) of normal subjects. [*See* BRAIN SCANNING/ NEUROIMAGING.]

IV. EXPERIMENTAL STUDIES

Right from the beginning of the modern era, a great deal of research effort has been devoted to claims that hypnotic suggestions enable individuals to transcend their normal voluntary capacities—to be stronger, see better, learn faster, and remember more. However, research has largely failed to find evidence that hypnosis can enhance human performance. Many early studies, which seemed to yield positive results for hypnosis, possessed serious methodological flaws, such as the failure to collect adequate baseline information. In general, it appears that hypnotic suggestions for increased muscular strength, endurance, sensory acuity, or learning do not exceed what can be accomplished by motivated subjects outside hypnosis.

A special case of performance enhancement has to do with hypnotic suggestions for improvements in memory—what is known as hypnotic hypermnesia. Hypermnesia suggestions are sometimes used in forensic situations, with forgetful witnesses and victims, or in therapeutic situations to help patients remember traumatic personal experiences. Although field studies have sometimes claimed that hypnosis can powerfully enhance memory, these anecdotal reports have not been duplicated under laboratory conditions.

A 1994 report by the Committee on Techniques for the Enhancement of Human Performance, a unit of the U.S. National Research Council, concluded that gains in recall produced by hypnotic suggestion were rarely dramatic and were matched by gains observed even when subjects are not hypnotized (in fact, there is some evidence that hypnotic suggestion can interfere with normal hypermnesic processes). To make things worse, any increases obtained in valid recollection are met or exceeded by increases in false recollec-

tions. Moreover, hypnotized subjects (especially those who are highly hypnotizable) may be vulnerable to distortions in memory produced by leading questions and other subtle and suggestive influences.

Similar conclusions apply to hypnotic age regression, in which subjects receive suggestions that they are returning to a previous period in their lives (this is also a technique used clinically to foster the retrieval of forgotten memories of child abuse). Although age-regressed subjects may experience themselves as children, and may behave in a childlike manner, there is no evidence that they actually undergo either abolition of characteristically adult modes of mental functioning or reinstatement of childlike modes of mental functioning. Nor do age-regressed subjects experience the revivification of forgotten memories of childhood.

One phenomenon that has received a great deal of attention is hypnotic analgesia—in large part because of the obvious clinical uses to which it can be put. A comparative study of experimental pain found that among hypnotizable subjects, hypnotic analgesia was superior to morphine, diazepam, aspirin, acupuncture, and biofeedback. Hypnotic analgesia relieves both sensory pain and suffering. It is not mediated by relaxation, and the fact that it is not reversed by narcotic antagonists would seem to rule out a role for endogenous opiates. There is a placebo component to all active analgesic agents, and hypnosis is no exception; however, hypnotizable subjects receive benefits from hypnotic suggestion that outweigh what they or their insusceptible counterparts achieve from plausible placebos.

Psychological explanations of hypnotic analgesia come in two primary forms. On the one hand, it is argued that hypnotized subjects use such techniques as self-distraction, stress-inoculation, cognitive reinterpretation, and tension management. While there is no doubt that cognitive strategies can reduce pain, their success, unlike the success of hypnotic suggestions, is not correlated with hypnotizability and thus is unlikely to be responsible for the effects observed in hypnotizable subjects. Rather, hypnotic analgesia seems to be associated with a division of consciousness which prevents the perception of pain from being represented in conscious awareness, without altering the physiological effects of the pain stimulus.

A great deal of research has also been devoted to the posthypnotic amnesia frequently displayed by hypnotizable subjects. This form of forgetting does not occur spontaneously and may be reversed by administration of a prearranged signal without the reinduction of hypnosis, so it does not represent a form of state-dependent learning. However, the reversibility of amnesia does indicate that its mechanisms may be located at the retrieval stage of memory processing, rather than at the encoding or storage stages. Posthypnotic amnesia does not prevent words studied during hypnosis from being used as free associates or category instances, indicating that posthypnotic amnesia is a disruption of episodic, but not semantic, memory. Moreover, the production of studied items as instances and associates is actually facilitated, resulting in priming effects. Similarly, posthypnotic amnesia does not affect retroactive inhibition or savings in relearning. Skills acquired during hypnosis are preserved afterward, even though the subject cannot remember the acquisition trials. This assortment of findings indicates that although posthypnotic amnesia disrupts explicit expressions of episodic memory (such as recall), it spares implicit expressions. [*See* AMNESIA.]

Other phenomena of hypnosis can also be understood in terms of the explicit–implicit distinction. For example, hypnotizable subjects given suggestions for deafness deny hearing anything; yet they show speech dysfluencies under conditions of delayed auditory feedback. And when given suggestions for blindness, they deny seeing anything, yet show priming effects from stimuli presented in their visual fields. With the analogy between explicit and implicit memory, we may say that hypnotic suggestions for blindness, deafness, and the like impair explicit perception while sparing implicit perception.

V. CLINICAL APPLICATIONS

Hypnosis has been used in clinics for both medical and psychotherapeutic purposes. By far the most successful and best documented of these has been hypnotic analgesia for the relief of pain. Clinical studies indicate that hypnosis can effectively relieve pain in patients suffering pain from burns, cancer and leukemia (e.g., bone marrow aspirations), childbirth, and dental procedures. In such circumstances, as many as one half of an unselected patient population can obtain significant, if not total, pain relief from hypnosis. Hypnosis may be especially useful in cases of chronic pain, where chemical analgesics such as morphine pose risks of tolerance and addiction. Hypnosis has also been used, somewhat heroically perhaps, as the sole analgesic agent in abdominal, breast, cardiac, and genitourinary surgery, and in orthopedic situations, although it seems unlikely that more than about 10% of patients can tolerate major medical procedures with hypnosis alone. [*See* PAIN.]

Hypnotic suggestion can have psychosomatic effects, a matter that should be of some interest to psychophysiologists and psychoneuroimmunologists. For example, several well controlled laboratory and clinical studies have shown that hypnotic suggestion can affect allergic responses, asthma, and the remission of warts. A famous case study convincingly documented the positive effects of hypnotic suggestion on an intractable case of congenital ichthyosiform erythroderma, a particularly aggressive skin disorder. Such successes have led some practitioners to offer hypnosis in the treatment of cancer. While there is some evidence that hypnosis can have effects on immunological processes, more research in this area is needed, and hypnosis should never be substituted for conventional medical treatments in such cases. [*See* PSYCHONEUROIMMUNOLOGY.]

Hypnosis has also been used in psychotherapy, whether psychodynamic or cognitive–behavioral in orientation. In the former case, hypnosis is used to promote relaxation, enhance imagery, and generally loosen the flow of free associations (some psychodynamic theorists consider hypnosis to be a form of adaptive regression or regression in the service of the ego). However, there is little evidence from controlled outcome studies that hypnoanalysis or hypnotherapy are more effective than nonhypnotic forms of the same treatment. By contrast, a 1995 meta-analysis by Kirsch and colleagues showed a significant advantage when hypnosis is used adjunctively in cognitive–behavioral therapy for a number of problems. In an era of managed mental health care, it will be increasingly incumbent on practitioners who use hypnosis to document, quantitatively, the clinical benefits of doing so. [*See* BEHAVIOR THERAPY; COGNITIVE THERAPY; PSYCHOANALYSIS.]

Hypnosis is sometimes used therapeutically to recover forgotten incidents, as for example in cases of child sexual abuse. Although the literature contains a number of dramatic reports of the successful use of this technique, most of these reports are anecdotal and fail to obtain independent corroboration of the memories that emerge. Given what we know about the unreliability of hypnotic hypermnesia, and the risk of increased responsiveness to leading questions and other sources of bias and distortion, such clinical practices are not recommended. Similar considerations obtain in forensic situations. In fact, many legal jurisdictions severely limit the introduction of memories recovered through hypnosis out of a concern that such evidence might be tainted. The Federal Bureau of Investigation has published a set of guidelines for those who wish to use hypnosis forensically, and similar precautions should be used in the clinic. [See CHILD SEXUAL ABUSE.]

Returning to strictly therapeutic situations, an important but unresolved issue is the role played by individual differences in the clinical effectiveness of hypnosis. As in the laboratory, so in the clinic: a genuine effect of hypnosis should be correlated with hypnotizability. It is possible that many clinical benefits of hypnosis are mediated by placebo-like motivational and expectational processes—that is, with the "ceremony" surrounding hypnosis, rather than with hypnosis per se. An analogy is to hypnotic analgesia, which appears to have a placebo component available to insusceptible and hypnotizable individuals alike, and a dissociative component available only to those who are highly hypnotizable. Unfortunately, clinical practitioners are often reluctant to assess hypnotizability in their patients and clients out of a concern that low scores might reduce motivation for treatment. This danger is probably exaggerated. On the contrary, assessment of hypnotizability by clinicians contemplating the therapeutic use of hypnosis would seem to be no different, in principle, than an assessment of allergic responses before prescribing an antibiotic. In both cases, the legitimate goal is to determine what treatment is appropriate for what patient.

It should be noted that clinicians sometimes use hypnosis in nonhypnotic ways—practices which tend to support the hypothesis that whatever effects they achieve through hypnosis are related to its placebo component. There is nothing particularly hypnotic, for example, about having a patient in a smoking-cessation treatment rehearse therapeutic injunctions not to smoke and other coping strategies while hypnotized. It is likely that more successful use of hypnosis as an adjunct to the cognitive–behavioral treatment of smoking, excessive weight, and similar habit

disorders would be to use hypnotic suggestions to control the patient's awareness of cravings for nicotine, sweets, and the like. Given the ability of hypnotic suggestions to control conscious perception and memory, such strategies might well have therapeutic advantage—but only, of course, for those patients who are hypnotizable enough to respond positively to such suggestions.

VI. THEORIES

The dual nature of hypnosis, in which alterations in consciousness occur in an interpersonal context, has meant that theoretical attempts to understand the phenomenon have been entangled in dichotomies. This has been the case since Mesmer, who thought his effects were due to a magnetic fluid, while the French royal commission attributed them to imagination. Charcot thought hypnotizability was a matter of neurology, while Liebeault and Bernheim emphasized suggestion. Sometimes these dichotomies are manifested within a single individual: Braid began with ideas about the paralysis of nerve centers and ended up emphasizing attention, imagination, expectation, and personality.

In the modern era these dichotomies are still visible, if somewhat obscured by theoretical nuance. Thus, the traditional (if perhaps somewhat tacit) view that hypnosis involves a "special" or "altered" state of consciousness is opposed by a variety of social–psychological or cognitive–behavioral views which assert that hypnotic behavior is a result of processes that are in every sense ordinary. However, there is considerable heterogeneity of viewpoint within each camp, which is sometimes ignored by the other side (a common feature of intergroup relations, according to social psychologists). Among those who are sometimes labeled as state theorists (including the present writer) are cognitive psychologists who think that hypnosis involves dissociative processes, psychoanalysts who invoke adaptive regression in the service of the ego, and neuroscientists who emphasize the inhibition of cortical structures. Among the critics of the state view are some who claim that hypnotic effects can be produced in the absence of a hypnotic induction, so long as subjects are appropriately motivated and instructed. There are others who emphasize the importance of prescriptive social roles played out by both hypnotist and subject, the self-fulfilling effects of expectancies, and the role of attributional processes and self-deception. While some social–psychological and cognitive–behavioral theorists have spent a great deal of time debunking exaggerated or erroneous claims about hypnosis, this has been no less true for some state theorists.

Although it is sometimes popular to portray this theoretical dispute as a kind of enduring debate, there is as much controversy within each camp as there is between camps, and in the final analysis most hypnosis research is designed more to illuminate the nature of specific hypnotic phenomena such as analgesia or amnesia than to provide evidence for any overarching theory of hypnosis. Nevertheless, scientists are trained to test hypotheses derived from theories, and, if possible, to test single hypotheses that will decide between competing theories, so that any empirical evidence obtained tends to be construed as evidence for one view or another.

In the early 1960s, J. P. Sutcliffe published a pair of seminal papers that contrasted a credulous view of hypnosis, which holds that the mental states instigated by suggestion are identical to those that would be produced by the actual stimulus state of affairs implied in the suggestions, with a skeptical view, which holds that the hypnotic subject is acting *as if* the world were as suggested. This is, of course, a version of the familiar dichotomy, but Sutcliffe also offered a third view: that hypnosis involves a quasi-delusional alteration in self-awareness—a delusion that is constructed out of the interaction between the hypnotist's suggestions and the subject's interpretation of those suggestions. Hypnosis is simultaneously a state of (sometimes) profound cognitive change, involving basic mechanisms of perception, memory, and thought, and a social interaction, in which hypnotist and subject come together for a specific purpose within a wider sociocultural context. A truly adequate, comprehensive theory of hypnosis will seek understanding in both cognitive and interpersonal terms. We do not yet have such a theory.

VII. PSYCHOLOGICAL UNCONSCIOUS

The psychological unconscious refers to the idea that mental states—cognitions, emotions, and motives— can influence ongoing experience, thought, and action outside of phenomenal awareness and voluntary control. Although the discovery of the unconscious is commonly attributed to Sigmund Freud, in fact, interest in unconscious mental states and processes goes back to the eighteenth century philosopher Leibnitz, who argued for the importance to perception of subliminal stimuli, and the nineteenth century psychophysicist Helmholtz, who argued that conscious perception results from unconscious inferences about environmental stimuli. Within contemporary cognitive psychology and cognitive science, interest in the psychological unconscious is almost entirely divorced from Freud and psychoanalysis.

In early cognitive psychology, the psychological unconscious was conceived as part wastebasket and part file cabinet. On the one hand, it was the repository for unattended inputs or for those contents of the sensory registers and short-term memory (STM) that had been rendered unavailable by virtue of decay or displacement. On the other hand, the unconscious was identified with the latent contents of long-term memory (LTM), which are brought into awareness when they are copied from LTM to STM. Later, acceptance of the distinction between automatic and effortful processes led to the idea that unconscious mental processes were executed automatically, without drawing on attentional resources. The upshot has been the identification of the unconscious with the unattended, and the rise of the notion that unconscious processing is limited to perceptual and other low-level, presemantic analyses.

More recently, unconscious processing has frequently been identified with the distinction between automatic and controlled mental processes. In some respects, the models for automatic processes are innate reflexes, taxes, instincts, and learned stimulus–response connections formed through classical and instrumental conditioning. Automatic processes are initiated independent of conscious intentions, are executed outside of awareness, and cannot be terminated until they have run to completion. Moreover, it appears that their execution consumes no attentional resources, so that they do not interfere with other ongoing perceptual–cognitive activities. Automatic processes are unconscious in the strict sense of the term: they are never directly available to conscious awareness and are known only by inference.

The automatic–controlled distinction refers to perceptual–cognitive processes engaged in the course of perceiving, remembering, and thinking. The implication is that percepts, memories, and thoughts themselves are available to conscious awareness. Logically, however, availability is no guarantee of accessibility, raising the possibility that mental contents as well as mental processes might be unconscious. In fact, a wealth of experimental evidence, involving both brain-damaged patients and normal subjects, supports a distinction between explicit and implicit memory. Amnesic patients or normal subjects who show preserved priming in the absence (or independent) of recall or recognition, constitute evidence for unconscious memory.

The explicit–implicit distinction can be extended to other psychological domains as well. In perception, for example, there is considerable evidence that stimuli which are subliminal, masked, or unattended can have effects on cognition and behavior even though the stimuli themselves are not consciously perceived. In cases of "blindsight," patients who have suffered damage to the striate cortex of the occipital lobe are able to respond appropriately to visual stimuli even though they are unable to see them. These experimental outcomes illustrate a distinction between explicit and implicit perception, analogous to the explicit–implicit distinction in memory. Explicit perception refers to the conscious perception of current events, as exemplified by the ability to locate and identify objects. By contrast, implicit perception refers to any effect of a current event on ongoing experience, thought, or action in the absence (or independent) of conscious perception, as exemplified by subliminal perception or blindsight.

The explicit–implicit distinction may also be relevant to discussions of thinking and problem solving. For example, intuitions about the solution to a problem, in the absence of conscious awareness of the solution itself, may be an example of implicit thought; incubation may reflect increases in activation associated with an implicit thought; and insight may occur once an implicit thought crosses the threshold required for conscious awareness.

It should be noted that the explicit–implicit distinction may be relevant to emotion and motivation as well as cognition. Many theorists distinguish among three components of an emotional response: subjective (or cognitive), referring to the person's conscious feeling state; behavioral, referring to overt motor activities associated with the emotion; and physiological, refer-

ring to associated covert somatic changes. Researchers have observed that these three components are not always positively intercorrelated, a situation known as desynchrony. A particular form of desynchrony, in which the subjective component of emotion is absent while the behavioral and physiological components persist, is tantamount to a dissociation between explicit and implicit emotion.

Implicit perception, memory, and thought serve as examples of preconscious cognition, in which the percepts and memories lie on the fringes of consciousness. Were the encodings deeper, or the retention interval shorter, or the retrieval cues richer, implicit memories might be consciously accessible. So, too, for implicit percepts: we would be conscious of them if only the stimuli contributing to implicit perception effects were of greater intensity or duration, or unmasked, or presented within the focus of attention. In general, the processing of preconscious percepts and memories is analytically limited. For example, the repetition priming effects obtained in the typical study of implicit memory are mediated by traces that represent the perceptual structure, but not the meaning, of the event in question. Semantic priming effects have been obtained in subliminal perception, but they are very weak and short-lived. Apparently, the conditions under which preconscious processing occurs do not permit very much to be done, cognitively, with these percepts and memories.

Hypnosis is relevant to the psychological unconscious because the phenomena of hypnosis appear to expand the boundaries of unconscious processing beyond the automatic and the preconscious. For example, the priming effects which are preserved in posthypnotic amnesia reflect semantic processing: the items in question were deeply processed at the time of encoding. Finally, the impairment in explicit memory is reversible: posthypnotic amnesia is the only memory disorder studied under laboratory conditions where implicit memories can be restored to explicit recollection. Taken together, then, these properties of priming in posthypnotic amnesia reflect the unconscious influence of semantic representations formed as a result of extensive attentional activity at the time of encoding. The priming itself may be an automatic influence, but it is not the sort that is produced by automatic processes mediated by a perceptual representation system or by presemantic or data-driven processing.

A second example is provided by posthypnotic suggestion, which appears to have a quasi-compulsive quality to it, especially when—as so often happens—the subject is unaware (by virtue of posthypnotic amnesia) that he or she is responding to the experimenter's cue. Thus it appears to be an automatic response to stimulation, but careful examination indicates that responding to the posthypnotic cue consumes attentional resources and interferes with other ongoing activities. Even though the posthypnotic suggestion is executed outside of the subject's awareness, and is experienced as involuntary, it is not automatic in the technical sense of being attention-free.

The identification of the psychological unconscious with automatic processing and with preconscious percepts and memories is popular, but if the phenomena of hypnosis are to be taken seriously, it is also misleading. Studies of hypnotic phenomena indicate that deep, semantic processing can occur without concurrent or retrospective awareness of what has been processed, and behavior executed outside of awareness can nonetheless consume attentional resources. The major contribution of hypnosis to our understanding of the psychological unconscious is the realization that there is more to consciousness than attention. At the very least, the phenomena of hypnosis seem to require another category, besides automatic processes and preconscious contents, in the taxonomy of unconscious mental life: subconscious contents. Subconscious percepts are in no sense subliminal or unattended; subconscious memories are in no sense weakly encoded. Yet neither are accessible to conscious awareness.

VIII. DISSOCIATION AND SUBCONSCIOUS PROCESSING

Hilgard and others have suggested that the phenomena of hypnosis and similar phenomena observed in other altered states indicate that consciousness can be divided, so that attentive, semantic processing can proceed outside phenomenal awareness. Hilgard's neodissociation theory of divided consciousness characterizes the mind as a set of modules that monitor and control mental functions in different domains. In the normal case, these modules are organized to be able to communicate with each other and with a central cognitive structure—what Hilgard calls the executive

ego—which serves as the end point for all conscious inputs and the point of origin for all conscious outputs. This executive ego provides the cognitive basis for the phenomenal experiences of awareness and intentionality.

However, neodissociation theory also asserts that certain conditions, one of which is hypnosis, can alter the integration of the various cognitive structures. If the lines of communication between two subordinate structures are cut, they may perform input–output functions in the absence of any coordination between them. If the communication between a subordinate structure and the executive ego is disrupted, the domain-specific module will perform its function in the absence of the phenomenal experience of awareness and intentionality. In descriptive terms, both cases constitute states of dissociation.

Neodissociation theory holds that responses to suggestions are executed by the subordinate cognitive substructures, alone or in combination, independent of involvement of the executive ego. In the case of posthypnotic amnesia, for example, the events and experiences of hypnosis are processed by modules dedicated to learning and memory; when the suggestion for posthypnotic amnesia is given, the normal communicative link between these modules and the executive control structure is disrupted. Thus, when the executive control structure tries to gain access to these memories in order to respond to an explicit memory test, it cannot do so. However, implicit memory functions such as priming, which do not require conscious access mediated by the executive control structure, are unimpaired. Similarly, posthypnotic suggestions are executed by the relevant substructures without involvement of the executive. Because the executive has no awareness of this activity, the behavior in question is experienced as automatic, even though it may be quite complex and cognitively demanding. Although some critics have interpreted dissociation theory as implying that dissociated activities should not interfere with other ongoing functions, it should be apparent that such a system of dissociated control may well make considerable demands on cognitive resources, resulting in decrements in the performance of simultaneous tasks.

How this dissociation occurs is not well understood. However, the neodissociation theory of divided consciousness, proposed in the context of hypnosis, has stimulated a revival of interest in various forms of dissociation observed clinically, such as psychogenic amnesia, fugue, and multiple personality (dissociative identity disorder). In addition to these clinical syndromes, which fall under the diagnostic rubric of "dissociative disorders," it has been noted that the various "conversion disorders," such as functional blindness, deafness, and paralysis, are essentially dissociative in nature. In each case, some aspect of perception or memory is split off from awareness. Research on the mechanisms of dissociation is at an early stage, but it is already clear that the phenomena of hypnosis, and the clinical syndromes which they resemble, expand the domain of the psychological unconscious and constitute major challenges to our understanding of the nature of conscious and unconscious mental life. [*See* DISSOCIATIVE DISORDERS.]

ACKNOWLEDGMENT

Preparation of this article was supported by Grant #MH-35856 from the National Institute of Mental Health.

BIBLIOGRAPHY

Bowers, K. S. (1976). *Hypnosis for the seriously curious.* Monterey, CA: Brooks/Cole.

Fromm, E., & Nash, M. R. (Eds.). (1992). *Contemporary hypnosis research.* New York: Guilford.

Gauld, A. (1992). *A history of hypnotism.* Cambridge, UK: Cambridge University Press.

Hilgard, E. R. (1965). *Hypnotic susceptibility.* New York: Harcourt, Brace, and World.

Hilgard, E. R. (1977). *Divided consciousness: Multiple controls in human thought and action.* New York: Wiley-Interscience.

Hilgard, E. R., & Hilgard, J. R. (1975). *Hypnosis in the relief of pain.* Los Altos, CA: Kaufman.

Lynn, S. J., & Rhue, J. W. (Eds.). (1991). *Theories of hypnosis: Current models and perspectives.* New York: Guilford.

Olness, K., & Gardner, G. G. (1988). *Hypnosis and hypnotherapy with children* (2nd ed.). Philadelphia: Grune & Stratton.

Rhue, J. W., Lynn, S. J., & Kirsch, I. (Eds.) (1993). *Handbook of clinical hypnosis.* Washington, DC: American Psychological Association.

Sheehan, P. W., & Perry, C. W. (1976). *Methodologies of hypnosis: A critical appraisal of contemporary paradigms of hypnosis.* Hillsdale, NJ: Erlbaum.

Spanos, N. P., & Chaves, J. F. (Eds.) (1989). *Hypnosis: The cognitive–behavioral perspective.* Buffalo, NY: Prometheus Books.

Spiegel, H., & Spiegel, D. (1978). *Trance and treatment: Clinical uses of hypnosis.* Washington, DC: American Psychiatric Press.

I

Impulse Control

Roy F. Baumeister

Case Western Reserve University

Abstinence Violation Effects A brief lapse or indulgence in some impulsive desire sets off a spiraling reaction that leads to further indulgences.

Activating Stimulus An environmental cue or opportunity that is relevant to a latent motivation and may lead to the creation of an impulse.

Delay of Gratification Processes Psychological mechanism by which people obtain larger but temporally distant rewards by refraining from choosing smaller, immediately available rewards.

Impulse A specific desire or urge to perform a particular action on some occasion.

Latent Motivation A chronic or ongoing desire that may not be active at a particular moment, such as a broad desire for money or sex.

Self-Regulation A broad term that encompasses all efforts by the organism to alter its own responses, including thoughts, feelings, and behaviors; akin to self-control.

IMPULSE CONTROL is the term used to describe attempts to control or regulate one's own motivated behaviors, particularly with regard to refraining from acts that might be strongly desired in the short run but that run counter to societal expectations or personal goals and standards in the long run. A person with good impulse control is one who behaves in the socially and personally appropriate fashion even when experiencing desires to act in other, contrary ways. This is not the same as someone who lacks such inappropriate desires. Poor impulse control is marked by spontaneous, motivated behavior that pursues short-term rewards and satisfactions, such as associated with sex, drugs, or violence, but that creates risks and problems.

Impulse control is thus one category of self-regulation, which is defined as all the efforts and processes people use to control themselves and alter their responses. Impulse control can be compared with affect regulation (i.e., control over emotional states), thought control, and some task performance processes (e.g., persistence in the face of frustration). Many features will be common to all four of these. Still, impulse control (especially in the form of resisting temptation) is the most widely familiar form of self-control.

I. INTRODUCTION

The term *impulse control* is misleading. What is controlled is not the impulse per se, but rather the behavior that carries out the impulse. A drug addict, for example, would probably respond to an opportunity by having a strong impulse to take a dose of his or her favorite drug. Impulse control in that setting is not a matter of altering or removing the desire to take the drug. Rather, good impulse control would entail resisting that desire in the sense of refraining from the drug-taking behavior.

The scientific study of impulse control received an early boost from research on delay of gratification processes. In a typical study, a child would be offered a choice between a small, immediate reward and a larger reward that required waiting. A fully rational, profit-maximizing individual would presumably prefer the larger reward, but this preference required the person to resist the impulse to obtain the pleasure that was immediately available. Educational, social, and occupational success often depends on the capacity to delay gratification, and indeed attending college may itself be considered a long exercise in delayed gratification insofar as the college student must live in poverty and low status in the hope of achieving well-paid work after graduation. By examining the causes and processes that allow people to take the larger, delayed reward instead of the immediate one, researchers began to learn about impulse control processes.

II. HOW IMPULSES OPERATE

It is generally agreed that each person carries around with him or her a multitude of ongoing motivations, only some of which are active at any given time. For example, a given person might have a passionate love of chocolate, baseball, and progressive political movements, none of which has any effect on the person's thoughts or acts while doing the laundry. At any given time, most motivations are latent.

These latent motivations are activated by encountering a situation that is relevant to them. Some stimulus in the environment provides a reminder or opportunity that invokes the motivation. Most commonly, the stimulus is the object of the desire, such as when a tempting display in the candy store window activates one's love of chocolate.

The encounter between an activating stimulus and a latent motivation gives rise to an impulse. An impulse thus differs from a motivation in terms of its specificity: The impulse is a desire to perform a specific

act on a particular occasion, whereas a motivation is a broad and general pattern of desire. To pursue the example, the person who has a general love of chocolate (motivation) and passes by a candy store (activating stimulus) will probably feel an impulse to obtain and eat a specific treat.

The everyday concept of temptation provides a good analog to the concept of impulse. The term temptation is used in ordinary speech to refer to the subjective wish to perform a particular, usually forbidden action, although sometimes it is used to refer only to the activating stimulus. Temptation thus encompasses the notion of a specific wish arising from the encounter between a broad, ongoing motivation (often an illicit or unacceptable one) and a particular opportunity.

As an alternative path, some impulses occasionally arise in the absence of an activating stimulus. If the latent motivation is sufficiently strong and attention is not held by current activities, an impulse may form spontaneously as an imagined act of satisfying the desire. Sexual daydreams are one example of this process. Such cases are exceptional, however, and because they do not involve a situational opportunity for action, they are largely irrelevant to the issue of impulse control.

III. THE FOCUS OF CONTROL

Strictly speaking, the impulse is not directly controllable because it follows automatically from the encounter between the latent motivation and the activating stimulus. Automatic responses are, by definition, largely immune to control. Successful impulse control thus requires finding some feature or step in the chain of responses that is not automatic.

The prime candidate for control is behavior, insofar as behavior is subject to conscious control. A person cannot presumably avoid wanting to perform some action, but he or she can refrain from actually performing it. In other words, the causal step from impulse to behavior is not fully automatic (in human beings, at least) and hence is the principal focus of impulse control.

In principle, another potential focus of impulse control would be prior to the formation of the impulse. That is, one can prevent the impulse from forming if one can successfully control the environmental stimuli (or one's own attention) so that the latent motivation is never activated. The religious effort to subdue sexual desires is an important example of this. Typically, sexual impulses are minimized in religious orders partly by depriving the individuals of exposure to sexual stimuli. Monks and nuns have generally lived in sexually segregated buildings that have been kept free from erotic art and other arousing stimuli. In a similar fashion, dieters may remove fattening foods from their homes so as to prevent temptations.

IV. THE ROLE OF ATTENTION

Like nearly all self-regulation processes, impulse control depends heavily on the management of attention. As a general principle, the more people attend to the forbidden (activating) stimulus, the less likely they will be to succeed at impulse control. In an important sense, the strategy of impulse prevention mentioned previously depends on preventing attention from encountering the activating stimulus, as in the example of religious institutions quelling sexual arousal by keeping sexual stimuli out of attention.

The simplest attentional strategy is distraction. If the mind can be kept focused on engrossing stimuli other than the forbidden ones, the impulses can be prevented or resisted.

Another attentional strategy is to keep attention focused on the benefits of resisting the impulse. Violent impulses may be resisted by contemplating the risks and dangers of acting on them, and the same goes for sexual impulses. Dieting may be facilitated by contemplating the desirability of losing weight and/or the costs of giving in to an impulse to eat. (Some dieters, for example, will tape a picture of a pig or a fat person to their refrigerator in order to remind themselves of the cost of giving in to temptation.)

All of these effects have been shown in studies of delay of gratification. The children in these studies generally succeed best at resisting the immediate temptation if they can keep their attention directed away from it, which in some cases entails closing their eyes or turning around to face the opposite direction. Self-distraction such as by singing or chanting has also been documented in these studies. Meanwhile, attending to the desirability of the delayed reward can help

strengthen self-control and increase the ability to resist the tempting stimulus.

V. WILLPOWER

Impulses vary in motivational strength, and so resisting them likewise requires some form of strength. The concept of ego strength dates back to Freud but has not figured centrally in most empirical studies of self-control, possibly because of the difficulty of measuring it. Nonetheless, it seems likely that ego strength will need to be studied and understood in order for a full and adequate theory of impulse control to emerge.

The concept of ego strength is akin to the colloquial expression "willpower," which implies that each person has some resource of power or energy that can be used to resist temptation. The term likewise implies that when this resource is depleted people will find it harder to resist and so impulse control will fail. Finally, it implies that people may be able to increase their capacity for impulse control by building up this strength, similar to how physical exercise increases physical strength.

Consistent with the notion of willpower, ample evidence indicates that people find impulse control more difficult (and fail at it more readily) when their strength has been depleted by situational demands. When people are under stress, such as due to impending deadlines in work or school or due to difficulties in family or romantic relationships, self-control breaks down in multiple ways. People in such circumstances are more likely to resume smoking or smoke more than usual, to consume more alcohol or drugs than they would otherwise, to break their diets, and to say or do unkind things that they may later regret. [*See* STRESS.]

By the same token, impulse control seems to break down when people are physically tired. Impulsive acts ranging from overeating to sexual misbehavior to violent (impulsive) crimes are most likely to occur late in the evening, after people presumably have used up much of their energy in the activities of the day. These patterns suggest that willpower is tied to physical energy.

Recent laboratory work has suggested that the energy or willpower available for self-control is quite limited. In one study, for example, subjects who spent

5 minutes resisting the temptation to eat chocolate later gave up much more readily on a difficult, frustrating task, indeed persisting only half as long as the subjects who had not had to resist temptation. Such findings suggest that impulse control takes a psychological toll in the short run.

VI. LEVELS OF THINKING

As philosophers of action have described, the same act can be described on multiple levels, ranging from specific, concrete, narrow ones up to broad, meaningful, abstract ones. Psychologically, people's awareness of what they are doing shifts among these levels. Perceived time span is correlated with level: Short time spans are associated with concrete, low-level thinking, whereas long-range perspectives are associated with the high-level, meaningful thought.

Impulses are specific and concrete, and so they tend to operate at low levels of awareness. Impulsive actions are characterized by a narrow time span ("spur of the moment"), a focus on concrete stimuli and acts as well as their immediate outcomes, and a lack of consideration of long-range or meaningful consequences. In contrast, the opposite of impulsive action is carefully planned, meaningful action that has been considered in terms of its long-range consequences and its relevance to broad goals and standards.

Impulse control can thus be helped or hindered by shifting the level of thinking. When attention drifts to low levels, impulse control is weakened, because the person attends primarily to immediate outcomes and stimuli. In contrast, keeping attention focused on long-range, high-level goals and standards will facilitate impulse control. In effect, this is another attentional strategy for impulse control.

VII. EMOTIONAL DISTRESS

It is well established that emotional distress undermines impulse control. Probably the most familiar example is that people drink more alcohol when they are upset, but similar patterns have been identified with smoking and overeating. When people are experiencing aversive emotional states they seem to give in much more readily to temptation, and so they say and do things that they may later regret. This can lead to a vicious circle in which emotional upset weakens impulse control, resulting in costly actions, resulting in further distress.

Some experts sort emotions by arousal as well as by pleasantness. Using this categorization, one can say that high-arousal unpleasant emotions are particularly associated with impulse control failure. Anger, anxiety, humiliation, frustration, and similar emotions lead to impulsive behaviors, whereas low-arousal feelings such as sadness, dejection, and grief do not consistently produce a similar effect. [*See* ANGER; ANXIETY.]

It is not known precisely how emotional distress undermines impulse control, and quite possibly there are several causal pathways. One of these is probably due to the common tendency to try to control one's own emotional distress. If willpower is indeed limited, then a person's limited resources will tend to be consumed by the effort of coping with his or her bad mood, leaving less left over to resist temptation or control impulses.

Emotion also has various effects on cognitive processing, and these effects may contribute to impulse control failure. High-arousal, unpleasant moods and emotions make people less inclined to think through the meaningful implications and long-term outcomes of their actions. The narrowing of attention to immediate outcomes may be associated with shifting to lower levels of thinking as well. These effects would increase impulsive actions by undermining the psychological factors that restrain them (e.g., consideration of long-term costs).

VIII. SELF-AWARENESS

Focusing attention on oneself has long been linked to self-regulation, and self-awareness does seem to facilitate impulse control. In an early study, for example, Halloween trick-or-treaters who were made self-aware by means of mirrors were less likely to filch extra candy for themselves from a tempting display. In another study, students who were made self-aware by means of hearing a recording of their own voice were less likely to cheat on an examination when an opportunity to do so presented itself (as compared with other students who were not made self-aware).

Self-awareness typically involves comparing oneself to standards of desirability or appropriateness. When people are self-aware, therefore, they are usually cognizant both of how they are acting and of how those actions measure up to how they should act. Such cognitions may facilitate impulse control, if only by directing attention to the meanings and implications of possible actions.

Loss of self-awareness is therefore a significant contributor to many instances of impulse control failure. Events that draw attention away from the self or allow people to forget themselves may facilitate impulsive behavior. Mob actions, in which people lose individual self-awareness and feel deindividuated, can be exceptionally violent or otherwise antisocial because the loss of self-awareness sweeps away the normal inner restraints against such impulses. Carnivals, in which people wear costumes or disguises, may produce similar effects. At a more mundane level, it is common to hear people describe impulsive acts by saying that they "forgot" themselves.

Sometimes people desire to lose self-awareness, because self-awareness has become unpleasant (e.g., due to a recent failure or rejection that makes the self look bad) or simply because constant self-awareness becomes oppressive and tiresome. Such efforts to escape from self-awareness often directly foster impulsive behavior. Thus, for example, eating binges often follow from a desire to forget oneself in response to anxieties and insecurities about one's competence or attractiveness to others. Escape from self-awareness can also result in novel, disinhibited sexual behaviors. At the extreme, suicidal behavior is often an impulsive act following an effort to escape self-awareness that has become painful as a result of recent humiliations.

IX. ALCOHOL

It is well established that impulse control is generally less effective among people who have recently consumed alcohol, particularly if they are intoxicated. Indeed, part of the appeal of alcohol seems to be that it weakens inhibitions, thereby allowing people to enjoy themselves and each other's company more robustly, such as at parties and celebrations. On the negative side, alcohol consumption increases aggressive responses to provocations and is implicated in a majority of violent crimes, probably because alcohol weakens the inner controls against violent impulses. Alcohol contributes particularly to impulsive crimes.

One relevant effect of alcohol is that it inhibits the inhibitors. An analysis of the findings of multiple studies showed that alcohol increases behavioral tendencies that are marked by inner inhibitory conflict—in other words, cases in which a person both wants to do and wants not to do some action. Alcohol does not appear to strengthen impulses or instill new ones (e.g., by giving rise to violent tendencies that were not already there). Instead, it undermines the person's capacity to resist his or her impulses.

Alcohol has also been shown to undermine self-awareness. Given the power of self-awareness to support inhibitions and strengthen self-control, anything that undermines self-awareness could easily lead to impulsive behavior. People who have consumed alcohol are less likely than others to reflect on the personal meanings and implications of possible actions, and as a result they are more willing to give in to temptations.

Finally, alcohol narrows the focus of attention, which may help bring it to the lower levels where impulse control is difficult. Intoxication may breed a here-and-now focus that makes tempting stimuli all the more salient while making potential sources of long-term regret less apparent. This too would foster impulsive behavior and undermine control. [*See* ALCOHOL PROBLEMS.]

X. SNOWBALLING

Contrary to popular belief, a single lapse in impulse control is only rarely a catastrophe. The most serious personal and social problems tend to arise when there is an extended failure of impulse control, such as in an eating or drinking binge. Eating the first cookie may in principle break one's diet, but the net effect of that one cookie on one's caloric intake and health is minimal—whereas continuing on to finish the entire bag of cookies is a much more serious matter.

It is therefore important to consider not only what causes people to suffer an initial lapse in impulse control but also how the initial lapse can "snowball" into a large-scale breakdown. Researchers have recognized that the initial lapse, although trivial in itself, can itself set off responses that cause self-control to fail in a broader fashion. Such *abstinence violation effects* can include attributions about oneself or about the situation that undermine further efforts at impulse control. For example, a recovering alcoholic may respond to a single drink by concluding that he has failed to defeat the addiction or is hopelessly in the power of a disease. Similarly, a single act of forbidden sex (e.g., with a partner from a forbidden category) can cause the person to label himself or herself as the sort of person who engages in such actions, and this view of self undermines efforts to resist further temptations.

Of particular importance are responses that explain the lapse on the basis of overpowering temptation. Such attributions may be appealing because they remove responsibility from the individual, such as by saying that the lapse involved an irresistible impulse or reflected the overwhelming allure of sex or drink or addiction. Once one has labeled the temptation as too powerful to resist, however, one may find oneself giving in to it the next time it materializes, because (one has already concluded) there is no point in fighting it.

XI. ACQUIESCENCE VERSUS IRRESISTIBLE IMPULSES

The concept of irresistible impulses raises a theoretical dilemma that is central to the understanding of impulse control: Do people voluntarily give in and indulge themselves, or are they overwhelmed by unstoppable desires despite their best efforts? This question has more than theoretical interest, because political issues and decisions about treatment depend on the answer. Various theorists, groups, factions, and individuals have asserted nearly the full range of possible answers to this question.

At one extreme is the view that major impulse control failures (especially addictions and violent crimes) are caused by irresistible impulses and so the individuals involved should not be held responsible for their actions but rather treated as victims of external forces. At the other extreme is the view that people are always free to choose their behavior and should always answer for the consequences. Many forms of compromise or intermediate views have been proposed. For example, the organization Alcoholics Anonymous asserts that alcoholism is a permanent disease and that people who suffer from it are powerless to resist the snowballing lure of alcohol, and so only constant vigilance and complete abstinence are acceptable. Yet AA also insists that its members accept responsibility for their actions, to the extent of seeking out people whom they disappointed or hurt during previous drinking episodes and apologizing to them.

There are undeniably some impulses that are irresistible. Certain bodily functions such as sleeping, breathing, or urinating cannot be resisted indefinitely, and resisting them simply makes the impulses grow stronger to the point at which further resistance is functionally impossible. Thus, there are cases in which impulses simply cannot be controlled.

On the other hand, the common focus of impulse control theory is on behaviors that are far more controllable, such as eating, drinking, sexuality, violence, and substance abuse. In these cases, people may want to claim that they were overwhelmed by irresistible impulses because such claims excuse them of responsibility, but the evidence to support such claims is weak. Indeed, there are ample signs of active acquiescence in such self-control breakdowns. For example, someone experiencing an eating or drinking binge is not passively letting the substances enter the body but rather is actively opening containers and putting the food or drink into the mouth. People will even exert considerable, intentional, planful actions to continue the binges, such as by going out to purchase more food or drink. These signs of active participation suggest that the person has to some extent acquiesced in the binge and is an active participant—contrary to the picture of someone who has simply been overwhelmed by an irresistible impulse.

Still, it would be excessive and dubious to assert that people freely choose to engage in seemingly impulsive behavior at every step. Someone having an eating or drinking binge does not consciously decide to have the binge, nor does the person freely choose at each step to continue the binge. People do describe their behavior as having the subjective feeling of being out of control, even though they may be exerting control in some ways (as already noted).

A full understanding of the question of acquiescence is not yet available and is likely to be complex. Given the present state of knowledge, it seems most plausible to propose that the process involves some form of disguised acquiescence that is not apparent to the individual but that sets off responses that maintain the feeling of being out of control. An initial lapse may occur for casual or trivial reasons, and it may result in a narrowing of attention, emotional distress, or attributional responses that contribute to a sweeping breakdown in control.

Cultural and situational factors may also contribute to acquiescence, particularly when a culture or subculture defines certain occasions as appropriate ones in which a typical person would lose control. Symbolic provocations such as verbal insults may be regarded by some cultures as trivial affairs to be laughed off but by other cultures as momentous occasions that require a lethally violent response. There is evidence that the effects of alcohol and drugs on impulsive behavior (including further consumption of same) depends on whether the culture specifies that people remain responsible for their actions after consuming them.

XII. SPHERES OF IMPULSE CONTROL

Research has examined various spheres of impulse control problems. Considerable information is available about eating, due to the pervasiveness of eating in daily life and to the ready availability of dieters, as well as societal and theoretical interest in eating disorders. For the majority of adults in all categories except young males, dieting is a recurrent feature of life and the most common impulse control dilemma is whether to eat some desired but fattening food.

Dieting is centrally concerned with impulse control because both inner and external cues prompt one to eat and so impulses are frequent. Food cues are pervasive and are the most commonly cited cause of dietary failure. Most dieters must rigidly monitor their caloric intake. Diets are often thwarted by eating binges, which are mediated by a cessation of monitoring, and indeed research suggests that many dieters cease keeping track of their food once their diet is broken for the day, with the result that they eat far too much. Dieting often depends on learning to ignore internal cues such as bodily sensations of hunger, with the unfortunate side effect that inner cues of satiety are ignored as well. Nondieters eat more when they have been deprived of food than when they have been "preloaded" with filling, tasty food, but dieters show the opposite pattern of paradoxically eating more after an initial tasty, filling snack than when deprived of food.

Dieting is generally futile in the long run. Some people fail to lose weight, and among those who succeed in losing weight, most regain the weight within a year and nearly all regain it within 5 years. Some evidence suggests that chronic or repeated dieting may result in weight gain, possibly because the body becomes efficient at storing and retaining fat in response to the periodic bouts of deprivation. [See DIETING.]

Eating conforms to the patterns of impulse control already described in this article. Stress and emotional distress seem to undermine or weaken willpower and lead to increased vulnerability to impulses to eat, although some forms of stress do undermine one's appetite and hence do not increase eating. Self-awareness facilitates monitoring and facilitates dieting, whereas loss of or escape from self-awareness leads to increased eating. Eating binges are characterized by low-level, here-and-now thinking and by snowballing. Alcohol consumption often leads to increased eating, and indeed weight gain associated with alcohol (e.g., a "beer belly") is generally caused by the food consumed along with the alcohol as opposed to any caloric effects of the alcohol itself. People describe eating binges as marked by subjective feelings of being out of control, but they do seem to acquiesce in the binges and will often go to some lengths to obtain and ingest more food.

Smoking represents one of the most difficult problems of impulse control, given its powerfully addictive nature. One study of people who were simultaneously addicted to nicotine and to cocaine or heroin found that majority said they could overcome their drug addiction more easily than their cigarette addiction. In the United States, most people are either nonsmokers or smokers, the latter marked by regular, chronic patterns of smoking that suggest addiction.

Although addiction to smoking entails that impulses often arise from purely internal cues, especially if the nicotine level in the blood is too low, external cues also affect smoking. Salient cues can capture attention and induce smokers to smoke more.

Some smokers seek to cut down by rigidly monitoring how many cigarettes they smoke, but these monitoring efforts are often undermined when smokers compensate for the reduced number of cigarettes by smoking them more thoroughly or by thwarting cigarette filters. For example, one practical means of making smoking less toxic is to manufacture cigarettes with vents that introduce fresh air into the tube to dilute the smoke. Unfortunately, many people who smoke vented cigarettes unconsciously learn to block the vents with their lips or fingers, resulting in intake of undiluted smoke. [See SMOKING.]

Stress and emotional upset are commonly cited

causes of increased smoking, consistent with other patterns of impulse control failure. The mechanisms linking smoking with stress and emotion may be different from other patterns, however. Stress and emotion cause bodily changes that reduce the proportion of nicotine that makes it from the lungs into the bloodstream, so that the smoker needs more cigarettes to maintain the habitual level of nicotine. Moreover, many smokers believe that smoking calms them down and thus helps them cope with stress or aversive emotion. Research suggests that smoking does not actually produce a calming effect (indeed, nicotine causes arousal), but an addict who has been temporarily deprived of nicotine will experience unpleasant symptoms of withdrawal, and so having a cigarette will relieve these symptoms and thereby simulate a feeling of relaxation or calm.

Like cigarettes, alcohol is addictive, although there are far more nonaddicted alcohol users than nonaddicted smokers. Also like smoking, alcohol consumption is responsible for many times more deaths every year than all illegal drugs combined, which suggests that alcohol and cigarettes must offer powerful satisfactions to justify the social cost.

Unlike cigarettes, alcohol is often used in erratic and binge patterns. It is strongly susceptible to snowballing, partly because it seems to undermine monitoring, so that drinkers lose track of how much they have drunk and even seem unable to gauge their own degree of intoxication. Also, heavy drinkers find that alcohol is increasingly appealing as they continue to drink, unlike light drinkers who begin to find alcohol distasteful after they have consumed a certain amount. The fact that drinking increases the desire to drink more is highly conducive to binges.

People sometimes consume alcohol as a deliberate response to emotional upset or stress, in the partly mistaken belief that alcohol is an effective cure for feeling bad. Alcohol is consumed particularly in response to stress that makes the self look bad, such as threats to self-esteem.

Gambling capitalizes on the understandable impulse to gain money quickly and easily, although rational, statistical analysis indicates that nearly all gamblers will end up with a net loss of money in the long run (because the casino keeps a percentage of all money bet). The social costs of gambling rarely extend to death (unlike alcohol and cigarettes) but impoverishment and debt can place severe, long-term strains on individuals and their families.

Gambling tends to have its worst effects in binges, such as marathon gambling sessions. During these binges, gamblers exhibit narrowed attention and low-level thinking, along with a sometimes euphoric cycle of intense emotion. Snowballing occurs particularly when gamblers try to recoup initial losses by making large bets. Like alcoholics, gamblers use various cognitive and self-deceptive strategies to conceal the problems caused by their addiction. Overconfidence and misperception of chance contribute to patterns of costly gambling. [See GAMBLING.]

Although some criminal activity is carefully planned and guided by rational profit-seeking activity, the majority of crimes appear to be impulsive. This is particularly true for violent crimes such as assault and murder, which frequently occur at the end of an escalating personal argument. Personal disputes give rise to anger and its attendant impulses to strike out at the other person, using any means at hand. The ready availability of guns in the United States entails that these impulses have fatal consequences more commonly than in other countries. [See CRIMINAL BEHAVIOR.]

Emotional distress and loss of self-awareness have been linked to increased tendencies to act out one's aggressive impulses. Cultural norms also enforce the belief that it is appropriate to lose control and lash out in response to certain kinds of provocations, such as an insult to one's gang or mother. Indeed, nearly all cultures have laws against violence but also have legal guidelines that make "crimes of passion" less reprehensible and less severely punished than other crimes. In other words, murder that results from a failure of impulse control is treated as less reprehensible than premeditated murder.

Violence is particularly prone to binges marked by snowballing, and indeed nearly all violent crimes begin with lesser acts of aggression (which are exchanged and function as mutual provocations). Attention focuses narrowly on the here and now, in which the opponent and provocation figure prominently. Alcohol often contributes to this narrowing of attention and indeed is implicated in a majority of violent crimes. Fatigue and depletion of willpower are also suggested by the fact that most violent crimes occur late at night, when people are tired. Still, there is evidence that people do acquiesce in their violent actions, at least to the extent of actively exercising volition about how to attack one's victim. [*See* AGGRESSION.]

BIBLIOGRAPHY

Baumeister, R.F., Heatherton, T.F., & Tice, D.M. (1994). *Losing control: How and why people fail at self-regulation.* San Diego, CA: Academic Press.

Gottfredson, M.R., & Hirschi, T. (1990). *A general theory of crime.* Stanford, CA: Stanford University Press.

Marlatt, G.A. (1985). Relapse prevention: Theoretical rationale and overview of the model. In G.A. Marlatt & J.R. Gordon (Eds.), *Relapse Prevention* (pp. 3–70). New York: Guilford.

Mischel, W., Shoda, Y., & Rodriguez, M.L. (1989). Delay of gratification in children. *Science, 244,* 933–938.

Peele, S. (1989). *The diseasing of America.* Boston, MA: Houghton Mifflin Co.

Polivy, J., & Herman, C.P. (1985). Dieting and bingeing: A causal analysis. *American Psychologist, 40,* 193–201.

Steele, C.M., & Southwick, L. (1985). Alcohol and social behavior I: The psychology of drunken excess. *Journal of Personality and Social Psychology, 48,* 18–34.

Individual Differences in Mental Health

Jorge H. Daruna

Tulane University School of Medicine

Patricia A. Barnes

Louisiana State University School of Medicine

Assortative mating The coupling of individuals based on their similarity on one or more characteristics.

Brain organization How the specific architecture of neural networks and their activity in time give rise to higher-order dynamic structures within the brain which, along with external stimulation, control responses.

Neural networks Neurons interconnected to form specific circuits that recur either within a given brain structure or across structures.

Social context The types of social interactions that one experiences by observing others as well as by directly relating to those in one's environment.

State space A multidimensional framework containing all possible configurations of the variables that define the state of a system or a complex entity.

Mental health is rooted in behavior interpreted within the context of culture. In this article, the concept of mental health is presented in dynamic terms. It is described as a region within a multidimensional framework (state space) that encompasses behavior, situation, and culture as determinants of mental health. **INDIVIDUAL DIFFERENCES IN MENTAL HEALTH** can then be represented as trajectories through such a state space. We review epidemiologic studies of mental disorder that allow estimates of the prevalence of mental health, and we argue that a biologic perspective is the most appropriate framework for understanding the relative importance of early social experience as well as for integrating all of the factors that affect mental health. Major psychological attributes that have been associated with mental health are presented. The roles of social context, relationships, and social support are emphasized with regard to attaining and sustaining mental health. We conclude by outlining the kinds of programs that are necessary to maximize mental health.

I. DEFINING MENTAL HEALTH

The concept of mental health is the result of discourse among individuals over time within evolving ideological contexts. The concept is rooted in the notion that individuals have minds which cause behavior. It constitutes a framework for assigning value judgments to behavior. If behavior appears aberrant, then the condition of the mind is called into question. By invoking the idea of health, typically used to refer to the body's functional status, a link between mind and body is implied. Mental health is not a universal concept, inasmuch as there is cultural variation in the extent to which it is thought to be applicable.

Mental health must be viewed in dynamic terms and not as a static concept. A framework that helps in this regard relies on the notion of behavioral state space. Behavioral state space encompasses all possible behaviors or responses of individuals within all imaginable situations across all conceivable cultures. This would of necessity be a space of very high dimensionality. However, it can be visualized by imagining a highly simplified three-dimensional version with behavior, situation, and culture each being represented by a single dimension. Any location in this space would constitute the intersection of a given behavior, a specific situation, and a particular culture. If members of that culture judged the behavior in the specific situation as not aberrant, then a point could be entered at that location. Repeating this procedure for each possible location would create a three-dimensional structure of points defining nonaberrance. The region of behavioral state space occupied by this three-dimensional structure could be regarded as the mental health subspace. The mental health subspace would be made more intricate and its boundaries would be blurred by incorporating a dimension of consensus within the culture, with points of varying intensity being used to depict agreement regarding aberrance. Finally, the mental health subspace could be further portrayed as a changing entity by introducing the dimension of time.

By relying on the notion of behavioral state space, one avoids getting bogged down in choosing between definitions of mental health. Essentially all definitions of mental health exist within behavioral state space. Taking a particular cultural perspective allows one to select the prevailing views of those within such a context. For instance, within Western cultural contexts mental health has been regarded as more than the absence of mental disorder. It has been stipulated that mental health requires that one view oneself positively and conduct one's life with purpose and direction. It is further stipulated that one's outlook should be realistic and not overly dependent on the assessments of others. Moreover, one needs to be well integrated and able to exercise mastery over the environment. These ideas tend to recur in all of the various attempts to formulate definitions of mental health, although some questions have been raised about the value of realism. There is also broad cultural variation regarding the value of independence (vs. interdependence) and mastery (vs. harmony). As a rule the terms used to describe mental health remain rather abstract, as any attempt to be concrete quickly leads to the realization that the significance of any given behavior is highly dependent on situation. It is this kind of complexity that can be best described within behavioral state space.

Individual differences in mental health can be con-ceptualized as trajectories through behavioral state space from early life to death. At any instant, individuals appear distributed throughout behavioral state space. Thus, if one samples the population periodically, one observes variability in that some individuals tend to maintain mental health, whereas others have a less stable course, and some may become stuck in maladaptive behavioral patterns. The vulnerability of individuals may be conceived of in terms of their location at any point in time vis-à-vis the boundaries of the mental health subspace.

II. QUANTIFYING MENTAL HEALTH

The number of individuals who exhibit mental health in a given population is entirely dependent on the definition and the procedures with which one chooses to evaluate each individual. Cultural and economic factors also play a role in determining the number of individuals who acknowledge or who are viewed as lacking mental health. For instance, in some societies where mental health services are scarce, people are more likely to portray themselves as physically ill or to view symptoms of mental disorder as reflecting supernatural causes in need of religious intervention. In countries such as the United States, where mental health services constitute a major industry, people are more likely to be diagnosed with a mental disorder; in particular, because those in the business of insurance require practitioners to diagnose mental disorder as a prerequisite to reimbursement. Moreover, the availability of disability payments and other forms of financial compensation to individuals afflicted with mental disorders lead some to portray themselves as chronically mentally disordered.

Epidemiologic studies of mental health have been primarily concerned with obtaining quantitative estimates of mental disorder in the general population. There has been comparatively little effort directed at quantifying positive mental health. Therefore, we rely on estimates of disorder in an effort to quantify the prevalence of mental health. [See EPIDEMIOLOGY: PSYCHIATRIC.]

The National Comorbidity Study (NCS) is the most recent attempt to characterize the prevalence of major mental health disorders as defined in the *Diagnostic and Statistical Manual of Mental Disorders III*

Revised (*DSM-III-R*). It is the first study to use a probability sample of the U.S. population and was conducted over an 18-month period beginning in September of 1990. The findings indicated that within the 12 months preceding the structured diagnostic interview, 30% of the population (ages 15 to 54) met criteria for at least one major psychiatric disorder (e.g., affective disorders, anxiety disorders, schizophrenia, antisocial personality, substance use disorder). Major depression was the most frequently encountered disorder (10%). The lifetime prevalence for any disorder was 49% for men and 47% for women. Major depression was again the most frequent diagnosis (17%) and was more often seen in women (21%) than in men (13%). The figures obtained in the NCS are higher than had been observed in the Epidemiological Catchment Area (ECA) study conducted approximately 10 years earlier. This study reported that 20% of the sample ($N = 20,000$) met criteria for at least one major psychiatric disorder in the preceding 12 months. Lifetime prevalence was 32%. Major depression was diagnosed in only 6% of the sample. These studies differed in a number of methodological features, but it is important to note that most of the discrepancy is due to differences in the diagnosis of major depression (NCS = 17%, ECA = 6%). International epidemiologic studies have also reported marked variability in the lifetime prevalence of major depression: Taiwan (1.5%); Korea (2.9%); West Germany (9.2%); Florence, Italy (12.4%); Paris, France (16.4%); and Beirut, Lebanon (19%). The fact that other affective disorders, such as bipolar disorder, do not show such marked variability (range 0.3% to 1.5%) suggests that major depression for whatever reason (cultural, methodological, genetic, situational) is a much more volatile condition. In this regard, it is noteworthy that psychological interventions (e.g., cognitive therapy) designed to alter outlook are particularly effective treatments for depression. [*See* COGNITIVE THERAPY; DEPRESSION.]

The most recent epidemiologic study of psychiatric disorders in children and adolescents conducted in the United States, the Method for the Epidemiology of Child and Adolescent Mental Disorders (MECA) study, gives a prevalence of 21% for the presence of at least one psychiatric diagnosis (e.g., anxiety disorders, depression, attention deficit hyperactivity disorder, oppositional defiant and conduct disorders), although

depending on the definition of functional impairment adopted, the figure can go as high as 51% or as low as 5.4%. This study found anxiety disorders to be the most prevalent diagnosis (13%), followed closely by disruptive behavior disorders (10%). Other recent epidemiologic studies of psychiatric disorders in children and adolescents conducted in the United States and in other countries indicate a mean prevalence of 17% (range 7 to 22%). These figures represent an increase from what was observed in the late 1970s when overall prevalence was closer to 12%. Earlier studies conducted in Asian countries also indicated a mean prevalence between 10% and 13%, depending on whether teachers or parents reported on the child's behavior. A study conducted in the Sudan between 1965 and 1980, found that although only 8% of the sample was judged to have psychiatric disorders in 1965, by 1980, the figure had increased to 13%. Moreover, the proportion of youngsters rated as well-adjusted decreased over the same period from 63% to 47%. [*See* ANXIETY; CONDUCT DISORDERS.]

The prevalence of mental disorder in older adults (65 and above) appears to be lower than in middle-aged and young adults according to the results of the ECA study. In that study, the lifetime prevalence for all ages was 32%, but for those 65 and older it was only 21%. Lifetime major depression was evident in only 2% of the 65 and over group, whereas the figure for the entire sample was 6%. The 12-month prevalence for the entire sample was 20%, but for the 65 and over group it was 17%. Evidently, only a small percentage of the 65 and over group had psychiatric disorders prior to the last 12 months. This could be partially a cohort effect, but it may also reflect that mental disorder earlier in life can adversely affect longevity.

Overall, the evidence suggests that (a) the more recent studies have obtained higher prevalence estimates of psychiatric disorders, raising the possibility that mental health in the general population may be declining; and (b) at any given moment approximately 20% of the population is afflicted by a psychiatric disorder and only about 50% of the population has never met criteria for a major mental disorder. Therefore, the number of individuals who may be regarded as mentally healthy at any moment must be less than 80%. Beyond this possible maximum, as one requires the presence of positive characteristics rather than simply the absence of symptoms, the figure will decrease significantly and is likely to fall well below 50%. Future epidemiologic research must incorporate procedures to allow more precise quantification of positive mental health.

III. BEHAVIOR, BIOLOGY, AND MENTAL HEALTH

It is not adequate to address the topic of mental health on the basis of behavior alone. It is necessary to venture into what underlies behavior, namely, the dynamics of neural networks. This is essential, because it is at the level of neural dynamics that one can appreciate how various factors that modify behavior, and thus mental health, exert their influence. It is also at this level that it becomes possible to have a clearer vision of an individual's development, a vision that recognizes that what transpires prenatally can be pivotal. It is not simply an unfolding of a program of assembly fully contained in the DNA. The prenatal brain is too complicated to be prespecified by the information available within the genome. Its structure, although obviously influenced by the individual's genotype, is also shaped by epigenetic factors, such as the mother's neuroendocrine responses to the social and nonsocial forces affecting her. This seems reasonable, because the mother's internal milieu, by exerting an influence on the developing brain, may impart to the infant some adaptive advantage, given the context which she inhabits.

There are a handful of studies that have provided evidence that the social circumstances and stressors affecting mothers during pregnancy may have a detectable effect on the offspring. These studies have typically focused on the presence of problems in the offspring. One interesting study examined the mental health records of adult individuals whose fathers had died in World War II, either during the prenatal period or within the first year of the individual's life. This study compared the timing of trauma to the mother on the mental health of the offspring in adulthood. The findings indicated that there was increased psychiatric morbidity for offspring whose mothers were pregnant at the time the fathers were killed. In particular, the prevalence of schizophrenia was significantly increased. The results could *not* be attributed to an increase in birth complications. However, what

was overlooked is the possibility that some exceptionally high functioning individuals might also have been found in the group whose fathers died before their birth. In other words, the adverse event might increase dispersion instead of simply increasing the odds of disability. [*See* Prenatal Stress and Life Span Development; Schizophrenia.]

A wide range of nonsocial factors can influence brain development by interfering with the chemical signaling that underlies cellular proliferation, migration, and differentiation. One well-documented adverse influence is the heavy use of alcohol or drugs during pregnancy. Viral infection during pregnancy is capable of adversely affecting brain development. Ionizing radiation can have devastating effects, particularly if exposure occurs during the time when cells are proliferating rapidly. Such factors cause changes in the developing brain that range from the relatively subtle (e.g., number of neurotransmitter receptors) to the not so subtle (e.g., abnormalities in the number or arrangements of neurons). These changes in turn may alter neural dynamic properties that manifest as behavioral tendencies. It is at the level of the variability in fine structure of neural networks that the behavioral individuality of infants (i.e., temperament) resides. Moreover, aberrations in the organization of neural networks are thought to underlie at least some cases of individuals who exhibit learning disorders or who eventually become afflicted with serious conditions such as schizophrenia.

The probable effect of the environment on brain organization during prenatal life is consistent with the fact that brain organization cannot be genetically specified in detail. This realization raises questions about current estimates of heritability, which typically do not take into consideration environmental influence during prenatal life. For instance, in the case of schizophrenia a genetic influence is inferred from the finding that identical twins have a higher concordance (48%) for the disorder than dizygotic twins (17%), who are in turn more concordant than siblings (9%). However, because dizygotic twins are no more genetically similar than siblings, their higher concordance raises the possibility of a gene–environment–time interaction. Eventually we will have direct measures of genetic makeup (i.e., the presence of specific alleles) and be in a better position to assess gene–environment interaction effects, although some alleles may be naturally more prevalent within specific contexts, making it difficult to separate effects without resorting to experimental manipulations. [*See* GENETIC CONTRIBUTORS TO MENTAL HEALTH.]

Brain growth and its organization by external stimulation continues postnatally at a rapid rate. An important aspect of this process is that as neural networks become functional their connectivity becomes less extensive. Essentially, they lose plasticity (or potential) in exchange for stability of functional characteristics selected in a context-dependent manner. The best studied examples of these processes are in the organization of sensory systems, particularly the visual system. One of the basic observations is that the neonatal visual cortex is hyperconnected. Normal stimulation of the visual system, during a sensitive period roughly coinciding with early visual experience, results in the irreversible elimination of some of the connections and the stabilization of others. Thus, it appears that patterns of neural activity occurring during sensitive periods lead to the establishment of stable neural networks with specific dynamic properties, which ultimately manifest in behavior. Herein lies the reason why early experience can be so important. Early experience is not simply stimulating a formed brain, it is actually shaping its structure in a dramatic and often irreversible manner. [*See* BRAIN DEVELOPMENT AND PLASTICITY.]

There is no reason to believe that early social experience is any less important than early visual experience with regard to selecting and stabilizing neural networks with particular response properties. Essentially, the fundamental guiding principles for interacting with other human beings begin to be established within the immediate social context of the infant. The brain cannot know that the patterns of interaction and social stimulation encountered at the outset may be atypical. What is immediate is taken as what is relevant in an automatic manner. The acquisition of language provides a good illustration of this point. Infants' early linguistic competence appears similar irrespective of the language environment into which they are born. However, soon thereafter their vocalization becomes progressively more attuned to the characteristics of the language being spoken in their surroundings. As this process progresses, they lose some ability to produce sounds that are not characteristic of their language. Their language-processing neural networks have been selected and stabilized in ways that hamper future learning. This is evident in learning a second language or in the age-dependence of language skill recovery when it is lost as a result of injury. The key point here is that the brain's maximal plasticity tends to be time-limited (i.e., characterized by sensitive periods) and that gaining competence implies a relative loss of plasticity that is highly dependent on the context at hand.

The caregiver–infant relationship is one of the forces capable of shaping brain structure within neural networks central to social behavior. One can expect that consistent patterns, whether they are characterized by nurturance, affection, neglect, or abuse, will promote a brain organization best suited for such circumstances. When interactional patterns are inconsistent, then brain organization is likely to retain unstable neural networks, which will manifest as erratic or seemingly incongruous behavior. Such early experiences may have enduring effects. Evidence supporting this possibility comes from work on the effect of early social experience on primate behavior. This work has dramatically illustrated the long-term impact of early experience. For instance, early social isolation causes a failure to develop a species-normative pattern of affiliation. When previously isolated animals are introduced to social groups, they engage in self-directed stereotypic activity, excessive or inappropriate aggression, are sexually incompetent, and, in the case of females, show abusive behavior toward offspring. However, these effects are not evident in all animals. As many as 30% of the isolated animals seem to be spared from aberrant behavior. It is also possible to induce some recovery if the isolated adult monkeys are allowed to interact for prolonged periods with infant monkeys. Rearing by inadequate caregivers (e.g., peers) produces more subtle effects. Such monkeys are not particularly deviant when observed in their habitual environment. However, when taken out of the familiar surroundings and housed in isolation, they react with behavioral and endocrine signs of extreme distress, and this tendency persists well into adulthood.

Detectable changes in brain organization continue to be evident well into adolescence in the form of synapse deletion and myelination of pathways. Changes in myelination continue to be detected even beyond adolescence. However, these changes are relatively subtle compared with what goes on prenatally and during early postnatal life. Obviously, new experiences remain capable of altering neural networks, but perhaps not as substantially as early on because of the more circumscribed areas of plasticity. It bears repeating at this juncture that by examining the level of neural organization, one is better able to appreciate that genes are only part of the story in the construction of the brain, because much of the sculpting of its organization occurs during sensitive periods in an experience-dependent manner. This process may be characterized as one of gaining the competence to deal with the circumstances at hand while losing some of the flexibility necessary to adapt to differing circumstances. It is this kind of awareness that seems most pertinent to fostering mental health.

Recognition that behavior is a manifestation of neural dynamic properties helps maintain the awareness that a variety of nonsocial factors are capable of affecting the activity of neural networks and thus mental health. Here, one encounters both factors that are detrimental as well as those that are helpful. The list of potential influences is lengthy and includes, on the negative side, toxic chemicals, radiation exposure, physical trauma, infection, nutritional deficiencies, and other organ dysfunction. On the positive side, there is evidence that pharmacological agents and electroconvulsive therapy are capable of improving mood and behavior in many individuals afflicted with specific psychiatric disorders. For instance, a compound as simple as lithium carbonate can have a profound beneficial effect on the propensity to exhibit marked affective instability. On the other hand, a metal such as lead, which can build up in individuals as a result of inadvertent exposure, can result in seriously disruptive social behavior, which exacerbates over time and can lead to an antisocial life style. Another nonsocial source of alteration in mental function that can also lead to psychological disturbance arises as a result of the activity of the immune system. Brain function can be altered by substances (e.g., antibodies, cytokines) released by the cells of the immune system, and this kind of mechanism has been implicated in the etiology of debilitating disorders that alter behavior (e.g., chronic fatigue syndrome) and disrupt thought processes (e.g., schizophrenia). [*See* PSYCHONEUROIMMUNOLOGY.]

In essence, throughout the life span, mental health, as defined by behavior, is a manifestation of neural dynamic properties shaped during sensitive periods by the ongoing interaction of genes, sensory-mediated experience, exposure to components of the physical environment, and the functional status of the individual's other organ systems.

IV. PERSONAL CHARACTERISTICS AND MENTAL HEALTH

Many individuals remain within the ranks of the mentally healthy. A minority of these do so despite unusually unfavorable circumstances, defined in terms of increased genetic risk for mental disorder, chronic health problems, or an excess of negative life events. The latter group has in recent times received much attention in the hope that lessons can be learned regarding personal characteristics that protect the individual from the ill effects of adversity.

How such characteristics are determined depends on age. Typically, the assessment of personal characteristics in infants and young children relies on reports by others (e.g., parents and teachers). In older children, input from peers may be solicited. In adolescents and adults, self-reports of behaviors and attitudes are most frequently used to assess personal characteristics. Other approaches rely on structured tasks and measure not only behavior but also physiological responses such as heart rate, blood pressure, skin conductance, blood chemistry, and brain activity. Here, we are primarily concerned with the behavior and personal outlook that appear to be associated with mental health. The term associated is preferred over predictive or protective because many of the personal characteristics that correlate with mental health sound very much like facets or aspects of mental health and are not distinct and independent entities. Therefore, we simply catalogue how individuals who maintain mental health tend to behave or describe themselves at various points over the life span.

Infant behavior can be characterized in terms of activity level, regularity, response to change, quality of mood, and attention span. The notion of temperament has been used to refer to such variability in infant behavior. Infants who have "easy" temperaments (i.e., tend to be regular, adaptable to change, and have a predominantly positive mood of mild to moderate intensity) appear less prone to develop behavior disorders than infants who exhibit "difficult" temperaments (i.e., are irregular, respond negatively to change, and sustain negative affect of high intensity). Thus, an easy temperament appears as one of the earliest constellations of behavior that has been associated with mental health. [*See* PERSONALITY.]

Research on children who have been able to maintain adaptive behavior despite adverse circumstances has shown that these children tend to be socially aware, possess a sense of humor, are less impulsive, and are more cognitively capable than children who develop behavior disorders. The recurring themes in the research in this area are that mental health in childhood is associated with positive self-esteem, feelings of control, a view of the environment as predictable, an attitude that life is basically a positive experience, social competence, and intelligence. Overwhelmingly, the research with children and adolescents points to social relationships as central to mental health, a topic that is addressed in more detail in the next section.

The concept of ego function deserves attention in this context because many of the characteristics found to be associated with mental health have been previously recognized as functions of the ego. According to Freud, the ego is that aspect of personality that ensures need satisfaction given the constraints imposed by the environment. Ego essentially refers to the mental activities that constitute adaptive problem solving. Ego functions develop with experience from a recognition that one has a separate existence to the eventual development of a sense of integrated identity in a diverse and complex world. Ego strength or resiliency are constructs that denote the stability of ego functions in the face of challenges. Self-report measures of ego strength have been developed and, as expected, negatively correlate with measures of psychological distress and mental disorder.

Hardiness is another construct that has been used to describe individuals who seem to manage adversity with minimal consequences to their health and sense of well-being. Hardy individuals are said to view life as meaningful (commitment). They believe that it is within their power to master situations (control) and that any situation, adverse or otherwise, constitutes an opportunity for personal growth (challenge). The construct of hardiness is typically assessed by self-report and correlates positively with ego-strength and negatively with measures of psychological disturbance. [See HARDINESS IN HEALTH AND EFFECTIVENESS.]

The notion of control subsumed within the construct of hardiness is also evident in earlier constructs, such as locus of control and self-efficacy, which have been proposed to explain differences in how people approach current situations given previous experience. Locus of control is the expectation of the individual concerning how good outcomes occur. Those who tend to believe that good outcomes are a matter of luck or result from the actions of others are said to have an external locus of control; whereas those who

view their own behavior as instrumental in bringing about good outcomes are said to have an internal locus of control. Self-efficacy is the conviction that one can successfully execute behaviors required to produce desired outcomes. Both an internal locus of control and high self-efficacy tend to be inversely related to psychological disturbance.

In general, an optimistic attitude regarding one's ability to deal with situations seems to permeate these constructs, as well as others such as global self-esteem and unconditional positive self-regard. Indeed, dispositional optimism has now been added to the list of constructs that tend to be associated with indicators of psychological well-being and health. What appears clear from much of this work is that certain beliefs about the causes of events and one's power as an agent of change tend to facilitate behavior that fosters well-being. When confronted with adverse circumstances or setbacks, the manner used to explain such events, that is, the individual's attributional style, becomes a determinant in the course of action that ensues. Causal attributions can be categorized along three basic dimensions: (a) internal–external, (b) stable–unstable, and (c) global–specific. For instance, after failing to get a job one could say to oneself, "The employer was not sure that my skills were right for that particular job" or "I am not capable of getting a job." The former attribution views the problem as residing with the employer (external), who was not sure (unstable), with regard to suitability for a particular job (specific). This leads to coping behaviors that are active and problem-focused. In contrast, the latter attribution views the individual as the problem (internal), who fundamentally lacks (stable) what it takes to get any job (global). This way of looking at the situation would tend to leave the individual with a more difficult challenge. [See OPTIMISM, MOTIVATION, AND MENTAL HEALTH.]

An important issue that relates to this kind of perspective on dealing with adversity concerns the extent to which being realistic actually proves to be adaptive, even though it has been considered by some to be a defining aspect of mental health. Often, those who are thought to possess mental health endorse overly positive views of the self, have exaggerated perceptions of personal control, and unrealistically high optimism. Indeed, there is significant evidence suggesting that realistic appraisals of situations tend to be more typical of depressed individuals. Thus, it appears as if the constructive distortion that allows one to sustain a positive outlook may be protective of mental health.

A final point concerns gender, which, as indicated earlier, tends to be associated with disorders such as depression and other psychological attributes that correlate with depression. There also appear to be gender differences prior to the onset of some disorders. For instance, studies have shown that before becoming depressed females tend to be anxious, easily upset, somatize, and lack self-esteem; whereas males engage in antisocial behaviors, are hostile, and give less direct evidence of feelings of inadequacy. Similarly, for individuals diagnosed with schizophrenia, females tend to have been characterized by better premorbid functioning. These findings simply underscore that gender is one of the factors that affects one's trajectory through behavioral state space. [*See* GENDER DIFFERENCES IN MENTAL HEALTH.]

In effect, individuals whose personal narratives incorporate a positive attitude toward the self and a conviction that they can master the challenges of life are basically acknowledging characteristics that are central to definitions of mental health. Thus, what the literature indicates is that being well within the mental health subspace helps to ensure that one remains there even if one's position changes along one or more dimensions as a result of shifting circumstances or the occurrence of disruptive events (e.g., illness, loss of job, divorce). The crucial question seems to be, how does one get into favorable positions from the outset? It is in this regard that relationships appear to be fundamental.

V. SOCIAL CONTEXT AND MENTAL HEALTH

It is customary to begin the exploration of how social context influences mental health with the mother–child relationship, as it is after birth that the infant can directly participate in a social relationship. However, social influences affecting the individual can be seen as operating before birth, certainly during prenatal life when interactions of the mother with her social world can have an impact on the fetus. It is even possible to begin the story of social context much earlier, that is, to consider how it is that the specific genes that will become the individual have been brought together at the moment of conception.

The simple answer is that social proximity is the determining factor. Unrelated individuals who are in frequent contact are most likely to mate. Social proximity occurs within specific cultural and economic contexts. People reside in neighborhoods with particular demographic characteristics and they interact within the institutions and settings that are part of the community. Within any such community the nature of social interactions is shaped by the density of individuals with particular relationship styles. Communities with a high proportion of individuals with poor relationship skills can be expected to constitute a disruptive social context. Social context in conjunction with assortative mating causes nonrandom self-reinforcing selection of genes. Genetic influences on behavior are in a sense a social phenomenon, the effect of which seems to be to increase phenotypic variability across the population, with positive and negative phenotypes concentrated at the extremes. Genetic and social forces are thus intertwined in self-perpetuating cycles that seem to sustain diversity.

Prenatal life ensues after genes have been selected within the constraints imposed by social context, and the process of genetic expression during this period remains susceptible to social forces either directly (e.g., neuroendocrine response to social stimuli) or indirectly (e.g., through drug abuse). Some evidence suggestive of social impact on brain development has already been cited. It has also been reported that interpersonal tensions of a chronic nature (e.g., marital discord) during pregnancy are associated with higher incidence of developmental and behavioral problems in infants and young children. Economic conditions per se do not appear to be a factor, although individuals with chronic relationship problems tend to be overrepresented in the low socioeconomic groups. Problems with relating are associated with economic disadvantage and also with an increase in the probability of negative outcomes in the health and behavior of offspring. Thus, the frequently observed association between low socioeconomic status and mental disorder is probably best viewed as indicative of the prevalence of maladaptive interactional patterns within such communities. [*See* SOCIOECONOMIC STATUS.]

However, it should be noted that individuals who lack relationship skills are not simply "drifting" into low socioeconomic status in a vacuum. Often, they are being nudged by others through values and attitudes that translate into specific economic policies. The end result is that a barrier (or zone of insensitivity) can form around such communities, making life within them difficult to endure or escape.

At birth, the infant begins to interact more directly

with the social context. Infant temperament becomes a factor in social interactions. As noted earlier, infants with difficult temperaments are more likely to exhibit behavioral disorders in childhood. However, this outcome is influenced by the caregivers' ability to manage their own frustration and remain responsive, consistent, and resourceful in their interactions with the infant. Here begins the process of child rearing. What transpires in the child rearing endeavor defines a most important aspect of the child's early social life. The accumulated knowledge makes it clear that poor outcomes are associated with inadequate parental monitoring, inconsistent discipline, absence of positive parenting, low levels of parental affection, low family cohesiveness, and high conflict and hostility.

Child rearing constitutes a central aspect of family life and is clearly affected by family intactness. Interactions within a family are complex and involve exchanges within the marital dyad, between parents and children, and between children. Family size is a factor in how much attention children receive, and it has been frequently found that first-born and only children fare better in terms of achievement.

Organization within the family is a factor in the ability of children to remain problem-free. Children from cohesive families (i.e., family members all feel close to each other) exhibit significantly fewer problems than children from families where children are excluded (detouring), caught in the middle (triangulated), or where closeness is lacking (separate).

Discord in the marital dyad is disruptive to child adjustment and may be differentially so as a function of gender. However, because disputes are inevitable within any human group, the issue is more one of what aspects of discord are deleterious. What seems most disruptive is discord that is frequent, affectively intense, involves the child, remains unresolved, and casts blame onto the child for the conflict. In this regard, it should be noted that child characteristics may indeed be a trigger for conflict in the marriage and may also moderate the impact of conflict on the child.

Early parenting, to the extent that it serves to foster secure attachment to the primary caregiver, promotes positive patterns of individual adaptation across the childhood years, even outside the family context. Secure attachment during the second year of life has been found to be associated in a prospective manner with indices of social competence across settings and over development well into adolescence. Infants with secure attachments more frequently grow up to be among those with positive expectations of others, who are self-confident, and who relate well to peers. It has been conjectured that this association is mediated by continuity of early emerging expectations about relationships and self-mastery over them. This leads to a style of social engagement that perpetuates relating in a manner that anticipates satisfaction. [*See* ATTACHMENT.]

Longitudinal data further suggest that parenting style during early childhood (at about age 4) proves to be significantly predictive of the degree to which individuals approach optimal adjustment in early adulthood. In essence, young children whose parents tend to maintain an authoritarian stance (i.e., who maintain rigid control with an element of hostility, disapprove of expression of negative affect, and view affection as making children weak) are seen in young adulthood as more anxious, defensive, easily disorganized by stress, and prone to give up when faced with adversity. They are viewed as lacking personal warmth, lacking the capacity for close relationships, and are generally less well liked or accepted by others. [*See* PARENTING.]

A particularly important aspect of parenting during early childhood concerns how parents help children deal with negative emotions. Parents who adopt an accepting approach to their children's negative emotions and who assist in the process of managing and expressing such emotions constructively tend to have children who, in middle childhood, achieve better in school, have positive peer relationships, and have good physical health.

By late adolescence, the characteristics of the individual's family environment are less directly associated with adult social competence than are the individual's personal beliefs, values, and lifestyle. Family influences appear to have an earlier impact on generating something akin to dispositional optimism, which stabilizes during early adulthood and serves to promote mental health.

An important aspect of family context is the presence of siblings who provide the opportunity for more complex interactions. The extent and style of parental intervention in intersibling interactions has been a topic of some debate. Some have favored no intervention by parents to avoid hindering the development of dispute resolution skills, whereas others believe sibling interaction to be a golden opportunity for instilling conflict resolution skills and the notion of fairness. These lessons may then be taken further and applied in other relationships such as those with peers, which are powerful indicators of life-long adaptive function.

Longitudinal studies of sibling relationships indicate that those with more positive relationships come from homes where the father, in particular, has more positive affect in his interactions and is equitable in his negative treatment of the children, family members view themselves as close (high cohesiveness), and the children tend to have temperaments that are not difficult. It has further been observed that differences in adjustment between siblings can at least partially be attributed to differential treatment by parents, usually in the form of more hostility directed at the less well-adjusted sibling. If there is high contrast in how siblings are treated, it exacerbates the negative influence on the less favored child. Sibling relationships are sensitive to the nature of parent–child interactions, the quality of the marital relationship, and the individual characteristics of the children. These are the same factors that consistently emerge as important with regard to mental health in childhood. Thus, one could argue that positive relationships with siblings is an aspect of mental health.

Relationships within the family set the stage for interactions with peers and nonfamilial adults. Parent–child interactions serve as a background for interactions with others. It is also the case that parents give direct instruction regarding how to relate to others. They can be instrumental in creating opportunities for their child's interaction with others. Interaction with others will in turn feed back and affect relationships within the family. The sheer complexity of interactions within this wider social context can lead to unanticipated outcomes. Peer relationships are especially important and have been found to be predictive of mental health. This is not to say that poor peer relationships play an etiological role; rather, they may be affected by early manifestations of impairments that will ultimately surface as bona fide disorders, ranging from schizophrenia to antisocial personality to milder forms of maladjustment.

The association of rejection by peers with maladjustment and mental disorder is consistent with extensive evidence documenting higher risk of mental disorder, physical illness, and even premature death in individuals lacking social support. Social support is typically indexed by the amount of contact one has with others, either in organized social settings (e.g., church, school, workplace) or within a network of friends and extended family. For instance, regularly attending religious services has been found to be protective of mental health at times of stress.

It is assumed that in the process of social support something positive transpires. Others are reassuring, provide a different perspective, give information, or offer concrete help. However, it is also possible that simply being able to talk to another person may be sufficient for benefit, as the act of disclosing important personal matters has been found to promote well-being.

Social support clearly depends on the relationship skills of those who happen to be interacting. At times, both social support and social undermining arise within the same relationship (e.g., married couples). The evidence suggests that social undermining proves to be the more powerful variable. Therefore, social encounters can have adverse effects, at least for some participants some of the time. Nonetheless, across large community samples, social support appears to be clearly beneficial. Unfortunately, it is not readily available to all. For instance, recent research has shown that some individuals who are highly distressed and who are most in need of social support are less likely to receive it because, as an expression of their distress, they tend to drive away potential supporters. Often, these individuals require professional assistance. In this regard it should be noted that psychotherapy in its many forms and various other types of mental health treatments can be viewed as specialized forms of social support. [*See* SOCIAL SUPPORT.]

VI. IMPLICATIONS FOR MAXIMIZING MENTAL HEALTH

Mental health is a dynamic concept subject to change as a function of cultural evolution. It was not long ago that homosexuality was regarded as a mental disorder. It is also the case that there is a core of abstract personal characteristics, such as the ability to maintain high self-esteem and sustain positive relationships, that consistently emerge as indicative of positive mental health.

How one comes to possess the personal characteristics that define mental health and that ensure its stability appears to be profoundly rooted in the social context that one happens to inhabit. Social context along with assortative mating constrains the genes that will come together at the moment of conception. Social context sets the stage for the probable social interactions of the mother during intrauterine development of the individual. Subsequently, social relationships within the family further shape the developing individual in a way that sets in motion particular expectations about relationships. Such expectations, along with social context, bias future interactions, leading to a cascade of experiences that ultimately may trap the individual in patterns of social interaction and behavior that are maladaptive within the broader society and may be regarded as mental disorder.

Clearly, social factors play a prominent role, but they cannot be viewed as the whole story, because, as was noted earlier, *all* behavior is biologically mediated and thus affected by numerous physical factors capable of altering brain function. Recognition of the biological underpinnings of mental life and behavior is indispensable to understanding the interactive influence of genes, social experience, and physical factors that operate during sensitive periods to steer the individual's course through life. Moreover, as a result of the brain's complexity, emergent phenomena are possible within an individual that are not reducible to genes, exposure, experience, or their interactions. The biological perspective makes it clear how disruption of mental health, for any reason, can make it more likely that one's vulnerability to other sources of disruption would increase. For instance, increased negative affect secondary to loss of social support can make one relatively immunosuppressed and more susceptible to infections or malignancies, which could in turn impair brain function and further compromise mental health. Another pathological scenario could lead the individual to alcohol or substance use to cope with distress, causing disruption of social support and toxic effects on the brain and other organs, which could ultimately lead to a more severe mental disorder.

Individual differences in mental health, or diverse trajectories through behavioral state space, reflect the action of multiple forces. It is clear that if one could stop the action at conception and represent individuals in something akin to genotype space, it would not be possible to project a life course trajectory with accuracy. This would also be generally true if one waited until the third trimester of gestation and represented the individual in terms of prenatal neural organization. However, by the time individuals are between 2 and 4 years of age, behavioral tendencies begin to be evident which appear to be predictive of subsequent behavior and mental health. This suggests that brain organization at this juncture may begin to be charac-

terized by relatively stable neural networks giving rise to patterns of activity, whose behavioral manifestations then elicit social responses which cause the patterns of activity to become further ingrained. For instance, an individual who anticipates aggression from others, and who then behaves aggressively and elicits aggression, will be compelled subsequently to aggression even more readily. [*See* AGGRESSION.]

Given our current understanding, efforts to maximize mental health should be primarily guided by the fact that development is characterized by sensitive periods during early life and that social forces are powerful organizers of neural networks and, thus, behavior. Therefore, services and programs to promote and safeguard mental health must begin quite early. Critical developmental events occur prenatally and efforts should be directed at the socioemotional condition of mothers and their families as an integral part of prenatal care. In this area, there is also a great need for well designed research that carefully documents prenatal events and subsequent individual outcomes. Moreover, it is essential that as part of standard neonatal care, relationships within the family be addressed. Interventions to promote mental health should continue to be available to families as a central feature of day care facilities and later within the schools. In the schools, the effect of social context should be supplemented by curricula about the social forces that affect individual development and behavior. Traditional mental health services must be made more readily available. They are indispensable for assisting individuals to overcome maladaptive tendencies, reformulate personal narratives, or manage psychological disabilities within a therapeutic context. In addition, there need to be outreach mental health services to address family crisis situations and to help reestablish constructive social interaction within families in turmoil. These services need to be available within neighborhoods on a scale similar to that of primary schools. Characteristics of the neighborhood should determine the capacity of such services. The central goal of these services is to prevent the stabilization of maladaptive behavioral patterns that erode mental health. Efforts to treat or alter maladaptive patterns after they have gained some measure of stability are relatively more difficult because, even though individuals retain a measure of plasticity and are capable of change, the task becomes one of reorganizing neural networks selected to self-perpetuate.

One must expect that the extensive services and

programs just outlined would be economically burdensome. Whether or not economic resources would be provided for such programs takes us back to culture and values. In this regard, it is noteworthy that at the level of individuals, maladjustment tends to be associated with ranking personal financial gain over community well-being. If this operates as well at the level of society, then one would expect that as mental health declines, the priority of personal financial gain becomes augmented at the expense of community well-being with the potential to undermine mental health even further. Are we seeing this dynamic at work in the constant threat of cutbacks for funding of mental health programs? One hopes not, but it is clear that action to promote mental health on a large scale has not been given adequate priority.

BIBLIOGRAPHY

Coan, R. W. (1977). *Hero, artist, sage, or saint? A survey of views on what is variously called mental health, normality, maturity, self-actualization, and human fulfillment.* New York: Columbia Press.

Desjardais, R., Eisenberg, L., Good, B., & Kleinman, A. (Eds.). (1995). *World mental health: Problems and priorities in low-income countries.* New York: Oxford Press.

Edelman, G. M. (1992). *Bright air, brilliant fire: On the matter of the mind.* New York: Basic Books.

Funder, D. C., Parke, R. D., Tomlinson-Keasy, C., & Widaman, K. (Eds.). (1993). *Studying lives through time: Personality and development.* Washington, DC: American Psychological Association.

Kauffman, S. A. (1993). *The origins of order: Self-organization and selection in evolution.* New York: Oxford Press.

Lubotsky-Levin, B., & Petrila, J. (Eds.). (1996). *Mental health services: A public health perspective.* New York: Oxford Press.

Mrazek, P. J., & Haggerty, R. J. (Eds.). (1994). *Reducing risks for mental disorders: Frontiers for preventive interventions research.* Washington, DC: National Academy Press.

Peterson, C., Maier, S. F., & Seligman, M. E. P. (1993). *Learned helplessness: A theory for the age of personal control.* New York: Oxford Press.

Plomin, R., & McClearn, G. E. (Eds.). (1993). *Nature, nurture, and psychology.* Washington, DC: American Psychological Association.

Rutter, M., & Rutter, M. (1993). *Developing minds: Challenge and continuity across the life span.* New York: Basic Books.

Infertility

Annette L. Stanton and Beth L. Dinoff

University of Kansas

Infertility Inability to achieve a pregnancy after 12 months of regular sexual intercourse without contraception.
Impaired Fecundity Difficulty or danger in achieving or carrying a pregnancy to term.

INFERTILITY typically is defined as the inability to achieve pregnancy after 12 months of regular sexual intercourse. Following a brief description of the problem of infertility, this article focuses on the psychosocial concomitants of infertility, including an examination of infertility's influence on individuals' mental health and couples' functioning. We go on to suggest factors that may promote or detract from adaptive psychological functioning in the face of infertility and to discuss psychological interventions in this area.

I. INFERTILITY: DEFINITIONS AND PREVALENCE

Based on National Survey of Family Growth interviews conducted in 1988 with a national sample of 8450 women aged 15 through 44 years, infertility is estimated to affect approximately 2.3 million married couples in the United States, or slightly fewer than 1 in 12. In primary infertility, for which the rate has increased in the past two decades from one-half million to one million couples, the couple has no history of conception, whereas those with secondary infertility (1.3 million in 1988) have had at least one biological child. Impaired fecundity, a broader category that includes difficulty or danger in carrying a pregnancy to term, affects an additional 2.6 million couples.

Although primary infertility has increased, the overall rate of infertility has changed little over the past two decades. However, the number of visits to physicians for infertility-related concerns has risen dramatically, nearly tripling from 1968 to 1988, in part owing to the rise in primary infertility, advances in medical treatments for infertility, and the decreased availability of adoption. The chance of achieving a viable pregnancy with medical treatment is approximately 50%, with distinct diagnoses and treatments carrying disparate success rates.

A biological cause for infertility can be diagnosed in 80 to 90% of cases, with approximately 10% remaining unexplained after medical evaluation. Female-factor infertility, which accounts for 40 to 50% of cases, commonly reflects pelvic abnormalities, ovulatory problems, and hormonal or immunological dysfunction. Male-factor infertility, accounting for 30 to 40% of cases, typically involves deficient sperm production or delivery. In approximately 20% of couples, both members carry a diagnosis.

II. IMPACT OF INFERTILITY ON THE INDIVIDUAL

Although psychosocial and environmental stress may play a role in the etiology of infertility, potentially affecting spermatogensis and ovulation, research in general has not revealed personality or other psychological factors to be causal in infertility. For example, no reliable evidence exists for the common belief that adoption facilitates subsequent conception. Empirical attention has shifted away from psychogenesis and toward specifying psychosocial consequences that infertile individuals and couples face.

The clinical literature portrays infertility as profoundly disruptive to psychosocial functioning. In 1991, Dunkel-Schetter and Lobel summarized the results of more than 30 qualitative descriptions of the effects of infertility, primarily authored by mental health professionals experienced in working with infertile couples. Psychological consequences were cited in four domains: (a) emotional effects, including grief, anger, guilt, shock, and anxiety; (b) loss of control and an inability to predict or plan for the future; (c) effects on self-esteem, identity, and core beliefs; and (d) social effects, such as those on marital, sexual, and interpersonal functioning. In the main, infertility was characterized as a life crisis, conferring negative impact in each of these domains.

Dunkel-Schetter and Lobel also examined the empirical literature on psychological functioning in infertile individuals, and their review was extended by Stanton and Danoff-Burg in 1995 to include 31 investigations in which infertile individuals' scores on standardized measures were compared with available norms or with data from a control group. Samples for the studies reviewed primarily consisted of women pursuing medical treatment for infertility. In contrast to the clinical descriptions, the empirical literature produced much less evidence of decrement in psychosocial functioning. Most individuals did not report distress that reached clinical levels on standardized measures. Although some studies revealed significant differences between infertile and fertile samples on psychological variables (e.g., depression, anxiety), these results were not uniform across studies. In fact, the finding of no significant between-groups difference was more common. This suggests that, on average, infertile individuals maintain adequate functioning in a number of psychosocial realms, including self-esteem, marital and sexual functioning, and distress and well-being.

Why do the clinical and the empirical bodies of work yield such disparate findings? Clinical writers may overestimate the psychosocial disruption produced by infertility because they are likely to encounter the most distressed individuals in clinical samples. Empirical researchers may underestimate psychosocial disruption because they use insufficiently sensitive or specific measures or because research volunteers represent the most well-functioning infertile individuals. We would suggest that both literatures are valuable in some regard. Infertility may pose an extreme crisis for some individuals, carrying severely negative consequences in a number of life domains. Clinical writings provide a rich description of these untoward effects, and they may offer guidance to those health care professionals who work with individuals in extreme distress and comfort to those infertile individuals who experience it. Perhaps the majority of those who face infertility, however, are able to negotiate its challenges such that it does not gravely compromise life quality. The importance of this finding is underscored by its consistency with those from groups who experience other serious medical problems. Even when diagnosed with life-threatening diseases such as cancer, many individuals demonstrate psychosocial resilience. We have much to learn about the personal and environmental resources that allow many individuals to confront infertility as a process that is stressful, yet manageable, as well as the risk factors that confer infertility's demands overwhelming for some.

III. IMPACT OF INFERTILITY ON THE COUPLE

Investigations of the impact of infertility on psychological health primarily have focused on the individual experiences of women and men rather than describing infertility's effect on the well-being of the couple as a unit. Although some individuals pursue single parenthood, most seek parenthood within a relational context, and the psychological burden of failing to conceive is assumed by the couple regardless of which partner carries the medical diagnosis. Within the dyadic context, researchers have explored marital and sexual satisfaction in infertile versus fertile couples, psychosocial functioning of partners relative to each other, and the trajectory of the infertility experience for couples.

A. Marital and Sexual Satisfaction of Infertile Relative to Fertile Couples

Most couples enter marriage assuming that they will become biological parents. Failure to accomplish this often central life goal potentially creates profound strain. Clinical reports suggest that attendant feelings of guilt, anxiety, isolation, anger, depression, grief, and unworthiness may influence infertile couples' functioning. Qualitative accounts of constrained communication and sexuality are commonplace. For example, couples often comment that the trials of undergoing treatment and the intense focus on the goal of reproduction serve to reduce spontaneity, decrease desire, and create concerns surrounding sexual performance. In some cases, sexual dysfunction causes or exacerbates infertility.

Few empirical studies have assessed relationship and sexual satisfaction of infertile couples versus a presumed fertile sample gathered specifically for comparison. The largest study incorporating such a comparison group is that of Abbey and colleagues in 1991. Their sample included 185 couples diagnosed with primary infertility, primarily recruited through medical practices specializing in infertility, and 90 presumed-fertile couples, primarily recruited through gynecological practices and marriage license applications. All couples were married and had no children but desired to do so (the presumed-fertile couples reported a desire for children within a few years). Marital quality and sexual satisfaction did not differ significantly for the infertile versus the presumed fertile couples.

These results converge with those of several studies using standardized measures that compare marital and sexual satisfaction in infertile couples with normative data, which reveal that these on average are within normal limits for infertile couples. Despite the exigencies of pursuing parenthood, couples are likely to report relatively high satisfaction in these domains, and partners' reports of their satisfaction tend to be correlated positively. How can partners remain resilient as they undergo an experience that presents so many challenges to intimate functioning? Perhaps the shared

nature of the stressor yields some positive outcomes. The few investigations assessing perceived benefits of the infertility experience reveal that participants often cite benefits with regard to enhanced dyadic communication and intimacy. Further, because partners are found to rely primarily on each other for emotional support regarding infertility, perhaps they are motivated to focus on the positive aspects of their relationship. In addition, it might be that more distressed couples are unlikely to elect the rigors of specialized fertility treatment, the primary source of research participants, or to volunteer for psychosocial study. These interpretations require empirical attention, as do the mechanisms whereby many infertile couples maintain satisfying relationships.

B. Psychosocial Functioning of Infertile Partners

Both partners experience the psychosocial consequences of infertility, and a number of studies have explored the relative adjustment of partners experiencing fertility problems. Although investigations in general do not indicate significant between-partner differences on indices of marital and sexual satisfaction, several studies reveal that women report greater distress and life disruption as a result of the infertility experience than do their partners. Several factors may account for these findings.

Women often carry the responsibility for initiating and participating in medical treatment, and research suggests that women are more likely than men to assume causal responsibility for infertility, even when the diagnosed problem does not reside with them. In addition, it is the woman who monitors her body for indicators of pregnancy and who each month confronts concretely the signal that she is not pregnant. Within a cultural context emphasizing motherhood as a central role, women also typically report that having a child is more important to them than do men. A greater discrepancy between infertile spouses on this variable has been associated with lower ratings of marital satisfaction by both partners. Finally, we should note the finding that negative events in general evoke more pronounced appraisals of stress in women than men. Empirical exploration of the mechanisms accounting for women's greater life disruption in the face of infertility, as well as development of interventions to promote couples' successful negotiation of the infertility process, are warranted. [*See* STRESS.]

C. The Trajectory of the Infertility Experience

With regard to the psychosocial experience of couples across the course of infertility, some cross-sectional studies suggest that the first year of medical investigation for infertility may be acutely stressful for couples, perhaps owing to new demands of medical involvement and concrete acknowledgment that a fertility problem exists. As the couple becomes accustomed to the infertility diagnosis and its treatment, distress may subside, to rise again as the stresses of infertility become chronic. However, other studies have not demonstrated an association between duration of infertility and psychological functioning or have suggested other patterns, and longitudinal studies that include assessments at multiple points across the course of the experience are necessary to elucidate the points at which infertility is maximally stressful and is typically resolved.

Although couples in general report satisfaction with the specialized medical services they receive for infertility and they approach new treatment attempts with optimism, medical interventions for infertility often are perceived as stressful by couples. These procedures often necessitate substantial commitments of time and money, as well as a willingness to reveal intensely personal aspects of one's functioning. Peaks in distress are likely, particularly for women, when the promise of a new treatment does not produce success. For example, couples have been found to overestimate substantially their likelihood for success with an in vitro fertilization attempt, and a failed trial of this costly and invasive procedure often yields sharp disappointment. Again, however, distress often remains at subclinical levels. In addition, we know very little about the psychosocial experience of those who do not elect medical treatment. Further, the advent of a number of technological advances in infertility treatments also raises questions regarding psychological consequences for couples who have limited access to them, as well as for those who feel it necessary to pursue every viable medical avenue, regardless of financial and psychological cost.

A few investigations have examined psychosocial consequences of becoming a parent after infertility.

The 1994 data of Abbey, Andrews, and Halman provide a longitudinal account of this transition. As often found for married couples in general, becoming a biological or adoptive parent was associated with a reduction in marital life quality for previously infertile couples. The numerous stresses of new parenthood, as well as idealistic expectations that may accompany this long-sought goal for infertile couples, may contribute to increased marital strain. It should be noted, however, that marriages remained satisfying on average. Further, becoming a parent was related to an increase in global life quality for infertile women, indicating that psychosocial rewards also accrue from the successful pursuit of parenthood.

In sum, as with the literature on individual functioning, the data highlight the variability in psychosocial consequences of infertility for couples. Although women on average may find infertility more stressful than do their partners, it is likely that both members of the couple will be able to sustain adequate quality of life. However, the demands of infertility may result in extreme life disruption for some couples, and it is essential to specify factors that enhance or detract from the well-being of those experiencing infertility.

IV. INFLUENCES ON PSYCHOLOGICAL ADJUSTMENT TO INFERTILITY

Attempts to delineate predictors of adaptive psychosocial functioning in infertile individuals and couples are rare relative to descriptive studies, and longitudinal examinations that allow statistical control of initial levels of adjustment are even fewer. In addition, research in this area often has not been theory-driven, or it has adopted a crisis model, which assumes uniformity in response. Stress and coping theories offer a model for understanding variability in reaction to negative encounters. According to these theories, both personal characteristics and situational factors are meaningful determinants of individuals' cognitive appraisals and coping processes, which in turn determine adjustment to situations experienced as stressful. Such theories have been applied successfully to the experience of health-related adversity in a number of realms, and researchers have begun to examine relevant constructs with reference to adjustment in infertile individuals. Within the context of these theories, three questions regarding psychological adjustment to infertility can be posed: (a) Which preexisting personal characteristics affect adjustment? (b) What situational factors influence individual outcomes? and (c) How do cognitive appraisals and coping strategies enhance or hinder adjustment to infertility? Because research on these questions is just beginning, some of the influences on adjustment to infertility suggested in the following sections are necessarily speculative. [See COPING WITH STRESS.]

A. Personal Characteristics as Predictors of Adjustment

Lazarus and Folkman cite personal commitments and beliefs as important determinants of cognitive appraisals in stressful situations. Commitments have enduring motivational attributes and reflect what is important or meaningful to the individual. Commitments relevant to the process of adjustment to infertility include central life goals, particularly meanings attributed to parenthood relative to other goals, and the nature of the bond between members of the couple attempting pregnancy.

Parenthood constitutes a central goal in life for many adults, and few anticipate difficulty accomplishing this aim. Should the goal be thwarted, the individual presumably will experience threat and life disruption commensurate with her or his commitment to parenthood. As mentioned previously, women's stronger commitment may in part explain their greater infertility-specific distress relative to men, and discrepancies between infertile partners in their commitment to parenthood may engender relationship strain. It has also been argued that, to the extent that the goal of parenthood is tied to other overriding life aims, such as finding happiness or a sense of purpose in life, the infertile individual will experience greater life disruption. An implication of this argument is that maintaining investment in other valued roles (e.g., career, community involvement) or finding alternative routes to one's central aims may buffer individuals from some of the threatening aspects of infertility.

The value one places on maintaining an intimate bond with one's partner may represent a commitment capable of shielding the individual from extreme distress in the face of fertility problems. Further, a shared commitment to parenting coupled with a strong com-

mitment to their relationship may allow partners to persist in what is often a lengthy, expensive, and intrusive diagnostic and treatment process. However, if this process begins to interfere with goals that are valued more highly than is becoming a parent, then adaptive termination of the pursuit of parenthood might occur. For example, if a couple highly cherishes their commitment to each other, with parenthood as a secondary goal, then they may decide to terminate infertility treatments if the ensuing strain on their relationship becomes great. Individuals' and couples' relative commitments and their impact on psychological adjustment to infertility deserve further empirical scrutiny.

Individuals' core beliefs represent another person variable that may influence adjustment to infertility. Tacitly held beliefs often become apparent when a person is confronted with a situation that presents a challenge to the belief system. Control and mastery beliefs represent an example. Couples identify loss of control as one of the most stressful aspects of infertility. As such, the experience of infertility may challenge one's generalized beliefs regarding mastery over the environment.

Work by Abbey and colleagues with samples of infertile and presumed-fertile couples revealed that general beliefs regarding personal control enhanced perceived quality of life over time for both infertile and fertile women and men, controlling for initial levels of life quality. Perhaps infertile individuals who maintain their generalized control beliefs reap psychological benefits through their abilities to devote energy to facets of life that are within their control (e.g., career pursuits) or to focus on the aspects of infertility that are relatively controllable, such as electing medical treatments.

Those who generalize their inability to control their fertility outcome to other life arenas, thus shattering generalized control beliefs, may be more likely to experience severe life disruption. It has been found that women experienced more depressive symptoms in response to in vitro fertilization failure if they reported a general loss of control over their lives as a result of infertility. A generalized expectancy for positive outcomes (i.e., dispositional optimism) was protective with regard to the experience of depression in these women.

Although the extant research has focused on beliefs regarding control, other core beliefs, such as belief in a higher power or beliefs in the fairness and predictability of life, also may be altered by the experience of infertility and in turn may influence psychological adaptation. The contributions of these and additional personal attributes to infertility-related adjustment require study.

B. Situational Characteristics as Predictors of Adjustment

Several properties of situations may shape individuals' appraisals, coping strategies, and adjustment. These include such factors as novelty, predictability, event uncertainty and ambiguity, duration, and timing with reference to the life cycle. Certainly, most individuals find infertility a novel, unpredictable, and unwanted experience; these attributes are likely to combine to produce greater perceived threat. Although there is no evidence on this point, it is possible that those who learn of their inability to have children prior to attempting conception (e.g., those who have diagnosed congenital anomalies) may adapt more readily to their status than those who invest considerable energy into attempting pregnancy, only then to meet with failure. Further, individuals may be aided to develop adaptive coping strategies through likening aspects of their infertility experience to those of other major stressors that they have managed successfully, thus reducing discomforting novelty.

Unless one receives a definitive diagnosis of permanent inability to conceive, infertility is inherently ambiguous in that there is no guarantee that one eventually will be able to have a child. Likelihood of success in pursuing alternatives such as adoption also is uncertain. Further, a burgeoning array of available fertility-enhancing technologies may bolster the likelihood of successful conception; however, they also may increase uncertainty with regard to whether and when to pursue or terminate treatment. Ambiguity and event uncertainty hold both the promise of hope that success will occur and the threat that it may not.

A factor relevant to ambiguity that has received some empirical attention is locus of cause for infertility. Although some research has revealed that individuals with unexplained infertility report greater distress than those with diagnosed causes, other studies have demonstrated greater distress in women or men when they carry the infertility diagnosis or have shown no association between locus of cause and distress. Perhaps it would be useful to assess both the locus of

cause and meanings attributed to the diagnosis or lack thereof, including perceived likelihood of success in treatment as well as extent of personal blame or connotation (e.g., attack on sense of masculinity/femininity) arising from the diagnosis. Objective characteristics of situations are filtered through individuals' perceptual lens in determining psychological impact.

Duration of the stressor is another situational quality that may influence appraisal, coping, and adjustment processes. Because an infertility diagnosis typically is not rendered until at least a year of unsuccessful attempts at conception has passed, infertility by definition may be regarded as a chronic stressor. Even more striking is that some research participants report pursuing parenthood for as many as two decades and that some elderly individuals comment on the lingering, profound disappointment that can accompany permanent infertility. For many, the intermittent, acute experience of recurrent treatment failure as signaled by menstrual onset is superimposed upon the chronicity of infertility.

Findings regarding the duration of infertility as related to psychological adjustment are mixed, with linear and quadratic relations obtained, as well as no demonstrated association between chronicity and adjustment. Again, whether exhaustion and increased distress or adaptive emotional habituation results from the chronic and acute stresses of infertility most likely is a function of meanings attributed to the experience, as well as internal and external resources brought to bear on its challenges.

Finally, the timing of the stressor in relation to the life cycle deserves mention. Individuals may be hypothesized to experience greater distress to the extent that they diverge from normative expectations for the timing of parenthood, owing to such factors as mounting social and familial pressures to begin a family, increased exposure to peers who are becoming parents, and the knowledge that potentially fertile years are dwindling. On the other hand, those who postpone childbearing may have developed other valued roles to buffer the strains of infertility, as well as resources to manage some of these pressures.

The foregoing analysis of personal and situational contributors to infertility-related adjustment illustrates both the potential impact that these factors may have on psychological functioning and the importance of considering them in the context of the meanings attributed to them by individuals and their interactions with other variables. For example, greater chronicity of infertility may predict extreme distress only in those who do not develop other valued roles. Or being diagnosed with male-factor infertility may be threatening only to those men who imbue the diagnosis with negative meaning for their sexual and masculine identities. It is important to consider cognitive appraisals and coping strategies that may mediate or moderate the relations of personal and situational qualities with adaptational outcomes in infertility.

C. Appraisals and Coping as Predictors of Adjustment

Cognitive appraisals of the extent to which a situation carries the potential for harm (i.e., threat appraisals) and benefit (i.e., challenge appraisals), as well as one's assessment of ability to manage its demands (e.g., secondary appraisals of control, efficacy), are important determinants of subsequent coping processes, which in turn influence adjustment. Researchers have found that infertile individuals perceive their status as conferring potential for both harm and benefit, and, at least among women, threat and challenge appraisals are related to adjustment in opposite directions. Abbey and colleagues also demonstrated that perceived infertility-specific stress predicted lower marital life quality and that finding positive meaning in infertility was associated with enhanced quality of life.

With regard to appraisals of adaptive resources, some researchers have assessed infertility-specific control appraisals. Campbell and colleagues found that women felt more control over some aspects of infertility than others. Women perceived some control over the likelihood that they would become pregnant and significantly greater control over their medical treatment choices and emotional responses to infertility. Perceived control over medical treatments and emotional responses was associated with better psychological adjustment. Similarly, it has been found that greater perceived control over the course of and alternatives to infertility was associated with more favorable adaptation. Abbey and colleagues found that generalized control beliefs, but not perceived control over the cause or solution to infertility, were related to enhanced life quality. Certainly, believing that one can control an outcome may be adaptive only in circumstances in which this belief is consistent with situational contingencies. Thus, it is reasonable that con-

trol assessments are related to adjustment only for dimensions of infertility that actually promise some measure of control (e.g., medical treatments) rather than those in which control is limited (e.g., fertility outcome).

Several studies have investigated the relations between coping processes and adjustment to infertility. Perhaps the most consistent findings across infertile women and men are that coping through avoidance and through self-blame are associated with greater distress and that obtaining emotional support from the partner or others in the social network predicts more positive adjustment. Avoidant coping, which involves cognitive and behavioral efforts to escape thoughts of the stressor, has been related significantly to maladjustment in many other studies of chronic stressful experiences. Evidence also indicates that attempts at avoidance are likely to be ineffective and indeed may be counterproductive, paradoxically increasing thought intrusion regarding the stressor. Additionally, some avoidant behaviors in themselves may be maladaptive (e.g., excessive drinking). Further, avoidant coping may involve limiting contacts with friends and family. For example, when baby showers or family gatherings involving children are painful, they may prompt nonattendance, resulting in deprivation of important sources of support. It should be noted that items to tap avoidance on coping scales in themselves may reflect manifestations of psychological dysfunction (e.g., the item "slept more than usual" may constitute a symptom of depression). Further, some studies have revealed gender differences in partners' coping processes, and their implications require further study.

In sum, to the extent that they have been tested, theories regarding cognitive appraisal and coping in chronic, stressful encounters have provided useful in understanding psychological adjustment to infertility. As Abbey and colleagues stated, "Psychosocial resources, such as personal control and social support, enhanced the perceived life quality of women and men, infertile and fertile, and couples with and without children." Thus, although infertility may present some unique challenges, it also holds substantial commonalities with other stressors. This implies that research and intervention with infertility can both contribute to and benefit from established stress and coping theory and research. Particularly in attempting to understand chronic stressors shared by intimate partners, infertility provides an excellent vehicle for study.

V. PSYCHOLOGICAL INTERVENTIONS FOR INFERTILE INDIVIDUALS

What implications do extant research and theory carry for psychological intervention for infertile individuals and couples? Clearly, mental health professionals should be aware of the evidence that those who face infertility in general are able to find benefit in their experience and to remain resilient with regard to global psychosocial functioning. As such, many who enter medical treatment may require no psychosocial service or only brief educational and supportive intervention. These may be of particular use as the couple is entering the diagnostic and treatment process or in advance of undergoing specific reproductive technologies and following treatment failure.

Mental health professionals also can expect substantial diversity in psychological response, and some individuals will experience extreme distress. Although many questions remain regarding risk factors for poor adjustment, those who view parenthood as an overriding life goal, who have low generalized expectancies for personal control and mastery of their environment, who are in unsupportive marriages and social contexts, who view infertility as a threat to many life realms and can cite no benefits in their experience, or who cope through self-blame and avoidance may be at risk for extreme distress. Accordingly, interventions designed to acknowledge and normalize the many stresses that couples may face as they negotiate the infertility process, to address the diverse personal meanings that infertility holds for individuals, to improve social support and intimate communication, to enhance perceptions of control for arenas in which control is possible, to provide alternative routes to central life aims tied to parenthood, and to decrease avoidant and self-blaming coping strategies may prove effective. However, we do not know the consequences of therapeutic attempts to alter long-used coping strategies, such as avoidance. It is important that such interventions be administered with care and monitored for effectiveness.

Because women are likely to experience more infertility-specific distress than their partners and because women are more likely to seek such psychosocial interventions as support groups, some services may be targeted productively toward women. However, because infertility is an intimately shared stressor and because adaptive communication and support are important contributors to adjustment, encouragement of couples' participation is warranted.

With regard to extant psychosocial services, a national network for information and support of infertile couples, RESOLVE, sponsors self-help support groups in many cities, and many specialized medical fertility practices offer psychological counseling. Very few controlled studies of psychosocial interventions directed toward enhancing adjustment to infertility have been reported. Other uncontrolled studies are promising in their demonstration of significant decreases in distress in infertile women after participation in group cognitive-behavioral treatment. This approach combines several elements such as relaxation training, stress management, cognitive restructuring, and social support. This has resulted in a reported 32% conception rate in participants 6 months after program completion; the potential reproductive advantage accruing from psychosocial intervention requires controlled study. Questions regarding who might benefit most from which sorts of psychosocial intervention offered at what points in the infertility process have yet to be examined.

VI. CONCLUSION

Certainly, psychosocial research in this area has progressed significantly from the time when women's personality deficits were blamed for causing infertility. We now know that many individuals and couples maintain psychosocial resilience in the face of infertility diagnosis. We also know that some infertile individuals are at risk for extreme distress and decrement in functioning. Some of the factors that confer risk for maladjustment have been identified, and stress and coping theories have proved fruitful in their suggestion of such factors.

We have far to go in continuing specification of risk and protective factors, however, particularly with regard to the consideration of the couple as a unit. Further, the majority of research in this area has been cross-sectional rather than longitudinal or experimental, and it has relied exclusively on questionnaire or interview data; conclusive research on risk and protective factors requires that we go beyond cross-sectional descriptive reports. In addition, samples studied have been predominantly White, relatively affluent individuals involved in specialized treatments. Generalization to couples with more diverse backgrounds, and particularly to those who have limited access to medical treatment, is necessary. Clearly, empirical demonstration of the most effective and efficient methods to influence preventable causes of infertility (e.g., sexually transmitted diseases) and to provide psychosocial aid to those facing infertility's challenges also is essential.

BIBLIOGRAPHY

Abbey, A., Andrews, F. M., & Halman, L. J. (1991). Gender's role in responses to infertility. *Psychology of Women Quarterly, 15,* 295–316.

Abbey, A., Andrews, F. M., & Halman, L. J. (1994). Psychosocial predictors of life quality: How are they affected by infertility, gender, and parenthood? *Journal of Family Issues, 15,* 253–271.

Berg, B. J., & Wilson, J. F. (1995). Patterns of psychological distress in infertile couples. *Journal of Psychosomatic Obstetrics and Gynecology, 16,* 65–78.

Domar, A. D., Zuttermeister, P. C., Seibel, M., & Benson, H. (1992). Psychological improvement in infertile women after behavioral treatment: A replication. *Fertility and Sterility, 58,* 144–147.

Lazarus, R. S., & Folkman, S. (1984). *Stress, appraisal, and coping.* New York: Springer.

Litt, M. D., Tennen, H., Affleck, G., & Klock, S. (1992). Coping and cognitive factors in adaptation to *in vitro* fertilization failure. *Journal of Behavioral Medicine, 15,* 171–187.

Mahlstedt, P. P., Macduff, S., & Bernstein, J. (1987). Emotional factors and the in vitro fertilization and embryo transfer process. *Journal of In Vitro Fertilization and Embryo Transfer, 6,* 242–256.

McQueeney, D. A., Stanton, A. L., & Sigmon, S. T. (1997). Efficacy of emotion-focused and problem-focused group therapies for women with fertility problems. *Journal of Behavioral Medicine, 21,* 313–330.

Mosher, W. D., & Pratt, W. F. (1990). Fecundity and infertility in the United States, 1967–1988. *Advance Data from Vital and Health Statistics,* no. 192. Hyattsville, MD: National Center for Health Statistics.

Rodin, J., & Collins, A. (Eds.). (1991). *Women and new reproductive technologies: Medical, psychosocial, legal, and ethical dilemmas.* Hillsdale, NJ: Erlbaum.

Seibel, M. (Ed.). (1990). *Infertility: A comprehensive text.* Norwalk, CT: Appleton-Lange.

Stanton, A. L., & Danoff-Burg, S. (1995). Selected issues in women's reproductive health: Psychological perspectives. In A. L. Stanton & S. J. Gallant (Eds.), *The psychology of women's health: Progress and challenges in research and application* (pp. 261–305). Washington, DC: American Psychological Association.

Stanton, A. L., & Dunkel-Schetter, C. (Eds.). (1991). *Infertility: Perspectives from stress and coping research.* New York: Plenum.

U.S. Congress, Office of Technology Assessment. (1988). *Infertility: Medical and social choices,* OTA-BA-358. Washington, DC: U.S. Government Printing Office.

Information Processing and Clinical Psychology

Patrick W. Corrigan and James A. Stephenson

University of Chicago

I. What Is Information Processing for a
   Clinical Psychologist?
II. Process Models of Human Development
III. Understanding Abnormal Behavior Cognitively
IV. Understanding Social Behavior Cognitively
V. Information Processing and Assessment
VI. Information Processing and Psychotherapy
VII. Information Processing and Rehabilitation

Abnormal Behavior Human cognitions and consequent behaviors are unable to assist the individual in coping with the demands of the environment.

Clinical Psychology The social science that seeks to evaluate, describe, assess, and treat maladaptive thoughts and behaviors.

Cognitive Development As the individual matures, cognitive functions improve commensurate with quantitative changes in corresponding biological structures.

Cognitive Rehabilitation The active treatment process in which patients who have suffered acute injuries or chronic disease regain necessary cognitive functions. Cognitive rehabilitation assumes that the central nervous system has a relative plasticity and that specific information processes can be remediated and compensated after being lost to disease or insult.

Cognitive Therapy Depressed individuals adopt negative beliefs about the self and world as a method for organizing and acting upon environmental stimuli.

Cognitive therapy seeks to alter these beliefs so that the individual can more effectively cope with environmental demands.

Information Processing A cognitive model in which macro aspects of sensory input are divided into discrete information bytes and the macro experience of human cognition is divided into composite functions which operate on the discrete bytes.

Serial Processing Information is processed in a stepwise fashion one byte at a time.

Social Cognition Social schemata act as templates through which social information is encoded and as blueprints that guide interpersonal responses. The most common social cognitive structures focus on situations, persons, and self.

INFORMATION PROCESSING models of human cognition have enabled clinical psychologists to better understand abnormal human behavior, and to better develop treatments for this behavior, by dividing the complex event of cognition into more readily discernible information bytes and processing functions. Specific abnormal behaviors may correspond with deficits in the information processing system which, in turn, may correspond with various deficits in the central nervous system. Interventions designed to compensate for, or circumvent, discrete losses of the information processing system aid clinical psychologists in developing more effective treatment plans for their patients.

I. WHAT IS INFORMATION PROCESSING FOR A CLINICAL PSYCHOLOGIST?

The manner in which humans perceive and comprehend their world has been shown to be one of the principle causes for how individuals act on it. Cognitive science assumes a central role in the psychologists' understanding of how individuals perceive and comprehend, and therefore, of how they behave. Clinical psychologists are particularly interested in the way in which human behavior has gone awry; i.e., how human cognitions and consequent behaviors no longer serve the individual well. Toward this end, clinical psychology is the social science broadly concerned with three endeavors.

1. Development and evaluation of descriptive and explanatory models of abnormal behavior. Frequently, these endeavors focus on derailed human development and limited social competence.
2. Development of assessment strategies that yield clinically useful descriptions of developmental and social problems.
3. Development of intervention strategies that ameliorate these problems.

Cognitive models in general, and information processing in particular, have been especially powerful paradigms for advancing these goals.

A. What Is Information Processing?

According to this model, the macro aspect of sensory input is divided into discrete information bytes (e.g., visual stimuli can be described in terms of color, contrast, depth, location, and relative size) and the macro experience of human cognition is divided into composite functions (like attention, memory, and response selection) that operate on these bytes and that interact in some meaningful order. Hence, the process of knowing can be understood by studying the various components of the information process individually and together. From a methodological standpoint, breaking down information and cognition into theoretical elements greatly enhances the study of these phenomena.

Information processing models are also appealing because of their apparent correspondence with central nervous system structures and functions. Research in neuropsychology has led to theories about associations between discrete information processes and structures in the central nervous system. For example, ongoing research has shown a significant association between functioning of the hippocampus and consolidation of information from short-term to long-term memory. Associations like these are especially exciting because an epistemological pathway has been identified between what have been parallel and independent sciences: psychology and biology.

We attempt to show in this article that understanding the endeavors of clinical psychology can be significantly enhanced by adopting an information processing framework. Information processing is not a unitary paradigm, however. Several models have been developed within this branch of cognitive science and are reviewed below.

B. Models of Information Processing

Early information processing theories were considered bottom-up, serial search models of cognition like the one illustrated in Figure 1. Information processing is serial in that it manipulates information in a stepwise fashion one byte at a time. The processing series comprises specific structures (e.g., short-term memory, long-term memory, response selection) and actions that operate on the information (e.g., encoding, consolidation, retrieval) as it moves along the series. These models are bottom-up in that processing is initiated by attention to incoming information rather than by a later stage in information processing.

As presented in Figure 1, the relative infinity of information in the subject's environment is significantly reduced by an attentional filter. Selected information then becomes the figural "snapshot" which is available in iconic memory for a very short time. Most of this information is lost as the icon decays. Remaining information is encoded vis-a-vis extant memory traces so that information has meaning beyond its stimulus qualities; e.g., that conglomeration of lines and curves, shades and hues is perceived to be the image of a human being.

The amount of information that can be held in short-term or working memory is relatively limited and decays quickly. Depending on the individual's previous experience with the incoming information, his or her mental set, and the environmental conditions, some information in short-term memory will be

Structures and actions

Products

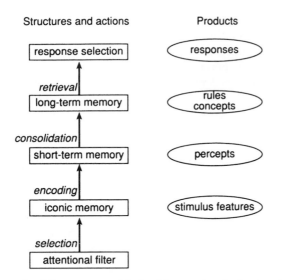

Figure I A bottom-up model of serial processing that begins with filtering the relative cacophony of stimuli impinging on the individual into a few bytes to be processed. Cognitive processes yield various products as the information bytes progress along the series.

consolidated into the long-term store. Information in long-term memory may eventually be retrieved. A response may then be elicited in reaction to external stimuli. The generated response may come from several motoric actions arranged hierarchically in the long-term store.

Different stages in the processing series imply different cognitive products (see Fig. 1). Exteroceptive and interoceptive stimuli are the raw data that impinge on the attentional filter. Selective attention results in the person attending to features of impinging stimuli. Comparing sets of stimulus features to previous information yields encoded percepts; "that mass of lines and curves is really my Aunt Lillian." Similarly, sets of percepts produce information categories or concepts. For example, Aunt Lillian, Brother Mike, Father, and Grandmother all make up the category of blood relatives. The relationship between concepts defines rules; "I am more intimate with my blood relatives than my friends."

The cognitive processes in bottom-up models, and their juxtaposition to neighboring processes, readily suggest their utility for clinical psychology. Structures, actions, and products may all serve as the foci of dysfunction. For example, according to Figure 1 cognitive deficits may result from: (1) an overly restrictive attentional filter that results in patients missing key

information, (2) inaccurate encoding of incoming information, (3) diminished consolidation to long-term memory, (4) overly inclusive concepts, (5) impoverished set of responses available for selection, and (6) random selection of responses from the response hierarchy. Deficits identified vis-a-vis an information processing model also suggest specific treatment strategies. For example, remediation of attentional deficits may include self-instructional strategies, repeated practice on attentional tasks, and differential reinforcement for attention to targeted stimuli.

Serial processing models, however, provide a cumbersome representation of cognition that does not correspond well with data about the manner in which information is actually processed. For example, given the time constraints of the functioning nervous system, perhaps only a hundred processing steps can be accomplished serially in the half second between perceiving and responding to an environmental stimulus. In actuality, however, this simple cognitive event probably requires hundreds or thousands of steps to complete. Parallel processing models suggest that several processes occur simultaneously during simple tasks.

In parallel distributed processing (PDP) models, cognitive events consist of multiple *interconnected units*; in the general case *all* units are interconnected, receive input from the environment, and send output to the environment. In the simplest models, connections between units are excitatory or inhibitory (on–off switches). In more restricted examples of the general case, some units may receive no input from nor give output to the environment and may be unconnected to other units. This model suggests that multiple processes occur simultaneously thereby surpassing the sluggish mechanism described by a serial processing model.

Transposition of PDP models to clinical psychology has thus far been limited. For example, it has only recently been used to describe the myriad of cognitive deficits found in schizophrenic patients. However, PDP models have an intimate history with neurobiology; investigators from that discipline have described neurological and cognitive events in terms of the network of units and connections. PDP models hold great promise for providing sophisticated neurocognitive formulations of abnormal behavior which may, in turn, lead to more sophisticated treatment prescriptions.

II. PROCESS MODELS OF HUMAN DEVELOPMENT

Clinical psychologists frequently explain adaptive and maladaptive behavior in terms of appropriate behavioral development, especially during childhood. Stage models have been popular for describing human development; individuals progress through significant life stages in which cognitive elements change qualitatively as corresponding biological processes activate. Contrast this view to information processing models of human development where biological structures underlying cognitive functions are believed to be present and functional from birth; development is better described as quantitative changes in these structures and their corresponding cognitive functions. As an example, a process model of memory development is reviewed.

A. The Ontogeny of Human Memory

Adult memory appears to progress through a complex course to maturity. Research has suggested that aspects of human memory are relatively intact from birth. For example, iconic memory operates at similar levels in both younger children and adults; research has shown that children's span of apprehension is quantitatively equal to that of most adults. The size of short-term memory store, however, is much smaller in young children. They recall far fewer items from a word list than older children. Similarly, the size of the long-term store is associated with age; people have more to remember as they add life experiences with age.

Retrieval strategies also differ with age. Older children and adults are more likely to retrieve information from long-term memory quickly. This pattern seems to be specific to recall memory, however. Rates of recognition are actually similar between adults and fairly young children. Strategies that facilitate the original consolidation of information into long-term memory is a significant factor for understanding recall. Research has shown that adults use mnemonic strategies like rehearsal, imagery, and chunking to assimilate information into the long-term store. Children under 5 years old have been shown to have these same strategies at their disposal but rarely use them spontaneously until older.

The process model also yields important descriptors about the elderly end of human development. Overall processing speed seems to diminish as adults pass 60. Therefore, retrieval of information diminishes in speed as people age. Moreover, short-term memory seems to diminish in many older adults, while long-term memory remains relatively intact.

B. The Utility of a Process Model of Native Development

A process model yields several benefits for the clinical psychologist attempting to understand human development. The structure, actions, and products subsumed by an information processing framework suggest specific foci which should change as the child develops. This correspondence is all the more powerful given the relationship between brain function and information processing construct. Future research in neuropsychology should be able to track changes in brain structures and physiology that correlate with the maturation of cognitive structures and actions.

In like fashion, a process model of development yields very specific expectations for guiding educational programs. Very young children lack the attention span and short-term memory to benefit from prolonged instruction. Therefore, class periods should be relatively shorter during the first few grades. Information processing models have also suggested that young children do not readily employ mnemonic strategies like imagery, chunking, and self-direction such that their ability to consolidate information into long-term memory is greatly hampered. Young children experience extreme limits to the breadth of information they can manage and learn as a result. Education during the primary years that includes an intensive focus on *how* to learn will help youngsters increase the amount to be learned.

Process models of development also lead to more specific recommendations for clinical intervention. Traditional cognitive assessment strategies are limited in their correspondence to effective interventions. Clinicians working with patients who are developmentally disabled as indexed by a low IQ score have few ideas about how to improve the person's cognitive functioning in the real world. However, individuals who are developmentally delayed in terms of memory retrieval dysfunction might improve by participating in treatment strategies that target mnemonic strategies. These issues are discussed more fully under Section VII. [*See* COGNITIVE DEVELOPMENT.]

III. UNDERSTANDING ABNORMAL BEHAVIOR COGNITIVELY

The Diagnostic and Statistical Manual of the American Psychiatric Association defines mental disorders as clinically abnormal behaviors that cause significant life distress and/or diminish independent adaptive functioning. Cognitive deficits are the major sequelae of many *DSM-IV* mental disorders. For example, schizophrenia has been characterized as a thought disorder and various organic brain syndromes have been described vis-a-vis discrete cognitive deficits. Information processing models have been especially fruitful for elucidating the component aspects of cognitive deficits in each of these psychiatric syndromes. The manner in which the information processing paradigm is useful for describing schizophrenia is described more fully as an example.

A. Schizophrenia Spectrum Disorders and Information Processing

Patients with schizophrenia show deficits in many information processes including selective and sustained attention, recall memory, retrieval, conceptual flexibility, and response selection. The abundance of cognitive deficits common to schizophrenia was a theoretical puzzle for clinical investigators such that early researchers sought to identify the *one* pathological dysfunction in the series of processing stages from which all other information processing deficits might result. Attentional deficits have been thought to be primary such that any subsequent processing dysfunctions result from skewed information entering the system. Conversely, the opposite end of the information process—response selection—has been thought to be the source of the pathognomonic deficit. During normal functioning, responses that surpass a hypothetical response threshold are most likely to be performed with response strength a function of previous experience and current arousal. Schizophrenic patients demonstrate collapsed response hierarchies such that, especially during hyperaroused situations, multiple

responses are above threshold and response selection is random.

More recently, the various cognitive deficits of schizophrenia have been explained within the framework of limited information processing capacity. Normal cognition is limited by the amount of information that can be processed simultaneously; for example, most individuals find it difficult to closely attend to a radio show, read the newspaper, and converse with a friend at the same time. The schizophrenic patient's cognitive capacity suffers even greater limits than normals such that their cognitive abilities are easily overwhelmed by demands of many everyday informational tasks. This model has been used to explain the diverse range of cognitive deficits in schizophrenia, including attention, memory, executive functioning, and response selection.

Alternative hypotheses have been offered to explain the schizophrenic patient's limited capacity. On the one hand, schizophrenic patients are thought to have insufficient capacity in steady "reserve," thereby unable to manage normal cognitive tasks.

Conversely, level of capacity is believed to be relatively equal between schizophrenic and normal groups, but less available from the patients. Capacity may be limited by the schizophrenic patient's arousal levels. The relationship between arousal and capacity is described by an inverted U such that during periods of underarousal or overarousal the normal individual experiences diminished capacity. Research suggests that schizophrenic patients demonstrate steady-state hyperarousal or both hypo- and hyperaroused patterns. [*See* SCHIZOPHRENIA.]

B. Traumatic Brain Injury and Information Processing

Traumatic brain injuries are by far the most prevalent form of brain damage for individuals younger than 40. Patients suffering from these injuries show a wide range of information processing deficits depending on the central nervous system locus of the injury. For example, individuals experiencing relatively discrete injuries to the frontal cortex are likely to demonstrate deficits in executive functioning. Therefore, information processing principles provide a neat outline for predicting the effects of specific brain injuries.

The specificity of traumatic insults on the brain depends in part on the type of injury. Closed head injuries tend to result in more global deficits attributed to the brain ricocheting around the skull after impact. Open head injury (perhaps caused by object penetration) tends to localize damage and cause a focal lesion. However, the correspondence between focal lesion and cognitive deficit is not always neat. Deficits in one information process may cascade into a general deficit because of the interrelatedness of the brain and its information processes.

IV. UNDERSTANDING SOCIAL BEHAVIOR COGNITIVELY

Just as long-term memory contains concepts and categories that define the world of objects, so too there exist knowledge structures that describe key interpersonal constructs. Social schemata are the templates by which social information is encoded as well as the blueprints that guide interpersonal responses. Research has focused on several distinct sets of schemata. Two are reviewed here: knowledge structures that represent situations and persons.

A. Situational Schemata

Several features have been identified that comprise schematic descriptions of situations including actions (the component behaviors that comprise an interpersonal event), rules (the expectations that govern behaviors in these situations), affect (emotions that coincide with these actions and rules), and goals (motivations underlying attempted actions). These features are related hierarchically such that definition of certain features restricts the range of subordinates. For example, goals defined by a specific situation narrow the set of rules that define the interaction. The goals implied by driving into a hamburger joint—to get sandwiches fast—preclude rules about social banter between waitress and customer that might be found at a coffee shop.

B. Person Schemata

Personality theorists presume that individuals have enduring traits that explain current functioning as well as predict future behavior across multiple situations. However, personality traits may represent epiphenomena that result from the prototypic manner in which individuals perceive others. Whether or not an individual acts consistently across situations, they are perceived to do so because their actions are understood in terms of various person schema. For example, an extroverted person schema defines individual exemplars as outgoing, chatty, and personable.

Cantor and Mischel have identified several characteristics of person schema including differentiation and concreteness. Differentiation refers to the amount of attributional overlap between two person schemata. A "pleasant person" and an "extrovert" share many attributes and therefore have low differentiation. Prototypic opposites like introverts and extroverts have little overlap and high differentiation. Person schema also vary in terms of quality of content or concreteness. Attributes have been divided into four groups: physical appearance or possessions, socioeconomic status, traits (e.g., happy or gloomy), and behavioral attributes (e.g., runs to the train, sloppy).

C. The Value of Social Cognitive Models

Models of social cognition are in many ways more ecologically valid representations of thinking than the more laboratory-based perspectives of information processing discussed above. Rather than describing remote processes like attention and iconic memory, schema theorists describe the manner in which real-world information is understood and stored. Findings from schema theory also provide fruitful heuristics for understanding psychopathology. Qualitative differences between specific schema may account for differential deficits in various neuropsychiatric populations. For example, research suggests that content of situational and person schemata affects the information processing of patients. Depressed populations have been shown to be more sensitive to the negative versus the positive content of schema. Patients with schizophrenia are better able to identify negative facial affect (e.g., angry, depressed, or worried) than more pleasant facial expressions.

In terms of treatment strategies, if the effects of interventions from information processing models generalize, then targeting discrete processing functions like attention, memory, and conceptual flexibility should lead to enhanced functioning in all knowledge domains. However, if rehabilitation strategies based on processing models do not effectively generalize (as the outcome literature suggests), then clinical investigators will need to develop more discrete training strategies specific to social cognitive constructs: e.g., differentially train patients to attend to and encode the features of a situation or the characteristics of a personality. Making social cognition the foundation of rehabilitation and therapy opens entirely new directions in treatment strategy.

V. INFORMATION PROCESSING AND ASSESSMENT

Standardized assessment of symptoms, disabilities, and dysfunctions is perhaps the *sine qua non* of the clinical psychologist's profession. In particular, clinical psychologists have developed exquisite strategies for measuring various behavioral, cognitive, and personologic constructs. The high standards required for good psychological assessment assure that tests are administered, scored, and interpreted in similar fashion to all patients. Moreover, good psychometric qualities diminish the confounds that patient and examiner variables may unknowingly wreak on test performance.

Assessment of cognitive abilities has traditionally been dominated by measurement of intelligence. Unfortunately, the intelligence quotient (IQ) is, at best, a generalized and static measure of cognitive functioning with little indication of specific deficits that might account for poor intelligence. Moreover, measurement of IQ yields few useful recommendations regarding strategies for remediating cognitive deficits. The structures and processes of an information processing model yield a broader range of measurement strategies for assessing cognitive deficits. Neuropsychologists, in particular, have been ingenious in developing assessment strategies that putatively represent specific cognitive deficits. These measurements usually take the form of performance tasks in which patients must, for example, recall a series of words from a test list read by the examiner, or recognize test words from the recitation of a paragraph. Performance on these tasks may, in turn, suggest various rehabilitation or therapeutic interventions that remediate the deficit. [*See* INTELLIGENCE AND MENTAL HEALTH.]

Despite the benefits that process-specific measures bring to the assessment enterprise, these strategies have their own set of caveats. Given the serial nature of cognitive structures, no single measure yields a unique description of a corresponding information process. For example, below average scores on the word list not only suggest deficits in verbal recollection, but also poor functioning in sustained attention, verbal encoding, and ability to maintain set. To counter this dilemma, neuropsychologists typically administer a battery of tests and look for dissociations among results to identify deficient information processes. Poor performance on a word list may be attributed to recall memory if the patient performs adequately on other measures in the battery that assess attention, encoding, and maintenance of set.

Like IQ measures, information processing tasks for the most part represent state descriptions of performance: How competent is a patient on a specific information process at the moment of testing? Summaries of cognitive deficits need to be mindful of the dynamic character of processing deficits and account for variables that describe the course of specific information processes. For example, cognitive deficits in schizophrenia are frequently exacerbated by psychotic symptoms. Therefore, description of symptom effects is a necessary component in preparing a treatment plan for these patients.

VI. INFORMATION PROCESSING AND PSYCHOTHERAPY

Psychotherapy is clearly a multifaceted and complex task in which countless patient, therapist, and intervention variables must be accounted for and affected to yield positive outcomes. Cognitive theories have been used to better conceptualize the therapeutic enterprise and improve the efficacy of interventions in the process. In particular, cognitive therapies have been found to be especially effective in the treatment of severe depression.

A. Aaron Beck's Model of Cognitive Therapy

Negative cognitions play a major role in the development and maintenance of depressive symptoms. In particular, individuals who are vulnerable to bouts of depression tend to interpret incoming (and often neutral) information based on their negative self-appraisals; these interpretations tend to be variations of themes about feeling helpless, hopeless, and worthless. In addition, depressed individuals are likely to attribute positive outcomes to external sources and negative outcomes to themselves. [*See* DEPRESSION.]

Distorted cognitions show marked lapses in logical representations of the environment. In general, patients tend to use the information against the self when such reality distortions occur. Some common examples of illogical representations are: arbitrary inference, the drawing of a conclusion from a situation when there is no evidence to support it; selective abstraction, focusing on details taken out of context; and overgeneralization, drawing conclusions about one's ability based on a single incident. Because distorted cognitions are automatic, out of awareness, and highly illogical, the patient has difficulty developing effective strategies for coping. Information processing approaches to the treatment of depression are designed to empower the patient with the knowledge and tools necessary to combat the various elements of distorted cognitions.

The therapeutic intervention developed by Aaron Beck teaches patients a form of hypothesis testing which allows them to challenge negative and distorted schemata. First, the therapist assists patients to identify the distorted cognitions and their corresponding effects on emotion. Once the distorted cognitions are identified, the patient subjects his or her beliefs to objective evaluation. It is important to educate the patient to the characteristics of distorted cognitions to facilitate the process of objective evaluation of beliefs. For example, distorted cognitions are automatic and involuntary suggesting that they are not based on logic or truth.

Once patients gain the capacity to question the legitimacy of their cognitions, they learn strategies to logically analyze distorted beliefs. Patients are encouraged to "check" their assumptions about a particular situation against "reality" by surveying others regarding the belief. Cognitions deemed to be invalid or inappropriate are neutralized by stating the reason for inaccuracy and by countering the distortion with a more appropriate belief. [*See* COGNITIVE THERAPY.]

VII. INFORMATION PROCESSING AND REHABILITATION

Rehabilitation defines an active treatment process in which patients who have suffered acute injuries (like a traumatic brain injury due to a car crash) or chronic diseases (like schizophrenia) regain necessary behaviors and cognitive abilities to live independently. Cognitive rehabilitation assumes that the central nervous system has a relative plasticity because specific information processes, and their corresponding central nervous system correlates, can be regained after lost to disease or insult.

A. Natural Recovery of Cognitive Processes

The manner in which rehabilitation strategies ameliorate patients' problems requires understanding of the natural process of recovery of brain function. For example, research has shown that destruction of certain areas of the brain does not result in total loss of the corresponding cognitive function. According to the theory of equipotentiality, other areas of the central nervous system might assume a function lost to a specific lesion. This phenomenon has been shown in language skills where some verbal processing abilities are assumed by the right hemisphere after significant damage to the left hemisphere. An alternate theory to equipotentiality is diaschisis; areas of the brain experience temporary shock, or diaschisis, when they are suddenly deprived of normal stimulation from neighboring, severely damaged regions. Frequently, undamaged tissue receives sufficient stimulation from other undamaged regions such that absent function returns.

Traditionally, it was thought that damaged neurons were irreplaceable. However, research has shown that certain neuronal tracts in the brain may regenerate in a manner similar to patterns of growth that have been demonstrated in the peripheral nervous system, though this regrowth may result in a muted return of cognitive functioning. Some neuronal tracts that lose stimulation from neighboring damaged areas become hypersensitive to the action potential of remaining axons. This hypersensitivity may diminish loss of function related to the damaged area. Interestingly, research has suggested that recovery functions related to denervation hypersensitivity may interact with other restorative processes. For example, research suggests that collateral sprouting may reduce the effects of denervation.

B. Models of Cognitive Rehabilitation

Various models of cognitive rehabilitation have been developed which guide clinical psychologists in developing comprehensive intervention programs specific to the patient's cognitive profile. An integrative model frames behavioral rehabilitation vis-a-vis a combination of relatively disparate professional perspectives: the neurologist's definition of the insult in terms of neuroanatomical foci and physiological sequelae, the neuropsychologist's test description of information processing deficits associated with the injury, and the behaviorist's treatment plans targeting the profile of behavioral problems. This view developed out of a professional consensus regarding the need for blending what had previously been the independent domains of each profession.

Contrast this model to a process model which views deficits as diminutions in specific information processes: e.g., a patient has poor memory because of diminished recall and recognition skills. The model, as presented here for cognitive rehabilitation, includes component processes that address three essential questions:

1. Acquisition. Why have fundamental information processes not developed appropriately? The answer to this question varies depending on the psychopathological category. Developmental disorders like mental retardation and autism imply that certain cognitive capacities are missing at birth or during early developmental periods. Similarly, information processing deficits of most psychiatric disorders may be predetermined as subtle vulnerability, albeit in dormant fashion, since infancy. Conversely, cognitive deficits in organically based patients represent recent loss rather than lack of acquisition. Implicit in the question about acquisition is the belief that some cognitive skills might be acquired that can replace or augment cognitive deficiencies. Of course, there are biological and behavioral limits to learning certain cognitive skills.

2. Performance. Why are certain cognitive skills that apparently exist in a patient's repertoire not regularly utilized? Could it be that incentive affects the patient's cognition? Patients who are not motivated to recall an event will not remember that situation. Lashley illustrated this point in a poignant example. He bet a patient, who in 900 trials had failed to learn the alphabet, 100 cigarettes that he could not learn the letters. Ten trials later the patient recalled them perfectly. Findings like these suggest that reinforcement strategies are necessary adjuncts to rehabilitation programs.

3. Generalization. Why does improved performance in one treatment milieu not generalize to other situations? All too often little change is observed at home in a patient even though significant improvement is noted in the treatment setting; successful changes accomplished in the treatment setting have not generalized to other environments. Clinicians must include strategies like homework and in vivo practice that help patients transfer newly (re)acquired cognitive skills into their world. The process model is useful for rehabilitation of cognitive deficits because treatment strategies are clearly wedded to the specific, deficient process in question: i.e., to the phenomena that brought about the behavioral excess and deficit, and to the phenomena that maintain these disabilities.

C. Cognitive Rehabilitation and Clinical Practice

Early proponents of cognitive rehabilitation were enamored with the potentials of computer hardware. In the prototypical rehabilitation program, patients were presented test stimuli repeatedly until they demonstrated the appropriate response (Fig. 2). Computers were especially attractive because precise adjustments of test stimuli could be controlled over thousands of iterations. The benefits of computers were frequently augmented by reinforcement strategies, in which patients might receive monetary rewards for correct responses, and by self-instruction, in which patients were taught to speak aloud the goal of the cognitive tasks (e.g., "I am supposed to key press to even numbers only").

Several investigations showed that patients who

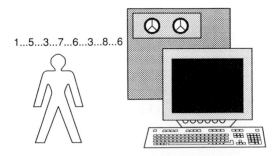

Press the key each time you see the number 3.

Figure 2 A computer-based rehabilitation program in which brain-damaged subjects learn to attend to a series of single-digit numbers. The subject receives a nickel reward for each correct identification.

completed rigorous computer-based cognitive training experienced significant improvements on the variables of interest. Rarely, however, has responding to computer-generated stimuli been shown to generalize to real-world information processing. Clinical investigators have raised questions like what does attending to matrices of test letters have to do with comprehending a request from a cab driver?

Investigators have grappled with the ecological validity of cognitive rehabilitation strategies in several ways. Social cognitive models have been used to develop rehabilitation strategies. For example, several studies have shown that the psychiatric patients' ability to learn from social skills training modules (a psychosocial rehabilitation technique in which severely mentally ill patients are taught specific interpersonal and coping skills) is highly associated with level of memory functioning. Therefore, memory enhancement strategies have been incorporated into the social skills training regimen and patients now show a much higher rate of acquiring interpersonal skills.

Alternately, experts in rehabilitation have recommended that environmentally based interventions may provide a useful means for circumventing cognitive deficits in the real world. For example, a straightforward command, "Speak slower," made to family and friends of a severely mentally ill adult will enhance this person's information processing capabilities sig-

nificantly. Similarly, strategically prepared signs that cue a brain-injured adult when to take his medicine or when she should cook her dinner provide a robust adjunct to short-term memory. Simple environmental changes like these may provide the best prostheses for rehabilitation of information processing deficits.

This article has been reprinted from the *Encyclopedia of Human Behavior, Volume 2.*

BIBLIOGRAPHY

Abramson, L. Y. (1988). "Social Cognition and Clinical Psychology." Guilford, New York.

Barlow, D. (1988). "Anxiety and Its Disorders." Guilford, New York.

Beck, A. T. (1976). "Cognitive Therapy and the Emotional Disorders." International Universities Press, New York.

Corrigan, P. W., & Yudofsky, S. C. (Eds.) (in press). "Cognitive Rehabilitation and Neuropsychiatric Disorders." American Psychiatric Press, Inc., Washington, DC.

Galambos, J. A., Abelson, R. P., & Black, J. B. (1986). "Knowledge Structures." Erlbaum, Hillsdale, NJ.

Ingram, R. E. (Ed.) (1986). "Information Processing Approaches to Clinical Psychology." Academic Press, New York.

Morris, R. G. M. (1989). "Parallel Distributed Processing: implications for Psychology and Neurobiology." Clarendon Press, Oxford.

Wedding, D., Horton, A. M., & Webster, J. (Eds.) (1986). "The Neuropsychology Handbook: Behavioral and Clinical Perspective." Springer, New York.

Intelligence and Mental Health

Moshe Zeidner
Haifa University, Mt. Carmel, Israel

Gerald Matthews
University of Dundee, Scotland

Donald H. Saklofske
University of Saskatchewan, Canada

Anxiety Feelings of apprehension and worry, accompanied by autonomic arousal, when individuals perceive they are under threat.

Attentional Resources A general-purpose reservoir of "energy" for processing, which may be flexibly allocated to specific processing routines.

Depression An affective disorder characterized by strong negative emotions, impairment of everyday social functioning, and negative beliefs such as hopelessness and lack of self-worth.

Personality Disorders Enduring pattern of inner experience and behavior that deviates markedly from the expectations of the individual's culture, is pervasive and inflexible, has an onset in adolescence or in early adulthood, is stable over time, and leads to distress or impairment.

Over the years, behavioral scientists have explored various avenues, linking human **INTELLIGENCE** to both personality factors and human adjustment. Researchers have attempted to unravel the theoretical and practical interface between human adjustment and mental health, on the one hand, and intelligence, on the other, hoping to shed light on how these two key constructs affect one another (and other variables) in the course of human development and in day-to-day functioning. Here, we examine the nexus of conceptual and empirical relationships between intelligence and mental health. Two senses of the term *intelligence* are important in this context. The first is the general factor of cognitive ability, *g*, identified by psychometric techniques, such as factor analysis, and measured by standard tests. The second aspect of intelligence is "practical intelligence": the person's ability to use cognitive skills adaptively in real-world contexts. Intelligence tests predict a variety of real-world criteria, such as occupational performance measures, so there is considerable overlap between the two aspects of intelligence, although the relationship between psychometric and "social" intelligence remains controversial. However, a person may sometimes have difficulty in applying his or her abilities within specific contexts, or, conversely, he or she may compensate for lack of ability through other means, such as context-specific learning. A general framework for relating intelligence to mental health is provided by cognitive models of well-being and maladjustment. Broadly, well-being tends to reflect people's cognitions about themselves and the social and physical worlds they inhabit. For example, depressed individuals tend to have low self-esteem, to retrieve predominantly negative memories of past events, and to commit errors in reasoning that exaggerate the negative side of life. Within this cognitive framework, there is scope for reciprocal relationships between intelligence and mental health. On the one hand, cognitions of the self may influence the development of intelligence and the behavioral expression of intelligence. Does a positive outlook on life foster the acquisition of the general-purpose cognitive skills central to psychometric intelligence and their application to real-life problems? On the other hand, intelligence may influence cognitions. Does knowledge of one's own ability and real-life competences encourage more positive attitudes? To address these questions, we examine some of the specific variables that frequently serve as markers of adjustment and mental health. We begin by examining variables that attempt to operationalize various self-beliefs directly: self-efficacy, perceived control, and self-concept. Intelligence may relate not just to beliefs, but also to the person's strivings for success and to the active attempts the person makes to deal with problems and obstacles.

I. INTELLIGENCE, PERSONALITY, AND ADJUSTMENT

It is commonly held that healthy human functioning is characterized, among other things, by a sense of self-efficacy and perceived control over the environment, positive self-regard, motivation to succeed in achieving salient personal goals, and adequate coping resources and strategies. In the following sections we review evidence bearing on the relationship between intelligence and selected markers of positive mental health and functioning. The variables we examine are in part personality factors in that they are associated with stable individual differences and in part reflect situational factors. For example, individuals differ in their general level of optimism, but any given individual will experience varying degrees of optimism or pessimism as they encounter differing situations.

A. Intelligence and Self-Agency

According to current social-cognitive theory, human action is governed not so much by the objective properties of the environment but rather by the perceived level of personal efficacy to effect changes by productive use of capabilities and sustained effort. Among the mechanisms of personal action control, or self-agency, none may be more central or pervasive than people's sense of self-efficacy. The term self-efficacy refers to the belief that one is able to master challenging demands by means of adaptive action. Self-efficacy can be conceptualized as a "can-do" cognition, which mirrors a sense of control over the environment, or as an optimistic view of one's capability to deal with stress and anxiety.

Both self-efficacy and positive outcome expectancies have been conceptualized as key precursors of mental health and low anxiety. Whereas efficacy expectancy is the conviction that one can execute behavior required to produce an outcome, outcome expectancy refers to a person's estimate that a given behavior will lead to certain outcomes. As the level of self-efficacy decreases, anxious arousal is expected to increase. Changes in anxiety level indicate there are changes in the way the person is appraising his or her relationship with the environment. Accordingly, as efficacy expectancies decrease and resources are judged to be less adequate for satisfying task demands, the relationship is appraised as holding the potential for less control and therefore it is perceived to be more threatening. Conversely, high efficacy is expected to reduce anticipatory distress, enhance coping with threat, and elevate performance when the person is confronted by a stressful task such as a major exam. Accordingly, it is only when persons cannot predict or exercise control over demanding situations that they have reason to fear them.

Thus, people with a firm belief in their self-efficacy figure out ways of exercising some measure of control in environments containing limited opportunities, whereas those who believe themselves to be inefficacious are unlikely to effect major changes even in environments that provide many potential opportunities. When setbacks occur, self-efficacious individuals recover more quickly and maintain a commitment to their goals. Personal goal setting is influenced, among other things, by self-appraisal of capabilities, including intelligence. The stronger the perceived self-efficacy, the higher the goal challenges people set for themselves and the firmer is their commitment to them.

Research from a social-cognitive perspective points to a meaningful relationship between self-efficacy and academic attainment and ability. Students who regard intellectual ability as a skill that can be acquired by gaining knowledge and competencies tend to adopt functional learning goals. These students seek challenges that provide opportunities to expand their knowledge and competencies. They regard errors as a natural part of the acquisition process, rather than as a source of distress. Thus, students who view ability as reflecting an acquirable skill foster a resilient sense of self-efficacy. Furthermore, healthy human functioning also appears to be affected by the beliefs people hold about how ability changes over time. Those who regard ability as a skill to be developed and practiced achieve higher attainments compared with those who regard intelligence or ability as a biological capacity that shrinks with age.

B. Perceived Control and Causal Attributions

Situational control appraisal is the extent to which the person believes he or she can shape or influence particular person–environment relationships. Perceived threat in a given situation may be conceptualized as a relational property between perceptions of the dangerous or threatening aspects of the environment, on the one hand, and perceived coping capabilities on the other. Thus, people who believe they can exercise control over immediate or potential threats do not engage in anxious and apprehensive thinking about these threats and are not perturbed by them. Situational appraisals of control are products of individual evaluations both of the demands of the situation and of personal ability to implement coping strategies. Those who believe they cannot manage threat experience high levels of anxiety arousal. These individuals dwell on their coping deficiencies and view many aspects of the environment as fraught with danger. They rehearse ways in which they may cope with feared situations, but uncertainty concerning coping capabilities fuels further anxiety. Behaviorally, perceptions of lack of control may lead to avoidance of threatening situations, which prevents the person from learning skills to deal with those very situations. Social phobics may be generally intelligent, but they lack the practical intelligence needed to handle social encounters because of their avoidance coping.

Perceived control may reflect, in part, people's need to seek a sense of control over their environment, often referred to as a motivation for "effectance." To achieve this environmental control, individuals spend considerable time and effort assessing environmental contingencies and contextual changes as well as analyzing their own powers to cope and excel in relevant contexts. Attribution theory posits that an essential motivation is to gain a measure of predictability and control over events, with emphasis on gaining an accurate appraisal of one's own personal characteristics.

Locus of causality is an attributional dimension of-

ten claimed to be related to cognitive ability, which refers to beliefs about the origins of behavior and the assignment of credit and blame for the results of one's behavior. Individuals with an internal locus of causality assume that their own behaviors and actions are responsible for the consequences that happen to them, whereas externally controlled people believe that the locus of causality is out of their hands and subject to the whims of fate. Internal locus of causality, especially for positive events, has commonly been associated with positive mental health and more adaptive functioning. Conversely, those who feel at the mercy of their environment and who feel they have little control over what happens to them may have low adaptive capacity.

Intelligence may affect the appraisal process by allowing more complex reasoning and consideration of alternatives and choices among options, thus affording greater control during both primary and secondary appraisal. People who believe they can control their own lives will put forth the effort to gain competencies and skills, thus enhancing their acquired or "crystallized" intelligence and abilities. Consistent with these hypotheses, intelligence has been reported to be moderately and inversely correlated with external locus of causality in junior and high school students. Also, some studies have specifically related deficits in mean IQ shown by black examinees to the phenomena of low controllability (learned helplessness), in which the motivation to cope with environmental contingencies is drastically diminished by preliminary exposure to uncontrollable aversive stimuli. Thus, people who have been successful at using their abilities come to believe that their abilities can control their destiny, so that locus of causality may shape the development of intelligence. However, it is not known for sure what the causal direction is: Do attributions affect cognitive test performance or do less intelligent people tend to rely more on luck and accidental or external factors than on their own abilities?

C. Self-Concept

People's self-image (how people come to see themselves) and their self-esteem (to what degree they feel positive about themselves) are crucial in determining their perceptions of the world, their goals and attitudes, the behaviors they initiate, the responses they make to others, and, generally, how they develop their potential for healthy functioning. Both theory and past research support the view that a positive self-concept and high self-esteem are related to higher academic ability and attainment, whereas negative beliefs about the self are associated with lower ability, scholastic underachievement, and failure. Individuals who have a poor self-image are likely to underestimate their own abilities, anticipate failure, and may well stop trying when difficulties arise.

The major determinant of the self-concept is generally thought to lie in the early and enduring patterns of parent–child relations that underpin the emotional security of the growing child. The child's self-concept is formed by interactions with significant others, with the child coming to see himself or herself as others do. Positive self-esteem is enhanced by positive parental regard for the child, respectful treatment of the child, and the definition of clear boundaries and realistic expectations for the child's achievement.

The causal dynamics underlying the modest correlations often reported between intelligence and self-concept are necessarily ambiguous. One commonly held view is that the causality flows from intelligence to self-esteem, with a positive self-concept and adjustment only reflecting past achievement and intellectual ability. Thus, the correlation of intelligence and self-concept may reflect little more than a person's subjective appraisals of his or her own social or educational standing and scholastic aptitudes. A second view is that a favorable self-image may lead to positive expectations of future success, which, in turn, produce increased effort and motivation to succeed and subsequent favorable outcomes on measures of both ability and achievement. Furthermore, measures of adjustment, such as self-concept, may tap values and attributes that facilitate achievement, and thus mediate the relation between ability and achievement. A plausible view is that there is a bidirectional relationship between the two constructs. Unfortunately, the available empirical evidence directly bearing on the relationship between self-esteem and ability is scant and often contradictory. [See SELF-ESTEEM.]

D. Motivation to Achieve

We have already seen, in the context of causal attribution theory, that cognitions and motivations may be intimately related. In this section, we put motivation center stage to consider how a person's motivations to strive for success relate to intelligence. Achievement motivation designates a general striving to perform one's best when the following two conditions hold: (a) the quality of one's performance is judged in terms of success or failure, (b) a relevant standard of excellence applies. According to achievement motivation theory, all individuals have both a basic motive to approach an achievement-related goal and an antagonistic motive to avoid failure, but the strengths of these motives vary from person to person, and from situation to situation.

Parental expectations and standards of performance are believed to underlie the development of two key motivational tendencies in children—to obtain praise and achieve success, on the one hand, and to avoid criticism and failure on the other. As children grow older, parental evaluations often become more demanding and critical and children become more sensitive to parental expectations. Thus, children strive harder to obtain parental praise and to achieve success, but also make an all-out effort to avoid criticism and failure. Low-anxious children tend to show a stronger motive to obtain praise than to avoid criticism, whereas anxious children show the opposite tendency. Because criticism frequently accompanies failure and praise typically follows success, motives to obtain praise and avoid criticism, respectively lead to motives to approach success and to avoid failure (which is often identified with test anxiety). Low-anxious children show persistence at working on cognitive tasks, a higher level of performance at complex tasks, and a distinct preference for tasks of intermediate difficulty. By contrast, in anxious children, the motive to avoid failure becomes more salient and compelling than the motive to achieve success. In fact, both motives, that is, fear of failure and the need to succeed, are stronger in high-anxious compared with low-anxious children. Accordingly, high-anxious children would be expected to persist longer under continued success as well as to leave sooner under continued failure compared with less anxious children. As anxious children progress through the educational system, they become even more strongly motivated to avoid failure than to achieve success. Less anxious children tend to orient to their own internal evaluations of their performance and to respond to the informational component of an adult's reactions rather than to social cues or contexts in which the reactions are made. By contrast, anxious children tend to avoid situations in which the likelihood of criticism is high.

The tendency to seek success and approach an achievement-related goal is postulated to be a product of three factors: (a) a relatively stable personality disposition to strive for success (need for achievement), (b) the (subjective) probability that one will be successful, and (c) the incentive value of success. If one of these values equals zero or near zero (e.g., the person feels his or her chances of success in a particular endeavor are nil or there is little point in doing well), the resultant multiplicative value will also be zero and no effort will be put forth by the individual to attain the goal. Similarly, the opposing force, the tendency to avoid failure, is posited to be multiplicatively determined by three factors: (a) the motive to avoid failure, (b) the probability of failure, and (c) the incentive value or negative affect (shame) associated with failure. Accordingly, achievement striving is postulated to be the result of an approach–avoidance conflict between the two opposing tendencies, with the stronger of the two tendencies being expressed in action.

Achievement motivation may influence intellectual development and performance in several ways. First, achievement motivation may determine the level of interest, striving, and effort that persons invest in the development of their intellectual skills throughout their life experiences prior to a test. Because a school environment emphasizes competitive intellectual strivings, students with strong competitive needs would be highly motivated to acquire intellectual skills to compete successfully with peers. Second, achievement motivation may help shape the level of attention, effort, concentration, and persistence applied in the actual evaluative or test situation. On the other hand, the hypothesized association of achievement motivation with intelligence may be the result of the adaptation of a person's motives to intelligence. Thus, a person high in quantitative ability is likely to develop a motive to achieve in math. Furthermore, highly intelligent students develop a strong motivation to acquire or develop various intellectual skills tapped by IQ tests and to perform well in a testing situation.

Motivation theory predicts that only persons of average intelligence should be strongly motivated either to achieve or to avoid failure, depending on the relative strengths of their motivations for success or motivation to avoid failure. The very bright or very challenged students would not be expected to have achievement-related dispositions aroused because the conventional competitive learning situation will be, respectively, either too easy or too difficult for them. Very bright students are expected to perform well in school and dull students poorly, regardless of motivation. Hence, performance differences as a function of motivation are relatively confined to groups intermediate in ability. Some reviews have reported modest positive relations between need for achievement and intelligence, but others conclude the correlation is not statistically reliable. Achievement motivation research may underestimate the context dependence of motivation. Successful entrepreneurs who left school with few qualifications may be highly motivated to succeed—but not at schoolwork. Achievement striving predicts a variety of indices of occupational performance.

E. Intelligence and Coping with Psychological Stress

Stress arises when the perceived demands of the environment tax or exceed the individual's perceived capacity to cope with these demands. Thus, perceptions of high intellectual capacity should reduce susceptibility to stress, provided that the person has the outcome expectancy that intelligent behavior will lead to more effective coping. Intelligence may be seen as a resource that facilitates personal growth and adjustment, as well as one that possibly buffers the effects of environmental stress on stress reactions. Thus, intelligence may affect each of the phases of the stress process. Given the view that intelligence is a global form of adaptation to the environment, intelligent people might also be expected to be better adjusted, both socially and emotionally, than their less intelligent counterparts.

Current cognitive-motivational-relational perspectives on emotion posit that if a person appraises his or her relationship to the environment in a particular way, then a specific emotion, which is tied to the appraisal pattern, always follows. It is conceivable that intelligence leads to more positive appraisals through more accurate diagnosis of causes of stress and through the ability to examine the situation from different viewpoints. For example, a more intelligent person subjected to inconsiderate treatment might be better able to consider alternative explanations for the event, such as the offending party was suffering from a personal tragedy. Furthermore, intelligence may enter into the actual process of coping, affecting both the choice and implementation of particular coping strategies in a stressful situation. The more intelligent person may have better problem-solving skills to use in deciding how to change themselves or their environment. Although problem- and emotion-focused strategies will likely be used by people of both high and low intelligence, those lower in intelligence may use emotion-focused coping more frequently because they will assess more situations as being the type they can do very little about.

However, intelligence is not necessarily beneficial in stressful situations. If the person is predisposed to worry about and ruminate on his or her problems, the more intelligent person may think of negative consequences of a difficult situation that would not occur to a less intelligent person. Awareness of a wide range of negative possibilities may contribute to a sense of being overwhelmed by the problem at hand, and so hinder coping. In other words, the relationship between intelligence and coping may be moderated by personality. The impact of intelligence may also depend on the extent to which the problem faced is amenable to reasoning and problem solving.

There is some empirical evidence that changes in intelligence from early adolescence to middle adulthood correlate positively with increased use of coping mechanisms, but correlate negatively with defense mechanisms. It is not clear from this research which particular experiences enhance and accelerate an individual's intellectual growth and freedom to cope with stress and which promote the development of defenses that close off the individual from experience and intellectual growth. Overall, there is little hard empirical evidence to back up the claims about the role of intelligence at various stages in the stress and coping process. Furthermore, although research in the stress domain has given lip service to the importance of intelligence as a coping resource, empirical research in this area has failed to assess directly and systematically the role of intelligence as a predictor of stress reactions or adaptational outcomes. [See COPING WITH STRESS; STRESS.]

II. NEGATIVE AFFECT AND INTELLECTUAL IMPAIRMENT

It is widely accepted that disturbances of affect or emotion tend to be associated with cognitive impair-

ment. Loss of intellectual function has been studied in both clinical patients suffering from mood or anxiety disorders and nonclinical samples whose levels of negative emotion are naturally or artificially elevated. In the sections which follow, several key issues arising from this research literature are discussed. Before proceeding, a number of caveats are in order. First, the observation that a negative emotion is correlated with intelligence test performance in some particular context is not in itself very informative. It is important to determine whether the emotional factor relates to specific intellectual functions and whether the relationship between emotion and intellectual functioning is invariant across different contexts, including real-world contexts such as the workplace and the classroom. Second, correlation does not imply causality. It seems plausible that emotional disorder should have a direct causal effect on intellectual functioning, but this hypothesis cannot be taken for granted. Negative emotions might arise from the person's appraisals of intellectual incapacity, or emotional disorder and mental illness might impact affect and intellect independently. Third, to the extent that emotion generates impairment, there are a variety of possible cognitive psychological underpinnings for the effect, which may vary in different emotional conditions.

Emotions are often categorized in terms of dimensions of negative affect and positive affect. From this perspective, there is considerable overlap between anxiety and depression. Both conditions are associated with negative affect, but depression is also associated with low positive affect. However, a more fine-grained approach is desirable for analyses of mood and cognitive function. Specifically, there are distinct bodies of work associated with (1) anxiety and tension, (2) depression and unhappiness, (3) anger, and (4) fatigue and lack of energy.

A. Anxiety

Anxiety is a signal that the individual is under threat. The threat evokes a fight or flight reaction, including such somatic reactions as increased heart rate, sweating, stomach aches, shaking, and trembling. Anxiety is perhaps the most intensively studied variable in personality research, and more reliable data seem to be available about its relationship to intelligence than for any other personality construct. Anxiety has received particular attention because it has long been recognized that high levels of anxiety may impair intellectual functioning and performance in a variety of contexts, ranging from intelligence test scores and school achievement to dating.

The literature suggests that the relationship between psychometric tests of intelligence and trait anxiety is negligible. Thus, neither pattern nor scatter analysis approaches to the Wechsler scales have showed any relation to a trait measure of anxiety. However, studies using situationally induced anxiety (i.e., state anxiety) reveal decrements in performance on the same measures of intellectual functioning. Only when we separate the currently anxious (state anxious) from the chronically anxious (trait anxious) can we show a decrement in intellectual performance due to anxiety. Furthermore, discriminating different components of anxiety shows that worry, but not emotionality, is related to impaired intelligence test performance under time pressure.

Anxiety may have somewhat more general effects on intellectual performance in real-world contexts. Meta-analytic studies suggest that there is an underlying correlation of about −.2 between anxiety measures and measures of performance and achievement at school and college. The relationship is stronger when measures of worry are used, and when the anxiety measure relates specifically to test anxiety and concerns about being evaluated. Test anxiety measures may be a stronger predictor of situational anxiety than general anxiety in such contexts. However, meta-analysis also shows that there is little difference between state and trait anxiety measures as predictors of educational performance criteria. Hence, detrimental effects of anxiety in the real world may represent more than just distraction from performance by the person's immediate worries about the test situation, which relates to state rather than to trait anxiety. The role of anxiety in job performance has been explored in less depth than for the educational context. The relationship between neurotic personality and occupational performance has also been estimated at about −.2 in studies in which there was an a priori rationale for performance being sensitive to neuroticism. It has been suggested, too, that neuroticism may be most detrimental to performance when the job is stressful, as in police work.

The causal status of anxiety is somewhat controversial, and there may be multiple mechanisms for observed associations between anxiety and performance impairment. Evidence that anxiety may directly impair intelligence test performance comes from studies

suggesting that state anxiety has a more adverse effect on difficult or complex tasks than on simple tasks. The worry component of state anxiety may use up working memory or attentional resources so that performance is impaired if the task is sufficiently demanding. Within current models of test anxiety, appraisals of personal competence are an important influence on worry. Demanding tasks, such as many intelligence tests, may be appraised as providing failure experiences, which leads to elevated anxiety. Such tasks may not only be particularly sensitive to worry-related impairment, but performing them may also be particularly prone to generate worries, especially in real-world evaluative situations. Subjects low in intelligence, for whom the task is objectively more difficult, may be especially vulnerable to anxiety-related impairments, a hypothesis confirmed by meta-analysis. However, there are alternative explanations for negative correlations between anxiety and intelligence. First, anxiety in the cognitive test situation may be generated by more or less veridical appraisals that failure is likely due to low ability or to a lack of preparation and study. In other words, anxiety is a marker for poor intellectual skills rather than a factor that directly affects performance. Second, to the extent that anxiety leads to beliefs of lack of self-efficacy in achievement-oriented situations, individuals high in anxiety may avoid activities that enhance intellectual growth, so that apprehension about academic contexts and lack of intellectual skills become mutually reinforcing. Third, the observed relationship of anxiety to intelligence may be the result of the artifactual influences of extraneous variables (e.g., social class, child-rearing patterns, test situation) affecting both variables. [See ANXIETY.]

B. Depression

Depressive disorders are characterized by strong negative emotions, impairment of everyday social functioning, and negative beliefs such as hopelessness and lack of self-worth. The relationship between depression and intelligence is rather underresearched, certainly in comparison with studies of anxiety. Relationships between depression and cognitive functioning may be investigated in both clinical and normal populations. In normal subjects, we can assess either immediate mood or the person's general level of depressive traits.

There is little evidence to suggest that subclinical

levels of depression reliably relate to impaired intelligence test performance in laboratory settings. For example, pretask pleasantness of mood is not reliably predictive of performance on verbal ability items. Deficits are found in clinical populations, however, especially on the performance subtests of the Wechsler Adult Intelligence Scale. Impairment of performance appears to generalize across a variety of high-level cognitive tasks, such as problem solving and reading comprehension. Causal effects of clinical depression on cognitive performance are generally accepted, especially for tasks requiring concentration or memory. However, other causal hypotheses have received little attention. It is conceivable that depression will result if low intelligence leads to a succession of performance failures, for example.

The significance of depression for intellectual functioning in the real world is presently unclear. The effects of neuroticism on occupational performance may be mediated as much by depression as anxiety, given that neuroticism relates to both conditions. There has also been little work on the manic symptoms central to some mood disorders, although low levels of symptoms (hypomania) may be associated with enhanced creativity. Most research on depression has been concerned with cognitive mechanisms for impairment, a theme to which we will later return. [*See* DEPRESSION; MOOD DISORDERS.]

C. Anger

Anger is commonly described as a negative emotion ranging in intensity from mild irritation to rage. Anger is often hailed as one of the most intriguing of human emotions and plays a central role in modern personality theory and research, having important implications for psychological practices in the clinical, health, occupational, and educational domains. It is closely linked to aggression, and therefore it can be a particularly destructive form of negative emotion. Excessive or inappropriate anger may appear as a symptom of both emotional and personality disorders (though it is particularly prevalent in the antisocial and borderline personality disorders discussed in the next section).

There is little research directly relating various facets of anger to cognitive ability or performance. There is considerable evidence to support the contention that there is an increased degree of delinquency and

crime, and even child and wife abuse, with lower IQ. Aggression may act over a long period of time to depress intellectual functioning. There are data suggesting that whereas intellectual competence has little or no influence on differences in aggression after about age 8, aggressive tendencies that exhibit continuity may act over a long period of time to depress intellectual performance.

How can we account for the general tendency for low IQ to go with increased aggression, impulsive behavior, and delinquency? Possibly, the correlation may be due to the effects of low intelligence on frustration and the inability to control impulses, delay rewards, and calculate one's own interest. The more intelligent person may seek further into the consequences of his or her behavior, build up more inhibitions, and acquire more socially desirable traits. Thus, high intelligence can aid a student in learning the realities of general and school culture and the physical world as part of an integrated learning process. By contrast, the less intelligent person will experience more frustration in the learning process and may therefore be more provoked to impulsive and antisocial activities. In short, intelligence may facilitate the ability to delay gratification, which may feed back into the further development of cognitive capacity. Conversely, excessive impulsivity may disrupt learning of intellectual skills. Aggression, impulsivity, and low intelligence may also be influenced by effects of additional variables, such as strict parental rearing patterns, social class, or quality of education. [*See* AGGRESSION; ANGER.]

D. Fatigue

Feelings of tiredness relate to energetic arousal, one of the fundamental dimensions of mood. Fatigue can, of course, be induced experimentally by prolonged work, although laboratory studies using manipulations of this kind typically show rather little effect on intellectual tasks. In the mental health context, we are primarily concerned with chronic fatigue conditions. Fatigue may contribute to the intellectual impairments seen in emotional disorders. It is a common symptom of depression, for example, and may occur in some anxiety conditions, in some cases as the result of insomnia. Recently, there has been considerable interest in chronic fatigue syndrome (CFS), associated with both muscle and mental fatigue. This syndrome is not infrequently accompanied by depression, but the extent to which it is psychogenic is controversial. Recent research investigating cognitive function in CFS patients showed wide-ranging deficits, including considerable impairment of full-scale IQ. In addition to loss of intelligence, the largest decrements were found on tests of attention, verbal memory, nondominant grip strength, and problem solving. Less dramatic but reliable attentional deficits are found in individuals whose mood is characterized by low energy, although there is no straightforward relationship between subjective tiredness and intelligence test performance.

E. Emotional Processing Mechanisms for Intellectual Impairment

In the preceding section, we discussed empirical findings that suggest that various negative emotions may be associated with intellectual impairment, at least under some conditions. However, causal relationships between emotional disturbance and intellectual function appear to be complex, certainly in the case of anxiety and probably also for other types of disturbance. In this section, we highlight two types of mechanisms that might mediate direct effects of negative emotion on intellectual performance. One type of mechanism is cognitive: the person's ability to process task-related information may be impaired. The alternative mechanism is motivational: the person may choose not to allocate effort to processing task stimuli, perhaps because of competing goals.

1. Cognitive Interference and Loss of Functional Resources

There is a reasonable consensus that worry has detrimental effects on cognition and information processing. In states of worry, attentional capacity or resources is diverted from the task at hand to processing cognitions associated with concerns about the task or other personal problems. Attentional resources are conceived as a general-purpose reservoir of energy for processing, which may be flexibly allocated to specific processing routines, and the loss of functional resources caused by worry is described as cognitive interference. The role of cognitive interference is demonstrated by a variety of studies showing anxiety-related decrements on attentionally demanding tasks. It appears that interference mechanisms may also explain detrimental

effects of other negative emotions. Recent reviews of studies of depression and performance deficit concluded that the tasks most sensitive to depression are those that require effortful or controlled processing rather than automatic processing. For example, Wechsler Adult Intelligence Scale subtests most sensitive to depression (Block Design, Comprehension) require more effort than those least sensitive (Vocabulary, Information). One of the defining features of controlled processing is its dependence on investment of attentional resources. Given that depression is often associated with rumination and self-reflection, it is plausible that cognitive interference contributes to its detrimental effects on intelligence. Ruminative worry may also contribute to observed deficits in controlled processing in obsessional-compulsive patients.

There are two other mechanisms for intellectual impairment which may also operate through their effects on the person's functional capacity for information processing. Research suggests that subjective energy is correlated with total availability of attentional resources. Energy may provide a marker for activity of arousal-related brain systems, the functioning of which is impaired in depression. Cognitive interference influences not so much attentional resources, but short-term memory. However, the short-term memory tasks most sensitive to anxiety tend to be those that also require active processing of information ("working memory" tasks) and may require attentional resources as well as short-term retention. In any case, it is important to realize that intelligence tests vary in their demands on attentional resources and working memory, and impairment in these information-processing functions does not necessarily result in impairment on any given intelligence test. We would expect emotional disturbance to be most detrimental to tests making high demands on controlled processing, attention, or working memory.

2. Motivational Deficits and Strategy Use

An alternative category of explanation for loss of intellectual functioning is motivation. Such explanations emphasize not so much changes in basic processing efficiency as the person's willingness to engage actively with the task. Motivation may influence both the overall effort applied to the task and the strategies applied to it: the motivated person may "work smarter" rather than work harder. It is generally accepted that depression is associated with a motivational deficit which contributes to performance deficit. In nonclinical groups, demotivating effects of depression are most evident when the task requires active restructuring of material. In 1994, Wells and Matthews developed a general model of attention and emotion that attributed performance deficits in affective disorder to replacement of task-focused goals by self-regulatory goals which generate worry and self-scrutiny. Consistent with this hypothesis, the intellectual performance of depressives is impaired by self-focus of attention and improved by a distracting secondary task. One study showed that depressives' deficit on the Porteus Maze intelligence test was eliminated when they also had to repeat digits back to the experimenter. This result is inconsistent with a simple resource theory explanation that the extra task would increase the requirement for resources and further disadvantage the depressives. Similarly, studies of driver stress have shown that negative emotions are most damaging to single-task driving; stress-vulnerable drivers appear to be able to mobilize sufficient effort to deal with dual-task situations.

The role of motivation in anxiety is more controversial, because there is no clear, overall motivational deficit. Eysenck and Eysenck have argued that anxious individuals may be motivated to compensate for their perceived deficit in performance through increased compensatory effort. Hence, anxiety may relate more strongly to processing efficiency than to observed performance effectiveness. The anxious individual can be compared to a car with a trailer hooked to it, additional acceleration is needed to reach a given level of speed compared with a car without a trailer. However, deficits in active strategy use have been observed in both trait-anxious subjects and neurotic subjects, implying that anxious individuals may have difficulty applying compensatory effort adaptively. Again, effects of anxiety on intellectual functioning may relate to self-regulatory goals which compete with task goals. There is a large experimental literature that shows that anxious subjects tend to focus selectively on threatening stimuli to the potential detriment of processing of nonthreatening stimuli. Such effects may relate to the general tendency of emotionally disturbed individuals to monitor for negative stimuli congruent with their personal concerns or to a hypervigilance for threat specific to anxiety).

In summary, it is likely that loss of both functional resources and motivational processes contribute to in-tellectual impairment in emotional disorders, although the relative importance of these processes may vary with emotional condition, information-processing demands of the task, and contextual factors which influence worry and personal goals. There is also likely to be some interaction between the two types of processes. Motivation may be affected by perceptions of lack of resources, but, conversely, lack of resources may impair the person's ability to carry out the processing that supports motivation.

III. INTELLIGENCE AND SEVERE MENTAL DISORDERS

The primary symptoms of severe or psychotic disorders are categorized as emotional in the case of depression, and cognitive in schizophrenics, although abnormality of emotion and cognition frequently coexist. If the person is unable to function in everyday life, we would expect most forms of psychological pathology to affect intellectual processes in some way. One of the effects of severe emotional stress and upheaval is to lower one's overall adaptive efficiency and to increase the rigidity of cognitive processes. Under severe emotional stress, it becomes difficult for the individual to assess the situation objectively, to differentiate rationally between relevant and irrelevant stimuli, to abstract crucial features, or to perceive and scan the range of available alternatives. In relatively mild cases, a distinction between performance and competence may be appropriate. Some individuals suffering from mild affective disorders act in an irrational manner and fail to think rationally in conflict-laden areas but otherwise show no impairment of intelligence. Thus, their underlying competence remains intact, but they fail to apply their intellectual capacity effectively in an emotionally laden field. In more severe affective disorders, cognitive interference and lack of motivation may seriously hinder the engagement of the rational processes involved in intelligence over a prolonged time, perhaps leading to competence deficits as well. [See EMOTION AND COGNITION.]

There has been considerable research on intellectual decline in schizophrenia, the most prevalent of the psychoses. Schizophrenic thought and judgment is seriously impaired as mental health deteriorates, with a growing tendency to confuse wish and reality. The schizophrenic mind, although unselectively registering everything in its field of vision, is unable to distinguish between relevant and irrelevant cues. In fact, disturbances in thinking (cognitive slippage) are thought to be the hallmark of schizophrenia. The intellectual abilities of manifest schizophrenia appear to fluctuate and the same person may obtain different scores on mental tests on different occasions.

A number of hypotheses exist in the literature with respect to the effects of schizophrenia on intellectual functioning. One common hypothesis is that all schizophrenics may go through a time-limited period of intellectual deterioration, after which intelligence stabilizes. A second hypothesis is that only some intellectual skills deteriorate (e.g., numerical, spatial), while others (e.g., verbal) do not. A third hypothesis states that the intellectual performance of some diagnostic groups deteriorates while those of others do not. Thus, both high IQ and low IQ schizophrenics may represent different subtypes, one of which is susceptible to intellectual deterioration and the other not. A fourth hypothesis states that intellectual skills do not decline, but personalities decompensate, thus creating the illusion of decline. It is also hypothesized that decrements in performance may partially be attributed to the subject's low motivation to perform, minimal cooperation, and impaired contact with the examiner.

Unfortunately, the direct empirical evidence of whether intellectual abilities of schizophrenics decline after the onset of psychosis, relative to their premorbid status, is conflicting and often confusing. Although the intelligence of severely schizophrenic individuals may be below average, one is struck by the preservation of average or even remarkable intellectual superiority in many schizophrenics, especially those diagnosed as paranoid. Some studies report substantial decline between high school (or military) and hospitalization, whereas some studies show that intellectual deficits among schizophrenics may be attributable to preexisting conditions and are not an inherent factor associated with the onset of schizophrenia. In one recent study, no significant decay in intelligence scores was observed for schizophrenics whose initial aptitude test scores were above average, with the observed decline in test scores being largely attributable to a drop in a specific skill—arithmetic performance. Because deterioration is limited to certain skills, it is best interpreted as a loss in particular intellectual functions rather than as a more generalized intellectual decay. Furthermore, the failure to report intellec-

tual loss in schizophrenia may often result because of instances of early IQ deterioration long before the illness became apparent.

Some research shows that intelligence deteriorates under schizophrenic attack, but under remission, performance on intelligence tests improves and goes up again. Chronic schizophrenic inpatients with long histories of hospitalization manifest greater intellectual deficit than do patients with recent onset or brief hospitalization. However, this may be due to changes in the composition of hospitalized cohorts over time rather than to the effects of hospitalization or processes intrinsic to psychosis. Longitudinal studies of hospitalized patients fail to find progressive decline. That is, chronics may be less bright than acutes because of an association between IQ and retention in and readmission to hospitals. There is some research to suggest that brighter patients are less often rehospitalized several years after discharge than patients of lower IQ. Thus, there appears to be a prognostic significance for IQ which contributes to the differences in intelligence between acute and chronic schizophrenics. [See SCHIZOPHRENIA.]

The effects of psychosis on intellectual functioning for children may be more pernicious than that for adults, and children suffering from certain personality dysfunctions and disturbances have been reported to suffer from a severe deterioration of abilities. Children with disintegrative psychosis usually have a period of normal development for the first 3 to 4 years, after which profound regression and behavioral disintegration occurs, intelligence declines, speech and language abilities deteriorate, and social skills diminish. In addition, children become restive, irritable, anxious, and overactive. Overall, the prognosis is poor. A child's level of ability may be related to a prognosis of childhood psychosis in a number of ways: (a) in families that are predisposed to schizophrenia, children with the lowest IQ are the most vulnerable; (b) the level of intelligence may be related to etiology, with psychotic children with nonorganic etiologies obtaining higher IQs than those with organic etiologies; and (c) the higher the intelligence the better the prognosis.

As previously discussed, intelligence may relate to one's current overall level of organization and integrative functioning. Hence, intelligence may play an important role in the prognosis of maladjusted individuals. Furthermore, on the assumption that intelligence involves the ability to cognize relations adequately (including social and emotional relations) and to correct cognitions on the basis of evidence, it might be hypothesized that high-intelligence patients would profit more from psychotherapeutic relations compared with their less intelligent counterparts and also show a better prognosis. Thus, on purely theoretical grounds, it may be predicted that greater effectiveness of intellectual functioning, revealing itself in IQ tests, should also be associated with greater modifiability in personality structure. Furthermore, because traditional psychotherapy involves verbal exchanges between therapist and patient, its success entails some verbal learning, such as acquisition and elimination of responses. Thus, success at psychotherapy should be related to general verbal learning ability and intelligence. In fact, there is some research to support the claim that intelligence is a significant predictor of success in psychological treatment and therapy, although not all studies substantiate the link. Furthermore, clients who remain in therapy are found to be more intelligent than those who terminate prematurely: Most of those who remain are of average IQ and above, and most of those who leave are below average IQ.

IV. COGNITIVE SUBSTRATES OF PERSONALITY DISORDERS

The domain of personality disorders provides an opportunity to examine the cognitive substrates of another important class of psychopathological disorders. The *DSM-IV* defines the personality traits underlying behavior as "enduring patterns of perceiving, relating to, and thinking about the environment and oneself" (p. 630). However, when these traits become inflexible, result in circular thinking, and undermine the structural integrity of one's personality, then a personality disturbance may be diagnosed. The *DSM-IV* multiaxial system separates clinical disorders (Axis 1) from personality disorders (Axis II). Personality disorders may be manifested in any two or more areas of cognition, affectivity, interpersonal functioning, and impulse control. The common features include "an enduring pattern of inner experience and behavior that deviates markedly from the expectations of the individual's culture, is pervasive and inflexible, has an onset in adolescence or early adulthood, is stable over time, and leads to distress or impairment" (p. 629). Endler and Summerfeldt's 1995 review of the litera-

ture concluded that characteristic ways of organizing and processing information and experience appear to play major roles in the genesis and perpetuation of personality disorders. In fact, self-consistent modes of perceiving, remembering, thinking, and problem solving are evident in each of the patterns identified in *DSM-IV*. The three clusters and ten specific personality disorders are

Cluster A
Paranoid personality disorder
Schizoid personality disorder
Schizotypal personality disorder
Cluster B
Antisocial personality disorder
Borderline personality disorder
Histrionic personality disorder
Narcissistic personality disorder
Cluster C
Avoidant personality disorder
Dependent personality disorder
Passive–aggressive disorder
Obsessive–compulsive personality disorder

Several brief examples from each of these clusters are used to illustrate the cognitive features of Axis II disorders. Cluster A disorders share in common the features of oddness and eccentricity. Underlying these defining behaviors is the way information is processed. For example, individuals diagnosed with schizotypal personality disorder have been described as cognitively autistic. This refers to perceptual and cognitive distortions that cause the boundaries defining reality to blur while attending to, or not being able to filter out, irrelevant or peripheral information. The inability to integrate information and experiences cognitively is implicated in the eccentric thought and behavior patterns seen in this cluster. Paranoid personality disorder is characterized by hostility and suspiciousness, in thinking and behavior. Persons diagnosed with this personality disorder see their world as hostile and threatening and view situations and human interaction with suspicion and distrust. This belief system is likely reinforced by attending to particular cues that can be interpreted as threatening or hostile. These persons are hypervigilant with regard to finding or interpreting persons or events as supporting their belief that the world is a hostile place. They expect to find examples of threat, look for them, interpret events as threatening, and thereby strengthen their beliefs. Hence, cluster A disorders tend to be associated with both intellectual impoverishment and a tendency for thinking to be driven by internal preoccupations rather than by external reality.

Cluster B disorders tend to share several defining features: behavior and thought are dramatic, emotional, and erratic. Antisocial personality disorder is most characterized by lack of insight and concrete and perseverative thinking that is manifest in behavior ranging from irresponsible to unlawful. There appears to be a deficiency in cognitive mediation; these persons are unable to see the consequences of their actions, both present and future. Their lack of planning ability goes hand in hand with a more concrete thinking style and high impulsiveness. Egocentric thought is the primary feature of narcissistic personality disorder. Information that reinforces the person's own grand opinion of himself or herself is attended to, in contrast to the more superficial attention and storage of information that is not central to this narcissistic sense of the self. Cluster B disorders are associated especially with difficulties in abstracting and integrating information, suggesting a general intellectual impairment.

Anxiety and fearfulness are the primary characteristics of the cluster C personality disorders. Once again, the defining features of the four disorders subsumed here clearly show the relevance of cognitive factors. The dependent and passive–aggressive personality disorders highlight the relevance of inflexible and dysfunctional beliefs as well as distortions in the interpretation of social stimuli. Avoidant personality disorder is characterized by oversensitivity and overestimation about disapproval and failure, as well as social insecurity and the fear of rejection. Such beliefs probably determine not only what is attended to but also the interpretation of experiences; these in turn become the schemata that define the self, self-efficacy, and the probability of experiencing failure and rejection. Obsessive–compulsive personality disorder is also identified by a number of cognitive factors. The manifest behaviors appear to reflect the need to impose structure and control on all aspects of experience. Various terms have been used to describe the cognitive style associated with this disorder: globally dichotomous thinking, certainty orientation, and noninclusive all-inclusiveness. It is the preoccupation with order, control, and perfectionism that determines and, in turn, is determined by the particular cognitive approaches for attending to and scanning, processing, and interpret-

ing information. Obsessionals may in fact score quite well on intelligence tests based on acquired information, but show impairment on performance-oriented tests. Cluster C disorders might also be associated with more general deficits on demanding intellectual tasks as a result of anxiety. [*See* Obsessive-Compulsive Disorder.]

There appears to be ample empirical and clinical evidence that the cognitive features of the various Axis II personality disorders are critical to understanding both their etiology and their resiliency. There is no clear answer to the question of whether these disorders stem from faulty or "different" cognitive factors at the input, process, or output levels, or occur and become consistent and persistent as a function of some other etiologic determinants. Nevertheless, the cognitive characteristics of these disorders hold considerable potential for differential diagnosis and treatment. There is rather little evidence on the consequence of personality disorders for intelligence from studies using psychometric tests. However, there is some clinical and experimental evidence showing that they tend to be associated with intellectual deficits, which vary from disorder to disorder.

V. CONCLUSIONS

This review suggests a rather complex reciprocal relationship between intelligence and emotional factors, with the two variables dynamically affecting each other in the course of development and in day-to-day behavior. On the one hand, personality dispositions and emotional disturbances may influence intellectual functioning. It is important to distinguish the effects personality may have on performance in the short term from effects on competence in the longer term. There is solid empirical evidence for various negative emotional states tending to impair intellectual performance to a moderate degree, especially when the task is demanding of attention or working memory. It is likely that both loss of functional resources and motivational processes contribute to intellectual impairment in both emotional disorders and in subclinical stress states. Conversely, styles of processing associated with mental health, such as beliefs in self-efficacy and personal control, may serve to maintain or enhance performance. Some of these effects may be context-dependent in that some kinds of disturbances may influence certain types of practical intelligence more strongly than psychometric intelligence.

It is less clear whether mental health influences basic competence, in addition to the person's performance on specific occasions. The cognitive framework for understanding mental health suggests that certain personality traits, such as low self-efficacy, poor self-concept, and aggression, may act over extended periods of time to depress intellectual functioning by reducing a person's motivation to acquire and develop specific intellectual skills. Psychotic conditions and personality disorders also may affect both temporary performance and underlying competence.

On the other hand, intelligence may affect mental health and affective states through encouraging more positive cognitions of personal competence. Thus, individuals high in intellectual functioning are frequently shown to be better adjusted, both socially and emotionally, than their less intelligent counterparts. High-IQ individuals frequently tend to evidence more positive self-concepts, greater perceived control over their environment, and greater impulse control. High intelligence can aid a student in learning the realities of general and school culture and the physical world as part of an integrated learning process, which helps the person acquire more socially desirable traits. Overall, intelligence may serve as a personal resource that can facilitate personal growth and adjustment and also serve as a buffer against the crippling effects of psycho-logical stress and disease. Negative moods may be generated by more or less veridical appraisals that negative outcomes are likely, as a result of low ability, and negative affects may result if low intelligence leads to a succession of performance failures. Thus, negative affect may be a marker for poor intellectual aptitude and past achievement as well as a factor that directly affects performance.

BIBLIOGRAPHY

American Psychiatric Association. (1994). *Diagnostic and statistical manual of mental disorders* (4th ed.). Washington, DC: Author.

Endler, N. S., & Summerfeldt, L. J. (1995). Intelligence, personality, psychopathology, and adjustment. In D. H. Saklofske & M. Zeidner (Eds.), *International handbook of personality and intelligence* (pp. 249–284). New York: Plenum Press.

Eysenck, H. J., & Eysenck, M. W. (1985). *Personality and individual differences*. New York: Plenum Press.

Schwean, V. L., & Saklofske, D. H. (1995). A cognitive-social description of exceptional children. In D. H. Saklofske & M. Zeidner (Eds.), *International handbook of personality and intelligence* (pp. 185–204). New York: Plenum Press.

Wells, A., & Matthews, G. (1994). *Attention and emotion: A clinical perspective*. Hillsdale, NJ: Lawrence Erlbaum.

Zeidner, M. (1995). Personality trait correlates of intelligence. In D. H. Saklofske & M. Zeidner (Eds.), *International handbook of personality and intelligence* (pp. 299–319). New York: Plenum Press.

Zeidner, M. (in press). *Test anxiety: The state of the art*. New York: Plenum Press.

Intrinsic Motivation and Goals

Judith M. Harackiewicz

University of Wisconsin, Madison

Achievement Goals   The general desire to develop, attain, or demonstrate competence at an activity in achievement situations.
Flow   Motivational state of total absorption and involvement produced by an optimal balance between a person's skill level and the challenge of the activity.
Intrinsic Motivation   Engagement in activities for their own sake.
Life Tasks   Goals for behavior that reflect individuals' general concerns at a particular point in time.
Overjustification Effect   Reduction of intrinsic interest when behavior is attributed to extrinsic factors.
Performance-Contingent Reward   A reward that is offered for attaining a specific level of competence.
Self-Determination   The perception that behavior is under internal, rather than external, control and autonomously motivated.
Task-Contingent Reward   A reward that is contingent simply on completing a task, without regard to competence.

INTRINSIC MOTIVATION reflects our desire to engage in activities for their own sake. We do some things simply because we love doing them. When we are intrinsically motivated, we are happier, become more involved in activities, persist longer at them, and perform at higher levels. Intrinsic motivation is therefore a critical component of adaptive functioning, and researchers have devoted considerable energy toward an understanding of the determinants and consequences of intrinsic motivation.

I. INTRINSIC MOTIVATION

Theorists have long placed competence and mastery at the heart of intrinsic motivation; for example, Robert White proposed in 1959 that interest in an activity derives from the opportunity it provides to master effectively or control the environment. Most contemporary theorists have continued in this tradition, emphasizing the central role of competence and control in intrinsic motivation. Csikszentmihalyi introduced the theoretical construct of *flow*, which is a motivational state characterized by positive affect and total involvement and absorption in an activity. He argued that individuals in this intrinsically motivated state are immersed in an activity to the point of losing self-awareness, forgetting the time, fatigue, and everything other than the activity itself. This state produces a genuine sense of satisfaction and it results from an optimal balance between a person's skill level and the challenge afforded by the activity. This balance can be difficult to attain, and flow experiences are not common in the course of daily life. When activities are too challenging, relative to an individual's skill level, anxiety results, and when skill levels are too high, relative to the challenge inherent in the task, boredom results. Thus, according to Csikszentmihalyi, the flow experience depends on the individual's competence and mastery of the activity.

In 1985, Deci and Ryan articulated a theory of intrinsic motivation that emphasized autonomy or a sense of personal control over behavior as a primary component of intrinsic motivation, in addition to perceived competence. According to this perspective, an individual must have a full sense of choice about engaging in an activity or perceive his or her behavior as self-determined (as opposed to externally pressured or coerced) to be intrinsically motivated. Thus, feelings of autonomy and self-determination are proposed to enhance intrinsic motivation, making a person more likely to enjoy activities and engage in them again in the future.

Intrinsic motivation represents an "inner resource" for performance and adjustment in a variety of social contexts, with clear implications for overall self-esteem and psychological functioning. It encompasses perceived competence (the confidence one has in oneself), self-regulation (the degree to which individuals self-direct and control their own behavior), and perceived control (one's beliefs about the causes of behavior in particular contexts). Deci and Ryan draw an important distinction between locus of control (which refers to expectations about the linkage of an individual's behavior and the outcome obtained) and *locus of causality,* which refers to the distinction between perceiving the source of initiation and regulation for motivated behavior as within the self (autonomous motivation) or outside the self (externally controlled motivation). Thus, individuals with an internal locus of control could be either autonomous or controlled in regulating their behavior, but it is the locus of causality that should have the strongest impact on motivation and adjustment. Each of these three components of intrinsic motivation (perceived competence, control, and self-regulation) has been found to be linked to performance and psychological adjustment in children, adolescents, and college students; intrinsic motivation contributes to active, productive engagement in work, academic, and leisure pursuits.

People are much more likely to become involved and remain interested in activities that they pursue for intrinsic, self-determined reasons. They will be happier and experience a sense of "flow" when they are optimally challenged and intrinsically motivated. Even when they are not intrinsically motivated, they some-

times strive to become so in an effort to generate interest and involvement to maintain motivation for important activities. In fact, research conducted in 1992 by Sansone and colleagues indicates that individuals actively regulate interest when performing an activity to maintain their performance. In that study, people performing a dull and repetitive activity were more likely to engage in strategies that made the activity more interesting (e.g., they chose to vary the procedures by which they performed the activity) when told there were health benefits from performing the task on a regular basis. Use of these strategies in turn was associated with greater motivation to perform the task in the future.

Researchers have examined intrinsic versus extrinsic orientations in the classroom (where learning is motivated by curiosity or interest vs. by rewards or evaluation, respectively) and have found that an intrinsic orientation is positively associated with perceived competence, competence valuation, task involvement, and continued interest. Extrinsic orientations have been found to undermine perceived competence and self-worth.

A large body of research conducted over the last 20 years has documented the benefits of autonomous versus controlled behavior in a number of physical and mental health domains. For example, individuals are more likely to adhere to exercise regimens if they are autonomously motivated. Other studies have found that autonomous behaviors are associated with greater cognitive flexibility, enhanced creativity, better adjustment, and more positive mental health. In 1996, Williams and colleagues reported that in a study conducted in the context of a weight-loss program for severely obese individuals, the degree of patients' autonomous motivation for participating in the program predicted attendance at weekly meetings and weight loss during the program period. Moreover, autonomous motivation also predicted the *maintenance* of weight loss at a 2-year follow-up. Similar findings have also been reported with the maintenance of smoking cessation and other behavioral changes produced by treatment.

II. DETERMINANTS OF INTRINSIC MOTIVATION

There is considerable knowledge about how intrinsic motivation can be fostered in others. For example, most theories of intrinsic motivation suggest that self-perceptions of competence promote subsequent interest in an activity. These perceptions of competence can develop from an individual's direct experience with an activity if a sense of mastery or improvement emerges during the course of task engagement. It should therefore be possible to structure materials in such a way to afford individuals an optimal challenge and promote self-perceptions of mastery as they work on a task. However, this task-based feedback is not always sufficient to promote perceived competence, because people often depend on social input to gain a clear sense of their competence. In other words, a person does not always know how good he or she is at something until someone else provides some external feedback about his or her performance. External communications and incentives may therefore be especially potent in promoting intrinsic motivation if they make people feel competent. For example, teachers or supervisors can evaluate performance and provide feedback about the quality of work completed, offer rewards for good performance, or set up competitions and identify winners. When these cues provide students or subordinates with positive feedback about their competence at the activity, it should enhance subsequent interest in the activity.

Performance feedback is often the end result of an individual's extended encounter with a task, however, and it is important to consider the situational contingencies and motivational processes that influence an individual's ongoing experience with a task. For instance, the availability of competence feedback usually implies some degree of external performance evaluation, and individuals may be aware of the upcoming external evaluation before they begin a task. The anticipation of performance evaluation can affect their motivational orientation and task involvement during task performance, and these motivational processes may influence subsequent interest in the task. Evaluation may therefore influence intrinsic motivation independently of any positive feedback that ultimately results. When teachers, coaches, and supervisors evaluate performance on an interesting and involving activity, their evaluation represents an extrinsic intrusion into what had been an intrinsically motivated activity, and may actually *undermine* subsequent intrinsic motivation, even if the eventual feedback produces feelings of competence.

These negative effects may occur because individuals feel that their behavior is externally controlled and thus lose their sense of self-determination or autonomy. In fact, many studies have shown that externally imposed rewards (e.g., task-contingent rewards) and other social contingencies (e.g., deadlines) that do not provide competence feedback reliably undermine intrinsic motivation. For example, a classic study conducted by Lepper, Greene, and Nisbett in 1973, demonstrated that children who were offered rewards simply for drawing pictures had lower levels of subsequent interest in the drawing activity, compared with a group that did not receive rewards for performing this interesting activity. This basic phenomenon, termed the overjustification effect (because people attribute their behavior to extrinsic rather than intrinsic causes, and discount intrinsic interest), has been replicated in a variety of settings, with a range of external contingencies and a wide range of subjects.

Subsequently, however, researchers have become more interested in external contingencies that are simultaneously controlling *and* informative about competence. Rewards can be promised for attaining certain levels of performance, or competitions can be set up when the external pressure to win is strong. Earning the reward or winning the competition signifies the attainment of excellence, but the feedback is received in a controlling context. In these cases, the theoretical analysis becomes more complex, because competence feedback comes at the cost of some loss of self-determination.

Evaluative situations have their effects on performance and motivation over the course of time, and it is important to consider the *process* of performance evaluation. Before beginning a task, individuals anticipate that their performance will be evaluated and they are aware of external evaluation while they perform. They may attribute their behavior to the external constraint or experience performance pressure, thus reducing their intrinsic interest in the task. While engaged in the task, individuals may worry about their performance, become distracted from the task, and may not have a clear sense of how they are doing. Performance feedback is not usually available during task performance, but external feedback may ultimately provide positive information about competence at an activity. When evaluative outcomes are positive, they should enhance subsequent intrinsic motivation. Thus, performance evaluation has both positive and negative implications for subsequent interest. It could have negative effects because of the cognitive and affective experience of evaluation during task performance, and positive effects because of the resultant (positive) evaluative outcomes.

Rewards often accompany positive evaluative outcomes, and when their attainment is contingent upon achieving a certain level of performance, they are performance-contingent (as opposed to task-contingent rewards, which are given simply for completing a task). When rewards are associated with competence, they can enhance interest independently of the competence feedback communicated in the evaluative situation. A reward can have *cue value* because it makes the potential evaluative outcome more salient, and it symbolizes a meaningful performance accomplishment. It can magnify the emotional significance of competence and make people more concerned about doing well in an evaluative situation. The effects of cue value may occur at the outset of performance, when individuals are motivated to achieve competence and earn the reward, and at task conclusion, when the receipt of performance-contingent rewards makes the positive evaluative outcome more salient.

In summary, evaluative situations possess three critical properties: the promise of performance evaluation, the competence feedback provided by evaluative outcomes, and the cue value of performance-contingent rewards. In 1984, Harackiewicz, Manderlink, and Sansone examined the effects of evaluation anticipation and cue value on intrinsic motivation in two comparisons. Evaluation groups expected their performance on a pinball game to be evaluated against an 80th percentile criterion, and then learned that they had surpassed it. Performance-contingent reward subjects were promised a movie pass if their performance exceeded the same criterion; they, too, learned that their performance was in the top 20th percentile and received the promised reward. Control subjects were not promised rewards and did not expect evaluation, but they did receive unanticipated feedback that they had scored above the 80th percentile. Thus, all subjects received positive competence feedback.

Evaluation subjects were less involved in the task while playing and played less pinball in a subsequent free choice situation than did control subjects, thus revealing the negative effect of evaluation anticipation on process measures as well as on subsequent intrinsic motivation. Performance-contingent reward subjects played more pinball than did evaluation subjects who were exposed to the same performance evaluation and feedback, thus revealing the positive effect of cue value.

These results demonstrate that material rewards that symbolize competence can enhance interest independently of the competence feedback they convey.

Clearly, teachers, therapists, and supervisors possess some power to foster intrinsic motivation in their students, clients, and subordinates, but there are risks as well. The key appears to be to provide positive competence feedback and make individuals care about doing well without threatening their sense of autonomy. One technique that may prove effective in this regard is goal-setting. External agents can suggest goals for performance without intruding on the individual's sense of self-determination, and individuals can then make these goals their own and use them to guide and evaluate their progress. Although relatively few studies have examined the effects of goals on intrinsic motivation, a large, more general goals literature is highly relevant to the study of intrinsic motivation.

III. GOALS AS A UNIFYING CONSTRUCT IN MOTIVATION RESEARCH

Goals are mental representations of what we want to do, who we want to be, or to what we are emotionally committed. Goals, and their implementation through plans, motivate and guide human behavior. A large body of motivational research concerns the determinants and consequences of the goals that people adopt and pursue in a variety of life settings. Accomplishing personal goals is fundamental to psychological adjustment. Even if goals are not attained, some theorists have argued that simply setting out to accomplish goals provides meaning and structure to life. Goals can range in a hierarchy from broad global aims ("I want to be the best I can be, every day, in every way") to domain-specific goals ("I want to be a good student"), and all the way down to the specific and mundane ("I want to get a 95 on this exam"). At the highest and most general level of this hierarchy, researchers have examined individuals' possible selves and self guides. At a somewhat lower level or midlevel, other researchers have concentrated on relatively more specific goals, such as personal projects, personal strivings, current concerns, and life tasks, which are conceptualized as idiographic units of study for personality research. Goals at these highest levels and midlevels transcend particular situations or contexts and reflect individuals' general concerns or goals at a particular period of time. For example, a college student might be working on the life task of getting good grades, making friends, or finding intimacy. These goals can be expressed and pursued in different ways by different people, and researchers are currently studying how people define and integrate their goals at different levels of specificity, how they decide to pursue their goals, and how these goals function in self-regulation.

IV. MIDLEVEL GOALS

The life task approach has proven useful as a conceptual tool for understanding personal goals that encompass both individuals' central motives and their more concrete expressions in daily life. This work begins with insights from life-span developmental theories about the normative developmental issues that individuals confront in the course of their everyday life (e.g., issues of identity, financial success), but assumes that individuals will have different personal construals of these issues. The theoretical models afford a powerful way of thinking about individuals in terms of their personal constructions of life tasks, personal projects, and so on, which allows for the integration of both individual (self-beliefs and interests) and situational or contextual factors (normative developmental issues, situational and contextual demands) in models of self-regulation.

A number of studies have identified relationships between these general goals and daily positive and negative affect, depression, life satisfaction, delinquency, and physical health. The aim of many studies has been to demonstrate that individuals who strive for and attain positive outcomes relevant to their personal goals, whatever their content, experience greater well-being and less emotional distress. More recently, researchers have begun to identify some negative consequences of some types of general goals. For example, one study found that personal strivings for power (the desire to control, impress, or manipulate others) were associated with more negative affect and distress. Other studies, by Cantor and colleagues, suggest that when individuals concentrate on the extrinsic outcomes of particular life tasks (e.g., when goal attainment and satisfaction depend on external rewards or on the reactions of other people, as when students are moti-

vated to get good grades to please their parents), goals are associated with decreased emotional involvement and negative affect in daily life.

One study found that college women who value academic achievement, but who worry about their performance, adopted a strategy of seeking approval and reassurance from their friends in social settings. This strategy, adopted to attain their higher-order goal of doing well in school, helped them achieve their academic goals, but it proved to have a social cost: these women experienced more negative affect and more dissatisfaction with their social life.

A study conducted by Kasser and Ryan in 1993 examined the extent to which individuals endorsed four general goals (self-acceptance, affiliation, community feelings, and financial success) and found that individuals who valued financial success (the aspiration to attain wealth and material success) above all other goals were more distressed, depressed, anxious, and lower in self-actualization and vitality. Having the goal of financial success per se should not necessarily affect psychological adjustment, but when people pursue this goal above others, they appear to be lower in psychological well-being. Comparable results were obtained in a sample of adolescents, where interview ratings of global functioning, social productivity, and symptoms of behavior disorders were associated with the centrality of financial success motives. These results clearly demonstrate the deleterious consequences of having money as an important "guiding principle" in life, and suggest that not all goals are equivalent in terms of their relationship to well-being.

V. ACHIEVEMENT GOALS

In contrast to focussing on individuals' global or long-term goals, other researchers have examined the general kinds of goals implicit in particular domains. One class of goals that has received considerable research attention is achievement goals, broadly defined by Dweck and others as the desire to develop, attain, or demonstrate competence at an activity. Theorists have recently converged on a distinction between *performance* goals, in which individuals seek favorable judgments of their competence, and *mastery* goals, in which individuals seek to increase their competence or master something new. Performance goals highlight normatively based standards and promote the *demonstration* of ability relative to others, whereas mastery goals are self-referential, focusing on the *development* of skill and competence relative to the task and one's own past performance.

Several researchers have compared these two goal orientations and examined their effects on affective, cognitive, and motivational processes. A consistent pattern of results suggests that mastery goals foster adaptive achievement behaviors, including a preference for optimal challenge, positive affect associated with effort, and persistence in the face of obstacles and failure. In contrast, performance goals produce a constellation of maladaptive achievement responses, including challenge avoidance, "giving up," and negative emotional states (e.g., anxiety, lowered self-esteem). These negative reactions are most pronounced when individuals encounter challenging tasks or experience difficulties when performing them. Individuals with the maladaptive pattern of achievement behavior are seriously hampered in the acquisition and display of cognitive skills when they encounter obstacles. Individuals with the adaptive pattern, however, respond to obstacles with renewed effort and often perform even better in the face of such challenges. Although individuals who display these different patterns of achievement behavior do not differ in their intellectual abilities, these motivational patterns can have profound effects on subsequent performance and adjustment.

Given the powerful effects of these goals on achievement behaviors, an effort has been made to identify the determinants of such goals. What makes someone more likely to adopt a performance versus a mastery goal in an achievement setting? Everyone pursues both types of goals at various times, and these goals may even be held simultaneously in some contexts. In other words, some situations afford the opportunity to both learn and perform. But what determines which goal is adopted when choices must be made? The choice of which goal to pursue has been shown to be a function of situational variables and personality factors.

A long history of personality research suggests that people differ in the extent to which they characteristically value and pursue competence, broadly construed. Defined normatively (demonstrating competence relative to others) or self-referentially (developing competence or skills), competence may be differentially valued depending on an individual's characteristic motivational orientation. Contempo-

rary research takes a more differentiated approach to achievement motivation, identifying personality characteristics that are related to these different goal orientations: the desire to attain mastery and the inclination to work hard in the face of challenge versus the more competitive desire to outperform others and surpass normative standards. Other research examines individual differences in performance versus mastery goal orientations in classroom settings and relates these variables to motivation and performance in the academic contexts.

Another approach relates achievement goals to individuals' implicit theories about the determinants of intelligence; specifically, when people hold an "incremental theory," believing that ability is malleable and can be improved, they are oriented to *developing* and improving that trait and thus are more likely to adopt learning goals in performance situations. Those who hold an "entity theory" believe that intelligence is a fixed, unchangeable trait and tend to orient toward gaining favorable judgments of that trait and to adopt performance goals. Moreover, they are motivated to *protect* positive judgments of intelligence and ability and are therefore less likely to take on difficult or challenging tasks if they risk losing a positive judgment in the process. A person who believes intelligence is malleable can better afford to risk negative feedback, because it simply means they should try harder the next time. Attributing failure to a lack of ability can have debilitating effects on motivation and performance, whereas attributing failure to effort promotes positive performance expectations and success-oriented behaviors. These findings suggest that causal attributions are a key variable in successful school performance. This approach has also been extended to the study of peer relationships and social skills, with clear implications for social skills, interpersonal relations, and adjustment.

These different goal orientations may also be implicit in a variety of situations, classroom structures, and settings. Some contexts may emphasize competition, interpersonal comparison, and the demonstration of competence; others may stress intrapersonal comparisons, personal improvement ("Just do your best"), and the development of competence. Thus the context can elicit the adoption of performance versus mastery goals, respectively. A large body of research has examined the environmental determinants of these goal orientations, either by experimentally manipulating situational features in laboratory studies or by studying classroom structure in field studies. Evaluative and competitive situations appear to engender the maladaptive achievement behaviors associated with performance goals, whereas situations that emphasize personal improvement and mastery promote adaptive achievement behaviors. One important line of research by Eccles and colleagues has related the structure of junior high school education, which represents a transition to a more evaluative and performance-oriented style of education, to the well-documented decrements in adjustment, performance, and motivation often seen in adolescents at this stage of development.

VI. ACHIEVEMENT GOALS AND INTRINSIC MOTIVATION

Given their mutual reliance on the competence construct, it is not surprising that there have been attempts to bridge the achievement goals and intrinsic motivation literatures. Most theorists have argued that performance and mastery goals should affect intrinsic motivation through the same processes that influence achievement behavior. Consequently, they predict that mastery goals will promote intrinsic motivation by fostering challenge seeking, persistence, and task involvement. Performance goals, on the other hand, should undermine intrinsic motivation by generating evaluative pressure or anxiety about performance. However, in 1993, Harackiewicz and Elliot suggested that the effects of performance goals on intrinsic motivation are more complex than this analysis implies. Performance goals may serve to highlight competence issues in situations where competence is not necessarily salient (e.g., enjoyable activities). If individuals typically define competence in terms of ability and normative comparisons, a performance goal orientation can make them more likely to think about or value their competence at an activity, thereby intensifying the positive impact of competence processes on intrinsic motivation. Thus, performance goals might even enhance intrinsic motivation when they lead people to notice, value, or appreciate their competence at an activity, at least when people are successful in attaining these goals. Recent studies indicate that a performance goal orientation can, in fact, enhance intrinsic motivation for some individuals, specifically for those who are characteristically oriented toward achievement. Thus

it is important to consider person–situation interactions in accounting for the effects of goals on motivation.

VII. TASK-SPECIFIC TARGET GOALS

In addition to achievement goals, researchers have been interested in the effects of even more specific goals on performance and motivation. There is evidence to suggest that clear, task-based standards for performance (e.g., solve at least three problems, stuff 14 envelopes) will enhance motivation and productivity. These lower-order goals act as targets for performance, and they are necessarily specific to a particular task in a particular context. As such, they allow the individual to compare performance with the goal and provide ongoing feedback through a feedback loop process. Individuals can monitor and adjust their behavior to bring it closer to their target goals. These goals can boost performance and intrinsic motivation through self-efficacy mechanisms; by helping individuals focus on the specific task at hand, they gain a sense of competence as they regulate their behavior.

Recent studies suggest that specific, attainable goals can enhance intrinsic motivation by providing individuals with ongoing feedback about their developing competence and by helping individuals become more involved in an activity. However, these effects have also been shown to depend on the individual's higher-order goals and to vary as a function of the goals implicit in the situation.

VIII. INTERPLAY OF GOALS

Recent findings emphasize the importance of considering a multiplicity of goals and the possibility that any given goal does not exist to the exclusion of other goals. In classrooms and in life, multiple goals may operate simultaneously, and more research is needed to explore the dynamic interplay among goals that are not necessarily mutually exclusive. For example, there is evidence that a multiple goals perspective may represent a more accurate picture of students in school contexts, and that holding both performance and mastery goals can be beneficial for classroom achievement, intrinsic interest in the course material, and social adjustment.

It is also important to consider the interplay of goals at different levels of specificity. Higher-order goals may establish the context in which an activity is performed and in which individuals regulate their ongoing behavior with respect to specific goals. One hierarchical model of goals and intrinsic motivation focuses on the match between the general goals that individuals pursue at the outset of task engagement and the specific competence information and feedback provided during the course of task performance. Achievement goals can establish a motivational context for task performance that can influence how people perceive and respond to the specific competence information they receive during the process of task engagement. According to this model, intrinsic motivation should be optimized when the process and outcome of task engagement is congruent with the initial achievement goal held by the individual. Both types of achievement goals have the potential to enhance intrinsic motivation, the critical determinant being whether or not the general goal is consistent with the specific type of competence information provided in the situation.

By considering the more general goals literature and analyzing the effects of goals (studied at several different levels in the goal hierarchy) on intrinsic motivation, we can examine intrinsic motivation in the context of what individuals are trying to accomplish in their lives. Moreover, the study of intrinsic motivation enriches the study of goals by providing a more detailed analysis of the *process* of task engagement and of individuals' experiences while pursuing their goals.

BIBLIOGRAPHY

Bandura, A. (1986). *Social foundations of thought and action: A social cognitive theory.* Englewood Cliffs, NJ: Prentice Hall.

Cantor, N., & Zirkel, S. (1990). Personality, cognition, and purposive behavior. In L. A. Pervin (Ed.), *Handbook of personality theory and research* (pp. 135–164). New York: Guilford.

Csikszentmihalyi, M. (1990). *Flow: The psychology of optimal experience.* New York: Harper Perennial.

Deci, E. L., & Ryan, R. M. (1985). *Intrinsic motivation and self-determination in human behavior.* New York: Plenum.

Dweck, C. S. (1986). Motivational processes affecting learning. *American Psychologist, 41,* 1040–1048.

Harackiewicz, J. M., & Elliot, A. J. (1993). Achievement goals and intrinsic motivation. *Journal of Personality and Social Psychology, 65,* 904–915.

Harackiewicz, J. M., Manderlink, G., & Sansone, C. (1984). Rewarding pinball wizardry: Effects of evaluation and cue value on intrinsic interest. *Journal of Personality and Social Psychology, 47,* 287–300.

Harackiewicz, J. M., & Sansone, C. (1991). Goals and intrinsic motivation: You can get there from here. In M. L. Maehr & P. R. Pintrich (Eds.), *Advances in motivation and achievement* (Vol. 7, pp. 21–49). Greenwich, CT: JAI Press.

Kasser, T., & Ryan, R. M. (1993). A dark side of the American dream: Correlates of financial success as a central life aspiration. *Journal of Personality and Social Psychology, 65,* 410–422.

Lepper, M. R., Greene, D., & Nisbett, R. E. (1973). Undermining children's intrinsic interest with extrinsic reward: A test of the overjustification hypothesis. *Journal of Personality and Social Psychology, 28,* 129–137.

Locke, E. A., & Latham, G. P. (1990). *A theory of goal setting and task performance.* Englewood Cliffs, NJ: Prentice Hall.

Sansone, C., & Harackiewicz, J. M. (1995). "I don't feel like it": The function of interest in self-regulation. In L. Martin & A. Tesser (Eds.), *Striving and feeling: Interactions between goals, affect, and self-regulation* (pp. 203-228). Hillsdale, NJ: Erlbaum.

Sansone, C., Sachau, D. A., & Weir, C. (1989). The effects of instruction on intrinsic interest: The importance of context. *Journal of Personality and Social Psychology, 57,* 819–829.

Sansone, C., Weir, C., Harpster, L., & Morgan, C. (1992). Once a boring task always a boring task? Interest as a self-regulatory mechanism. *Journal of Personality and Social Psychology, 63,* 379–390.

Williams, G. C., Grow, V. M., Freedman, Z., Ryan, R. M., & Deci, E. L. (1996). Motivational predictors of weight loss and weight-loss maintenance. *Journal of Personality and Social Psychology, 70,* 115–126.

L

Legal Dimensions of Mental Health

Ross A. Thompson

University of Nebraska

I. Introduction
II. Mental Health and Responsibility
III. Mental Health and Liberty
IV. Mental Health and Compensation
V. Mental Health and Prevention
VI. Conclusion

Civil Commitment The involuntary treatment (typically hospitalization) of individuals who are deemed by courts to be mentally disordered and thus requiring care, and sometimes confinement, because they can be dangerous to themselves or to others.

Forensic Professional practices associated with a court of law.

Guardianship/Conservatorship The delegation of decision-making authority concerning the care and protection of the person (*guardianship*) or possessions (*conservatorship*) of individuals who are deemed, by courts, to be incompetent to make these decisions.

Mental State at the Time of the Offense (MSO) A determination by a mental health professional concerning a criminal defendant's psychological condition related to criminal culpability or intent, which may result in pleas of "not guilty by reason of insanity," "guilty but mentally ill," or assertions of diminished capacity.

Therapeutic Jurisprudence A new theoretical orientation for examining the integration of law and mental health, based on the view that the law is a powerful social force with potentially therapeutic impact on those it influences.

Tort Law A body of law to provide compensation for damages suffered by one person by another; in ad-

dition to traditional torts of battery, assault, slander, and false imprisonment, more recent torts such as "intentional infliction of emotional distress" encompass more explicitly mental and psychological harms.

Worker's Compensation A system of regulations designed to provide financial relief to workers who are accidently injured on their jobs to compensate for the loss of future earning power; mental or psychological factors may figure prominently in "worker's comp" claims.

LEGAL DIMENSIONS OF MENTAL HEALTH encompass the variety of legal problems requiring mental health perspectives, as well as the legal regulation of mental health practice. These issues require the thoughtful interaction of mental health practitioners with legal actors and agency representatives, as well as considerable multidisciplinary competency and ethical sensitivity by the clinician. This article presents a selective overview of legal dimensions of mental health, focusing especially on psycholegal questions of (a) mental health and responsibility, (b) mental health and liberty, (c) mental health and compensation, and (d) mental health and prevention, to illustrate the breadth of issues that jointly engage mental health specialists and legal actors.

I. INTRODUCTION

When considering the legal aspects of mental health, practitioners typically (and unsurprisingly) think first of legal liability concerning malpractice and other aspects of professional regulation. While these are important features of professional practice, for most mental health practitioners they do not constitute their primary avenues of contact with the legal system. Instead, mental health specialists may be enlisted in a variety of other ways into legal forums, whether as expert witnesses concerning the assessment of mental disability or psychological trauma in the context of a civil lawsuit, as forensic evaluators in the determination of an individual's capacity to make legally relevant choices and decisions, in guardianship and conservatorship proceedings, in judicial hearings concerning a child's best interests in conflicts over child custody or allegations of abuse, and even in criminal proceedings when the specialist's assessment of criminal responsibility and culpability may be essential. In a surprisingly diverse variety of forums, mental health specialists offer crucial expertise that is relevant to judicial determinations concerning competency, responsibility, culpability, self-determination, capability, and even future potential.

Recognizing that mental health practice intersects with the legal world in various ways apart from concerns with professional liability and malpractice means that the skills required of the mental health practitioner extend far beyond knowing and complying with legal standards of professional conduct. In addition, mental health specialists must become skilled at working collaboratively with legal actors and agency representatives who have perspectives and goals that may be much different from their own. It requires understanding the legal process and the appropriate (and inappropriate) roles of mental health specialists in offering expert testimony and other forms of evidence. It involves maintaining a current grasp not only of the professional clinical literature but also of cognate research findings that are relevant to clinical expertise, as well as professional standards related to forensic assessment. It requires distinguishing the questions for which psychological expertise is relevant from the ultimate legal questions that are reserved for the court. Moreover, working in the legal world requires also an acute sensitivity to the breadth and limitations of professional expertise: an ability to clearly distinguish what is known with confidence from what is unknown or uncertain in psychological research findings or clinical experience, and the ability to convey these limitations candidly and accurately in legal forums. Finally, the intersection of

law with mental health requires also an ethical awareness of the multiple and sometimes conflicting roles of the mental health specialist, and the knowledge of how best to address the challenges of professional ethics in legal settings.

This article is written to provide a general overview of the diverse questions, roles, and challenges entailed in the legal dimensions of mental health. This discussion is organized in terms of several constellations of legal questions requiring the expertise of psychological specialists. First, questions of mental health and responsibility are considered because these constitute the core of criminal and mental health law. These include the contributions of mental health specialists to the assessment of criminal responsibility and the relevance of clinical theories to legal questions of culpability, but they also extend to questions of the determination of a person's capacity to exercise legal rights as well as responsibilities. Second, questions of mental health and liberty are considered because these constitute many of the practical contexts in which psychological specialists offer substantive expertise to courts. These questions include the determination of incompetency related to civil commitment, the ability to consent to or to refuse treatment, and even the termination of parental rights. Third, questions of mental health and compensation are briefly considered because these constitute primary problems of forensic assessment of disability and injury, especially with respect to mental and psychological trauma and its effects on future capability. Fourth, and finally, questions of mental health and prevention are considered because these constitute crucial considerations in the prevention of psychological dysfunction and the promotion of mental health. These questions include developmental considerations that pertain to determining children's "best interests" in custody disputes or their future in the context of allegations of child maltreatment. More broadly, they also encompass issues concerning the role of legal policies and procedures in the promotion of mental health, which has been addressed recently in theories of "therapeutic jurisprudence."

Although this selective survey emphasizes diverse issues of forensic assessment and estimates of disability and competency, it is important to recognize that issues of professional liability and malpractice remain important legal issues for mental health practitioners. Indeed, with the current expansion of the roles and responsibilities commonly assumed by mental health practitioners, professional and legal issues associated with exercising due care in the diagnosis and treatment of a client's illness or disability have become correspondingly more complex and multidimensional. Professional organizations have helped to articulate expected standards of conduct and to provide enforcement processes for clinical specialists. Although there will be little further consideration of these legal dimensions of professional liability, the remaining topics in this chapter indicate the variety of complex responsibilities that have become part of many mental health specialists' professional obligations in recent years, requiring greater understanding of professional expectations, ethics, and standards of expertise. Moreover, issues of professional responsibility assume added meaning in the context of the mental health professional's assistance to courts, where ethical issues concerning the interaction of psychological and legal authority can be profound. Taken together, therefore, the breadth with which the topic of "legal dimensions of mental health" is currently defined has important implications for issues of professional liability and responsibility, as well as reflecting the broadened roles of mental health specialists in the legal system.

II. MENTAL HEALTH AND RESPONSIBILITY

In the law, individuals are responsible for their actions when they are competent to make choices. As a consequence, questions of competency in relation to responsibility permeate criminal and civil law, whether they pertain to a person's competency to stand trial, competency to enter into a contract, competency to consent to (or decline) medical treatment, or responsibility for criminal conduct based on their mental state at the time of the offense (MSO). Not surprisingly, mental health specialists are commonly enlisted in legal forums to conduct such competency assessments. The manner in which they do so—and the professional responsibilities they assume—depend on the nature of the actions for which an individual might be held responsible.

A. Competency to Stand Trial

One of the most frequently adjudicated competency issues concerns the determination of a defendant's competency to stand trial for a criminal offense. It is not difficult to understand why: defense attorneys may request competency evaluations because of their concerns about a client's mental condition, but they do so for other reasons also, such as to obtain other information concerning the defendant's condition that might be useful to the defense, and to delay court proceedings. Attorney requests for competency evaluations are usually granted by courts, and this typically results in an assessment by one or more clinicians in conditions that may range from an extended inpatient evaluation at a state institution to a more brief, outpatient assessment procedure. This variability in the typical duration and intensity of competency assessment procedures is striking in view of the fairly straightforward legal standard that must be satisfied. Essentially, mental health specialists are to assist the court in determining whether the individual is capable of consulting competency with his or her attorney and whether he or she sufficiently understands the legal proceedings.

This assessment of competency is both minimal and functional: it does not require a psychiatric diagnosis, an evaluation of the defendant's state of mind at the time of the offense, or a comprehensive portrayal of the individual's mental status or personality functioning. Indeed, it may be unhelpful for clinicians to approach the legal standard of competency from the standpoint of psychiatric diagnosis, because diagnostic syndromes are not typically directly relevant to legal standards of competency. For example, the fact that an individual is clinically depressed or psychotic may or may not be relevant to their ability to participate rationally in their legal defense. Because the legal criteria are minimal, however, it is perhaps unsurprising that the large majority of individuals who are assessed are found to be competent to stand trial. Those who are found incompetent are typically characterized by a history of involvement with both the criminal justice and mental health systems. Perhaps equally unsurprising is growing research evidence that competency evaluations do not necessarily require inpatient evaluation, extended assessment procedures, or even the participation of a medical or doctoral-level forensic evaluator. Instead, a variety of assessment procedures (including structured interviews and questionnaires) with demonstrated validity and reliability can be used either as primary evaluation tools or, equally usefully, as screening instruments to identify the subset of individuals requiring more detailed forensic evaluation. There is also evidence that these assessments can be used effectively by psychiatric social workers and other clinically experienced individuals who do not have medical or doctoral-level training.

B. Competencies to Confess, Plead Guilty, Waive Counsel, and Sentencing Considerations

Somewhat more complex considerations accompany other kinds of competency evaluations in criminal proceedings. For example, determinations of an individual's competency to confess to a crime is typically based on an assessment of whether that person knowingly, intelligently, and voluntarily waived their rights against self-incrimination, or alternatively whether their confession is inadmissible because of intoxication, intimidation, or mental impairment. This can be a challenging evaluation because the clinician must retrospectively assess a previous state of mind that may be much different from the defendant's current condition. Analogous considerations apply to determinations of an individual's competencies to plead guilty or to waive the right to counsel, except that a somewhat different constellation of rights must be demonstrably understood in order for the person to be deemed competent in their waiver.

After a criminal verdict has been rendered, moreover, the mental health professional's contributions to the court may be extended to sentencing considerations. Clinical assessments may figure prominently in identifying mitigating circumstances related to culpability and punishment; assessing the potential for rehabilitation; assisting the court in sentencing repeat offenders, youthful offenders, individuals found guilty of capital crimes, and other special cases; contributing to the complex determinations involved in special sentencing provisions for individuals deemed "mentally disordered sex offenders" and "guilty but mentally ill"; and (after sentencing) assisting in evaluating treatment needs for convicted defendants. Although the contributions of clinical specialists to these different sentencing considerations can vary widely, in each case they entail presenting to the court specialized information concerning the defendant's mental status and how this particular offender may compare with others the court has previously seen.

C. Mental State at the Time of the Offense

Clearly, the most controversial competency determination in criminal courts concerns a defendant's mental state at the time of the offense (MSO), which may lead to various defense pleas: not guilty by reason of insanity, diminished capacity, or "guilty but mentally ill." Insanity pleas are controversial because of public perceptions that they are commonly used in criminal courts, and result in the acquittal and subsequent release of large numbers of individuals who remain extremely dangerous. By and large, these perceptions are inaccurate: insanity pleas are rarely used in criminal cases and are rarely successful (and successful cases often result from plea bargains in which prosecutors agree that the defendant was incompetent), and individuals who are so acquitted are usually confined for treatment for a sustained period. But public concern over the potentially inappropriate overuse of such defenses does not ease the clinician's assessment task.

There are also important distinctions between various defenses related to an individual's mental state at the time of the offense. A successful insanity defense, for example, addresses the defendant's fundamental responsibility for criminal conduct, and results in acquittal and commitment for treatment. By contrast, a "diminished capacity" defense is concerned with more specific questions of criminal intent, and may result in acquittal without requiring treatment or conviction on a lesser charge. As an alternative to these two defenses that may result in release of the defendant or treatment in a noncorrectional setting, "guilty but mentally ill" defenses have more recently been authorized by state legislatures to permit judges and juries to find a defendant guilty but suffering from mental illness and can require treatment in the context of incarceration.

In general, insanity defenses require evidence that the defendant suffered from a "mental disease or defect" at the time of the offense that was directly related to culpability for criminal conduct. This can include cognitive impairment that rendered the individual incapable of knowing the nature and wrongness of the criminal act, or a psychiatric or medical condition that produced a loss of control over actions. This is a dauntingly complex determination not only because of the importance of assessing mental functioning and its relevance to criminal culpability, but also because of the necessity of doing so retrospectively—that is, drawing conclusions about the defendant's mental state at the time of the offense, not the present moment. The limited relevance of many standard clinical assessment procedures to such a retrospective analysis, especially in the context of criminal proceedings (in which a legal, not a psychiatric or medical, standard must be addressed), exacerbates the clinician's difficulties. Moreover, because the defendant has a large stake in the outcome of this determination, the MSO investigation may be encumbered by concerns with the defendant's credibility, the defendant's distrust of the clinician, or the impact of the stresses of recent events on his or her mental state, as well as the ethical dilemmas for the mental health professional that may arise from the importance of the evaluation for the defendant in the context of these uncertainties concerning the reasons for the defendant's behavior.

Consequently, a typical MSO investigation is more comprehensive and complex than many conventional clinical assessments. It often relies heavily on third-party sources of information, such as knowledge about the crime itself drawn from police and attorneys, records of prior psychiatric hospitalization and/or treatment, prior court proceedings, interviews with witnesses and codefendants, and conversations with family members. The interview with the defendant is also likely to be atypical (compared to a usual clinical assessment) because greater effort must be devoted to explaining the reasons for the evaluation and establishing rapport, as well as discussing specific aspects of the alleged offense. Efforts to test the credibility of the defendant's presenting symptoms or reports of disturbance, or to penetrate memory lapses of the alleged offense, can also complicate the interview. In addition, certain psychobiological assessments may be necessary to confirm or eliminate consideration of the influence of organic disorders on the defendant's mental state, such as brain damage. It is not surprising, therefore, that Melton, Petrila, Poythress, and Slobogin have characterized clinical examiners in MSO assessments as "investigative reporters." Although there have been efforts to streamline and systematize this comprehensive information-gathering procedure (most notably, in the Rogers Criminal Responsibility Assessment Scales [RCRAS], which require ratings of key dimensions of the MSO assessment), it can often be an extended, complex process for the clinician. However, there is also fairly good evidence that well-conducted MSO investigations yield not only reliable but also reasonably valid determinations.

In the end, the mental health professional should avoid offering a final judgment of whether the defendant was (or was not) legally insane at the time of the offense. Instead, the clinician's responsibility is to provide all pertinent forensic information that will enable the court to make this final determination. This is important because a judgment concerning whether a defendant's mental state at the time of the offense reduces or excuses culpability is a legal determination for which courts have sole as well as ultimate responsibility. While the mental health professional's expert testimony may figure prominently in this legal determination, it is important not to confuse the clinician's psychological assessment of this mental state from the legal judgments of the judge or jury. By failing to distinguish these, the clinician risks assuming a more authoritative role than she or he can legitimately claim and, at worst, may mislead the legal authorities responsible for such a judgment.

III. MENTAL HEALTH AND LIBERTY

The issues discussed above concerning mental health and criminal culpability highlight a number of ethical issues that make clinical assessments for the courts a complex professional responsibility. In addition to the challenges of addressing legal standards of competency using clinical tools, mental health specialists encounter more fundamental dilemmas concerning the nature of their professional roles. One dilemma concerns identifying who is the client. In therapy, the client's identity is clear. He or she is the person receiving therapy, and clinical evaluations are intended to contribute toward that person's eventual health and well-being. By contrast, in legal contexts clinicians may experience competing obligations toward the defendant who is being evaluated and the court and/or attorney(s) requesting the evaluation, each of whom may be regarded as the mental health professional's client. While the forensic evaluation may assist the court in making judgments concerning the defendant's criminal culpability or competency to stand trial, these judgments have much different significance for defendants that may (from their perspective) either significantly enhance or undermine their well-being. Thus the mental health professional's typical helping role toward the client is significantly complicated, and often conflicted, when psychological evaluations are performed for the court.

Other ethical dilemmas concern the assurance of confidentiality to promote trust in the clinician, and respect for individual privacy (including the freedom to participate or not in clinical assessments). Each of these assurances is essential to successful therapy but also to effective psychological evaluation, since free and confidential disclosure is necessary to the candor required in assessments of mental state and psychological functioning. But clinical specialists cannot guarantee confidentiality in forensic assessments because their reports will be read by various attorneys and court officials, nor can defendants easily exercise their freedom to choose or decline to participate, or to resist privacy intrusions, as clients typically do in most clinical settings. Consequently, mental health specialists often experience considerable uncertainty in considering how best to create a psychological climate that is well-suited to an effective psychological evaluation in the midst of legal procedures that instead foster skepticism, distrust, anxiety, or dishonesty in the client. Mental health specialists also experience conflicts when they seek to generalize to forensic evaluations the roles they typically assume in clinical contexts as trusted confidantes who are unreserved advocates for the client. In many respects, they are instead (in the words of Melton and colleagues) "double agents" whose obligations to the courts can create conflicting loyalties.

These ethical dilemmas are apparent not only in the context of criminal investigations and trials, but also in civil courts where issues concerning mental health and liberty are contested. By contrast with questions concerning criminal responsibility, legal questions pertaining to liberty concern the circumstances in which individuals who have committed no crime can nevertheless be coerced into conditions that are not of their choosing, often entailing the abridgement of fundamental rights. These issues include the determination of incompetency related to civil commitment, the appointment of a guardian or conservator, the ability to consent to or to refuse treatment, or even to retain parental rights to the care of offspring.

A. Civil Commitment

In civil commitment proceedings, a court must determine whether an individual is mentally disordered to the extent that involuntary treatment (typically hospitalization) is required to provide care and, perhaps equally important, prevent the person's possible harm to themselves or others. Civil commitment can require inpatient hospitalization, but recent years have witnessed increasing outpatient civil commitment in most states. Not surprisingly, mental health professionals assume a significant, often preeminent, role in these legal actions because of their expertise in assessing both the nature and consequences of an individual's mental condition, as well as predicting the risk of future harm. Moreover, the relatively vague legal standards governing civil commitment make the mental health professional's contribution especially important because of the self-acknowledged limitations in judges' and juries' capabilities to assess these psychological processes in mentally disordered individuals. Finally, because civil commitment is a civil rather than criminal procedure, the relative informality and diminished adversarial nature of the proceedings enhance the clinician's influence, but this makes the responsibility for cautious, ethically informed contributions equally important.

Although state statutes vary, civil commitment is typically based on several determinations concerning an individual's mental condition that, taken alone or in combination, may result in a civil commitment order. First, individuals may be shown to suffer from a substantial mental disorder with significant consequences for their capacity to function effectively on their own (some states include a provision that the individual is, as a consequence, unable to recognize the need for treatment). This requires a clinical assessment that resembles the typical process of psychiatric diagnosis. Second, individuals may be shown to be a danger to themselves and/or others as a result of the mental disorder. This requires an estimation from the mental health professional concerning current or future proneness to harm. Concerning potential danger to self, evidence concerning suicidal ideation or past attempts may be pertinent. Concerning potential danger to others, the clinician must (as in sentencing hearings described above) consider homicidal motives or intent, prior history of violent behavior, potential circumstances in the future that might increase (or diminish) violent tendencies, and other characteristics of the individual that are directly relevant to predictions of future dangerousness. As earlier noted, such estimations of dangerousness are difficult, even for skilled clinicians, because of the complexity of human behavior and the indeterminacy of estimating future conditions provoking violence. Third, in most states, individuals may be shown to be unable to care for themselves as a consequence of their mental disorder, and that they need treatment. Although this is related to the diagnostic process that is enlisted into other aspects of the civil commitment determination, it requires also the clinician's judgment concerning the relevance of the mental disorder to the capacity to function effectively in society, and the treatment required if individuals are unable to do so. In some states, moreover, explicit consideration of the location of treatment is also encompassed within civil commitment proceedings, usually with respect to identifying the setting that best affords assistance to the person. Thus, for example, comparing the advisability of hospitalization rather than outpatient or community-based treatment may be required.

Civil commitment procedures can be inaugurated by an emergency hospitalization resulting from a perceived need (by family, friends, police, a clinician, or others acquainted with the individual) to act quickly to prevent harm to the person or to others. There is considerable clinical and judicial discretion in the conditions warranting such immediate, emergency hospital admissions. Before long (within 2 to 3 days in most jurisdictions, but after a considerably longer duration in some), however, a commitment hearing must occur that involves representation by counsel, the opportunity to call and cross-examine witnesses, and the chance to present and examine other evidence concerning the individual's mental state. Although these procedures are adversarial in nature—with both parties allowed to present and rebut relevant evidence—these procedures are considerably less formal than are criminal trials, and may be adversarial in name only if the respondent's attorney (who is frequently court-appointed) is convinced of the need for hospitalization of her or his client. The same is true of the review hearings that must be held periodically after a commitment order has been made in order to determine whether the individual continues to satisfy the criteria for civil commitment. In all cases, considerable deference is accorded the mental health professional who, after having examined the person in question, offers an authoritative judgment concerning that individual's mental condition and other characteristics that is often unquestioned by the judicial decision makers involved.

Deference to mental health specialists occurs both because of the "medicalization" of civil commitment procedures—in which issues of psychiatric diagnosis, capacity for self-care, and clinical estimates of dangerousness are paramount—combined with the ambiguity of statutory terms like "mental disorder" and "danger to oneself or others." The intuitive belief of judges and jurors that psychiatrists and psychologists know best whether individuals are disordered, and whether they should be civilly committed, heightens the mental health specialist's influence over civil commitment procedures, but also the ethical need for caution in their determinations. Quite often, considerations such as whether an individual who suffers from a psychiatric condition is nevertheless capable of living effectively in society, or whether treatment but not hospitalization is required, are unlikely to be raised in civil commitment hearings except by the clinical professional. Moreover, the uncertainties inevitably attending a psychological evaluation of an individual who is under considerable stress and (potentially) confusion, is distrustful of others, experiences considerable powerlessness, and is anxious and uncertain about his or her current circumstances and future are unlikely to be voiced except by the mental health professional. In the end, because the clinician's judgment is very likely to be dispositive in civil commitment proceedings, the mental health professional bears a weighty ethical reponsibility for appropriately cautious, thoughtful judgments.

B. Guardianship and Conservatorship

Civil commitment can be followed by the appointment of a guardian over individuals who are deemed incompetent to care for themselves. But in other circumstances, guardians are appointed for people who are living in the community with assistance, but who are incompetent to manage their own care and/or their possessions. In these instances, courts may appoint *guardians* who have decision-making authority to provide for the care and protection of the person, or *conservators* who have authority to manage their possessions and estate, when individuals have been determined incompetent to make these decisions. Such appointments can either entail general authority over these issues of care and management or, alternatively, may entail more limited authority over specific decisions (such as giving consent to nonroutine medical treatment, or specific real estate transactions). In each case, the guardian or conservator is required to act in the best interests of the person for whom they have been appointed.

Mental health professionals assume a central role in guardianship and conservatorship proceedings for the same reasons they do so in civil commitment proceedings. The statutory standards for such appointments are rather general, requiring determinations concerning both mental competency and the capacity for self-care or management of one's possessions. The judicial procedures associated with guardianship/conservatorship appointments may be relatively informal, often lacking the vigorous advocacy that characterizes criminal proceedings. And lawyers and judges may be relatively inexpert in assessing the skills required for self-care or management of one's estate. For these reasons—and because of the impact of guardianship/conservatorship determinations on an individual's autonomy and well-being—mental health professionals must be as conscientious as possible in their assessment of the capabilities of the person in question. In contrast to civil commitment determinations, in which a psychiatric diagnosis figures prominently in judicial considerations, the assessments associated with the appointment of a guardian or conservator are functional in nature. In essence, the clinician must determine what the person can and cannot do, and what capabilities exist with assistance and support from others. This requires proceeding beyond diagnostic considerations to a detailed assessment of a person's specific skills associated with managing medical care, money, diet, and hygiene, as well as competencies in creating and maintaining satisfactory living arrangements, using transportation, communicating effectively with others, maintaining the household, engaging in financial planning and, for some, managing a complex estate. These functional assessments are important not only because (as earlier noted) these capabilities may not be well-reflected in a general diagnostic assignment, but also because they require different evaluative procedures by the clinician, such as visiting the individual at home, than are typical for clinical assessments. Such an evaluation is crucial, however, because of its relevance to the determination not only of whether guardianship/conservatorship is necessary, but also whether a general or limited appointment is warranted. For this reason, clinicians should refrain from addressing the ultimate legal question of whether a guardian or conservator should (or should not) be appointed, and instead provide

courts with as much detailed information concerning the individual's competencies as possible.

C. Other Kinds of Liberty

Psychological evaluations pertaining to civil commitment are necessarily broad because of the comprehensive infringement on individual liberty that is entailed in a person's commitment. Somewhat narrower evaluations are entailed in guardianship/conservatorship determinations because of the more limited domains of personal freedom that are delegated to the authority of another, especially under limited guardianships. When mental health professionals evaluate individuals concerning even more specific competencies, such as those entailed in freedom of choice, their assessments are narrower still. For example, when determining the competency of individuals to consent to or decline treatment for medical or psychological disorders, the clinical expert must assess specifically (a) the extent to which consent/refusal has been truly informed (i.e., all pertinent information has been provided), (b) the extent to which consent/refusal has occurred with understanding and a reasonable decision-making process (i.e., focusing on the cognitive and motivational processes of the individual), and (c) the extent to which consent/refusal has been voluntary (i.e., was not coerced). These determinations rely less on conventional diagnostic classifications than on specific competencies related to treatment decision making and the social–psychological context in which they are exercised. Related considerations apply to psychological evaluations of competency to consent to research participation and other activities. Significantly more challenging are psychological evaluations associated with testamentary capacity—that is, an individual's competency to exercise the reasoned choices entailed in executing a will. Especially if the individual in question is deceased at the time this assessment is requested (which is usually the case), the clinician assumes the role of an investigator who uses diverse sources of indirect evidence bearing on the extent to which that person was "of sound mind" and was not improperly influenced by others in making her or his will.

As these considerations suggest, the mental health professional must often conduct psychological evaluations in conditions of indeterminacy, when clinical judgments of complex mental and psychological conditions are uncertain and probabilistic rather than confident. This is especially true when assessments of liberty in relation to the mental or psychological state of juveniles is concerned. One controversial area in which this may occur concerns the competency of female minors to choose abortion when faced with an unwanted pregnancy. In most jurisdictions, statutes require parental consent whenever a female under the age of majority chooses an abortion, with exceptions for juveniles deemed to be "mature," emancipated, and in other specific, extenuating circumstances. Yet the ambiguity of the statutory definitions of "mature minor" together with the conceptual uncertainty of the psychological criteria of maturity render the clinical expert's opinion in these cases fairly speculative.

In these and other areas of psychological assessment, a candid (and sometimes humbling) acknowledgment to the court of the limitations of psychological expertise and, consequently, the limited authority of the clinician in the courtroom is not only reasonable but perhaps ethically necessary. This is most aptly illustrated in a final area in which the mental health professional advises courts concerning mental health and (the deprivation of) liberty: the termination of parental rights. When parents have been found culpable of child maltreatment, or when their adequacy as caregivers is questioned by legal authorities because of mental illness, mental retardation, chronic substance abuse, or for other reasons, courts often turn to clinical experts for assessments of parental "fitness" and of the quality of the parent–child relationship in determining whether parental rights should be terminated. This is one of the weightiest forensic evaluations for the clinician because of the seriousness of the circumstances and the importance of their judgments for the future well-being of the children, yet it is weighty also because of the inherent ambiguity of the standard for assessing parental competence. How is parental "fitness" assessed? How should the mental health professional weigh aspects of parental incompetency against the emotional attachment that commonly exists between children and their marginally adequate parents? How should evidence of attachment and adequate care be balanced against undesirable qualities of the home environment and parental lifestyle? Because of the limitations in relevant research on these topics and the absence of reliable, well-standardized clinical assessments, mental health professionals are wise to be careful and cautious in their psychological evaluations in

termination of parental rights proceedings, providing detailed description of strengths and weaknesses in parental functioning and the parent–child relationship (without addressing the ultimate legal question of parental "fitness"), and acknowledging to the court the limitations that exist in relevant research and clinical knowledge.

IV. MENTAL HEALTH AND COMPENSATION

Mental health specialists often appear in courtrooms to address the harms suffered by individuals as the result of accidental, negligent, or intentional behavior by others. In worker's compensation claims, for example, workers seek financial awards because of accidental injury or disability resulting from employment, or beneficiaries seek compensation because of the accidental death of a family member. In private lawsuits, individuals seek damages because of harms caused by the action or inaction of another person under tort law. When these claims involve allegations concerning mental injury, emotional distress, or psychological disability, clinical experts are enlisted to provide psychological evaluations concerning the nature of the harm that has been suffered, its relation to the actions (or negligence) of another (such as an employer), and its significance for the plaintiff's future. Although worker's compensation regulations and tort law have traditionally been slow to recognize the importance of mental and psychological harm independent of other types of damage, this is changing with the growth of tort claims like "intentional infliction of emotional distress" and other kinds of compensable causes of action. The increasing incidence of such claims and the importance of forensic evaluations to their disposition make the mental health professional a central figure in such disputes. This is especially so in private lawsuits, when the clinician's assessment can be crucial not only to the determination of culpability, but also to the amount of damages awarded.

Psychological evaluations associated with compensation claims are extraordinarily difficult, however, because of the multifaceted assessment that is required. The clinician must not only determine what kind of mental or psychological injury has occurred (and what kind of harm), but must also conduct a retrospective reconstruction of the individual's condition prior to the incident to determine whether the injury arose from a specific alleged event. In addition, a prospective assessment is required: in worker's compensation claims it pertains to the impact of the injury on the person's future wage-earning capability; in tort law, it concerns the extent to which the individual is incapable of functioning in the future as he or she did previous to the incident. Consequently, a wide-ranging inquiry is required involving a detailed history, examination of preexisting psychological problems, prior employment performance, an assessment of potentially related harms (e.g., medical problems) also suffered in the incident in question, a complete assessment of current psychological functioning, as well as detailed information concerning postincident behavior in work and elsewhere with special attention to its prognostic import. This complex, multilayered investigation is made additionally difficult by the pressures on the clinician to provide an account that is amenable to the party enlisting her or his services, which increases the importance of careful reflection about personal biases as well as social influences, and ethical sensitivity to the role of the mental health professional in the legal determination of liability and compensation.

These considerations are pertinent also to a different area of law in which clinical experts assume a somewhat similar professional role. Mental health practitioners are often asked to contribute to determinations related to a person's entitlement to services and assistance as a result of disability. For example, the Social Security Disability Insurance (SSDI) and Supplemental Security Income (SSI) programs comprise much of the federal government's effort to assist individuals who are incapable of working. When mental or psychological impairments are in question, clinical experts are often asked to determine whether an individual suffers from one or more of a range of eligible disabilities or, if not, whether their disabilities render them otherwise incapable of employment. Pertinent regulations require that the clinician conduct a detailed psychological evaluation (involving diagnostic assessment as well as behavioral observations) in the context of a detailed history, with attention to the severity of disability as well as its amenability to treatment.

These assessment considerations foreshadow an increased role for mental health practitioners in determinations related to disability, discrimination and compensation under the provisions of the Americans with Disabilities Act and other statutes. Moreover, the significant changes in mental health services with the growth of managed care raise other important issues for clinical experts concerning the availability and financing of mental health service delivery systems for individuals with demonstrated need and eligibility for mandated services.

V. MENTAL HEALTH AND PREVENTION

One important feature of a clinician's professional role is to create conditions fostering well-being and the prevention of mental illness, and this is also true in psycholegal contexts. While mental health professionals are most commonly enlisted into legal forums to conduct assessments related to disability, incompetency, and/or dangerousness, they are also often asked to provide judgments concerning the factors contributing to a person's future mental health. This is most apparent in the evaluations associated with determining treatment needs for individuals who have been found not guilty by reason of insanity or guilty but mentally ill, but it is also implicitly apparent in psychological assessments associated with determining compensation in tort actions arising from prior injury or distress. More broadly, it is arguable that clinical experts can also contribute to the introduction of more humanistic and therapeutic approaches to jurisprudence because of their expertise as mental health practitioners. In these ways, mental health experts have a proactive role in the courtroom in fostering the prevention of psychological disability as well as their more typical reactive role in assessing mental dysfunction.

The association between mental health and prevention issues is most evident in a variety of judicial considerations pertaining to children and youth. Earlier, we considered the role of clinical experts in the termination of parental rights, when weighty considerations concerning parental fitness and the best interests of offspring are applied to estimating whether children should remain in the care of their biological parents, or be released to the care of others. One reason why mental health experts find psychological assessments concerning the termination of parental rights so vexing is that they entail vague legal standards (e.g., parental "fitness") that require weighing and balancing inestimable factors, such as the strength of a young child's attachment to a marginally adequate caregiver, or the detriments to a child's long-term well-being by remaining with—or being taken from—an alcoholic parent. This can make judgments concerning the conditions fostering the child's future well-being inherently speculative, and can make determinations intended to prevent future harm highly uncertain.

Similar difficulties apply to another area of law in which psychological assessments are enlisted into estimations of future well-being: child custody decisions when parents divorce. Although the large majority of custody decisions are made jointly by parents when they agree to part, legally contested custody disputes can easily consume financial resources, court time, and emotional energy because of the heated and complex considerations they inevitably entail. When mental health professionals become involved in these disputes, they must also confront both the ambiguity of the legal standard governing custody determinations and the difficulties in its assessment. In most jurisdictions, the legal standard requires awarding custody according to the "best interests of the child," an expression that simultaneously articulates the overarching goal of an ideal custody award and glosses over the specific meaning of these interests. Inarticulate in this standard is, for example, a delineation of whether short-term or long-term interests are paramount, or the relative importance of residential stability, economic prosperity, and the child's own wishes, or how to weigh the child's different relationships with each parent. Equally complex are the psychological assessments by which these interests must be appraised and weighed, which should include interviews with each parent (and stepparent) and the child(ren), as well as other informants (e.g., teachers, extended family members) who can provide insight into family dynamics, and other relevant information. However, given that these assessments must occur in the context of the inherent ambiguity of the "best interests of the child" standard, it is perhaps inevitable that such assessments will be shaped by the clinician's own values concerning desirable developmental outcomes in children and the parental practices that foster those outcomes. More than most other psychological topics discussed in this article, therefore, it is important for the mental health practitioner to be careful and cautious in identifying the assumptions underlying his or her evaluation, and articulate with the court concerning these values and their effects on the psychological evaluation.

To be sure, clinical experts can offer useful contri-butions in custody disputes by identifying and summarizing research findings concerning family dynamics relevant to the court's decision (e.g., the impact of marital conflict on child adjustment; the predictors of successful joint custody arrangements; and so forth), as well as by gathering information concerning the family that is relevant to the custody determination. In doing so, of course, mental health professionals should avoid directly addressing the ultimate legal issue of whether the child's "best interests" mandate custody to either parent (or to both parents jointly) both because this is the court's legal judgment to make, and also to avoid introducing into such a judgment the clinician's personal opinions that extend beyond professional expertise. However, when such caution is observed, mental health practitioners can significantly enhance decision making concerning child custody by alerting the court to psychological factors that might not otherwise be considered by the judge.

Indeed, some have argued recently that psychologists have a broader responsibility to bring therapeutic issues into the courtroom in a variety of legal contexts besides child custody disputes. Proponents of "therapeutic jurisprudence" argue that the law is a powerful social force with potentially therapeutic (or antitherapeutic) impact on those it touches. By contrast with a traditional focus on legal doctrine, therapeutic jurisprudence focuses on legal process in an effort to refashion legal procedures, rules, judgments, and roles in order to promote therapeutic as well as legal goals. Working within the framework of therapeutic jurisprudence, for example, some researchers have examined whether individuals are helped or harmed by involuntary hospitalization in the context of civil commitment, and whether legal procedures can be refashioned to make involuntary commitment a more humane and healing experience. Others have proposed how attorneys can promote therapeutic goals for their clients by encouraging alternative forms of dispute resolution, such as by fostering mediated resolutions to child custody disputes when parents divorce. Others have adopted a therapeutic jurisprudence orientation to examining whether worker's compensation procedures and tort compensation approaches promote health or further suffering, or how termination of parental rights proceedings might be approached differently with a paramount focus on children's needs, or how legal standards might encourage rather than discourage incompetency in criminal trials.

In creating a new integration of mental health and the law, proponents of therapeutic jurisprudence (like David Wexler) emphatically underscore how mental health and the prevention of psychological dysfunction can be allied in psycholegal settings. While this approach has been justifiably criticized for neglecting important conceptual problems entailed in the integration of law and mental health, this reorientation to the roles and responsibilities of mental health professionals in the courtroom has already generated exciting new research and theoretical reflection on legal dimensions of mental health.

VI. CONCLUSION

When entering the courtroom, the mental health professional encounters roles and responsibilities that are both familiar and unfamiliar. While the procedures of psychological evaluation are similar to those encountered in the typical therapeutic setting, the questions to be addressed in these courtroom evaluations are often quite different, as are the legal standards that frame the evaluation. Furthermore, clinical experts cannot expect to generalize the experience of trust and confidential self-disclosure of the therapeutic encounter to their forensic evaluations, where they are more likely to be greeted with suspicion, anxiety, and dissembling. In contrast to the therapeutic environment where the clinician is clear concerning who is the client, and can create an atmosphere conducive to psychological healing, mental health practitioners often have several clients in psycholegal contexts, each of whom may evoke competing loyalties because of their different needs and goals. Furthermore, clinical experts must work collaboratively with other legal actors and agency representatives who have interests that are different from their own. In the therapeutic setting, the clinician can rely on the assurance derived from years of training and clinical experience in offering insights to clients seeking assistance, but in forensic evaluations clinicians constantly encounter the limitations in their expertise and authority that derive from seeking to address ambiguous legal standards with assessment tools that may or may not be directly relevant, and that often yield uncertain and indeterminate answers, while mindful also of the differences between their authority as psychological experts and the ultimate authority of the court. Finally, the ethical

dilemmas encountered in forensic settings also often differ from those of the typical therapeutic context, especially in the conflicting responsibilities to the parties to the litigation, lawyers, and ultimately to the court.

Balanced against these challenges in forensic assessment are the essential contributions of the mental health practitioner to the determinations and judgments that range throughout the law, whether concerning issues of criminal culpability, competencies related to the exercise of personal liberty, compensation for personal harm and eligibility for special services, the "best interests" of children, or the wide variety of other psycholegal issues that characterize legal inquiry. Beyond the specific areas of mental health expertise that the clinician can offer, moreover, is the possibility of introducing to the court considerations related to human welfare and psychological well-being that might otherwise be neglected or misconstrued by legal actors. When mental health practitioners approach their forensic responsibilities with care and caution, aware of the limitations of their expertise and authority in the courtroom, and with ethical sensitivity, there is every reason to expect that their contributions to the law can be instrumental in advancing the human needs that are central to law.

ACKNOWLEDGMENTS

I am grateful to Gary Melton and Mario Scalora for thoughtful exchanges on the issues discussed in this article. I am also grateful to Steve Penrod, Tom Hafemeister, and Mario Scalora for very helpful comments on an earlier version of this article.

BIBLIOGRAPHY

Bull, R., & Carson, D. (Eds.). (1995). *Handbook of psychology in legal contexts*. Chichester, UK: Wiley.

Kagehiro, D., & Laufer, W. (Eds.). (1992). *Handbook of psychology and law*. New York: Springer-Verlag.

Melton, G. B., Petrila, J., Poythress, N. G., & Slobogin, C. (in press). *Psychological evaluations for the courts* (Rev. Ed.). New York: Guilford.

Monahan, J., & Walker, L. (1997). *Social science in law: Cases and materials* (4th ed.). Westbury, NY: Foundation.

Reisner, R., & Slobogin, C. (1990). *Law and the mental health system* (2nd ed.). St. Paul, MN: West.

Wexler, D. B., & Winick, B. J. (Eds.). (1996). *Law in a therapeutic key: Developments in therapeutic jurisprudence*. Durham, NC: Carolina Academic Press.

Limbic System

R. Joseph*

Neurobehavioral Center and Palo Alto Veterans Affairs Medical Center

Adipsia A failure to drink and lack of thirst.

Agnosin An inability to recognize or to achieve understanding.

Aphagia A failure to eat and lack of hunger.

Cognition A mental process involved in speech, thought, and achieving knowledge.

Enkephalins Opiate-like chemical substances.

Evoked Potentials Electrical activity of the brain elicited in response to flashes of light or sounds, which is then measured and detected by electrodes placed in the brain or on the surface of the skull.

Neural Ganglia A collection of nerve cells (neurons) which perform similar functions.

Neuron A cell specialized to receive, process, or express sensory or motor information.

Nuclei A collection of nerve cells which perform similar functions.

*R. Joseph is presently at the Brain Research Laboratory, San Jose, California.

Pheromone A chemical substance secreted by glands in the skin and detected by specialized neurons and which can indicate one's sexual, social, and emotional status.

The **LIMBIC SYSTEM** is buried within the depths of the cerebrum and consists of a collection of ancient brain structures which are preeminent in the mediation and expression of emotional, motivational, sexual, and social behavior. The limbic system is involved in learning and the formation of new memories, monitors internal homeostasis and basic needs such as hunger and thirst, controls the secretion of hormones involved in pregnancy and reactions to stress, and even makes possible the ability to experience orgasm, depression, fear, rage, and love.

Broadly, these limbic system nuclei include the hypothalamus, amygdala, hippocampus, septal nuclei, and cingulate gyrus (see Fig. 1). Also related to limbic system functioning are portions of the reticular activating system, the orbital frontal and inferior temporal lobes, as well as parts of the thalamus and cerebellum. The limbic system is exceedingly ancient and originally provided the foundation for the development and evolution of much of the brain. [*See* Brain.]

I. THE EVOLUTION OF THE OLFACTORY/LIMBIC SYSTEM

About 700 million years ago a cellular metamorphosis of paramount importance resulted in the creation of a completely unique type of cell, the neuron. These nerve cells in turn were especially responsive to light as well as chemical (olfactory and pheromonal) messages.

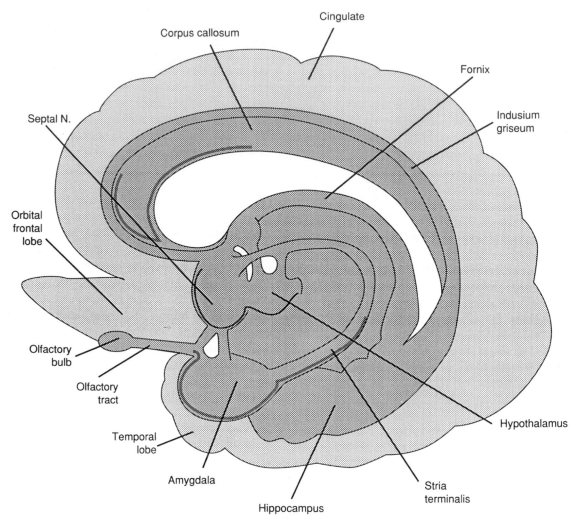

Figure 1. The limbic system: the amygdala, septal nuclei, hippocampus, hypothalamus, and cingulate gyrus. [Reproduced with permission from Joseph, R. (1990). "Neuropsychology, Neuropsychiatry, Behavioral Neurology." Plenum, New York.]

Over the course of evolution, as the number of secreting and transmitting nerve cells that creatures possessed increased, a network of interlinked neurons, called the "nerve net" was fashioned. Soon tiny neural ganglia, composed of colonies of similarly functioning nerve cells began to form in the anterior head region of various ancient and primitive creatures.

By the time the first vertebrates and fish began to swim the oceans, around 500 million years ago, the first primitive lobes of the brain had also become fashioned through the collectivization of these neural ganglia. This included the olfactory–limbic lobe (the forebrain), which was concerned with the detection of olfactory/pheromonal chemicals that might betray the presence of predators, prey, or a mate; the optic lobe/tectum of the midbrain which was responsive to visual messages; and the hindbrain which was concerned with movement. By 450,000 years ago, the first sharks had acquired a limbic system, which they, like modern humans, still possess today.

II. HYPOTHALAMUS

The hypothalamus is an exceedingly ancient structure and unlike most other brain regions it has maintained a striking similarity in structure throughout phylogeny and apparently over the course of evolution. The hypothalamus is fully functional at birth and is highly involved in all aspects of endocrine, hormonal, visceral, and autonomic functions and mediates or exerts controlling influences on eating, drinking, and the experience of pleasure, rage, and aversion. The hypothalamus is the central core from which all emotions derive their motive force. The hypothalamus is also sexually differentiated. That is, structurally and functionally the hypothalamus of men and women is sexually dissimilar.

A. Lateral and Ventromedial Hypothalamic Nuclei

Although the hypothalamus consists of several distinct regions and subgroups, the lateral and medial (ventromedial) hypothalamic nuclei play particularly important roles in almost all aspects of emotion and internal homeostasis. They also appear to share a somewhat antagonistic relationship and act to exert counterbalancing influences on each other.

For example, the medial hypothalamus controls parasympathetic activities (e.g., reduction in heart rate, increased peripheral circulation) and exerts a dampening effect on certain forms of emotional/motivational arousal. The lateral hypothalamus mediates sympathetic activity (increasing heart rate, elevation of blood pressure) and is involved in controlling the metabolic and somatic correlates of heightened emotionality.

B. Hunger and Thirst

The lateral and medial region are highly involved in monitoring internal needs such as hunger and thirst. For example, both nuclei contain receptors which are sensitive to the body's fat content (lipostatic receptors) and to circulating metabolites such as glucose, which together indicate the need for food and nourishment. The lateral hypothalamus also appears to contain osmoreceptors which determine if water intake should be altered. Both hypothalamic nuclei also become highly active immediately prior to and while the organism is eating or drinking.

For example, the lateral region alters its activity when the subject is hungry and simply looking at food. If the lateral hypothalamus is electrically stimulated a compulsion to eat and drink results. Conversely, if the lateral area is destroyed there results aphagia and adipsia so severe animals will die of

starvation. If the medial hypothalamus is surgically destroyed, inhibitory influences on the lateral region appear to be abolished such that hypothalamic hyperphagia and severe obesity result.

Overall, it appears that the lateral hypothalamus is involved in the initiation of eating and acts to maintain a lower weight limit such that when the limit is reached the organism is stimulated to eat. Conversely, the medial regions seem to be involved in setting a higher weight limit such that when these levels are approached it triggers the cessation of eating. That is, the medial area seems to act as a satiety center, but, a center that can be overridden. In part, these nuclei exert these differential influences on eating and drinking via motivational/emotional influences they exert on other brain nuclei (e.g., via reward or punishment).

C. Pleasure and Reward

In 1952, R. G. Heath reported what was then considered remarkable. Electrical stimulation near the septal nuclei elicited feelings of pleasure in human subjects: "I have a glowing feeling. I feel good!" Subsequently, in 1954 James Olds and Peter Milner reported that rats would tirelessly press a lever in order to receive electrical stimulation via tiny electrodes planted in this same region. Olds and Milner, in fact, concluded that stimulation in this region of the brain "has an effect which is apparently equivalent to that of a conventional primary reward." Even hungry animals would demonstrate a preference for self-stimulation over food.

Feelings of pleasure have since been obtained following electrical excitation to a number of diverse limbic areas including the olfactory bulbs, amygdala, hippocampus, cingulate gyrus, the basal ganglia, thalamus, reticular formation, medial forebrain bundle, and orbital frontal lobes. However, the greatest area of concentration and the highest rates of self-stimulatory activity were found to occur in the lateral hypothalamus. Indeed, according to Olds, animals "would continue to stimulate as rapidly as possible until physical fatigue forced them to slow or to sleep."

More recently, the lateral hypothalamus (as well as the amygdala and other limbic nuclei) have been found to have nerve cells which produce and are responsive to opiate-like substances, i.e., enkephalins. Hence, when an individual is injected with various narcotic substances, it is these limbic nuclei which respond with feelings of pleasure.

In contrast to the lateral hypothalamus and its involvement in pleasurable self-stimulation, activation of the medial hypothalamus is so aversive that subjects will work to reduce it—apparently so as to obtain relief (e.g., active avoidance). In this regard, when considering behavior such as eating, it might be postulated that when upper weight limits (or nutritional requirements) are met, the medial hypothalamus becomes activated which in turn leads to behavior which terminates its activation (e.g., cessation of eating). In fact, it is probably in this manner that the hypothalamus is able to exert considerable influence on a variety of behaviors, acting either to reward one's actions or to generate feelings of aversion so that one is less likely to act in a similar manner in the future.

D. Emotional Incontinence: Laughter and Rage

Although highly involved in all aspects of emotion and motivational functioning, the emotional states elicited by the hypothalamus are very primitive, diffuse, undirected, and unrefined, being limited to pleasure in general, or aversion/unpleasure in general. It is for this reason that ancient and primitive animals are also very limited in their ability to express and perceive emotion. Higher order emotional reactions (e.g., desire, love, hate, etc.) require the involvement of other limbic regions as well as the participation of the more recently evolved regions of the brain, the neocortex (i.e., "new brain").

Nevertheless, due to its involvement in the generation of positive and negative emotions, not surprisingly, when the hypothalamus has been injured or is made to function abnormally, extremely positive or negative reactions can also be elicited, including rage and uncontrolled laughter. For example, laughter has been noted to occur with hilarious or obscene speech—usually as a prelude to stupor or death—in cases where a tumor has infiltrated the hypothalamus. In several instances it has been reported that in the course of neurosurgery involving the hypothalamus, patients "became lively, talkative, joking, and whistling each time the hypothalamus was manipulated." In one case, the patient became excited and began to sing. Some individuals with hypothalamic damage have in fact died laughing. However, such patients claim that their laughter does not reflect their true feelings. Hence, laughter in these instances has been referred to as "sham mirth." Moreover, the

type of emotional reaction elicited is dependent on which region of the hypothalamus has been injured or activated.

Stimulation of the lateral hypothalamus, for example, can induce extremes in emotionality, including intense attacks of rage accompanied by biting and attack upon any moving object. If this nucleus is destroyed, aggressive and attack behavior is abolished. Hence, the lateral hypothalamus is responsible for rage and aggressive behavior, including attack and predatory actions, which coincides with its involvement with eating. In contrast, stimulation of the medial region counters the lateral hypothalamus such that rage reactions are reduced or eliminated. If the medial region is destroyed there results lateral hypothalamic release and the triggering of extreme savagery. [See AGGRESSION.]

Nevertheless, like "sham mirth," rage reactions elicited in response to direct electrical activation of the hypothalamus immediately and completely dissipate when the stimulation is removed. As such, these outbursts have been referred to as "sham rage."

III. PSYCHOLOGICAL MANIFESTATIONS OF HYPOTHALAMIC ACTIVITY

Phylogenetically and from an evolutionary perspective, the appearance and development of the hypothalamus predates the emergence and differentiation of all other limbic nuclei, e.g., amygdala, septal nucleus, hippocampus. It constitutes the most primitive, archaic, reflexive, and purely biological aspect of the psyche.

Biologically the hypothalamus serves the body tissues by attempting to maintain internal homeostasis and by providing for the immediate discharge of tensions in an almost reflexive manner. Hence, as based on studies of lateral and medial hypothalamic functioning, it appears to act reflexively, in an almost on/off manner so as to seek or maintain the experience of pleasure and escape or avoid unpleasant, noxious conditions.

Emotions elicited by the hypothalamus are largely undirected, short-lived, and unconnected with events occurring within the external environment, being triggered reflexively and without concern or understanding regarding consequences. Direct contact with the real world is quite limited and almost entirely indirect as the hypothalamus is largely concerned with the internal environment of the organism. It has no sense of morals, danger, values, logic, etc., and cannot feel or express love or hate. Although quite powerful, hypothalamic emotions are largely undifferentiated, consisting of feelings such as pleasure, unpleasure, aversion, rage, hunger, thirst, etc.

As the hypothalamus is concerned with the internal environment much of its activity occurs outside conscious–awareness. Moreover, being involved in maintaining internal homeostasis, via, for example, its ability to reward or punish the organism with feelings of pleasure or aversion, it tends to serve what Sigmund Freud described as the "pleasure principle."

IV. AMYGDALA

In contrast to the primitive hypothalamus, the amygdala is preeminent in the control and mediation of all higher order emotional and motivational activities, including the capacity to form emotional attachments and to feel love. Neurons located in the amygdala are able to monitor and abstract from the sensory array stimuli that are of motivational significance so as to organize and express appropriate feelings and behaviors. This includes the ability to discern and express even subtle social–emotional nuances such as friendliness, fear, affection, distrust, anger, etc., and at a more basic level, determine if something might be good to eat. In fact, amygdaloid neurons respond selectively to the flavor of certain preferred foods, as well as to the sight or sound of something that might be especially desirable to eat.

Moreover, some neurons located in the amygdala are responsive to faces and facial emotions conveyed by others. Many neurons are also able to respond to visual, tactual, olfactory, and auditory stimuli simultaneously. Hence, many amygdaloid neurons are predominantly polymodal, responding to a variety of stimuli from different modalities. It is in this manner that the amygdala has come to be involved not only in emotion, but attention, and learning and memory, for multimodal assimilation of various sensory impressions occurs in this region.

A. Medical and Lateral Amygdala Nuclei

The amygdala is buried within the depths of the anterior–inferior temporal lobe and consists of two major nuclear groups. These are a phylogenetically ancient anteromedial group (or medial amygdala) which is involved in olfaction, pheromonal perception, and motor activity (via rich interconnections with the basal ganglia), and a relatively newer basolateral division (lateral amygdala) which is maximally developed among humans.

Like the lateral and medial hypothalamus, the medial and lateral amygdala are rich in opiate receptors and cells containing enkephalins and both subserve different functions. For example, the medial amygdala is highly involved in motor, olfactory, and sexual functioning, whereas the lateral division is intimately involved in all aspects of higher order emotional activity including the generation of selective attention. That is, the amygdala acts to perform environmental surveillance and can trigger orienting responses as well as mediate the maintenance of attention if something of interest or importance were to appear. Hence, electrical stimulation of the lateral division can initiate quick and/or anxious glancing and searching movements of the eyes and head such that the organism appears aroused and highly alert as if in expectation of something that is going to happen.

Indeed, via its rich interconnections with the inferior, middle, and superior temporal lobes, as well as other neocortical regions, the lateral amygdala is able to sample and influence the auditory, somesthetic, and visual information being received and processed in these areas, as well as scrutinize this information for motivational and emotional significance. It is through the lateral division that emotional meaning and significance can be assigned to as well as extracted from that which is experienced.

B. The Amygdala and Hypothalamus

The amygdala, overall, maintains a functionally interdependent relationship with the hypothalamus. It is able to modulate and even control rudimentary emotional forces governed by the hypothalamic nucleus. However, it also acts at the behest of hypothalamically induced drives. For example, if certain nutritional requirements need to be met, the hypothalamus signals the amygdala which then surveys the external environment for something good to eat. On the other hand, if the amygdala via environmental surveillance were to discover a potentially threatening stimulus such as a predator, it acts to excite and drive the hypothalamus as well as the motor centers, so that the organism is mobilized to take appropriate action.

When the hypothalamus is activated by the amygdala, instead of responding in an on/off manner, cellular activity continues for an appreciably longer time period. The amygdala can tap into the reservoir of emotional energy mediated by the hypothalamus so that certain ends may be attained.

C. Fear, Rage, and Aggression

Initially, electrical stimulation of the amygdala produces sustained attention and orienting reactions. If the stimulation continues fear and/or rage reactions are elicited. When fear follows the attention response, the pupils dilate and the subject will cringe, withdraw, and cower. This cowering reaction in turn may give way to extreme fear and/or panic such that the animal will attempt to take flight.

Among humans, the fear response is one of the most common manifestations of amygdaloid electrical stimulation. Moreover, unlike hypothalamic on/off emotional reactions, attention and fear reactions can last up to several minutes after the stimulation is withdrawn. In addition to behavioral manifestations of heightened emotionality, amygdaloid stimulation can also result in intense changes in emotional facial expression. This includes facial contortions, baring of the teeth, dilation of the pupils, widening or narrowing of the eye-lids, flaring of the nostrils, tearing, as well as sniffing, licking, and chewing. In fact, epileptic seizure activity in this area (i.e., temporal lobe epilepsy) often induces involuntary chewing, and smacking of the lips and licking.

In many instances, rather than fear, stimulation of the amygdala results in anger, irritation, and rage which seems to gradually build up until finally the animal or human will attack. Unlike hypothalamic "sham rage," amygdaloid activation results in attacks directed at something real, or, in the absence of an actual stimulus, at something imaginary. Moreover, rage and attack will persist well beyond the termination of the electrical stimulation of the amygdala. In fact, the amygdala remains electrophysiologically active for long time periods even after a stimulus has been removed (be it external–perceptual or internal–electrical) such that it appears to continue to process—in the abstract—information even when that information is no longer observable. Moreover, tumors in this area can trigger violent rage attacks. A famous example of this is Charles Whitman, who in

1966 climbed a tower at the University of Texas carrying a high powered hunting rifle and for the next 90 minutes shot at everything that moved, killing 14, wounding 38. Postmortem autopsy of his brain revealed a glioblastoma multiformed tumor the size of a walnut compressing the amygdaloid nucleus. [*See* ANGER.]

D. Social–Emotional Agnosia

Among primates and mammals, bilateral destruction of the amygdala significantly disturbs the ability to determine and identify the motivational and emotional significance of externally occurring events, to discern social–emotional nuances conveyed by others, or to select what behavior is appropriate given a specific social context. Bilateral destruction of both amygdalas (located in the right and left temporal lobe) usually results in increased tameness, docility, and reduced aggressiveness in cats, monkeys, and other animals and humans. It also lowers responsiveness to aversive and social stimuli, and reduces fearfulness, competitiveness, dominance, and social interest. Indeed, this condition is so pervasive that subjects seem to have tremendous difficulty discerning the meaning or recognizing the significance of even common objects—a condition sometimes referred to as "psychic blindness," or the "Kluver–Bucy syndrome." However, it is important to note that although Drs. Kluver and Bucy reported this in 1937, this condition had first been reported in 1888 by Drs. Brown and Shaefer.

Like an infant (who similarly is without a fully functional amygdala), individuals with bilateral amygdala destruction engage in extreme orality and will indiscriminately pick up various objects and place them in their mouth regardless of its appropriateness. There is a repetitive quality to this behavior, for once they put it down they seem to have *forgotten* that they had just *explored* it, and will immediately pick it up and place it again in their mouth as if it were a completely unfamiliar object.

Hence, humans as well as animals with bilateral amygdala destruction, although able to see and interact with their environment, respond in an emotionally blunted manner, and seem unable to recognize what they see, feel, and experience. Things seem stripped of meaning. This condition pervades all aspects of higher level social–emotional functioning including the ability to appropriately interact with loved ones.

As might be expected, maternal behavior is severely affected. According to Dr. A. Kling, mothers will behave as if their "infant were a strange object to be mouthed, bitten and tossed around as though it were a rubber ball."

Among primates who have undergone bilateral amygdaloid removal, once they are released from captivity and allowed to return to their social group, a social–emotional agnosia becomes readily apparent as they no longer respond to or seem able to appreciate or understand emotional or social nuances. Indeed, they appear to have little or no interest in social activity and persistently attempt to avoid contact with others. If approached they withdraw, and if followed they flee. Indeed, they behave as if they have no understanding of what is expected of them or what others intend or are attempting to convey, even when the behavior is quite friendly and concerned. Among adults with bilateral lesions, total isolation seems to be preferred.

It is thus apparent that the amygdala, in conjunction with other limbic tissue, such as septal nuclei and the more recently evolved transitional limbic cortex, the cingulate gyrus, is highly involved in all aspects of social and emotional functioning. It has been argued that the differential maturation of these limbic structures, in particular, that of the amygdala, septal nuclei, and cingulate gyrus, is responsible for seeking contact comfort and forming of emotional and loving attachments during infancy.

V. SEPTAL NUCLEI

The septal nuclei appears to develop out of the hypothalamus. Phylogenetically and presumably, ontogenetically, it seems to mature following the development of the amygdala, but at about the same time as the hippocampus, a limbic system structure involved in the formation of memory. The septal nuclei also increases in relative size and complexity as we ascend the ancestral tree, attaining its greatest degree of development in humans.

The septal nuclei lies in the medial portions of the hemispheres, just anterior to the hypothalamus, and maintains rich interconnections with all regions of the limbic system. Unfortunately, unlike other limbic tissue, the functioning of the septal nuclei is still not well understood. Nevertheless, it appears to maintain a complementary relationship with the hippocampus, but an oppositional, and sometimes antagonistic relationship with the amygdala. For example, the amygdala appears to act so as to either facilitate or inhibit septal functioning whereas septal influences on the amygdala are largely inhibitory. However, in large part, the amygdala and septal nuclei appear to exert the majority of their counterbalancing influences on the emotional functioning of the hypothalamus with which they both maintain rich interconnections.

A. Rage and Quiescence

A primary activity of the septal nucleus appears to be that of reducing extremes in emotionality and arousal, and maintaining the organism in state of quiescence and readiness to respond. Stimulation of the septum acts to reduce blood pressure and heart rate, induces adrenocortical secretion, counters lateral hypothalamic self-stimulatory activity, inhibits aggressive behavior and suppresses the expression of rage reactions following hypothalamic stimulation.

If the septal nucleus is destroyed, these counterbalancing influences are removed such that initially there results dramatic increases in aggressive behavior. In fact, bilateral lesions of the septal nuclei can trigger explosive emotional reactivity to tactile, visual, or auditory stimulation such that the animal may attempt to attack or run away. However, if the amygdala is subsequently destroyed, the septal rage and emotional reactivity are completely attenuated. However, when the amygdala remains intact, septal lesions appear to result in a loss of modulatory and inhibitory restraint.

B. Contact Comfort and Septal Social Functioning

Although initially destruction of the septal nuclei results in rage reactions, within a few weeks this aggressiveness subsides and/or completely disappears. However, a generalized tendency to overrespond and a generalized failure to inhibit emotional responsiveness persists, and animals so affected tend to demonstrate an extreme and indiscriminate need for social and physical contact. That is, in contrast to amygdaloid lesions which produce a severe social–emotional agnosia and social avoidance, septal lesions produce a dramatic and persistent increase in social cohesiveness.

These findings suggest that the normal, intact amygdala appears to promote social behavior whereas the septal nucleus seems to counter socializing tendencies. Hence, with destruction of the septal nuclei (which results in a release of the amygdala), the drive for social contact appears to be irresistible such that persistent attempts to make physical contact occurs—even with species quite unlike their own.

For example, septal lesioned rats, unlike normals, will readily seek out mice (to which they are normally indifferent) or rabbits (which they usually avoid). If presented with a choice of an empty (safe) chamber or one containing a cat, septal lesioned rats persistently attempt to huddle and crawl upon this normally feared creature, even when the cat is acting perturbed. If a group of septally lesioned animals are placed together, extreme huddling results. So intense is this need for contact comfort following septal lesions, that if other animals are not available they will seek out blocks of wood, old rags, bare wire frames, or walls.

Among humans with right-sided or bilateral disturbances in septal functioning (such as due to seizure activity being generated in this region), a behavior referred to as "stickiness" is sometimes observed. Such individuals seek to make repeated, prolonged, and often inappropriate contact with anyone who is available or who happens to be near by so as to tell them stories, jokes, or merely pass the time. Moreover, they refuse to take a "hint," and do not depart unless given a direct request to do so.

VI. EMOTIONAL ATTACHMENT AND AMYGDALA–SEPTAL INTERACTIONS

Physical, social, and emotional interaction and contact during infancy is critically important to the child's well-being as well as his or her neurological, sensory, cognitive, intellectual, social, and emotional development. Indeed, babies need their "mamas" and all the love and attendant physical and emotional interaction they can get. The more an infant is held, stroked, and spoken to, and the greater the visual divergence of his surroundings, the greater will be its resilience and capability to adapt to negative emotional and physical onslaughts and to withstand stressful extremes later in life. In fact, the very cells of the nervous system will prosper by growing larger and more complex.

So great is the need for stimulation that until 6–7 months of age most children will eagerly and indiscriminately seek social and physical contact from anyone including complete strangers. Indiscriminate social interaction is not merely a manifestation of friendliness but serves a specific purpose: it maximizes opportunities for social and physical contact and interaction. Like hunger and the desire for food (which is mediated by the hypothalamus) there is a physical drive and hunger for social, emotional, and physical stimulation (which is mediated by the amygdala).

At about 7 months of age the infant becomes more discriminate in his or her interactions and it is during this time period that a very real and specific attachment (e.g., to one's mother) becomes progressively more intense and stable. This does not mean that prior to this period the mother is not highly important to the infant, but rather maximal social interaction takes precedence during the first critical months of life. Often a baby needs more contact than a single mother is capable of providing.

After these specific attachments such as to mother have been formed, most children increasingly begin to show anxiety, fear, and even flight reactions at the approach of a stranger. By 1 year of age 90% of children respond aversively to strangers. This also serves a purpose for it maximizes the bond with mother and ensures that a child who can crawl and maneuver through space does not indiscriminately attach to and wander off with a stranger.

Thus, the infant's initial seeking of indiscriminate social contact is followed at a later age by progressively narrowed contact seeking. According to a theory developed by Dr. R. Joseph, these stages of emotional development coincide with the maturation of different nuclei in the limbic system of the brain; the amygdala, septal nuclei, and cingulate gyrus.

As noted, the septal nucleus and amygdala often act in balanced opposition. That is, the septal nuclei appears to be highly involved in social and intimate contact seeking, but in a fashion quite different from the amygdala. The *normal* amygdala, which matures before the septal region promotes social contact seeking, whereas the *normal, undamaged* septal nuclei, which matures later, acts to inhibit and restrict these tendencies so that they are directed and focused (such as upon one person), rather than being generalized and indiscriminate. These two regions of the brain, in conjunction with the cingulate gyrus, are highly interactive and crucially important in the formation of our first and earliest attachments, as well as those later in life.

It is these same limbic nuclei which later in life are involved in the ability to feel love (as well as hate and anger) for, and attachment to, a loved one. That is, the limbic system controls the basic aspects of emotion, such as love, hate, anger, rage, fear, pleasure, the desire to bond together, as well as biological drives, including hunger, thirst, and even the capacity to experience orgasm during sex. Often all these impulses and needs at one time or another becomes associated with mother or the primary caretaker, and later in life (to a considerable degree), with a spouse. Even the presence or absence of mother can at one time or another elicit these responses (e.g., rage when the infant is not being held or fed).

Similarly, due to limbic attachment, the rejecting actions of a mate elicit limbic reactions including infantile feelings of rage and abandonment. That is, the amygdala striving to maintain the bonds of love responds with rage when the bond is severed, and the hypothalamus, feeling likewise, responds similarly. Even the murderous desire to kill one's spouse can be elicited. Indeed, loss of love, such as occurs when a relationship ends, seconded only by jealously and money, is a prime elicitor of such murderous feelings and is due to the high involvement of the limbic system in all affairs of the heart.

A. Limbic Abnormalities in Love and Socialization Skills

If contact with others is restricted during the early phases of infant development, then the ability to interact successfully with others at a later stage of life is retarded. That is, the infant and child must experience love and nurturance during this time period, otherwise these limbic nuclei will not develop and interact normally. If these interactional needs are not met during this critical period of development, gross abnormalities can result. Children will lose the ability to form emotional attachments with others, sometimes for the rest of their lives.

This is even true among non-human animals. Kittens which are not handled or stroked by humans soon become "wild" and unapproachable even when they have otherwise been exposed to people on a daily basis. Similarly, young children and infants who are separated from their parents and who fail to receive necessary loving and social stimulation are also affected adversely. They have difficulty forming emotional attachments and even their brains may not properly develop. If not adequately physically and emotionally stimulated, the child may even die.

In other words, if a child is not firmly attached to a mother figure and has been neglected early in life, the ability to form attachments increasingly narrows and then disappears, possibly forever. The child becomes attached to no one and its ability to form loving attachments later in life will be abnormal if drastic countermeasures are not taken. This is because cells in the amygdala, not receiving sufficient and appropriate stimulation begin to die and atrophy from disuse; just like a muscle if unused: "Use it or lose it." Once these limbic neurons die or if certain interconnections between different regions are not maintained, they are no longer able to respond appropriately to physical, emotional, and social interaction.

VII. THE CINGULATE GYRUS

A. The Evolution of Maternal Care

As noted, most creatures, including sharks, amphibians, reptiles, and fish, possess a limbic system, consisting of an amygdala, hippocampus, hypothalamus, and septal nuclei. It is these limbic nuclei which enable a group of fish to congregate together, i.e., to school, or for reptiles (creatures who first began to roam the planet about 300 million years ago) to form territories and very loosely organized social aggregates consisting of an alpha male and female, several subfemales, and a few juveniles. Such creatures, however, although sometimes showing parental investment, generally do not provide long-term care for their young and do not produce complex meaningful vocalizations, although, like amphibians they do produce very limited socially meaningful sounds, which in turn appear to be generated and perceived by limbic nuclei such as the amygdala.

Nevertheless, although in possession of a limbic system, reptiles and other non-mammalian species are lacking the more recently acquired cingulate cortex which appears to have begun to evolve around 250 million years ago when reptiles diverged to form repto-mammals (the therapsids) who in turn evolved into mammals and then primates. It was with the appearance of the repto-mammals that the first evidence of suckling of infants and long-term maternal care came into being. Indeed, it has been postulated by Paul Maclean (who in fact coined the term "limbic system"), as well as by Dr. R. Joseph, that the cingulate (in conjunction with the amygdala and septal nuclei) is largely responsible for the appearance of maternal feelings and the evolution of the family.

However, primates and other mammals, in addition to limbic and transitional limbic cingulate cortex, are also equipped with the six- to seven-layered neocortex which evolved approximately 100 million years ago and which covers the old brain like a shroud. However, like the amygdala, the cingulate has reached its maximal size among humans and maintains rich interconnections with the neocortex as well as with the older portions of the limbic system such as the amygdala and hippocampus.

Among humans and lower mammals, destruction of the anterior cingulate results in a loss of fear, lack of maternal responsiveness, and severe alterations in socially appropriate behavior. Humans will often become initially mute and socially unresponsive, and when they speak, their vocal melodic–inflectional patterns and the emotional sounds they produce sound abnormal. Animals, such as monkeys who have suffered cingulate destruction will also become mute, will cease to groom or show acts of affection, and will treat their fellow monkeys as if they were inanimate objects. For example, they may walk upon and over them as if they were part of the floor or some obstacle rather than a fellow being. In other words, their behavior is more typical of a reptile than a primate. Maternal behavior is also abolished following cingulate destruction, and the majority of infants soon die from lack of care.

More importantly, when the cingulate cortex is electrically stimulated, the separation cry, similar if not identical to that produced by an infant, is elicited. In fact, it appears that the cingulate, in conjunction with the amygdala and other limbic tissue, is responsible for not only the development of long-term infant care, but also the initial production of what would become language. This has been referred to by Joseph as "limbic language." In fact, be it humans or reptiles the limbic system is preeminent in the mediation, produc-

tion, and comprehension of emotional–social sounds, including sex differences in their production.

VIII. LIMBIC LANGUAGE

Phylogenetically and ontogenetically, the original impetus to vocalize springs forth from roots buried within the depths of the ancient "limbic lobe" a term coined by Paul Broca in the 1800s. Although nonhumans do not have the capacity to speak, they still vocalize, and these vocalizations are primarily limbic in origin being evoked in situations involving sexual arousal, terror, anger, flight, helplessness, and separation from the primary caretaker when young.

The first vocalizations of human infants are similarly emotional in origin and limbically mediated, consisting predominantly of sounds indicative of pleasure and displeasure. Indeed, these sounds and cries are produced soon after birth, indicating they are innate, and are produced even by infants born deaf and blind. Similarly, apes and monkeys reared in isolation or with surgically muted mothers also produce appropriately sounding complex emotional calls in order to convey a wealth of information, including the presence of danger. Moreover, they will respond to these same calls with appropriate reactions, even when they had never before been heard.

A. Limbic Localization of Emotional Sound Production

Emotional cries and warning calls have been produced via electrode stimulation of wide areas throughout the limbic system. Nevertheless, the type of cry elicited, in general, depends upon which limbic nuclei has been activated. For example, portions of the septal nuclei, hippocampus, and medial hypothalamus have been repeatedly shown to be generally involved in the generation of negative and unpleasant mood states, whereas the lateral hypothalamus and amygdala, and portions of the septal nuclei, are associated with pleasureable feelings. Not surprisingly, areas associated with pleasurable sensations often give rise, when sufficiently stimulated, to pleasurable calls, whereas those linked to negative mood states will trigger cries of alarm and shrieking. However, of all limbic nuclei, the amygdala and cingulate gyrus appear to be the most vocal.

In humans and animals a wide range of emotional

sounds have been evoked through amygdala activation, including those indicative of pleasure, sadness, happiness, and anger. Conversely, in humans, destruction limited to the amygdala, the right amygdala in particular, has abolished the ability to sing, convey melodic information, or enunciate properly via vocal inflection and can result in great changes in pitch and the timbre of speech. Even the capacity to perceive and respond appropriately to social–emotional cues is abolished.

However, in the cingulate gyrus, completely different emotional calls can be elicited from electrodes which are immediately adjacent, and the calls do not always correlate with the mood state. This suggests considerable flexibility within the cingulate which also appears to have the capability of producing emotional sounds that are not reflective of mood. This suggests a high degree of voluntary control within the cingulate. However, of the many sounds produced, the separation cry of the infant is one of the most significant, particularly in regard to the evolution of language. It is from the cingulate where the separation cry is most frequently elicited.

B. Limbic Language and Mother–Infant Vocalization

Among social terrestrial vertebrates the production of sound is very important in regard to infant care, for if an infant becomes lost, separated, or in danger, a mother would have no way of quickly knowing this by smell alone. Such information would have to be conveyed via a cry of distress or a sound indicative of separation fear and anxiety. It would be the production of these sounds which would cause a mother to come running to the rescue. Hence, the first forms of limbic social–emotional communication was probably produced in a maternal context.

Indeed, considerable vocalizing typically occurs between human and non-human mammalian mothers and their infants, and the infants of many species, including primates, will often sing along or produce sounds in accompaniment to those produced by their mothers. In fact, among primates, females are more likely to vocalize and utter alarm calls when they are near their infants versus non-kin, and vice versa, and adult males are more likely to call or cry when in the presence of their mother or an adult female vs an adult male. Similarly, infant primates will loudly protest

when separated from their mother so long as she is in view and will quickly cease to vocalize when isolated. It thus appears that the purpose of these vocalizations are to elicit a response from the mother.

Hence, the production of emotional sounds appears to be limbically linked and associated with maternal–infant care, and with interactions with an adult female. In fact, human females in general tend to vocalize more so than males and their speech tends to be perceived as friendlier and more social.

It is important to note, however, that the hypothalamus, septal nuclei, and the periquaductal gray (which is located in the midbrain) are also important components in the formulation of limbic language. Given the role of these limbic nuclei in sex related differences in cognition and behavior, it is perhaps highly likely that they may contribute to sex differences in language as well.

IX. SEXUAL DIFFERENTIATION OF THE HYPOTHALAMUS AND AMYGDALA

As is well known, sexual differentiation is strongly influenced by the presence or absence of gonadal androgen hormones during certain critical periods of prenatal development in many species including humans. However, not only are the external genitalia and other physical features sexually differentiated but certain regions of the brain have also been found to be sexually dimorphic and differentially sensitive to steroids, particularly the amygdala and the preoptic area and medial nucleus of the hypothalamus. Specifically, the presence or absence of the male hormone, testosterone, during this critical neonatal period directly affects and determines the pattern of interconnections between the amygdala and hypothalamus, between axons and dendrites in these nuclei, and thus the organization of specific neural circuits. In the absence of testosterone, the female pattern of neuronal development occurs.

That various limbic regions, such as the preoptic and medial (ventromedial) hypothalamus are sexually differentiated is not surprising in that it has long been known that this area is extremely important in controlling the basal output of gonadotrophins in females prior to ovulation and is heavily involved in mediating cyclic changes in hormone levels (e.g., estrogen, progesterone). Chemical and electrical stimulation of these nuclei also triggers sexual behavior and even sexual posturing in females and males. Moreover, in primates, electrical stimulation of the preoptic area increases sexual behavior in males, and significantly increases the frequency of erections, copulations, and ejaculations, as well as pelvic thrusting followed by an explosive discharge of semen even in the absence of a mate. Conversely, lesions to these nuclei eliminate male sexual behavior and result in gonadal atrophy.

Similarly, electrical stimulation of the amygdala, the medial division in particular, results in sex related behavior and activity. In females this includes ovulation, uterine contractions, and lactogenetic responses, and in males penile erections.

Conversely, damage to the amygdala bilaterally, often results in heightened and indiscriminate sexual activity. For example, primates and other animals (while in captivity) will engage in excessive masturbation and genital manipulation and will repeatedly attempt to copulate even with species other than their own (e.g., a cat with a dog, a dog with a turtle, etc.) regardless of their sex. Hence, with bilateral destruction, animals are not only overly active sexually, but also unable to identify appropriate partners. Conversely, with abnormal activity involving the amygdala, such as due to temporal lobe epilepsy, sensations of sexual excitement, and even sexual behavior sometimes leading to orgasm, may also occur as a function of seizures originating in the temporal lobe.

A. Sex Differences in Language and Cognition

Hence, it thus appears that the limbic system not only is involved in all aspects of emotion, including sexual behavior and the production of emotional speech, but that these same limbic nuclei may be responsible for sex differences in thought, feeling, and even language. For example, it has been argued that sex differences in language, emotion, and cognitive capability may represent the differential effects of early hormonal influences on various limbic system nuclei as well as within the neocortex. Indeed, the administration of testosterone to females during these early critical periods or the castration of males will completely reverse sex differences in behavior and cognition.

For example, it is well known that men, boys, and even male rats demonstrate superior spatial-perceptual abilities, such as in maze learning, as compared to fe-

males. If testosterone is not present during these early critical periods, these superiorities are reversed. On the other hand, women and young girls have shown some superiority in regard to various aspects of language, including those related to social and emotional functioning. It may be that these results are also related to early hormonal influences on limbic organization.

Consider for example intonation and pitch. Women tend to employ five to six different variations and to utilize the higher registers when conversing. They are also more likely to employ glissando or sliding effects between stressed syllables, and they tend to talk faster as well. Men tend to be more monotone, employing two to three variations on average, most of which hover around the lower registers. Even when trying to emphasize a point males are less likely to employ melodic extremes but instead tend to speak louder.

B. Sex Differences in Emotion

As has been demonstrated in a number of recent studies, women are also more emotionally expressive, and are more perceptive in regard to comprehending emotional verbal nuances. This superior female sensitivity even includes the comprehension of emotional faces, and the ability to feel and express empathy. In fact, from childhood to adulthood women appear to be much more emotionally expressive than males in general. Indeed, given woman's role in rearing children, and the role of the limbic system in promoting maternal care and communication, it seems rather natural that they are much more sensitive to and expressive of these nuances. These differences may reflect sex-related differences in the structure and function of the male vs female limbic system.

Indeed, although sex differences in the structure of the cingulate have not yet been reported, consider for example, the anterior commissure, a bundle of fibers which acts to interconnect the two amygdalas and inferior temporal lobes. This fiber pathway is 18% larger in the female vs the male brain. Given the preimmanent role of the amygdala in emotionality and sound production, as well as evidence indicating that this nuclei is sexually dimorphic, this latter finding of an enlargement in the anterior commissure may be yet another reason why females are more emotionally expressive, receptive, and tend to employ a wider range of melodic pitch when they speak. Moreover, given the intimate role of the amygdala with the hippocampus, it is possible that sexual differentiation of this and other limbic nuclei may be responsible for sex differences in spatial–perceptual abilities and other cognitive differences as well.

X. HIPPOCAMPUS

A. Arousal, Attention, and Inhibition

The hippocampus is an elongated structure located within the inferior medial wall of the temporal lobe, posterior to the amygdala, and is shaped somewhat like a telephone receiver. It consists of an anterior and posterior region, and is richly interconnected with the septal nuclei (which in some ways acts as a relay nucleus for the hippocampus), as well as the cingulate gyrus and amygdala. Among animals it has also been found to be sexually differentiated.

Various authors have assigned the hippocampus a major role in information processing, including memory, new learning, spatial mapping of the environment, and voluntary movement toward a goal, as well as in attention and behavioral arousal. For example, hippocampal cells greatly alter their activity in response to certain spatial correlates, particularly as an animal moves about in its environment. It is also intimately involved in the encoding and memory storage of spatial, as well as verbal, emotional, and other forms of information. However, few studies have implicated the hippocampus in emotional functioning per se, although responses such as "anxiety" or "bewilderment" have been observed when directly electrically stimulated.

Over the course of evolution the hippocampus has become modified and many of its functions have come to be hierarchically mediated, controlled, or at least, influenced by activity occurring within the neocortex, with which it maintains rich interconnections. Due to this interrelationship the hippocampus is able to monitor as well as exert reciprocal influences over neocortical functioning which it monitors.

For example, when the neocortex becomes highly activated, the hippocampus functions at a much lower level of arousal in order not to become overwhelmed. When the neocortex is not highly aroused, the hippocampus presumably compensates by increasing its own level of arousal so as to tune in to information that

is being processed at a low level of neocortical intensity. However, in situations where both the neocortex and the hippocampus become highly aroused and activated, the individual becomes easily distracted, hyperresponsive, and overwhelmed, confused, and disoriented. Attention, learning, and memory functioning are also decreased due to this interference in the ability to selectively maintain attention. Situations such as this sometimes occur when individuals are highly anxious or upset.

There is also evidence to suggest that the hippocampus may act so as to reduce extremes in neocortical arousal. For example, whereas stimulation of the reticular activating system augments cortical arousal and EEG evoked potentials, hippocampal stimulation reduces or inhibits these potentials such that cortical responsiveness and arousal are dampened.

On the other hand, if neocortical arousal is at a low level, hippocampal stimulation often results in an augmentation of the neocortical evoked EEG potential, thus increasing arousal levels. It is presumably in this manner that the hippocampus can exert influence on what is being processed in the neocortex so as to control selective attention and maintain concentration. Again, this aids in learning and the retention of significant information via selective attention or the filtering of irrelevant forms of input that might otherwise become processed and attended to.

The hippocampus thus prevents the neocortex from becoming overwhelmed or inattentive, and may act to increase neocortical arousal so that it is sufficiently activated. This is because very high or very low states of excitation are incompatible with alertness and selective attention as well as the ability to learn and retain information. When the hippocampus is damaged or destroyed, animals have great difficulty inhibiting behavioral responsiveness or shifting attention. The ability to shift from one set of perceptions to another or to change behavioral patterns is disrupted and the organism becomes overwhelmed by a particular mode of input. Learning, memory, and attention, are greatly compromised.

B. Learning and Memory

The hippocampus is thus associated with learning and memory encoding (e.g., long-term storage and retrieval of newly learned information), particularly the anterior regions. Of course, many other brain areas such as the mammillary bodies, dorsal medial nucleus of the thalamus, etc., are also important in memory functioning. Nevertheless, the hippocampus, in conjunction with the amygdala, appears to be preeminent in this regard.

It is now well known that bilateral destruction of the anterior hippocampus results in striking and profound disturbances involving memory and new learning, i.e., anterograde amnesia. For example, one such individual who underwent bilateral destruction of this nuclei (H.M.) was subsequently found to have almost completely lost the ability to recall anything experienced after surgery. If you introduced yourself to him, left the room, and then returned a few minutes later he would have no recall of having met or spoken to you. Dr. Brenda Milner has worked with H.M. for almost 20 years and yet she is an utter stranger to him. However, events that occurred for up to 2 years before his surgery were also somewhat disrupted. [See AMNESIA.]

Nevertheless, H.M. is in fact so amnesic for everything that has occurred since his surgery that every time he rediscovers that his favorite uncle died (years after his surgery) he suffers the same grief as if he had just been informed for the first time. Even so, although without memory for new (nonmotor) information, H.M. has adequate intelligence, is painfully aware of his deficit, and constantly apologizes for his problem. "Right now, I'm wondering" he once said, "Have I done or said anything amiss?" You see, at this moment everything looks clear to me, but what happened just before? That's what worries me. It's like waking from a dream. I just don't remember. . . . Every day is alone in itself, whatever enjoyment I've had, and whatever sorrow I've had . . . I just don't remember."

As noted above, presumably the hippocampus acts to protect memory and the encoding of new information during the storage and consolidation phase via the gating of afferent streams of information and the filtering/exclusion (or dampening) of irrelevant and interfering stimuli. When the hippocampus is damaged there results input overload, the brain is overwhelmed by irrelevant stimuli, and the consolidation phase of memory is disrupted such that relevant information is not properly stored or even attended to. Consequently, the ability to form associations (e.g., between stimulus and response) or to alter preexisting schemas (such as occurs during learning) is attenuated.

C. Hippocampal and Amygdaloid Interactions: Memory

The amygdaloid nucleus via its rich interconnections with other brain regions is able to sample and influence activity occurring in other parts of the cerebrum and add emotional color to one's perceptions. As such it is highly involved in the assimilation and association of divergent emotional, motivational, somesthetic, visceral, auditory, visual, motor, olfactory, and gustatory stimuli. Thus, it is very concerned with learning, memory, and attention, and can generate reinforcement for certain behaviors. Moreover, via reward or punishment it can promote the encoding, storage, and later retrieval of particular types of information. That is, learning often involves reward and it is via the amygdala (in concert with other nuclei) that emotional consequences can be attributed to certain events, actions, or experiences, as well as extracted from the world of possibility so that it can be attended to and remembered. Indeed, the amygdala, in conjunction with the hippocampus, is extremely important in learning and memory, and both are richly interconnected.

The amygdala thus seems to reinforce and maintain hippocampal activity via the identification of motivationally and emotionally significant information and the generation of pleasurable rewards (through action on the lateral hypothalamus). This is because reward increases the probability of attention being paid to a particular stimulus or consequence as a function of its association with reinforcement. As such, events which are positively or negatively reinforced are more likely to be remembered.

Hence, the hippocampus acts to reduce or enhance extremes in arousal associated with information reception and storage in memory, whereas the amygdala acts to identify the social–emotional motivational characteristics of the stimuli as well as to generate (in conjunction with the hippocampus) appropriate emotional rewards so that learning and memory will be reinforced. Thus, we find that when both the amygdala and hippocampus are damaged, striking and profound disturbances in memory functioning result.

D. Visual and Verbal Memory

It is now very well known that lesions involving the inferior temporal lobes and the amygdala/hippocampus of the left cerebral hemisphere typically produce significant disturbances involving verbal memory. Left-sided damage disrupts the ability to recall simple sentences and complex verbal narrative passages or to learn verbal paired-associates or a series of digits.

In contrast, right temporal amygdala–hippocampal destruction typically produces deficits involving visual and spatial memory, such as the learning and recall of geometric patterns, visual mazes, human faces, or even where some object was placed the night before. Right-sided damage also disrupts the ability to recall olfactory stimuli, emotional sounds and passages, or sounds from the environment.

Hence, the left amygdala/hippocampus is highly involved in processing and/or attending to verbal information, whereas the right amygdala/hippocampus is more involved in the learning, memory, and recollection of nonverbal, visual–spatial, environmental, emotional, motivational, and facial information. However, as noted above, the limbic system, including the hippocampus, is sexually differentiated, which in turn appears to affect the ability to attend to and recall spatial vs emotional and verbal information. In this regard, the male limbic system appears to have conferred an advantage in the processing of spatial information, whereas the female limbic system is more adept at expressing, processing, and possibly recalling emotionally laden visual and verbal stimuli.

This article has been reprinted from the *Encyclopedia of Human Behavior,* Volume 3.

BIBLIOGRAPHY

Aggleton, J. P. (1992). "The Amygdala." Wiley-Liss, New York.

Gerall, A. A., Molttz, H., & Ward, I. L. (Eds.) (1992). "Sexual Differentiation." Plenum, New York.

Joseph, R. (1990). "Neuropsychology, Neuropsychiatry, and Behavioral Neurology." Plenum, New York.

Joseph, R. (1992). The limbic system: Emotion, laterality, and unconscious mind. *Psychoanal. Rev.* **79,** 405–456.

Joseph, R. (1992). "The Right Brain and the Unconscious." Plenum, New York.

Joseph, R. (1993). "The Naked Neuron: Evolution and the Languages of the Body and Brain." Plenum, New York.

Joseph, R. (1996). "Neuropsychiatry, Neuropsychology, and Clinical Neuroscience." Williams & Wilkins, Baltimore, MD.

Kling, A. S., Lloyd, R. L., & Perryman, K. M. (1987). Slow wave changes in amygdala to visual, auditory, and social stimuli following lesions of the inferior temporal cortex in squirrel monkey. *Behav. Neural Biol.* **47,** 54–72.

MacLean, P. (1990). "The Triune Brain in Evolution." Plenum, New York.

Olds, M. E., & Forbes, J. L. (1981). The central basis of motivation: Intracranial self-stimulation studies. *Annu. Rev. Psychol.* **32,** 523–574.

Steklis, H. D., & Kling, A. (1985). Neurobiology of affiliative behavior in nonhuman primates. In "The Psychobiology of Attachment and Separation." (M. Reite and T. Field, Eds.). Academic Press, Orlando.

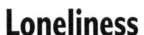

Loneliness

Daniel Perlman

University of British Columbia

Letitia Anne Peplau

University of California, Los Angeles

Discrepancy Model A conceptual model positing that loneliness occurs when there is a significant mismatch or discrepancy between a person's actual social relations and his or her needed or desired social relations.

Emotional Loneliness The type of loneliness that occurs when a person lacks an intimate attachment figure, such as might be provided for children by their parents or for adults by a spouse or intimate friend.

Loneliness The subjective psychological discomfort people experience when their network of social relationships is significantly deficient in either quality or quantity.

Social Isolation The objective situation of being alone or lacking social relationships.

Social Loneliness The type of loneliness that occurs when a person lacks the sense of social integration or community involvement that might be provided by a network of friends, neighbors, or co-workers.

LONELINESS is the unpleasant experience that occurs when a person's network of social relationships is significantly deficient in quantity or quality. This article examines loneliness and its implications for mental health. It begins with a brief historical perspective on loneliness and then provides a conceptual model for understanding loneliness and the phenomena associated with it. Subsequent sections discuss the nature and types of loneliness, examine the life cycle development and demographics of loneliness, review the mental and physical health correlates of loneliness, and discuss coping strategies and professional interventions for overcoming loneliness.

I. HISTORICAL PERSPECTIVES ON LONELINESS

One may think of loneliness as a modern condition, born of urbanization and technology, and further intensified by postmodern trends. Yet, the desire for companionship (or cooperation) versus the fear of social rejection (or hostility) undoubtedly operated in prehistoric times. Themes of aloneness can be found in Greek mythology and drama. For instance, Jung and others have interpreted Prometheus's stealing fire from the Gods as symbolic of his raising himself above and thereby alienating himself from his fellow humans. Although the *Odyssey* focuses on Homer's geographical wanderings, this tale implies that he was socially adrift as well. In their analytic writings, Greek philosophers had similar concerns: Aristotle saw humans as social animals, needing friendship. In the seventeenth century, Hobbes characterized human life not only as "nasty, brutish, and short" but also as "solitary." Since then philosophers such as Descartes, Nietzsche, and Sartre have written extensively on social isolation and solitude.

Social science examination of loneliness dates back at least as far as T. L. Stoddard's 1932 volume entitled

Lonely America. In 1938, Gregory Zilboorg published an article linking loneliness, which he saw as stemming from early childhood experiences, with three personality attributes: narcissism, megalomania, and hostility. In the 15-year period after World War II, there was a small trickle of publications on loneliness, mostly by clinical psychologists who gained insights into loneliness from their observations of clients. Probably the best known of these authors were Frieda Fromm-Reichmann and Harry Stack Sullivan. Fromm-Reichmann believed that real loneliness plays a role in the genesis of mental disorders including psychosis and schizophrenia. She contended that loneliness is such a frightening experience that people in its grip cannot discuss it and will do almost anything to avoid it. Harry Stack Sullivan saw loneliness as an exceedingly unpleasant experience arising when humans are unable to satisfy their need for intimacy.

Available bibliographies list only a dozen or so psychologically oriented, English language publications on loneliness prior to 1960. Another 64 articles and books appeared in the 1960s. In that decade, empirical research on topics such as loneliness among older adults became more prominent, and systematic efforts to measure individual differences in loneliness began. Moustakas published his popular book, *Loneliness*, on existential loneliness. A widely read sociological analysis, *The Lonely Crowd*, by David Riesman and colleagues, focused attention on the societal underpinnings of loneliness, a paradoxical emphasis on being a team player and yet simultaneously distinguishing oneself individually.

Approximately 170 publications on loneliness appeared in the 1970s, and nearly 650 more between 1980 and June 1996. Thus, there has been a noticeable increase in the rate of publication on loneliness. The early 1970s mark what might be called the beginning of the contemporary era for loneliness research,

the era that will be covered in this article. In 1973, Robert Weiss published his influential book, *Loneliness: The Experience of Emotional and Social Isolation*. Since then, there have been other noteworthy edited volumes and reviews. The knowledge gained during this quarter century of research and theory development is summarized here.

II. A MODEL FOR UNDERSTANDING LONELINESS

Before reviewing empirical findings, it is helpful to have a general framework for conceptualizing loneliness. Although the experience of loneliness is different for each individual, common elements in loneliness can be identified. Figure 1 presents a model for undererstanding loneliness and the phenomena associated with it. Central to this discrepancy model is the idea that loneliness occurs when there is a significant mismatch between a person's actual social relationships and his or her needed or desired social relations. A man who longs to be married but who is still single will feel lonely. Loneliness theorists differ in how they conceptualize the nature of this discrepancy. Some theorists posit basic human social needs and believe that loneliness occurs when these enduring needs are not met. This approach is called the social needs perspective on loneliness. Other theorists take a more cognitive perspective, emphasizing the match between a person's desires or expectations for relationships and the reality of his or her social life. This is known as the cognitive discrepancy model of loneliness.

The model in Fig. 1 also includes the more distal antecedents of loneliness, distinguishing between predisposing factors that make people vulnerable to loneliness and precipitating events that trigger the onset of loneliness. Diverse predisposing factors can increase a

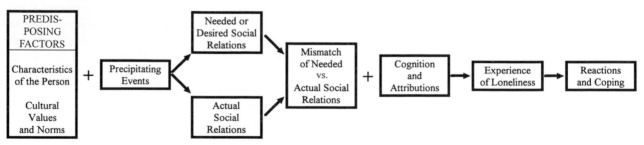

Figure 1 A model of the experience of loneliness.

person's risk of loneliness. Individual differences in personality and behavior such as extreme shyness or the lack of social skills may interfere with creating or maintaining satisfying social relationships and thereby set the stage for loneliness. Cultural values and norms can also affect a person's vulnerability to loneliness. American culture has been characterized as being highly individualistic; our values encourage personal independence and the pursuit of individual goals even at the expense of social ties. In contrast, other cultures in Asia, Africa, and Latin America are more collectivistic; their values encourage loyalty to family, adherence to group norms, and the preservation of harmony in social relations with members of one's own group. Although research on this point is needed, it seems likely that cultural differences in values such as individualism and collectivism affect the experience of loneliness. Within a society, social norms may also affect the tendency to feel lonely. For instance, American high school students report more intense feelings of loneliness if they are alone on a weekend evening (which teen culture defines as a time for socializing) than if they are alone on a school night during the week. [*See* SHYNESS.]

The person's immediate social situation can also affect loneliness. Situations vary in the opportunities they provide for social contact. Some situational factors are very basic, e.g., time, distance, and money. The hardworking medical student may have little time for sleep, let alone making friends. The traveling salesman who spends most days on the road may find it hard to find a spouse. The stress of unemployment may strain marital satisfaction and increase conflict. Situational constraints can also limit the pool of available partners. For example, because women live considerably longer than men, older widowed women have fewer prospects for remarriage and are significantly less likely to remarry than are older widowed men. When situational factors persist over time, they can increase the risk of loneliness.

The onset of loneliness is often initiated by a precipitating event, usually a change in a person's actual or desired/needed social relationships. Examples include the loss of an important relationship through death or divorce or the disruption of social relations created by moving to a new school, town, or job. Figure 1 also shows that how a person perceives and thinks about his or her life situation—cognitive processes such as social comparison and causal attribution—affects the expe-

rience of loneliness. The intensity of loneliness may be increased if people evaluate their own situation as worse than that of their peers, or if they attribute the causes of their loneliness to personal inadequacies. Finally, Fig. 1 calls attention to differences in the ways that people react to being lonely.

This model is not a specific theory of loneliness but rather a general framework that highlights important elements of the loneliness experience. The components of this model could be analyzed from diverse theoretical perspectives. The next sections of this article review empirical evidence relevant to various aspects of loneliness.

III. NATURE, TYPES, AND MEASUREMENT OF LONELINESS

Several different definitions of loneliness have been given. Often, these definitions reflect a particular theoretical approach to loneliness. For example, behavioral theorists emphasize loneliness as a response to an absence of social reinforcement, cognitive theorists emphasize the perception of a discrepancy between desired and achieved social contacts, and psychodynamically oriented theorists such as Weiss and Sullivan focus on the lack of need fulfillment. Although definitions of loneliness vary, most assume that loneliness results from social deficiencies, that loneliness is a subjective phenomenon not synonymous with objective social isolation, and that it is aversive.

A. The Nature of Loneliness

When laypeople are asked what characteristics they associate with a person being lonely, their answers can be grouped into three clusters. The dominant cluster includes the thoughts and feelings directly related to the experience of loneliness: feeling different, excluded, isolated, unloved, and inferior. Laypersons also have a cluster of images about why individuals experience loneliness: being reserved and avoiding social contacts, working too hard, and being introspective. Finally, observers also see the lonely person as having other negative feelings: paranoia, anger, and depression. Complementing how others see lonely people, lonely individuals themselves report such feelings as sadness, a sense of estrangement and rejection by others, a lack of self-confidence, boredom, anger against others, and depression.

B. Types of Loneliness

Although they have searched for universal facets of loneliness, researchers have also tried to identify different types of loneliness. One typology uses the duration of loneliness to classify people as experiencing short-lived or state loneliness versus long-lived or trait loneliness. Trait and state loneliness differ in several important ways other than chronicity. A first difference is that *trait loneliness* has cross-situational generality; *state loneliness* is more situation-specific. Available evidence also suggests that trait-lonely individuals, compared with state-lonely people, are more likely to have deficient social skills, to attribute their loneliness to undesirable, unchangeable aspects of their personality, and to have difficulty overcoming their social deficits.

A second typology of loneliness was suggested by Weiss (1973), based on his analysis of what relationships provide. He distinguished between emotional and social loneliness. *Emotional loneliness* stems from the absence of emotional attachments provided by intimate relationships. Bereavement, divorce, or empty-shell marriages are likely antecedents of this form of loneliness. *Social loneliness* stems from the absence of an adequate social network. Moving, loss of a job, being excluded by peers, and not belonging to community organizations are likely antecedents of this form of loneliness. The symptoms of emotional loneliness include anxiety, a sense of utter aloneness, vigilance to threat, and a tendency to misinterpret the hostile or affectionate intention of others. The symptoms of social isolation are feelings of boredom, restlessness, and marginality. The affective sequelae of emotional loneliness are generally more intense and unpleasant than the sequelae of social loneliness. A recent study of Israeli university students suggests that it may be possible to divide emotionally lonely individuals into two subgroups—those of the "paranoid" type with angry feelings who believe they are the targets of others' hostility and those who feel depressed. [*See* BEREAVEMENT.]

C. Measures of Loneliness

Beyond describing phenomena and delineating subtypes, social scientists are eager to operationalize constructs. In 1978, Daniel Russell and his associates published the University of California, Los Angeles (UCLA) Loneliness Scale. This 20-item paper-and-pencil measure helped to spur an increase in loneliness research. Since then, psychometric work has moved steadily forward. These advances include revision of the UCLA scale to simplify the wording and to balance the response pattern so that agreeing with some items and disagreeing with others reflects loneliness; demonstration of the UCLA scale's discriminant validity vis-à-vis constructs such as depression, social desirability, self-esteem, and anxiety; translation of the UCLA scale into several different languages (e.g., French, German, Greek, Japanese, Persian, Portuguese, Russian, Spanish); the development of other scales besides the UCLA measure; the development of scales for measuring trait versus state loneliness and for social versus emotional loneliness; and the construction of scales for children.

At least a dozen studies have examined the factorial structure of the revised UCLA Loneliness Scale. Often, two or three factors are statistically identified, although some investigators find just one factor and others believe that underlying the multiple factors there is a single main or higher-order factor. In any case, the Cronbach alpha of the UCLA Loneliness Scale is high, therefore research-oriented use of overall loneliness scores is justified.

IV. DEVELOPMENT AND DEMOGRAPHICS OF LONELINESS

A. Emergence of Loneliness in Childhood

The exact age at which children begin experiencing loneliness is open to debate. Some have argued that loneliness emerges in early childhood, even as early as the first 3 months of life. Attachment research demonstrates that within roughly the first 6 months, infants form specific attachment bonds and shortly thereafter develop separation anxieties; by 10 months, children resist being separated from caregivers. Others, however, have argued that loneliness does not emerge until children are older. Harry Stack Sullivan believed that children need to be able to form intimate chumships before the absence of such bonds can trigger loneliness. According to his analysis, this stage is not reached until the preadolescent period. [*See* ATTACHMENT.]

In trying to resolve this controversy, some authorities claim that infants experience separation anxiety but that this is different from loneliness per se. Weiss's analysis is compatible with this view; he believes that loneliness has more ramifications than separation anxiety. Two pieces of evidence, however, are consistent with the position that loneliness exists well before preadolescence. First, symptoms of social (as opposed to emotional) loneliness (e.g., malaise, boredom, and alienation) have been observed in preschool children of age 3. Second, psychometric analyses of data from children as young as 5 show that these children can reliably and validly complete loneliness measures. If they were not already experiencing loneliness, it seems unlikely that their answers would form meaningful patterns.

Whenever loneliness begins, it appears to have roots in experiences in the family. A Manitoba study of 130 female undergraduates and their parents demonstrated that daughters' loneliness scores were modestly correlated with both their mothers' ($r = .25$) and their fathers' ($r = .19$) loneliness scores. This association could be due to either genetic or social factors. A number of studies have shown that lonely individuals have (or at least report that they have) cold, less nurturant parents. For instance, in one large-scale study, lonely adults were more likely than nonlonely adults to remember their parents as having been remote, untrustworthy, and disagreeable. In another study on adolescence, greater loneliness was associated with participants feeling that their parents had done little to encourage them to strive for popularity and had been dissatisfied with their choice of friends.

B. Prevalence of Loneliness in Adulthood

In a representative sampling of U.S. citizens, 26% said that they had felt "very lonely or remote from other people" in the past few weeks. Naturally, the results vary as a function of the exact wording of the question posed to respondents. When asked whether they have ever been lonely in their lives, more people answer affirmatively. When asked whether they see themselves as a "lonely person," fewer respond affirmatively. During adulthood, loneliness also varies as a function of several demographic variables and life experiences.

C. Nationality Differences

Sociological explanations of loneliness emphasize that societal-level variables contribute to loneliness. Thus, one would expect nationality differences in loneliness.

Data from the World Values Survey on how often people feel lonely support this expectation. Among adults in 18 countries interviewed in the early 1980s, Italians and Japanese respondents reported the most frequent feelings of loneliness; Danish and Dutch respondents reported the least frequent feelings of loneliness. Consistent with the analysis of American culture by Riesman and others, respondents from the United States ranked high (fourth) in the extent of their loneliness. Within the United States, a large National Institute of Mental Health (NIMH) study of two communities (Kansas City, Missouri, and Washington County, Maryland) found that African Americans were more apt to report loneliness than white Americans.

D. Socioeconomic Factors

Several studies have shown that loneliness is more prevalent among lower-income groups. For instance, in a survey of 8634 households in a large, predominantly urban Southwestern U.S. county, members of families with incomes under $10,000 (in 1986) were 4.6 times more likely to report loneliness than members of families with incomes of $75,000 or more. In that study, education also showed an inverse relationship to loneliness.

One might expect that in most societies unemployment is associated with loneliness. One small-scale project studied Oklahomans' use of the services of their state unemployment center. It showed that participants who had been unemployed longer and who were ineligible (or no longer eligible) for unemployment benefits were more lonely than those who had been unemployed for a shorter period and who had benefits. More extensive testing is needed of the relationship between unemployment and loneliness. [See SOCIOECONOMIC STATUS.]

E. Gender Differences

An early meta-analysis found that gender differences in loneliness are measure-specific. When scores on the UCLA Loneliness Scale were analyzed, typically no difference in the scores of men and women was found. In the few studies (3 of 28) where differences were obtained, men tended to have higher UCLA loneliness scores than women. This scale does not directly ask respondents if they are lonely. In contrast, when respondents have been directly asked if they are lonely, women generally reported more loneliness than men. Thus a gender difference occurs when people are asked to identify or label themselves as lonely but not when other, less direct questions are posed.

More recent findings seem consistent with these patterns. For instance, in two representative surveys of residents of Edmonton, Alberta, men showed a nonsignificant trend toward greater loneliness on a short form of the UCLA scale. In the development of the third version of the UCLA scale, gender differences were found in only one of four samples. Again, when gender differences did emerge in UCLA scores, men were more lonely than women. Turning to studies which explicitly asked about feelings of "loneliness," analyses of the data from 18 countries participating in the World Value Survey provide global results. In all 18 countries, women more frequently than men acknowledged feeling lonely.

There are several possible explanations for sex differences in self-labeled loneliness. One possibility that has gained attention and support in the literature is that it is more socially acceptable for women to express their difficulties than it is for men. According to this view, the negative consequences of admitting loneliness are less for women than for men. This possibility has been tested by having university students read a standard description of a lonely person. When the lonely person was identified as a woman rather than a man, participants rated the lonely person as better adjusted, more socially acceptable, and more effective in performing various roles. Thus, the stigma of loneliness appears greater for men than for women. An interesting prediction for future testing is that the stronger the traditional sex-role expectations in a society, the larger the gender difference in reluctance to acknowledge loneliness. [*See* GENDER DIFFERENCES IN MENTAL HEALTH.]

F. Health Status and Age

A Canadian survey examined the effects of health status on loneliness. The investigators obtained a representative sample of disabled adults ($N = 731$) from 10 counties in southwestern Ontario, and then obtained an equivalent sample of nondisabled subjects ($N = 850$) matched on age, sex, and area of residence. At all age levels, disabled respondents were more likely to report loneliness than were members of the matched sample.

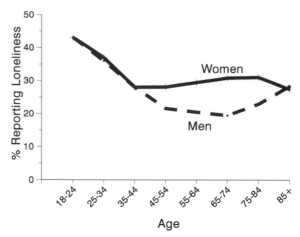

Figure 2   Age trends in loneliness.

The media often portray old age as a time of loneliness. Consistent with this view, 65% of younger adults aged 18 to 64 in a National Council on Aging survey said they thought loneliness was a "very serious problem for most people over 65." In contrast, only 45% of the older adults aged 65 or older in this study concurred in this belief.

To explore how loneliness actually varies over the life cycle, data sets of respondents under and over age 65 are needed. Figure 2 is based on an unweighted aggregation of male and female respondents ($N = 18,682$) from six surveys containing similar self-labeling questions about loneliness. The incidence of loneliness starts high, drops from young adulthood through middle age, and then seems to increase again slightly. In the data aggregated across gender, 43% of 18- to 24-year-olds reported loneliness. This dropped to 25% for respondents 45 to 64, and then rose again to 26%, 28%, and 28% for individuals in the 65 to 74, 75 to 84, and 85+ age groups, respectively.

Three nuances of the association between age and loneliness are worth noting. First, the exact shape of the curve is influenced by gender, with sex differences being greater in midlife than in young adulthood or old age. From their 40s until their 80s, women reported more loneliness than men. Second, age accounts for only a small proportion of the variance in loneliness (e.g., as little as 1%). Third, in other studies restricted to just older adults (aged 55+), findings on the association between age and loneliness vary, some studies showing marked increases, others showing none at all. The magnitude of any possible increase in loneliness among older adults may depend on the proportions of widowed and incapacitated persons in older subgroups. Finally, with slight variations, the same basic age trend also emerged when other measures of loneliness were used.

How can age trends in loneliness be explained? One approach is to consider why loneliness might be high or low in specific stages of the life cycle. For instance, some authors have claimed that separation from parents, the challenges associated with forming a personal identity, and other social transitions all contribute to the likelihood of adolescents becoming lonely. To explain the modest upturn in loneliness at the opposite end of the life cycle, others have argued that a decline in the social ties of the elderly makes them susceptible to loneliness. Research provides evidence that older adults do indeed have smaller social networks and do spend less time with others than do either adolescent or middle-aged Americans. On the other hand, a general decline in the experiencing of emotions (including loneliness) may diminish the loneliness that older adults would otherwise feel. The presence of two such countervailing forces may be useful in understanding why the changes in later life are modest. [*See* Aging and Mental Health; Social Networks.]

According to the cognitive discrepancy perspective described earlier, loneliness results when there is a discrepancy between people's desired and achieved levels of contact. Many factors may alter desired or achieved levels of contact, but it is the gap between these parameters that is identified as the immediate antecedent of loneliness. If the syllogism "being old = being alone = being lonely" is faulty, this cognitive model suggests it may be because older adults have lowered desired levels of social ties. Research demonstrates that throughout the life cycle, the desired–achieved gap is a good predictor of loneliness. Whatever explanation one endorses, the idea that the retirement years are typically fraught with loneliness appears to be more myth than reality.

G. Correlates of Loneliness across the Life Cycle

These possible explanations of age changes in loneliness are related to another similar question: Are the predictors of loneliness the same across the life cycle or do they change? The answer appears to be that both views are correct. Several variables (e.g., personality factors such as self-esteem, people feeling that their relationships are not as good as those enjoyed by their friends) are associated with loneliness throughout the life cycle. Similarly, the quality of people's relationships is generally a better predictor of loneliness than the number of social ties they have. In the interpersonal domain, however, age-specific correlations have been found. For instance, as children go from preadolescence to late adolescence to young adulthood, there is a shift in the type of relationship that is most closely linked with loneliness. In the middle elementary years, it is the quality of children's relationships with their mothers. In late adolescence, for example, it is the quality of college students' relationships with their peers. In early adulthood, romantic relationships become crucial. In midlife, family relations, especially marital relationships, predict loneliness. Among the elderly, friends and neighbors assume considerable importance.

H. Marital Status

Data from respondents in more than 20 nations document that loneliness is less common among married than nonmarried individuals. This finding is so consistent that it has been called a sociological law. Furthermore, in one study comparing the strength of association between eight common demographic factors and loneliness, marital status was the strongest predictor. When the unmarried are categorized as never married versus divorced or widowed, the results vary somewhat by study. The general tendency appears to be for never-married people to be less lonely than the divorced or widowed.

In addition to these group differences, loneliness is also part of the process of ending relationships. When young adult romantic relationships end, both partners experience the loss of their bond. Yet the person who is left behind is more likely to experience loneliness than the person who initiates the breakup. This finding can be interpreted from a discrepancy model perspective as the result of a sense of control over the breakup tempering the psychological impact of loss.

The role of loneliness in the experience of divorce is illustrated by a study of 74 recently divorced men and women from Oklahoma. Individuals who were more lonely at the time of data collection (1 week to 3 years postdivorce), as compared with those who were less lonely, blamed more of their marriages' problems on their former spouses. They also reported that they had more difficulties in their relationships with their ex-partners (e.g., arguments over child rearing), drank more, experienced greater depression, felt more cut-off from their friends, and were less likely to become romantically involved with a new partner. In essence, people who are lonely appear to experience more difficulties in the process of separation. Similar findings have been obtained for widows in the period leading up to and after the loss of their spouses.

Although marital status is important, one should not be lulled into believing that it is a steadfast guarantee against loneliness. Within-group analyses demonstrate that some factors increase loneliness among married individuals and other factors decrease it among the nonmarried. Looking first at married individuals, those who are unhappy with their marriages and name another person besides their spouse as their closest relationship partner are vulnerable to loneliness. From the reverse vantage point, a recent Dutch study showed that older adults without partners can be relatively free of feelings of loneliness when they are well supported by friends, are more accepting of their single status, and see opportunities for changing their status if they wish.

In summary, loneliness emerges early in life. It is especially prevalent in late adolescence and early adulthood. Loneliness is affected by one's demographic characteristics. Some categories of people including the poor, the disabled, and the nonmarried are at greater risk for loneliness than others. Many psychological predictors of loneliness operate at all ages, but the strength of some interpersonal correlates of loneliness is age-related. Loneliness is interwoven with how people pass through life transitions. Social transitions such as divorce can create loneliness. At the same time, people who are especially lonely during such transitions may find them more stressful and difficult than do nonlonely individuals.

For anyone concerned with community programs and preventive mental health, people in high-risk categories for loneliness warrant special attention. For example, evidence that loneliness emerges in childhood and that marriage reduces the risk of loneliness suggests the importance of preventive and supportive interventions for families. For practitioners working with lonely individuals, interventions may be enhanced by attention to life cycle considerations such as parenting programs to benefit young children indirectly, marital enrichment programs for individuals at midlife, and the promotion of companionship among

the elderly. Finally, demographic findings suggest that loneliness is caused not only by psychological and interpersonal dynamics but also by larger social factors.

V. MENTAL AND PHYSICAL HEALTH

Transitory loneliness, such as the distress of being separated from loved ones or the difficulties of making friends after moving to a new town, are part of the routine fabric of human life in modern society. In contrast, when loneliness is severe and persists for a long time, it has more serious implications for psychological well-being. Two types of research have linked loneliness to psychological problems: self-report studies of nonclinic samples and clinical studies of individuals in treatment.

A. Self-Report Studies

A growing number of empirical studies have used paper-and-pencil self-report measures to assess loneliness, personality characteristics, and psychological problems in samples of adolescents and adults. Several patterns have been found. An association between loneliness and depression is well established. Lonely people often report feeling sad and depressed, and they score higher than the nonlonely on standardized measures of depression. Loneliness is also correlated with low self-esteem, social inhibition or shyness, and anxiety. In men, loneliness has been linked to hostility and to a greater potential to rape. Some studies have found an association between loneliness and neuroticism. Lonely people are more likely than the nonlonely to report extensive use of tobacco, alcohol, and illegal drugs. Among adolescents, loneliness has been associated with poor grades in school, running away from home, stealing, and vandalism. [See ANXIETY; DEPRESSION; SELF-ESTEEM.]

B. Clinical Studies

Beginning in the 1950s, therapists began to publish accounts linking loneliness to such psychological problems as schizophrenia and alcohol abuse. Since then, more systematic studies of clinical samples have been conducted. Elevated levels of loneliness have been found among people in counseling and psychotherapy, and also among patients in residential psychiatric facilities. Among Israeli soldiers, loneliness has been associated with mental breakdowns during or immediately after battle. Individuals who have attempted suicide and those in treatment for alcoholism also show greater loneliness. Research finds that prisoners and patients hospitalized for medical problems experience loneliness, perhaps as a result of being separated from their typical social networks. [*See* SCHIZOPHRENIA.]

C. Causal Mechanisms

Although much is known about the correlates of loneliness, relatively little is known about the causal mechanisms producing these patterns of association. Consider the case of loneliness and alcoholism. One possibility is that loneliness leads to alcohol abuse. Some people may drink to drown their sorrows and to cope with chronic feelings of loneliness. A second possibility is that problem drinking leads to loneliness. Alcoholism may disrupt a person's social life, driving away friends and loved ones or leading to the loss of a job; these events may then result in loneliness. A third possibility is that some people experience many life problems such as unemployment, poor physical health, or inadequate social skills which simultaneously lead them to feel lonely and to abuse alcohol. It is likely that all of these possible causal pathways occur. More generally, the links between loneliness and psychological problems are probably reciprocal and interactive. [*See* ALCOHOL PROBLEMS.]

D. Physical Health

Loneliness is also associated with physical health problems. Compared with nonlonely peers, lonely people are more likely to report such symptoms as sleep disturbances, headaches, backaches, and poor appetite. In some cases, lonely people tend to worry more about their health and to visit physicians more frequently. In addition to these self-report findings, research has also linked loneliness to physicians' ratings of patients. There is some evidence that physicians perceive lonely people as lower in general health and less likely to comply with medical regimens than nonlonely patients.

There is also evidence linking loneliness to an increased risk of death. For example, a recent longitudinal population-based study of Finnish men over the age of 40 found that the risk of death from all causes was greater among men who rated their social relationships as inadequate and who were divorced or never married. During a 5-year period, men who rated their social relationships as inadequate (bottom quartile) were 1.83 times more likely to die than men who rated their social relationships positively (top quartile). More direct evidence linking loneliness (measured by a short form of the UCLA Loneliness Scale) and health comes from research on adults age 65 or older living in rural Iowa. Over a 2-year period, lonely people were significantly more likely to move to a nursing home and to die than were the nonlonely. This effect was found even when other risk factors, such as depression, were controlled. For example, the mortality rate was 4.5 per hundred among the least lonely, but 17.5 per hundred among the most lonely.

The mechanisms linking the subjective experience of loneliness to physical health outcomes are not well understood. Many factors may be involved. For instance, lonely people may take poorer care of their health or may cope with loneliness in health-compromising ways. Nonlonely people may benefit from friends and loved ones who offer advice and assistance. Several empirical studies suggest that physiological factors may also mediate the loneliness–health association. In these studies, researchers have assessed loneliness and immune functioning among diverse samples, including medical students, spouses of cancer patients, psychiatric patients, and men testing positive for HIV. For example, lonely medical school students have been shown to have poorer cellular-immune control of the latent Epstein-Barr virus and lower natural killer cell activity than nonlonely medical students. Although results have not been entirely consistent, most studies have found that lonely people show lower immunocompetency than nonlonely people. [*See* PSYCHONEUROIMMUNOLOGY.]

VI. OVERCOMING LONELINESS

During the journey from birth to death, few people escape the misery of loneliness. The problems leading to loneliness are varied; there is no single universal cause of loneliness. A recognition of this diversity is essential for understanding how people cope with loneliness and for designing effective interventions to assist the lonely. It is useful to distinguish problems concerning the initiation of new relationships, the maintenance of satisfying relationships over time, and the dissolution of relationships.

A. Initiating Relationships

A central problem for many lonely people is how to establish new relationships—how to make friends, find a confidant, fall in love. For some people, the successful initiation of relationships is hampered by poor social skills, social anxiety, and shyness. Cognitive factors may also be important: individuals with low self-esteem, distorted perceptions of themselves, or unrealistic standards for eligible partners may have difficulties. Yet most people manage on their own to make friends and find partners. Parents, teachers, and other adults often try informally to help children learn social skills, and young people often give considerable thought to these issues as well. Clubs, sports teams, and social and religious organizations are often places to meet new people with common interests and values. Recently, advances in computer technology and the accessibility of the Internet have provided new opportunities for people to get acquainted electronically.

Several therapeutic interventions can assist people having problems initiating relationships. For example, social skills training programs have been designed for both children and adults. Such programs use a variety of techniques (e.g., modeling, role playing, self-observation) to improve communication skills and self-presentation. Shyness groups and assertion training groups have also been developed to help individuals overcome social inhibitions. Cognitive–behavioral therapies are helpful to people whose self-defeating thought patterns impede the formation of relationships. [See BEHAVIOR THERAPY; COGNITIVE THERAPY.]

It is also worth noting that cultural norms and values can affect the ease or difficulty of initiating relationships. In many parts of the world, for example, marriages arranged by parents ensure that young adults find partners. Americans have the freedom of personal choice, but also the dilemma of finding a compatible mate. Finally, situational factors such as a person's financial resources and work obligations can also affect the ability to initiate relationships. The firespotter who lives in a remote part of the forest has few opportunities to meet people. Overcoming this problem may require a change in jobs, rather than a change in social skills. Loneliness can result not only from the absence of

relationships, but also from having a restricted or impoverished network of social relations. Social needs theorists such as Robert Weiss believe that people need a network of social relationships, including ties to friends, a loved partner, and family. From this perspective, a happily married woman might feel lonely if she lacks close friends or has troubled relations with her co-workers. A growing body of research on loneliness, social support, and multiple roles demonstrates that people benefit from having a rich and diverse social network.

B. Maintaining Satisfying Relationships

As noted earlier, being married or having friends is no certain guarantee of avoiding loneliness. Although we tend to think of lonely people as lacking relationships, this is not always the case. Separation from friends and loved ones can create loneliness. Events such as going away to school, moving to a new town, serving in the military, or working away from home can cause loneliness. Some institutions, such as colleges, recognize the social challenges faced by newcomers and offer orientation programs designed to ease the transition to a new social environment.

Loneliness can also arise from dissatisfaction with the quality of existing relationships. Research has only begun to identify the specific features of relationships that are most closely tied to loneliness. Likely candidates include conflict; a lack of intimacy, reciprocity, and companionship; and low levels of rewards. Family research describes empty-shell marriages that provide few benefits to the partners but persist because of children or other barriers to divorce. Efforts to help unhappy couples might involve couple or family counseling. Marital enrichment programs such as those offered by religious groups also address this problem. For troubled relations in the workplace, conflict resolution or mediation might be appropriate.

C. Ending of Relationships

A major cause of loneliness is the loss of a loved one through death, divorce, or breaking up. Loneliness that results when a significant social relationship ends differs from other types of loneliness. It may be associated with grief, anger, and a variety of other intense emotions. Widowhood and divorce can lead to other major life changes in financial resources and housing, as well as to changed social networks. Effective strategies for helping individuals who are experiencing the ending of relationships are tailored to the nature of the social loss. Specific programs have been created to help those experiencing divorce or widowhood. Rather than being cast as therapy, such groups often have titles such as "Seminars for the Separated" and include lectures by experts as well as small group discussions by people going through the same type of experience. It is important to recognize that although professional interventions and supportive friends can help ease the loss created by death or divorce, they cannot eliminate this distress entirely or quickly. It often takes considerable time for the emotional loneliness created by losing an important attachment figure to diminish. [*See* DIVORCE.]

D. Self-Help: Coping with Loneliness

Most lonely people do not seek professional help. A study of the transition to college found that less than 10% of first-year students had seen a counselor or therapist about how to overcome loneliness. Studies of widows find that few bereaved individuals turn to the clergy and fewer still to doctors or therapists. Relatively little is known about the ways in which people cope with loneliness, or how these coping strategies differ depending on the problem that caused the loneliness. One self-report study of adults identified four major coping patterns:

1. Sad passivity. A state of lethargy associated with watching television, sleeping, taking tranquilizers, overeating, drinking alcohol, or sitting and doing nothing.
2. Active solitude. Finding constructive ways to spend time, such as reading, exercising, or working.
3. Spending money. Finding ways to distract oneself from feeling lonely.

4. Social contact. Making efforts to reduce loneliness by calling or visiting a friend.

Many questions about coping with loneliness remain. How common are responses such as the four just described? How do reactions to loneliness change over time? Which coping strategies are most effective for particular types of loneliness?

This article has reviewed the current research on loneliness. Rather than being a sign of weakness, loneliness reflects our human need for social relationships, needs that all people share. This is why the only real cure for loneliness is to establish relationships that meet our desires for a sense of intimacy and connectedness with others.

BIBLIOGRAPHY

Hojat, M., & Crandall, R. (1987). Loneliness: Theory, research, and applications. *Journal of Social Behavior and Personality*, 2(2).

Jones, W. H., & Carver, M. D. (1991). Adjustment and coping implications of loneliness. In C. R. Snyder & D. R. Forsyth (Eds.), *Handbook of social and clinical psychology: The health perspective* (pp. 395–415). New York: Pergamon Press.

Marangoni, C., & Ickes, W. (1989). Loneliness: A theoretical review with implications for measurement. *Journal of Social and Personal Relationships*, 6, 93–128.

Peplau, L. A., & Perlman, D. (Eds.). (1982). *Loneliness: A sourcebook of current theory, research, and therapy.* New York: Wiley Interscience.

Rook, K. S. (1984). Promoting social bonding: Strategies for helping the lonely and socially isolated. *American Psychologist*, 39, 1389–1407.

Russell, D., Peplau, L. A., & Cutrona, C. E. (1980). The revised UCLA Loneliness Scale: Concurrent and discriminant validity evidence. *Journal of Personality and Social Psychology*, 39(3), 472–480.

Weiss, R. S. (1973). *Loneliness: The experience of emotional and social isolation.* Cambridge, MA: MIT Press.

Love and Intimacy

Elaine Hatfield and Richard L. Rapson

University of Hawaii, Manoa

Attachment   An emotional bond between infants and their caretakers. Infants are considered to be attached to their caretakers if they appear to be comfortable in their presence, cling to them when threatened, and become anxious if they are separated.

Commitment   Decision/commitment refers, in the short term, to a couple's decision that they love one another, and in the long term, to their commitment to maintain that love.

Companionate Love   The affection and tenderness men and women feel for those with whom their lives are deeply entwined. Companionate love is a complex functional whole including appraisals or appreciations, subjective feelings, expressions, patterned physiological processes, action tendencies, and instrumental behaviors.

Intimacy   A process in which couples, who feel close and who trust one another, reveal personal information and feelings to one another and, as a consequence, come to feel cared for, known, and validated.

Passionate Love   A state of intense longing for union with another. Reciprocated love (union with the other) is associated with fulfillment and ecstasy. Unrequited love (separation) with emptiness, anxiety, or despair. Passionate love is a complex functional whole including appraisals or appreciations, subjective feelings, expressions, patterned physiological processes, action tendencies, and instrumental behaviors.

Scientists distinguish between two forms of **LOVE**—passionate love and compassionate love. Both kinds of love are based, in part, on the parent/child attachment experience. Researchers interested in passionate love tend to focus on infants' attachments to their caretakers as the prototype of later passionate attachments. Those interested in compassionate love tend to focus on maternal and parental attachments to one another and their children as the prototype of compassionate love. Of course, love relationships can involve both passion and companionship.

I. DEFINING AND MEASURING LOVE

Love is a basic emotion. It comes in a variety of forms. Most scientists distinguish between two kinds of love—passionate love and compassionate love. *Passionate love* is a "hot," intense emotion. It is sometimes also labeled obsessive love, puppy love, a crush, lovesickness, infatuation, or being-in-love. It has been defined as

> A state of intense longing for union with another. Reciprocated love (union with the other) is associated with fulfillment and ecstasy. Unrequited love (separation) with emptiness, anxiety, or despair. Passionate love is a complex functional whole including appraisals or appreciations, subjective feelings, expressions, patterned physiological processes, action tendencies, and instrumental behaviors. (Hatfield and Rapson, 1993)

The Passionate Love Scale was developed to assess the cognitive, emotional, and behavioral components of such love.

Companionate love is a "cooler," far less intense emotion. It is sometimes also called true love or conjugal love. It combines feelings of deep attachment, commitment, and intimacy. It has been defined as

> The affection and tenderness people feel for those with whom their lives are deeply entwined. Companionate love is a complex functional whole including appraisals or appreciations, subjective feelings, expressions, patterned physiological processes, action tendencies, and instrumental behaviors. (Hatfield and Rapson, 1993)

Psychologists have used a variety of scales to measure compassionate love. One of the most popular scales is the measure of Companionate Love, which includes measures of commitment and intimacy.

Social psychologists have observed that in close, compassionate, relationships, couples' thoughts, emotions, actions, and lives are profoundly linked. The close relationship is one of strong, frequent, and diverse interdependence that lasts over a considerable period of time. Researchers have developed scales to measure how close couples' thoughts, emotions, actions, and lives are profoundly linked. The close relationship is one of strong, frequent, and diverse interdependence that lasts over a considerable period of time. Researchers have developed scales to measure how close couples are—i.e., how closely linked their organized action sequences are.

Other scientists have proposed still other typologies of love. Some scientists contended that people could adopt any of six different styles of loving. The Love Attitudes Scale was designed to measure these love styles: *Eros* (passionate, intense, disclosing love), mania (obsessive, dependent, insecure love), *storge* (friendship-based, steady, secure love), *pragma* (practical, logical love), *agape* (altruistic, giving, spiritual love), and *ludis* (game-playing, cool, playful love). Robert Sternberg proposed a triangular model of love. He argued that the different kinds of love differ in how much of three different components—passion, intimacy, and the decision/commitment to stay together—they possess. Passionate love (which he labeled infatuation), for example, involves intense passionate arousal but little intimacy or commitment. Companionate love involves less passion but far more intimacy and commitment. The most complete form of love is consummate love, which combines passion, intimacy, and commitment.

II. PASSIONATE LOVE

A. Predictors of Romantic Attraction

Researchers have identified four factors which affect couples' interactions: "person" factors, "other" factors, "Person × other" factors, and "environmental" factors. Let us consider how the first two factors can affect men's and women's readiness for love and their preferences for various kinds of partners.

1. "Person" Factors

There is evidence that certain kinds of people, at certain times, are especially susceptible to passionate love.

a. Attachment Theory and Passionate Love   Mary Ainsworth observed that infants and toddlers form different kinds of attachments to their caretakers. Some infants are securely attached. They are tightly bonded to their mothers. They feel comfortable in her presence. They are confident that she will be there when they need her; that she will support them when they feel brave enough to explore the world. (These infants may also be genetically predisposed to have an even temperament.) Other infants possess an anxious/ambivalent attachment to their caretakers. Their mothers may have been more responsive to her own rhythms than to their infants'. As a consequence, sometimes they "smother" their infants with unwanted affection; sometimes they ignore them. Since these infants have learned they cannot count on their mothers, they tend to be anxious and uncertain in their interactions with her. (Of course, some infants are simply born with a fearful disposition.) Finally, some infants develop an avoidant attachment with their caretakers. Perhaps their mothers generally ignored them. Perhaps the infants were simply lacking whatever it takes to form close relationships with anyone. In any case, such infants are unemotional and unresponsive.

Social psychologists proposed that children's early patterns of attachment should influence their adult attachments. They found that children who were securely attached did tend to mature into adults who were able to trust and depend on those they cared for and who were comfortable with intimacy. Those who were anxious/ambivalent tended to fall in love easily, seek extreme levels of closeness, worry that they would be abandoned, and have short-lived love affairs in later life. The avoidant tended to become adults who were uncomfortable getting too close and who had difficulty depending on others. There is considerable evidence that childhood attachments do serve as a model for later passionate love relationships.

If passionate love is rooted in childhood attachments, it follows that anything that makes adults feel as helpless and dependent as they were as children, anything that makes them fear separation and loss, should increase their passionate craving to merge with others. There is some evidence that this is so. For example, researchers have found that when men and women's self-esteem is threatened, when they are anxious and afraid, when they feel insecure or are dependent on others, they tend to be especially vulnerable to falling in love. [See ATTACHMENT.]

b. Additional Person Factors There are other "Person" factors that affect susceptibility to passionate love. For example, in love, timing is often everything. There are certain times when people are ready for love; times when they are not. If young people are not in a romantic relationship and wish they were, they are especially vulnerable to potential romantic partners. Conversely, if they are already dating someone, they are unlikely to feel much attraction toward others; they may even devalue others in order not to be tempted.

2. "Other" Factors

Most people prefer dates and mates who are reasonably good looking, personable, warm and intelligent, and similar to themselves in background characteristics (such as age, race, socioeconomic class, religion, and educational level), as well as in attitudes and values, and perhaps even more. People reject potential dates who are arrogant, conceited, rude, boring, or consistently make life difficult.

B. The Emotional Consequences of Falling in Love

The previous section, dealing with the roots of passion, has painted a somewhat dismal picture. It focused on the bruised self-esteem, the dependence, and the insecurity that make people hunger for love. When people fall in love with someone and feel loved in return, however, they may well experience intense happiness and excitement. Interviews with lovers suggest that they may experience five kinds of awards. Moments of passionate bliss; feeling understood and accepted; sharing a sense of union; feeling secure and safe; and transcendence. Of course, passionate love may have its costs too. When hopes are dashed, or relationships fall apart, people's self-esteem may be shattered; they may feel lonely and miserable and may experience intense jealousy.

All in all, for most people, passionate love is a bittersweet experience. People from individualistic studies (such as America and Western Europe), which tend to idealize passionate love, generally have a fairly optimistic view of passionate love. They expect it to go well. People from collectivistic societies (such as Eastern Europe, Asia, and the Middle Eastern countries), generally assume "unrestrained" love is a threat to social order. They tend to be more pessimistic about the possibilities of passionate love.

C. How Long Does Passionate Love Last?

Passionate love is generally fleeting. Researchers surveyed dating couples, newlyweds, and couples married varying lengths of time to ascertain how passionately they loved one another. Initially, it was often passion that drew men and women together. As the relationship matured, however, passion began to fade into the background. After a while, what seemed to matter most was compassionate love, commitment, and intimacy.

III. COMPANIONATE LOVE

A. Evolutionary Antecedents

Theorists have often taken an evolutionary approach to explain the origins of compassionate love. They argued that emotional "packages" are inherited, adaptive patterns of emotional experience, physiological reaction, and behavior. At every phylogenetic level, they pointed out, organisms face the same problems. If they are to survive and reproduce they must find food, avoid being killed, mate, and reproduce. Many theorists believe that companionate love is built on the ancient circuitry evolved to ensure that animals mate, reproduce, and care for their young. Recently neuroscientists, anthropologists, and developmentalists have begun to learn more about compassionate love.

1. The Chemistry of Love

Neuroscientists have begun to speculate about the biological bases of compassionate love and tenderness. They have identified a hormone, oxytocin, which seems to promote sexual and reproductive behavior and to facilitate affectionate, nurturant, close, intimate bonds between caretakers (usually mothers) and their infants.

2. The Looks, Sounds, and Postures of Love

Some theorists have argued that love's ancient heritage can be read today in the looks, gazes, and sounds of compassionate love. Emotions researchers have found that the universal emotions—such as joy, love, sadness, fear, and anger—reveal themselves in certain characteristic facial expressions. Some speculate that when men and women are feeling compassionate love and tenderness they tend to display traces of the expressions caretakers often instinctively display when they are gazing happily and tenderly at their young infants. They gaze downward (at the child). Their faces soften, and a slight, tender smile may play about their lips.

French psychophysiologists have argued that compassionate love is associated with certain breathing patterns and sounds. Mothers often coo or croon softly with their mouths held near the infant's head. They speculated that such tender maternal sounds become the forerunners of the breathing patterns associated with compassionate love and tenderness.

Desmond Morris argued that after birth, mothers instinctively try to recreate the security of the womb. They kiss, caress, fondle, and embrace their infants; they cradle them in their arms. In the womb, neonates hear the steady beat of the mothers' hearts—pulsing at 72 beats per minute. After birth, mothers instinctively hold their babies with their heads pressed against their left breasts, closest to the maternal heart. When their infants fret, mothers rock them at a rate of between 60 and 70 rocks per minutes, the rate that is most calming to infants. Morris points out: "It appears as if this rhythm, whether heard or felt, is the vital comforter, reminding the baby vividly of the lost paradise of the womb." Of course, in adulthood, these same kisses, tender caresses, and embraces continue to provide security for men and women—unconscious of their early origins.

Anthropologists have observed that primate mothers and infants and adults in all cultures reveal their close attachments in much the same ways. For instance, newborn infants rhythmically rotate their heads from side to side as they root for their mothers' nipples. As adults playfully nuzzle someone they love, they sometimes find themselves using motions, rhythms, and gestures from the distant past: holding the beloved's head and rubbing their lips against the other's cheek with a sideways movement of their head. They argue that such primitive kissing, mutual feeding, and embracing bonds people together.

Now that we have discussed the antecedents of compassionate love, let us focus on what scientists have learned about three of its components—affection and liking, intimacy, and commitment.

B. Affection and Liking

1. Reinforcement Theory

Many psychologists use reinforcement theory principles to explain why people love and like others. According to reinforcement theory, men and women come to care for those who provide them with important rewards and dislike those who punish them. They also come to feel the same way about people who are merely associated with pleasure or pain. For example, people judged members of the other sex to be more physically attractive if they made their assessments while they were listening to pleasant rock music rather than harsh avant-garde tones. Both men and women were more attracted to people they met in pleasant surroundings than to those they met in rooms that were too hot or too cold, too humid or too dry, crowded, or dirty.

Social psychologists contrasted the behavior of happily married couples with those who were distressed. Happy couples generally had positive exchanges. They smiled, nodded, and made eye contact. They spoke to each other in soft, tender, happy voices. They leaned forward to catch one another's words. Distressed couples had corrosive patterns of interacting. They tried to bludgeon one another into agreements by complaints and punishment. They sneered, cried, and frowned at one another. Their voices were tense, cold, impatient, whining. They made rude gestures, pointed, jabbed, and threw up their hands in disgust; or they simply ignored one another. As soon as one partner resorted to these tactics, the other began to respond in the same way, leading to an escalation of reciprocal aversiveness.

Unfortunately, as couples settle into a routine, kind words are often replaced by harsh evaluations, thoughtful courtesies by neglect. For some reason, married couples frequently treat one another worse than they treat strangers.

2. Equity Theory

Couples care both about how rewarding their relationships are and how fair they seem to be.

A few theorists have argued that lovers and marital partners do not really care very much about fairness. A few social psychologists, for example, asserted that couples have very different ideas as to the nature of appropriate behavior in *communal* relationships (such as love relationships, family relationships, or close friendships) as opposed to *exchange* relationships (such as encounters with strangers or business associates). In communal relationships, they argued, couples feel responsible for one another's well-being. They wish to show their love and affection; to help those they love. They expect nothing in return. In exchange relationships, on the other hand, acquaintances do not feel particularly responsible for one another. They care very much about "what's in it for me?"

Most theorists, however, take the equity perspective. Elaine Hatfield and her colleagues, for example, assumed that couples must be careful to ensure that their partners feel loved, rewarded, and fairly treated. Otherwise, love relationships will suffer and possibly dissolve. Persons generally believe that if their partners loved them they would *wish* to treat them fairly; but it doesn't always work that way. If men and women get too much or too little from their relationships for too long a time it leads to serious trouble. In a number of studies, equity considerations have been found to be important in determining who gets into relationships in the first place, how those relationships go, and how likely they are to endure. Researchers have found that couples in equitable relationships are more likely to fall in love and become sexually involved. When couples who were sexually intimate were asked why they had decided to have sexual relations, those in equitable relationships were most likely to say that *both* of them wanted to have sexual inter-

course. Couples in inequitable relationships were more likely to admit that sex had not been a mutual decision; often, one person had pressured the other into having sexual relations. It is not surprising then, that couples in equitable relationships had more satisfying sexual lives.

Equitable relationships tended to be happier and more satisfying. When researchers interviewed dating couples, newlyweds, and couples married for various lengths of time, they found that equitable relations were the most comfortable relations at every stage. If lovers gave too much and received nothing in return (not even gratitude), they eventually began to feel uneasy. Did the other really *love* them? If so, why didn't he or she seem to appreciate their sacrifices? The selfish usually began to have their doubts too. What kind of men or women would allow themselves to be made a doormat? Didn't they have any pride? Not surprisingly, those who feel they were receiving less than they deserved from their dating relationships and marriages were especially dissatisfied.

Couples were most committed to their relationships when they felt equitably treated. When undergraduates were asked to write an essay on "Why we broke up," 12% of them mentioned the lack of equity as a precipitating factor. Women were most likely to mention inequity as the reason they wanted out. (Perhaps many women keenly feel the injustice of having to work outside the home and then coming home to work a "second shift" cooking, shopping, doing housework, and caring for children.) Equitably treated men and women have also been found to be especially reluctant to risk their marriages by getting sexually and emotionally involved with someone else.

Researchers disagree as to how important equity is in determining whether couples remain together, separate, or divorce. Most agree, however, that it plays at least some part in such decisions.

C. Intimacy

The word intimacy is derived from *intimus,* the Latin term for "inner" or "inmost." Scientists reviewed the way most theorists have used this term. They found that almost all of them assumed that intimate relationships involved affection and warmth, self-disclosure, and closeness and interdependence. Most people mean much the same thing by intimacy. Some scientists asked college men and women to tell them about times when they felt especially intimate with (or distant from) someone they cared about. For most people, intimate relations were associated with feelings of affection and warmth, with happiness and contentment, talking about personal things, and sharing pleasurable activities. What sorts of things put an impenetrable wall between couples? For most, distant relationships were associated with anger, resentment, and sadness as well as criticism, insensitivity, and inattention. Men and women seemed to mean something slightly different by "intimacy." Women tended to focus primarily on love and affection and the expression of warm feelings when recounting "intimate moments." They rarely mentioned sex. For men, a key feature of intimacy was sex and physical closeness.

Clinical psychologists developed the Personal Assessment of Intimacy in Relationships (PAIR) to measure intimacy. They identified five types of intimacy: Emotional, social, intellectual, sexual, and recreational intimacy.

I. The Components of Intimacy

The threads of intimacy—affection, trust, emotional expressiveness, communication, and sex—are so entwined that it is almost impossible to tease them apart.

a. Love and Affection Men and women generally feel more love and affection for their intimates than for anyone else; such mutual affection is probably the first condition of intimacy.

b. Trust People seldom risk exposing their dreams or fears unless they know it is safe to do so.

c. Self-Disclosure When men and women are able to reveal their inner feelings and experiences to others, relationships bloom. Caring and trust may be the soil in which self-disclosure thrives, but self-disclosure, in turn, nourishes love, liking, caring, trust and understanding.

Researchers reviewed a series of studies on the "social penetration process." They made two major discoveries: (1) intimacy takes time. As couples began to get better acquainted, they began to disclose more. (2) Acquaintances tend to match one another in how intimate their disclosures are. In some relationships, both participants are willing to reveal a great deal about themselves. In others, both confine themselves to small talk.

Intimates confide two very different kinds of information—feelings and facts—to one another. On a first encounter, acquaintances usually reveal only the bare facts of their lives; they talk little about their feelings. New acquaintances are careful not to reveal too much too soon and not to reveal much more than their partners do. Daters tend to warm up fairly quickly, however. After 6 weeks or so, people are already confiding in one another at about as high a level as they ever will. It is in long-term love relationships that intimates can be *most* relaxed and trusting. Once couples know each other well, the recital of mere facts counts for little; it is the communication of feelings that is critical to dating and marital satisfaction. In long-term relationships, moment-to-moment reciprocity becomes unimportant. Things can wait. When relationships are about to end, however, the pattern of self-disclosure changes. Now, words can be used to wound. In terminal relationships, couples often begin to spew out the ugly accusations that they have kept hidden. They begin to spill out years of hatred, anger, and exaggerated grievances. Couples may begin to talk through the night, trying to figure out what went wrong and if there is any chance to set things right.

d. Nonverbal Communication Intimates feel comfortable in close physical proximity. They sneak little looks at their mates to convey shared understandings, gaze at one another, touch, stand close, and even lean on one another. Of course, people can reveal how alienated and distant they feel from one another via the flip side of these same techniques. If a person feels that a potential date they have just met is moving too fast and they are starting to feel cornered, they can reduce intimacy in several ways—by averting their gaze, shrinking back, shifting their body orientation, or simply by changing the subject and steering clear of intimate topics. We all know how enemies behave when they want to sever all contact. They glare, clench their jaws, sigh in disgust, or walk on ahead.

2. Perspectives on Intimacy

Theorists have taken a trio of approaches to intimacy:

a. Life-Span Developmental Models Developmental theorists have observed that young people must learn how to be intimate. Erik Erikson pointed out that infants, children, adolescents, and adults face a continuing series of developmental tasks. If loved and nurtured, infants develop a basic trust in the universe. They develop the ability to hope. In early, middle and late childhood, children learn to be autonomous, to take initiative, and to be industrious. They develop a will of their own, a sense of purpose, and a belief in their own competence. The next two stages are those in which we are primarily interested. In adolescence, teenagers must develop some sense of their own identity. Only when adolescents have formed a relatively stable, independent identity are they able to master their next "crisis"—to learn how to become intimate with someone, to learn how to love. Mature relationships, then, according to Erikson, involve an ability to balance intimacy and independence.

b. Motivational Approaches Psychiatrists and psychologists have pointed out that people are *motivated* to be intimate. Developmental psychologists point out that some people are high in intimacy motivation. They tend to be more loving and affectionate, warmer, more egalitarian, less self-centered, and less dominant than their peers. They spend more time thinking about people and relationships, more time talking and writing to others; they are more tactful and less outspoken. They stand closer to others. Not surprisingly, others like them, too.

c. Equilibrium Models Researchers point out that people prefer an optimal level of intimacy. Too much or too little intimacy makes everyone uncomfortable. When people get close to us, we become physiologically aroused. If we feel positive about this arousal we will move closer to them. If it is "too much" we will back off. We literally back up when someone gets too close too fast. We move forward when they seem to be slipping away. Two features of this model are worth noting. First, researchers view intimacy from a dialectical perspective. They see people as constantly adjusting the level of their intimate encounters. Second, they point out that once the intimacy equibilibrium has been disturbed, any of several different techniques can be used to set things right. People differ markedly in how much intimacy they desire. Attaining the "right degree" of intimacy often requires a delicate balancing act.

3. Why People Seek Intimacy

If seems a bit odd to ask *why* people wish for intimacy. When scientists ask men and women what they most desire in life, they generally mention a close intimate relationship. People can feel sad and lonely for two very different reasons. Some lonely people are experiencing *emotional loneliness*; they hunger for one special intimate. Others are experiencing *social loneliness*; they merely lack friends and casual acquaintances. Of the two, it is emotional loneliness that is the more painful. Contentment is better predicted by the existence of intimacy (i.e., lack of loneliness) than popularity, the frequency of contact with friends, or the amount of time spent with acquaintances. Theorists contend that intimacy has the three following major beneficial effects.

a. Its Intrinsic Appeal If people were happily in love, over 90% of them were also "very happy in general." If they were generally unhappy, most thought that love was the one thing that they needed to be happy. So people long for intimacy in and of itself.

b. Its Links to Psychological Well-Being A number of studies document that intimacy and psychological health seem to go hand-in-hand. Intimacy has been shown to be associated with happiness, contentment, and a sense of well-being. Happy (intimate) marriages provide social support.

c. Its Links to Mental and Physical Well-Being A number of medical researches have confirmed that intimacy and mental and physical well-being are connected. Intimate relationships apparently buffer the impact of stress. Intimacy problems are closely linked to many mental health disorders. If persons have a chance to disclose emotionally upsetting material to someone who seems to care, they exhibit improved mental and physical health in follow-up physical examinations. Most of our knowledge about the ties between intimate relationships and physical health comes from studies of the impact of a husband or wife's death on the survivor's mental and physical health. Investigators find that bereavement increases the likelihood of a host of mental and physical problems. Bereavement increases vulnerability to mental illness; produces a variety of physical symptoms (these include migraines, headaches, facial pain, rashes, indigestion, peptic ulcers, weight gain or loss, heart palpitations, chest pain, asthma, infections, and fatigue); aggravates existing illnesses; causes physical illness; predisposes a person to engage in risky behaviors—

such as smoking, drinking, and drug use; and increases the likelihood of death. Of course, a "close" relationship filled with hatred and strife can be worse than no relationship at all for couples' mental and physical health. [*See* BEREAVEMENT; COPING WITH STRESS.]

4. Why People Avoid Intimacy

Given all the advantages of intimate relationships, why would people ever be reluctant to become intimate with others? Men and women admit that they are hesitant to get too deeply involved with others for a variety of reasons: Some people feared that if they get too close to someone they will end up "stuck" with them; having to take care of someone worse off than themselves. Some people fear that if they begin to confide in others, they will end up feeling worse—aware of how sad, frightened, or angry they really are. Some fear that if they reveal too much about themselves, others will criticize them, be disappointed in them, or get angry at them. Some worried that if a relationship were to end, vindictive dates or mates would confide the innermost details of their lives to subsequent dates, mates, or business associates. Close relationship researchers developed the Perceptions of Risk in Intimacy scale to measure people's fear of intimacy.

5. Are There Gender Differences in Intimacy?

Researchers have observed that there is a gap between men's and women's ideas of what constitutes intimacy. Researchers interviewed 130 married couples at the University of Texas. They found that for the wives, intimacy meant talking things over. The husbands, by and large, were more interested in action. They thought that if they did things (took out the garbage, for instance) and if they engaged in some joint activities, that should be enough. Huston found that during courtship men were willing to spend a great deal of time in intimate conversation. But after marriage, as time went on, they reduced the time for close marital conversation while devoting increasingly greater time to work or hanging around with their own friends. Ted Huston observed:

> Men put on a big show of interest when they are courting, but after the marriage their actual level of interest in the partner often does not seem as great as you would think, judging from the courtship. The intimacy of courtship is in-

strumental for the men, a way to capture the woman's interest. But that sort of intimacy is not natural for many men. Women complain about men's "emotional stingyness."

Huston suggested a compromise: Couples should try to engage in the sort of intimate conversation which springs spontaneously from shared interests. This requires, of course, that couples share some interests—that they read books, or watch films, or plan trips to Europe together, and so forth.

Researchers pointed out that men are taught to take pride in being independent while women take pride in being close and nurturant. Erik Erikson contended that as men mature, they find it easy to achieve an independent identity; they experience more difficulty in learning to be intimate with those they love. Women have an easy time learning to be close to others; they have more trouble learning how to be independent. There is considerable evidence that men are less comfortable with intimacy than women.

Researchers find that in casual encounters, women disclose far more to others than do men. In our culture, women have traditionally been encouraged to show feelings. Men have been taught to hide their emotions and to avoid displays of weakness. In a study of college students, social psychologists found that women's friendships were more deeply intimate than were men's. Women placed great emphasis on talking and emotional sharing in their relationships. Men tended to emphasize shared activities; they generally limited their conversations to sports, money, and sex.

In their deeply intimate relationships, however, men and women differ little, if at all, in how much they are willing to reveal to one another. Researchers, for example, asked dating couples how much they had revealed to their steady dates. Did they talk about their current relationships? previous affairs? their feelings about their parents and friends? their self-concepts and life views? their attitudes and interests? their day-to-day activities? Overall, men and women did not differ in how much they were willing to confide to their partners. They did differ, however, in the kinds of things they shared. Men found it easy to talk about politics; women found it easy to talk about people. Men found it easy to talk about their strengths; women found it easy to talk about their own fears and weaknesses. Interestingly enough, traditional men and women were most likely to limit themselves to stereotyped patterns of communication. More modern men and women were more relaxed about talking about all sorts of intimate matters—politics, friends, their strengths and their weaknesses.

Women receive more disclosures than do men. This is not surprising in view of the fact that the amount of information people reveal to others has an enormous impact on the amount of information they receive in return. In any case, both men and women seem to feel most comfortable confiding in women. Modern tradition dictates that women should be the "intimacy experts."

Some authors have observed that currently neither men nor women may be getting exactly the amount of intimacy they would like. Women tend to desire more intimacy than they are getting; men may prefer more privacy and distance. Couples tend to negotiate a pattern of self-disclosure that is bearable to both. Unfortunately, this may ensure that neither of them gets what they really want. Of course, as men and women's roles become more alike, this double standard of intimacy might be expected to decline.

6. A Prescription for Intimacy

Most humans appear to flourish in a warm intimate relationship. Yet, intimacy is risky. What then is the solution? What advice do social psychologists give as to how to secure the benefits of deep commitment without being engulfed by its dangers? A variety of therapists and researchers have developed programs to teach young people intimacy skills. Generally, they focus on teaching men and women four types of skills: (1) encouraging people to accept themselves as they are; (2) encouraging people to recognize their intimates for what they are; (3) encouraging people to express themselves; and (4) teaching people to deal with their intimate's reactions.

D. Commitment

1. Perspectives on Commitment

It is not always easy for people to know how committed they and others are to one another. Researchers have begun to elaborate on how the commitment process works. Researchers proposed that a close relationship's cohesiveness (stability) can be defined as "the total field of forces which act" on the pair to keep them in the marriage." There are three kinds of forces that influence cohesiveness: (1) Attractiveness of the relationship. Is the relationship more (or less) rewarding than the couple expected? The more rewarding and the less costly the relationship, the more stable it will be. (2) Alternative attractions. Is this relationship more attractive than other relationships or than living alone? The more attractive the alternatives, the more likely the marriage is to dissolve. (3) Barriers against leaving the relationship. These are the "psychological restraining forces" that keep people in marriages. They include religious, legal, economic, and social barriers as well as responsibilities to children. Other researchers proposed a similar model to explain who likely will persevere in a relationship as opposed to those most likely to separate or divorce. They argued that the more satisfied couples are, the more eager they will be to preserve their relationships; the more they have invested in their relationships (in time, money, and effort) and the more limited their alternatives, the more reluctant they will be to sacrifice everything by leaving.

Recently, scientists attempted to test the relative importance of the factors that attract people to relationships (love and reward) versus the factors that prevent them from leaving (feelings of commitment and a knowledge that they have invested a great deal in the relationship) in keeping couples together in times of stress. They found that although love and rewards are important, even more important are the commitments couples feel they have made to the relationship and the practical investments they have made in it.

E. How Long Does Companionate Love Last?

Researchers have studied the fate of passionate and companionate love. One researcher interviewed couples married one month to 36 years. Initially, it was passion that drew men and women to one another. As the relationship matured, passion began to fade into the background. "Passion is the quickest to develop, and the quickest to fade," he observed. After a while, what mattered most was companionate love—which comprises commitment and intimacy. It took longer for couples to feel fully committed to their marriages and to become intimate with one another, but in love, these were the things that seemed to last.

This article has been reprinted from the *Encyclopedia of Human Behavior, Volume 3.*

BIBLIOGRAPHY

Ainsworth, M. D. S. (1989). Attachments beyond infancy. *Amer. Psychol.* **44,** 709–716.

Erikson, E. (1982). "The Life Cycle Completed: A Review." Norton, New York.

Gottman, J., Notarius, C., Gonso, J., & Markman, H. (1976). "A Couple's Guide to Communication." Research Press, Champaign, IL.

Hatfield, E., & Rapson, L. R. (1993). "Love, Sex, and Intimacy: Their Psychology, Biology, and History." HarperCollins, New York.

Kelley, H. H., Berscheid, E., Christensen, A., Harvey, J. H., Huston, T. L., Levinger, G., McClintock, E., Peplau, L. A., & Peterson, D. R. (Eds.) (1983). "Close Relationships." Freeman, New York.

Morris, D. (1971). "Intimate Behavior." Triad: Grafton Books, London.

Shaver, P. R., & Hazan, C. (1988). A biased overview of the study of love. *J. Soc. Pers. Relationships,* **5,** 474–501.

Sternberg, R. J., & Barnes, M. L. (Eds.) (1988). "The Psychology of Love." Yale University Press, New Haven.

Managed Care

Michael A. Hoge

Yale University School of Medicine

Behavioral Health Care The provision of mental health and substance abuse services to individuals suffering from psychiatric, psychological, or addictive disorders.

Capitation A financing strategy in which an organization receives in advance a predetermined, per person payment for delivering a specified range of services, as needed, to an identified group of individuals. The organization assumes financial risk for costs of services that exceed the negotiated prepayment.

Care Management The process of receiving requests for services, establishing the medical necessity of such services, authorizing a specific modality and duration of service, and connecting an individual in need with an appropriate provider.

Carve-Out The process in which a payer purchases managed behavioral health services separate from all other healthcare. The vendor for such services is typically a specialty managed behavioral health organization.

Medical Necessity Refers to services judged to be essential to assess, diagnose, and/or treat a psychiatric or substance abuse disorder.

Prior Authorization The process in which the medical necessity of services is reviewed in advance and a provider is given authorization by a managed care organization to deliver a specific type, frequency, and duration of service.

MANAGED CARE consists of a series of strategies for controlling costs and improving the appropriateness, quality, and outcome of health care. This is typically accomplished by interjecting a managed care organization (MCO) and its care management staff between the purchaser of health care and the providers. Managed care is forcing dramatic changes in the financing and practice patterns of mental health and substance abuse service delivery.

I. HISTORICAL OVERVIEW

Managed behavioral health care emerged in the early 1980s in response to dramatic increases in the utilization and cost of mental health and substance abuse treatment. As a product of government deregulation promulgated by the Reagan administration, constraints on the development and operation of hospitals were diminished. This led to explosive growth in the number of for-profit mental health and substance abuse facilities, many operated as part of large chains.

The increase in availability of services was accompanied by substantial increases in utilization. These trends were most dramatic and most disturbing with respect to the psychiatric hospitalization of adolescents. The number of adolescents hospitalized increased by approximately 400% between 1982 and 1987, reaching an annual total of a quarter of a million individuals. This increase appears to have been driven, in large part, by aggressive marketing campaigns launched by the hospitals, designed to capitalize on parents' worst fears about their children. The advertisements often cautioned parents not to ignore their children's anger, defiance, changes in habits, or school problems as "just another phase," and warned of possible dire consequences such as school failure, runaway, arrest, addiction, or suicide. Scandals occurred in California, Florida, and Texas regarding the unethical and illegal recruitment and the admission, treatment, and billing practices of psychiatric hospitals. Insurers filed suits against providers for such practices, and the federal government issued an increasing number of indictments for Medicare and Medicaid fraud.

In addition to these egregious problems, there were other difficulties with the financing and delivery of behavioral health services. Unrelated to unethical or illegal practices, the costs of mental health and substance abuse services were escalating at a marked pace. In the absence of clear standards or guidelines regarding admission criteria, lengths of stay, and provider credentialing, it was difficult for purchasers of behavioral health benefits to judge the value or appropriateness of what they were purchasing. Lastly, benefit plans typically gave the best coverage for inpatient care, inadequate coverage for outpatient care, and no coverage for treatments of intermediate intensity, often referred to as "alternatives to hospitalization." Such benefit plans encouraged individuals to use hospitals, which are the most intensive and expensive services, while affording only marginal care during the critical period immediately after such hospitalizations.

All of these forces converged in the early 1980s to foster the creation of managed care organizations (MCOs) specializing in behavioral health. These companies, at times referred to as managed behavioral health organizations, were mostly entrepreneurial start-ups that contracted directly with self-insured employers who were seeking to control costs and increase the value of the behavioral health services that they were purchasing. Using managed care processes that will be elaborated below, these MCOs developed provider networks and employed utilization management strategies to direct care and control costs. After

a decade of rapid growth, these MCOs have now begun to merge, and many have been acquired by large insurance companies.

II. DEFINING MANAGED CARE

Managed care is difficult to understand because it has had a very brief history, and has gone through numerous developmental stages. Drawing on previous conceptual models offered by Albert Waxman of Merit Behavioral Care and Michael Freeman and Tom Trabin of the Behavioral Health Alliance, it is possible to identify five generations of managed behavioral health care.

The first generation, referred to as *managing benefits,* actually predates the advent of modern managed care. This involved a series of techniques used by insurers to design benefits so as to limit reimbursement for care. The techniques included excluding coverage of certain disorders and treatments, instituting annual and lifetime maximums on coverage, and implementing high deductibles and copayments. Insurers tended to use these techniques more frequently and more aggressively in regard to psychiatric versus other medical benefits.

The second generation focused on *managing access.* The thrust of this activity was to restrict access to care, even if the care was covered by an individual's benefit plan. This was accomplished through the use of gatekeeping techniques such as prior authorization and through concurrent review of the need for continued care for those in treatment. This generation, which occurred in the 1980s, is often considered the dark days of managed behavioral health care, in which the focus was largely on reducing costs through simply denying requested access to services.

The third generation focuses on *managing care.* Rather than simply limiting access, the emphasis is on balancing cost and quality by matching clients with the most appropriate form of care and an appropriate provider. This is accomplished by creating a provider network that encompasses a continuum of care comprised of treatments of varying levels of intensity, and then utilizing more refined assessment criteria for matching a client to a treatment level. This generation is the predominant form of managed behavioral health care in operation at the current time.

The fourth generation, which has begun to emerge

over the last several years, is that of *managing outcomes.* Here the focus shifts to an emphasis on the "cost effectiveness" of care, examining the outcome of what is delivered in relationship to its cost. The notion behind this emphasis on outcome is that inexpensive care may actually be more costly if it does not produce intended clinical effects. Unfortunately, outcome measurement in behavioral health is still an imprecise science, and thus has limited impact on the management of behavioral health care at the present time. However, its impact in the future is expected to increase substantially.

The fifth generation focuses on *managing health.* Here the emphasis shifts from treatment to prevention and health promotion, based on the premise that avoiding health problems is not only better for an individual, but also reduces treatment costs. Common strategies include health risk screening, intervention with "at risk" individuals, education and skill-building programs such as stress management, and self-help groups. Such interventions are most commonly utilized by employers who have long-term responsibility for the health of their employees.

Understanding these five generations serves to clarify the differing stages of managed care. In addition, it also leads to a more integrated definition of the concept, for each generation, in essence, represents one or more objectives of a comprehensive approach to managing care. Thus managed care, in an ideal form, can be defined as the organization and management of *comprehensive, accessible,* and *accountable* behavioral systems of care that *flexibly deploy resources* to *promote health* and match *covered individuals* with *appropriate, cost-efficient,* and *clinically effective* services.

III. ORGANIZATIONAL MODELS AND CONCEPTS

There is a range of concepts and organizational models that form the groundwork for health care delivery in a managed care environment. Selected concepts and models are outlined below.

A. Parties to the Health Care Transaction

Historically, health care delivery involved only two parties. A provider delivered the care and the patient was responsible for payment. With the advent and growth of health insurance, responsibility for paying for health care was largely assumed by employers, unions, and governments, these entities often being referred to in such transactions as *third party payers.* These payers often retained *insurers,* and more recently *managed care organizations,* to facilitate the delivery of health care and the payment for services rendered. These entities become an *intermediary* or a *fourth party* to the health care transaction.

B. Carve-outs versus Integrated Models

When a third party payer decides to contract with another entity to manage its health care it faces a fundamental decision regarding behavioral health. Behavioral health care differs on many dimensions from general health care; the health benefit tends to be less generous, there is a broad range of treatments that have not been well standardized across the country, and utilization management issues are unique and often complex. Thus many payers opt to *carve out* or separate their contracting for behavioral health from other medical care, and retain a specialized managed behavioral health organization to manage mental health and substance abuse benefits. If a payer does not carve-out behavioral health then it *integrates* contracting for the management of mental health, substance abuse, and other medical services. However, it is important to note that while a payer may decide on an integrated approach to contracting for health care, the organization that receives such a contract may subcontract the management of behavioral health services to a managed behavioral health company, thus creating a carve-out.

C. Employee Assistance Programs (EAPs)

Historically, employee assistance programs focused on helping individuals who were suffering from substance abuse. Currently, EAPs tend to offer assistance with a broad range of problems including stress, work performance, parenting, legal and financial difficulties, and caring for elderly parents. EAP services are often made available at the worksite, and are presented as nonthreatening, nonpsychiatric interventions in order to circumvent the stigma often associated with seeking psychiatric help. EAP counselors are often the gatekeepers for more traditional mental health and substance abuse treatment, screening all requests for such assistance.

D. Managed Behavioral Health Organization

As described above, managed behavioral health organizations developed as for-profit entrepreneurial ventures that contracted directly with payers to manage the utilization of mental health and substance abuse benefits through contracted provider networks. According to a recent report in the industry newsletter *Open Minds,* 121.7 million of the 141.6 million Americans who have managed behavioral health benefits, have these benefits managed by such an organization, while the remaining 16.9 million Americans have their benefits managed through the health maintenance organization in which they are enrolled.

E. Health Maintenance Organization (HMO)

A health maintenance organization is one of the most common and most established forms of managed care. An HMO contracts with a payer to deliver needed medical services to individuals or *members* covered by the health plan, and does so at a preset, per-member monthly charge. Thus an HMO assumes financial risk for health care utilized, and is responsible for delivering that care as well. Service delivery can be established by creating a *staff model HMO* in which the HMO employs providers directly, or by forming a network of contracted individual or group providers. It is very common for HMOs to carve out the responsibility for mental health and substance abuse services to managed behavioral health care organizations.

F. Preferred Provider Organizations (PPOs)

PPOs consist of groups of providers that have agreed to comply with utilization review and management procedures and to deliver services at discounted rates. In exchange, they are promised an increased flow of referrals and more timely payment for services rendered. These providers are "preferred" in that members of a health plan are given incentives to use them. Typical incentives involve decreased deductibles or copayments.

G. Physician Hospital Organizations (PHOs)

In a PHO, hospitals and other providers form a comprehensive provider system and then negotiate as a single entity with payers, insurers, or managed care organizations. The providers most often continue to deliver services in their separate practice locations.

IV. FINANCING MODELS

Understanding managed behavioral health care involves understanding the flow of money from payer to provider, and the various incentives involved in each method of payment. The following are the predominant models that currently exist.

A. Salary

This is the traditional form of employment for many providers, in which an employer pays a provider an agreed upon amount for each week or month of work. This offers a level of security and certainty of income for the provider, but historically has not encouraged the provider to increase productivity or efficiency. It has become more common for salaried providers to be offered performance incentives in which some portion of their income is tied to productivity.

B. Fee-for-Service and Discounted Fee-for-Service

Fee-for-service is the financing method on which independent practice has typically been based. Providers receive a preset fee for each unit of service delivered. The incentive to providers under this system is to deliver more care and more expensive care. The more care delivered, the greater the income of the provider. Under discounted fee-for-service arrangements, providers agree to a lower price per unit of service. In exchange, they may receive continued referrals from a health plan or guarantees regarding referral volume. These arrangements may include *withholds,* which involve the retention by a health plan of a certain percentage of a provider's payments. Whether the provider ever receives this withhold is typically contingent on either a review of the efficiency of the provider or on the financial health of the health plan as a whole.

C. Case Rates

Under this method of financing, providers receive a predetermined rate for delivering a service and must absorb any costs that exceed the amount of payment for that intervention. For example, a fixed case rate may be offered for a complete course of inpatient, acute treatment, from admission to discharge, or for a course of ambulatory detoxification that involves multiple visits. Under this arrangement, providers have a strong incentive to complete the course of treatment efficiently, controlling or reducing the amount of services delivered since cost savings are retained by the provider.

D. Capitation

This form of financing involves a prepaid payment to an organization for each member covered by a health plan. In exchange for this payment, the organization is responsible for delivering a defined set of services to those members as needed, and is at financial risk for any losses incurred if utilization of services is greater than expected. This also creates an incentive to reduce the use of services, and particularly the use of costly services, since savings typically can be retained by the organization. Capitation contracts can be issued directly to provider organizations, but more typically are issued to large organizations such as MCOs or PHOs, which are positioned to take the financial risk. Such organizations can minimize the probability of catastrophic financial losses by serving a large number of members. With a large pool of covered members, unexpectedly high utilization of services by a small number of individuals does not greatly effect the average cost of care *per patient,* and thus the financial health of the organization is not adversely impacted.

V. KEY ELEMENTS OF MANAGED CARE

The organizational models described above form the structures through which health care is delivered, and the financing models govern payment and reimbursement for services rendered. While there are many different organizational and financial models within managed behavioral health care, most rely on a common set of elements and processes to manage service delivery. Since managed care organizations, or more specifically managed behavioral health care organizations, dominate the delivery of such services, they will be used to illustrate the elements and processes outlined below.

A. Networks, Contracting, and Credentialing

The delivery of managed behavioral health services routinely occurs through networks of mental health and substance abuse providers. The MCO selectively recruits and contracts with a range of providers in order to accomplish several objectives. Ambulatory mental health and substance abuse services must optimally be available within 20 miles of each member served by the MCO. Diversity must be achieved so that trained providers are available to meet the needs of children, adolescents, adults, and the elderly, and for most if not all diagnostic conditions. The network should optimally encompass a full range of service types and levels of care so that members can receive the most appropriate and least restrictive form of treatment. Finally, selected providers must be willing to accept the fee schedule or case rates offered by the MCO.

The contracts offered to providers by MCOs tend to be detailed and fairly restrictive. Typically a provider must contact the MCO prior to rendering any care, may not deliver care without authorization, must discontinue care when the authorization lapses or is withdrawn, and may not serve a member outside of this contractual arrangement even if the member expresses a willingness or desire for such an arrangement.

Once agreement is reached on a contract, providers and provider organizations must be *credentialed.* This process involves the submission of detailed information by the provider regarding issues such as education, training, licensure, accreditations, services offered, staffing, insurance, and malpractice history. MCOs are obligated to review and verify the submitted information since they have a contractual obligation with the payer to ensure that network providers meet a range of minimum standards.

B. Continuum of Care

During the past decade, it was common for at least 70% of expenditures on behavioral health services to be used for inpatient care. Managing behavioral health benefits has been based on two assumptions:

first, that substituting less intensive "alternatives" to inpatient treatment saves considerable money, and second, that these alternatives are less restrictive and hence clinically better for the patient. The nature of this clinical argument is that these alternative treatments do not disrupt contact with natural social supports such as family and outpatient treaters, and are less likely to foster regression or to build dependence on the treatment system.

The most established alternative to inpatient care is partial hospitalization. Developed in the 1940s to address hospital overcrowding in Russia, these programs typically involve a minimum of 4 hours of structured programming per day, 5 days a week. The most financially viable form of partial hospital care is referred to as day hospitalization, and involves intensive medical, psychological, and social interventions for acutely ill individuals. Such programs have average lengths of stay that range from a few days to several weeks, and serve as an alternative to inpatient admission or as a rapid step down from inpatient care. In a variant of standard day hospitalization, this modality is at times combined with an overnight, supervised residence and used as a 24-hour crisis program for acutely ill psychiatric patients, or as an alternative to a 28-day inpatient substance abuse program for those suffering from serious addictive disorders. Less intensive forms of partial hospitalization, such as day treatment and day care, have focused on rehabilitation and maintenance functions. These programs have become less common as MCOs have refused to reimburse such services, claiming that these fall outside of the "medically necessary" services covered by most health plans.

Beginning approximately 5 years ago, there was a dramatic increase in partial hospitalization usage as MCOs aggressively shifted care from inpatient to day hospitals in an attempt to reduce costs. However, the interest in utilizing day hospitals has waned considerably over the past few years as MCOs have increasingly questioned the necessity, lengths of stay, and costs of this modality. Partial hospital stays are often double in length compared with inpatient stays, offsetting or eliminating cost savings. Further, partial hospitals are often used after an inpatient stay, leading to concerns that total costs per episode actually increase when this modality is employed.

MCOs have now shifted their interest to intensive outpatient programs (IOPs), which are often operated in day hospitals with a modified schedule, typically 3 hours per day and 1 to 3 days per week. IOP treatment tends to be heavily group based and very time limited. Increasingly, such programs are now being offered in ambulatory group practice or clinic settings.

Also gaining in popularity with MCOs are a range of outreach and diversion programs. Assertive community treatment (ACT) involves multidisciplinary treatment teams that provide a comprehensive range of services to severe and persistently ill clients, mostly in community settings or in the patient's home. ACT teams are commonly used in public sector programs with patients identified as high utilizers of service. The use of home care has also been on the rise for severely ill psychiatric patients who typically do not keep follow-up outpatient appointments after hospitalization, tend to discontinue their medications, or are unable to leave their place of residence. Diversion programs that conduct outreach to patients' homes and to emergency rooms are also being increasingly used as a mechanism of crisis intervention to divert impending hospitalizations.

Standard ambulatory or outpatient services are now required to manage fairly acute patients and to reduce lengths of treatment through the use of brief therapy. For addicted individuals, ambulatory detoxification, managed through a series of outpatient visits, has largely replaced inpatient hospitalization for detoxification.

C. Access to Care

Ready access to care by patients is a fundamental principle of managed care. Mechanisms must be in place such that a health plan member can make a request for services 24 hours per day. Ambulatory providers in the network must comply with access standards which typically require that routine initial visits occur within 72 hours of the request, and urgent initial visits occur within 8 hours. All providers must maintain a 24-hour system of on-call coverage so that patients can reach their providers or covering clinicians in times of crisis.

D. Care Management

The process of fielding requests for services and connecting patients with appropriate care is typically referred to as *care management*. Care managers are usually master's-prepared mental health professionals employed by the MCO. They can be reached through a toll-free phone line, and respond to calls from members seeking service, evaluate the nature of the presenting problem, and verify the individual's eligibility and benefit coverage. Using a set of utilization management guidelines or algorithms which have been developed by the MCO, care managers match the needs of the enrollee with a specific level of care (e.g., outpatient, partial hospitalization, or inpatient) and with a specific network provider. They then issue an *authorization* or *certification* for the provider to deliver the service for a specified duration of sessions or days. Providers see the patient and submit to the care manager written documentation regarding the clinical assessment and treatment plan. This is followed by a process of *concurrent review* in which care managers review the need for continuing treatment at the level initially authorized, and typically press for the patient to be moved through less intensive levels of care, and toward a timely termination if clinically appropriate.

The application of utilization management guidelines to service requests is often a conflict-ridden process. Patients and providers often resent the intrusion of care managers into the treatment process, particularly when requests for care or a specific type of care are denied. Providers often resent the control exercised by care managers who may have considerably less training or experience than the provider. Appeal and grievance mechanisms are essential to an MCO so that patients and providers can obtain a review of care management decisions that they believe to be unjustified.

To monitor practice patterns in their networks, MCOs engage in *provider profiling*. This involves tracking data by provider on key variables such as the average time between referral and initial visit, lengths of stay, patient satisfaction and complaints, and the complaints lodged by care managers about the provider's compliance with the policies, procedures, and decisions of the managed care organization. Profiling may be augmented by data collection strategies that involve the formal measurement of patient satisfaction, clinical processes, and clinical outcomes. Providers have often argued that MCOs use provider profiling to identify and remove from the network those providers who object to the company's policies or practices and aggressively advocate for the patient and his or her treatment needs. MCOs, to the contrary, argue that profiling is a useful strategy for identifying those providers whose practice patterns deviate from accepted professional standards and norms. Clearly provider profiling is used to compare providers, shape referral patterns, and groom provider networks.

VI. MANAGED CARE IN THE PUBLIC SECTOR

In its early stages, managed behavioral health care focused almost exclusively on the commercial or private sector. The focus on the young, entrepreneurial MCOs was to contract directly with employers to manage the benefits of employees and their families. However, several forces have converged over the past several years to create a strong interest in public sector managed care: competition in the commercial sector has been fierce, the majority of medium-sized and large employers have now contracted with an HMO or MCO to manage their behavioral health benefits thus reducing the number of new business opportunities, and finally, the federal and state governments have begun to search for ways to cut the rapidly rising public sector health costs. Several forms of public sector managed care have emerged.

A. State Employee Health Care

Faced with rising costs of health care, the executive and legislative branches of many state governments have moved to purchase various forms of managed health care for state employees. Such opportunities provided an easy transition for HMOs and MCOs to gain experience and comfort in contracting with the government entities given that the health plan members were employed individuals quite similar to those covered through the MCOs' existing commercial accounts.

B. Managed Medicaid

A much more radical departure for HMOs and MCOs has been a move into managing behavioral health benefits for Medicaid recipients. This health insurance program for the poor and disabled is funded through a combination of state and federal funds. The costs of Medicaid have grown dramatically in recent years, leading the federal government to grant waivers of regulations that had previously prohibited initiatives to restrict patient choice of providers and to manage the Medicaid benefit. Some states have chosen to carve out the management of behavioral health care for Medicaid beneficiaries to MCOs while others have selected an integrated approach by contracting with HMOs to manage all health care. Similarly, there are differences among states as to whether they have moved to manage the care only of the poor, who as a group have fewer and less severe behavioral health problems, or alternatively, have included the poor and disabled in their managed care initiatives. At the present time the vast majority of states have either moved to manage at least a portion of Medicaid health care benefits or have submitted waiver requests to the federal government to do so.

C. Managed Medicare

Medicare is a principal source of health insurance for the elderly. As the costs of Medicare have continued to increase, the federal government has sought ways to control these costs. Medicare enrollees have also sought ways to cover or control the costs of services for which they are responsible, such as prescriptions, deductibles, and copays. Managed Medicare involves voluntary programs in which Medicare recipients can enroll. In exchange for agreeing to utilization management procedures and to a restricted choice of providers, enrollees typically receive coverage for some or all of the expenses that they would have had to cover under the standard Medicare program. The number of enrollees in such HMO programs is growing steadily, particularly in those states where the Medicare premium paid to the HMO is relatively generous. There is some evidence that only the healthiest of Medicare enrollees are signing up for such programs, leaving the highest utilizers in the standard Medicare program.

VII. THE IMPACT OF MANAGED BEHAVIORAL HEALTH CARE

In examining the outcome of managed behavioral health care there appear to be three general and recurrent findings. First, costs are almost always reduced either from (a) the actual costs of care in the year before managed care was introduced, or (b) from the costs predicted had managed care not been intro-

duced. These cost savings are often quite substantial. Second, access to care as measured by the number of individuals who receive some form of mental health or substance abuse services tends to increase with the introduction of managed care, although the amount and intensity of services received, on average, may go down. Third, these changes occur without apparent negative consequences in quality of care or decreased enrollee satisfaction. Since the technology for measuring the quality of behavioral health care is still fairly crude, questions remain regarding the potential negative and yet undetected impact of managed care. However, the absence of glaring negative effects on quality and outcomes is notable. Below are examples from industry and the public sector that illustrate these findings.

A. Impact in the Private Sector

The Washington Business Group on Health represents large employers who are major purchasers of health care. This organization has reported on the early successes of its members in utilizing managed behavioral healthcare. The McDonnell Douglas Helicopter Company in 1989 introduced an EAP program, care management, and select provider network. In the first year of implementation the number of employees who used their behavioral health benefit rose from 10% to 17%, while the costs of these benefits, per employee, declined 34%. Cost savings resulted from several factors. The number of inpatient admissions declined by 50% for psychiatric disorders and 29% for addictive disorders, while admissions that did occur declined in average length of stay by 47%. Further, negotiated discounts by providers resulted in additional cost savings. All of this was accomplished without any employee complaints about the quality, accessibility, or quantity of care.

The Chevron Corporation serves as a similar example from corporate America. Concerned that employees had inadequate coverage for mental illness and addictive disorders, the company expanded the range of covered benefits, created incentives for the use of ambulatory versus hospital services, and introduced utilization management and a select provider network. For the first year following these changes, EAP use increased 60% while the number of inpatient admissions decreased 21%. The plan nearly doubled in terms of the number of eligible employees, while the cost of the plan rose only slightly, from $9.2 to $9.8 million.

B. Impact in the Public Sector

The most striking example from the public sector is the Massachusetts Medicaid experiment. As reported by James Callahan and colleagues who conducted an evaluation of this initiative, it was the largest capitated, managed behavioral health care carve-out when it began in 1992. With the approval of a federal 1915 waiver from the federal government, Massachusetts contracted with a private MCO to manage the mental health and substance abuse care for 375,000 Medicaid recipients, including both disabled and nondisabled individuals.

The MCO was charged with reducing costs and changing practice patterns by introducing utilization management, negotiating discounted rates with a select provider network, and increasing the use of interventions designed to divert Medicaid recipients from inpatient care. The latter included aggressive case management and crisis intervention. The financial outcomes for the 1993 fiscal year were striking. Predicted costs for that year, had managed care not been introduced, were $210 million. Actual costs with the implementation of managed care were $163 million, resulting in a $47 million (22%) savings.

The details of how these savings were achieved are illustrative of the managed care process. The cost of administering the Medicaid program went up significantly with managed care, from a predicted $2 million to an actual $12 million in 1993. Payments to providers went down by $57 million, a substantial 27% decline. Of the $57 million reduction in provider payments, $44 million (78%) was related to decreased 24-hour care, which included inpatient, detoxification, and residential treatments. By far the greatest reduction in provider payments came in the substance abuse arena where 48% of the cost of care was cut in a single year, largely by eliminating almost all utilization of standard 28-day inpatient substance abuse programs. In contrast, mental health care costs declined by 19%.

Accompanying these cost savings in this Massachusetts managed Medicaid program was a 10.6% increase in the number of enrollees receiving outpatient mental health treatment. Surveys of providers about the impact of managed Medicaid suggested that, in their opinion, access to care was relatively unchanged, and that diversionary care was more available. Their overall rating of clinical quality was favorable with respect to the MCO's treatment recommendations, after-care plans, length of stay decisions, and the selection of appropriate treatment settings. However, one-quarter of respondents stated that clinical decisions were usually inappropriate. This was particularly true among providers of services to children who were concerned with, among other things, a 10.1% increase in the hospital readmission rate for children and adolescents.

VIII. FUTURE TRENDS

A. Focus on Cost Effectiveness

The examples cited above illustrate the potential positive effects of managed behavioral health care, particularly with respect to cost savings. While major negative effects on clinical quality have not been demonstrated, there is lingering concern that the dramatic shifts in the locus of care, from inpatient to ambulatory, combined with the large decreases in payments to providers, are having significant and potentially long-term, harmful effects on the health of enrollees in managed care plans. As a result, there is increasing attention being paid to the measurement of clinical outcomes. Unfortunately, the science and technology for measuring outcomes is still in infant stages of development in behavioral health as well as most other areas of medicine. As this science and technology is developed further, there will likely be a shift from a near-exclusive focus on cost, which predominates in the behavioral health marketplace at this moment, to an emphasis on cost effectiveness. From this latter perspective, the cost of a service will be evaluated in relationship to the clinical outcome that it produces.

B. Public and Provider Protests

In the meantime, there are increasingly negative reactions among the public to managed care, including managed behavioral health care. The executive and legislative branches of state governments have begun, in small ways, to regulate managed care practices. Managed mental health has been the focus of exposes such as the segment titled *"Managed or Mangled*

Care" that was televised recently by the CBS news program *60 Minutes*. There are also a growing number of lawsuits against managed behavioral health care organizations alleging illegal practices such as restraint of trade and interference with professional medical decisions. It is unclear whether this backlash against managed care will result in significant constraints on managed care practices, or is instead a final, half-hearted gasp of protest as providers and recipients of health care adjust to a loss of control over the health care that they deliver and receive.

C. MCO and Provider Integration

As provider organizations have become more sophisticated in the techniques of managed care, managed care organizations have shifted financial risk and care management responsibilities directly to some of these providers. This has led to speculation that provider organizations might be able to assume many if not all of the MCOs' functions, possibly eliminating the MCOs (and their costs) as middlemen in the health care transaction. There is now a clear trend in the country for providers to develop their own health plans and to contract directly with purchasers. In the area of behavioral health, the most common variation on this theme has been for MCOs and providers to form joint ventures that meld provider delivery capacities and MCO management expertise. These partnerships have occurred between MCOs and national provider chains, such as the recent merger between Greenspring and Charter Medical, and have also involved smaller scale ventures between MCOs and local providers, usually in response to state specific opportunities regarding managed Medicaid. The future likely holds an ever increasing number of such partnerships, and growth in the role of providers in managing as well as delivering behavioral health care services.

D. Long-Term Care and the Uninsured

While the debate about managed care continues, it is important to note that managed care has not, to date, addressed in significant measure two critical issues. First, managed behavioral health care has focused primarily on acute care, leaving long-term care to state departments of mental health. Long-term care contin-

ues to consume a significant percentage of the health-care dollar and must be addressed in the future for reasons of cost, and because of the need to develop better continuity between short-term and long-term services. Second, managed care applies to those who have health benefits. Unfortunately, a large proportion of the American population remains uninsured. The cost savings from managed care could serve as one potential source for expanding the pool of individuals covered by health care benefits. However, significant trends to expand coverage are not occurring, and the recent cuts and restrictions in welfare, entitlement, and disability programs may increase the number of individuals who have no access to mental health and substance abuse services.

E. An Uncertain Future

From the perspective of improving the behavioral health of the American population it is crucial that there be a shift from the almost exclusive emphasis on financing and cost control to a more balanced focus on costs, quality, and access for all individuals in need. Managed care at its best can be a mechanism for making explicit, data-driven decisions about the use of scarce health care resources in order to maximize the positive effects of prevention and treatment efforts. At its worst it can be a ruse for denying needed services and for draining the health care system of essential resources. From a developmental perspective, managed behavioral health care has entered an age of adolescence. Its mature form and functions remain uncertain.

BIBLIOGRAPHY

Austad, C. S., & Berman, W. H. (1991). *Psychotherapy in managed health care: The optimal use of time and resources.* Washington, DC: American Psychological Association.

Feldman, J. L., & Fitzpatrick, R. J. (1992). *Managed mental healthcare: Administrative and clinical issues.* Washington, DC: American Psychiatric Press, Inc.

Feldman, S. (Ed.). (1992). *Managed mental health services.* Springfield, IL: Charles C. Thomas.

Freeman, M. A., & Trabin, T. (1994). *Managed behavioral healthcare: History, models, key issues, and future course.* Rockville, MD: U.S. Center for Mental Health Services.

Hoge, M. A., Davidson, L., Griffith, E. H., Sledge, W., & Howenstine, R. (1994). Defining managed care in public-sector psychiatry. *Hospital and Community Psychiatry, 45,* 1085–1089.

Lazarus, A. (1994). *Controversies in managed mental health care.* Washington, DC: American Psychiatric Association Press, Inc.

Schreter, R. K., Sharfstein, S. S., & Schreter, C. A. (Eds.). (1996). *Allies and adversaries: The impact of managed care on mental health services.* Washington, DC: American Psychiatric Association Press, Inc.

Schreter, R. K., Sharfstein, S. S., and Schreter, C. A. (Eds.). (1997). *Managing care, not dollars.* Washington, DC: American Psychiatric Association Press, Inc.

Marital Health

Adrian B. Kelly and Frank D. Fincham

University of Wales, Cardiff

Affect The subjective experience of a partner's behavior or the marital relationship (evidenced through self-report, observed behavior, or physiological arousal during interactions).

Attributions Explanations for partner behavior and marital difficulties.

Attribution Style Variability in attributional response patterns.

Coercive Escalation The reciprocation and increasing aversiveness of behavioral responses between interacting spouses.

Marital Quality A spouse's overall evaluation of his or her marital relationship (in this entry, this term is used interchangeably with marital satisfaction, marital adjustment, and marital distress).

Marital Stability The status of a marriage (whether it is continuing or whether the spouses have separated or divorced).

Physiological Linkage The degree to which each spouse's physiological activity can be predicted from the other's activity, controlling for the autocorrelation within each spouse's physiological responses.

In the mass media, marriage is portrayed as providing lifelong companionship, romance, support, sexual fulfillment, and commitment. For a large number of couples these positive qualities erode over time, and some couples reach the point where they evaluate their relationship as unhappy overall, which may, in turn, lead to its termination. The proportion of couples who end their relationship through separation or divorce is high (e.g., about 42% of marriages in the United Kingdom, 55% of marriages in the United States, 35% of Australian marriages, and 37% of German marriages end in divorce). However, not all distressed couples make the decision to separate. For some, the barriers to separation, or the perceived absence of alternatives, may result in remaining married despite being unhappy with the relationship. Relationship distress, separation, and divorce are associated with numerous adverse physical and mental health problems in spouses and their children. Not surprisingly, more people seek professional help in the United States for marital problems than for any other problem. Understanding why some couples remain happy while others deteriorate is therefore a critical public health issue. The overall goal of this entry is to advance understanding of what constitutes **MARITAL HEALTH.** Toward this end, the first section attempts to document what is currently known about healthy marriages. Although seemingly straightforward, this task is complicated by the fact that attempts to study the positive features of marriage are rare. The second section therefore attempts to build on the first and offers an expanded view of marital health. The last section summarizes the main themes and identifies promising avenues for future research and clinical interventions with couples.

I. WHAT DO WE CURRENTLY KNOW ABOUT MARITAL HEALTH?

Since the early part of this century, hundreds of scholarly studies on marriage have been conducted, the vast majority of which have focused on marital satisfaction, adjustment, success or some synonym indicative of the quality of marriage. It would therefore be reasonable to expect that the characteristics of healthy marriage have been thoroughly documented. However, this does not appear to be the case. In order to understand this state of affairs we need to examine research on the central construct of marital quality and uncover some of the assumptions made in marital research.

A. Marital Quality

In *Anna Karenina,* Tolstoy states that "All happy families resemble one another; every unhappy family is unhappy in its own way," and marital researchers appear to have accepted Tolstoy's observation. Marital research has focused on "unhappy" marriages, assuming perhaps that "happiness" in marriage is self-evident or does not require examination. With rare exceptions, marital quality has been studied by means of spouse self-reports. What are the self-reported characteristics of marriages that overcome the odds and stay happy over long periods of time?

1. Quantitative Self-Report Measures of Marital Quality

Two major approaches have been used to document in quantitative terms the features of marital quality. On the one hand, some researchers view marital quality as a multidimensional construct that indexes dimensions of the relationship. These researchers tend to favor the use of such terms as marital adjustment to indicate that their measures include items that assess relational characteristics such as communication and conflict. On the other hand are researchers who view marital quality in terms of spousal sentiments about the marriage. To understand these two viewpoints, it is useful to examine traditional and widely used measures of marital quality.

The most widely used quantitative measures of marital quality are the Dyadic Adjustment Scale (DAS) and the Marital Adjustment Test (MAT). The first striking feature of such measures is that they contain a mixture of differentially weighted items, ranging from reports of specific behaviors that occur in marriage to evaluative inferences regarding the marriage as a whole. For example, on the MAT, items include ratings of disagreement on eight issues (most, but not all, of which are scored from 0 to 5) and questions such as "Do you ever wish you had not married?" (scored as 0, 1, 8, or 10 depending on responses). The inclusion of behavioral and judgment categories and the number and weighting of items used to assess each category varies across measures of marital quality, making it unclear as to what these tools actually measure. The aggregation of various dimensions of marriage in omnibus measures of marital quality (e.g., interaction, happiness) also precludes meaningful study of the interplay among such dimensions (e.g., interaction may influence happiness and vice versa). Consequently, while such omnibus measures have proven useful in identifying distressed and nondistressed couples, they do little to throw light on the nature and critical components of marital quality.

In light of such observations, several researchers have argued that marital quality should be limited to spouses' overall evaluations of the marriage. Although this approach to marital quality is conceptually clear, it too tells little about the content of high- versus low-quality relationships. This is perhaps hardly surprising as quantitative research on marital quality has been motivated more by practical than theoretical concerns. Nonetheless, the quantitative approach triggers an important theoretical issue concerning the properties of marital quality.

In contrast to Tolstoy's remark, implicit in most previous research on marital quality is the view that a couple's score on a questionnaire indexes their marital quality. Marital quality has traditionally been conceived of as a unidimensional continuum, ranging from the divorcing couple to the blissfully married couple. Is marital quality a continuum, or are happy couples qualitatively distinct from distressed couples?

Some researchers have questioned the construct and heuristic validity of the assumption that marital quality is continuous and unidimensional. Several phenomena are difficult to explain from this perspective. For example, couples with the same score on the DAS may be ambivalent (both very positive and very negative) or indifferent (neither positive nor negative) about the marriage. Also, why do some couples experience high variability in their moment-by-moment marital experience, whereas others do not? In clinical practice, it is easy to recall instances where a couple might show great sensitivity and affection at one moment and then intense hostility the next, whereas another couple might show stable levels of sentiment toward each partner. Defining marital quality unidimensionally therefore fails to capture the richness of marital quality and its variation.

Marital theorists have argued that conceptual understanding of marital quality is enhanced by reconceptualizing it as multidimensional. For example, Fincham and colleagues advocate a bidimensional approach in which marital quality is conceived of in terms of positive and negative components. They offer empirical information to show that these components provide nonredundant information about relationship quality. In a similar vein, Snyder developed the Marital Satisfaction Inventory (MSI), a psychometrically sophisticated instrument that offers a profile of marital quality much like the Minnesota Multiphasic Personality Inventory (MMPI) offers a profile of individual functioning. Like the MMPI, the MSI offers actuarial data to assist in its interpretation. Although promising for understanding marital quality, such tools have been underutilized in comparison to the DAS or the MAT.

Unidimensional quantitative measures of marital quality such as the DAS have been used extensively to provide anchors (e.g., to form distressed and nondistressed groups) for the study of other self-reports thought to be important to happy marriages, such as love, commitment, and acceptance. Before reviewing findings from such research, it is important to note that the heterogeneity of items in measures like the MAT or DAS may result in spurious findings. To illustrate, it is not surprising that self-report measures of commitment correlate highly with these measures, as the DAS and MAT contain items that measure related constructs (e.g., MAT—"If you had your life to live over, do you think you would marry the same person/a different person/not marry at all"; DAS—"Which of the following statements best describes how you feel about the future of your relationship?"). Some "correlates" of marital quality may emerge therefore simply because they are not independent at either the conceptual or empirical levels. We turn to research on self-reported correlates of marital quality with this caveat in mind.

2. Self-Reports of Distressed and Nondistressed Couples

By using quantitative measures of marital quality as criteria for group membership, a variety of studies have attempted to pinpoint self-report characteristics that differentiate happy and unhappy marriages. One way of achieving a richer view of marital health is to provide an unstructured setting within which couples can report on what they think are the important aspects of their relationship. A basic premise here is that we are best able to increase our understanding of marital quality by examining the characteristics of couples who have demonstrated "expertise" in the maintenance of high marital quality. Despite its intuitive appeal, such methods have rarely been used in the study of marital relationships. Happy couples married for more than 20 years identify several components of happy marriage, the most commonly reported components being commitment, love, loyalty, and companionship.

There is some convergent evidence to suggest that constructs such as commitment and love are important aspects of happy marriages. Commitment, defined as one's willingness to tolerate adversity in a relationship, significantly predicts marital satisfaction for both sexes, but most strongly for women. Rusbult and her colleagues define commitment as a psychological state consisting of beliefs and emotional components, representing one's long-term orientation toward a relationship. They provide an impressive array of research suggesting that markers of commitment are significantly related to marital quality. Love, not surprisingly, has been shown to be associated with marital satisfaction. However, as already noted, the conceptual redundancy in these measures is likely to be high.

3. Summary

The majority of research has focused on quantitative conceptions of marital quality. Although there are some qualitative studies, quantitative and qualitative approaches have had very little impact on each other and are seldom cross-referenced. The focus on marital quality reflects the applied origins of marital research and most likely continues to motivate interest because self-reported marital quality is thought to be the "final common pathway" that leads couples to seek professional help. However, self-reported marital quality gives little information on what processes lead to this path and reflects a number of assumptions that require careful evaluation. Indeed, there are inherent limits as to how much information the study of self-reported marital quality can provide about marital health.

Before examining such limits, we provide a brief overview of the large body of research that attempts to account for variance in marital quality. Much of this research evolved from a behavioral perspective of marriage. According to this perspective, rewarding or positive spouse behaviors increase reports of satisfaction and aversive spouse behaviors lead to reports of dissatisfaction. Although the focus of research shifted to observation of couple behaviors, behaviorally oriented research retained self-reported marital quality as a central construct, using observed behaviors to account for variability in marital quality. Since the 1980s, however, the focus on observed behavior expanded to include the study of intrapersonal variables such as cognition and emotion. In the next three sections, we briefly summarize what has been learned about behavioral, cognitive, and affective correlates of marital quality, recognizing that the distinctions among these three constructs are in many ways artificial.

B. Behavior and Marital Quality

Attempts to identify the behavioral correlates of marital quality have taken two primary forms. Using spouses as observers of their partners' behaviors, researchers have attempted to examine behaviors that co-vary with daily reports of marital satisfaction. A second strategy entails laboratory observations of the behaviors of couples who report high and low marital quality. What does this research show about the behaviors associated with marital health?

The first point to note is that agreement between spouses in reports of daily marital behaviors is modest and is not greatly improved by training spouses. Such findings raise questions about the epistemological status of spouse reports of partner behavior, suggesting that they may reflect more about the reporter's perceptions than the observed spouse's behavior. With this caveat in mind, it has been found that reported spouse behaviors co-vary only slightly with daily reports of satisfaction (the two variables share about 25% of their variance), the covariation remains slight, even when lists of behaviors are customized for each couple. Behaviors classed as affective are more highly

related to satisfaction than other classes of behavior (e.g., instrumental), events experienced as displeasing (e.g., "spouse interrupted me") are more highly related to satisfaction ratings than events that are "pleasing," and the association between daily behaviors and satisfaction is higher in dissatisfied than satisfied couples.

Although their status as veridical reports of partner behavior are questionable, some of the results obtained for spouse reports of behavior are remarkably consistent with the findings that emerge from observed couple interactions. For example, negative behaviors appear more consistently to distinguish couples classified as satisfied versus dissatisfied on traditional measures of marital quality. In summary, distressed couples, when compared with nondistressed couples, show a range of dysfunctional communicative behaviors when they are observed discussing problem issues, including higher levels of specific negative behaviors such as criticalness, hostility, defensiveness, and disengagement, such as not responding or tracking the partner. Distressed couples also fail to listen to each other actively when interacting. These negative interactional behaviors are also more likely to occur in some contexts than in others. Diary studies show that stressful marital interactions occur more frequently in couples' homes on days of high general life stress, and at times and places associated with multiple competing demands. Furthermore, the topics of marital disagreements often coincide with the activities the partners are engaged in at the time.

There are also particular sequences of behavior that tend to occur in distressed couples. For example, they show coercive escalation and gender-skewed effects of female demand behaviors coupled with male withdrawal behaviors. Gender-based demand–withdraw patterns occur in many couples, regardless of marital satisfaction, but are notably strong in distressed couples.

Although there is considerable agreement on the behaviors displayed by unhappy couples, much less is known about the behaviors of happy couples. Compared with distressed couples, short interactions on problem issues in nondistressed couples show more positive behaviors, such as empathy, pinpointing and verbalizing problems in a noncritical way, and generation of solutions to the problems. It is likely that rewarding and intimate verbal interactions and activities are critical components of happy couple relationships. Happy couples report that spending positive shared time together is a major reason for the rewarding nature of their relationship, and happy couples also actively share and build on experiences communicated by their mate.

In summary, research on marital behavior has focused primarily on microbehaviors during communication tasks and couple activities. A considerable amount is known about the behavioral characteristics of distressed couples, but much less is known about the behavioral processes or dynamics that occur between happy partners. The available research has focused on the frequencies of specific behaviors and is only just beginning to investigate processes such as active sharing of positive memories and events.

Although the study of interactional behavior has proven to be fruitful in understanding marital quality, its explanatory power is limited. The association between measures of interactional behavior and measures of marital satisfaction is relatively small and, as noted, spouses do not agree well on the occurrence of positive and negative behaviors. These findings point to the importance of how couples perceive and interpret each other's behavior. We therefore turn to what is known about cognition in marriage.

C. Cognition and Marital Quality

The role of cognition in understanding marital quality has received considerable empirical attention in the last decade. Most research has studied the content of cognitions. For example, dysfunctional and unrealistic relationship beliefs (e.g., that disagreements are destructive, partners cannot change, as measured in the *Relationship Beliefs Inventory*) are related to observed spouse behavior and significantly predict therapy outcome. However, like global measures of marital quality, such measures have been criticized because they blur conceptual distinctions between different cognitions.

In contrast to a focus on dysfunctional unrealistic beliefs, a few studies focus on functional unrealistic beliefs or idealized views of the partner or relationship (e.g., kindness, affection, openness, patience, understanding, responsiveness, tolerance, and acceptance). For example, happy couples view their partners in a more positive light than their partners view themselves, and individuals are happier in their relationships when they idealize their partners and their part-

ners idealize them. However, very little is known about how idealization of the partner develops or erodes over the course of a relationship.

The most extensively investigated cognitions in marriage are the attributions or explanations spouses offer for marital events. A large number of studies have shown that distressed spouses, relative to nondistressed couples, make maladaptive causal attributions that accentuate the impact of negative marital events and minimize the impact of positive events. For example, a distressed spouse may attribute his or her partner's failure to complete a chore to a stable and global factor located in the partner (e.g., laziness), whereas a nondistressed partner may attribute such behavior to an unstable, specific, external factor (e.g., an unusual work demand). The distinction between causal attributions (who or what produced an event) and responsibility attributions (who is accountable for the event) has also proved useful in differentiating distressed from nondistressed spouses; distressed spouses are more likely than their nondistressed counterparts to attribute negative partner behavior to selfish motives, to see it as intentional and blameworthy. Finally, attribution style or variability in attributions has been linked to marital quality. Less variable responses have been associated with marital distress, although attempts to replicate this finding have only been partially successful.

The importance of attributions in understanding marital quality is further highlighted by evidence that attributions may play a role in the initiation and maintenance of marital distress. Establishing the causal role of attributions in marital distress is a difficult task as ethical and practical considerations rule out experimental studies. Perhaps the closest one can reasonably get to establishing causality is to demonstrate that attributions predict later satisfaction, while controlling for initial satisfaction. Attributions, but not unrealistic beliefs, have been found to predict marital satisfaction 12 months later, after statistically controlling for earlier satisfaction. This longitudinal association has been replicated and has been shown to be independent of spousal depression and marital violence. Any causal relation between attribution and marital satisfaction is hypothesized to occur through the influence of attributions on behavior. It is therefore noteworthy that maladaptive attributions are related to less adaptive problem-solving skills observed during discussion, to greater anger and blame during a problem-solving discussion, and to greater rates of negative behavior and increased reciprocation of negative behavior. Attributions account for approximately the same amount of variance in behavior as marital satisfaction and depression. Finally, it is noteworthy that the attribution–behavior link is independent of level of marital satisfaction or depression.

Although the study of behavior and cognition in couples has proven fruitful, intuitively we know that these phenomena fail to capture the full experience of marriage. What is missing from our picture thus far is what is often most evident in couple interactions, the smiles, laughs, affection, and warmth that happy couples show, and the anger, tears, distress, agitation, and coldness often shown by distressed couples. In the next section, we therefore briefly turn to the literature on emotion in marriage.

D. Emotion and Marital Quality

A variety of indices of emotion have been applied in the study of married couples. These indices vary in the aspect of subjective emotional experience that is tapped (self-reported affect, observed affect, physiological arousal), the degree to which affect is tied to actual interactions (global self-report questionnaires vs. "on-line" ratings of behavior), and the complexity with which emotion is conceived (e.g., the dimensionality of emotion, the individual vs. the dyad as the unit of analysis). This variability perhaps reflects the range of theories regarding emotion, a review of which is beyond the scope of this article. To simplify this section, we provide a brief overview of the most common methods used to assess emotion and review central findings about the role of emotion in the phenomenology of happy and unhappy relationships.

An index of emotion that has long been used in the assessment of marital dyads is nonverbal behavior. Simple coding systems, where voice tone, facial expressions, and body posture are used to code affect as positive, neutral, or negative, are an integral part of several coding systems. Although such assessment of affect is clearly simplistic, several fascinating findings support the centrality of affect in couple relationships. For example, affect codes are more powerful than verbal codes in discriminating distressed and nondistressed couples. Furthermore, distressed and nondistressed couples differ in their use of neutral and negative, rather than positive, affect. Finally, distressed

couples are able to alter verbal behavior if instructed to pretend to be happily married, but they are unable to change their nonverbal behavior. [See NONVERBAL COMMUNICATION.]

Several other indices hypothesized to capture aspects of emotion have been applied to the marital dyad, including verbal report methods, "on-line" affect rating methods, and most recently physiological measures such as heart rate. What do studies using these methods find?

Arising from the observation that married individuals believe that love (or the overall level of positive affect an individual feels for his or her spouse) is an important characteristic of a good marriage, paper-and-pencil measure of this variable have been developed. These measures discriminate between clinic and nonclinic couples, and share about one half of their variance with the MAT, suggesting that love is an important component of marital satisfaction (although this latter finding is not surprising given that affect-related items appear in the MAT). Such measures probably focus on more stable and global affect-laden beliefs (e.g., honesty, trustworthiness, attraction, and friendship), and the degree to which these measures reflect the experience of couples while they interact is unknown.

To investigate affective experience during interactions, couples have been asked to make continuous ratings of how they feel (ranging from very negative to very positive) as they review a videotape of their interaction. These ratings reliably discriminate between distressed and nondistressed couples, with happy couples experiencing problem-solving interactions as more positive than distressed couples. These studies also show that spouses' negative feelings are likely to be followed by negative feelings from their partners, whereas nondistressed spouses are likely to validate their partners when they have expressed negative feelings.

These findings have been extended to the domain of physiological measures of affect. This research assumes that the sympathetic branch of the autonomic nervous system (which controls four physiological systems—heart, vasculature, sweat glands, and muscle activity) controls affect during marital interactions. Research on the patterns of physiological responses between couples provides good preliminary evidence on the role of emotion in understanding couple interactions. Gottman and colleagues have taken on-line measurements of autonomic nervous system activity during the course of low- and high-conflict discussion tasks and temporally matched them with self-reported affect ratings (with the affect rating dial system) taken while the couple viewed a videotape subsequent to the interaction. Physiological interrelatedness (or physiological linkage) occurred at the times when negative affect was reported as occurring and being reciprocated. It was higher in the high-conflict task compared with the low-conflict task, and was inversely related to marital satisfaction. Perhaps the most salient finding is that physiological linkage during the high-conflict task explained 60% of the variance in marital satisfaction, and self-reported affect explained an additional 16%. When compared with the 25% of variance in marital satisfaction explained by observed behavior, this finding is impressive.

Gottman and colleagues assessed the role of current self-reported affect in determining future marital quality. Marital satisfaction 3 years after the initial assessment was predicted by specific gender-imbalanced patterns of affective exchange or reciprocity. Declines in satisfaction were predicted by more reciprocity of the husband's negative affect by the wife, and by less reciprocity of the wife's negative affect by the husband. These findings suggest that as marital satisfaction declines, partners may increasingly behave in a way that further decreases marital satisfaction. Husbands may become more emotionally withdrawn, leading to expressions of increased dissatisfaction by wives, which results in increased negative affect reciprocity. This pattern of affect reciprocity may have a considerable negative impact on marital quality in the long term. Although intriguing, these findings still await replication.

In summary, happy couples score higher on measures of affect-laden relationship beliefs such as love, affection, trustworthiness, and honesty. With regard to observed affect, even highly simplified coding systems show that unhappy couples are not only characterized by negative affect, but also find it difficult to turn off or modify negative affect. Happy couples are distinguished from unhappy couples more by their relatively few displays of negative affect, rather than by excesses in displays of positive affect. Although the mapping of observed and reported affect onto physiological measures is far from perfect, affective processes (both self-reported affect and physiological indices) are strong predictors of concurrent marital quality and long-term marital quality.

E. Conclusion

In this section, we examined the construct that dominates research in the marital literature and reviewed research on its correlates. Although it receives considerable attention, the construct of marital quality is poorly understood, which reflects, in part, the atheoretical nature of much marital research. Notwithstanding the relative lack of theoretical development, a number of behavioral, cognitive, and emotional correlates of marital quality have been identified. Although important, research on marital quality provides limited information on marital health owing to some of the assumptions made in the research literature.

The problem with conceptualizing marital quality as a continuum is that marital health may not simply be the opposite of marital distress. A closely related problem is the assumption that marital health is not just the opposite of marital dissatisfaction, but the *absence* of marital dissatisfaction. Weiss and Heyman recently stated that such a conclusion is illogical, noting that "Marital harmony is not just the absence of whatever it is that dissatisfied couples do." Although the focus on the pathological aspects of marriage has been helpful in defining what happy couples do not do, we know remarkably little about what happy couples do that is functional.

Even if some of the assumptions underlying research on marital quality withstand close scrutiny, there are inherent limits in the extent to which self-reports of marital quality can be informative about marital health. This is because marital health presumably consists of more than spousal reports. In the next section, we attempt to offer a more complete view of marital health.

II. TOWARD A MORE COMPLETE PICTURE OF MARITAL HEALTH

In marital therapy and in marital prevention and enrichment programs attempts are made to intervene in a couple's life to bring about or enhance marital health. These attempts are presumably based on explicit models of the healthy marriage; therefore, we begin by examining these literatures to expand the definition of marital health.

A. Marital Therapy Literature

Marital therapy is the professional application of psychological theories and psychotherapeutic techniques to move couples from a state of marital dysfunction to one of marital health. Therapeutic change, therefore, presumably provides a key to understanding marital health. Emanating from a variety of theories of marriage (e.g., behavioral marital theory, family systems theory, insight-oriented marital theory), several major therapies have been proposed, but relatively few have been subjected to controlled and replicated experimental scrutiny. An exception is behavioral marital therapy (BMT), the efficacy of which is thought to be well established. This mode of therapy therefore places us in a strong position to evaluate the keys to moving couples from a state of distress to a state of marital health.

Behavioral marital therapy is built on the premise that if the natural contingencies in couples' interactions are changed, then couples' relationships will become more reinforcing. Traditionally, however, BMT has only partially fulfilled this premise, as it has tended to focus more on extinguishing destructive interactional patterns and much less on imparting skills aimed at enriching interactions (although promising behavioral interventions focusing on enhancing tolerance and acceptance are currently under trial). It appears that BMT has focused on a model of pathology rather than on a model of marital health.

Although such a model is inadequate for our purposes, this state of affairs enables us to address an important issue raised earlier: Is marital happiness the inverse of marital distress? For example, if therapeutic intervention results in partners who are nonviolent, who do not have regular escalations of negative behaviors and affect, and who do not have dysfunctional patterns of demand–withdraw behavior, are the couples happy? In other words, does BMT produce marital happiness?

Numerous empirical reviews have evaluated more than 20 controlled trials of BMT in which it has contained combinations of behavior exchange, communication, and problem-solving training. It is clearly more effective than either no treatment or nondirective counseling. However, a significant proportion of couples (25 to 30%) do not improve by the end of therapy, and only about one half of those who do improve can be said to be maritally satisfied. For those couples who do show improvements in marital satisfaction, there is substantial relapse, with less than half of presenting couples maintaining clinically significant gains longer than 2 years after therapy.

One possible reason for the limited efficacy of BMT is that it has failed to provide adequately for the development of the skills or characteristics of happy couples, and instead has focused on eliminating distressing characteristics. Perhaps for a high proportion of distressed couples, BMT interventions move couples in the right direction (i.e., by removing negatives), but fall short by not fostering whatever characterizes happy relationships. For example, little research attention has been paid to how commitment and love might be enhanced in distressed couples who wish to stay together, constructs which, as noted earlier, are associated with high marital quality. However, interventions that focus on couple intimacy have been shown to be comparable in treatment effects to conventional BMT. Also, other research has found that one of the primary issues raised by marital therapy clients is their waning love for their partner. To date, there has been no clear demonstration that clinical change in these constructs occurs.

Even the interventions in conventional BMT, which ostensibly enhance positive dimensions of marital experience (e.g., positive communication skills), are of questionable face validity. Do happy couples naturally use open-ended questions, reflective statements, summarize their partners' point of view, and check for understanding? Probably not as much as one thinks they might. The limited efficacy of BMT and its focus on extinguishing interactional patterns characteristic of distressed couples reinforces the need to take a step back and pay more attention to qualities that make for happy relationships. What we can conclude from the BMT literature is that removal of dysfunctional behavioral patterns does not seem to work well in the long term, and this suggests that there is more to marital health than the absence of features that characterize distressed relationships. [*See* BEHAVIOR THERAPY; COUPLES THERAPY.]

B. Prevention and Enrichment Programs

Work on the prevention of marital distress and the enrichment of existing happily married couples is somewhat more promising, with a large body of research demonstrating that prevention programs are efficacious in the short term and possibly in the long term. Examination of this literature may help to explain the core processes important for the maintenance or enhancement of high marital quality.

A meta-analytic study of some 85 prevention and enrichment programs found that the average participant improved more from pretest to post-test than did 67% of those in a control condition. This effect represents a modest increment of 17% improvement relative to an ineffective treatment (in which the average participant is better off than 50% of the controls). Although these results show us that, broadly speaking, prevention and enrichment programs are effective in the short term, our primary interest is in the specific interactional processes associated with sustained marital quality. We need to examine studies that describe intervention content in sufficient detail and that follow couples for a period of many years (because marital distress is most likely to occur in the first 7 years of marriage).

Very few studies have examined the long-term benefits of prevention and enrichment programs. Markman and colleagues evaluated a prevention program that consisted of therapy techniques used in communication-oriented marital enhancement programs (e.g., training in speaker and listener skills, expressing negative feelings and managing conflict, problem solving, expectations and relationship beliefs, and sexual enhancement). The emphasis of this program was on the future of the relationship rather than on directly addressing current problems. Although the group receiving the program and a no-treatment control did not differ immediately after the intervention, couples receiving the intervention reported significantly higher relationship satisfaction 19 months later. These effects were maintained at later follow-ups. At 3 years, couples receiving treatment reported significantly higher sexual satisfaction, less intense marital problems, and higher relationship satisfaction than control couples. Five years after the intervention, couples receiving treatment reported more positive and fewer negative communication skills and less marital violence than control couples. It appears that imparting skills for dealing with future potential problems may be an important aspect of enhanced marital well-being.

What degree of confidence can we have in the conclusion that these sorts of preparative interventions contain skills important to the maintenance of satisfying relationships? Unfortunately, the Markman et al. study lacked an attention-only control condition, making it unclear whether the interventions used were responsible for the effects or whether the effects were caused by some general attention factor. Several researchers have also raised questions about the selection biases that occur in these programs and question whether they reach those at high risk of marital deterioration.

Other work has evaluated prevention programs specifically targeting couples at risk of marital distress. Using a program similar to Markman's, Van Widenfelt and colleagues recruited couples who were currently mildly maritally distressed, and where at least one partner had experienced parental divorce (two previously identified risk factors). At both 9-month and 2-year follow-ups, participation in the intervention did not prevent decline in relationship functioning for couples in which at least one partner had experienced parental divorce.

The literatures on marital therapy and on prevention/enhancement offer comparatively little guidance as to what constitutes marital health or even what comprises a happy marital relationship. It appears that there are a variety of characteristics and skills that may be *necessary* for high marital quality, including good communication skills, the ability successfully and mutually to anticipate and resolve problem issues, the ability to anticipate and prepare for future marital stressors, and the ability to maintain a high ratio of positive to negative interactional behaviors. There is no convincing evidence, however, to suggest that these characteristics are *sufficient* to produce high marital quality. Behavioral marital interventions designed to rectify or prevent problems have modest effects in producing high marital quality that is maintained over time. A significant problem with determining the critical components of prevention programs relates to ambiguity regarding the degree of risk of future marital problems shown by couples participating in them. We therefore offer some building blocks for a more complete picture of marital health.

C. Building Blocks for an Expanded View of Marital Health

Although existing literatures on marriage fail to provide a clear conception of marital health, they do provide valuable ideas for future research in this area. In this section we present some essential elements for an expanded view of marital health, guided, in part, by extant research findings.

1. Marital Quality

It is difficult to imagine a definition of marital health that does not include spouse reports of marital quality. At a minimum, then, we argue that marital health will include a subjective sense of well-being about the relationship. This is a theoretically simple index of marital quality that can be used as a component of marital health; however, subjective reports of marital quality are, by themselves, insufficient as an index of marital health. What else might be needed?

2. Commitment

In view of its emergence in research on positive dimensions of marriage, it is prudent to include commitment in any definition of marital health. Although there is widespread agreement regarding the phenomena accounted for by commitment, the construct of commitment has been the subject of considerable debate among social psychologists. In the present context, it suffices to note that many of the conceptions can be traced to social exchange theory and, crudely stated, amount to variations concerning the definition of and ways of combining the pros and cons of remaining in the relationship. However defined and combined, the pros of being in the relationship must outweigh the cons for commitment to exist. Marital health would be incompletely specified if we did not go further and state that the commitment must be realized in the form of a marriage that lasts over time for it to be considered healthy.

3. Marital Stability

At a minimum, then, marital health includes not only subjective marital satisfaction and commitment, but also marital harmony of success over time (indexed, in part, by positive spouse reports). Although most research on marital quality is motivated by the attempt to understand marital success, studies of marital quality are, by themselves, inadequate for gaining insight into the causes and consequences of marital success and failure; marital quality and marital stability may be related but they are not synonymous. Unfortunately, the substantial literature that has developed on marital stability adds little to the understanding of marital health. Practical concerns again lead to an emphasis on the negative in research on marital stability,

with most studies focusing on predictors of relationship dissolution, reflecting the assumption that these same variables lead to an understanding of marital stability.

Research on marital stability is only part of a broader and emerging emphasis on the longitudinal study of marriage. This emphasis has grown out of the recognition that concurrent correlates of marital quality may be different from those that predict marital quality over time. A recent review of 115 longitudinal studies of risk factors for marital distress found that couples with a lower age at marriage, lower income, lower education, parental divorce, lower marital satisfaction, higher levels of neuroticism, and higher levels of stress may be more likely to experience marital difficulties than couples without these factors.

4. Adaptation to Stress: The Centrality of Spousal Support

In their recent analysis of longitudinal predictors of marital distress, Karney and Bradbury suggest that marital outcomes are a joint function of enduring vulnerabilities, exposure to stress, and adaptation to the stress. Because few couples can avoid exposure to stress, which is a significant risk factor for declines in marital quality, we argue that marital health must include consideration of a couple's adaptation to stress.

Couples vary in their ability to adapt to stress. For example, some couples might report that their relationship was severely and negatively affected by a stressful event, whereas others might report a healthy adaptation to significant stress, and may even report an enhanced relationship as a consequence. Moreover, an event considered to be highly stressful to most people may be perceived as minimally stressful by certain couples. What leads to differences in outcomes for couples?

Although individuals differ in their ability to cope with stress, we argue that supportive behavior from a partner is central to the couple's adaptation to stress. In view of this claim, we briefly examine social support in marriage. Within the marital context, it has proven difficult to isolate the topography of behaviors thought to be "supportive." Clearly, social support in marriage contains a behavioral element, and the list of potentially supportive behaviors is endless. Providing problem-focused coping strategies aimed at managing or eliminating the source of stress (such as providing information about coping options, planning coping strategies, providing instrumental assistance) as well as emotional support (such as providing opportunities to debrief, responding with unconditional regard to distress, and physical affection) are all potential examples of supportive acts within the marital context. However, the essential element of social support, the sense of being supported, or "perceived support," is not well captured in purely behavioral topographies of social support.

This problem has led marital researchers to consider the role that cognitive representations of partner behavior have in determining perceived support. Marital theorists argue that the reason inferred for a partner behavior is likely to be a major factor in determining whether it is perceived as supportive. For example, if a spouse in need perceives a supportive partner behavior as something that was involuntary, unlikely to occur again, and selfishly motivated, perceived support may be low or absent. Conversely, if the same behavior was perceived as freely and unselfishly performed, perceived support may be high.

In summary, we make two points about the role of social support in marriage. First, perceived support (i.e., behavior independently coded as supportive, as well as attributions about the behavior) is likely to covary with marital satisfaction and facilitate successful adaptation to stress. Second, a couple's capacity to provide support in the event of stress may not be readily evident until stress arises. For example, marital satisfaction may be high, but partners' resources for coping with stress and providing support may be poor when significant stress occurs. [See COPING WITH STRESS; SOCIAL SUPPORT.]

Thus far we have identified three central components of marital health and have briefly noted what is known about each from the available literature. None should be seen in isolation, as each takes on its meaning for marital health in the context of the others. Thus, marital quality, marital success or stability, and adaptation to stress have all been identified as important elements of marital health. But do these components alone define marital health?

5. Individual Well-Being: Psychological and Physical Health

We argue that a complete account of marital health requires consideration of individual well-being. Until recently, the interaction of marital and individual well-being has been underplayed. We hypothesize that the degree to which a marital relationship promotes or impedes individual well-being is a critical component of marital health. A functional and healthy marital relationship is one that contributes to individual well-being for both partners. In contrast, an unhealthy relationship is one that detracts from or impedes individual well-being in one or both partners. We offer an overview of evidence (most of which is limited to the investigation of marital quality) to support this view.

Psychological health is related to marital quality. Disorders as diverse as schizophrenia, agoraphobia, and depression have been linked to marital quality. The largest body of research has focused on depressive symptoms. Longitudinal studies suggest that marital quality and interactional behavior may have a causal role in the etiology and maintenance of depressive symptoms. In community samples, high proportions of women who experience a significant negative marital event, and who have no history of depression, evidence depressive symptomatology 1 year subsequently. Also, marital therapy interventions appear to be an effective intervention for depressed individuals and marital therapy added to existing treatment regimes (e.g., pharmacotherapy) shows added improvements in marital quality. [See DEPRESSION.]

There is also evidence that marital quality may be associated with prolonged and dependent use of alcohol. People presenting for marital therapy report high levels of substance abuse, and people presenting for alcohol dependency treatment report high levels of marital distress. Marital distress is often a precipitant of problem drinking and increases the chance of relapse in recently treated alcohol-dependent women. Incorporating conjoint maritally focused interventions for heavy drinking males has short-term efficacy (at 6 months posttreatment), providing further support for the potential role of marital problems in maintaining alcohol problems. However, the effects of these interventions are less clear in the long term (at 2-year follow-up). [See ALCOHOL PROBLEMS.]

Physical health also appears to be related to marital quality. Marital problems may impact health through several mechanisms. The first, and perhaps most obvious, is the accentuated risk of verbal and physical violence and associated physical and psychological trauma. Although the frequency of physical aggression is similar across genders, the risk of physical and psychological sequelae are the most serious for female partners, and the frequency of violence is accentuated where alcohol abuse is present in one or both partners.

Marital interactions may also impact physical health less directly through social control (regulation, modeling, selective reinforcement) of positive and negative health-related behaviors such as smoking, drinking, diet, exercise, and leisure time. Such social control factors may provide useful indices to aid in the prevention and early detection of health problems.

A third possible mechanism by which marital quality affects health is through persistent alterations to cardiovascular functioning and endocrine functioning that mediates immunological changes. Predominant psychosomatic models of cardiovascular disease suggest that cardiovascular responses to environmental stressors are an important mediating mechanism. These models assume that individuals with consistently more pronounced, frequent, or enduring increases in blood pressure or heart rate in response to stressors are more likely to develop cardiovascular diseases.

What support is there for the association of marital quality with cardiovascular responses and the subsequent development of cardiovascular disease? The work of Kiecolt-Glaser and colleagues suggests a positive correlation between marital distress, conflict, and marital termination and biological indices of stress and physical health problems. For example, Kiecolt-Glaser and colleagues compared degree of loneliness, physical health (frequency of illness), and immunodeficiency in separated/divorced and married men (both distressed and nondistressed). Separated/divorced men were more distressed and lonelier, had more recent illness, and had poorer values on two indices of immunity (antibody titers to two herpes viruses) compared with married men. Among married men, poorer marital quality was associated with greater distress and poorer response on one immunological measure.

Other work in this laboratory has examined the association of marital quality (poor, high, separated/divorced) with physiological indices of stress and psychological functioning among women. Using a cross-sectional design and controlling for negative life events, they associated poorer marital quality with greater depression and a poorer response on these qualitative measures of immune function. Women who had been separated for 1 year or less had poorer immune functioning than their matched married counterparts. This study selected for those who did not abuse alcohol or drugs, addressing the criticism that nonmarried individuals may have riskier lifestyles than married people. Without longitudinal data, we do not know how the presumably consistent decreases in immunological functioning in this study affect actual health.

Although marital quality is associated with various indices of stress and stress-related health problems, we know little about the sorts of marital factors that are associated with these problems. Physiological mechanisms have been proposed, but interactional mechanisms have not. A problem with these models is that they do not allude to the processes or mechanisms by which marriage affects physical and psychological health. A few recent studies help to give a clearer idea of what types of marital problems might have an impact on physiological stress responses. [*See* Stress.]

There is preliminary evidence that specific types of marital interaction processes are associated with cardiovascular response. For example, the effects of exerting social influence or control within marital interactions impacts systematically on cardiovascular response. Compared with female partners, male partners who attempt to influence, dominate, or persuade their wives display higher systolic blood pressure before and during interactions. These physiological effects are associated with increases in anger and a more hostile interpersonal style. Female partners who engage in social control behaviors do not show these elevations in systolic blood pressure. Kiecolt-Glaser and colleagues replicated this "nasty versus nice" effect on blood pressure, its gender-biased pattern, and also found that the effect holds for immune responses.

Two important observations need to be made in interpreting the research reviewed. First, the links between marital quality, interactional behavior, physiological arousal, immune functioning, and the development of physical health problems are clearly in need of replication with larger samples across different laboratories. Second, the relationship between marital quality and well-being may be spurious, as previous states may affect both the tendency to get married and current well-being. Without controls for preexisting psychological states, the possibility that people with the best psychological health are selected into marriage, with the most distressed remaining unmarried, cannot be ruled out.

Nevertheless, the research on marital quality and physical well-being points to some exciting areas for future research. There is some preliminary support for drawing together two fields of marital inquiry that have until now been explored independently. The first field is research on the nature of marital quality. The second field is the findings of differential physiological responses across different interactional styles (e.g., "nasty" vs. "nice," overt hostility and dominance vs. withdrawal). Applying more recent conceptualizations of marital quality as bidimensional (relatively orthogonal dimensions of positive and negative behavior/affect) may clarify the relationship between marital quality and physical health. Different dimensions of marital quality may be more closely linked to physiological arousal and resultant physical stress than others, and, while there is evidence that specific interactional patterns are associated with high arousal, research to date has retained a unidimensional view of marital quality.

In the discussion so far, we have highlighted several components of a healthy relationship. These include subjective report of marital quality, commitment, marital success or stability, adaptation to stressful events, and a positive or at least neutral impact on physical and psychological well-being. It is reasonable to hypothesize that the weight accorded to each dimension will vary according to the marital life cycle. While a percentage of couples will remain in a state of overall satisfaction with their relationship, the nature of marital quality may change according to developmental phases of marriage (e.g., having no children and few financial obligations, becoming parents, retirement). Also, changes in social networks, work patterns, leisure activities, and physical changes as partners grow older may lead to variation in the phenomenology of marital experience. In the next section we briefly address the changing picture of marital health over the life span.

D. Changing Picture of Marital Health over the Life Span

Does the initial glow that accompanies the beginning of a relationship remain for those couples who stay together and who are happy in the long term? To evaluate this question, numerous studies have examined marital satisfaction in different age groups, or have examined marital satisfaction retrospectively. However, methodological problems, such as the confounding of age/ years married, cohort differences, and memory bias, are best avoided by following couples longitudinally. Interestingly, these methods yield different findings.

For example, cross-sectional research of age group cohorts shows that marital satisfaction is high initially, lower in midlife, and in later life shows a partial return to initial levels. When long-term marriages are investigated prospectively, however, this U-curve of marital satisfaction becomes less pronounced. What does seem to vary longitudinally is perceptions of the ease with which disagreements are resolved, with female partners reporting that this becomes more difficult with time.

Again, by using cross-sectional studies of age cohorts, researchers have compared the moment-by-moment interactions of younger and older couples. Couples have been found to vary in the overall level of interactional positivity and negativity as years of marriage increase. Two studies have found that behavioral negativity tends to decrease as couples age together, and there is evidence that negative sentiment is a variable that may act independently of relationship satisfaction in older happily married couples.

These findings have been extended to the study of self-reported affect and autonomic and somatic physiology during positive, neutral, and aversive discussions in distressed and nondistressed couples. Compared with younger couples, older couples report more positive affect during marital interaction and find discussion of difficult issues less physiologically arousing, even after controlling for overall greater positivity. Finally, the degree to which partners are able to provide emotional and practical support to a spouse may become increasingly important in older couples, especially as the risk of illness increases.

It appears that there may be changes in reports of marital quality, the topography of behavior, physiological arousal, and so on across the life span. Thus, we should not expect the components of marital health to remain static but to reflect changes in the marital life cycle. For example, that fact that older couples, compared with their younger counterparts, show less negative affect, more positive affect, and less physiological arousal independent of marital satisfaction, suggests that any definition of marital health requires flexibility to accommodate developmental differences among married couples.

III. CONCLUSION

In an attempt to understand marital health, we reviewed a large body of research on marriage, much of which focused on marital quality. Our examination of marital quality and its behavioral, cognitive, and emotional correlates provided some useful clues regarding marital health, but overall it appears that we know a considerable amount about marital distress and relatively little about marital health. We argued that this reflects, in part, the tacit but mistaken view that healthy marriages are the inverse or opposite of distressed or unhealthy marriages. As a consequence, we concluded that marital health needs to be investigated as an end in itself.

We have attempted to develop a more complete picture of marital health. Our starting point was the literature on couple therapy and on prevention/enrichment as the involvement of professionals in couple relationships that is presumably designed to bring about, maintain, or enhance a state of marital health. There is some evidence that anticipation and preparation for future, perhaps inevitable, marital problems are an important dimension of marital health, as highlighted in research on prevention of marital distress. Overall, however, professionals' activities did not appear to be informed by explicit models of marital health, but instead seemed to be based on a tacit view similar to that found in basic research; that is, that marital health is achieved by the removal or avoidance of factors associated with marital distress (e.g., poor communication). Although this may be necessary for marital health, research data do not provide convincing evidence that this strategy is sufficient for ensuring marital health.

Drawing on the basic and clinical research literatures, we went on to offer some building blocks for an expanded view of marital health. First, we identified marital quality as an important component. Its centrality for understanding marital health suggests that the examination of richer self-report measures of marital quality will pay handsome dividends. Not only will it inform more fully our conception of marital health, but it will also facilitate the development of more sophisticated and clinically informative assessments of marital quality. Second, several constructs (e.g., love, idealization) investigated in social psychological research on relationships appear to be relevant to marital health and we included one of them, commitment, as an important building block in our analysis. A possible problem here, though, concerns the variety of approaches that have been taken to investigate this construct; we therefore recommend a clear focus on the ideas common to them.

Third, the need to realize commitment in an ongoing relationship led us to identify time as a relevant factor for understanding marital health and to propose marital stability as another important building block. As with the preceding two building blocks, this one is meaningful for understanding marital health only when it is viewed in the context of the others. Fourth, we argued that marital health can only be understood when marriage is viewed in a broader environmental context that includes examination of stressors and couples' adaptation to them. We proposed that such a view necessarily leads to consideration of spousal support, as such support seems central to successful adaptation. Fifth, our attempt to develop a more complete view of marital health led us to propose that the influence of the marriage on individual psychological and physical health needs to be considered. Although the mechanisms linking marital functioning to individual health are complex and underexplored, there is enough evidence to justify individual health variables as a potential marker of marital quality and, in our view, of marital health.

Finally, the broader view emphasizes the need for marital health to be considered in terms of the stage of development in the marital life cycle. For example, it is quite likely that the presence of stressors external to the relationship, resources and skills for dealing with stress and the impact of individual health problems, are all linked with the longitudinal development of marital health. It is also likely that the differential weights of each component of marital health vary according to the developmental stage of a couple.

In this article we emphasize the need to enrich and widen our conception of marital quality. Although traditional conceptions of marital quality have proven fruitful, it is now time to consider using richer measures of marital quality, turning attention to marital health in addition to marital pathology, to assess more systematically the ways in which broad environmental forces impinge on marital relationships, the ways in which couples respond to these forces, and the mechanisms by which marital problems affect individual health.

ACKNOWLEDGMENT

This article was written while the authors were supported by a grant from the Economic and Social Research Council of Great Britain.

BIBLIOGRAPHY

Bradbury, T. N., & Fincham, F. D. (1991). A contextual model for advancing the study of marital interaction. In G. J. O. Fletcher & F. D. Fincham (Eds.), *Cognition in close relationships* (pp. 127–150). Hillsdale, NJ: Lawrence Erlbaum.

Burman, B., & Margolin, G. (1992). Analysis of the association between marital relationships and health problems: An interactional perspective. *Psychological Bulletin, 112,* 39–63.

Cutrona, C. E. (1996). *Social support in couples: Marriage as a resource in times of stress.* Thousand Oaks, CA: Sage.

Fincham, F. D., Beach, S. R. H., & Kemp-Fincham, S. I. (1997). Marital quality: A new theoretical perspective. In R. J. Sternberg & M. Hojjat (Eds.), *Satisfaction in close relationships* (pp. 275–306). New York: Guilford Press.

Gotlib, I. H., & McCabe, S. B. (1990). Marriage and psychopathology. In F. D. Fincham & T. N. Bradbury (Eds.), *The psychology of marriage: Basic issues and applications* (pp. 226–257). New York: Guilford Press.

Gottman, J. M. (1995). An agenda for marital therapy. In S. M. Johnson and L. S. Greenberg (Eds.), *The heart of the matter: Perspectives on emotion and marital therapy* (pp. 256–296). New York: Brunner-Mazel.

Hahlweg, K., & Markman, H. (1988). The effectiveness of behavioral marital therapy: Empirical status of behavioral techniques in preventing and alleviating marital distress. *Journal of Consulting and Clinical Psychology, 56,* 440–447.

Karney, B. R., & Bradbury, T. N. (1995). The longitudinal course of marital quality and stability: A review of theory, method, and research. *Psychological Bulletin, 118,* 3–34.

Rusbult, C. E. (1983). A longitudinal test of the investment model: The development (and deterioration) of satisfaction and commitment in heterosexual involvements. *Journal of Personality and Social Psychology, 45,* 101–117.

Weiss, R. L., & Heyman, R. E. (1997). A clinical-research overview of couple interactions. In W. K. Halford & H. J. Markman (Eds.), *The clinical handbook of marriage and couples interventions* (pp. 13–41). New York: Wiley & Sons.

Meditation and the Relaxation Response

Richard Friedman, Patricia Myers, and Herbert Benson

Harvard Medical School

Fight-or-Flight Response Physiological arousal of the sympathetic nervous system which prepares an organism to either fight or run away from a perceived threat.

Central Nervous System Neural activity that occurs within the brain and the spinal cord.

Meditation Any activity that focuses conscious attention.

Peripheral Nervous System Neural activity that occurs outside the brain and spinal cord including the sympathetic branch of the autonomic nervous system.

Relaxation Response An integrated physiological response that is the opposite of the fight-or-flight response—i.e., it reduces physiological arousal. The relaxation response is elicited by two simple steps: (1) focusing attention on a word, sound, prayer, phrase, image, or physical activity, and (2) passively ignoring distracting thoughts and returning to the repetition.

Sympathetic Nervous System A branch of the human body's autonomic nervous system. In response to stress, sympathetic nervous system activity automatically increases resulting in the fight-or-flight re-

sponse. During meditation or other mental focusing techniques, sympathetic nervous system activity is decreased, resulting in the relaxation response.

Over the past several decades, hundreds of scientific studies have documented the deleterious effects of psychological stress on the psychological, behavioral, and physiological functioning of humans. Upon exposure to psychological stress a series of central and peripheral nervous system changes occurs that compromise our ability to think effectively and behave appropriately. psychological stress also causes physiological changes that can cause and exacerbate somatic illness. Not surprisingly, attempts have been made to develop strategies to minimize the adverse effects of stress. Some of these management strategies are related to cognitive restructuring and other therapeutic approaches within the context of Western psychology; others, such as **MEDITATION**, are related to older Eastern traditions. This article discusses meditation; its psychological, behavioral, and physiological effects; and how it can be effectively incorporated into the routine care of individuals who require mental and medical interventions.

I. HISTORICAL PERSPECTIVE

The concept of meditation, as well as its therapeutic value, is frequently misunderstood. For centuries meditation has been associated with positive psychological benefits. Although many Eastern cultures have embraced the concept that regular meditation practice can alter one's state of consciousness or enhance one's perception of reality, the mystical or metaphysical overtones associated with meditation have inhibited Western societies from adopting it more extensively.

Twenty-five years ago, Benson and his colleagues began to examine the psychological and physiological components of meditation within a Western scientific and medical framework. After studying the cultural, religious, philosophical, and scientific underpinnings of meditation, Benson and his colleagues concluded that meditation requires only two specific steps: (1) focusing one's attention on a single repetitive word, sound, prayer, phrase, image, or physical activity; and (2) passively returning to this focus when distracted. When one engages in these two steps, a set of predictable physiological events occurs within and outside the central nervous system (CNS) that promote a sense of calm and behavioral inactivity. Benson labeled this set of physiological events the *relaxation response*. The relaxation response is the biological consequence of a wide variety of mental focusing techniques, one of which is meditation. This widely applicable and beneficial concept should be routinely integrated into psychological, behavioral, and medical treatments.

To appreciate the short- and long-term effects of eliciting the relaxation response and its clinical use it is necessary to understand the physiology of stress.

II. PHYSIOLOGY OF STRESS AND THE RELAXATION RESPONSE

More than 50 years ago, Cannon observed that mammals faced with life-threatening situations respond with predictable physiological arousal of the sympathetic nervous system (SNS) that prepares them to either face the threat or run away from it. He labeled this the now-familiar *"fight-or-flight response."* This response stimulates physiological changes to facilitate vigorous skeletal muscle activity. SNS arousal, mediated by the release of epinephrine and norepinephrine, increases heart rate and blood pressure, which in turn accelerates blood circulation to meet the increased demand for oxygen, nutrients, and waste removal. Platelet activity also increases to enhance coagulation in the event of potential injury with blood loss.

Numerous psychological events (e.g., the perception of physical danger) can automatically elicit the fight-or-flight response. For primitive man, this response was necessary for survival. Today, faced with everyday stresses, such as being kept waiting in line or on the phone, we experience the same response to varying degrees.

The behavioral and physiological opposite of the fight-or-flight response is the relaxation response which is believed to be an integrated hypothalamic response that depresses SNS activity in a generalized manner. Forty years ago, Hess described this effect as the trophotropic response. By electrically stimulating the anterior hypothalamus of cats Hess was able to elicit signs of reduced sympathetic nervous system arousal including decreases in muscle tension, blood pressure, and respiration. This response was the opposite of what he termed "ergotropic" responses, which corresponded to the heightened state of SNS activity described by Cannon as the fight-or-flight response.

The early experimental work of Cannon and Hess, combined with the more recent observations of Benson and his colleagues, suggests that these two responses are actually symmetrical. Although both involve central and peripheral nervous system changes, the fight-or-flight response prepares the organism for action while the relaxation response prepares the organism for rest and calmness, behavioral inactivity, and restorative physiologic changes. Whereas repeated or prolonged elicitation of the fight-or-flight response has been implicated in illness related to stress and SNS arousal, repeated elicitation of the relaxation response appears to prevent or ameliorate stress-related disorders. [*See* STRESS.]

III. MEDITATION, THE RELAXATION RESPONSE, AND PHYSIOLOGICAL CHANGES

Benson and his colleagues were among the first to use Western experimental standards to study the physiology of meditation and its potential clinical benefits. In experiments involving Transcendental Meditation conducted at the Harvard Medical School and at the University of California at Irvine, physiological parameters were monitored in subjects in both meditative and nonmeditative states. Measures of blood pressure, heart rate, rectal temperature, and skin resistance as well as electroencephalographic (EEG) events were recorded at 20-minute intervals. During the meditative states oxygen consumption, carbon dioxide elimination, respiratory rates, minute ventilation (the amount of air inhaled and exhaled in a 1-minute period), and arterial blood lactate levels (an indication of anaerobic metabolism) were reduced. These acute changes are all compatible with reduced SNS activity and were not evident when the subjects simply sat quietly. Since these initial demonstrations, others have documented that elicitation of the relaxation response results in important physiological changes that are mediated by reduced SNS activity.

In addition to the SNS effects of the relaxation response, its central nervous system effects have been dramatically illustrated in a controlled study of frontal EEG beta-wave activity. Novice subjects listened to either a tape designed to elicit the relaxation response or a control tape that provided a discussion of the relaxation response and its benefits. Using topographic EEG

mapping, researchers found that elicitation of the relaxation response appeared to reduce cortical activation in anterior regions of the brain (see Fig. 1).

Another study has also provided evidence of the effect of the relaxation response on CNS indices of arousal. Jacobs, Benson, and Friedman examined the efficacy of a multifactor behavioral intervention for chronic sleep-onset insomnia. The interventions included education about sleep (e.g., sleep states, sleep architecture) and sleep hygiene (e.g., abstaining from alcohol, caffeine, and nicotine use in the evening), sleep scheduling, and modified stimulus control (restricting use of the bed to sleeping). The subjects were taught relaxation-response techniques and were instructed to practice them at bedtime. Those insomniacs exposed to the intervention exhibited significant reductions in sleep-onset latency and were indistinguishable from

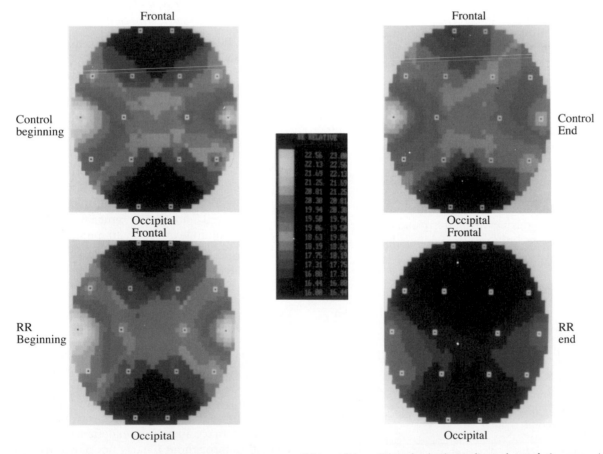

Figure 1 Beta relative power for control and relaxation response (RR) conditions. Vertical color bar indicates beta relative power (white highest, black lowest). Topographic maps are displayed in relative spectral power for greater resolution. *Note:* At RR end (lower right), beta relative power is significantly (*p* < .0164) decreased in frontal areas.

normal sleepers. More importantly, the insomniacs showed a marked reduction in cortical arousal, as assessed EEG power spectra analyses; specifically, the percentages of beta total power decreased from pre- to posttreatment.

The relaxation response training most likely mediated these reductions in cortical arousal and were therefore probably responsible for the dramatic decrease in sleep-onset latency. These findings in insomniacs support the contention that regular elicitation of the relaxation response leads to physiological changes opposite to those seen during the fight-or-flight response (i.e., decreased vs increased cortical arousal, respectively).

Since the physiological changes and therapeutic effects of the regular elicitation of the relaxation response lead to significant beneficial physiological changes and these effects appear to be the same as those associated with rest and sleep, what extra benefits does this practice offer above and beyond those derived from sleeping? Actually, the two activities are quite different. Although oxygen consumption plummets within the first few minutes of eliciting the relaxation response (in this example through meditation), oxygen consumption during sleep decreases appreciably only after several hours (see Fig. 2). The concentration of carbon dioxide in the blood increases significantly during sleep, whereas during meditation it decreases. The electrical conductivity of the skin tends to increase during sleep, indicating reduced sympathetic activity. However, the rate and magnitude of sleep-related increases in skin conductivity are much smaller than those observed during meditation and other relaxation-response techniques. Researchers have demon-

strated that CNS effects of the relaxation response also differ from those observed during sleep. [*See* SLEEP.]

IV. RATIONALE AND TECHNIQUE FOR ELICITATION OF THE RELAXATION RESPONSE

A variety of techniques can be used to elicit the relaxation response, including meditation, progressive muscle relaxation, autogenic training, yoga, exercise, repetitive prayer, and the presuggestion phase of hypnosis. Although all of these strategies result in the same physiological response, two components appear to be essential to achieving the relaxation response: mental focusing and adopting a passive attitude toward distracting thoughts.

The following is an instructional set developed by Benson and his colleagues for elicitation of the relaxation response.

Step 1. Pick a focus word or short phrase that's firmly rooted in your belief system.
Step 2. Sit quietly in a comfortable position.
Step 3. Close your eyes.
Step 4. Relax your muscles.
Step 5. Breathe slowly and naturally, and as you do, repeat your focus word, phrase or prayer silently to yourself as you exhale.
Step 6. Assume a passive attitude. Don't worry about how well you're doing. When other thoughts come to mind, simply say to yourself, "Oh, well," and gently return to the repetition.
Step 7. Continue for 10 to 20 minutes.
Step 8. Do not stand up immediately. Continue sitting quietly for a minute or so, allowing other thoughts to return. Then open your eyes and sit for another minute before rising.
Step 9. Practice this technique once or twice daily.

Sample focus words, prayers, phrases include: One, Ocean, Love, Peace, Calm, Relax, "The Lord is my shepherd," "Shalom," "Insha'allah," or "Om."

Regular practice at eliciting the relaxation response has been shown to produce chronic physiological changes by at least two research groups. With repeated practice, patients can experience the benefits of relaxation throughout the day not only during actual practice periods.

It is the clinician's responsibility to help the patient develop a personally relevant and effective technique.

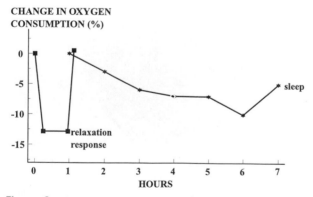

CHANGE IN OXYGEN CONSUMPTION (%)

Figure 2 O$_2$ consumption during sleep and the relaxation response.

It is important to emphasize that adherence to relaxation regimens will be maximized by selecting a strategy that is compatible with the patient's belief system and customary practices. It is useful to ask patients about their belief systems and to adapt an approach compatible with them. For example, a religious person might be more comfortable focusing on a familiar repetitive prayer, while someone interested in physical exercise might be more comfortable performing a repetitive exercise. The manner in which the response is elicited is immaterial since the psychological and physiological results are the same.

V. THE RELAXATION RESPONSE IN PSYCHOTHERAPY

For many patients with psychological disturbances, who might be hesitant to enter therapy, relaxation-response training is a nonthreatening intervention that can be introduced prior to other more rigorous forms of therapy such as cognitive therapy or medication. Meditation and other modes of eliciting the relaxation response can be a means of preparing for standard psychotherapy by allowing the patient to observe thoughts and mental events.

In 1985, Kutz and colleagues were the first to systematically study the relationship between psychotherapy and meditation. They studied the change in psychological well-being and the impact on psychotherapy of a 10-week meditation program in 20 patients. The intervention consisted of weekly 2-hour group sessions and daily home practice. Patients showed significant decreases in psychological symptoms from pre- to posttreatment as measured by the Symptom Checklist 90 Revised (SCL-90R), a standard psychological inventory, and the POMS. Subjects experienced the largest decrease in depression and anxiety. These results suggested that meditation facilitated the goals of the psychotherapeutic process. It is worth considering why such meditation training may have been helpful.

Patients were instructed in mindfulness meditation and were taught how to become detached observers of their thoughts. This form of meditation helps patients increase their insight regarding how mental categories are developed. With the enhanced awareness patients can detach themselves from their habitual ways of thinking, and through therapy they can progress to greater cognitive flexibility and more adaptive self-im-

ages and lifestyle changes. Much of what occurs in psychotherapy is intended to bring about these changes. While meditation alone cannot obviate skilled therapy and is no substitute for a therapeutic alliance, it may be the case that the CNS changes that occur when meditation is used to elicit the relaxation response set the stage for more rapid and persistent psychotherapeutic change.

For many types of disorders such as anxiety and other stress-related disorders, elicitation of the relaxation response via meditation or other techniques can help reduce sympathetic nervous system activity, which can be a part of the treatment. Researchers have examined the effectiveness of meditation-based stress reduction program in a pilot study on patients with anxiety disorders.

Patients participated in an 8-week course in which they attended weekly 2-hour classes. In the sixth week they also attended an intensive 7.5-hour retreat. Patients showed significant reductions in anxiety, panic symptoms, and depression from pre- to posttreatment and results were maintained 3 years later. It has been suggested that, unlike those who participate in cognitive therapy, patients who practice mindfulness meditation are not asked to substitute one thought pattern for another. Instead, patients observe the "inaccuracy, limited nature, and intrinsic impermanence of thoughts in general and anxiety-related thoughts in particular." [See ANXIETY; DEPRESSION; PANIC ATTACK.]

While meditation and other techniques used to elicit the relaxation response can play an important role in the treatment of some psychological problems, such interventions might not be recommended for patients with certain personality disorders, dissociative disorders, or schizophrenia. [See DISSOCIATIVE DISORDERS; PERSONALITY DISORDERS; SCHIZOPHRENIA.]

VI. THE RELAXATION RESPONSE AND BEHAVIOR CHANGE

Relaxation-response training can be used to facilitate behavior modification goals. Most patients who begin a diet or a smoking cessation program are able to stay with the program for short periods of time. When stresses arise, however, it generally becomes more difficult to maintain the new routine. Coping with stress and anxiety has a "psychic cost" that takes the form of a diminished capacity for self-regulation. Presumably, the cause of this "stress disinhibition effect" is a depletion in the cognitive and emotional resources required to maintain self-regulation. Increased stress and anxiety lead to immediately gratifying, but ultimately damaging behaviors, such as dietary indiscretions, alcohol or drug abuse, and an increase in smoking. Relaxation training has proved to be effective as an acute coping strategy to reduce anxiety. [*See* COPING WITH STRESS.]

The extent to which stress-related relapses are prevented is directly related to the degree to which relaxation-response training alleviates stress and anxiety. For example, smoking-cessation programs are unsuccessful in about 60 to 80% of cases and stress has been identified as a major contributor to this high rate of failures. In a recent study, smokers who had completed a smoking-cessation program were assigned to either a relaxation training or a control group each of which met for 3 months. The relaxation-based intervention included audiotapes for home training in guided imagery techniques. The relaxation group was asked to practice 20 minutes a day at least four times a week. Relaxation-trained subjects reduced stress, enhanced imagery effectiveness, and, perhaps most importantly, were more successful in abstaining from smoking compared with control subjects who were not exposed to the training. During a 3-month follow-up only 28% of the relaxation-trained subjects relapsed whereas 49% of the control subjects resumed smoking. [*See* SMOKING.]

Since relaxation training is often taught as a part of behavior-change programs with multiple components it is difficult to measure to what degree the beneficial effects are attributable to relaxation training alone. The effect of relaxation training was evaluated in one of the most successful behavior-change programs, the Lifestyle Heart program, developed by Ornish. In this program relaxation training is combined with diet and exercise regimens as well as group support to reduce symptoms in patients with coronary heart disease. In a controlled trial patients attended a week-long retreat followed by two 4-hour sessions each week thereafter. They performed 1 hour of aerobic exercise and participated in 1-hour sessions of stress management techniques which consisted of relaxation, yoga, stretching, breathing techniques, meditation, and guided imagery.

Among the participants the mean degree of coronary artery stenosis regressed from 61.1 to 55.8%. These results were compared with those in a group of nonparticipating patients in whom the mean degree of stenosis actually progressed from 61.7 to 64.4%. Analysis also showed that diet alone could not account for the beneficial effects. While almost all the patients maintained a healthier diet, those who practiced stress management more often showed greater stenotic regression. [*See* HEART DISEASE: PSYCHOLOGICAL PREDICTORS.]

In another study involving 156 patients who had had a myocardial infarction, relaxation response training augmented the effects of concurrent therapeutic strategies. Patients were randomized into two groups: one was given physical exercise training alone and the other was given both physical exercise and relaxation training. Several questionnaires were administered: the State-Trait Anxiety Inventory (a 40-item standardized anxiety inventory); a sleeping habits questionnaire (a 10-item questionnaire concerning hours of sleep, sleep quality, etc.); a functional complaints questionnaire (a 25-item inventory concerning complaints frequently expressed by cardiac patients); and the Heart Patients Psychological Questionnaire (HPPQ) (including scales on well-being, subjective invalidity, displeasure, social inhibition). Patients in the exercise-only group reported no change in psychological measures, whereas the group who received relaxation training reported less anxiety and subjective invalidity. The two groups also differed on physical outcomes as measured by exercise testing. Improvement was defined as the absence of signs of cardiac dysfunction that required treatment and was greater in the relaxation-training-and-exercise group compared with the exercise-only group.

VII. INTEGRATING THE RELAXATION RESPONSE INTO HEALTH CARE

The relaxation response has been associated with improvements in many medical conditions including: hypertension, cardiac arrhythmias, chronic pain, insomnia, side effects of cancer therapy, side effects of AIDS therapy, infertility, and preparation for surgery and X-ray procedures. It is also important to indicate that more recently, the overall implications of integrating relaxation response in routine clinical treatments has been examined. Some relevant examples will be discussed.

The effect of a behavioral group intervention that included relaxation response training on chronic pain patients. One hundred and nine patients who were members of an HMO participated in the study. The average duration of pain among the patients was 6.5 years. The interventions consisted of 90-minute group sessions, which were held once a week. At the end of the 10-week intervention period, participants in the group showed decreases in negative psychological symptoms including anxiety, depression, and hostility. This study also showed that such an intervention could result in significant cost savings. Group participants showed a 36% decrease in clinic use during the first and second year following the intervention. This latter result is particularly pertinent. There is a growing interest in the use of nonpharmacologic interventions such as elicitation of the relaxation response to not only facilitate psychological and medical goals but to help reduce medical utilization and costs. The above study is simply an example of the way in which such interventions can have this positive economic effect while at the same time have beneficial clinical outcomes.

Relaxation-response training was shown to improve outcomes among a group of patients with peripheral vascular disease who underwent femoral angiography. Forty-five patients participated in the study. Patients listened to either a relaxation tape that included instruction in progressive muscle relaxation and cognitive relaxation involving mental focusing or to a tape of recorded music. A third group of patients listened to a blank tape. Patients who listened to a relaxation-response tape experienced less anxiety and pain during the surgical procedure and requested significantly less medication that those patients who listened to the tape of recorded music or the blank tape. This study also showed that relaxation-response training can be administered very inexpensively and in ways that are practical for staff and patients.

Clearly, there is substantial research that shows that meditation and other relaxation-response techniques can be effective components in psychotherapy, behavior-change programs, and in medical treatment. Resistance to adjunctive use of such treatments, especially elicitation of the relaxation response, appears to be waning. A recent survey of medical schools found that approximately two-thirds now include discussions of relaxation techniques in their medical training. Knowledge of relaxation-response training can be helpful to physicians not only for the physiological benefits to patients but because many patients who present with medical problems really have a psychological disorder.

Such patients may feel uncomfortable about seeing a mental health professional or participating in psychotherapy. Relaxation techniques can be a means for the physician to start a dialogue about dealing with psychological disorders.

While the use of relaxation training is unquestioned in psychological treatment, there are still barriers to its use in medical settings. One barrier is a misunderstanding of the relaxation-response interventions and why they are used. Meditation and other introspective procedures bring about important central and peripheral physiological changes because they elicit the relaxation response. These central and peripheral changes are compatible with better mental and physical well-being. However, no single intervention can work for everyone. More research to define under what specific circumstances relaxation-response training would be most beneficial and cost effective for which patients still needs to be completed.

Many practitioners, insurers, and patients remain confused about the differences between the use of such services and psychotherapy. Relaxation training alone and when used with other types of behavioral therapies is more focused than traditional psychotherapy. It is often conducted in groups settings, and sessions are limited to 8 to 10 sessions. The important difference is that while the goal of psychotherapy is to change psychological symptoms, the goal of relaxation-response training with medical conditions is to change somatic manifestations. Relaxation training should be better understood, more routinely used, integrated, as well as paid for in medical settings. Such integration is imperative to the clients/patients and society.

BIBLIOGRAPHY

Benson, H. (1975). *The relaxation response.* New York: Morrow.

Benson, H. (1996). *Timeless healing: the power and biology of belief.* New York: Scribner.

Benson, H., & Stuart, E. M. (1992). *The wellness book.* New York: Simon and Shuster.

Friedman, R., Sobel, D., Myers, P., Caudill, M., & Benson, H. (1995). Behavioral medicine, clinical health psychology, and cost offset. *Health Psychology, 14*(6), 509–518.

Jacobs, G. D., Benson, H., & Friedman, R. (1996). Topographic EEG mapping of the relaxation response. *Biofeedback and Self-Regulation, 21*(2), 121–129.

Kabat-Zinn, J. (1994). *Wherever you go there you are: Mindfulness meditation in everyday life.* New York: Hyperion.

Kutz, I., Borysenko, J. Z., & Benson, H. (1985). Meditation and psychotherapy: A rationale for the integration of dynamic psychotherapy, the relaxation response and mindfulness meditation. *American Journal of Psychiatry, 142,* 1–8.

NIH Technology Assessment Panel on Integration of Behavioral and Relaxation Approaches Into the Treatment of Chronic Pain and Insomnia. (1996). Integration of behavioral and relaxation approaches into the treatment of chronic pain and insomnia. *JAMA, 276(4), 313–318.*

Sakakibara, M., Takeuchi, S., & Hayano, J. (1994). Effect of relaxation training on cardiac parasympathetic tone. *Psychophysiology, 31,* 223–228.

Wallace, R. K., & Benson, H. (1972). The physiology of meditation. *Scientific American, 226,* 84–90.

Menopause

Linda Gannon

Southern Illinois University, Carbondale

Androgen A general class of hormones that stimulates the development and continued activity of the sexual and reproductive organs of the male.

Estrogen A general class of hormones that stimulates the development and continued activity of the sexual and reproductive organs of the female.

Hormone A complex chemical substance produced by endocrine glands in one part of the body and carried through the blood stream to initiate or regulate the activity of an organ or a group of cells in another part of the body; secretion of hormones is regulated by a negative feedback system in which an excess of target organ activity signals a decreased need for the hormone.

Hormone Therapy Pharmaceutical preparations of estrogen or estrogen and progesterone, most commonly used as oral contraceptives or as a palliative for discomforts of menopause.

Menopause Permanent cessation of the menstrual cycle and fertility in the female.

Osteoporosis A reduction in the quantity or quality of bone and increased vulnerability to fractures, usually limited to elderly persons.

Progesterone Hormone produced by the corpus luteum and the adrenal cortex during the luteal phase of the menstrual cycle.

Testosterone The most potent, naturally occurring androgen.

Although **MENOPAUSE** refers to the cessation of menstruation, a clearly biological event, the experience of menopause encompasses far more than biology. In our culture, menopause has considerable symbolic meaning. This life transition is often approached with feelings of dread and loss, as traditionally, women have been valued for their biological capacity for being attractive and bearing and raising children. Similarly, menopause is presented by the medical profession and the popular media as a tragedy, but a tragedy that can be postponed by plastic surgery and hormone therapy. Given this cultural context, women are likely to view menopause negatively, and these attitudes can and do create adverse psychological consequences. The feelings of helplessness when faced with the biological inevitability of menopause and of aging, the cultural focus on the negative and neglect of the positive aspects of menopause, the absence of health-related information and research on aging in women, and the risks associated with "cures" generate an atmosphere that is likely to exacerbate mental health problems in aging women.

I. PHYSIOLOGY OF MENOPAUSE

An overview of the typical menstrual cycle in women between ages 18 and 40 provides a background against which to appreciate the changes that surround menopause. The menstrual cycle relies primarily on the activities of the hypothalamus, the anterior pituitary, and the ovaries. Beginning arbitrarily at menstruation, the hypothalamus produces a hormone (gonadotropin-releasing hormone), which, in turn, stimulates the anterior pituitary to release two hormones: follicle-stimulating hormone (FSH) and luteinizing hormone (LH). Follicle-stimulating hormone triggers the initial growth of follicles in the ovary, and these follicles begin to produce estrogen. Eventually, one follicle assumes dominance and continues to develop and produce estrogen while the others are absorbed. The estrogen exerts negative feedback on further production of FSH, causes the lining of the uterus (endometrium) to grow or proliferate, and stimulates the anterior pituitary to release a surge of LH. This, in turn, is followed by ovulation—the release of the mature ovum from the follicle. Luteinizing hormone also transforms the ruptured follicle into the corpus luteum, a short-lived organ that produces estrogen and progesterone. Progesterone exerts negative feedback on the pituitary, inhibiting the release of FSH and LH, and acts on the endometrium causing the blood supply to increase and the cells to store nutrients in preparation for pregnancy. In the absence of fertilization, the corpus luteum is absorbed, accompanied by decreasing levels of estrogen and progesterone. Without stimulation from estrogen and progesterone, the endometrium returns to its quiescent stage, shedding the built-up layers as menstruation.

Menopause, strictly speaking, refers to the cessation of this cycling activity. The cause of menopause is not known; hypotheses include a reduction in the number of remaining follicles, a lessened responsiveness to FSH in those remaining, and an accelerated rate of follicle loss prior to menopause. Given the fine-tuning of the hypothalamic-pituitary-ovarian system required to maintain the regular ovulatory cycles just described, an alteration in any part of this system could initiate the changes that culminate in menopause.

The underlying physiological process of menopause is not a sudden one in natural menopause but a gradual decrease in the percentage of cycles during which ovulation occurs. This is accompanied by gradually increasing levels of LH and FSH, and gradually decreasing levels of estrogen and progesterone. Usually between the ages of 45 and 55, menstruation and ovulation cease completely. The relationships among the various hormones and the relationships among hormones, menstruation, and ovulation do not follow a universal pattern but vary considerably across individual women. Generally, menopause is defined as the absence of menstruation for 1 year. In contrast to this typically gradual process, surgical removal of the ovaries in premenopausal produces an abrupt menopause. Shortly after surgery, estrogen and progesterone levels fall dramatically and FSH and LH levels gradually increase. This discussion is limited to natural menopause.

The ovaries of postmenopausal women continue to be active in terms of hormone production. The outer cortex of the ovary contains cells that are the primary source of ovarian estrogen, and although these cells decrease in number and productive capacity during menopause, estrogen continues to be secreted in small amounts. Androgens (hormones typically secreted in greater quantities in men) continue to be produced by inner cells of the ovary and by the adrenal cortex after menopause. A portion of the estrogen detected in the blood of postmenopausal women may be estrogen that has been converted from androgens. Adipose tissue (fat) is a primary site of conversion of androgens to estrogens. This process is believed to be the underlying cause of the consistent research finding that estrogen levels are associated with body weight and excess fat in postmenopausal woman and that thin postmenopausal women report a higher incidence of hot flashes than the obese. The reduced levels of estrogen and the increased levels of androgens may contribute to a minor androgenic state, including balding on the scalp, hair growth on the face and chest, and changes in fat distribution in a minority of postmenopausal women.

To summarize briefly, the normal hormonal profile before menopause consists of high levels of estrogen and progesterone, and low levels of FSH and LH, and these hormones fluctuate in a predictable, rhythmic cycle. During the menopausal transition, the normal hormonal state is one of gradually decreasing levels of estrogen and progesterone, and gradually increasing levels of FSH and LH. Although cyclic fluctuations continue, they become unpredictable and disassociated with fertility. After the menopausal transition and during the postmenopausal years, the normal hormone profile is one of low and stable levels of estrogen, an absence of progesterone, and high and stable levels of FSH and LH.

II. THEORETICAL MODELS OF MENOPAUSE

Menopause has become the scapegoat of any negative change that occurs during midlife in women. The popularized version of menopause associates this life change with a variety of unpleasant symptoms and changes, including hot flashes, profuse sweating, headaches, increased weight, dryness and thinning of the vaginal walls, increased incidence of vaginal infections, depression, insomnia, wrinkled skin, loss of breast firmness, dizziness, sensations of cold in the hands and feet, loss of interest in sexual activity, irritability, constipation, cardiovascular disease, and osteoporosis. Menopause, however, is only one of many processes and changes in middle age that may predispose an individual to physical and psychological difficulties. Women of this age and older may experience temporarily debilitating stress in terms of parental deaths, divorce, and children leaving home; they may be experiencing the cumulative effects of a lifetime of poor health habits; they may have been devoted to the roles of mother and wife and find these increasingly unfulfilling; and/or they may feel the loss of fertility and youthful attractiveness in a society that equates these with womanhood. Essentially, they are aging women in a culture that does not value aging or women.

Midlife changes in women are appropriately studied in several disciplines, including psychology, medicine, sociology, and anthropology, and each discipline offers a unique perspective within which to study and explain the developments of midlife. Various theoretical models have emerged from these disciplines: (a) medicine views midlife changes in women as caused by decreasing levels of estrogen; (b) psychology attributes transitional difficulties to stress, poor coping responses, and/or personality problems predating menopause; (c) a sociological perspective focuses on changing roles, poverty, physical health, and institutionalized sexism; and (d) anthropologists study midlife developments in the context of a culture's valuation of women, aging, and fertility. In the last decade, there has been a surge of interest in the biological or medical view of menopause. This is not because the medical perspective is necessarily more valid, more relevant, or more rationale than the other models, but because the medical community and the related pharmaceutical industry have invested considerable financial resources in promoting menopause as a medical disorder requiring physician assistance and pharmaceutical remedies.

These models, or ways of understanding middle age, are not mutually exclusive; that is, a particular midlife change may be the consequence of numerous causes interacting with one another. For example, some women suffer from low bone density in midlife. This could be caused by decreasing levels of estrogen, aging processes (all women and men experience some decrease in bone density with aging), a lifetime of poverty precluding adequate medical care and good nutrition, and a cultural imperative for women to be thin—resulting in a calcium-deficient diet—and passive—resulting in a high value being placed on a sedentary lifestyle. As is frequently the case for topics that cross disciplinary boundaries, there has been little attempt among researchers to create an integrated model. The resulting narrowness of vision has hindered progress in explicating and understanding this complex life transition.

Research has been conducted within the context of each of these models with surprisingly consistent results. In general, the evidence suggests that hot flashes, slowed sexual arousal, and, to some extent, osteoporosis are caused by the changing hormonal environment of menopause; whereas other physical and psychological complaints, such as depression, irritability, fatigue, and wrinkles, are the result of aging and historical, cultural, social, and stress factors. Furthermore, many changes and complaints of midlife have multiple causes. For example, some women find that if they experience frequent and severe hot flashes during the night, they develop insomnia, and that in turn may cause depression and irritability.

Within each discipline or model, the research literature focuses almost solely on the negative changes associated with menopause and midlife. This is because, in our culture, women traditionally and primarily have been valued for their fertility and youthful attractiveness, and the elderly are seen as forgetful, slow, and a burden to society. In this context, a woman who is no longer fertile and no longer looks or is young, is thought to be developing only in negative and deteriorating ways. In fact, menopause and midlife are clearly associated with positive changes and benefits. The decreasing levels of estrogen are associated with a lesser risk of breast cancer, uterine fibroids, and endometriosis, as well as with a general, overall health improvement with elimination of the risks associated with fertility: birth control methods, pregnancy, abortion, and birth. Similarly, within the realm of psychology, in spite of the potential for new and severe stressors, midlife is frequently associated with an emerging sense of freedom that is likely to improve psychological well-being; the freedom from caring for young children and the freedom from conforming to the cultural ideal of womanhood may be liberating and enlightening. The sociology model predicts a sense of motivated energy and increases in self-esteem due to facing and overcoming the challenges of role and career changes. Finally, anthropologists have noted that menopause and midlife are associated with negative changes in cultures that value women primarily for their beauty and fertility, whereas in societies where aging increases one's status and perceived wisdom, and where the desexualization associated with menopause renders women less threatening to men, aging women experience a rise in self-esteem and an elevation of status.

The focus on negative developmental changes during menopause is exemplified most clearly in the medical model. Physicians with their high visibility and "expert" status have overwhelmed the public and the media with a "disease" perspective of menopause. This limited view of menopause, if accepted by the menopausal woman, may actually influence her experience. Psychologists have for decades acknowledged the impact of attitudes and expectations on experiences: if an individual expects an experience to be positive, that individual is more likely to have a positive experience than one who expects the experience to be negative. Within this context, researchers have noted that women who expect menopause to be a negative experience report more complaints and difficulties associated with menopause than do women who expect menopause to be a positive experience. Researchers then asked, why do women expect a negative experience? In one study, individuals expressed their attitudes and expectations concerning menopause when menopause was presented as a symbol of aging, a life transition, or a medical problem. The medical context yielded the most negative view of menopause. Indeed, menopause is no more a medical problem than is puberty. Although puberty may be associated with skin problems and emotional distress, and these may require professional treatment, adolescence is not viewed as a medical event or a medical disorder. Similarly, menopause may be accompanied by hot flashes and the emotional turmoil associated with identity and role is-

sues, and the individual may choose to seek professional help for specific difficulties. However, the majority of women transiting menopause, as well as the majority of teenagers transiting puberty, do so with minimal difficulty.

III. MENTAL HEALTH IN THE MENOPAUSAL AND POSTMENOPAUSAL WOMAN

Menopause may be associated with mental health problems. Some women report feeling depressed or irritable, others report problems surrounding various aspects of sexuality, and still others may experience mental health problems as a consequence of physical problems caused either by the normal aging process or by the cumulative effects of a lifetime of poor health habits. These are discussed individually, although the reader is reminded that these areas are not mutually exclusive, but rather, are mutually interactive.

A. Depression, Irritability, and Anxiety

Historically, menopause and midlife in women have been assumed to be associated with depression, irritability, and anxiety. Indeed, an early twentieth century psychiatric term, "involutional melancholia," referred specifically to midlife depression in women. In the last decade, this term was eliminated from the official diagnostic system because depression in midlife women appears to have the same causes, symptoms, and effective treatments as depressions occurring at any other time of life. Furthermore, surveys of psychological problems in women across the life span have found the ages typically associated with child-bearing and child-rearing, rather than menopause, to have the highest incidence of mental health problems, including depression. Research suggesting that menopause, per se, does not increase a women's vulnerability to mental health problems is rather convincing: (a) information from large surveys of women of premenopausal, menopausal, and postmenopausal age indicates that the incidence of depression does not change with menopausal status; (b) studies of the association between hormone levels and mental health have reported that the severity of psychological difficulties is not associated with levels of estrogen, progesterone, LH, or FSH; and (c) hormone therapy has not been demonstrated to be effective in relieving irritability, depression, anxiety, or any other mental health problem. These findings inform the conclusions that menopause is not associated with an increased vulnerability to psychological problems and that those mental health problems that are reported by midlife women are not caused by the changing hormonal environment and are not alleviated by hormone therapy.

This is not to deny that some mid- and old-age women, at some times, feel depressed, irritable, and anxious. Mid- and old-age women are likely to face the type of traumatic stress that is known to increase vulnerability to depression, such as loss of a loved family member or friend. The cumulative effects of chronic stress and the consequences of a life-time of poverty, loneliness, sexism, racism, and/or poor health may well lead to deteriorating mental health. In a society in which women have traditionally been valued for their roles as lovers and mothers, menopause is likely to diminish self-esteem, which in turn could lead to depression. This devaluation of aging women is exacerbated by the professional communities' priorities. The medical and psychological communities have devoted far greater energy, interest, and finances to understanding and treating the reproductive problems of women than to the developments and difficulties associated with aging. This is evident in the considerable scholarly attention devoted to pregnancy compared with the relative neglect of menopause and aging. To the medical professional, the whims and demands of the pregnant woman are to be indulged and are thought to be normally "feminine," whereas the idiosyncrasies of mid- and old-age women are a source of irritation. [*See* DEPRESSION; STRESS.]

Traditional psychological and behavioral methods for treating depression, anxiety, and low self-esteem may appropriately be used with menopausal and postmenopausal women suffering from these symptoms. Cognitive therapies may be particularly appropriate in modifying attitudes toward menopause, and the behavioral therapies may help women find new and satisfying roles or careers and new sources of social support. In addition, as many of the events occurring around the time of menopause are particularly stressful, stress reduction and training in coping strategies might be effective. The clinician may also benefit menopausal women by promoting a wellness view of menopause. As educators, lecturers, writers, and interviewers, professionals can encourage the view that menopause is a natural life transition which conveys benefits as well as difficulties and that associated problems are expected and temporary. Changes in attitudes and attributions in the direction of improved mental health may occur on an individual level in psychotherapy, on a group level in consciousness-raising groups, on an educational level in the classroom, and/or on a mass media level. [*See* COGNITIVE THERAPY.]

B. Sexuality

Stereotypes of women's sexuality in our society are deeply influenced by an overriding belief that women are biologically determined. That is, it is a common, although erroneous, belief that a woman's behaviors, values, attitudes, and competencies are strongly influenced by the sex hormones, estrogen and progesterone. This idea originated in professional scholarship as a theory or a proposal, but has become widely accepted among lay persons as a "law" of nature and permeates many of our beliefs and values regarding womanhood. For example, an angry woman is often said to have premenstrual syndrome rather than a legitimate cause for anger: her emotions are viewed as determined by her hormones rather than by her environment. In contrast, an aggressive man is not thought to have excess testosterone but to have justifiable cause for his aggression. In this context, many professional and lay persons assume that throughout a woman's life her sexuality is directed, determined, and governed by hormones, particularly estrogen. In this context, many believe that women's sexuality changes when their hormones change—at puberty, across the menstrual cycle, during pregnancy, and at menopause. Consequently, the menstrual cycle and menopause have been the focus of considerable research on sexuality in women.

Although our concern here is menopause, the research on sexuality and the menstrual cycle can provide information regarding the relationship between sexuality and hormones. Typically, researchers have measured some aspect of sexuality—self-reported or physiological sexual arousal, frequency of sexual activity, intensity of sexual desire—or some variable thought to be related to sexual arousal—mood, recency of sexual experience, vividness of imagery—and compared these measures at different points in the menstrual cycle. The general conclusion has been that the hormonal fluctuations of the menstrual cycle do not influence sexuality in any noticeable or important manner. Similarly, numerous surveys since the 1950s of mid- and old-age women indicate that changes in sexuality with age do not follow a set pattern. When questioned during or after the menopausal transition, some women report a diminished interest in sex and less sexual activity, others report an increased interest and more sexual activity, whereas still others do not notice a change. Again, the conclusion is that hormones have little or no impact on sexuality.

Contributing to this knowledge base, researchers have studied the effects of estrogen therapy on sexuality in mid- and old-age women. The overall conclusion from this research is that estrogen increases vaginal lubrication during sexual arousal. However, in spite of this, women taking estrogen reported no changes in sexual frequency, satisfaction, or desire. An alternative hormonal treatment is based on the assumption that sexuality in both men and women is influenced primarily by testosterone (the primary androgen). Although there is little or no evidence to support this assumption, and although there is no evidence that menopause creates a testosterone deficiency, testosterone therapy is sometimes recommended to mid- and old-age women with the goal of increasing sexual activity. There has been minimal research designed to evaluate the effectiveness of testosterone therapy and, at this time, there is little or no evidence for its effectiveness. Furthermore, advocates of testosterone therapy have paid insufficient attention to the possibility of undesirable side effects, such as growth of facial hair, lowered voice, increased risk of cardiovascular disorders, and redistribution of fat.

Overall, researchers and practitioners have concluded that sexual activity in postmenopausal women is more highly associated with factors other than menopausal status and hormone levels. Conditions that have been found to influence sexuality during midlife and beyond are the availability of a partner, adequate emotional support from the partner, alcoholism in the partner, chronic psychological problems, anger, fatigue, and relationship problems. Disregarding these research findings, many professionals continue to believe that women's sexuality is hormonally determined and to recommend some form of hormone therapy in order to "treat" sexuality in menopausal and postmenopausal women.

The reader may gain another perspective on the topic of sexuality in aging women by considering the overwhelming cultural influence on sexual customs. In the mid-nineteenth century, medical and religious leaders believed any type of sexual activity or sexual desire in mid- and old-age women to be the result of either a sinful life or an illness. Today, proper and healthy aging seems to be defined as "not changing": the goal is to maintain the energy level, the figure, the skin, and the sexual activity of a 25-year-old. Thus, in contrast to nineteenth century beliefs, today the absence of sexual activity in mid- and old-age is seen as illness caused either by psychological inhibitions or by physical failings. These changing views on sexuality in the aging are not the consequence of medical or psychological research but are the opinions and values of the culture influencing the practice of medicine and psychology. Unless individuals report distress about their sexuality and request help, the expression and enjoyment of sexuality should not be of concern to physicians or psychologists, nor should they dictate proper or healthy sexual behavior. Some elderly women will place a great emphasis on sexuality, others will choose to abstain—in either case, professionals need not assume the presence of a problem. [See SEXUAL BEHAVIOR.]

C. Psychological and Behavioral Consequences of Physical Changes

There are a variety of physical changes that accompany menopause and aging. Although the professionals disagree as to which changes are due to menopause, which to aging, and which to poor lifestyle habits, there is agreement that many of these physical changes are accompanied by, are caused by, or cause significant mental health difficulties.

1. Hot Flashes

The most common complaint of menopausal women in the United States is vasomotor instability or hot flashes. Hot flashes are characterized by sensations of heat usually in the face, neck, and chest and sometimes followed by perspiration, shivering, or both. Among those women who experience this phenomenon, hot flashes most commonly begin prior to the complete cessation of menses and continue through the early years after menopause. The frequency, intensity, and duration of hot flashes vary greatly among individuals. Although there seems to be no simple relationship between hot flashes and estrogen levels, estrogen therapy alleviates hot flashes in the majority of menopausal women who suffer them. Unfortunately, estrogen treatment may postpone, rather than eliminate the problem, as when the treatment is stopped, the hot flashes often return. Many herbal, vitamin, and mineral therapies are advocated as treatment for hot flashes, although there is little information available on their effectiveness. In the absence of treatment, hot flashes tend to diminish over time and eventually cease altogether. Hot flashes have been found to increase under stressful life conditions and, in some women, are exacerbated by high environmental temperatures, caffeine, and alcohol.

Hot flashes do not usually present a threat to a woman's physical or psychological well-being and, thus, do not require treatment. On the other hand, hot flashes may be of such severe frequency or intensity as to cause considerable discomfort. They may occur during the night, causing sleep disruption by decreasing the efficiency and quality of sleep; and/or they may cause considerable embarrassment to some women, seriously interfering with their work performance and their social life. Embarrassment is most intense and disabling for those women who have difficulty accepting the aging process and whose self-esteem may depend on apparent youthfulness.

Although hormone therapy is effective in treating hot flashes, such treatment is unacceptable to many women, because of a medical condition, discomfort with the side effects, or a personal preference not to take drugs. A variety of psychological therapies to treat hot flashes are available. Relaxation training and stress reduction have been used successfully to reduce the frequency and intensity of hot flashes, as has temperature biofeedback, which is designed to aid women in exerting conscious control over their body temperature. Other forms of psychotherapy have been used with the goal of modifying attitudes, transforming self-concept, and increasing self-esteem. When successful, these therapies have the impact of reducing the anxiety, fear, and embarrassment associated with hot flashes by modifying the symbolic meaning of menopause. This approach to treatment is consistent with a cross-cultural perspective on menopause. In cultures where women's status and freedom increase with menopause, rather than decrease as in the United States, menopause is not "difficult." For example, in one study of Indian women who were from a society in which premenopausal women were forbidden certain activities, whereas menopausal and postmenopausal women were allowed considerably more freedom,

menopausal women offered no complaints of depression or incapacitation. Thus, modifying attitudes, beliefs, roles, and values in behavioral or dynamic psychotherapy may, in some women, be sufficient to render the hot flashes minor and inconsequential.

2. Osteoporosis

Throughout life, new bone is continually formed and existing bone continually reabsorbed or lost. In the young, particularly during the years of growth, more bone is made than is lost. Peak bone mass is reached at about age 35, after which time, resorption exceeds formation, and all persons lose bone with advancing age. If the bone loss is excessive or if the peak bone mass was inadequate, then bone density decreases to such an extent that bones break easily; this proclivity to fractures caused by low bone density is referred to as osteoporosis. Osteoporotic fractures most commonly occur in the vertebra, the forearm, and the hips.

Because the two primary determinants of osteoporosis are peak bone mass and rate of bone loss, either or both can contribute to an eventual problem. Peak bone mass is determined by genetics, diet, weight-bearing load, and exercise, whereas the rate of bone loss is determined by weight, exercise, diet, and sex hormones in both men and women. The body makes bone in response to need, so if the bone needs to support weight in the form of fat or in the form of muscle, the bone will be stronger. Gravity-bearing exercise places stress on bones and causes the bone to increase in density. Diet contributes by supplying the necessary bone-making ingredients of calcium, magnesium, and vitamin D.

Although the medical community and the popular media of the last decade have defined osteoporosis as a symptom of menopause, in fact, both men and women experience decreasing levels of bone density as they age, and osteoporosis may occur in either sex. If osteoporosis were clearly and strongly associated with menopause, then aging women of all cultures would be vulnerable to osteoporosis. However, in some cultures men are more susceptible to osteoporosis than are women. In the U.S. culture, those of African descent (both men and women) suffer from osteoporosis far less often than do those of European descent, and women of both descents are diagnosed with osteoporosis more often than are men. Persons of both genders and all races experience diminished levels of their respective sex hormones (estrogen in women, testosterone in men) as they age, and this is assumed to be one cause of accelerated bone loss in midlife. However, women are far more likely to have had their ovaries surgically removed than are men to have had their testicles surgically removed. Women are, therefore, more likely than men to experience a sudden and drastic reduction in hormones.

Although the sex difference in osteoporosis has been attributed to differences in diminishing rates of sex hormones, this does not seem plausible given that all women experience menopause, yet a minority experience osteoporosis, and in light of the cultural and racial differences in the incidence of osteoporosis. Cultural values and practices provide a partial, but important, explanation for the differences in the incidence of osteoporosis between women and men in the United States. Men are less likely to be concerned about their weight and are, therefore, heavier than women. The heavier weight of men requires stronger bones and, as men tend to eat more to maintain their heavier weight, they are more likely to have adequate calcium intake. Before the 1950s, many women were required to exercise in order to survive—they were farmers, factory workers, or housewives who lived without modern appliances. When the role of women became more housewifely and the home became mechanized, the white, middle-class American woman became the "little woman" and femininity was defined as being frail and small and was epitomized by someone who did not exercise or sweat. Finally, our society has promoted traditional gender-related activities and careers. For those who have conformed, a woman's career diminishes considerably when her children leave home, which usually occurs when she is in her 40s, and a man's career when he retires, usually in his 60s. Both of these events may be accompanied by a drastic reduction in physical activity, leading to increased vulnerability of osteoporosis occurring at different ages for women and men.

The cultural expectation that all women be mothers may also place women at risk. Pregnant and lactating women have higher calcium needs because of the demands of the fetus and infant, and, if these needs are not met with diet or supplements, a woman's bones will be depleted of calcium in order to supply the need. This demand apparently has long-term consequences, leading to the finding that the more children a woman has borne, the less dense are her bones as she ages. Thus, women who were 20 to 30 years of age in the 1950s are today 60 to 70 years of age, and their bones may be suf-

fering the consequences of poor exercise, poor diet, and too many children. Since the 1970s, with much help from the women's movement, women do not "retire" when their children leave home, women athletes are recognized and rewarded, aerobics for women are not only socially acceptable but desirable, and the cultural demand to produce children has lessened. Perhaps, the current generation of women will not suffer similar consequences with regard to osteoporosis.

There are numerous recommendations from the medical and alternative health communities concerning the prevention and treatment of osteoporosis. The medical profession highly recommends hormone therapy. However, in order for estrogen to influence the rate of bone loss, the treatment must be initiated concurrently with the beginning of menopause and the benefits last only as long as the woman continues to take the medication. If the woman stops taking the hormones, the bone loss will occur to the same extent and at the same rate as it would have had the hormones never been taken. Because fractures are most likely to occur when a woman is in her 70s, if she is suffering from osteoporosis, she would need to take daily medication for 20 years to reduce the risk of fractures.

Osteoporosis is a mental health issue because the best prevention and one of the effective treatments is to ensure a healthy diet and adequate exercise. The development and maintenance of these habits involves issues of motivation, self-esteem, time management, and assertiveness. If women in their 20s were concerned about osteoporosis and developed lifestyles that minimized the risk, osteoporosis would be an extremely rare problem. If peak bone mass is sufficiently high, then the bone loss caused by aging and menopause would not be a serious problem, as the bone density would remain above the fracture threshold. If women become concerned with osteoporosis only when they reach midlife, diet and exercise continue to be one of the best methods to reduce or reverse the bone loss, although attempting to correct a lifetime of poor health habits requires considerable motivation.

Persons of both sexes have difficulty developing and maintaining a healthy lifestyle; however, women's difficulties are exacerbated by the cultural stereotype of the "perfect woman." This is, of course, a wife and mother, and part of the role is to consider the husband and children as more important than the self. Thus, a woman's diet is often determined by the type of food demanded by her family; she may be aware of the need for certain nutrients but does not consider herself sufficiently important to impose these on her family. Or a woman may allow her diet to suffer for the sake of her desired physical appearance if she is intensely committed to the cultural definition of a beautiful woman, which includes extreme thinness. If the woman is the primary caretaker of young children, then she may not feel she has the right to demand the freedom and the opportunity to exercise outside the home. Thus, the feminine stereotype that dictates that the perfect woman is one who is giving, dependent, and subservient, who places herself second, who does not make demands, and who does not "lose her figure" as she grows older contributes to the development of poor health habits which, in turn, causes an increased risk of osteoporosis.

Although the medical community has been quick to advocate hormone therapy to prevent osteoporosis, the benefits require a lifetime commitment to this regimen, and long-term hormone therapy is associated with rather serious side effects (see the next section). On the other hand, the benefits of calcium supplements and weight-bearing exercise can be realized with only positive side effects. The beneficial effects of weight-bearing exercise on bone density and size as well as the detrimental effects of immobility have been known for decades; they are certainly known by anyone who has broken a bone and been dismayed at the emaciated limb that emerged from the cast. Perhaps this information has not been applied to osteoporosis in the elderly because it has been assumed that to be effective, the exercise has to be strenuous and prolonged and beyond the capabilities of elderly persons. However, a moderate but regular exercise program has been found to be effective in increasing bone density in elderly people. The benefits are even more remarkable when examining life-long exercise patterns. One researcher found runners, aged 50 to 72, to have 40% higher bone density than sedentary persons of the same age and weight. Osteoporosis is not a disorder of menopause in women but a disorder affecting persons of all ages, both genders, and all races whose lifestyles preclude healthy bone. [*See* EXERCISE AND MENTAL HEALTH; PHYSICAL ACTIVITY AND MENTAL HEALTH.]

3. Cardiovascular Disorders

Advocates of hormone therapy have, in the last decade, promoted the idea that the hormonal changes accompanying menopause increase the risk of cardiovascular disorders and that hormone therapy can prevent this increased risk. The initial impetus for investigating this area was an attempt to understand the difference in the incidence of cardiovascular disorders between men and women. Prior to middle age, men suffer from far more cardiovascular disorders than do women. Beginning at 40 to 50 years of age, the gap between men and women decreases, although men continue to experience more cardiovascular problems than do women throughout life. This narrowing of the gap between women and men in midlife has been attributed by gynecologists to diminished estrogen in women. Cardiologists, on the other hand, attribute the narrowing of the gap to lowered levels of testosterone in men, testosterone having negative effects on the cardiovascular system.

Although the presentation of information by the popular media would lead one to believe that hormone therapy reduces cardiovascular risk in menopausal and postmenopausal women, there is no published experimental research to document such a claim. The survey research that is often cited to support the benefits of hormone therapy on cardiovascular risk simply note that women who have been taking hormones for 5 to 10 years have fewer cardiovascular events than those who have not. However, these groups not only differ in their use of hormones; women reporting fewer cardiovascular events also smoke less, exercise more, have higher incomes, have attained higher levels of education, and have less body fat. Any or all of these factors may be the "cause" of the differing risk for cardiovascular disorders. In the absence of controlled studies, the scientist cannot simply pick out one of the many differences and claim that this is the important and relevant factor that influences cardiovascular risk. What has been interpreted as evidence for a benefit on the cardiovascular system from hormone therapy is most likely due to a tendency for already healthy women to take hormones.

As with osteoporosis, cardiovascular disease in women most likely has the same or similar causes and calls for the same or similar effective treatments as those for men. Although cardiovascular disorders in men continue to be treated aggressively with drugs and surgery, there is an increasing appreciation for the value of lifestyle changes, including an improved diet, increased aerobic exercise, reduced use of nicotine, caffeine and alcohol, and modifying certain personality traits, particularly hostility and aggressiveness. Both the medical and psychological professions are recognizing that not only are such lifestyle changes extremely effective, but the individual derives additional benefits: improved overall health, greater self-efficacy and feelings of control over one's life, improved social relationships, and less job pressure. The rate of cardiovascular mortality declined 37% between 1963 and 1983. This decline has been similar for women and for men, and is usually attributed to cultural changes resulting in healthier lifestyles.

D. Psychological and Behavioral Side Effects of Hormone Therapy

The medical community has defined menopause as a disease. The reasoning behind this definition is that if women are biologically determined and driven, then their appropriate or useful roles are limited to those of wife, sex partner, and mother. Consequently, the standard, normal, optimal biology for women is that which allows and facilitates these roles—menstruation and pregnancy, with "normal" hormonal levels being defined as those typical of the premenopausal, postpuberty woman. The menopausal or postmenopausal woman can no longer fulfill her reproductive role. If that is the only role society allows her, then her defining biology is seen as a deficiency disorder. And the medical community recommends that this deficiency be "corrected" with hormone treatment.

Hormone therapy has gone through several transformations in the last 30 years. In the 1960s, hormone therapy was in the form of estrogen supplements and was promoted as treatment for those complaints that were then viewed as menopausal problems—obesity, wrinkles, depression, memory problems, as well as most other symptoms associated with aging. Research during this time and later, clarified that hormone therapy was an effective treatment for only hot flashes and vaginal lubrication. Far more damaging to the promotion of hormone therapy was the link established between estrogen supplements and an increased risk of uterine cancer. When this association became widely known in the 1970s, the use of estrogen diminished considerably. The medical–pharmaceutical industry then developed a new hormone therapy: estrogen for 28 days with progesterone added on days 18 to 28, followed by a week free from medication to allow a "period." This newer regimen does not increase the risk of uterine cancer.

Both forms of hormone therapy increase a woman's

vulnerability to mental health problems. Scientists have noted that not only does hormone therapy not relieve depression, but in some women may cause depression. The effects of estrogen on mood has been likened to those of oral contraceptives—another hormone treatment found to cause depression in some women. The hypothesis is that estrogen therapy (used either for contraception or menopause) will, within a year, use up stores of vitamin B6, increasing one's vulnerability to depression. This effect can often be alleviated by taking vitamin B6 supplements. Since adding progesterone to the treatment regimen, there has been a growing awareness that the progesterone component may magnify mental health problems. A common complaint of women on this regimen is that during the progesterone phase of their medication cycle, they experience symptoms similar to those commonly associated with premenstrual syndrome—depression, irritability, anxiety, bloating, and weight gain. For many women, these symptoms are of such severity that they abandon the medication.

The decision to take or not to take hormone therapy is, itself, stressful for menopausal women. The benefits of the therapy are the alleviation of hot flashes, increased lubrication during sexual arousal, and a reduction in the rate of bone loss—the latter true only as long as the woman continues to take the medication. The disadvantages are the documented increases in the risk of breast cancer, maintaining or increasing the risk of uterine fibroids, and a continued risk of endometriosis. Although less thoroughly studied, other reported side effects include increased risk of asthma, ovarian cancer, migraine headaches, lupus, and urinary tract infections. The popular media do not accurately present the whole picture and frequently simply quote spokespersons from the medical profession who claim that hormones are essentially wonder drugs—eliminating wrinkles, prolonging life, curing depression. A woman suffering from low self-esteem who has little respect for her own ability to find and evaluate relevant information will readily accept a recommendation from an "expert." A woman who valued, above all else, her youthful beauty and fertility may all too readily believe that there is a magic pill that prevents aging. Thus, this decision is not an easy or straightforward one and may be facilitated by informal or formal support and professional help in examining motives and goals.

Medical and pharmaceutical professionals are strong and verbal advocates of the "menopause as deficiency disease" idea. The consequence of widespread acceptance of this perspective are considerable. The psychological impact of being informed at age 50 that one has a chronic disease that is not curable but can be "controlled" with drugs and will require regular medical visits for the rest of one's life, could be overwhelming. We have several decades of laboratory and clinical research documenting the importance of perceived control on psychological health. Although most people will experience a diminished sense of control as they age, those who have chronic physical problems necessitating a strong dependence on medical help will experience a particularly intense loss of control. Indeed, the impact of loss of control over a major part of one's life increases as one ages—perhaps because the elderly have, in reality, less control as they age so they may be more sensitive to the loss of what little they have. Our society has increasingly encouraged the practice of taking a pill for a quick cure of every physical and psychological problem. If a menopausal woman believes that she can take a pill rather than accept the inevitability of aging and death and rather than develop healthy lifestyle habits, she is relinquishing control over important aspects of her life.

IV. CONCLUSIONS

To understand the mental health issues of menopause, it is necessary to appreciate fully the specific contributions from the various disciplines that provide a meaningful context for studying menopause. Although the hormonal fluctuations accompanying menopause do not directly impact a woman's mental health, mental health issues may arise from physical symptoms that characterize menopause. Hot flashes are the most frequent complaint of menopausal women, and those women who experience particularly severe and frequent hot flashes or who suffer insomnia and/or embarrassment as a consequence of hot flashes, may report feeling depressed or irritable and may experience a negative impact on their professional and social lives. The treatment modality may focus on reducing the frequency and severity through hormone therapy or through relaxation, stress reduction, biofeedback, or cognitive therapy. A second physical consequence of hormonal changes is a reduced lubrication to sexual stimuli. This symptom is also alleviated with hormone therapy, although, in general, menopausal and postmenopausal women do not report sexuality to be a

problem. If a woman is considering treating either of these difficulties with hormone therapy, she may seek mental health support for help making this difficult decision and for alleviation of potential side effects of the treatment.

The medical community and the media have portrayed osteoporosis and cardiovascular disease as symptoms of menopause, although the research is more consistent with the view that these disorders are the consequences of aging and are exacerbated by poor health habits. Regardless of the causes of these two potentially debilitating disorders, mental health professionals may aid prevention and treatment by facilitating lifestyle changes that include a healthy diet rich in calcium and aerobic exercise. Treatments designed to focus attention toward a context of health rather than adherence to gender stereotypes and to promote the motivation, assertiveness, and self-esteem necessary to accomplish these changes are appropriate.

Natural menopause occurs at an age when there exists a high probability of traumatic stressors of the type that predispose women to depression, specifically, the loss of a loved friend or relative. This is also the age when many women find that the personal, social, and professional roles that suited them for the pervious decades are no longer challenging, meaningful, and fulfilling. These changes are exacerbated by the symbolic meaning of menopause. In a culture that places little value on women and aging, menopause signals the closure of fertility and beauty and the inevitability of death. In this context, menopause is necessarily negative, and depression, listlessness, and pessimism may result and may require professional treatment.

BIBLIOGRAPHY

Coney, S. (1993). *The menopause industry: A guide to medicine's "discovery" of the midlife woman.* Claremont, CA: Hunter House.

Doress-Worters, P. B., & Siegal, D. L. (1994). *Ourselves, growing older.* New York: Simon & Schuster.

Gaby, A. (1994). *Preventing and reversing osteoporosis.* Rocklin, CA: Prima.

O'Leary Cobb, J. (Ed.). *A friend indeed newsletter.* Champlain, NY.

Northrup, C. (1994). *Women's bodies, women's wisdom: Creating physical and emotional health and healing.* New York: Bantam Books.

Notelovitz, M., & Tonnessen, D. (1993). *Menopause and midlife health.* New York: St. Martin's Press.

Vines, G. (1993). *Raging hormones: Do they rule our lives?* London: Virago Press.

Mental Control Across the Life Span

Becca Levy and Ellen Langer

Harvard University

Competency The belief that one is capable of carrying out a behavior that leads to a specific outcome, or "I can do X."

Contingency The belief that an action will lead to a specific outcome, or "If X occurs, Y will happen."

Entity Theory The belief that intelligence is beyond mental control and thus a fixed entity. Thus, when entity theorists fail at a task, they tend to make negative self-attributes to ability, express negative affect, and show debilitated performance.

Incremental Theory The belief that intelligence is subject to mental control and thus malleable. When incremental theorists encounter failure, they tend to focus on where the process might have gone wrong and try to develop conclusions about strategies or effort that will allow future mastery.

Mental Control The belief that one has choice among responses that are differentially effective in achieving a desired outcome.

Primary Control Changing one's environment to bring about a desired outcome. This frequently requires a behavior.

Secondary Control Leaving one's environment unchanged but obtaining goals through alternative paths such as altering one's perspective on existing realities so as to derive meaning from them and accept them.

MENTAL CONTROL, the belief that one can bring about a desired outcome, contributes to one's physical and mental health in many ways. In 1959, Robert White first described the central motivational force for individuals to find competence in their interactions with the environment. He called this force "effectance motivation." Since his description of this force, researchers have documented the positive association of mental control with academic achievement in childhood, life satisfaction, feelings of self-worth, the ability to engage in positive and creative work, the capacity to care about others, physical health, memory performance in old age, and longevity. Also, researchers believe that the lack or absence of mental control can cause depression, particularly when one encounters a stressful event.

I. OVERVIEW OF MENTAL CONTROL

Some theorists argue that mental control is a personality trait that remains stable throughout the life span. Much of the control research suggests that instead it is a dynamic construct that responds to development. It is the latter view that we explore here. As individuals grow from infancy to old age, their experiences of control can change as a result of both cognitive development and the way in which cultures define certain control-related behaviors and events as age-appropriate.

As a result of these changes, humans tend to alter the control domains of concern and the strategies they use to exert control. This entry gives an overview of some of the changes that occur in mental control across the life span and reviews the related research. We argue that when researchers and clinicians ignore how individuals in a particular stage experience mental control, it can lead to various misinterpretations. This article does not deal directly with the related concepts of leaned helplessness, attributional style, and self-efficacy. For reviews on these topics, the reader should consult Bandura (1995), Berry and West (1995), and Peterson (1995).

Here, mental control is defined as the belief that one has choice among responses that are differentially effective in achieving a desired outcome. Several aspects of this definition are worth nothing. First, although they are strongly related, research suggests that the *belief* that one can bring about an outcome is more important for one's mental health than the *act* of achieving a desired outcome. Early research on control focused on one's ability to produce a desired outcome. Today control researchers concentrate on the importance of the *interpretation* of one's ability. To believe control exists does not require that one engage in actions designed to exercise that control. To believe that we could be great Olympic swimmers does not necessitate that we ever dive into the water.

The second notable aspect of the definition is that the notion of differentially effective choices suggests that some degree of uncertainty must exist in the alternatives. If the achievement of an outcome is guaranteed, such as pressing a gas pedal to move a car, people will act mindlessly and thus not have the phenomenological experience of control. If too much uncertainty exists, control will also not be experienced. Individuals in this case will not trust that their acts can produce desired outcomes. Thus, individuals tend to activate mental control in the course of meeting what for them are reasonable challenges.

In addition, mental control may be particularly adaptive in times of crisis. It can buffer against stressful life events. Some individuals in stressful situations tend to develop feelings of mental control as a coping mechanism. For example, one study revealed that individuals who just found out they have levels of the human immunodeficiency virus (HIV) known to cause acquired immunodeficiency syndrome (AIDS), tended to develop greater feelings of control over AIDS than

similar individuals who found out that they are not HIV seropositive. The researchers also found that among a group of men who chose not to find out their HIV status, those who were HIV seropositive did not differ on their reported levels of control over AIDS from those who knew that they were HIV seronegative. Thus, the control belief seemed to follow the knowledge that one has the beginning symptoms of AIDS. [*See* COPING WITH STRESS; HIV/AIDS.]

As mentioned, it is not so important whether an individual exerts or can exert control. In fact, individuals often believe that they can exert control in situations that from an observer's perspective seem unrealistic, such as playing the lottery. Langer originally called this phenomenon of holding a false expectation of being able to influence a future event an "illusion of control." Although many researchers continue to call this optimistic thinking an illusion of control, Langer revised her thinking about this phenomenon: she now believes that the illusion of control is only an illusion from the observer's perspective. If the probability of success from the observer's perspective is zero, the observer may see the actor as operating under an illusion of control. For the actor, it is not an illusion but rather an informed prediction based on her assessment of herself and the situation. Thus, actors and observers faced with different situations and different information available to them are responding to different perceived probabilities of success. To say an event is uncontrollable suggests a type of knowledge that cannot be had. All events are uncontrollable until a way is found to control them. To believe an event is inherently uncontrollable robs one of the motivation to look for ways to control it.

Thus, it may be strategically efficacious to treat the attainment of all desired outcomes as controllable. If one holds onto a control belief, then one potentially has much to gain in achieving a desired outcome. But if one gives up a control belief, one has little to gain and potentially much to lose, such as falling into a state of learned helplessness. An example of how holding onto a control belief, however unrealistic it seems to an observer, may alter the probability of the event occurring can be found in control beliefs over AIDS. Individuals who test positive for HIV who have feelings of control over AIDS may be more likely than individuals without feelings of control over AIDS to sign up for a randomized drug trial with the hope that the new drug can treat their illness. Until recently, most scientists would have argued that it is impossible to eradicate the virus. Recent trials of tens of thousands of individuals with HIV have resulted in the successful removal of all detectable viruses from their bodies. One of the AIDS researchers involved in the trials remarked that if someone had asked him several months before the discovery if HIV infection could be eradicated, "I would have laughed in your face. But now we have been able to demonstrate that we can effectively suppress viral production. And that is leading to a dramatic change in how we think of this disease. Until today, we have not even thought of eradication" (p. 13, The Boston Globe, June 4, 1996).

Thus, one's mental control has important implications for one's behavior and mental health. To better understand how individuals experience mental control across the life span, we first summarize two longitudinal studies of control and then examine the dynamics of mental control in three phases of development: childhood, adolescence and young adulthood, and old age.

II. LONGITUDINAL STUDIES OF CONTROL

The importance of considering a life span approach to understanding the dynamics of mental control is highlighted by two studies, one with rats and one with humans. The study with rats suggests that early control experiences can influence one's adult health. Seligman and Vistainer found that the rats' neonatal experiences with shocks influenced their ability to fight off tumors in adulthood. They started with three groups of rats. At 27 days of age, when the rats were weanlings, the rats in the helpless group were given inescapable shocks, and those in the mastery group were given shocks with the ability to stop the shocks. The rats in the control group were not given shocks. When the rats reached adulthood, the experimenters injected all of the rats with tumor cells and gave them additional shock experiences. Normally, 50% of rats reject tumors. In this study, most (about 68%) of the rats that received escapable shocks as weanlings rejected the tumors regardless of whether they received the escapable or inescapable shocks as adults. Significantly fewer (about 28%) of the rats in the inescapable shock or helpless group as weanlings rejected the tumors regardless of whether they received the escapable or inescapable shocks as adults. Thus, it appears that the

early control experiences determined how the rats responded to later shocks and how well they could fight off the virus.

Another longitudinal study also found a relationship between earlier control beliefs and later health. Peterson, Seligman, and Valliant extracted control explanations of bad events from the writings of male students in the classes of 1942 through 1944 at Harvard University, when the students were approximately 25 years old. The explanatory styles of the students ranged from pessimistic (e.g., I am an inept human being therefore I cannot prevent undesirable outcomes) to optimistic (e.g., It was a fluke.). They found that the control reasoning used when the participants were young adults did not significantly correlate with their health at this age. However, the participants' control reasoning at about age 25 predicted their health ratings and longevity at ages 45 and 60, even when initial physical and mental health were held constant. Thus, the influence of control on health may not always take place immediately, but instead may take place years later.

III. CONTROL DYNAMICS IN CHILDHOOD

It is important to consider childhood mental control both because children experience control differently from adults and because childhood control has profound implications for later life. Starting in childhood, individuals who believe that they generally have control will have the confidence to select optimally challenging tasks and will concentrate on achieving success and confirming their beliefs in their competency. In contrast, people who believe that they have little control may act in ways that undermine success and thereby confirm their belief that they lack control. For example, a boy who believes that he does not have control over performing well at math may not ask questions in class or exert much effort in his algebra homework. His resulting bad grade on a math test will confirm his earlier beliefs and discourage future studying. Thus childhood beliefs about control may determine adult realities and the beliefs endemic to those realities.

Much of the research on children's perception of control has been conducted from an observer's perspective. Researchers have assumed that the control measures that were developed with adults are also valid with children. Although the language may be simplified for the children's versions of these scales, the scales tend to reflect adult models of control. For example, many control studies rely on the Norwicki-Strickland Locus of Control Scale or similar scales which assume control is a unidimensional bipolar construct that can be measured by forced choice responses. This extension of adults' concepts of control to children makes little sense considering the growing evidence that children think differently about control than adults. In this section we will first review how the cognitive changes of childhood influence the development of mental control, then we will briefly consider how when observers fail to consider the control experiences of children it can lead them to conclude that children's control beliefs are unrealistic. Finally, we review how culture may influence mental control.

A. Influence of Cognitive Development on the Experience of Mental Control

During childhood, the domains of control, the strategies to exert control, the cultural expectations, and the cognitive hardware differ from later life. An individual needs the cognitive hardware to operate the conceptual software. The hardware includes a sense of self, the ability to recall, and metacognition, all of which develop in the first decade of life. For example, metacognition or the awareness of one's thinking allows the child to act intentionally through developing strategies and trying to problem solve, skills that are needed to think through choices to achieve the desired outcome.

Many cognitive psychologists have documented how children undergo systematic cognitive changes with development. Weisz believes that two concepts which develop during the school years are crucial to the development of mental control: contingency and competency. He feels that these two realms follow distinct developmental trajectories and do not fully integrate until the end of childhood or the beginning of adolescence. Contingency, also called means–ends relations and response–outcome expectancies, is the belief that an action will lead to a specific outcome, or "If X occurs, Y will happen." An individual must perceive that an outcome results from his or her actions to develop a belief in mental control. Competency, also called self-efficacy expectation and agency, is the belief that one is capable of carrying out a be-

havior that leads to a specific outcome, or "I can do X." Competency requires one to assess the difficulty of a task, judge the effort one must exert, and then compare one's own behavior to that of others. Feelings of competency encourage one to persist at a task. Children first develop an awareness of contingencies, later they develop a sense of competency, and still later they integrate these beliefs to establish fully functioning mental control beliefs.

One theory is that the development of mental control is dependent on the development of the concept of self. Self can only emerge when the individual starts to notice that control is behaviorally determined. But one needs a sense of self, or a sense that one is an agent causing acts, to develop a mature sense of mental control. Infants are born without a sense of self or control beliefs but gradually construct them throughout the life span. One could argue that there are three major steps in the development of mental control in relation to the emerging sense of self.

In the first stage, infants develop event–event contingency schemas. That is, infants start to realize in a vague way that events are connected to their activities, although they do not recognize them as such. From their first weeks of life, babies begin to discriminate and to respond to social and physical contingencies. Perhaps the first contingency is established during feeding. Newborn babies accommodate their sucking to the shape of their mother's nipple. Their sucking muscles are among the only muscles that are under voluntary control. Piaget describes 2-month-old babies noticing and showing a fondness for event–behavior contingencies, as long as the interval between the event and behavior is less than 6 seconds and is in a restricted domain of activity. For example, babies at this age will increase nonnutritive sucking to move a mobile seconds later.

In the second stage, young children develop self-event schemas. They start to play with causal schemas. Piaget believes that children in their first month of their second year start to alter their actions with the aim of varying the effects. When babies are about 18 months old, they start to develop a sense of self to which they can attribute outcomes. The chid starts to realize that outcomes originate with one's actions and that these actions are part of oneself. At about 2 years of age, children start to use feedback to evaluate their competence. At about 3 years of age, children develop emotions related to self-event schemas: they may experience pride in success and shame or embarrassment in failure. They also start to refuse to help in carrying out tasks because they want to feel the pride that comes from knowing they acted alone.

The third stage, which takes place during the elementary school years, involves developing a sophisticated sense of mental control by differentiating the control-related concepts of ability, task difficulty, and chance. Children do not tend to use social comparison or evaluate how well they can perform in relation to their peers until about 7 years. They also tend to confuse random and nonrandom events. In about fifth grade, children start to notice the compensatory relationship between effort and ability such that a person with high ability may not need to exert a lot of effort.

Several researchers of childhood control have written about how children tend to overestimate control beliefs. For example, Flammer found that until children are about 10 years of age, they tend to overestimate control beliefs because they confuse effort and ability. This interpretation may be due to the actor–observer bias mentioned in the introduction. In the view of children, they are not overestimating the control beliefs but rather they are interpreting situations to the best of their knowledge. It particularly makes sense to hold optimistic views of control in childhood, when children are acquiring new skills and abilities so rapidly.

During the first decade of life, as the child's control-related concepts differentiate, the number of domains over which the child believes he or she can exert control slowly expands. It seems that infants start out with general undifferentiated feelings of control. As the self-event schema build up, the child slowly develops specific control domains in such areas as school, social interaction, and sports.

As the number of control domains expand, research suggests that children tend to start life using primary control strategies and then slowly develop secondary control strategies. The model of primary and secondary control was first introduced by Rothbaum, Weisz, and Snyder in 1982. Primary control involves changing one's environment to bring about a desired outcome. It frequently requires a behavior. Secondary control involves leaving one's environment unchanged but obtaining goals through alternative paths, such as altering one's perspective on existing realities "so as to derive meaning from them and accept them" (p. 956).

In support of the later development of secondary control strategies, Altshuler and Ruble gave children aged 5 to 12 years old positive and negative scenarios. For example, a positive scenario consisted of a child waiting for a birthday party to occur a day later, and a negative scenario consisted of waiting to receive an injection. The researchers asked the participants how the child in each of the scenarios should respond. The researchers then coded these answers. The 5- to 6-year-olds were significantly more likely then the older children to mention escaping, a primary control strategy. The 7- to 11-year-olds were significantly more likely than the younger children to mention cognitive distraction, a secondary strategy. Although the youngest children revealed an awareness of secondary control strategies, they tended to increase their use of them with age. The delayed development of secondary control strategies may be due to the relative subtlety of these strategies and the difficulty of observing the gains that can be achieved with them.

B. Influence of Culture on Mental Control Development

In addition to the cognitive changes that determine how children experience control, cultures differ in the expectancies they have for how children should behave. Asian countries tend to stress secondary control strategies more than the United States. Asian parents tend to teach secondary control strategies, such as yielding decision making to one's elders, by emphasizing greater interdependency with one's family. For example, in Japan, when parents want to punish their children, they lock them out of the house, whereas in the United States, parents ground their children or prevent them from going out.

John Weisz and his colleagues compared control-related behavioral problems among children in Thailand to children in the United States by analyzing the types of behavior parents reported when they took their children to mental health clinics. They hypothesized that overcontrolled behaviors (e.g., social inhibition, headaches, sadness, worrying) would be categorized as more of a problem than undercontrolled behaviors (e.g., impulsivity, swearing, disobedience, fighting) in the Thai culture. They based their hypothesis on the assumption that within a culture, psychopathology tends to model culturally prevalent patterns of adaption. That is, they thought that in the

United States, parents and schools tend to socialize children to exert primary control and act independently, whereas in Thailand, the culture socializes children to act modestly, avoid disturbing others, and exert secondary control. As predicted, the researchers found that the 12 most common referral problems in the American clinics were undercontrolled behaviors, whereas 7 of the 12 most common referral problems in Thailand were overcontrolled behaviors.

IV. CONTROL DYNAMICS IN ADOLESCENCE AND YOUNG ADULTHOOD

Most of the research on mental control has been conducted with adolescents and young adults. Two factors contribute to these age groups dominating the literature: (a) researchers who tend to work in academic settings find college students a convenient sample, and (b) control is a particularly important construct for this age group. In this section, we outline some of the control changes that occur in adolescence and young adulthood. We examine how observers who ignore the control experiences of adolescent actors may be causing teenagers to lose motivation and lower their academic performance when they make the transition from elementary school to junior high school. Finally, we look at how researchers who have concluded that control can become maladaptive may also be ignoring the mental control experiences of adolescents and young adults.

Erik Erikson, perhaps one of the most eloquent clinicians and theorists of adolescence, writes about some of this life stage's central issues, many of which influence the dynamics of mental control:

> In the later school years young people, beset with the physiological revolution of their genital maturation and the uncertainty of the adult roles ahead, seem much concerned with faddish attempts at establishing an adolescent subculture with what looks like a final rather than a transitory or, in fact, initial identity formation. They are sometimes morbidly, often curiously, preoccupied with what they appear to be in the eyes of others as compared with what they feel they are, and with the question of how to connect the roles and skills cultivated earlier with the ideal prototype of the day (Erikson, 1968, p. 128).

Subsequent research supports that several of the elements Erikson mentions seem to be important in the mental control dynamics of the teen years. These relevant elements include the integration of earlier ele-

ments, the search for a new identity, the concern with others' impressions, and the need to fit in with the demands of society.

Several control elements integrate in adolescence. Whereas in childhood, individuals expand their domains of control, in adolescence, individuals tend to integrate domain-specific beliefs to form a general perception of control that becomes the basis of their identity. Mental control contributes to self-esteem throughout the life span, but may be particularly important in determining individuals' self-image during adolescence, when any individuals question their identities. As part of their search for a new identity, many adolescents not only integrate previous control realms but branch out into new control domains that continue to develop throughout adulthood. These new realms can include work, civic responsibilities, sexual relations, and political action.

In addition, it may not be until adolescence that young adults can integrate contingency and competency beliefs. Weisz found that younger children tend to rely on beliefs about competency rather than contingency to make control judgments. It is not that children do not have contingency beliefs, but rather that for many individuals, adolescence is the first time they are able to think about several complex pieces of information simultaneously.

A. Lack of Mental Control and Decreases in School Motivation

When students move from elementary school to middle school, many show a drop in control beliefs. Parents and teachers used to blame the raging hormones of puberty and the increased self-consciousness of this stage for the declines in motivation, performance, and self-assurance about their abilities. Now, research suggests that these declines may be caused by "a developmental mismatch" between control beliefs of adolescents and the school environment. Junior high schools tend to focus more on performance and less on learning tasks than elementary schools. Whereas elementary school teachers tend to focus on fostering their students' strengths and creativities, junior high school teachers tend to stress grades and competition. Junior high school may be where a nurturing environment that stresses learning rather than performance is most needed. It is in junior high school that adolescents develop their self identities and increased sensitivity of how they appear to others and how to fit in to social norms. Many researchers and educators agree that it is important to reevaluate educational environments.

Dweck argues that children's implicit control theories can determine their academic and social functioning. These theories, which seem to develop as early as nursery school, may have the most dramatic effects in early adolescence. Dweck believes that individuals tend to adopt one of two types of control styles for confronting challenges. Those with an entity orientation believe that intelligence is a fixed entity. Thus, when they fail at a task, they tend to blame their inadequate ability, express negative affect, and show debilitated performance. Individuals with mastery or incremental orientations view intelligence as malleable. When they encounter failure, they tend to focus on where the process might have gone wrong and try to develop conclusions about strategies or effort that will allow future mastery. Dweck and colleagues have found that children of all intelligence groups are represented in the two styles, also that these styles operate in the social domain both in evaluating one's social ability and in judging the behavior of others. When faced with social failure, children with entity theories blame their general social ability and tend to judge others who display negative behaviors more harshly and rigidly than children with incremental theories.

The importance of one's implicit control theory becomes especially significant during the transition to junior high school. Dweck et al. found that although confidence best predicts grades in elementary school, an interaction of confidence and control styles takes over in junior high school. In a study of 165 seventh-grade students making the transition into junior high school, Dweck et al. found that although many students lowered their grades during the transition, some students improved their grades. They found that grades dropped the most for the high-confidence entity theorists, whereas the low-confidence incremental theorists tended to excel in their new school environments. It appears that when entity theorists encounter new challenges, they view them as a threat and tend to decrease their efforts, so their performance suffers. In contrast, the incremental theorists seem to be invigorated by the challenges and then increase their efforts, so their performance is enhanced.

Young women may be particularly vulnerable to the adolescent drop in control beliefs. This may be due in part to cultural expectations that female teenagers should achieve independence while maintaining relationships. The psychologist Carol Gilligan believes that in the United States at about the age of 12, many girls lose their voice or their feelings of competency that they can live up to society's expectations for women. Girls tend to be more likely than boys to adopt entity theories or helpless performance styles, and boys tend to adopt incremental theories or mastery styles. This dynamic combined with socialization factors may explain why boys tend to perform better than girls at math, a discipline that tends to rely on mastering new elements.

In a study examining whether this dynamic may relate to sex differences in academic achievement, Licht and Dweck studied the interaction between control style and type of learning situation. They gave a learning task to all of their participants, but then also gave half of the students an added section with confusing irrelevant information that was difficult to master. They found that when the task contained the confusing piece, those with a mastery style outperformed those with a helpless style, but when the task did not include it, both groups performed similarly. This suggests that differences in motivation rather than differences in ability account for the mastery-style students outperforming the helpless-style students. The researchers also found that gender and intelligence interacted: the brightest girls tended to be most debilitated by the confusing material, whereas the brightest boys tended to excel when faced with this same material. Thus, maladaptive control styles may particularly impede intelligent young women's potential to achieve.

Negative feedback may help establish control patterns in children and adolescents. It is likely to lead the individual to believe that intelligence is a stable, uncontrollable factor if, at a young age, parents and, at an older age, teachers make comments that are critical of a child's intellectual ability. Ames found that a large-scale intervention designed to nurture learning goals in elementary school children led to positive changes in the children's learning strategies, self-conceptions of ability and competence, and motivation. Therefore, environments can reform children's achievement and motivation.

B. Mental Control and the Observer's Perspective

Several researchers have argued that mental control can be maladaptive at times by citing studies conducted with adolescents or young adults. There are three behaviors these authors tend to refer to as evidence: self-handicapping, control over serious illness, and leadership roles given to individuals uncomfortable with this increase in potential control. Each of these cases when considered from the perspective of the young adult do not support the argument that mental control is maladaptive.

Some adolescents and young adults intentionally appear as if they are giving up control in a process called self-handicapping or defensive pessimism, which is to intentionally give oneself a disadvantage in a performance situation. For example, some adolescents would rather go to a party and get drunk than study the night before an exam so that they can blame their failure on their inebriation rather than on their poor abilities. Self-handicapping cannot take place in early childhood because self-handicapping requires an understanding that effort and ability are often negatively related or that lower effort tends to be associated with higher ability. As mentioned, this concept does not emerge until fifth grade.

If one takes the perspective of adolescents, it becomes clear that self-handicapping youth are not giving up mental control. For many teenagers, the desired outcome is to preserve self-esteem and identity. Researchers have demonstrated that individuals are more likely to self-handicap when they think they will do poorly if they make an effort. In support of the idea that self-handicapping occurs when individuals want to lower public accountability, researchers have demonstrated that if individuals are offered a debilitating drug, they tend to take it only when it will be known by others that they took a drug. When the drug is offered in anonymity, individuals tend to refuse the drug. Also, individuals high in social anxiety tend to show self-handicapping more than those low in social anxiety. One could categorize self-handicapping as a secondary control strategy, because it indirectly achieves the desired outcomes. Among those who set low expectations, self-handicapping can lead to more motivation, a lowering of performance anxiety, and a greater enjoyment of a performance situation than for those who do not use this strategy.

Several authors have argued that strong control beliefs in the face of serious illness can lead to a host of bad outcomes, including depression and an inability to start coping with the misfortune. These authors or others in the role of observer may think that persons with fatal diseases cannot manipulate their environment and the disease. A study often cited to show that perceived control over illness can be maladaptive is one by Affleck, Pfeiffer, Tennen, and Fifield. They studied 92 patients with rheumatoid arthritis, a progressive illness with intermittent periods of painful flare-ups. Among the patients with severe disease, they found an association between a belief of control over the course of the disease and more mood disturbance and poor psychosocial adjustment, as rated by members of the patients' medical team. If one takes the actors' perspective or the perspective of the patients with arthritis, the desired outcome may not be a good mood or good evaluations by the medical staff, but rather it may be to try to lessen the impact of the illness and to know that they have tried everything.

A study of children and young adults with chronic illnesses found an association between a greater belief in control and a more sophisticated conceptual understanding of the disease. Conceptualizations of their illnesses were rated as more sophisticated if the participants referred more frequently to bodily cues, used greater realism, and used more complex descriptions of physiological processes. A more sophisticated understanding of a disease can lead to improved coping strategies, greater compliance with treatment plans, and a more active role in pursuing new treatments. Because of the correlational nature of the study, it is not known whether more control leads the participants to take a more active role in acquiring information about their diseases or whether greater knowledge of the diseases leads to more control. Perhaps both are true.

Another example that is sometimes cited to show that more control is maladaptive is the case of individuals who when placed in leadership roles tend to feel anxiety about social disapproval. If someone is feeling insecure, an increase in responsibilities—even if they carry with them an increase in potential control—may lead to negative reactions, such as a perceived loss of control and anxiety about social approval. A promotion may highlight for individuals an awareness of all they do not know and all the contingencies they feel they cannot control. That is, while for the observer the promotion leads to the perception that the actor has an increase in control, for the actor, it may lead to a feeling of loss of control. Thus, the situation does not demonstrate that control is maladaptive, but rather that how one gains control may differ for different individuals and different situations.

V. CONTROL DYNAMICS IN OLDER ADULTHOOD

A perception exists in the research and among the lay public that control declines in old age. This perception may be due to an actor–observer bias. This assumption is based on what appears to be uncontrollable events that tend to occur in later life, such as deaths of loved ones, chronic disease, loss of one's job, and one's own approaching death. Most researchers and clinicians who specialize in the elderly are younger than their clients and research participants. The younger observer tends to perceive these occurrences as inevitable negative life events, whereas the older actor may not experience these events as losses. For example, the observer may categorize retirement as a loss of control, whereas the older actor may perceive it as a chance to start a second career or as time to devote to oneself.

In addition, some of these events, such as the death of a spouse, might be experienced as uncontrollable tragedies if they happened to individuals earlier in their lives, but when they occur in old age they may have less of an impact because older actors tend to expect these events to occur during the last stage of their life. In support of the more positive interpretation older individuals give to these life events, research demonstrates that older individuals tend to report life satisfaction equal to or greater than their younger counterparts.

There is also a tendency of younger individuals to label older individuals as lacking in control and thus unintentionally turning this label into a self-fulfilling prophecy. By helping older individuals, the young may deprive their seniors of opportunities to feel mastery and confirm control beliefs. Avorn and Langer demonstrated that when experimenters directly assisted old participants, they performed worse than when the experimenters gave them verbal encouragement or left them alone. Frequently the decision to help older people is based on criteria such as speed that may not be as relevant to the older person as it is to the younger observer. A young nurse may help an old patient get dressed to save time when the patient is capable of dressing and is in no rush.

The assumption about the decline in mental control in old age may be due to the switch in strategies that sometimes occurs in old age from primary to secondary control. Schulz, Heckhausen, and Locher

(1991) believe the switch is due to culture. They believe that as individuals reach old age, most cultures downplay attributes related to primary control, such as physical abilities and emphasize attributes related to secondary control, such as giving control to powerful others. In nursing homes, the advantageous strategy may be to become dependent, a way of operating secondary control. One study found that older adults who primarily used internal control benefitted from an intervention designed to increase internal control, but those with a more secondary control strategy tended to benefit most from a placebo intervention that involved dependence on others. There is a need to fit the person's desire for primary control and the type of control an intervention affords.

Another study demonstrated that the perception that control declines in old age may be due to actor/observer differences. The researchers asked a group of young adults and older adults to fill out questionnaires about locus of control when thinking about themselves and when thinking about the other age group. They found that the younger group tended to rate the older adults as more external in their control beliefs than the older group rated themselves, and that the old adults tended to rate the younger adults as more internal in their control beliefs than the young rated themselves. In addition, the old rated themselves as more internal than the young rated themselves. Thus, the assumption that control declines in old age may originate in younger adults imposing societal expectations of the life course rather than based on any reality.

This study and others have found that contrary to the stereotype, reported perceived control increases with age. This could be due to developmental changes, such as the accumulation of wisdom over the years. It could also be caused by cohort changes. The amount of mental control individuals feel tends to vary according to the decade in which they live. One study found a decrease in internality of control from 1966 to 1975. It seems possible that those who grew up in the early 1900s, during the Depression and the two World Wars when independence and self-efficacy were stressed, would be higher in control than those who grew up in the decades after World War II.

Although a general decline in mental control may not occur with age, certain domains of control seem to decline. Mental control over intellectual functioning, health, and development seems to decline, whereas overall control and control over interpersonal function remain stable. The ability of individuals to maintain general feelings of control may be due to a shift in focus to the control domains not lessened by cultural expectations and to the tendency to engage in downward social comparison or to compare themselves to those older people who are doing worse.

As Peterson and Stunkard point out, "Cultural norms concerning collective control are perhaps the single most important determinant of personal control" (p. 822). In old age, these cultural norms about control seem to be particularly strong. Unfortunately, the control domains that society expects to decline in old age are intellect and health, two highly valued domains in old age. Research conducted by the authors supports the idea that cultural stereotypes of how older individuals behave influences how the elderly experience control and how well they can use their intellectual abilities. In China, a culture that tends to hold more positive views of aging than held in the mainstream population in the United States, there seems to be less memory decline in old age. This may be because there is less of an expectation for a loss of control over memory in old age in China than in the United States.

Further support for the influences of cultural stereotypes on control and memory comes from an intervention study. Levy also found that when older American individuals were primed with negative stereotype words associated with old age (e.g., senility), they tended to experience a decline in memory abilities. The older participants who were primed with positive stereotype words associated with age (e.g., wisdom) tended to improve their memory performance. Young individuals, who are not exposed to cultural expectations that they lose control over their memory, primed with the same words did not tend to demonstrate any change in memory abilities.

There have been several intervention studies with nursing home residents that support the idea that declining control is not inevitable in old age. Nursing homes tend to create iatrogenic problems, including increased dependency, reduced feelings of mental control, and social isolation. Margaret Baltes has demonstrated in a series of studies that nursing home staff tend to reward dependent behaviors and discourage independent behaviors.

Ellen Langer and Judith Rodin observed what would happen when they increased mental control among nursing home residents. They increased mental control in one group by encouraging them to take an active role in such activities as caring for a plant and making mundane decisions such as whether and when they wanted to see a movie. They gave the same amount of attention to the comparison group but encouraged them to feel that the staff would take care of their needs; for example, they gave the comparison group members plants as well but told them the staff would care for them. The authors studied the residents immediately after and 18 months after the intervention. They found that the intervention group tended to be more alert, active, and reported feeling happier than the comparison group. According to the doctor's evaluations, the intervention's positive effect on health increased over the 18 months. Most important, mortality rates differed at 18 months. The intervention group showed a 15% mortality rate, whereas the comparison group showed a 30% mortality rate.

Schulz and colleagues found that giving residents control over the frequency and duration of visits from college students had a significant impact on the activity, satisfaction, and health of nursing home residents immediately after the intervention. But they found that about 2 years after they terminated the study, those in the intervention group showed a greater decline in health than those never exposed to it. It seems that the intervention did not give the residents in the decision-making group the ability to continue their new realm of control and thus the cessation of the intervention made the loss of control salient.

These two studies demonstrate the importance of emphasizing process rather than outcome in control studies. That is, the long-term positive effects probably occurred in the Langer and Rodin study because they gave the residents an ongoing decision-making treatment that the residents could continue on their own after the study ended. The Schulz study, on the other hand, only gave the residents a limited control task with a specific outcome of controlling the college students' visits that had no meaning after the researchers left. As mentioned in the beginning, one's belief that one can bring about a desired outcome is more important than the act of bringing about that outcome. Thus, the residents in the Langer and Rodin study continued to believe that they had the capability to bring about various outcomes, such as when to water a plant; whereas once the visits were over and the desired goals were obtained in the Schulz study, the residents no longer believed that they had control over certain aspects of their lives.

VI. CONCLUSION

Researchers have demonstrated the importance of life stage and culture to the dynamics of control. More may be understood about the functioning of control across the life span when researchers and clinicians consider actor–observer differences in perspective. The differences between the actor and the observer highlight the distinction between process and outcome that arose in the studies reviewed. For example, in junior high school, the adolescents who stressed process, the incremental theorists, tended to outperform their peers who stressed outcome, the entity theorists. This brings us back to perhaps the most important finding in the research on mental control: one's own beliefs about control are crucial. It is not as important that others interpret our situation as one that can be controlled as it is that we believe that our responses will make a meaningful difference.

BIBLIOGRAPHY

Affleck, G., Pfeiffer, C., Tennen, H., & Fifield, J. (1987). Attributional processes in rheumatoid arthritis patients. *Arthritis Rheum, 30,* 927–931.

Altshuler, J., & Ruble, D. (1989). Developmental changes in children's awareness of strategies for coping with uncontrollable stress. *Child Development, 60,* 1337–1349.

Bandura, A. (1995). Exercise of personal and collective efficacy in changing societies. In A. Bandura (Ed.), *Self-efficacy in changing societies.* New York: Cambridge University Press.

Berry, J., & West, R. (1995). Cognitive self-efficacy in relation to personal mastery and goal setting across the life span. *International Journal of Behavioral Development, 16,* 351–379.

Dweck, C., & Leggett, E. (1988). A social-cognitive approach to motivation and personality, *Psychological Review, 95,* 256–273.

Heckhausen, J., & Schulz, R. (1995). A life span theory of control. *Psychological Review, 102,* 284–305.

Lachman, M. (1991). Perceived control over memory aging: Developmental and intervention perspectives. *Journal of Social Issues, 47,* 159–175.

Langer, E., & Brown, J. (1992). Control from the actor's perspective. *Canadian Journal of Behavioral Science, 24,* 267–275.

Levy, B. (1996). Improving memory in old age through implicit self-stereotyping. *Journal of Personality and Social Psychology, 71,* 1092–1107.

Peterson, C., & Stunkard, A. (1989). Personal control and health promotion. *Social Science and Medicine, 28,* 819–828.

Rothbaum, F., Weisz, J., & Snyder, S. (1982). Changing the world and changing the self: A two-process model of perceived control. *Journal of Personality and Social Psychology, 42,* 5–37.

Schulz, R., Heckhausen, J., & Locher, J. (1991). Adult development, control and adaptive functioning. *Journal of Social Issues, 47,* 177–196.

Taylor, S., & Brown, J. (1988). Illusions and well-being: A social psychological perspective on mental health. *Psychological Bulletin, 103,* 193–210.

Weisz, J. (1990). Development of control-related beliefs, goals, and styles in childhood and adolescence: A clinical perspective. In J. Rodin, C. Schooler, & K. W. Schaie, *Self-directedness: Cause and effects throughout the life course.* Hillsdale, NJ: Lawrence Erlbaum.

Mental Health Services Research

Lucy Canter Kihlstrom

University of California, Berkeley

Access to Care The timely receipt of appropriate care.

Cost Sharing Methods, such as deductibles and co-insurance, that are used to spread the cost of a program among interested parties and/or to contain the costs of a program.

Deinstitutionalization A movement that began in the mid-1950s and continued through the mid-1970s, the goal of which was to shift individuals suffering from mental disorders out of the state hospitals into community-based treatment settings.

Diversion Programs Mechanisms and personnel used to (a) screen and evaluate individuals for mental health disorders while they are detained in jail; (b) negotiate with other agents within the legal and mental health system to produce a disposition that facilitates treatment rather than mere detention; and (c) link detainees with follow-up services in the community.

Health Maintenance Organization (HMO) As originally conceived in 1972, this type of organization offered health care services with five key features that

differed from the traditional fee-for-service practice: (a) Contractual responsibility was built-in to provide or assure the delivery of a stated range of health services; (b) the population to be served was defined by enrollment in a specific plan; (c) enrollment was voluntary; (d) the enrollee or consumer paid a fixed annual or monthly payment that was independent of the services used; and (e) the organization assumed at least part of the financial risk or gain in the provision of services.

Managed Care A generic term for organized systems of care that include precertification requirements, a limited network of providers, and risk-based payment.

Offset Effects Mental health services that when used reduce costs in other service areas provided by the insurance plan.

Outcome Changes in adaptive behavior and role status that are logical consequences of mental health services.

Prevention Research Research that is designed to yield results that are directly applicable to interventions that prevent the occurrences of disease or disability or the progression of detectable asymptomatic disease.

Quality of Care The degree to which mental health services for individuals and populations increase the likelihood of desired mental health outcomes in a manner that is consistent with current professional knowledge.

MENTAL HEALTH SERVICES RESEARCH is both a basic and an applied multidisciplinary field that explores issues of access to care, utilization, cost, organization, financing, delivery, quality of care, and outcomes of mental health care services. Its purpose is to elucidate the structure, processes, and effects of mental health services that are provided to individuals and special populations.

I. EVOLUTION OF MENTAL HEALTH SERVICES RESEARCH

Mental health services research, which evolved from the social and behavioral sciences as well as from the field of psychiatric epidemiology, draws from a large body of theoretical and empirical research in these fields. It seeks to answer questions about basic individual, organizational, and systemic behaviors as well as practical questions that managers and policymakers may ask.

Before the 1950s, much of this research focused on state-operated hospitals and the care provided within them. Early behavioral science research that examined familial responses to mental illness and the precipitating factors that lead to an individual's hospitalization is still considered important to the field. The epidemiologic studies conducted before the 1960s focused on issues such as how individuals entered treatment, how long they remained in treatment once a referral was made, and the ways in which individual characteristics interacted with the type of treatment provided and the setting in which it occurred.

Between 1955 and 1975, the policy of deinstitutionalization facilitated a change in the way mental health services were provided. Much of the research conducted in the 1970s and early 1980s addressed two broad empirical questions: (a) whether the services provided in the community could effectively replace the services provided in the custodial hospital, and (b) whether the cost of community treatment was less than the cost of treatment in the institution. [See MENTAL HOSPITALS AND DEINSTITUTIONALIZATION.]

During the late 1970s and in the 1980s, as the focus shifted more toward the cost, financing, and reimbursement of services, economists entered the field of health services research. However, many economists were somewhat reluctant to enter the mental health services research field, because the definitions of mental illness were often unreliable and the effec-

tiveness of many of the treatments had not been demonstrated. Currently, economic models and economic analyses are used increasingly to examine the effects of financial incentives on providers, organizations, and consumers of mental health services and the extent to which alternative methods of organizing and providing services are efficient.

At the same time, clinical researchers in psychology, social work, and psychiatry focused their efforts on systematically defining and measuring the components of mental health and illness. Both clinical drug trials and psychotherapy research expanded the knowledge base with respect to the effectiveness of particular mental health interventions. In the late 1980s and early 1990s, managed care became a predominant force in the field and much of this work evolved into clinical outcomes research. [See MANAGED CARE.]

A final shift in the focus of mental health services research included vulnerable populations such as children, the elderly, and individuals who suffer from both mental disorders and substance abuse disorders (dual diagnoses). There is a growing number of studies that address issues unique to these populations.

Although the strength of the field is that it requires a multidisciplinary approach to mental health and illness, adopting such an approach to scientific inquiry is problematic. Traditional disciplinary boundaries, competing theoretical and methodological approaches, and even the terminology used by the various disciplines often present impediments to truly collaborative research. In an attempt to overcome these barriers, interdisciplinary programs in services research evolved within academic institutions, private sector research organizations and units, and funding agencies.

II. ROLE OF PREVENTION RESEARCH

The fact that prevention research has been separated both conceptually and within funding agencies from services research is unfortunate, as the main purpose of prevention efforts is to inhibit or delay the onset of a mental disorder, and the success of such efforts can affect the use of services in the future.

Prevention efforts began as early as 1909 when the Mental Health Association was founded. Reducing risk is central to prevention research, but for any individual, risk factors may include characteristics and variables that increase the likelihood that a particular individual will develop a disorder, such as biological, psychological, and social factors in the individual, family, and environment.

As demonstrated by the research, many individuals who may be at risk for mental disorders have factors in their lives that serve to protect them. One approach to research has been to use a risk reduction model that incorporates protective factors and then to target clusters of risk and protective factors for examination. Identifying the causal risk factors that can be altered through intervention is the next step. The final step may be to test the effects of interventions through controlled trials.

The Institute of Medicine's review of prevention research programs discusses the following major findings in this area. (a) There is no evidence that the incidence of mental disorders is reduced by preventive interventions; however, findings are encouraging about the prevention of the onset of some disorders, for example, major depressive disorder and alcohol abuse. (b) Prevention programs are frequently directed toward young children and adolescents, but very few programs target the needs of adults or the elderly. (c) Education, physical health care, employment, and mental health care are clearly related and therefore collaboration among agencies must occur to a greater degree. (d) When risk factors are evident in several domains of an individual's life, interventions must take place in each one. [See ALCOHOL PROBLEMS, DEPRESSION.]

Much is known about risk factors associated with several mental disorders, but in spite of the advances that have been made and in spite of the fact that prevention efforts began early in the century, progress has been limited. One reason for this lack of progress is that mental disorders have long carried a stigma that is so pervasive that even agencies supporting certain types of interventions do not use the phrase "mental disorder." In addition, research results that demonstrated the existence of effective interventions are not widely understood by the general public. Moreover, there seems to be a belief that the prevention of disorders is possible only if treatments for them are highly effective. Another problem in the prevention of mental disorders has been the lack of an overriding theoretical framework. Finally, with respect to successful in-tervention efforts, barriers have occurred because of the difficulties in identifying, defining, and classifying mental disorders.

III. MENTAL HEALTH SYSTEM CHARACTERISTICS

A. Organizations

A vast array of organizations, both in the private and public sectors, provide mental health services. The organizations range from outpatient mental health clinics that provide only ambulatory services to psychiatric hospitals (either public or private) that provide inpatient care. In between, the forms of organizations cover the entire spectrum. They include residential treatment centers for children with serious emotional disturbance, mental health organizations that offer only day or night partial care, multiservice mental health organizations that may include community mental health centers, and, finally, general hospitals that offer separate psychiatric services. Also, services may be provided by facilities operated by the Department of Veterans Affairs or other federal agencies.

Over the period 1970 to 1990, the characteristics of the mental health system changed dramatically in the number, capacity, structure, and operation of the organizations that provide service. As an example, during this period, the total number of mental health organizations increased steadily, with almost all of the increase occurring in the number of private psychiatric hospitals, separate psychiatric services of general hospitals, and residential treatment centers for children with serious emotional disturbance. By contrast, the number of state and county mental hospitals and freestanding psychiatric outpatient clinics decreased.

In addition to these types of organizational forms, mental health services may also be provided to individuals through various managed care organizations. These organizational forms emerged in the 1970s and developed largely in the private sector, primarily serving the employed population.

The health maintenance organization (HMO), the most familiar type of managed care organization, provides mental health services through a variety of approaches, including the direct provision of mental health services through internal, formal departments as well as through a variety of external mechanisms, such as referral agreements and contractual arrangements with private providers, specialized managed mental health care organizations, and arrangements with community agencies. Beginning in the late 1980s, the types of managed care organizations began to proliferate. As the forms began to change, so too did the contracting arrangements and other mechanisms within these organizations for providing mental health services.

In the late 1980s and early 1990s, managed care organizations began contracting with states to provide mental health services to Medicaid beneficiaries. These arrangements can assume a variety of forms. For example, a state may choose to integrate mental health services into comprehensive systems of care or it may separate these services from the rest of health care benefits. Debate continues about the optimal way to design these approaches and about which approach will best meet the mental health needs of the Medicaid population.

B. Professions

Mental health services are provided both in formal psychiatric and health care organizations as well as in office-based practice settings by a variety of professionals, including psychiatrists, clinical psychologists, clinical social workers, marriage and family therapists, psychiatric nurses, and mental health counselors.

Mental health services researchers have examined the relationships among skills, financing patterns, and treatment use. Early studies indicated that the total number of hospitalization days was highest among patients of psychiatrists, but that these patients were more impaired on several health status measures. On the other hand, psychologists' clients seemed to average a higher number of visits when compared with those of psychiatrists. Service patterns of the other professionals were not included.

In addition to these professionals, primary care clinicians have become an important part of the mental health services delivery system. These types of clinicians, for example, office-based physicians and associated health providers in general internal medicine, general pediatrics, and family practice, are often the primary source of health care of any kind for many individuals who suffer from mental disorders.

The existing research points to several findings that should be explored to a greater degree. In general, pri-

mary care clinicians provide services to a large number of individuals; however, these clinicians generally underrecognize, underdiagnose, and undertreat clients with mental disorders. Although interventions to alter the current situation have been made, further research is required to determine whether these interventions would change mental health service delivery in primary care. The literature on mental health services that are provided in primary care settings is generally descriptive in nature and focuses on the process or clinical aspects of care; it has not generally examined the organizational and financial factors that affect service delivery.

IV. COST OF CARE

As a salient example of how difficult estimating the costs of mental health coverage can be, in 1995, Frank and McGuire reviewed the process that was used to estimate costs during the 1993 Clinton health care reform debate. Three general areas created intense disagreement among those attempting to project the cost of mental health services, and these same areas will in all likelihood continue to be points of contention.

The first broad area involves the impact that managed care will have on costs. During the health care reform debates, experts differed over the projected number of individuals who would be enrolled in the managed benefit plans that were emerging. Because managed benefit plans generally have a variety of mechanisms that are designed to contain costs, the number of individuals enrolled in these types of plans would greatly affect the cost estimates. For example, if it is assumed that a large number of individuals would enroll in these plans, then the cost of mental health services may be lower as a result of the cost containment mechanisms in these plans. Cost estimates also differed because of the assumptions that were made regarding the effects of management practices on costs. Managed care may contain a variety of techniques that affect costs, however, the research literature that examines the impact of these techniques on managed mental health care is sparse. As a result, the assumptions that are often made remain speculative.

A second broad area involves the impact on the estimates of insuring those individuals who have no insurance coverage. One of the major problems in the 1993 health care reform effort was that differing data sources were used to make baseline estimates of mental health care utilization by the uninsured. In addition, different assumptions were made by various experts regarding the ways in which utilization would change after uninsured individuals obtained coverage.

Finally, the issue of offset effects was critical to the health care reform debate, and it remains an important concern. Advocates of mental health coverage claim that increased coverage will result in lower general medical costs. Although the argument that offsets are real and important is certainly plausible, Frank and McGuire pointed out the methodological difficulties associated with developing an unbiased estimate of this effect.

V. FINANCING

In *Mental Health, United States, 1994,* Frank and McGuire detail three major categories of financing arrangements for mental health services: federal, state, and private insurance. These particular categories were selected because they account for a large proportion of mental health payments and because the responsibility for payment varies among them.

Most individuals in the United States are covered by private health insurance offered through employers, and this arrangement represents the primary payment method for mental health services (1991 data). Usually, individuals must pay a monthly premium in order to receive employment-based health insurance. This insurance often imposes limits on both inpatient and outpatient coverage. Although these limits may vary by employer, typical limits include 30 days of inpatient care and 25 outpatient visits with 50% cost sharing.

Historically, mental health care has been subject to coverage restrictions in private health insurance for a variety of reasons, including its perceived ineffectiveness, the high levels of demand for mental health care when compared with other medical conditions, the risk of attracting more individuals who need services to plans that provide good coverage for mental health services, and the fact that the public, in general, seems to hold unfavorable stereotypes about mental illness and about those individuals who suffer from mental disorders.

Although subject to federal mandates and oversight, Medicaid, the second type of financing system,

is a state-run program financed through a combination of federal and state contributions. The program varies widely by state in terms of benefit design and payment system provisions.

With respect to the coverage of mental health services, states may define particular services that will be paid for within general, broader categories of services. Therefore, services required to treat mental illness may not be covered even if services for other conditions are. Moreover, states may specify the amount and duration of each of the services, and mental health treatment services may have different limits in the number of visits, periods of coverage, reimbursement amounts, and types of providers.

Recently it has been argued that the Medicaid system of care for individuals with severe mental disorders is fragmented, and, as a result, individuals could actually be harmed because many fail to receive needed services or they receive inappropriate services. To rectify this situation, a growing number of states have begun, starting in 1986, to reimburse mental health providers for managing the services required by these individuals. Currently, the majority of states pay for this type of service coordination.

The third type of financing system involves state governments, primarily through state mental health agencies. As might be expected, the responsibilities and programs of state mental health agencies vary widely across the states. These agencies may be responsible for various types of services, ranging from children's mental health to domestic violence services. The delivery of services may be provided through central statewide organizations or may be controlled by local authorities.

With respect to expenditures, in 1990, 58% of the funds controlled by state mental health authorities were used for services provided by state mental hospitals, while 38% went to programs operated in the community; in 1981, the proportions were 67% and 29%, respectively. Since 1981, the trend toward more community-based care has accentuated the role played by the more local levels of government such as city, county, or catchment area authorities.

Beginning in the early 1990s, states began to rely increasingly on privately owned providers (such as HMOs or subcontracted specialized firms) to manage mental health services in the public system. While it is too early to assess the impact of managed mental health care in the public system, early data suggest that problems in implementation and funding often slow the development and growth of managed care in this sector.

VI. ACCESS TO CARE

Early findings reported in 1995 by Berk, Schur, and Cantor from the National Access to Care Survey sponsored by The Robert Wood Johnson Foundation (RWJF) suggest that 1.4% of those surveyed reported that they were unable to obtain mental health care. Although this is a relatively low percentage, it is much higher than reported in previous studies. The RWJF investigators advise that the estimate of 1.4% must be interpreted with caution, because it represents only those individuals who realize they require mental health services and who actively seek such services. The catchment area studies that have been conducted indicate that a much larger proportion of the population may require services but may not be receiving them.

Services research has attempted to focus on differences in access to care across income levels, racial groups, age, and so on. Financial barriers, including the lack of insurance coverage, have been of particular interest to service researchers. However, barriers to appropriate care may also include sociocultural and organizational factors, as well as other nonfinancial factors such as geographic availability.

In many of the studies conducted, however, service utilization seems to be equated with access to care. That is, if service use is low for a particular group, then the low utilization often seems to be explained as an accessibility issue. In reality, access to service may be more of an underlying construct, the indicators of which may be concretely measured by the length of waiting times, the difficulty in obtaining appointments, and the distance to a service site. However, access to care also involves individual perceptions and attitudes about such indicators. For example, for one individual, waiting for an appointment for 2 weeks may seem reasonable, whereas for a second individual, 2 weeks may be perceived as inordinately long. For the second individual, the waiting period may have become a barrier to receiving timely, appropriate care.

Access to mental health care is a multifaceted issue that involves individual perceptions, demographic characteristics, organizational practices, and delivery system attributes. While it may be true that low levels of service utilization can be indicative of an access problem, service utilization cannot be causally linked to access without further analyses. What is troublesome is that too often in the literature the analyses have stopped with an examination of levels of service use.

VII. QUALITY OF CARE

From the mid-1960s to the mid-1980s, studies that focused on quality of care were conducted by hospital accreditation and peer review committees. The classic conceptual framework used to examine quality of care included the use of structural, process, and outcome measures.

Within this classic framework, two broad categories of studies were conducted and reported during the early 1970s and into the 1980s. The first category described peer review programs in various types of settings, for example, hospitals, community mental health centers and state and national professional associations. Critics of these peer review programs complained that in many cases investigators failed to use external, predetermined standards. The second type of study addressed the appropriateness of psychotropic medication prescribing practices. Critics of this type of study argued that appropriateness was evaluated largely by relying on implicit rather than explicit criteria.

Beginning in the late 1980s, quality of care studies were incorporated into services and policy research for two primary reasons. First, emerging reimbursement strategies, such as prospective payment, raised issues about quality of care. For example, if these strategies encouraged clinicians to limit the quantity of care, what would the impact be on the quality of care? Second, several studies in the late 1970s and early 1980s documented variations in the cost, process, and outcomes of care across hospitals and providers.

Services research tended to examine two major aspects of the delivery process: the technical process (the amount, type, and way in which resources are used) and art of care (the interaction between the provider of care and the individual who seeks care). Each of these aspects can be examined in a variety of ways depending on the disciplinary training of the investigator.

Several important types of this kind of research can

be identified. First, governmental agencies, insurers, and employers are interested in whether the outcomes achieved justify the expenditures. This is referred to as the cost–quality trade-off issue and can be conceptualized in the following manner. Initially, using more resources will probably result in higher levels of quality, but after a period of time, using additional resources will not increase the quality of care provided. Furthermore, at some point, using more resources (and increasing expenditures) may actually negatively affect the quality of care provided. Second, researchers examine the impact on the health and functional status of individuals when aspects of the delivery system change so that the individual's ability to obtain needed care is altered. Finally, a developing body of literature addresses the extent to which interventions are used appropriately. In the research on psychotherapy, clinical researchers in psychology have begun to assess, both through meta-analytic reviews of the literature and by clinically based investigations, which interventions are efficacious for particular disorders.

In the late 1980s and 1990s, various organizations, such as the American Psychological Association, the American Psychiatric Association, and the Joint Commission on Accreditation of Healthcare Organizations (JCAHO), became actively involved in shaping both the guidelines used to assess the quality of care and the evaluation process itself.

In summary, for three decades, research on defining, measuring, and examining various aspects of quality has occurred, and as a result of these efforts, the field of mental health services research has made great strides. However, to continue the progress, the field requires (a) more data on the variation within clinical practices, (b) adoption of a variety of techniques by which studies may be designed and complex data analyzed, and (c) a greater degree of collaboration among researchers from the various disciplines.

VIII. OUTCOME-BASED EVALUATION

The evaluation of programs and services began in the 1960s after the number of social programs grew and requests for evaluations of them emanated from both funding sources and governmental institutions. The purpose of evaluation is to inform decision makers, to outline available options, and to provide feedback about programs or services. Recently, a growing num-

ber of evaluation theorists have argued that evaluation projects are able to produce more useful information when they are grounded in a theoretical framework. Theories that guide evaluation projects may focus on the selection of an intervention, the intervention process itself, or the underlying theory or theories of the disorder under investigation.

The growth of managed systems of mental health care triggered a shift in the way in which evaluation is conceptualized and in the techniques that are used. In the world of managed care, evaluation became outcome-based. The vague question of whether the individual is doing better is no longer acceptable. More precise questions must be answered, such as, Does treatment work in ways that are measurably valuable to the individual, the payor of services, the clinician, and the managed care organization? However, it must be emphasized that in the mid 1990s, outcomes research in the mental health field is still in its infancy.

In general, in 1995, McLellan and Durell noted that there are several pragmatic guiding principles that should be followed when outcome-based evaluations are designed and conducted. First, it is necessary to assess an individual before the actual program or treatment begins as well as after the course of care has terminated. Second, the outcomes to be examined must include indicators of health, adaptive behavior, and role-specific social functioning and should not be limited simply to the diagnostic categories of illness. Third, whenever possible, outcome evaluations should use standardized measures that are appropriate for the specific group being studied. Fourth, in follow-up contacts with individuals who have completed a program, the contact rate must be relatively high (above 70%) for the results to be valid. Finally, assessments of change and outcome status offer differing perspectives; therefore, both a measurement of change in function from pre- to postintervention, as well as an assessment of actual functional status must be part of the evaluation.

The World Health Organization proposed a mental health outcomes framework that includes five broad elements and the major types of outcomes to be examined:

1. *Physical health* includes general health as well as the physiological effects produced by intervention. Outcomes focus on physical symptoms, mortality, medication side effects, and physical development and health.

2. *Psychological health* includes well-being, self-esteem, affective states, and sensory and cognitive functioning. Outcomes encompass measures of psychological and cognitive development, symptoms and side effects, level of distress, and sense of well-being.

3. *Level of independence* encompasses activities of daily living, capacity for communication, work, adaptive growth, and dependence on substances. Outcomes may include performance in work and school, reliance on restrictive services, independent living, level of impairment from substance use, and criminal activity.

4. *Social relationships* involve intimacy and loving relationships as well as participation in giving and receiving social support. Outcomes encompass measures of the presence and strength of social supports, relationships with peers, family functioning, and parenting ability.

5. *The environmental* domain includes an examination of both the community and residential environment, as well as safety issues, material resources, and the availability of adequate services. Outcomes include the adequacy and stability of housing and income as well as the level of protection from victimization.

Schalock offers three broad types of outcome-based analyses that can be done depending on the purpose of the evaluation and the availability of information or data.

1. *Effectiveness analysis.* This type of analysis addresses the question of whether the program or intervention met the intended goals and objectives. Its major purposes include describing results, establishing a feedback mechanism, and offering information that facilitates program or treatment change.

2. *Impact analysis.* This type of analysis determines whether the program or intervention made a difference compared with either no intervention or an alternative intervention. An absolute requirement is that a comparison group or condition be present. The purpose of this type of analysis is to focus on the impacts of the intervention, to determine whether the impacts can be attributed with reasonable certainty to the intervention or service being evaluated, and to provide feedback. This type of analysis includes controlled clinical trials.

3. *Cost–benefit analysis.* The primary issue addressed by cost–benefit analysis is whether the impacts of the program are large enough to justify the costs needed to produce them. It relies heavily on the clear delineation and measurement of impacts and of the costs involved in generating them.

The research on mental health outcomes is difficult to summarize effectively because much of the work focuses on particular groups with specific disorders (e.g., outcomes of juvenile-onset depression), on particular drug therapies for specific disorders (e.g., relapse of individuals with mood disorders who are taking lithium), or on the use of particular treatment modalities or treatment settings (e.g., community-based treatment vs. inpatient treatment). The annual Faulkner and Gray *Behavioral Outcomes and Guidelines Sourcebooks* provide an extensive review of the literature and include state-of-the-art approaches to outcomes research.

IX. FUTURE OF MENTAL HEALTH SERVICES RESEARCH: NEEDS OF SPECIAL POPULATIONS

The groups discussed in this final section represent growing segments of society and/or segments of society that have received too little attention from researchers in the past.

A. Children

Although concern about children and adolescents with serious emotional disturbance has existed for more than 10 years, it has only recently emerged as a critical issue in mental health policy. There are two broad areas in which advances have been made. First, progress has been made in developing instruments for assessing emotional disturbance in children. Second, it has been possible to determine treatment efficacy for specific mental disorders. However, in *Mental Health, United States, 1994,* Hoagwood and Rupp have noted that the extent of emotional disturbance among children, the actual but unmet need for care, the types of services used, and the ways in which children enter the mental health system are issues that will require additional research.

The reasons for such gaps in our collective knowledge about children's mental health needs and service patterns are numerous. For example, the way in which serious emotional or behavioral disturbances are defined with respect to children vary by profession, by federal agency, and by state. As might be predicted, these variations confound any attempt to coordinate care across the different levels of government.

In addition, the responsibility for children's mental health services is dispersed across many service systems, including schools, welfare, the justice system, and so on. Children with mental health needs are scattered across these systems, and the needs of the children do not necessarily coincide with the system that provides the service; for example, children with learning difficulties are not necessarily treated for learning difficulties in the educational system.

Despite the somewhat bleak picture presented, changes are occurring and research efforts are underway under the auspices of the National Institute of Mental Health to answer several important questions, such as What is the extent of unmet needs for services by children and their families? What are the barriers to obtaining these services? What are the costs of care across program elements in the various service sectors? How are mental health services for children and adolescents financed? And, what impact will managed mental health systems of care have on the delivery of services to children?

B. The Elderly

In general, older adults are more likely to use inpatient rather than outpatient services. They are more likely to use general hospitals rather than other treatment sites, and are likely to be treated by general medical practitioners rather than by mental health professionals. In addition, the underutilization of mental health services by the elderly has been documented and attributed to a number of factors, including reluctance to seek treatment because of the stigma attached to mental illness, inadequate detection of mental disorders among the elderly by clinicians, relatively low referral rates by general practitioners, and limited knowledge on the part of the elderly regarding the availability of mental health services.

In 1995, Estes identified a lengthy research agenda for the future. The structure and performance of mental health delivery affects access, cost, and quality and therefore these relationships must be examined. More information is needed about the extent to which the elderly are served by varying types of organizations (e.g., for-profit, not-for-profit, or public) and about

the effects of various financing mechanisms, such as capitation, on service use and access to care. Further research is required on the types of interorganizational relationships that are forming between local mental health providers and other types of providers of services to the elderly.

The number of elderly is predicted to increase in the next two decades and the demand for services by this group will more than likely increase as well. Very little is known about the effects of mental health policy on the elderly; therefore, this area must be one that receives special attention in the future.

C. Ethnic Minorities

In 1996, Takeuchi and Uehara reviewed the existing research and suggested areas that will require more attention from researchers. They noted that although the details may vary across ethnic groups, in general, the research indicates that the mental health needs of ethnic minorities are largely unmet. In addition, when services are available, they are, more often than not, inappropriate.

Assessing the prevalence of mental disorders and the need for services among ethnic minority groups has proved to be problematic. Treatment data have often been used in an attempt to estimate the prevalence and need for service. Early studies seemed to indicate that African Americans have been overrepresented and Asian Americans underrepresented in mental hospitals. The evidence for Latino Americans remains ambivalent. It is important to point out that most epidemiologists believe that service use is an unreliable indicator of actual need, and this may be particularly true for ethnic minority groups as many members of these groups have difficulty accessing and using services as they are currently designed.

Although methodological problems hamper the generalizability of the community studies that have been conducted on the extent of mental health problems in ethnic minority populations, two general points can be made. First, several of the community studies contradict the evidence derived from treatment data. For example, about one half of the community studies conducted in recent years have demonstrated that African Americans had a higher rate of psychopathology (supporting the conclusions that were drawn from treatment studies); however, the other half of the studies reported that the rate of psychopathology was comparable to or even lower than that found in white Americans.

Second, there seems to be controversy surrounding the issue of whether the differences in prevalence rates should be attributed to ethnic minority status or to social class phenomena. Two theoretical frameworks are used to attempt to explain the ethnic minority-white American differences in psychological distress and psychopathology. The first framework suggests that forms of psychopathology and distress, in general, derive from the fact that society tends to stratify individuals according to their ethnic and racial backgrounds, thereby creating serious obstacles to equality in economic, occupational, and educational opportunities. The second framework argues that race differences in psychopathology disappear when social class is taken into account in the study design. This framework suggests that barriers created by lower incomes, not ethnicity per se, can result in debilitating effects on individuals or groups.

Finally, a number of empirical studies suggest that ethnic minorities do not seek professional treatment for mental health issues as often as other groups do. Moreover, when ethnic minorities use mental health services, treatment tends to be inappropriate or inadequate. Minority service providers and researchers have suggested that the mental health system must become more sensitive and responsive to the needs of ethnic minorities. However, few studies have described what such sensitivity entails or identified what factors might contribute to a more effective mental health system. [See ETHNICITY AND MENTAL HEALTH; SOCIOECONOMIC STATUS.]

D. Persons with Severe Mental Illness

In 1989, the National Institute of Mental Health in collaboration with the National Center for Health Statistics provided supplementary information to the National Health Interview Survey. The purpose of the project was to update the estimates of the number of persons with severe mental illness in the household population of the United States and to examine the use of various mental health services.

The survey findings suggest that the number of persons with severe mental illness can be conservatively estimated to include 2.1 to 2.6% of the adult population. This estimate has various components, including individuals living in households, nursing homes, mental hospitals, and state prisons, and individuals who are homeless.

A 1991 report, *Caring for People with Severe Mental Disorders: A National Plan of Research to Improve Services*, prepared by the National Advisory Mental Health Council (NAMHC), offered recommendations for research designed to improve the quality of care for individuals suffering from severe mental disorders. However, even if knowledge from this line of research is available, there are still issues of providing such services in an efficient, economical, and equitable manner.

The dilemma of how to develop effective service systems for persons with severe mental illness, as well as for persons with both severe mental and substance abuse disorders (dual diagnoses), will continue to confront service providers, planners, and service researchers. The NAMHC's report identifies crucial areas that require the attention of mental health service researchers. For example, given the number of agencies, eligibility criteria, and recertification requirements that exist for programs attempting to serve these groups, what are the optimal organizational and procedural arrangements for providing health insurance coverage, housing, income maintenance, and rehabilitation? In many parts of the country, adequate resources are simply unavailable. Moreover, the delivery system, as it exists, may not have adequate staffing levels or financing arrangements. As the report indicates, research on the development and evaluation of strategies for improved community and state systems of care for individuals with severe mental illness must be given priority.

E. Persons with Mental Illnesses Who Have Been Arrested

The number of persons incarcerated who also exhibit mental disorders is increasing. Persons with mental disorders who have been arrested for serious offenses should, it has been argued, remain in jail, but they should receive mental health treatment while incarcerated. How best to provide the needed array of services, both while the individual is in jail and especially after he or she is released, remains controversial.

It has also been argued that individuals with mental disorders who have been arrested for nonviolent crimes may benefit more from diversion programs than from incarceration. Although these programs begin to address the issue of the growing number of persons with severe mental disorder who are incarcerated for minor offenses, in general, the literature offers little assistance with respect to definitions or guiding principles for developing effective programs. Additional longitudinal studies are required that use client-based and organizational outcome measures.

X. CONCLUSION

In the final analysis, although particular vulnerable populations require the attention of mental health service researchers, there is much work to be done in all of the areas discussed in this entry. Two broad obstacles inhibit progress. First, mental health service researchers themselves must acknowledge the multidisciplinary nature of mental illness and must be more willing to collaborate across disciplines. Perhaps the key to successful collaboration lies with the interdisciplinary training programs that have developed in academic institutions over the last decade. Second, funding for service system research must be stabilized. To combat the collective lack of knowledge about the effective organization, delivery, and financing of services, continuous and more reliable funding mechanisms for research are required.

BIBLIOGRAPHY

Bergin, A. E., & Garfield, S. L. (1994). *Handbook of psychotherapy and behavior change* (4th ed.). New York: Wiley & Sons.

Berk, M. L., Schur, C. L., & Cantor, J. C. (Fall 1995). Ability to obtain health care: Recent estimates from The Robert Wood Johnson Foundation National Access to Care Survey. *Health Affairs, 14* (3), 139–146.

Estes, C. L. (1995). Mental health services for the elderly: Key policy elements. In M. Gatz (Ed.), *Emerging issues in mental health and aging* (pp. 303–327). Washington, DC: American Psychological Association.

Field, M. J., Tranquada, R. E., & Feasley, J. C. (Eds.). (1995). *Health services research: Work force and educational issues.* Washington, DC: National Academy Press.

Frank, R. G., & McGuire, T. G. (Fall 1995). Estimating costs of mental health and substance abuse coverage. *Health Affairs, 14* (3), 102–115.

Manderscheid, R. W., & Sonnenschein, M. A. (Eds.). (1994). *Mental health, United States, 1994.* Washington, DC: U. S. Government Printing office.

McLellan, A. T., & Durell, J. (1995). Outcome evaluation in psychiatric and substance abuse treatments: Concepts, rationale, and methods. In K. J. Migdail, M. T. Youngs, & B. Bengen-Seltzer (Eds.), *The 1995 behavioral outcomes and guidelines sourcebook* (pp. 389–402). New York: Faulkner & Gray.

Mrazek, P. J., & Haggerty, R. J. (Eds.). (1994). *Reducing risks for mental disorders: Frontiers for preventive intervention research.* Washington, DC: National Academy Press.

National Advisory Mental Health Council. (1991). *Caring for people with severe mental disorders: A national plan of research to improve services.* Washington, DC: U. S. Government Printing Office.

Schalock, R. L. (1995). *Outcome-based evaluation.* New York: Plenum Press.

Takeuchi, D. T., & Uehara, E. S. (1996). Ethnic minority mental health services: Current research and future conceptual directions. In B. L. Levin & J. Petrila (Eds.), *Mental health services: A public health perspective* (pp. 63–80). New York: Oxford University Press.

Taube, C. A., Mechanic, D., & Hohmann, A. A. (Eds.). (1989). *The future of mental health services research.* Washington, DC: U. S. Government Printing Office.

Trickett, E. J., Dahiyal, C., & Selby, P. M. (1994). *Primary prevention in mental health: An annotated bibliography, 1983–1991.* Rockville, MD. National Institute of Mental Health.

Mental Hospitals and Deinstitutionalization

H. Richard Lamb

University of Southern California

Aftercare After hospitalization, a continuing program of treatment and rehabilitation designed to reinforce the effects of therapy and to help patients adjust to their environment.

Board-and-Care Home A congregate living facility in the community for persons with mental illness. Board-and-care homes provide room, board, minimal staff supervision, and, in some states, the dispensing of medications.

Deinstitutionalization The mass exodus of mentally ill persons from living in hospitals to living in the community.

Gravely Disabled A condition in which a person, as a result of a mental disorder, is unable to provide for his or her basic personal needs for food, clothing, or shelter.

Institutes for Mental Disease In California, community facilities that are usually, but not always, locked. They provide 24-hour structured care, close medication supervision, and at least 27 hours per week of therapeutic activity for every resident.

Institutionalism A syndrome characterized by lack of initiative, apathy, withdrawal, submissiveness to authority, and excessive dependence on the institution.

There has been a profound change in the lives of chronically and severely mentally ill persons. Institutionalization has given way to **DEINSTITUTIONALIZATION** and living in the community for most of this population. In the four decades of this process, we have learned a tremendous amount about the needs and methods of treatment and rehabilitation in the community for these persons. Although there have been problems, the overall result has been a significant enhancement of their lives.

I. BACKGROUND

Before the current era of deinstitutionalization, chronically and severely mentally ill persons were usually institutionalized for life in large state mental hospitals. This often began with these persons' first acute mental breakdown in adolescence or in early adulthood. Sometimes, these patients went into remission in the hospital and were discharged, but at the point of their next psychotic episode were rehospitalized, often never to return to the community.

In the 1960s, British social psychiatrist John Wing and others observed that persons who spent long periods in mental hospitals developed what has come to be known as institutionalism, a syndrome characterized by lack of initiative, apathy, withdrawal, submissiveness to authority, and excessive dependence on the institution. Sociologists such as Erving Goffman argued that in what he called "total institutions," such as state mental hospitals, impersonal treatment can strip away a patient's dignity and individuality and foster regression; the deviant person is locked into a degraded, stigmatized, deviant role. Goffman and others believed that the social environment in institutions could strongly influence the emergence of psychotic symptoms and behavior. Other investigators, however, observed that institutionalism is probably not entirely the outcome of living in dehumanizing institutions; it may in large part be characteristic of the schizophrenic process itself.

With deinstitutionalization, these latter researchers observed that many chronically and severely mentally ill persons who were liable to institutionalism seemed to develop dependence on any other way of life in the community that provided minimal social stimulation and that allowed them to be socially inactive. They gravitated toward a lifestyle that allowed them to remain free from symptoms and painful and depressive feelings.

Is this dependent, inactive lifestyle bad? For many deinstitutionalized persons, it may lead to unnecessary regression and impede their social and vocational functioning; thus for these patients it should be discouraged. On the other hand, this restricted lifestyle may meet the needs of many deinstitutionalized severely mentally ill individuals and help them stay in the community. Mental health professionals, and society at large, are coming to recognize the crippling limitations of mental illnesses that in many cases do not yield to current treatment methods. It is important to provide adequate care for this vulnerable group so that the end result is not like the fate of the mentally ill in the back wards of state hospitals. For those who can be restored only to a degree, many mental health professionals advocate lowered expectations and pro-

viding reasonable comfort and an undemanding life with dignity.

II. FUNCTIONS OF THE STATE HOSPITAL

Valid concerns about the shortcomings and antitherapeutic aspects of state hospitals in the United States often overshadowed the fact that the state hospitals fulfilled some crucial functions for the chronically and severely mentally ill. The term "asylum" was in many ways appropriate; these imperfect institutions did provide asylum and sanctuary from the pressures of the world with which, in varying degrees, most of these patients were unable to cope. Furthermore, they provided medical care, patient monitoring, respite for the patient's family, and a social network for the patient, as well as food, shelter, and needed support and structure.

In the state hospitals, the treatment and services that did exist were in one place and under one administration. In the community, the situation is very different. Services and treatment are under various administrative jurisdictions and in various locations. Even the mentally healthy have difficulty dealing with a number of bureaucracies, both governmental and private, to get their needs met. Patients can easily get lost in the community; in a hospital, they may have been neglected, but at least their whereabouts were known. These problems have led to the recognition of the importance of case management. For instance, many of America's homeless mentally ill would probably not be on the streets if they were on the caseload of a professional or paraprofessional case manager trained to deal with the problems of the chronically mentally ill, monitoring them (with considerable persistence when necessary) and facilitating services.

The use of the word asylum, which has taken on such a negative connotation in the United States, needs further elaboration. The fact that the chronically mentally ill have been deinstitutionalized does not mean they no longer need social support, protection, and relief, either periodic or continuous, from external stimuli and the pressures of life. In short, they need asylum and sanctuary in the community.

Unfortunately, because the old state hospitals were called asylums, asylum took on an almost sinister connotation. Only in recent years has the word again become a respectable part of our language in signifying the *function* of providing asylum, rather than asylum as a *place*.

The concept of asylum and sanctuary in the community becomes important in postdischarge planning because although some chronically mentally ill persons eventually attain high levels of social and vocational functioning, others have difficulty meeting simple demands of living on their own, even with long-term rehabilitative help. Whatever degree of rehabilitation is possible for each person cannot take place unless support and protection in the community—whether from family, treatment program, therapist, family care home, or board-and-care home—are provided at the same time. Moreover, if society does not take into account this need for asylum and sanctuary in the community from many of the stresses of life, living in the community may not be possible at all for many chronically and severely mentally ill persons.

III. ORIGINS OF DEINSTITUTIONALIZATION

In 1955, when the numbers of persons in state hospitals in the United States reached their highest point, 559,000 persons were institutionalized in state mental hospitals out of a total national population of 165 million. Now there are 72,000 for a population of at least 250 million. In about 40 years, the United States has reduced its number of occupied state hospital beds from 339 per 100,000 population to 29 per 100,000 on any given day. Some individual states have gone even further. In California, for example, there are now fewer than 7 state hospital beds per 100,000 population, not including forensic patients (those committed through the legal system).

Before deinstitutionalization, state mental hospitals had fulfilled the function for society of keeping the mentally ill out of sight and thus out of mind. At the same time, before the advent of modern psychoactive medications, the controls and structure provided by the state hospitals, as well as the granting of asylum, may have been necessary for many of the long-term mentally ill. Unfortunately, the ways in which structure and asylum were achieved, and the everyday abuses of state hospital life, left scars not only on the patients but also on the mental health professions and on the reputation of state hospitals. Periodic public outcries

about the deplorable conditions, documented by journalists such as Albert Deutsch in his influential 1948 book, *The Shame of the States,* set the stage for deinstitutionalization. These concerns, shared by mental health professionals, led to the formation by Congress of the Joint Commission on Mental Illness and Health, which issued recommendations for community alternatives to state hospitals.

When the new psychoactive medications appeared in the 1950s, along with a new philosophy of social treatment, the majority of the chronic psychotic population seemed to have been left in an environment that was no longer necessary or even appropriate.

Other factors also came into play. First, the conviction that mental patients receive better and more humanitarian treatment in the community than in state hospitals far removed from home was a philosophical keystone of the community mental health movement. Another motivating force was concern that the system of indefinite commitment and institutionalization of psychiatric patients in many ways deprived them of their civil rights. Finally, many financially strapped state governments wished to shift part of the fiscal burden for these persons to federal and local government, that is, to federal Supplemental Security Income (SSI) and Medicaid, and to local law enforcement and emergency health and mental health services.

The process of deinstitutionalization was accelerated in 1963 by two developments at the federal level. Under the provisions of categorical Aid to the Disabled (ATD), the mentally ill became eligible (by administrative fiat of the Secretary of Health, Education, and Welfare) for federal financial support in the community; moreover, Congress passed legislation to facilitate the establishment of community mental health centers. With ATD, psychiatric patients and mental health professionals acting on their behalf now had access to federal grants-in-aid, in many states supplemented by the state, which enabled patients to support themselves or to be supported either at home or in such facilities as board-and-care homes (boarding homes) or old hotels at little cost to the state. Aid to the Disabled is now called Supplemental Security Income (SSI) and is administered by the Social Security Administration. Instead of maintaining patients in a state hospital, the states, even those that provided generous ATD supplements, found the cost of maintaining these patients in the community to be far less than had been the cost of maintaining them in state hospitals. Although the amount of money available to patients under ATD was not a princely sum, it was sufficient to pay for a board-and-care home or to maintain a low standard of living elsewhere in the community.

Many individuals in the community discovered that they could earn substantial additional income by taking former state mental hospital patients into their homes, even at the rates allowed by the ATD grants. Some entrepreneurs set up board-and-care homes for as many as 100 persons or more in large, old houses and converted apartment buildings and rooming houses. Although these board-and-care home operators were not skilled in the management of psychiatric patients, they could accommodate tens of thousands of persons who had formerly been in state hospitals, but who were not now major behavior problems, primarily because these persons were being treated with the new antipsychotic drugs.

In 1963, Congress passed the Mental Retardation Facilities and Community Mental Health Centers Construction Act, which was amended in 1965 to provide grants for the initial costs of staffing newly constructed centers. This legislation was a strong incentive for developing community programs with the potential to treat people whose main recourse had been the state hospital. However, although rehabilitative services and aftercare services were among the 10 services eligible for funding, an agency did not have to offer them to qualify for funding as a comprehensive community mental health center. Many community mental health centers chose to focus on persons with neuroses and problems of living—the healthy but unhappy. The chronically and severely mentally ill were often just as neglected in the community as they had been in the hospitals.

Sweeping changes in the commitment laws of the various also contributed to deinstitutionalization. In California, for instance, the Lanterman-Petris-Short Act of 1968 provided further impetus for moving patients out of state hospitals. Underlying this legislation was a concern for the civil rights of the psychiatric patient. (Much of this concern came from civil rights groups and individuals outside the mental health professions.) The act made the involuntary commitment of psychiatric patients a much more complex process. Holding psychiatric patients indefinitely against their will in mental hospitals became much more difficult. Thus, the initial stage of what was formerly the career of the long-term hospitalized patient—namely, an involuntary, indefinite commitment—became a thing of the past. California's Lanterman-Petris-Short Act soon became a model for states across the nation, many of which passed even more restrictive laws that made involuntary psychiatric treatment more difficult to obtain in those states than in California.

IV. HOSPITAL VERSUS COMMUNITY

In the view of some, deinstitutionalization has gone too far in terms of attempting to treat long-term mentally ill persons in the community. Some long-term mentally ill persons clearly require a highly structured, locked, 24-hour setting for adequate intermediate or long-term management. The great majority of mental health professionals, those who actually treat patients, believe that for those who need such care, society has an obligation to provide it, either in a hospital or in an alternative setting, such as California's locked Institutes for Mental Disease.

Where to treat need not be an ideological issue as it has become because of the ideologies of the community mental health and civil rights movements. Where to treat is a decision that is best based on the clinical needs of each person. Unfortunately, deinstitutionalization efforts have, in practice, too often confused locus of care and quality of care. Where mentally ill persons are treated has been deemed to be more important than how or how well they are treated. Care in the community has often been assumed almost by definition to be better than hospital care. In actuality, poor care can be found in both hospital and community settings. But the other issue that requires attention is appropriateness. The long-term mentally ill are not a homogeneous population; what is appropriate for some is not appropriate for others.

For instance, what of those persons who are characterized by such problems as assaultive behavior; severe, overt major psychopathology; lack of internal controls; reluctance to take psychotropic medications; inability to adjust to open settings; problems with drugs and alcohol; and self-destructive behavior. When attempts have been made to treat some of these persons in open community settings, it has required an inordinate amount of time and effort from mental health professionals, various social agencies, and the criminal justice system, and even then these attempts have met with only limited success. Many have been lost to the mental health system and are on the streets and in the jails.

Moreover, this less than satisfactory result has often been seen as a series of failures on the part of both mentally ill persons and mental health professionals. One consequence has been an alienation of a number of long-term mentally ill persons from a system that has not met their needs, and some mental health professionals have become disenchanted with their treatment as well. Unfortunately, the heat of the debate over this issue of whether or not to provide intermediate and long-term hospitalization for such patients has tended to obscure the benefits of community treatment for the great majority of the long-term mentally ill who do not require such highly structured 24-hour care.

V. NEW GENERATION OF CHRONICALLY MENTALLY ILL PERSONS

Perhaps the most important lesson to be drawn from the American experience is that the most difficult problem is not the fate of those patients discharged into the community after many years of hospitalization. Rather, the problem that has proved most vexing was almost totally unforeseen by the advocates of deinstitutionalization, namely, *the treatment of the new generation of severely mentally ill persons that has emerged since deinstitutionalization.*

For instance, it has been largely from this generation that the homeless mentally ill have been drawn. Thus, the large homeless population with major mental illness—that is, schizophrenia, schizoaffective disorder, bipolar illness, and major depression with psychotic features—has tended to be young. [*See* DEPRESSION; MOOD DISORDERS; SCHIZOPHRENIA.]

How did this come to be? The chances are that most of the current long-stay hospitalized patients who are most inappropriate for discharge—because of a propensity to physical violence, very poor coping skills, and marked degree of manifest pathology—will not be discharged, or if they are discharged and fail, will not be sent out again.

Those who have been hospitalized for long periods have been institutionalized to passivity. For the most part, they have come to do what they are told. When those for whom discharge from the hospital is feasible

and appropriate are placed in a community living situation with sufficient support and structure, most, although by no means all, tend to stay where they are placed and to accept treatment.

This sequence has not been true for the new generation of severely mentally ill persons. They have not been institutionalized to passivity. Not only have they not spent long years in hospitals, they have probably had difficulty just getting admitted to an acute hospital (whether they wanted to be or not) and even greater difficulty staying there for more than a short period on any one admission.

To understand the plight of this new generation of the chronically and severely mentally ill, their problems need to be considered from an existential point of view. A study of long-term severely disabled psychiatric patients (in a board-and-care home in Los Angeles) showed that significantly more patients under the age of 30 had goals to change anything in their lives as compared with patients over the age of 30. How can we understand this finding? Perhaps, as these persons with limited capabilities have become older, they have had more time to experience repeated failures in dealing with life's demands and in achieving their earlier goals. They have had more time to lower or set aside their goals and to accept a life with a lower level of functioning that does not exceed their capabilities. Thus, in the same study, a strong relationship was found between age and history of hospitalization; three fourths of those under age 30 had been hospitalized during the preceding year as compared with only one fifth over age 30.

When one is still young and just beginning to deal with life's demands and trying to make a way in the world, one struggles to achieve some measure of independence, to choose and succeed at a vocation, to establish satisfying interpersonal relationships and attain some degree of intimacy, and to acquire some sense of identity. Lacking the ability to withstand stress and the ability to form meaningful interpersonal relationships, the mentally ill person's efforts often lead only to failure. The result may be a still more determined lead to another failure accompanied by feelings of despair. For a person predisposed to retreats into psychosis, the result is predictably a stormy course with acute psychotic breaks and repeated hospitalizations often related to these desperate attempts to achieve. The situation becomes even worse when such persons are in an environment where unrealistic expectations emanate not just from within themselves, but also from families and mental health professionals.

Before deinstitutionalization, these "new chronic patients" would have been chronically institutionalized, often starting from the time of their first breakdown in adolescence or early adulthood. Sometimes, these persons reconstituted in the hospital and were discharged, but at the point of their next decomposition were rehospitalized, often never to return to the community. Thus, these mentally ill persons, after their initial failures in trying to cope with the vicissitudes of life and of living in the community, were no longer exposed to these stresses: they were given a permanent place of asylum from the demands of the world.

Such an approach now tends to be the exception, not the rule; since large scale deinstitutionalization began, hospital stays tend to be brief. In this sense, the majority of "new" long-term patients are the products of deinstitutionalization. This is not to suggest that we should turn the clock back and return to a system of total institutionalization for all chronically and severely mentally ill persons, in the community, most of these patients can have something very precious, their liberty, to the extent they can handle it. Furthermore, they can realize their potential to pass successfully some of life's milestones. Nevertheless, in the United States, it is this new generation of chronically and severely mentally ill persons that has constituted the greatest concerns about deinstitutionalization. They have posed the most difficult clinical problems in treatment and by swelling the ranks of the homeless mentally ill and the mentally ill in jail, they have created serious social problems for the community.

VI. PROBLEMS IN TREATMENT OF THE NEW LONG-TERM PATIENTS

As recently as 1950, there were no psychotropic drugs to bring persons out of their world of autistic fantasy and help them return to the community. Even today, many patients fail to take psychotropic medications because of disturbing side effects, fear of tardive dyskinesia, denial of illness, or in some cases to avoid the dysphoric feelings of depression and anxiety that result when they see their reality too clearly; grandiosity and a blurring of reality may make their lives more bearable than a relative drug-induced normality.

A large proportion of the new chronically mentally ill patients tend to deny a need for mental health treatment and to eschew the identity of chronic mental patient. Admitting mental illness seems to them to be admitting failure. Becoming part of the mental health system seems to many of these persons like joining an army of misfits. Many of these persons also have primary substance abuse disorders and/or medicate themselves with street drugs.

These problems become worse for those whose illness is more severe, for failure to engage these persons in treatment may result in serious problems such as homelessness. Thus, evidence has begun to emerge that the homeless mentally ill have a greater severity of illness than the mentally ill generally. At Bellevue Hospital in New York City, approximately 50% of inpatients who were homeless are transferred to state hospitals for long-term care as opposed to 8% of other Bellevue psychiatric inpatients.

VII. BASIC NEEDS OF CHRONICALLY AND SEVERELY MENTALLY ILL PERSONS IN THE COMMUNITY

Clearly, a comprehensive and integrated system of care for the chronically and severely mentally ill with designated responsibility, accountability, and adequate fiscal resources needs to be established in the community. With such a system in place, the level of functioning and quality of life can be greatly enhanced. The following are the components of such a system (see Table I).

Adequate, comprehensive and accessible psychiatric and rehabilitative services need to be available and, when necessary, be provided assertively through outreach services. First, there needs to be an adequate number of direct psychiatric services that provide (a) outreach contact with the mentally ill in the community, (b) psychiatric assessment and evaluation, (c) crisis intervention, including hospitalization, acute and sub-acute day treatment, (d) individualized treatment plans, (e) psychoactive medication and other somatic therapies, and (f) psychosocial treatment. Second, there needs to be an adequate number of rehabilitative services that provide socialization experiences, training in the skills of everyday living, and social and vocational rehabilitation. Third, both treatment and rehabilitative services need to be provided assertively, for instance, by going out to patients' living settings if they do not or cannot come to a centralized program

Table I Components of a Comprehensive System of Care for the Chronically and Severely Mentally Ill

Direct Psychiatric Services
- Psychiatric assessment and evaluation
- Crisis intervention including acute hospitalization
- Acute and sub-acute day treatment
- Psychoactive medications
- Assertive Outreach
- Psychosocial treatment
- Individual and group therapy
- Social and vocational rehabilitation
- Adequate number of trained professionals and paraprofessionals

Housing
- Supervised housing needed for most of this population
- Range of supervision and structure

Case Management
- One mental health professional or paraprofessional responsible for care of each patient

Families
- Important allies in the treatment
- Families need adequate support

Legal and Administrative Procedures
- Acute care—commitment laws need to be less restrictive
- Long-term care—increased use of conservatorship, guardianship, commitment to outpatient treatment and treatment as a condition of probation

Increased Coordination and Integration of Community Agencies

General Social Services

Ongoing Structured Intermediate and Long-Term 24-Hour Care When Indicated

location. Fourth, the difficulty of working with some of these patients should not be underestimated.

Crisis services need to be available and accessible. Too often, the chronically and severely mentally ill who are in crisis situations are put into inpatient hospital units when rapid specific interventions, such as medication or crisis housing, would have been more effective and less costly. Others in need of acute hospitalization are denied it because of shortages of hospital beds.

An adequate number of professionals and paraprofessionals need to be trained for community care of the chronically and severely mentally ill.

An adequate number and ample range of graded, stepwise, supervised community housing settings need to be established. Some small portion of the severely and chronically mentally ill can graduate to independent living. For the majority, however, mainstream low-cost housing is not appropriate. Most housing settings that require people to manage by themselves are beyond the capabilities of most chronically and se-

verely mentally ill persons. Instead, settings are needed that offer different levels of supervision, both more and less intensive, including quarterway and halfway houses, board-and-care homes, satellite housing, foster or family care, and crisis or temporary hostels. [See COMMUNITY MENTAL HEALTH.]

A system of responsibility for the chronically and severely mentally ill living in the community needs to be established, with the goal of ensuring that each patient has a therapeutic relationship with one mental health professional or paraprofessional (a case manager) who is ultimately responsible for his or her care. In such a case management system, each patient's case manager would do the following: ensure that the appropriate psychiatric and medical assessments are carried out; formulate, together with the patient, an individualized treatment and rehabilitation plan, including the proper pharmacotherapy; monitor the patient; and assist the patient in receiving services.

Clearly, the shift of psychiatric care from institutional to community settings does not in any way eliminate the need to continue the provision of comprehensive services to mentally ill persons. As a result, society needs to declare a public policy of responsibility for the mentally ill who are unable to meet their own needs, governments need to designate programs in each region or locale as core agencies responsible and accountable for the care of the chronically and severely mentally ill living there, and the staff of these agencies need to be assigned individual patients for whom they are responsible.

For the more than 50% of the chronically and severely mentally ill population living at home or for those with positive ongoing relationships with their families, programs and respite care need to be provided to enhance the family's ability to provide a support system. Where the use of family systems is not feasible, the mentally ill person needs to be linked with a formal community support system. In any case, the entire burden of deinstitutionalization should not be allowed to fall on families.

Basic changes need to be made in legal and administrative procedures to ensure continuing community care for the chronically and severely mentally ill. In the 1960s and 1970s, laws that made commitment more difficult to obtain and patients' rights advocacy remedied some very serious abuses in public hospital care. At the same time, it became more difficult for many persons who need involuntary treatment to receive it.

Involuntary commitment laws need to be made more humane to permit prompt return to active inpatient treatment for mentally ill persons when acute exacerbations of their illnesses make their lives in the community chaotic and unbearable. Involuntary treatment laws should be revised to allow the option of outpatient civil commitment, whereby the court orders mandatory treatment at a mental health outpatient facility rather than commitment to a hospital; in states that already have provisions for such treatment, that mechanism should be more widely used. Finally, advocacy efforts should focus on making available competent care in the community, rather than simply focus on "liberty" for mentally ill persons at any cost.

For outpatients who are so gravely disabled or who have such impaired judgment that they cannot care for themselves in the community without legally sanctioned supervision, conservatorship status needs to be easier to obtain. For instance, in California, conservatorship has become an important therapeutic modality for such persons. Conservatorship is sought for individuals who are considered to be "gravely disabled." Gravely disabled means "a condition in which a person, as a result of a mental disorder . . . is unable to provide for his or her basic personal need for food, clothing, or shelter" (California Welfare and Institutions Code, Sections 5000–5466).

The conservator may be granted a number of powers over the mentally ill person. Most commonly granted are powers related to the conservatee's residential placement, his or her involvement in psychiatric treatment, and management of the conservatee's money. That is, the conservator has the power to place the conservatee in any setting (e.g., at home or in a board-and-care facility, or a psychiatric hospital) and to require that the conservatee participate in psychiatric treatment and take medications to remedy or prevent the recurrence of being gravely disabled.

Conservatorship is particularly effective when conservators are psychiatric social workers or persons with similar backgrounds and skills who use their court-granted authority to become a crucial source of stability and support for chronically mentally ill persons. Conservatorship thus can enable persons who might otherwise be long-term residents of hospitals to live in the community and to achieve a considerable measure of autonomy and satisfaction in their lives.

A system of coordination among funding sources and implementation agencies needs to be established.

Because the problems of the chronically and severely mentally ill need to be addressed by multiple public and private authorities, coordination, so lacking in the deinstitutionalization process, needs to become a primary goal. Territorial and turf issues have often been at the root of this problem, and different agencies serving the same patients have often worked at cross-purposes. The ultimate objective needs to be a true system of care rather than a loose network of services, and an ease of communication among different types of agencies (e.g., psychiatric, social, vocational, and housing) as well as up and down the governmental ladder, local through federal.

General social services need to be provided. In addition to the need for specialized social services, such as socialization experiences and training in the skills of everyday living, there is a pressing need for generic social services. Such services include arranging for escort services to agencies and potential residential placements, help with applications to entitlement programs, and assistance in mobilizing the resources of the family.

Ongoing structured 24-hour care should be available for that small proportion of the chronically and severely mentally ill who do not respond to current methods of treatment and rehabilitation. Some mentally ill persons, even with high-quality treatment and rehabilitation efforts, remain dangerous or gravely disabled. For these persons, there is a pressing need for ongoing structured 24-hour care in long-term settings, whether in hospitals or in locked, highly structured community alternatives to hospitals such as California's Institutes for Mental Disease.

Unfortunately, not enough of this knowledge about the needs of severely mentally ill persons has found its way into practice. Where it has, however, it has led to a much richer life experience and higher quality of life.

VIII. FAMILIES OF THE CHRONICALLY AND SEVERELY MENTALLY ILL

Mental health professionals have learned that the chronically and severely mentally ill and their families need advice. Many mentally ill persons lack the ability to cope with the routine stresses of life and need specific guidance about what to do in many areas of their lives. For instance, a chronically and severely mentally ill person may find himself or herself in a situation which will, if not resolved, precipitate an exacerbation of acute psychosis. Although it may be very clear to a mental health professional what the mentally ill person needs to do, the person may be overwhelmed and immobilized by what he or she perceives as the complexity of it all. Advice and assistance from mental health professionals are crucial and must be given.

Managing major mental illness in a relative at home is an immensely difficult task. Families can, and often do, learn by trial and error over a period of years how to help stabilize their mentally ill relatives by encouraging the avoidance of excessive stress, having realistic expectations, setting appropriate limits, understanding the patient's problem in tolerating social stimulation, learning how to react to psychotic symptoms, and encouraging the taking of medications. But families learn this at great emotional cost that could have been avoided had they been assisted by knowledgeable professionals. Clearly, families deserve better. If mental health professionals themselves learn how to manage chronically and severely mentally ill persons at home, they can then advise the families and make their lives, and the lives of their mentally ill relatives, immeasurably better.

Mental health professionals can also use families' abilities to play an important role in the treatment process. Mental health professionals have to learn to help families set limits and take charge of their households, to feel comfortable in telling the family that schizophrenia and other major mental illnesses are biological illnesses and that the family has not caused them, to be unambivalent about the use of psychoactive medications and in advising families to urge their relatives to take them, and to work with the families and their mentally ill relatives to determine what are realistic goals. Mental health professionals need to help relatives understand that social withdrawal may be a necessary defense for mentally ill persons against too much stress or social stimulation, that excessive withdrawal may lead to a form of institutionalism in the home, and that a balance must be struck.

IX. THERAPEUTIC BUT REALISTIC OPTIMISM

Experience with deinstitutionalization has shown that nothing is more important than therapeutic optimism for those who work successfully with the long-term mentally ill. But equally important, it has become apparent that there is a need for a realistic appraisal of these persons. Such an appraisal will make possible the necessary vigorous treatment and rehabilitation efforts for those with the potential for high levels of functioning, and make possible the striving for other goals, such as improving quality of life, for those whose potential is less.

An important issue with regard to goal setting is that the kinds of criteria used by theorists, researchers, policy makers, and clinicians in assessing social integration have a distinct bias in favor of values held by these professionals and by middle-class society generally. Thus, holding a job, increasing one's socialization and relationships with other people, and living independently may be goals that are not shared by a large proportion of the long-term mentally ill.

Likewise, what makes the mentally ill person happy may be unrelated to these goals. They may want (or need) to avoid the stress of competitive employment, or even sheltered employment, and of living independently. They may experience more anxiety than gratification from the threat of intimacy that accompanies increased involvement with other people. Furthermore, many relatives may be primarily interested in the simple provision of decent custodial care.

Moreover, if the only model used is expectations applicable to that proportion of the long-term mentally ill who are higher functioning, there will be neglect of the large population who are lower functioning and who cannot respond to these expectations. In fact, in many jurisdictions this has happened.

A major obstacle to understanding and addressing the problems of deinstitutionalization and the long-term patient has been a failure by many mental health professionals to recognize that there are many different kinds of long-term mentally ill persons, who vary greatly in their capacity for rehabilitation and for change. Long-term mentally ill persons differ in their ability to cope with stress without decompensating and developing psychotic symptoms. These persons also differ in the kinds of stress and pressure they can handle; for instance, some who are amenable to social rehabilitation cannot handle the stresses of vocational rehabilitation, and vice versa. What may appear to be, at first glance, a homogeneous group turns out to be a group that ranges from persons who can tolerate almost no stress at all to those who can, with some assistance, cope with most of life's demands.

Such a view is supported by the very marked variations of course and outcome in both the shorter term follow-up studies of schizophrenia and the longer term studies discussed later. For some chronically and severely mentally ill persons, competitive employment, independent living, and a high level of social functioning are realistic goals; for others, just maintaining their present level of functioning should be considered a success.

Dependency, and the reactions of professionals to it, may well be another important factor. To gratify dependency needs and to nurture are crucial activities in the helping professions. And professionals learn to do this in such a way that patients do not experience a loss of self-esteem from knowing that they need help and support. Not only may this process be draining, but in addition, when professionals nurture, they expect growth and are sorely disappointed when they do not get it, despite the fact that the potential for the growth they seek may not be there. As a result, lower functioning patients may receive less professional attention, priority, and resources.

Moreover, most professionals, as products of our culture and our society, tend to have a moral disapproval of persons who have "given in" to their dependency needs, who have adopted a passive, inactive lifestyle, and who have accepted public support instead of working. Perhaps this moral disapproval helps to explain why programs with the goal of rehabilitation to high levels of functioning, or "mainstreaming," have attracted the most attention and the most funding. Such programs have been very much needed. If, however, attempts are made to reverse low-functioning adaptations to the pressures of life without making a realistic appraisal of the capabilities of each individual, an acute exacerbation of psychosis may result. Probably no problems have been more difficult to overcome in the treatment of the long-term mentally ill than those of professionals having to come to terms with the fact that some persons are unable and/or unwilling to give up a life of dependency.

The matter of independence presents similar problems. Society generally, including mental health professionals, highly values independence. And yet, nothing has been more difficult for many long-term mentally ill persons to attain and sustain. The issue of supervised versus unsupervised housing provides an example. Professionals want to see their patients living in their own apartments, managing on their own perhaps with some outpatient support. But the experience of deinstitutionalization has been that most long-term severely mentally ill persons living in unsupervised settings in the community find the ordinary stresses of managing on their own more than they can handle. After a while they tend to not take their medications, to neglect their nutrition, to let their lives unravel and become disorganized, and eventually to find their way back to the hospital or the streets.

Mentally ill persons themselves highly value independence, but they very often underestimate their dependency needs. Professionals need to be realistic about their patients' potential for independence, even if the patients are not.

Still another factor has been a lack of appreciation by some of the rewards of treating the lower-functioning members of the long-term mentally ill population and of forming a relationship over many years with both the mentally ill person and the family. Even when the potential for higher functioning is limited, mental health professionals can derive an immense amount of satisfaction from helping to transform chaotic, dysphoric lifestyles into stable ones with at least some opportunity for pleasure and contentment—for both the mentally ill person and the family.

X. HOMELESS MENTALLY ILL

The homeless mentally ill have become one of the greatest challenges to public mental health and to society in general. The two American Psychiatric Association Task Forces on the Homeless Mentally Ill (1983 to 1984 and 1991 to 1992) concluded that this problem is the result not of deinstitutionalization per se, but of the way it has been implemented; homelessness among the chronically and severely mentally ill is symptomatic of the grave problems facing this population generally in this country. Thus, the problem of homelessness will not be resolved until the basic underlying problems of the chronically and severely mentally ill generally are addressed and a comprehensive and integrated system of care for them is established. The solutions, then, for homelessness among the mentally ill are the same solutions enumerated earlier in the section on basic needs of chronically and severely mentally ill persons in the community.

How do the chronically and severely mentally ill become homeless? Obviously, there are many pathways to the streets, but it is useful to look briefly at some of them. The chronically and severely mentally ill are not proficient at coping with the stresses of the world; therefore, they are vulnerable to eviction from their living arrangements, sometimes because of an inability to deal with difficult or even ordinary landlord–tenant situations and sometimes because of circumstances in which they play a leading role. In the absence of an adequate case management system, they are out on the streets and on their own. Many, especially the young, have a tendency to drift away from their families or from a board-and-care home; they may be trying to escape the pull of dependency and may not be ready to come to terms with living in a sheltered, low-pressure environment. If they still have goals, they may find an inactive lifestyle extremely depressing; or they may want more freedom to drink or to use street drugs. Some may regard leaving their comparatively static milieu as a necessary part of the process of realizing their goals, but this is a process that exacts a price in terms of homelessness, crises, decompensation, and hospitalizations. Once the mentally ill are out on their own, they will more than likely stop taking their medications and, after a while, they will lose touch with the Social Security Administration and will no longer be able to receive their Supplemental Security Income checks. Their poor judgment and the state of disarray associated with their illness may cause them to fail to notify the Social Security Administration of a change of address or to fail to appear for a redetermination hearing; in this way they lose their financial support. The lack of medical care on the streets and the effects of alcohol and other drug abuse are further serious complications. They may now be too disorganized to extricate themselves from living on the streets—except by exhibiting blatantly bizarre or disruptive behavior that leads to their being taken to a hospital or jail.

XI. CRIMINALIZATION

As a result of deinstitutionalization, there are now large numbers of mentally ill persons in the community. At the same time, there is a limited amount of community psychiatric resources, including hospital beds. Society has a limited tolerance of mentally disordered behavior, and the result is pressure to institutionalize persons who need 24-hour care wherever there is room, including in jail. Indeed, a growing number of studies have found criminalization of mentally disordered behavior—a shunting of mentally ill

persons in need of treatment into the criminal justice system instead of into the mental health system. Instead of receiving hospitalization and psychiatric treatment, the mentally ill often are subject to inappropriate arrest and incarceration. Legal restrictions placed on involuntary hospitalization also probably result in a diversion of some mentally ill persons to the criminal justice system.

Societal pressure to remove those with psychotic behavior from the community is not the only reason for criminalization of mentally ill persons. Another important factor is that when chronically and severely mentally ill persons were living out their lives in state hospitals, they were not exposed to situations in the community in which they might run afoul of the criminal justice system. Now, they are in the community, and, especially for those who go untreated, all that has changed.

It is possible that the less serious misdemeanor offense is frequently a way of asking for help. For instance, in one study of the mentally ill in jail, more than one half of those charged with misdemeanors had been living on the streets or on the beach or in missions or in cheap hotels. Persons living in such places obviously have a minimum of community supports and need a thorough psychiatric evaluation and referral to psychiatric treatment and rehabilitation. In many cases, they are in need of intermediate or long-term hospitalization.

Still another factor causing criminalization may be that many of this group of uncared-for mentally ill persons are being arrested for minor criminal acts that are really manifestations of their illness, their lack of treatment, and the lack of structure in their lives.

XII. CONCLUSIONS

Deinstitutionalization is now an accomplished fact. We have taken away from the chronically and severely mentally ill the almost total asylum from the pressures of the world and the care, however imperfect, that they received in state hospitals. The central problem that now needs to be addressed is society's obligation to provide the care and treatment they need but in the community setting. With the advent of the modern antipsychotic medications and psychosocial treatments, the great majority are able to live in a range of open settings in the community, with family, in their own apartments, in board-and-care homes, in halfway houses, and so on. Nevertheless, there remains a minority of persons with chronic and severe mental illness who need highly structured, 24-hour care, often in locked facilities. The fact that a significant proportion of this minority are now living in our jails, in the streets, and in other squalid conditions is evidence that adequate community care has not been provided for the most severely ill. Moreover, it may be that we have deinstitutionalized some mentally ill persons who cannot be effectively treated in the community. But overall, the lives of most chronically and severely mentally ill persons have changed permanently, from institutionalization to community living. With adequate treatment and support, this change can be a great improvement, leading to a much richer life experience and a higher quality of life.

BIBLIOGRAPHY

Bachrach, L. L. (1996). The state of the state mental hospital in 1996. *Psychiatric Services, 47,* 1071–1078.

Lamb, H. R. (Ed.) (1984). *The homeless mentally ill: A task force report of the American Psychiatric Association.* American Psychiatric Association, Washington, DC.

Lamb, H. R., Bachrach, L. L. Kass, F. I. (Eds.) (1992). *Treating the homeless mentally ill: A task force report of the American Psychiatric Association.* American Psychiatric Association, Washington, DC.

Lefley, H. P., Johnson, D. L. (Eds.) (1990). *Families as allies in treatment of the mentally ill: New directions for mental health professionals.* American Psychiatric Press, Washington, DC.

Thornicroft, G., Bebbington P. (1989). Deinstitutionalization—From hospital closure to service development. *British Journal of Psychiatry, 155,* 739–753.

Torrey, E. F. (1997). *Out of the shadows: Confronting America's mental illness crisis.* New York: Wiley & Sons, Inc.

Mental Institutions: Legal Issues and Commitments

Linda E. Weinberger and Etan Markowitz

University of Southern California

Decompensation   A breakdown of organized psychological functioning.

Due Process   Procedural safeguards to ensure fundamental fairness with respect to a person's life, liberty, and property.

Forensic Mental Patient   A mentally impaired individual over whom the court has jurisdiction.

Intervention   A way to treat an individual's impairment.

Least Restrictive Alternative   The treatment effective for the disorder that infringes in the least possible manner on the patient's life and liberty.

Recidivism   The commission of another criminal act.

Social Control   A legal means by which an individual's freedom is restricted.

MENTAL INSTITUTIONS are a modern development. Although born of society's sense of need and scientific advances in psychiatry, their purpose and function have remained controversial since inception. Much of the controversy arises from the legal aspects of placing people in mental institutions. The expectations that society and the judiciary have about the ability of mental health professionals to treat persons committed to mental institutions have produced great debate. This article reviews the history of mental institutions and describes the types of legal commitments that exist for the mentally impaired. Legal issues pertaining to patients' commitment and treatment are also presented.

I. HISTORY OF MENTAL INSTITUTIONS

Compassion and concern for the mentally ill and mentally retarded date at least to the sixth century Babylonian Talmud. For centuries, families cared for their mentally impaired relatives at home. Sometimes, the community and religious charities assisted poor families in the care of impaired members. A mentally impaired individual with neither family nor other means of support was allowed to wander about the open country or joined bands of transients. However, violent individuals were often imprisoned. As towns became more populous, tolerance decreased for deranged people who were poor or without family.

The first workhouse was established in England in 1697; many destitute mentally ill were committed to it. The mentally impaired were not separated from criminals and paupers in prisons and workhouses; the purpose of these institutions was detention, not treatment. As these institutions became overcrowded with criminals, troublesome family members, the poor, and the mentally impaired, a new institution was created out of necessity and in response to financial incentive: the private asylum. In eighteenth century England, anyone could invest in a facility housing the mentally ill and charge a fee. Private madhouses boarded individuals whose fees were paid either by their families or by charities, mentally impaired officers and seamen whose fees were paid by the Royal Navy, and some poor who were admitted at reduced rates. There was little regulation and supervision of the facilities; many kept the residents in filthy and neglectful conditions. The English government established licensing safeguards and guidelines, and by 1807 there were 45 licensed houses. Complaints about inadequate housing and care, as well as a lack of facilities for the mentally ill in many counties, led Parliament to pass the Act of 1808, authorizing asylums for both private and public patients, with priority for the poor mentally ill.

The first general hospital in the United States was established in Pennsylvania in 1752 by the Quakers for the mentally ill and poor physically ill. The first hospital exclusively for the mentally impaired was built in Virginia in 1773. These asylums were created with good intentions. There was a belief that placing mentally impaired people in tranquil settings away from slums and crowded cities would help them recuperate. Although a result of humanitarian concern, asylums were not always used benevolently. Asylums came to be known as "convenient places for inconvenient people." People who acted strangely and were viewed as a threat to the community or to themselves, or who were in need of care in the form of food, clothing, or hygiene were committed against their will. Detention in mental institutions was justified not only for the dangerous but for those whose mental impairment rendered them unable to manage their affairs. It was not unusual for family members to initiate commitment for a relative who might make imprudent business decisions.

Although asylums were used for custodial purposes and did not offer formal interventions, other than seclusion and restraints for unruly or assaultive patients, they were usually motivated by kindness rather than punishment. Patients were placed in mental institutions in the hope that their care and the environment would produce recovery. Patients were detained as

long as necessary; however, as many as half recovered and were discharged within 12 months of admission.

In the late nineteenth century, the patient population in mental institutions grew enormously. Overcrowding and understaffing led to a loss of individual attention, more mixing of mentally ill criminals with those who were not criminals, and poor physical conditions. In addition, former patients, most notably Mrs. E. P. W. Packard, and reformers, most notably Dorothea Lynde Dix, wrote exposés about mental institutions and the loss of liberty and property and the lack of formal guidelines justifying commitment and ensuring due process rights. At the same time, the field of psychiatry emerged and some of its leaders called for a change in the commitment process and in the purpose of hospitalization. Consequently, mental institutions changed from custodial facilities to treatment facilities. In addition, laws affecting the rights of the mentally impaired were enacted.

In 1873, Isaac Ray, a patriarch of American psychiatry, petitioned the Pennsylvania legislature to establish separate institutions for mentally impaired individuals who committed crimes and for those who had not. He believed that people whose mental illness caused them to commit criminal acts should not be hospitalized in civil mental institutions because these patients were difficult to treat and would adversely affect the other patients. This distinction between criminal and noncriminal mentally impaired is the basis of the two types of individuals who are committed to mental institutions: those who are not involved in the criminal justice system (civil commitment patients) and those who are (mentally disordered offenders).

II. CIVIL COMMITMENT

Treatment in a psychiatric hospital may be categorized legally as voluntary or involuntary. Voluntary patients are those who seek psychiatric treatment and consent to obtaining it in mental institutions. They retain the right to accept or reject treatment, as well as to leave the hospital without legal constraints. Although the patient has these rights, many psychiatric hospitals do not admit voluntary patients unless the individual is willing to accept the treatment provided and not request discharge before a specified period of time deemed necessary for adequate treatment. While voluntary patients make up the majority of those in psychiatric hospitals today, with approximately 70% of patients in public mental institutions voluntarily admitted, this is a relatively recent occurrence. Civil commitment historically and legally involved involuntary psychiatric commitment.

There were no statutes in colonial times governing placement in asylums for the mentally impaired. The justification for institutionalizing these individuals was a belief that they required it but were so impaired as to not realize this and voluntarily seek treatment. Family or friends usually initiated the commitment, which was readily accepted by the hospital staff. Medical personnel authorized the admission of the patients, as well as their discharge. There were no formal procedures to safeguard the rights and liberty interests of the mentally impaired. These circumstances were true for both private and public mental institutions. The rationale offered for involuntary commitment to mental institutions was based on two doctrines of law: *parens patriae* power and police power.

Parens patriae, literally "father of the country," was originally used by sovereigns, who had the power and duty to protect the interests of their subjects. With the formation of democracies, *parens patriae* referred to the authority of the state to act on behalf of those citizens who were unable to provide for their own best interests and care, such as the mentally and physically impaired, the elderly, and minors without guardians. These people were deemed incapable of making sound decisions on their own behalf, so their consent to the state's intrusion in their lives was not considered necessary. The fear that the government's actions might be viewed as coercive in cases where the individual refused interventions obligated the state to justify its actions.

Police power refers to the state's responsibility to protect its citizens' welfare and safety. While *parens patriae* power is directed toward protecting the individual, police power is directed toward protecting society. Police power is implemented when the state acts on an individual who is dangerous or who poses a threat of harm to others.

The rationales justifying commitment to mental institutions based on *parens patriae* power and police power were articulated in statutes and court decisions. In 1842, laws in New York authorized the state to confine immediately "all lunatics, not only the dangerous ones." Laws allowed the commitment of the mentally ill so that they "might be cured of their disease."

An 1845 Massachusetts case illustrates the justification for institutionalizing a 67-year-old man. Josiah Oakes' family confined him in McLean Asylum because he had a "hallucination of mind," did not act as one would upon the death of a spouse, and became engaged to a young woman of questionable character a few days after his wife's death. Mr. Oakes contested his involuntary detention; however, the Massachusetts Supreme Court held that the "right to restrain an insane person of his liberty is found in the great law of humanity, which makes it necessary to confine those whose going at large would be dangerous to themselves or others." Moreover, the court opined that, "The restraint shall last . . . until he experiences relief from the present disease of mind."

As these statutes were enacted and court cases decided, reformers were crusading to change commitment laws. In 1860, Mrs. E. P. W. Packard was institutionalized in the Illinois State Hospital for 3 years based on her husband's petition. At the time, the law allowed married women and children to be confined at their husband's or father's request, without the evidence of mental impairment necessary in other cases. Upon Mrs. Packard's discharge, she and social reformers like Dorothea Lynde Dix exposed the conditions under which the mentally impaired were confined, which led to the gradual enactment of judicial procedures for guarding against wrongful commitments and protecting the patient's liberty interest. These procedures included questioning the inviolability of the medical staff in admission and discharge decisions; specifying commitment criteria more clearly; objecting to the use of certain treatment interventions, such as electroshock therapy and psychosurgery; challenging indefinite periods of hospitalization; and granting patients due process rights, including the right to hearings, the right to present evidence, the right to legal counsel, and the right to treatment offered through least restrictive alternatives.

When changes were made in the commitment laws, they were directed more toward *parens patriae* and police power issues than toward individual liberty interest issues, until the 1960s and 1970s. Civil commitment laws for the mentally impaired changed dramatically as a result of the civil rights movement, the emergence of psychiatric medications to treat the mentally impaired, and the medical professions' self-criticism toward treating involuntary patients. During this time, the state's power to commit mentally impaired persons against their will was narrowed, with a contemporaneous broadening of patients' rights.

One of the first limitations imposed judicially was the doctrine of least restrictive alternative, applied to involuntary psychiatric hospitalization. In the District of Columbia case, Lake v. Cameron (1966), the court's decision directed that it be determined whether there were alternative courses of treatment other than hospitalization. Only if less restrictive alternatives, such as outpatient treatment or placement in a halfway house or residential care facility, were unavailable or insufficient to meet the individual's treatment needs, could psychiatric hospitalization be considered. Another landmark case challenged the civil commitment process in Wisconsin. In Lessard v. Schmidt (1972), the District Court held that Wisconsin's civil commitment procedures were constitutionally defective. The decision established a number of necessary procedures. Among them were the patient's right to a jury trial, to a full hearing on the necessity for commitment when the detention period was longer than 2 weeks, and to representation by counsel. In California, as a result of the legislature's distrust of the decision-making process in civil commitment, a new set of statutes was enacted in 1969 to end "inappropriate, indefinite involuntary civil commitments." The laws in California were a model for other states because they clearly delineated the purpose and intent of involuntary hospitalization as well as the procedures that must be followed "to safeguard individual rights through judicial review" and "to guarantee and protect public safety."

During the 1970s, the individual liberty interests of patients extended beyond issues related to confinement and judicial review to those involving the "right to treatment." In Wyatt v. Stickney (1971), the District Court held that involuntarily committed patients "unquestionably have a constitutional right to receive such treatment as will give each of them a realistic opportunity to be cured or to improve his or her mental condition." The court found that the patients at an Alabama mental institution were being denied their right to treatment. Consequently, the court mandated that all Alabama state hospitals implement minimum constitutional standards for adequate treatment; these standards were appended to the decision. The constitutional right to treatment, designed to help involuntarily committed mental patients improve their mental

condition or be cured, was again upheld in 1974 in a District Court case in Florida (Donaldson v. O'Connor). Beginning in the early 1980s, the patient's "right to refuse treatment" was upheld by the courts. In Rennie v. Klein (1983), the U.S. Court of Appeals held that involuntarily committed patients have a right to refuse antipsychotic drugs and that administration of such drugs against the patient's will should follow "accepted professional judgement." In the case of Rogers v. Commissioner of the Department of Mental Health et al. (1983), the Massachusetts Supreme Court stated that the involuntary commitment of mental patients was not determinative of their competence to make treatment decisions; if they were found incompetent judicially, the judge would approve the treatment plan. However, patients who insist on exercising the right to refuse treatment may subject themselves to prolonged institutionalization.

With the advent of case law and legislation balancing the rights of society against those of the individual, involuntary civil commitment now fulfills a multipurpose role. It provides a means by which mentally impaired persons can be treated in a safe and therapeutic environment while being protected from inappropriate detention. Moreover, it is also a means by which the community can be protected from a mentally impaired individual's conduct before the person commits a dangerous act.

Those who remain subject to involuntary civil commitment today are the mentally impaired. They include the mentally ill and the mentally retarded. However, the mentally retarded are frequently treated separately from the mentally ill, and the commitment procedures may also differ. Moreover, states may permit the involuntary commitment of alcohol and drug abuse disordered individuals. As before, the doctrines of *parens patriae* and police power continue to govern the criteria under which an individual is committed involuntarily to psychiatric hospitals, that is, persons who have a mental disorder that causes them to be a danger to themselves or others, or causes them to be gravely disabled. Some states require an actual showing that the individual performed an act demonstrating their dangerousness; others require only a "likelihood." Some states allow commitment for mentally disordered individuals who present a danger to property. The terms "gravely disabled" or "inability to care for self" usually refer to mentally disordered persons who, because of their mental impairment, cannot provide for their own basic needs such as food, clothing, or shelter.

Involuntary civil commitment is still usually initiated by family members or friends of mentally impaired individuals; however, all states permit peace officers to petition for commitment. The hospital staff is responsible for determining whether the individual meets admission criteria. There are distinct phases for involuntary psychiatric hospitalization. The first phase is usually called emergency detention and is designed to deal with urgent situations. Depending on the length of time allowed for this initial phase, some states require that the individual be observed and treated so that they are no longer a danger to self, a danger to others, or gravely disabled. The length of an emergency detention or an initial observation and treatment period ranges from 24 hours to 15 days. If the initial commitment period is longer than a few days, most states have statutes that allow for independent review by officials other than the hospital staff to determine whether the patient continues to meet the commitment criteria. If the patient is not discharged during this period, there is a second, more lengthy, observation and treatment period. For nearly all states, it ranges from 3 days to 6 months. The hospital has the responsibility to file a renewal of the patient's commitment with the court. Judicial review of this commitment phase is either automatic or the patient is informed of the right to an independent review by a judge or, in some cases, a jury. Again, if the patient is not discharged during this second phase, an extended commitment period is available. Usually, if the person is gravely disabled, someone (relative, friend, or public guardian) is judicially appointed to act as the patient's conservator, which may hasten the patient's discharge from the hospital into a less restrictive alternative. The extended commitment term requires an independent hearing as well as periodic review of the patient's need for involuntary commitment. In some states, the extended commitment term may last up to 1 year and can be renewed. As the patient enters progressively longer periods of institutionalization, the criteria become more stringent and the burden of proof necessary for supporting continued involuntary commitment increases.

The legal guidelines imposed on civil commitment and the granting of due process rights to the mentally impaired have greatly reduced the number of involuntary commitments. In 1956, more than 550,000 patients occupied state hospital beds in the United States (333 beds per 100,000 population); today, there are fewer than 100,000 (fewer than 40 beds per 100,000 population). It can be argued that these low numbers also reflect the impact of the medical profession on treating involuntary psychiatric patients in mental institutions, namely, the development of antipsychotic and antidepressant medications, which allow for treatment in less restrictive settings, and the profession's protest about its lack of expertise and accuracy in predicting an individual's dangerousness. Moreover, during the 1960s, the movement toward deinstitutionalization and the establishment of community mental health centers reduced the number of involuntarily hospitalized patients as well as their length of stay.

Although community mental health treatment was intended to provide an alternative to hospital treatment, it never reached its goal. Financial resources were scarce and mental health care was not a high priority. There was much public resistance to the treatment of mentally impaired individuals in the community. Deinstitutionalization and the lack of appropriate treatment or housing for mentally disordered people led in some cases to a worsening of an individual's mental condition such that he or she acted out and was arrested. Those who might have formerly received services through the civil mental health system were now offenders and placed in mental institutions through the criminal justice system. [See MENTAL HOSPITALS AND DEINSTITUTIONALIZATION.]

States vary in the care and treatment facilities offered a mentally disordered offender. The mentally disordered offender may be sent to a local psychiatric hospital, a regional hospital in the state, or a centralized forensic facility. The psychiatric hospital may allocate only one or a few wards for legally committed patients, or the entire hospital may be designated as a forensic institution. The freedom of movement allowed patients differs among institutions and is based on security and treatment needs as well as the length of time a patient remains in the institution. Some provide only short-term treatment or diagnostic services; others are designed to treat long-term and difficult patients. Some mental institutions admit both civil and criminal psychiatric patients, whereas others admit only civil or only criminal patients. The mental institutions are usually funded and operated by the county or state departments of mental health or hygiene or human services. Institutional services include treatment and periodic court evaluations of certain offender populations, for example, persons incompetent to stand trial, insanity acquittees, and sexual psychopaths. In some states, hospitals provide pretrial and presentencing evaluations for attorneys and courts. The purpose of forensic mental institutions is not to deliver punishment, but to provide a secure setting for mentally disordered offenders who are dangerous and in need of treatment that would reduce their threat of recidivism.

III. COMPETENCY TO STAND TRIAL

Competency to stand trial was formulated in England. English common law tradition not only prohibited the criminal prosecution of defendants who were physically absent during the trial, but also those who were "mentally absent." This arose from the fundamental principle that individuals charged with a criminal offense are entitled to a fair trial and to fulfill their role as a defendant. Prosecuting, convicting, and sentencing individuals who are unaware of what is happening to them or who are unable to participate in the trial process would appear unjust and unseemly. The model for the current standard of competency to stand trial was developed in England in the early nineteenth century. It defined competency as the ability to understand the nature and purpose of the proceedings taken against the defendant, as well as the defendant's ability to assist counsel in presenting a defense. This standard continues to be used in England and other countries, including Canada and the United States. In Dusky v. United States (1960), the United States Supreme Court clarified and unified across states the criteria for competency: "the 'test must be whether he [the defendant] has sufficient present ability to consult with his lawyer with a reasonable degree of rational understanding— and whether he has a rational as well as factual understanding of the proceedings taken against him.'" Although this case did not specify that a defendant's inability rationally to understand, communicate, or make decisions about the legal proceedings was limited to mental conditions that cause such impairment, most states require a mental disease or defect.

An inquiry about the defendant's competency to stand trial may be brought up at any point during the legal proceeding: pretrial, during the trial, and, if convicted, at the time of sentencing. The question of competency may be raised by the judge or the prosecuting attorney; the majority are raised by defense counsel. A 1992 study by Miller and Kaplan found that the majority of cases with a question of competency were in situations where the defendants' mental disorder caused significant difficulty in communication between them and their attorney. If doubt is raised about the defendant's competency to stand trial, the trial proceeding stops and a mental examination must be performed by a psychiatrist or psychologist.

Competency evaluations are usually conducted in forensic mental institutions, where the defendant is committed for examination and observation for a period of time (usually 30 to 90 days); however, many states have the resources to provide competency evaluations while the defendant is in jail or at liberty in the community. Placement in a forensic institution has the advantage of having defendants observed by trained staff for a reasonable length of time in order to rule out malingering. It also exposes the defendants to measures, such as individual and group meetings simulating courtroom procedures and stresses, that test their capacity to meet the competency criteria. Finally, psychiatric hospitalization permits the treatment of mentally ill defendants.

Approximately 1 in 15 criminal defendants is referred for a competency evaluation, and about 25 to 30% of them are found incompetent to stand trial. These individuals are usually diagnosed as psychotic and have few social and economic resources. Most have never been married and a high proportion do not have steady employment. In addition, a large percentage have previous arrests and psychiatric hospitalizations. Although mental retardation may contribute to an individual's incompetency to stand trial, few mentally retarded defendants are found incompetent and, thus, their legal proceedings continue.

When defendants are found incompetent to stand trial through a judicial hearing, the legal proceedings are interrupted until competency is restored. If and when the defendant regains competency, the trial resumes at the point where it stopped. Defendants who are declared incompetent are, in almost all cases, ordered to undergo treatment in a maximum security hospital. Until the landmark Supreme Court case of Jackson v. Indiana (1972), the incompetent defendant's length of hospitalization was indefinite. Defendants remained hospitalized until their condition improved; for some, this could amount to a life sentence even if charged with a minor infraction. Theon Jackson was a 27-year-old mentally defective, illiterate, deaf mute who was charged with two separate robberies of women, consisting of a purse and $9 in contents. The doctor's opinion was that Mr. Jackson's condition "precluded his understanding of the nature of the charges against him or participating in his defense" and that his prognosis was "rather dim" in that his intelligence "was not sufficient to enable him ever to develop the necessary communication skills." It was argued that Mr. Jackson's commitment was "tantamount to a 'life sentence' without his having been convicted of a crime." The Supreme Court decided that "a defendant cannot be held more than the reasonable period of time necessary to determine whether there is a substantial probability that he will attain competency in the foreseeable future. If it is determined that he will not, the State must either institute civil proceedings applicable to indefinite commitment of those not charged with crime, or release the defendant." Although the court did not state what a "reasonable period of time" was, this opinion prompted many states to revise the length of commitment for mental incompetents. Most states now limit the period of treatment for restoration to competency to the maximum sentence the individual would receive if convicted of the crime charged. In some states, the maximum term of commitment is the maximum sentence for the crime or a specific number of years (e.g., 1, 2, or 3), whichever is less. In states with a definite period of commitment, there is usually a provision for continued institutionalization through civil commitment. This can be used for persons who have not regained their competency at the conclusion of the commitment term and who meet civil commitment criteria. Whether the individual's criminal charges are dismissed when they are civilly committed varies among the states. Most persons found incompetent to stand trial, in fact, are restored to competency within a short period of time, usually less than 90 days, through treatment interventions.

When a defendant is committed to a forensic mental institution as incompetent to stand trial, the purpose of the commitment is to treat the individual to restore competency. Most people are declared incompetent because of a severe mental illness; consequently, psychiatric medication is the most common

form of treatment. Some courts have addressed the issue of "forced medication for competency purposes." Does the incompetent defendant have a right to refuse antipsychotic medication and perhaps remain incompetent indefinitely? In U.S.v. Charters (1988), the Federal Court of Appeals opined that incompetent defendants could be medicated against their will at the discretion of medical personnel if a judicial review was available. The U.S. Supreme Court in Riggins v. Nevada (1992) held that for nonconsenting persons, the state would have to demonstrate an overriding justification for the medication, as well as demonstrate that no less intrusive alternative was available.

Medication is not the only form of treatment, particularly for defendants whose incompetency is the result of mental retardation or other cognitive disorders. Educational programs, exercises, and therapy are additional approaches designed to address psychological and behavioral factors, such as perceptual and thought disturbances, delusions, hyperactivity, belligerence, slow or concrete thinking, attention deficit problems, and memory impairment, related to the defendant's incompetency. Videotapes, problem-solving group sessions, simulated courtroom proceedings, role-playing, group instruction, stress management, and individual and group therapy are techniques used to expose, teach, and enhance the patients' abilities in relevant competency issues, such as the roles and functions of courtroom personnel, various pleas and their consequences, the defendant's criminal charges and possible sentence, the sequence of events in a trial, appropriate courtroom decorum, and active participation with their attorney.

Within the criminal justice system, competency to stand trial is the question most frequently posed to mental health professionals. Persons examined for competency and those declared incompetent make up the largest category of forensic patients in mental institutions. The most publicized forensic population, however, consists of those who are found "not guilty by reason of insanity."

IV. NOT GUILTY BY REASON OF INSANITY (NGRI)

Although the insanity defense is one of the most controversial areas in forensic mental health, it is fraught with misconceptions. The insanity defense is not used exclusively in serious felony cases, but is used in less serious charges as well; however, violent or potentially violent crimes constitute the majority of charges for which this defense is invoked. The rate the insanity defense is raised and the rate it is successful vary widely among the states. A 1991, eight-state study by Callahan et al. reports that felony cases in which the defense was raised ranged from 0.3 to 5.7%; of these cases, defense success ranged from 7.3 to 87%. It is most often accepted through plea bargaining between the prosecuting and defense attorneys without going to trial. Many insanity acquittees have a history of psychiatric hospitalization. While the majority of insanity acquittees are extremely disturbed and suffer from schizophrenia or other psychoses, or from mood disorders, there are some cases where the individual has only a personality disorder. Finally, persons found not guilty by reason of insanity (NGRI) are usually hospitalized as long as, if not longer, than the period of time they would have served had they been convicted and sentenced. Although the insanity defense has aroused much mistrust and disapproval because of political, social, and legal factors related to its application, it has a lengthy history and purpose within the criminal justice system.

The insanity defense dates to the ancient Hebrews, who believed that certain people should not be held criminally responsible for their acts, namely, children and insane persons. This exculpation of criminal responsibility was based on the belief that people who committed criminal acts intentionally should be distinguished from those whose acts were unintentional. The ancient Greeks recognized that conduct based on ignorance and compulsion was less blameworthy than conduct based on free will. If punishment is to be perceived as just, and is to be a deterrent, a distinction must be made between people who are capable of free and rational choice of behavior and those who are incapable of conforming or of comprehending their actions.

The elements essential for holding persons criminally responsible for their acts require proving that the individual not only committed the illegal act but that they did so with *mens rea*. *Mens rea*, literally "guilty mind," has been interpreted as a person who commits an act with criminal intent. In twelfth century England, the insanity defense was established in common law; if successful, it resulted in complete acquittal. In 1265, the jurist Henry de Bracton defined an insane person as "one who does not know what he is

doing, who lacks in mind and reason and is not far removed from the brutes." In 1724, the English judge Robert Tracy expanded on de Bracton's definition, holding that not all madmen should be considered insane, only those who are "totally deprived of understanding and memory, and doth not know what he is doing, no more than an infant, than a brute, or a wild beast." The insanity defense was extended further to include persons harboring delusions. In 1800, James Hadfield was acquitted by reason of insanity when he attempted to assassinate King George III because of a delusion that Hadfield himself was destined to attain a martyr's death.

In 1843, a standard for insanity was created in English law that continues to be the test in many countries to this day. Daniel M'Naghten, a Scottish woodturner, attempted to assassinate Sir Robert Peel, the prime minister of England, because of persecutory delusions. However, M'Naghten mistook Edward Drummond, the prime minister's secretary, for Peel and killed him instead. A jury acquitted M'Naghten by reason of insanity, but an outraged Queen Victoria and public demanded that the defense of insanity be more clearly defined, along with the specific circumstances in which it would apply. An assembly of common law judges determined that for a person to be found NGRI, the defendant must be "laboring under such a defect of reason, from disease of mind, as not to know the nature and quality of the act he was doing; or if he did know it, that he did not know he was doing what was wrong."

The M'Naghten standard or its modified form was the predominant test for insanity in the United States until the appearance of the American Law Institute's (ALI) rule that was drafted in 1955 and adopted in 1962. This test was developed in an effort to acknowledge that exculpation for criminal behavior should not be based on the impairment of cognitive processes alone, that is, an inability to understand the nature and quality of one's acts or understand its wrongfulness. The ALI standard recognized that a person's illegal behavior may be the product of either a cognitive disturbance or a behavioral one. It stated that a person is NGRI if "as a result of mental disease or defect he lacks substantial capacity either to appreciate the criminality [wrongfulness] of his conduct or to conform his conduct to the requirements of the law." It further recommended that the mental disease or defect not "include an abnormality manifested only by repeated criminal or otherwise anti-social conduct." Currently, the M'Naghten rule or a modification of it is used in slightly more than half the states in the United States, three states (Idaho, Montana, and Utah) have no insanity standard, and the rest use the ALI test or a variation of it. The three states without a specific insanity standard nevertheless accept that mentally ill persons who commit a crime but who do not have *mens rea* should be treated and not punished.

Defendants who raise an insanity defense are examined by mental health professionals who opine whether the person meets the insanity standard. In some states, this examination is conducted in mental institutions. The examination is a retrospective analysis of the defendant's state of mind when the crime was allegedly committed, in contrast to the incompetency to stand trial examination, which is an examination of the defendant's current mental condition. These opinions regarding the defendant's sanity may then be used for plea bargaining or may be submitted at trial.

Before the 1800 Hadfield case, defendants who were found NGRI were acquitted and released back into the community. Within a month of Hadfield's trial, however, England passed the Criminal Lunatic's Act of 1800, by which all persons found NGRI were "to be kept in strict custody, until his Majesty's pleasure be known." Most of those were detained in jail until 1814, when separate facilities were constructed in the Hospital of St. Mary of Bethlehem ("Bedlam"). In the United States, acquittees found NGRI were also detained in asylums or prisons for "safekeeping." Today, while insanity acquittees are not committed to correctional facilities, the commitment laws vary among the states. Some provide for outright acquittal and release with no social control, such as conditions of probation or mandatory outpatient treatment. The majority require a hearing shortly after the person is found NGRI to determine whether the individual should be committed to a mental institution. Commitment is based either on that state's civil commitment criteria or on some form of dangerousness (to self, others, or property). Once an individual is committed to a mental institution as an insanity acquittee, the commitment is periodically reviewed judicially. The length of hospitalization differs among jurisdictions. In some states, it is definite and no longer than the maximum period of time the individual would have served for the crime if found guilty; in other states, it is indefinite. There are two standards by which an insanity acquittee may be discharged from a psychiatric hospital: either the insanity acquittee is no longer mentally ill, or the insanity acquittee is no longer mentally ill and dangerous. In those states that have definite commitment terms, the acquittee's commitment may be extended beyond the maximum period if the individual meets civil commitment criteria or continues to be mentally ill and dangerous. Both discharge and commitment extensions are accomplished by judicial hearings.

The emphasis on the insanity acquittee's mental illness and dangerousness illustrates society's response to such individuals. Although society may not hold the individuals criminally responsible for their illegal act, the community wants to protect itself from these disordered persons. This can be accomplished by treating and protecting mentally impaired people, and by isolating them from the public until they are judged safe. In this context, forensic mental institutions do not exist for punishment but for "therapeutic restraint." The treatment for insanity acquittees is directed toward their mental impairment in order to reduce their threat of illness-related dangerousness. Psychiatric medications, drug and alcohol rehabilitation programs, and individual and group psychotherapy are the predominant forms of treatment. In addition, skills necessary for successful adjustment to living in the community are emphasized while the person is hospitalized. Although many insanity acquittees are released into the community with no further social control, many states have provisions for conditional discharge. In conditional discharge, the insanity acquittee is perceived as sufficiently nondangerous as long as he or she is under treatment and supervision in the community, usually through mental health programs; if there is any noncompliance or significant decompensation, the insanity acquittee is returned to the forensic institution.

The use of mental institutions for the dual purposes of treating mentally disordered offenders who are dangerous and protecting society from future criminal acts by these individuals is demonstrated not only by commitment laws related to insanity acquittees but to other offenders as well, such as those who are found "guilty but mentally ill," sexual psychopaths, and mentally ill prisoners.

V. GUILTY BUT MENTALLY ILL (GBMI)

As stated earlier, the insanity defense provokes a great deal of public outrage and frustration because of the belief that there are too many insanity acquittees and that their confinements are too short. In response,

Michigan introduced a new defense in 1975: guilty but mentally ill (GBMI). The goals of the defense were to decrease the number of persons found NGRI and to recognize a defendant's mental impairment but still theoretically hold him or her criminally responsible. Through these goals, society would be protected and treatment could be available for mentally disordered offenders. After John Hinckley was acquitted by reason of insanity of the attempted assassination of President Reagan in 1981, other states either modified their insanity standard or introduced the GBMI plea. There are 13 states that have GBMI pleas. In addition to the GBMI plea, the NGRI plea is also available to a mentally impaired defendant; thus, the GBMI plea is a supplement to, and not a substitute for, the insanity defense.

The GBMI standard is that the defendant is guilty of the crime and was not insane at the time of committing the offense but was suffering from mental illness or mental retardation. If the defendant is found guilty, a hearing is conducted to determine whether the defendant was insane or GBMI during the commission of the crime. States vary as to what happens to those found GBMI. In some states, the GBMI individual is confined to the Department of Corrections and evaluated for treatment, which might be provided in a prison setting. In other states, the GBMI individual is evaluated by corrections personnel, but then transferred to a mental institution for treatment. In still other states, the GBMI individual is committed directly to the Department of Public Health/Mental Health and evaluated and treated in a mental institution. Not all states provide for mental health treatment for GBMI individuals; they are treated like other prisoners and are only evaluated by corrections personnel if their mental impairment becomes problematic while imprisoned. For those states providing treatment in correctional settings or mental institutions, the GBMI are often treated until they are no longer mentally impaired and dangerous to others or self. When they do not require further treatment, they are returned to the general prison population or transferred to prison to serve the remainder of their sentence.

Despite the hope that the GBMI verdict would resolve problems created by the insanity defense, this has not occurred. The number of insanity verdicts has not declined markedly, nor have many individuals been provided any special treatment to address their mental impairment and dangerousness different from what any other mentally disordered offender in prison would have received.

VI. SEXUAL PSYCHOPATH LAWS

Offenders who commit sex crimes comprise another category that may receive treatment in mental institutions. In 1937, Michigan was the first state to enact sexual psychopath laws; California followed in 1939. By 1972, 25 states had sexual psychopath laws. Specific laws for sex offenders often arose from a publicized case that outraged the community, which then demanded special approaches for dealing with such offenders. In addition, mental health professionals claimed the high recidivism rate in sex offenders could be reduced if they were provided with treatment. Thus, the purpose of these laws was to treat mentally disordered sex offenders in special treatment programs until they were no longer believed to be a danger to others. Because of treated sex offenders who re-offended, limited financial resources for specialized treatment programs, and the mental health professions' disillusionment with treatment outcomes, many states repealed their sexual psychopath laws. Ten states continue to distinguish sex offenders from other types of offenders.

In states that retained sexual psychopath statutes, the laws generally apply to persons who commit a sex offense involving force or violence, primarily child molestation and rape, and who are unable to control their sexual impulses, as characterized by repetitive or compulsive behavior. The laws may state that the offender suffers from a mental disorder that predisposes the individual to commit such crimes and to be dangerous. In cases where a defendant is found guilty of a sex crime and meets the statutory criteria for a sexual psychopath, his or her sentence will involve treatment. Treatment may be administered in a correctional facility; however, in most states, mentally disordered sex offenders are committed to a mental institution where they remain until no longer sexually dangerous, and then they are either released into the community or transferred to a correctional facility to complete their prison term. A few states permit indefinite treatment in a psychiatric hospital, justified by the goals of care and treatment, rather than punishment. There are periodic judicial reviews for sex offenders committed to forensic mental institutions.

The more common psychiatric diagnoses of individuals committed as sexual psychopaths are psychotic and mood disorders, mental retardation, substance abuse, sexual disorders, and personality disorders. Treatment interventions consist of medication for the mental illness or to inhibit sexual arousal and drive; individual, group, and family psychotherapy addressing the patient's psychological problems; alcohol and drug rehabilitation programs; stress and anger management; social skills training; sex education and human sexuality classes; and behavior modification aimed at changing deviant sexual arousal patterns. Despite intensive efforts to modify and redirect the patient's inappropriate sexual behavior, the nature of a forensic mental institution limits the conclusions mental health professionals can draw about a patient's successful response to treatment. Mental institutions are usually maximum security facilities, where there is little opportunity to observe and test the patient in a setting resembling the community. Therefore, many mental institutions include long-term programs of careful monitoring and supervision as the patient is gradually reintroduced to the community. [*See* Substance Abuse; Mental Retardation and Mental Health; Mood Disorders.]

VIII. MENTALLY IMPAIRED PRISONERS

Studies in various countries have found that many mentally impaired individuals are sent to prison. In Scotland, almost one half of the prison population could be considered psychiatrically abnormal, and in England, approximately one third of the men in prison are regarded as in need of psychiatric treatment. Canada, Australia, and New Zealand also have a large proportion of prisoners who are mentally disordered. In the United States, rates range from 10% for mentally retarded persons and 14% for psychotic individuals to 50% for prisoners with behavioral disorders. Correctional institutions must address the needs of this special population to maintain order, security, and safety for all inmates, as well as to assure mentally impaired prisoners their eighth amendment right to reasonable care and treatment.

States vary as to the site for psychiatric care provided inmates. In some states, convicted felons are evaluated and treated by mental health professionals within the correctional system. They are treated as outpatients who live in the general prison population

and see a mental health professional regularly, or they live in a hospital ward inside the prison, or they are sent to a hospital operated by the Department of Corrections. In other states, they are evaluated by the correctional staff, but transferred for treatment to a mental institution operated by the Department of Mental Health/Human Services. There are neither general rules regarding the length of time a prisoner may be hospitalized nor rules about whether prisoners transferred to mental institutions are returned to prison or placed on parole after receiving treatment. These decisions are based on state laws and the length of time the prisoner has thus far served. Treatment is provided either on a voluntary or involuntary basis. In Washington v. Harper (1990), the U.S. Supreme Court held that treatment may be imposed on a prisoner against his or her will if the prisoner was "dangerous to himself or others and treatment was in the prisoner's medical interest." In addition to addressing the prisoner's dangerousness, another purpose of psychiatric hospitalization for inmates is to reduce their psychiatric symptoms and stabilize them so that they may be returned to the general prison population. Psychiatric medication and the therapeutic structure of hospitalization are the most common forms of treatment.

There are some states that permit confinement beyond the prisoner's sentence if the individual was convicted of a violent offense, suffers from a mental disorder that was related to the commission of the crime, and is not in remission at the time of parole or expiration of their prison term. In such cases, the "violent mentally disordered offender" or the "sexually violent predator" is usually sent to a mental institution for treatment until the mental disorder is in remission and the individual no longer poses a substantial danger of physical harm to others.

Although all states are obligated to evaluate mentally disordered prisoners to determine whether they require psychiatric treatment, few prisoners actually receive the treatment they need. There are many reasons for this; however, a primary factor is limited availability of resources. [*See* Criminal Behavior.]

VIII. TREATMENT FOR LEGALLY COMMITTED PATIENTS

Mental institutions that treat legally committed patients usually differ from psychiatric hospitals treating voluntary patients. They tend to be more secure facilities, because of issues of custody and elopement. In addition, they are staffed by professionals who know the laws pertaining to mental health commitments. The staff-to-patient ratio for institutions that treat mentally disordered offenders is usually larger than that found in other psychiatric hospitals. The treatment staff tends to include physicians, psychiatrists, psychologists, social workers, nurses, and rehabilitation/occupational therapists. Students in medicine and mental health-related fields are frequently involved in providing services if a school or university is affiliated.

Except for those committed as incompetent to stand trial, the goals for all patients in forensic mental institutions can be summarized as increasing self-esteem, responsibility, and independence; reducing maladaptive and dangerous behavior; improving communication skills and interpersonal functioning; recognizing warning signs of decompensation; and learning coping mechanisms and strategies. Treatment goals for those committed as incompetent to stand trial are restoring and stabilizing them to a level of rational psychological function such that they may be able to understand the legal proceedings and cooperate with their counsel.

There are many treatment modalities directed toward these goals. The treatment administered depends on the nature of the disorder; psychiatric medication is one of the most common treatments. Medication is used for persons suffering from mental and emotional disorders as well as for persons who demonstrate violent, aggressive, or self-injurious behavior.

Individual and group therapy are other frequently reported interventions. Individual and group therapy can provide support, insight, socialization, and education. The particularly therapy used depends on the patient's mental condition, for example, insight-oriented therapy for less impaired individuals, reality-supportive therapy for more impaired individuals. A patient's treatment may include special groups such as anger management, social skills development, assertiveness training, sexual dysfunction, sex education, relaxation training, and substance abuse. Narcotics Anonymous and Alcoholics Anonymous usually hold regular meetings in mental institutions. Behavior modification programs are also effective. These programs can be designed for mentally retarded patients, persons with aggressive or violent behavior, and individuals who have deviant sexual arousal. For example, biofeedback

is an effective technique in changing sexual arousal patterns. Family therapy may also be part of the treatment plan. If the family is able and willing to be involved, treatment may focus on dysfunctional patterns among family relationships in an attempt to correct them. In addition, family therapy may provide family members with insight and instruction to help the patient make a satisfactory adjustment when released from the mental institution.

A group intervention that is useful for the highly impaired mentally ill and mentally retarded patient is one that targets problems of daily living. In these groups, the staff helps the patients develop or improve skills that are necessary for meeting everyday challenges, such as personal hygiene, communication, food preparation, handling money, and use of transportation.

The hospital setting can also be therapeutic. The hospital ward provides structure, order, and rules for all patients. There are interactions among patients and between patients and staff, the early detection and amelioration of problems by trained professionals, and daily activities. Many psychiatric wards conduct "community meetings" or "ward government," where patients and staff discuss issues relevant to the ward and where patients are encouraged to perform some functions of self-government, such as determining the use of the television, selecting ward leaders who assist other patients, making work assignments, airing grievances, and planning parties.

Educational, occupational, and recreational activities are common services found in forensic mental institutions. These activities enhance patient self-esteem and independence, encourage economic security, address important areas of social interaction, provide acceptable outlets for stress or excess energy, and assist in making the successful transition from the institution to the community. Educational programs may include classes that prepare patients for a general education diploma (the equivalent of a high school diploma), college courses, or special interest classes. Occupational training develops job skills and good work habits and attitudes, practices meaningful work activities, and presents information on obtaining a job. Some patients are reinforced by payment for their work. Recreational programs may include team and individual activities, such as team sports, table games, and arts and crafts projects.

Other interventions used in forensic hospitals are seclusion and restraint. These are only warranted when patients are unmanageable and it is necessary to prevent them from harming themselves or others, or from causing substantial property damage. These methods are frequently the last resort for patients whose behavior cannot be managed by other means. The use of seclusion and restraint both require extensive documentation and monitoring.

Although these treatment interventions are appropriate for forensic patients, they are not always available. Moreover, many mentally disordered individuals in mental institutions do not receive a course of treatment that is sufficiently individualized for them. In some instances, the mental institutions do not properly differentiate mentally retarded patients from others; therefore, they are treated with methods designed for the mentally ill, which are not effective for them. There are some patients who are not amenable to treatment because of their motivational level, severity of mental disorder, or chronic behavioral management problem.

IX. DISCHARGE INTO THE COMMUNITY

The final consideration for mentally impaired patients who are hospitalized in forensic psychiatric hospitals is their discharge from the hospital into the community. Some patients may no longer require hospitalization but are not suitable for outpatient treatment. They may be placed in day-hospital treatment, where they spend their days in a treatment facility and their nights in the community.

Before discharge from a hospital, the clinician must consider the patient's readiness for return to the community. Variables clinicians should analyze include the patient's mental disorder, behavioral problems, medication compliance, treatment participation and attendance, awareness and acceptance of, and insight into their mental disorder, and the relationship between their disorder and their problematic behavior. It is likely that patients who have been committed to forensic hospitals will need further interventions when released to the community; therefore, additional factors to consider are the patient's acceptance of the need to continue treatment and comply with any imposed restrictions, awareness of warning signs and methods to avert decompensation, and ability to behave appropriately in a less structured setting.

It is very difficult to predict with confidence whether a patient will make a successful transition into the community based on their performance in the mental institution. Life in a psychiatric hospital is not an adequate simulation of life in society. The hospital's security, structure, supervision, and therapeutic orientation contribute to treating the patient, but they do not necessarily test patients for normal life situations. There should be a stage during treatment when the patient is resocialized to provide adequate training and assessment for community living. Some mental institutions have special wards devoted to these goals, or they place the patient in specialized transitional residential programs before complete discharge; some psychiatric hospitals use trial furloughs where the patient has an opportunity to live in the community without stringent supervision.

Many mentally disordered patients discharged from psychiatric hospitals require outpatient treatment and special living arrangements. It is imperative that those involved in the treatment services and living situations know about and are comfortable with this special population. They should understand and be experienced with the needs of these individuals and what they can do to help them live successfully in the community. Therapists should be aware of the patient's need for limit setting and treatment compliance, as well as the need to act swiftly at the first signs of a patient's decompensation. Therapists can also include the family in the patient's treatment to improve relationships among family members and the patient and to educate the family in more effective stabilization of the patient. Whoever provides the patient's housing should know the proper administration of the patient's medication, as well as provide adequate structure and supervision. Therapeutic activities that structure most of the patient's day are very helpful for the more mentally impaired individual.

Another important component of successful transition to and living in the community is case management. Each patient has a designated professional who is responsible for his or her overall care. The case manager formulates an individualized plan for the patient, which should include treatment, living situation, adequate funds, and vocational rehabilitation. Case managers monitor the patient's access to these resources, as well as progress and the need for any further services. An individual who is not only aware of the patient's adjustment in the community but who has knowledge of available resources and uses them on behalf of the patient is a significant factor in relapse prevention.

X. CONCLUSION

Many more people today are far less concerned with the mental health needs of others than in previous times. Some may argue that we have become more accepting of deviant behavior and respectful of individual liberty rights and are reluctant to impose treatment on those who refuse it. However, it is also true that society has remained just as concerned, if not more so, about the threat of violence and the need for protection from those who are dangerous. Although equating mental illness and mental retardation with dangerousness is an exaggeration, in fact, there are mentally impaired individuals who engage in aggressive behavior and who pose a threat of harm. Thus, although treatment resources may be diminishing for the psychiatric population in general, they are increasing for mentally disordered offender patients. The expanding use of mental institutions to treat legally committed patients is a reflection of society's values and needs. It is incumbent on mental health profes-

sionals to be proficient in understanding and treating this population, while balancing the rights of patients with those of society.

BIBLIOGRAPHY

Appelbaum, P. S., & Gutheil, T. G. (1991). *Clinical handbook of psychiatry and the law* (2nd ed.). Baltimore, MD: Williams & Wilkins.

Bartol, C. R., & Bartol, A. M. (1994). *Psychology and law* (2nd ed.). Pacific Grove, CA: Brooks/Cole.

Goldstein, A. S. (1980 reprint). *The insanity defense.* Westport, CT: Greenwood Press.

Heilbrun, K., Nunez, C. E., Deitchman, M. A., Gustafson, D., & Krull, K. (1992). The treatment of mentally disordered offenders: A national survey of psychiatrists. *Bulletin of the American Academy of Psychiatry and the Law, 20,* 475–480.

Poythress, N. G. (Ed.). (1993). Forensic treatment in the United States: A survey of selected forensic hospitals. *International Journal of Law and Psychiatry, 16,* 53–132.

Reisner, R. (1994). *Law and the mental health system: Civil and criminal aspects* (1995 Suppl.). St. Paul, MN: West.

Rosner, R. (Ed.). (1994). *Principles and practice of forensic psychiatry.* New York: Chapman & Hall.

Way, B. B., Dvoskin, J. A., & Steadman, H. J. (1991). Forensic psychiatric inpatients served in the United States: Regional and system differences. *Bulletin of the American Academy of Psychiatry and the Law, 19,* 405–412.

Mental Retardation and Mental Health

Sharon A. Borthwick-Duffy

University of California, Riverside

Adaptive Skills An array of age-appropriate behavioral competencies required to function in and adapt to the environments encountered in daily living.

Age-Appropriate Typical of one's chronological age peers.

Aversive Intervention Any intervention that is applied in a behavior-contingent manner with the expected effect that the future rate of the behavior will decline as the individual seeks to avoid the stimulus.

Diagnostic Overshadowing When the presence of mental retardation decreases the perceived significance of problem behavior and reduces the likelihood of the behavior being linked to a psychiatric disorder.

Dual Diagnosis Individuals who have both mental retardation and a psychiatric disorder.

Etiology Cause or causes of a given condition.

Maladaptive Behavior Observed problem behavior that may or may not be symptomatic of a psychiatric disorder.

Psychotropic Drug Any agent prescribed for the purpose of bringing about behavioral, cognitive, or emotional change.

Self-Injurious Behaviors Acts directed toward oneself that result in tissue damage.

Stereotyped Behaviors Self-stimulatory behaviors that are repetitious motor behaviors or action sequences that are not contingent on reinforcement and are considered pathological.

MENTAL RETARDATION is characterized by low intelligence and deficits in adaptive skills that are observed before the age of 18. The majority of people with mental retardation are mentally healthy and free of serious behavior problems, although the prevalence of psychiatric disorders is higher than in the general population. This entry discusses the factors that contribute to the risk of behavior problems and emotional disorders, as well as the assessment, treatment, and implications of mental health problems among persons with mental retardation.

I. DEFINITION OF MENTAL RETARDATION

According to the most recent (1992) definition of the American Association on Mental Retardation (AAMR), people with mental retardation are characterized by significantly subaverage intellectual functioning (IQs lower than 70 or 75) and by concurrent limitations in two or more adaptive skill areas. Mental retardation is defined as a fundamental difficulty in learning (intellect) and an ensuing difficulty in performing daily life skills (adaptation). Consistent with a developmental perspective, mental retardation is manifested before age 18. Although certain aspects of this new definition depart from previous conceptions of mental retardation, the dual criteria of low IQ and deficits in adaptive behavior have been critical elements of most definitions for many years. Defining mental retardation in terms of adaptive behavior deficits is especially important when considering the presence of co-occurring mental health problems. [*See* INTELLIGENCE AND MENTAL HEALTH.]

A. Evolution of the Definition of Mental Retardation

There has never been a universal consensus as to what mental retardation actually is. Moreover, at any time in history, the definition of mental retardation has reflected the current status of scientific knowledge and prevailing views on social issues related to mental retardation. From the turn of the century until the first formal AAMR definition in 1959, mental retardation was widely believed to be a biologically based condition of the central nervous system, existing from birth, that was incurable and probably irremediable. The 1959 AAMR definition was less restrictive, focusing on current functioning rather than constitutionality, and not explicitly stating that mental retardation was incurable.

The assumption of a theoretically normal distribution of intelligence suggests that most people will have IQs that are closer to the mean score of 100 (i.e., scores close to the cutoff) and that the number of people who are expected to have more severe forms of mental retardation decreases as IQs deviate farther from the mean. Thus, mild retardation comprises the largest group of people with mental retardation.

The arbitrariness of the concept of mental retardation is illustrated by the AAMR definitional change in 1973, which moved the upper IQ limit from approximately 85 (one standard deviation from the mean of 100) down to 70 (two standard deviations from the mean). With this change, approximately 13% of the population "lost" their potential membership in the mental retardation category. For individuals with severe forms of mental retardation, these definitional differences were irrelevant; they would probably have been identified no matter what definition was used. But, for those with IQs between about 70 and 85, who had been previously identified as having mental retardation, this decision changed their diagnosis.

Today, the majority of children with mild forms of retardation do not have known pathology (biologic origins). They are more likely to come from adverse economic and living situations that contain risk factors, such as poor nutrition, poor medical care, low motivation for personal achievement, and parents who have below average IQs. For some children, these factors will result in depressed intellectual functioning, poor development of adaptive skills, and a diagnosis of retardation.

Most formal organizations (e.g., American Psychiatric Association, World Health Organization, state and federal agencies) have historically used approximations of the AAMR definitions in their definitions or eligibility criteria for mental retardation. But because the 1992 AAMR definition and classification system is still rather new and has introduced some conceptual shifts, its long-term impact on the definitional criteria used by other organizations is unknown.

B. Sociological Perspective on Deviant Behavior and Mental Retardation

For those people whose IQs are close to the cutoff, adaptive functioning is the key determinant in their diagnosis. It is the lack of adaptive competence, rather than low IQ, that usually leads to referral for evaluation and diagnosis. Thus, many individuals with IQs below the cutoff will never be referred for evaluation if their levels of adaptive competence do not draw attention. The measurement of adaptive functioning is subjective, as it involves a determination of what constitutes "normal" or competent behavior within specific environments. From a sociological perspective, then, the values and expectations of each society determine how mental retardation is to be defined, that is, by identifying the types and degree of deviant behavior that is not tolerated. This suggests that a diagnosis of mental retardation is assigned when an individual with subaverage intelligence deviates too far from the behavior standards dictated by societal norms. Thus, two people with the same IQ score and the same repertoire of adaptive competencies could presumably end up with different diagnostic outcomes (with or without mental retardation) if their environments produce different demands and behavioral expectations.

C. Mental Retardation Distinguished from Mental Illness

In the earliest civilizations mental retardation was not differentiated from other handicapping conditions, and it was common for adults with mental retardation to be institutionalized with people with mental illness. Both groups were believed to be insensitive to cold, heat, hunger, and pain, thus justifying the harsh treatment they often received in their confinement. Later attempts to distinguish between mental retardation and mental illness included Paracelsus's definition during the Renaissance period and Esquirol's classification system in the early nineteenth century, which designated mental retardation as *amentia* and mental illness as *dementia*. Despite the fact that mental retardation was scientifically acknowledged in the early 1800s to be an important social problem distinct from mental illness, many people today still do not recognize that the majority of persons with mental retardation are mentally healthy and are free of significant behavioral problems.

The distinction that eventually was made, to associate mental retardation with low intelligence and to associate mental illness with emotional disorders, has been identified as one explanation for current tendencies toward dismissing the possible presence of behavior disturbance among persons with mental retardation. In other words, once it was clear that mental retardation was not synonymous with mental illness, the pendulum swung back such that these conditions were not even expected to co-occur.

D. Dual Diagnosis

The term dual diagnosis is now applied to persons who have intellectual deficits (mental retardation) along with emotional impairment (psychiatric disorders). As noted previously, people with mental retardation experience difficulty functioning independently in their environments but they do not necessarily have psychological disturbances. When psychiatric disorders are present, they are usually of the same types and are diagnosed by the same criteria as for persons of normal intelligence. The dual diagnosis term grew out of the recognition that individuals with both conditions present unique needs to mental retardation and mental health service systems.

Professionals have established the fact that the presence of these two conditions creates a complex set of issues that may complicate the diagnostic process and may require unique methods of treatment. The utility of the dual diagnosis term has been questioned by some clinicians who believe it adds another stigmatizing label to persons who already experience difficulties ob-

taining services from agencies that resist taking responsibility for them. Others suggest this reflects problems with the service systems, rather than with labels or assessment per se.

II. PSYCHOPATHOLOGY AND BEHAVIOR PROBLEMS

Although mental retardation and psychopathology are believed to be functionally independent, studies of the prevalence of psychiatric disorders among individuals with mental retardation have shown, almost without exception, rates that are much higher than those found in the general population. The rates reported in the literature range from less than 10% to more than 80% for persons with mental retardation, depending on methods of sampling, eligibility criteria, and types of assessment. The two largest epidemiological population studies conducted in the Isle of Wight, Wales (Rutter & Graham, 1970) and in Aberdeen, Scotland (Koller, Richardson, Katz, & McLaren, 1982) concluded that the prevalence of psychiatric disorders among children with mental retardation was about four times greater than in the general population. The prevalence rates of psychiatric disorders for children with normal intelligence in those studies ranged from 5 to 10%.

A. Specific Psychiatric Disorders with Mental Retardation

Although the incidence of psychiatric disturbance has been found to be higher among persons with mental retardation, the literature consistently affirms that the majority of symptoms do not differ in kind from people without mental retardation who are referred for psychiatric evaluation.

1. Affective Disorders
Affective disorders, including depressive and bipolar disorders, have been found to occur with much greater frequency among children and adults with mental retardation than in the general population. Contrary to earlier hypotheses that people with mental retardation are devoid of feelings, the results of some studies suggest that adults with mild mental retardation appear to experience even higher rates of de-

pression than their peers without mental retardation. [*See* DEPRESSION; MOOD DISORDERS.]

2. Schizophrenia

Schizophrenia has been found to be present in about 2 to 3% of persons with mental retardation, a prevalence that is much higher than in the nonretarded population. The symptoms of schizophrenia are generally similar across groups, although they may be simpler in form among persons with mental retardation. [*See* SCHIZOPHRENIA.]

3. Autism

It has been estimated that 75% of children with autism will perform at a level within the regarded range throughout their lives; however, less than 3% of persons with mental retardation have autistic behavior. Contrary to early theories that autism was caused by "cold" parenting styles, a variety of biological problems are now thought to explain the central nervous system dysfunction that characterizes this disorder. [*See* AUTISM AND PERVASIVE DEVELOPMENTAL DISORDER.]

4. Anxiety Disorders

Anxiety disorders have received less attention than other psychiatric disturbances among persons with mental retardation. Although prevalence estimates are scarce, several authors have reported higher rates of anxiety among persons with mental retardation than in the general population. A 22-year longitudinal population study conducted in Aberdeen, Scotland, for example, found that more than one fourth of the children exhibited problems with nerves and anxiety by early adulthood. No differences were observed between boys and girls, but a higher prevalence was found among those with more severe levels of retardation. [*See* ANXIETY.]

5. Phobias

Studies have shown that persons with and without mental retardation experience the same types of fears. Several studies suggest that mental age is a factor in comparisons of fears across these groups, where fears of older people with mental retardation tend to be more similar to fears of younger nonretarded people. Social phobias are expected to be high among persons with mental retardation; in the presence of cognitive limitations, social skill deficits are common and lead to increased vulnerability for peer rejection, low levels of social support, and social anxiety. [*See* PHOBIAS.]

B. Estimating Prevalence of Psychopathology

Two primary factors have been associated with the discrepancy (less than 10% to more than 80%) in prevalence rates of psychiatric disorders that have been reported for people with mental retardation.

I. Assessment

An accurate count of individuals who have a dual diagnosis is dependent on valid and reliable assessments of both mental retardation and psychiatric disorder. Difficulties associated with obtaining valid estimates of adaptive behavior deficits have been noted since this criterion was first included in the definition of mental retardation. Prevalence studies have also been based on definitions of mental retardation that vary from the AAMR definition. Some widely cited studies (e.g., Isle of Wight) have even used definitions that considered low IQ, but not adaptive behavior deficits, as the criterion for mental retardation.

Reliable diagnosis of mental health problems in persons with mental retardation also presents a major challenge to clinicians. Identification of psychiatric disorders depends on the clinical method, the source of information, and the taxonomy of disorders used to assign diagnoses. For example, one multimethod study of people with mental retardation found that the prevalence rates of mental disorders ranged from about 12 to 59%, depending on the method of assessment that was used.

2. Sampling Bias

Prevalence estimates are also affected by sampling bias. A large number of studies have been based on samples of individuals who have either been referred to clinics for psychiatric assessment or have resided in institutions where behavior problems led to their placement. Not surprisingly, these studies overestimate the presence of mental health problems among the population of persons with mental retardation. Service system registries comprise another major sampling source, wherein individuals receiving state-funded services are included in databases containing records of client characteristics and services provided. Because people with mild mental retardation are less likely to require state services if they do not have serious health or behavior-related problems, these databases probably overestimate the prevalence of dual diagnoses among people with mild mental retardation in the population. Finally, because many states have separate agencies providing services for persons with mental retardation and mental health problems, prevalence estimates may be affected by the determination of which agency tends to serve persons with both conditions.

C. Relationships with Age

Although age has not been found to be related to the overall distribution of psychiatric impairment, studies of specific disorders suggest that some conditions may be age-related. Moreover, in studies of behavior problems that have not been restricted to those with formal psychiatric diagnoses, age differences have been identified in rates of observed problem behavior in people with mental retardation, with lower rates found for children than for adolescents and adults. [*See* AGING AND MENTAL HEALTH.]

D. Relationships with Intellectual Level

The relationship between the overall frequency of psychiatric disorder and severity of retardation has not been established; however, the available evidence suggests that specific types of psychiatric disorder appear to be more commonly found among certain levels of mental retardation. Most studies show that the types of psychiatric syndromes observed among children and adults with mild or moderate levels of mental retardation are similar to those found in the general population, for example, major affective disorders; schizophrenia; obsessive–compulsive disorder; disorders of conduct; anxiety, activity levels, and attention; and mood and affect disorders. In contrast, some disorders are more commonly manifested by persons with severe levels of mental retardation, such as autism and other pervasive developmental disorders, aggression, stereotypic behaviors, and self-injurious behavior. Stereotypy (repetitive motor behaviors) and self-injury may occur in isolation or in conjunction with major neuropsychiatric disorders among persons with severe or profound mental retardation.

E. Relationships with Gender

Most studies have found no significant relationships between overall behavior disturbance and gender. However, gender differences have been observed within certain types of disturbance. For example, consistent with findings in the nonretarded population, antisocial behavior has been found to be more preva-

lent among males, while emotional disturbance has been observed more frequently among females. [*See* GENDER DIFFERENCES IN MENTAL HEALTH.]

F. Relationships with Etiology of Mental Retardation

The evidence suggests that certain genetically related causes of mental retardation, such as Prader Willi syndrome, Cornelia de Lange syndrome, Lesch-Nyhan disease, fragile X syndrome, and Williams syndrome are associated with the presence of specific behavior problems and psychological disorders in persons with mental retardation. Lesch-Nyhan disease is best known for the manifestation of self-injurious biting. The minority of individuals with Lesch-Nyhan who do not bite indulge in some other form of self-injurious behavior, such as head banging. Aggressive behavior is also directed against others, and most of these individuals vomit, which interferes with nutrition. Lower incidences of self-injurious behavior than those in Lesch-Nyhan have been observed among persons with Cornelia de Lange syndrome, Tourette's syndrome, and fragile X syndrome. The majority of self-injuring individuals, however, have nonspecific diagnoses of mental retardation and display this behavior in self-stimulating or stereotypic patterns.

Fragile X syndrome is the most common known inherited cause of mental retardation and developmental disabilities. Attention deficit disorders, autistic disorders, and socially related and anxiety-based disorders appear to be associated with fragile X syndrome, although these disorders are not present in all persons who have fragile X. Food preoccupation, hyperphagia, and obesity are most often associated with Prader Willi syndrome. Recent studies have also linked maladaptive symptoms that are not related to food, such as obsessive–compulsive disorder, temper tantrums, internalizing problems, and oppositional-defiant disorders to individuals with Prader Willi syndrome. Recent data suggest increased risks of anxiety disorders and attention deficit hyperactivity disorder among people with Williams syndrome. Adults with Down syndrome appear to be at a higher risk of depression relative to other adults with mental retardation. Researchers have also discovered links between Down syndrome and Alzheimer's disease, with people with Down syndrome having a greater than average risk of developing this disease after the age of 45. [*See* GENETIC CONTRIBUTORS TO MENTAL HEALTH.]

G. Behavior Problems Distinguished from Psychiatric Disorders

Observed behavior problems do not by themselves indicate psychopathology. Interrelationships between deficits in adaptive behavior, maladaptive or problem behavior, and psychiatric disorders among persons with mental retardation are complex. Maladaptive behavior is a term that has been used in the field of mental retardation to refer to problem behaviors that are sometimes categorized as personal (e.g., self-injury, depression) or social (e.g., aggression, property destruction). In general, the terms maladaptive behavior and behavior problems are used interchangeably. Despite the definitional criteria that require deficits in adaptive skills to be present in persons with mental retardation, these deficits are not always associated with maladaptive behavior. Adaptive and maladaptive behavior represent two distinct, independent constructs and deficient interpersonal skill development (i.e., lack of adaptive skills) is not always associated with undesirable or pathological behavior.

Psychopathology is only indicated when behavior problems are part of an overall pattern of behavior. Although persons with a dual diagnosis are at a higher risk of evincing destructive behavior patterns (e.g., self-injury, aggressive behavior, and property destruction), it is clear that these destructive behaviors are also present among a significant proportion of people whose only diagnosis is mental retardation.

III. ASSESSMENT OF MENTAL HEALTH

Although the diagnosis of mental retardation is determined in part by deficits in adaptive functioning, the behaviors that one must display in order to be considered competent cannot be clearly delineated for every situation and age group. Measures of social competence must, for practical reasons, sample only selected behaviors that are used to represent typical functioning. Decisions that rely on measurement of adaptive and maladaptive behavior are highly dependent on the method of assessment used. Moreover, behavior is not expected to be "normal" for persons with mental retardation. Because base rates of behavior may be compared either to the general population or to the subset of people with mental retardation, the selection of a comparison group can also influence the identification of pathology.

A. Applicability of Taxonomies Used for the General Population

There is a general consensus that the full range of mental disorders observed in the general population is found among persons with mental retardation. Psychopathology is typically reported according to established diagnostic systems, such as the American Psychiatric Association's Diagnostic and Statistical Manual (DSM-IV), that are also used to classify disorders in persons with normal intellectual ability. Early versions of the DSM classification system were thought to lack reliability and validity for persons with mental retardation, but the heightened awareness of dual diagnosis in the 1980s led to vast improvements in defining DSM categories that were appropriate for persons with mental retardation. Some clinicians still contend, however, that the expression of psychopathology among persons with severe and profound mental retardation may take on different forms and require separate classifications.

B. Consideration of Quality and Reliability of Mental Health Information

1. Multimethod Approach to Assessment

Multiple informants and multiple methods of data collection are typically used to provide a clinical picture of abnormal behavior among persons with mental retardation. These methods, which may include abstracting information from case records, systematic observations, interviews, formal instruments, and medical examinations, provide ratings that may differ according to the rater's familiarity with the individual, contexts in which behaviors are observed, rater or situational tolerance of the behavior, behavioral expectations, and response styles on rating scales.

2. Complications Caused by Communication Deficits

Communication deficits that are associated with low intelligence complicate the evaluation process in several important ways. The simplistic emotional expressions and concrete thought patterns that are characteristic of these individuals can lead to clinical misinterpretations of their behavior or mental health conditions. The identification of some syndromes also depends on information obtained by interview with the individual or observation of his or her speech (e.g., hallucinations, complaints of pain, or fears). With individuals who are nonverbal or who lack expressive language, it may be impossible to diagnose reliably certain conditions. Finally, individuals who lack the communication skills necessary to make their needs known or to interact socially with others may develop problem behaviors that represent attempts to communicate and do not stem from emotional disturbance.

3. Effect of Behavior on IQ Test Performance

Although the extent of its impact is difficult to determine, it is possible that severe behavior disorders, especially those present from early childhood, lead to poor performance on intelligence tests, which can result in a false diagnosis of mental retardation. The importance of knowing whether behavior disturbance has depressed a person's behavioral functioning to such a degree that his or her IQ falls within the retarded range, or whether in fact the person has both mental retardation and a severe emotional disorder, has been questioned in terms of its relevance to treatment. Nevertheless, this distinction affects prevalence rates of dual diagnosis and may also determine which bureaucratic system (mental retardation or mental health agency) will assume responsibility for the provision of services to that individual.

C. Diagnostic Overshadowing

Diagnosticians are less likely to identify psychiatric illness in individuals with mental retardation, even when their observed behaviors are identical to those displayed by persons of average intelligence. This phenomenon, which has been referred to as diagnostic overshadowing, suggests that behavioral problems evinced by persons with mental retardation tend to be attributed to the retardation rather than to a concomitant behavior disorder. Because adaptive skill deficits partly define mental retardation, this attribution is understandable; however, it is likely to affect prevalence rates and may also lead to different profiles of persons with and without mental retardation who are given the same psychiatric diagnosis.

D. Measures Developed for Individuals with Mental Retardation

Historically, attempts were made with limited success to adapt instruments developed for the general population for use with people with mental retardation. The

1980s was a period in which the lack of adequate assessment instruments for identifying and classifying psychopathology among persons with mental retardation emerged as an important clinical and research priority. In 1991, Aman published a comprehensive review for the National Institute of Mental Health of instruments that had been specifically developed for or tested with samples of people with mental retardation. He identified 23 instruments that were appropriate as general purpose diagnostic tools. Of these, most were developed after 1984, indicating a flurry of activity in the past decade. Despite what appears to be a wide selection of available measures, however, the numbers are greatly reduced when they are broken down by relevant age groups, levels of mental retardation, specific conditions covered, type of rater used (self-ratings, other informant, or clinician), and whether adequate psychometric testing (e.g., reliability and validity) has been reported.

I. Clinical Dimensions across Instruments

A moderate degree of consistency has been found across factor analytic studies of the clinical dimensions of psychopathology, suggesting that similar dimensions are being tapped by different instruments. Aman noted, however, that the dimensions that emerge from factor analysis of items on an instrument are highly dependent on the collection of items or questions that it contains. For example, if an instrument contains few or no questions about self-injury, factor analyses cannot produce a separate dimension related to this problem. This point is particularly relevant if some behaviors that are unique to persons with severe and profound retardation are not included on measures that were originally developed for people with normal intelligence.

2. Validity of Instruments

Many instruments have not been evaluated for their validity, that is, their ability to identify accurately the psychopathology, and especially specific diagnostic categories. When the correctness of classifications has been examined, the current version of the DSM has typically been used as the criterion or standard (i.e., representing the true diagnosis). If the concerns that have been noted with regard to the appropriateness of using DSM systems to identify all disorders found among persons with severe and profound mental retardation are valid, then using the current version of the DSM as the criteria to establish the validity of new instruments may be problematic. It is also possible that certain disorders might exist in such persons but may be presented quite differently than presented in the general population, which would further compromise use of the DSM. Future work in this area of assessment should focus on the need for adequate standardization samples, carefully designed studies of classification accuracy and reliability, developmentally appropriate measures for persons of all ages and levels of mental retardation, and establishment of validity with respect to external criteria (differential response to treatment, long-term outcome, etc.).

E. New Evaluation Techniques

The development of neuroimaging technology in recent years presents new opportunities to understand certain psychiatric disorders and to provide rationales for treatment methods. Brain imaging techniques, for example, examine brain structure and anatomy, and include the use of computerized tomography (CT) and magnetic resonance imaging (MRI). Positron-emission tomography (PET) technology emphasizes brain function and provides sophisticated computer images of brain activity that can help to explain causes of emotional states in individuals with and without mental retardation.

IV. TREATMENT AND INTERVENTION

A. Historical Perspective on the Treatment of Behavior Disorders

With the recognition in recent years that a significant number of people with mental retardation have dual diagnoses, there has come a shift in approaches to treatment. Historically, maladaptive behavior was thought to be primarily a management of care issue and was treated by mental retardation professionals who used behavioral methods. Reduction of behavior problems meant more opportunities for educational, vocational, and residential placements in less restrictive settings, as well as increased involvement in community activities. Recent attention to dual diagnosis, combined with a broadened interest in affective and other internalizing behavior disturbances, has led to a greater involvement of mental health professionals in treatment efforts. Unlike behaviorally oriented therapists who view the specific diagnostic category as less

important than observable behaviors, mental health professionals are more likely to believe that the best possible treatment requires the identification of a specific disorder and an accurate psychiatric diagnosis.

B. Relationship of Causal Factors to Treatment Methods

I. Causal Factors

Selected treatments of problem behaviors and psychiatric disorders were historically determined in conjunction with specific causal theories (e.g., organic, behavioral, developmental, and sociocultural) that were assumed to explain the behavior. In contrast to this single-factor approach, more recent efforts have focused on the complex interactions of multiple causes (e.g., biological and psychosocial) and on interdisciplinary approaches to treatment.

a. Low Intelligence and Environmental Factors Reduced intellectual capacity, along with a limited repertoire of skills for coping with environmental demands, expose children with mental retardation to a wide range of stressful experiences. Some situations, although not unique to persons with mental retardation, are exacerbated by intellectual disability. For example, individuals with mental retardation are more likely to encounter teasing, social rejection, communication handicaps, academic failure, parental guilt and overprotectiveness, and overall rejection than their nonhandicapped peers. Lower intelligence, combined with environmental demands to adapt to novel situations or to modify established patterns of behavior, may also result in higher levels of anxiety. It is not surprising that difficult social situations, combined with limited abilities to handle them, result in an increased vulnerability to develop emotional problems.

b. Developmental Explanations Based on the premise that persons with mental retardation develop along the same general patterns but at slower rates than their nonhandicapped peers, behaviors of individuals who are at similar levels of cognitive development are expected to respond in similar ways to environmental events and demands. Moreover, some behaviors that are considered appropriate when displayed by young children could also be considered "appropriate" (not pathological) among older persons with mental retardation who function at lower cognitive levels. In general, current developmental theories of disordered behavior consider genetic background, family history, neurological conditions, and life experiences along with cognitive levels of development.

c. Behavioral Theory As noted earlier, behavioral theory has tended to dominate the treatment of maladaptive behaviors that are disruptive or harmful. Behavioral models focus on observed behaviors and on the interactions between people and their environments. Operant conditioning models concentrate on the effects of various types of reinforcement on both prosocial and problem behaviors. The importance of reinforcing appropriate behavior and of discovering and removing unintentional reinforcement of problem behaviors is emphasized. Classical conditioning and social learning theories have been used to explain connections between fears, phobias, and past experiences among persons with and without mental retardation. Although behavioral methods used in isolation have been successful in the reduction of problem behaviors among many persons with mental retardation, the importance of considering possible interactions between specific organic problems and behavioral contingencies has been noted.

d. Genetic Links to Behavior Current research efforts have focused on the relationship of psychopathology to psychosocial and genetic factors, suggesting that knowledge of behavioral phenotypes (behaviors associated with specific genetic mental retardation syndromes) may help the development of optimal therapy and intervention for people with different disorders. For example, studies linking molecular genetics to behavioral variables are finding associations between psychopathology, cognition, and specific aspects of the fragile X gene. Other work has shown promising results that relate skin-picking and other compulsions to features of chromosome 15. Although there appears to be a link between affective disorders and Down syndrome, researchers have not yet determined that it is the genetic disorder that leads to depression. Current findings in genetic research suggest that the identification of causal relations between specific genetic syndromes and problem behaviors will make rapid progress during the next decade.

e. Family Influences The evidence suggests that family processes are contributory factors in some cases of

behavioral disturbance in children with mental retardation. Notwithstanding the fact that many families with children with retardation function quite well and provide emotional support to their children, the additional stresses associated with the child's disability may lead to home environments and parent–child interactions that contribute to the development of behavior problems or more serious psychopathology. [*See* FAMILY SYSTEMS.]

f. The "New Morbidity" Advances in medical care over the last several decades have greatly reduced the incidence of children's mortality and morbidity (illness) from serious infectious disease. At the same time, however, a "new morbidity" has been described that affects a significant number of children in the United States and it appears to be strongly related to socioeconomic status, family constellation, and other social characteristics. These behavioral, social, and school-related problems in American society are thought to be health risks, because they are known to contribute to poor adjustment, handicaps, physical illness, mental retardation, and mental health problems in children. The risk factors associated with the new morbidity tend to operate interactively, causing children to become psychologically and biologically vulnerable to failure in environments that lack the supports necessary to promote their successful adaptation. The concept of a new morbidity has immediate implications for the prevention of dual diagnoses. For example, Fetal Alcohol Syndrome is a preventable condition that is known to be related to emotional disability. It is also one of the most commonly identified causes of mental retardation. Low birthweight babies, more common in poor economic and social environments, are also at high risk of mental retardation and emotional disorders. The concept of a new morbidity suggests that medical advances will not be sufficient to reduce the risk of dual diagnosis. A significant investment is also necessary in research and prevention efforts directed toward the social and behavioral aspects of the new morbidity.

g. Consideration of Multiple Causes: Self-Injury As an Example Causal theories of self-injurious behavior have been studied extensively and can illustrate the ways in which multiple pathways can result in the same observed behavior. Self-injury, which is associated with several types of psychiatric disorder but is also observed independent of mental illness, appears to result from a variety of mechanisms. Among the noted origins are direct biochemical causes such as metabolic error (e.g., in persons with Lesch-Nyhan disease), increased levels of B-endorphin that increase tolerance for self-injury, and environmental factors (e.g., inadvertent reinforcement from attention received during behavior-stopping efforts, attempts to communicate needs or feelings). Research studies have also noted that even though one mechanism may serve as the initial cause of self-injury, a shift may occur later to a different mechanism that maintains more serious forms of the behavior. These different origins of self-injurious behavior suggest different approaches to treatment. Therefore, researchers have suggested that the most effective prevention and treatment approaches for behavior problems are determined by an understanding of the history and sequence of causal factors in each individual.

2. Treatment

Whereas clinical researchers studying treatment issues traditionally concentrated on problems affecting behavior management and treatment of severe behavior disorders (e.g., self-injurious behavior) in institutional settings, increased attention in recent years to such conditions as depression, schizophrenia, and anxiety disorders reflects a mental health movement that also considers the emotional well-being of all individuals with mental retardation, regardless of their residential placements. Current practices also reflect an interdisciplinary strategy that integrates behavioral, psychopharmacological, developmental, and other approaches to intervention.

a. Matching Treatment to Genetic Causes of Mental Retardation The recent literature on syndrome-related differences in psychopathology suggests that improved accuracy in the identification of genetically caused mental retardation syndromes may have important implications for treatment. It has been suggested, for example, that "etiology-specific early intervention" may optimize treatment outcomes for some disorders. This approach assumes that some aspects of treatment are useful for all individuals with a given behavior; whereas other aspects of treatment may be unique to particular etiologies. It should be noted, however, that although certain genetically caused forms of mental retardation show associations with

certain behavioral patterns, the behaviors are usually not exhibited by every person with the syndrome. This area represents a relatively new area of study that is being conducted in connection with the identification of new genetic disorders.

b. Behavior Therapies Behavioral procedures have been identified as one of the most effective techniques for eliminating problem behaviors and replacing them with alternative, acceptable, and functional behaviors. Behavioral interventions focus on specific observable behaviors, rather than on syndromes. In a functional analysis of a target problem behavior, the environmental conditions that serve as antecedents or consequences of that behavior are identified. For example, functional analysis might reveal that inappropriate behaviors serve a communication or social function, a self-regulatory function, or a self-reinforcing play function. Similar behaviors can serve different functions across and even within children. Knowledge of this type informs therapists about the design of behavioral interventions. Intervention plans may involve teaching alternate, more appropriate responses to antecedent conditions, improving communication skills, rearranging the environment by removing or reducing stimuli related to problem behavior, or rearranging contingencies associated with the behavior.

Functional analyses can be used to modify instructional and environmental variables that affect student behavior at school. Altering antecedent stimuli, such as student choice and variation of tasks, instructional pace, sequencing tasks and breaking them into component parts, and modifying task difficulty have all been shown to reduce the occurrence of problem behavior among students with mental retardation. Although these methods may be less effective for more severe forms of disordered behavior, they are likely to promote learning and improved interpersonal relationships among a large percentage of students who exhibit behavior that is incompatible with effective instruction.

Similar behaviors that have different causal factors have been found to be differentially responsive to behavioral treatments. In general, behavioral interventions will be appropriate for learned behaviors, but may not be effective with behaviors that are organically or biologically caused. For example, whereas self-injurious biting among persons with Cornelia de Lange syndrome has been successfully treated by operant conditioning, this same behavior in Lesch-Nyhan patients tends to be resistant to behavioral approaches. Because Lesch-Nyhan disease is characterized by a defective enzyme that appears to influence the balance of neurotransmitters in the central nervous system, it is not surprising that behavioral methods are less effective in treating self-injury in these individuals. [*See* BEHAVIOR THERAPY.]

c. Ethics of Aversive Interventions Behavior reduction programs may use a combination of positive reinforcement and aversive procedures. Aversive interventions have been defined narrowly (e.g., interventions that cause physical or emotional pain or discomfort) and broadly (e.g., interventions that are not "positive," including timeout, physical, or chemical restraints). Although pain or discomfort is commonly associated with aversive interventions, an aversive stimulus is simply a stimulus that a person seeks to avoid, defined by its consequences on the targeted behavior. Questions about the moral justification for the use of these procedures has caused considerable controversy among direct-care workers, clinicians, and professional organizations. Whereas a "freedom from harm" position holds that aversive intervention is morally wrong in all instances, the "right to effective treatment" position contends that unpleasant or painful treatments are ethical if they lead to outcomes that involve less overall physical damage than would be the case without the intervention. The latter position suggests that aversiveness must be judged in the context of long-term suffering experienced by the individual, not just in relation to the immediate effects of the aversive program. In other words, nonaversive interventions that are ineffective or only effective for the short-term, may, in fact, result in more prolonged suffering. Those who support the right to effective treatment base their arguments on an assumption of the effectiveness of aversive interventions; if these procedures are more immediately effective, then their use is justified from the beginning. The argument becomes more complicated in the absence of compelling evidence on the expected efficacy of treatment or degree of harm for specific individuals. Yet, individual circumstances and ethical considerations in studies designed to gather this information make it extremely difficult to gather the information. Other concerns about aversive treatments have been noted regarding the powerful role of the therapist, maintenance and generalization issues, lack of social acceptability, and emotional side effects.

d. Psychopharmacological Interventions Clinical experience and experimental studies have provided promising evidence that psychopharmacological interventions can effectively treat psychiatric disorders among persons with mental retardation. Moreover, researchers are now finding that many behavior problems that have been resistant to behavioral or other treatment efforts have biological etiologies. There is some optimism that this knowledge will lead to successful prevention and effective neurochemical treatments for at least some of these conditions. For example, self-injurious behavior has been reduced in some individuals by as much as 50% through treatment by drugs that inhibit endorphin release and that appear to lower pain thresholds. Research findings on vulnerable neurotransmitter systems in nonhandicapped adults with Alzheimer's disease have also led to pharmacological strategies that could alleviate cognitive impairments. Several studies have shown that behavioral symptoms associated with autistic disorders, including self-injury and stereotyped behavior, aggression, hyperactive behavior, and affective disorders, can be successfully treated with psychotropic medication. For some conditions, such as schizophrenia, responsiveness to pharmacological treatment has been found to be generally similar to that found among persons with mental retardation.

Claims of overuse and misuse of psychotropic drugs in institutional settings (often prescribed without regard to diagnosis and without close monitoring), along with evidence of high rates of the tardive dyskinesia (involuntary movement) side effect during the 1960s and 1970s, created a heightened awareness and even fear of psychopharmacological treatment. Psychopharmacology tended to be directed at the suppression of behavioral symptoms, rather than at matching drug therapies to well-defined syndromes. The antidrug sentiment was probably exacerbated by the exposure of a prominent researcher who was found to have falsified his research on drug therapies. This period was followed by dramatic decreases in psychotropic drug treatment. Although still the subject of controversy, current attitudes are generally more favorable toward drug therapy. Many clinicians are now trained to (a) differentiate psychiatric symptoms from maladaptive behavior, (b) consider the implications of behavioral syndromes, (c) pay attention to the psychological and physical costs of drug therapy, and (d) plan drug withdrawal programs that monitor the effects of withdrawal. The importance of close monitoring of pharmacological treatments, especially for persons residing in community-based settings, is emphasized. Continued scientific study with controlled procedures and standardized assessments is also needed to answer questions about disorders and medications that have received less attention in previous research, potential side effects, identification of clinical factors that predict who will respond favorably to medical interventions, and the relative importance of linking pharmacological treatment to identified psychiatric disorders (rather than to isolated behavioral symptoms). [*See* PSYCHOPHARMACOLOGY.]

e. **Skill Development** Functional skill development, initiated at early ages, has been hypothesized to play an important role in the prevention of serious behavior problems among persons with mental retardation. State-of-the-art services providing infant and preschool training in communication and social skills represent a comprehensive approach to teaching functional responses that might otherwise be replaced by problem behaviors. This approach to understanding behavior problems focuses on the lack of functional skills, rather than on the presence of behavioral excesses. Researchers and clinicians advocating this approach acknowledge that it may not be applicable to some severe problem behaviors that have physiological origins.

The communication function served by problem behaviors among many persons with mental retardation is well established. Communication training provides a mechanism for replacing inappropriate behavior with alternate means of expressing intentions and ideas. Research has demonstrated that even persons with severe degrees of mental retardation can be taught communication skills. Pragmatic theory, which focuses on the social function of language, has been emphasized to teach people with mental retardation to communicate.

Social skills training, which is based on the theory that social competence relies on specific skills necessary for social interactions, has been used successfully with many individuals with mental retardation. The need for training in social skills has been emphasized in numerous studies that have found people with mental retardation to lack the skills required to promote social acceptance and friendships in integrated settings. These studies have concluded that social skills training may be the key to the successful integration of people with mental retardation with their nonhandicapped peers. This training typically focuses on either context-specific skills (e.g., school, workplace, or residential setting) or on reducing social fears among persons with diagnosed social phobias.

V. PROMOTION OF MENTAL HEALTH

The President's Committee on Mental Retardation has emphasized the need for national prevention programs in relation to mental health issues of people with mental retardation. Although national prevention programs have received less attention than other mental health issues in terms of federal support, research not specifically aimed at prevention has led to a sense of optimism about preventing or reducing the impact of mental health problems.

A. Prevention and the New Morbidity

Recognition of social and economic factors that cause or influence degrees of mental retardation and psychiatric disorders, that is, the new morbidity, has important implications for prevention. Prevention efforts that focus on subgroups with characteristics (e.g., low socioeconomic status, high prevalence of drug and alcohol use) that place them at a high risk for mental retardation and mental health problems will have the greatest impact. For example, improved prenatal care and health-oriented treatment of drug and alcohol abuse during pregnancy are obvious targets of prevention efforts.

B. Genetic Mapping

Recent scientific advances in the identification of causal factors related to mental health problems among persons with mental retardation have provided a sense of optimism about the eventual prevention of these conditions. More than 50% of severe and profound mental retardation is caused by genetically determined disorders. The application of DNA technology to studies of mental retardation has made it possible to map abnormal genes to specific chromosome regions. Within the next decade or so, researchers expect to define all of the disorders that are associated with severe mental retardation. Ultimately, researchers hope to identify DNA alterations that cause abnormal genes to malfunction. This research is progressing quickly and there is a sense of great optimism, because the capacity to develop DNA markers for genetic causes of mental retardation has important implications for prevention. It will soon be possible to identify persons who are at risk of having children that will be affected with genetic conditions that can result in mental retardation. Moreover, it is possible that in the long range it will be possible to develop complex gene therapies to treat genetic disorders. These developments in genetic mapping have provided new hope with regard to future cures or reversals of effects of inherited diseases that cause both mental retardation and mental illness.

C. Early Intervention Programs

Part H of the federal special education law, the Individuals with Disabilities Education Act, mandates that states provide coordinated early intervention services to children with disabilities from birth through 36 months. One component of Part H is the Individualized Family Service Plan, which identifies specific needs of the child and family and designates the services to be provided to meet those needs. Services can include psychological services, family training, counseling, and home training if their purpose is to prevent or reduce the impact of disabilities on the child and family. This recently mandated program, along with other federal and state-sponsored programs that target low income and disadvantaged children, should lead to reductions in the incidence of mental health problems among children with mental retardation.

VI. IMPLICATIONS OF MENTAL HEALTH CONSIDERATIONS

A. Cost of Mental Health Care

The cost of providing services to individuals in the United States with mental retardation who also dis-

play destructive behavior (e.g., aggression, self-injury, property destruction) was estimated in a 1991 study by the National Institute of Child Health and Human Development to exceed $3.5 billion per year.

B. Residential Placement

The presence of behavior problems among people with mental retardation has a direct influence on how and where they will live. In the wake of the deinstitutionalization movement, the majority of people who still reside in large, segregated, residential facilities are either those who are medically fragile or whose behaviors are not tolerated in less restrictive settings. Thus, the presence of challenging behaviors, especially those that are harmful to self, others, or property, limits opportunities for individuals with mental retardation to live with their families or in smaller community placements that provide for increased levels of independence. Studies of individuals living in community-based residences who are in jeopardy of being moved to more restrictive settings have noted that unmet needs for support, such as mental health services, professional counseling, and behavioral intervention services, contribute to the vulnerability of their residential status. Despite these systematic trends in placement selections, challenging behaviors are present among people in all types of living arrangements. The availability of resources, including well-trained and adequately paid staff, to serve the mental health needs of these individuals, will be a key to their living as independently as possible. [See COMMUNITY MENTAL HEALTH; MENTAL HOSPITALS AND DEINSTITUTIONALIZATION.]

C. Family Issues

Research on families of children with mental retardation has established the important role that families play in the development and adjustment of their children. Contrary to earlier stereotypes of these families as typically having serious marital problems, parental psychopathology, and psychosocial adjustment problems, more recent research indicates that families with children with mental retardation are equally likely to function well. Trends toward a more positive perception of these families have not ignored the fact, however, that the presence of children with mental retardation adds additional parenting responsibilities and may contribute to higher levels of emotional and physical stress than is found in other families. Caregiving of children with mental retardation, who also have severe behavior problems or psychological disorders, presents additional responsibilities as families encounter more difficulties obtaining needed educational, medical, psychological, or other services. Depending on the condition that is identified as the primary diagnosis, the family may end up working with either or both mental health and mental retardation service systems, where professional attitudes toward parental involvement may differ and conceptual approaches toward treatment are also likely to differ. Although families are no longer implicated as the primary cause of psychological disturbance in their children, various factors related to the home and family context (e.g., marital relationships, parental depression, parent–child interactions, sibling relationships) have been identified as contributory factors for some children. Further research on these relationships is needed.

D. Educational Implications

1. Guarantee of Public Education

The Individuals with Disabilities Education Act (PL 94-142) requires public education systems to serve all children with mental retardation and severe behavior disorders. To the greatest extent possible, these students must be educated in what is believed to be the least restrictive environment, that is, by spending as much time as possible with their nonhandicapped peers. The law has also been interpreted in such a way as to limit the school system's power to expel a student whose behavior is thought to be part of his or her disability. Each student must have a written Individualized Education Plan (IEP) that describes the major goals of his or her educational program. For children with mental retardation and severe behavior problems, the IEP should address remediation of behavioral excesses and deficits. It should designate opportunities to learn appropriate behaviors and document methods of discipline to be used. The use of intrusive or restrictive disciplinary procedures is prohibited unless there is compelling evidence that they represent least restrictive alternatives.

2. Written Safeguards in Schools

The legal guarantees for special education students have also led to the need for administrative procedures that safeguard both teachers and students in relation to responses to unacceptable behaviors exhibited in school. Constitutional rights and full informed parent/guardian consent required by PL 94-142 provide the basic protections to treatment of students. In addition, many schools have established behavioral specialist teams and human rights review committees, along with specific written safeguards that protect the rights of students, teachers, and educational administrators.

E. Service Delivery Systems: Two Handicaps—Two Service Delivery Systems

In the 1970s, most states recognized that the service-related needs of individuals with mental retardation and mental illness are different and they created two separated bureaucracies to serve them, that is, a department of mental retardation and a department of mental health. Concerns were expressed at the time that the needs of individuals who had both mental retardation and mental health problems might be left unserved, as they fell through the cracks between service delivery systems. Concerns were also voiced about the importance of cross-training competent professionals who would understand the complex mental health issues of people with a dual diagnosis. These concerns remain a high priority today.

Historically, efforts were made to distinguish between primary and secondary handicaps, thus determining the agency that would assume primary responsibility for provision of care. Services provided focused on the primary handicap, with little or no attention given to the secondary handicap. The concept of a dual diagnosis represents an alternative to the primary versus secondary handicap distinction, in which presumably all service needs can be addressed. This group of people requires specialized services that involve high levels of agency intercollaboration and interdisciplinary treatment programs; this is clearly an instance where the whole (dual diagnosis) is greater than the sum of its separate parts (mental retardation and mental health needs). Because doctors tend to be trained in either mental retardation *or* mental illness, but not both, our service systems currently lack professionals specifically trained to treat individuals with dual diagnoses. The federal Department of Health and Human Services has recently recognized this, citing the mental health needs of individuals with developmental disabilities (including mental retardation) as one of its top funding priority areas.

F. Legal Issues

The presence of both mental retardation and mental illness poses difficult legal and ethical issues. For example, individuals with mental retardation and serious mental illness may find it difficult, or even impossible, to make informed, legally appropriate decisions. In this case, a third-party decision maker may assume this responsibility. Although this is legally defensible and is intended to benefit the individual, ethical issues remain when personal autonomy is substituted for proxy consent. Thus, according to a "substitute judgment doctrine" invoked by the legal system, the task of the decision maker is to attempt to determine how the individual would have decided if he or she were competent in this role, rather than to judge what is best for him or her. Analysts of this doctrine explain that this rule treats people with dual diagnoses (who are determined incompetent in the legal sense) the same as it treats individuals who can decide for themselves, that is, with respect, autonomy, and dignity of choice.

Individuals with dual diagnoses are protected by the due process clauses in the Fifth and Fourteenth Amendments. Therefore, they have the right to the same procedural safeguards as people without mental retardation. This right has particular relevance when individuals with dual diagnoses are accused of crimes, refuse medical treatment, or are placed in state residential facilities. Numerous court cases have confirmed the constitutional rights of this group; neither punishment, nor medication, nor residential confinement without safety and personal freedom can be denied on the basis of a person's limited intellectual capacity. [*See* LEGAL DIMENSIONS OF MENTAL HEALTH.]

BIBLIOGRAPHY

Aman, M. G. (1991). *Assessing psychopathology and behavior problems in persons with mental retardation: A review of available instruments.* [DHHS Publication No. (ADM) 91-1712]. Rockville, MD: U.S. Department of Health and Human Services, Public Health Service, Alcohol, Drug Abuse, and Mental Health Administration, National Institute of Mental Health.

Bregman, J. D. (1991). Current developments in the understanding of mental retardation: 2. Psychopathology. *Journal of the American Academy of Child and Adolescent Psychiatry, 30,* 861–872.

Dibble, E., & Gray, D. B. (Eds.). (1988). *Assessment of behavior problems in persons with mental retardation living in the community.* Bethesda, MD: National Institute of Mental Health.

Koller, H., Richardson, S. A., Katz, M., & McLaren, J. (1982). Behavior disturbance in childhood and the early adult years in populations who were and were not mentally retarded. *Journal of Preventive Psychiatry, 87,* 386–395.

Luckasson, R. (Ed.). (1992). Mental retardation: Definition, classification, and systems of supports (9th ed.). Washington, DC: American Association on Mental Retardation.

Matson, J. L., & Barrett, R. P. (Eds.). (1993). *Psychopathology in the mentally retarded.* Needham Heights, MA: Allyn & Bacon.

Matson, J. L., & Mulick, J. A. (Eds.). (1991). *Handbook of mental retardation.* New York: Pergamon Press.

Nezu, A. M. (Ed.). (1994). Mental retardation and mental illness. *Journal of Consulting and Clinical Psychology, 62,* 4–62.

Repp, A. C., & Singh, N. N. (Eds.). (1990). *Perspectives on the use of nonaversive and aversive interventions for persons with developmental disabilities.* Sycamore, IL: Sycamore.

Rutter, M., & Graham, P. (1970). Epidemiology of psychiatric disorder. In M. Rutter, J. Tizard, & K. Whitmore (Eds.), *Education, health, and behavior* (pp. 178–201). London: Longman Group.

Stark, J. A., Menolascino, F. J., Albarelli, M. H., & Gray, V. C. (Eds.). (1988). *Mental retardation and mental health: Classification, diagnosis, treatment, services.* New York: Springer-Verlag.

Thompson, T., & Gray, D. (Eds.). (1994). *Destructive behavior in developmental disabilities.* Thousand Oaks, CA: Sage.

Middle Age and Well-Being

Carol D. Ryff

University of Wisconsin, Madison

Burton Singer

Princeton University

Allostasis The biological imprint of the body's attempt to equilibrate in the face of challenge. The sympathetic nervous system, the immune system, and the hypothalamic–pituitary–adrenal axis all respond to challenges, attempting to bring the organism back into an effective operating range.

Autonomy A component of psychological well-being in which one is self-determining and independent, able to resist pressures to think and act in certain ways, regulates behavior from within, and evaluates self by personal standards.

Environmental Mastery A component of psychological well-being in which one has a sense of mastery and competence in managing the surrounding environment, controls a complex array of external activities, makes effective use of surrounding opportunities, and is able to choose or create contexts suitable to personal needs and values.

Personal Growth A component of psychological well-being that comprises feelings of continued development, seeing one's self as growing and expanding, being open to new experiences, having the sense that one's potential is being realized, seeing improvement in self and behavior over time, and being able to change in ways that reflect more self-knowledge and effectiveness.

Positive Relations with Others A component of psychological well-being in which one has warm, satisfying, trusting relationships with others, shows concern for the welfare of others, is capable of strong empathy, affection, and intimacy, and understands the give and take of human relationships.

Purpose in Life A component of psychological well-being that includes having goals in life and a sense of directedness, feeling there is meaning in one's present and past life, holding beliefs that give life purpose, and having aims and objectives for living.

Resilience Capacity to withstand adversity and stress; assessed in terms of the *maintenance* or *recovery* of mental and physical health following life challenges; with positive indicators of health, it is possible to demonstrate human ability to thrive and flourish after challenge.

Self-Acceptance A component of psychological well-being that includes having a positive attitude toward one's self, acknowledging and accepting one's good and bad qualities, and feeling positive about one's past life.

This article discusses **MIDDLE AGE AND WELL-BEING.** Psychological theory and philosophical perspectives provide the basis for an explicit operational definition of positive mental health that encompasses multiple components of well-being. Empirical studies show how these qualities are distributed by age, gender, class, and culture. The influence of particular life experiences on well-being is illustrated with research on parenthood. How life histories are linked with mental health is also examined, with a specific focus on psychological resilience in the face of cumulating adversity. A final section explores linkages between mental and physical health through elaboration of the physiological substrates of positive quality of life.

I. WHAT IS POSITIVE MENTAL HEALTH?

There is a long-standing imbalance in the mental health field whereby greater knowledge has been amassed about illness than well-being. Indeed, operational definitions of mental health have persistently targeted the *absence of illness* (e.g., depression, anxiety, other neuroses and psychoses) as the hallmark of adaptive functioning. Such approaches ignore the person's capacity for going beyond illness into wellness, which requires an explicit characterization of the *presence of the positive* in life. Numerous psychological theories as well as philosophical accounts have described the nature of the positive, or the good life. These are briefly summarized here to distill key elements that define psychological well-being.

Life-span developmental psychology offers numerous formulations of positive functioning conceived as progressions of continued growth across the life course. Erikson's model of psychosocial development, for example, described the challenges of identity, intimacy, generativity, and integrity as adolescent and adult routes to ever higher levels of functioning. Buhler's characterization of basic life tendencies that work toward the fulfillment of life gave emphasis to creative expansion and upholding internal order as adult forms of proactive engagement with life. Neugarten also described the executive processes of personality development in midlife and the turning inward in the later years as avenues of continued development.

Clinical psychology provides further accounts of positive functioning, such as Maslow's detailed description of the characteristics of self-actualizers whose lives are governed by being rather than by deficiency needs. Roger's characterization of the fully functioning person and Jung's description of the process of individuation provide other examples of comprehensive efforts to understand the optimal human condition. The elaboration of maturity by Allport repre-

sents still another attempt to formulate the positive. Of particular note in the mental health literature is the claim by Jahoda nearly 40 years ago of the unsuitability of the absence of mental disease as a criterion for health. Instead, she formulated six criteria of positive mental health: positive self-attitudes, growth and self-actualization, integration of personality, autonomy, reality perception, and environmental mastery.

Philosophical accounts on the meaning of the "good life" provide additional literature of relevance for defining the contours of positive human functioning. Diverse philosophies emphasize the individual's potential to choose and carry out projects; that is, to have active pursuits that give life dignity. Self-command, mastery, and decision making are also prominent in expositions of criterial goods, along with ideas of self-love, self-esteem, and self-respect. Writings about the importance of the interpersonal realm—benevolence, concern and affection for others, companionship, love, deep personal relations—are central to philosophical perspectives. Ideas of human excellence, human flourishing, and the realization of one's true potential are fundamental to Aristotle's eudaemonistic accounts of ethics and the good life. Finally, philosophers have emphasized the focus on *whole lives*; that is, looking at all aspects of an individual's life through time, rather than examining only particular domains of life, fixed in time.

Interestingly, philosophers have been critical of happiness or pleasure as the key target for a good life, noting well-known figures who experienced pleasure in life, but who were unjust, evil, or pointless in their pursuits. Alternatively, the personally desolate lives of those of profound nobility, creativity, courage, or self-sacrifice (e.g., Albert Schweitzer) are elevated in philosophical descriptions of the good life. John Stuart Mill stated, for example, that happiness is not to be attained if made an end in itself, but is the byproduct of other more worthy pursuits.

Taken together, these many lines of psychological theory and philosophical argument converge in their depiction of the good, healthy, positively functioning life as one that involves multiple components of well-being: possessing positive self-regard, setting and pursuing goals, realizing one's unique potential, experiencing deep connections to others, effectively managing surrounding demands and opportunities, and exercising self-direction. These core dimensions comprise central components of the model of psychological well-being that guides the empirical program of research described here.

A. Self-Acceptance

The most recurrent criterion of well-being evident in the previous perspectives is the individual's sense of self-acceptance (see glossary definition). Such positive self-regard is a central feature of mental health as well as a characteristic of self-actualization, optimal functioning, and maturity. Life-span theories also emphasize acceptance of one's self and one's past life, and philosophical criterial goods underscore the importance of self-love, self-esteem, and self-respect. Thus, holding positive attitudes toward oneself emerges as a central feature of psychological well-being.

B. Positive Relations with Others

Many psychological theories emphasize the importance of warm, trusting interpersonal relations. The ability to love is viewed as a central component of mental health. Self-actualizers are described as having strong feelings of empathy and affection for all human beings and as being capable of greater love, deeper friendship, and more complete identification with others. Warm relating to others is a criterion of maturity, and adult developmental stage theories also emphasize the achievement of close unions with others (intimacy) and the guidance and direction of others (generativity). The interpersonal realm (caring for others, benevolence, companionship, affection, deep connections) is elaborated in philosophies of the good life. Thus, many formulations of positive human functioning emphasize quality ties to others.

C. Autonomy

Psychological theories speak of qualities such as self-determination, independence, and the regulation of behavior from within. Self-actualizers are described as showing autonomous functioning and resistance to enculturation. The fully functioning person has an internal locus of evaluation and does not look to others for approval, but evaluates himself or herself by personal standards. Individuation involves a "deliverance from convention" in which one no longer clings to the collective fears, beliefs, and laws of the masses. The process of turning inward in the later years is also seen by life-span developmentalists as giving the individual a sense of freedom from the norms governing everyday life. Philosophical accounts have emphasized the importance of self-command. Taken together, autonomy is repeatedly articulated as a key characteristic of positive functioning.

D. Environmental Mastery

The individual's ability to choose or create environments suitable to his or her psychological needs is defined as a characteristic of mental health. Maturity requires participation in a significant sphere of activity outside of oneself. Life-span development incorporates the ability to manipulate and control complex environments. These theories thus emphasize the individual's ability to act on his or her surrounding worlds, perhaps changing them through physical or mental activities. Successful aging has also been described in terms of the capacity to take advantage of environmental opportunities. Criterial goods in the philosophical literature include capacities for decision making and taking action. In combination, these descriptions point to active participation in and mastery of the environment as key ingredients to positive psychological functioning.

E. Purpose in Life

Mental health in Jahoda's formulation includes the belief that one's life has purpose and meaning. The definition of maturity also emphasizes clear comprehension of life's purpose, a sense of directedness, and intentionality. The life-span developmental theories refer to a variety of changing purposes or goals in life, such as being productive and creative, or achieving emotional integration in later life. Thus, one who functions positively has goals, intentions, and a sense of direction, all of which contribute to a feeling that life is meaningful. The philosophers emphasize the individual's potential to choose and carry out projects that are valuable and give life dignity. Purpose and meaning have also been elaborated in explaining survival under extreme conditions, such as in Victor Frankl's (1969) account of Nazi concentration camps. The role of meaning in understanding positive physical health has been further explicated by Antonovky's (1987) sense of coherence.

F. Personal Growth

Optimal psychological functioning requires not only that one achieve the aforementioned characteristics, but also that one continue to develop talents and potentials, to grow and expand as a person throughout life. The need to actualize oneself and realize one's potential is central to clinical perspectives on personal growth. Openness to experience, for example, is a key characteristic of the fully functioning person. Such an individual is continually developing, rather than achieving a fixed state in which all problems are solved. Life-span theories also give explicit emphasis to continued growth and the facing of new challenges or tasks at different periods of life. And Aristotle's conceptions of human flourishing gave central emphasis to eudaimonia—the imperative to know oneself (one's daimon) and to turn it, as completely as possible, from an ideal to an actuality. Thus, continued growth and self-realization are prominent themes in multiple conceptions of well-being and quality of life.

Despite the extensiveness of these theoretical and philosophical writings about positive human functioning, remarkably little empirical research has been guided by these formulations of well-being. Calls to shift the focus in the positive direction have been sounded as, for example, by the declaration by the World Health Organization nearly 50 years ago that health is a "state of complete physical, mental, and social well-being and not merely the absence of disease or infirmity" (WHO, 1948). Regrettably, there has been scant progress in carrying this conception to the realm of scientific research or practice. Typical indices of health, mental and physical, continue to focus on disease, illness, and negative concepts, *not* on well-being. The following program of empirical research summarizes attempts to focus on the positive.

II. AGE, GENDER, CLASS, AND CULTURAL VARIATIONS IN WELL-BEING

Definitions of the six key dimensions of psychological well-being are provided in the glossary. For the program of empirical research, self-descriptive statements were written to operationalize each of these dimen-

sions and extensive item and scale analyses were conducted to evaluate their psychometric properties (e.g., internal consistency, test-retest reliability, convergent and discriminant validity, confirmatory factor analyses). The original scales consisted of 20 items for each of the six dimensions; subsequent assessments involved reduced depth of measurement (e.g., 14-item scales, 3-item scales), with the shortest version created to include measures in surveys of nationally representative samples. The findings presented here are from multiple studies, including community volunteer samples, local probability samples, national samples, and cross-cultural samples. The research program also encompasses cross-sectional as well as longitudinal designs, the latter of both short-term and long-term intervals (see original studies for measurement and sampling details).

A. Age and Gender Differences

In a series of studies, young, middle-aged, and old adults rated themselves on each of the six dimensions of well-being. Findings revealed a diverse pattern of cross-sectional differences. Certain aspects of well-being, such as environmental mastery and autonomy, showed incremental patterns with age, particularly from young adulthood to midlife. Other aspects, such as personal growth and purpose in life, showed decremental patterns, especially from midlife to old age. Still other aspects, notably positive relations with others and self-acceptance, showed no significant age differences. The consistency of these findings, based on community volunteers ($N = 321$) and the full 20-item scales, was subsequently demonstrated with a national probability sample ($N = 1108$) and dramatically reduced 3-item scales. In both studies, environmental mastery revealed incremental patterns with age, purpose in life and personal growth showed decremental age patterns, and self-acceptance revealed no age differences. Across these studies, women consistently rated themselves higher on positive relations with others than men, and on some studies they also scored higher on personal growth relative to men (including a Korean sample). The remaining aspects of well-being showed no significant differences between men and women.

Recently, the MacArthur Research Network on Midlife Development conducted a national survey (MIDUS: $N = 3032$) of adults aged 25 to 74. Age patterns from this study continue to document the consistency of previous findings (see Figure 1). Specifically, environmental mastery remains significantly higher among older respondents than among young adults or middle-aged persons. Purpose in life and personal growth show declines from young adulthood to midlife to old age. And again, self-acceptance showed no significant age differences. These age patterns held true for both men and women. For men only, positive relations with others was significantly higher among

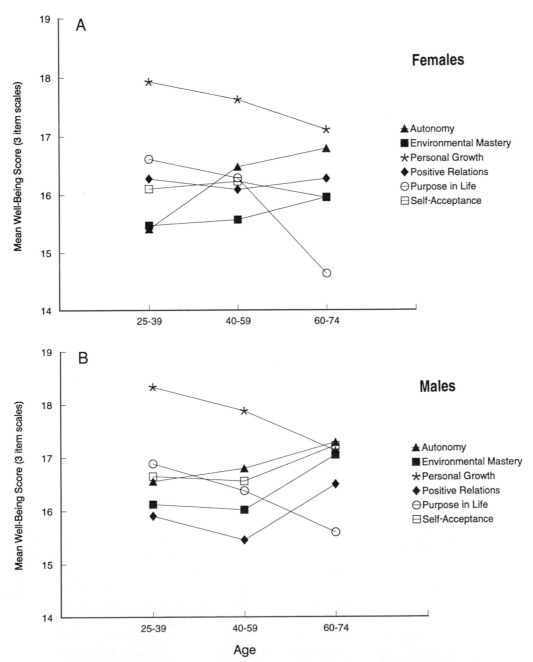

Figure 1   Age and psychological well-being. Source: MIDUS (MacArthur National Survey).

the older compared with the two younger age groups.

Viewed in concert, these cross-sectional studies show apparent gains, losses, and stability for different dimensions of psychological well-being. It is impossible to know, in the absence of longitudinal data, whether these patterns represent aging, maturational processes, or enduring cohort differences. Whatever the interpretation, midlife, compared with earlier and later periods of the life course, reflects truly *middle standing* on positive aspects of psychological functioning. That is, middle-aged respondents show comparable standing to the other age groups on certain aspects of well-being (e.g., self-acceptance), better standing than young adults on some dimensions (e.g., autonomy) and worse on others (e.g., purpose in life, personal growth), and better standing than old adults on some dimensions (e.g., purpose in life, personal growth) and worse on others (e.g., environmental mastery).

Gender differences in this national survey continued to show that women score higher on positive relations with others compared with men. However, in this investigation, which included a wider socioeconomic spectrum of respondents, men, but *only* those with lower levels of education (high school or less), were found to score higher than women on environmental mastery and self-acceptance. The remaining scales continued to show largely similar profiles for men and women, with select exceptions for particular age groups (e.g., old-aged women had significantly lower scores on purpose in life than old-aged men; young adult women had significantly lower scores on personal growth than young adult men; among the young adult and aged respondents, women had lower scores on autonomy than men).

These findings are usefully juxtaposed with previous mental health research, which has repeatedly documented a higher incidence of certain psychological disorders, particularly depression, among women. When positive well-being is considered, however, women show greater strengths compared with men on some aspects of positive functioning (positive relations with others) and comparable profiles for most age groups on most other dimensions. Moreover, when men score higher than women, such differences were frequently restricted to individuals with lower levels of education. Women with higher levels of education show comparable profiles with men on multiple components of psychological functioning. To neglect this portrayal of the positive is to tell an in-

complete and overly negative story about the mental health of women. [*See* GENDER DIFFERENCES IN MENTAL HEALTH.]

B. Class Differences

Is psychological well-being linked with social class standing (typically measured in terms of education, income, and occupational status)? Illustrative findings are reported from the Wisconsin Longitudinal Study (WLS), begun in 1957 with a random sample of more than 10,000 Wisconsin high school graduates. Well-being among a subsample ($N = 6306$) of these individuals, who have been followed from their senior year in high school into midlife (about age 53), shows higher profiles of well-being for those with higher educational attainment (see Figure 2), particularly for purpose in life and personal growth for both men and women. Education for these individuals remains strongly linked with well-being, even after controlling for life history variables (e.g., high school IQ, parental education, income, and occupational status). Those with a higher occupational status in the WLS also show higher well-being. Findings from the National Survey of Families and Households, a nationally representative U.S. sample, also show large educational differences on the six measures of well-being.

The MIDUS national survey further underscores educational differences in well-being and their particular significance for women. For dimensions of environmental mastery, positive relations with others, and self-acceptance, those with college educations rate themselves higher than individuals with less than a college education, with the differences being particularly pronounced for women. For purpose in life and personal growth, there were strong linear educational differences among both men and women. Autonomy was the single dimension of well-being showing no educational differences.

Taken together, these findings speak to the growing literature on class and health, which has documented that those in lower socioeconomic positions have greater likelihood of negative health outcomes. Research on positive psychological functioning extends this tale by demonstrating that lower class standing, indexed here primarily by education, *decreases the likelihood of experiencing well-being*. Because these positive characteristics likely provide important protective factors in the face of stress, challenge, and adversity, their absence suggests other vulnerabilities

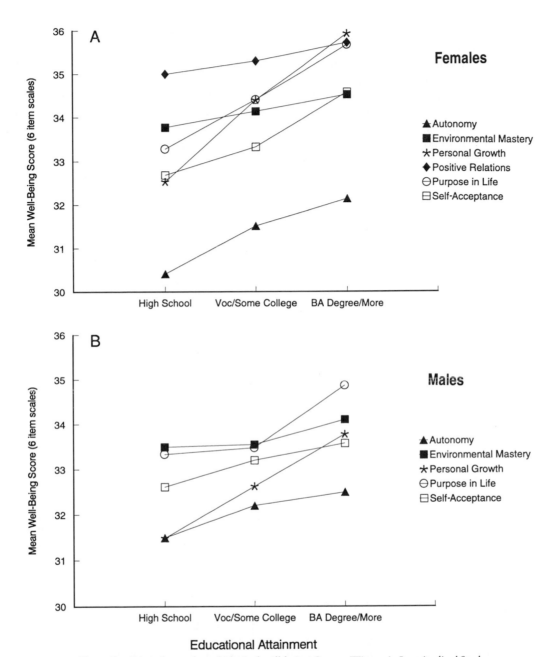

Figure 2 Education and psychological well-being. Source: Wisconsin Longitudinal Study.

among those lower in the socioeconomic hierarchy. [*See* SOCIOECONOMIC STATUS.]

C. Cultural Differences

How culture influences both definitions of and distributions of mental health has received extensive consideration with regard to the negative end of functioning (mental disorders). Far less is known about cultural variations in conceptions and experiences of positive functioning. Extensive work has elaborated differences between individualistic/independent cultures and those that are collectivistic/interdependent. These ideas suggest that more self-oriented aspects of well-being, such as self-acceptance and autonomy, may have greater play in Western cultural contexts, whereas others-oriented dimensions, such as positive relations with others, may be of greater significance in Eastern cultures with collectivist/interdependent orientations. To explore these possibilities, Ryff and colleagues investigated psychological well-being with a midlife sample of American adults and a sociodemographically comparable sample of adults from South Korea.

American adults were found on the whole to rate themselves more highly on these positive qualities than Koreans, a finding consistent with cultural differences in tendencies toward modesty and self-effacement. Despite these large contrasts, analyses of data *within* culture showed that the Koreans, as predicted, scored highest on the measure of positive relations with others and lowest on self-acceptance and personal growth. Among American respondents, personal growth was rated highest, especially for women, and autonomy was rated lowest. In both cultures, women rated themselves higher on positive relations with others and personal growth than men. The study also included qualitative data, which revealed, contrary to prevailing characterizations of Western and Eastern cultures, themes of selfhood (e.g., self-realization, self-knowledge, self-reliance) as well as connection to others (e.g., faithfulness, responsibility, kindness, trust) in *both* Korean and American respondents. Taken together, the findings suggest, contrary to many current characterizations, that individualistic and interdependent aspects of well-being were evident in both cultural contexts.

III. EVENTS, EXPERIENCES, AND WELL-BEING: THE CASE OF PARENTHOOD

The preceding summary of sociodemographic variations in psychological well-being, despite the systematic, replicable nature of effects, account for surprisingly little (usually less than 10%) of the overall variance in positive psychological functioning. To sharpen understanding of how well-being is fostered or hindered, we also look at the actual substance of people's lives, that is, their life events and experiences. Some of these are discrete transitions, such as community relocation in later life, an increasingly typical event for aged women, many of whom outlive their

husbands and move, at some point, to an apartment or retirement community. Other experiences are more enduring, such as growing up with an alcoholic parent. Some are common and normative, such as raising children, whereas others are uncommon and not normative, such as caring for a child with mental retardation. Physical health problems in later life have also been studied with regard to their impact on psychological functioning. Across these inquiries, we investigate theory-based, sociopsychological processes that help explain how individuals give meaning to and are influenced by their experiences. These include social comparisons, reflected appraisals, attributions, and assessments of importance or centrality.

Findings from the research on parenting are briefly summarized to illustrate the particular linkage of life experience and well-being in midlife. Parenthood is a common experience among midlife adults, including approximately 90% of those between the ages of 35 and 64. Although an extensive body of literature has examined the effects of parents on the development and well-being of their children, much less research has elaborated how parents themselves are affected by having and raising children, and what research does exist details largely the negative effects of children on marital satisfaction, parental depression, and so on. Our question was whether children contribute, for example, to parents' feelings of self-regard and their sense of purpose and meaning in life.

Parenthood is an experience of lengthy duration, and its effects on parents' well-being may differ depending on the age and caregiving demands of the children. We chose to examine parental links with psychological well-being at a particular point, namely, when children are emerging as adults in their own right and parents have a sense of how they have "turned out." In looking at the products of their parental investment, what do parents see and how does it relate to their assessments of multiple aspects of their own well-being? Midlife parents ($N = 215$) were asked to evaluate the lives of their grown children in terms of their personal and social well-being as well as their educational and occupational achievements.

We found that parents' assessments of children's personal and social adjustment were strongly predictive of their own well-being—those who saw their children as well-adjusted had higher levels of many aspects of well-being, but especially environmental mastery, purpose in life, and self-acceptance (and lower levels of depression). These findings were true for midlife mothers and fathers, although mothers' well-being was more strongly predicted by the adjustment of sons rather than daughters. Children's educational and occupational achievements were weaker predictors of parental well-being.

We also found that parents' well-being was further predicted by social comparison ratings (i.e., how well parents felt they compared with their adult children) and attribution ratings (i.e., the extent to which they saw themselves as responsible for children's life outcomes). Contrary to our predictions, but consistent with previous social comparison research, parents had *lower* well-being if they perceived that their children had done *better* than themselves, with such effects restricted largely to the domain of children's personal and social adjustment. Parents also had lower well-being if they saw themselves as having children who had not turned out well *and* simultaneously believed they had exercised little responsibility for these outcomes. Presumably, such parents suffer from the combined effects of their children's difficulties in adulthood and their own regrets as parents.

Overall then, parenthood emerges as a realm of experience having clear linkage to the well-being of midlife adults: how one's children turn out, how one compares with them, and the degree of responsibility taken for their children's lives are all tied to multiple aspects of mothers' and fathers' psychological self-evaluations. [*See* PARENTING.]

IV. LIFE HISTORIES AND WELL-BEING: UNRAVELING THE MYSTERIES OF RESILIENCE

Although single life event/experience studies are informative in establishing specific linkages between the nature of the experience and well-being, they capture only a small part of an overall life. To understand the influence of multiple events and experiences across multiple life domains, it is necessary to adopt a life history approach to the study of well-being. We explore this richer, more complex array of unfolding experience with life histories of members of the Wisconsin Longitudinal Study.

Our approach draws on numerous conceptual frameworks, including the limited differences theory, which examines the events to which individuals are exposed over their lives and their reactions to these events. Over short intervals, events and reactions to them produce small, or limited differences in outcome measures. Such small differences tend to accumulate, however, and over the life course, these cumulative effects can substantially influence diverse outcomes, including mental health. These ideas, and others, are elaborated as *organizing principles* to guide the task of working with multidomain (e.g., work, family, leisure, community, health) life history data that span more than three decades (high school to midlife). Such principles draw on the extensive existing literature. They are stated here as hypotheses of factors influencing the health outcomes of interest.

1. *Adversity and its cumulation over time has negative health consequences.* That negative events and chronic life conditions contribute to physical and mental health problems is an idea of long-standing presence in health research, particularly in the human and animal literatures on stress. The life history approach calls for tracking of negative experience (events and chronic conditions) in multiple life domains, thereby capturing patterns of "pileup" (simultaneous problems in work, family, neighborhood, etc.). Cumulation also points to the enduring, persistent features of life strains, which are key to understanding the physiological substrates involved in illness and disease, or, more generally, the connections between mental stress and physical health.

2. *Advantage and its cumulation over time has positive health consequences.* Because our approach seeks to explicate not just states of mental or physical illness, but also positive health, we also track the positive features of individual lives. These may come in multiple forms: starting resources (e.g., intact family, high socioeconomic status parents), personal capacities and abilities (e.g., high IQ, optimism), and positive events (e.g., job promotions, births of desired children). Although adversity is believed to compromise health, experiences of advantage are hypothesized to provide protective and buffering resources.

3. *Reactions to adversity and advantage exacerbate or ameliorate the impact of life experiences.* Consistent with extensive previous research on how individuals perceive and cope with stressful life experiences, we see reactions to and interpretations of what happens in life as central to understanding mechanisms that affect mental and physical health. However, because our life histories include not only unexpected life

events, but also chronic conditions, normative life transitions, and general life evaluations, we broaden the scope of what is typically examined as reactive responses.

4. *Position in social hierarchies across life domains has health consequences.* Social hierarchies are viewed as ubiquitous features of human and animal life. We adopt an expansive view of hierarchy that includes traditional socioeconomic status (SES) classifications (e.g., education, income, occupational status), but also consider ability hierarchies, positions of influence in the family and community, and degree of autonomy and authority in the workplace. We propose that negative health results from the cumulative effects of low social standing across diverse domains, and, alternatively, that high social standing in stable hierarchies and its cumulation over time has positive health consequences. Assessment of hierarchy is conducted at both social structural and individual levels; the former captures actual position in a distribution (e.g., occupational status hierarchy), and the latter involves subjective evaluations of one's lot in life relative to others (e.g., social comparison processes).

5. *Social relationships can exacerbate or ameliorate the impact of life experience and enduring conditions.* This principle reflects the vast literature on social supports and their role in reactivity to life stress. Following in this tradition, we examine the helping or hindering role of quality relationships in the face of difficult life experiences; in addition, we also consider the presence of quality ties to significant others as enhancing experiences (psychologically, emotionally, physiologically) that protect and maintain the integrity of the organism.

In WLS, we draw on these principles to understand the mental health profiles of the respondents, as assessed in midlife (approximate age, 52/53). We briefly describe findings for one select group of respondents: resilient women. To be classified as resilient, respondents had to have reported a prior episode (or episodes) of serious depression (assessed with a subset of items from the Composite International Diagnostic Interview) at some time in their life, but also to have reported high levels of psychological well-being (using the previously described six dimensions) at the time of data collection in 1992 and 1993, when respondents were approximately age 52 or 53—168 women in the study fit this description.

We begin with detailed biographies of randomly selected cases from this group and progressively thinned the 250 variables with which the analysis began to a reduced subset that covered multiple aspects of their early life resources (e.g., parental education, intact family, IQ, high school grades), chronic conditions (e.g., alcohol problem at home, stressful work conditions) and the age intervals over which the conditions occurred, acute events and the age of the respondent at the time of their occurrence (e.g., death of parent, occupational advancement), quality of social relationships, social integration, and social comparisons with parents and siblings. Complex strings of life characteristics or conditions were created in the form of Boolean statements (logical AND/OR statements). We note that although rich in information about chronic conditions and acute events across multiple life domains and position in SES hierarchies, WLS data are relatively weak in assessment of reactions to life experiences and quality relationship indicators (new data collection designed to alleviate these deficiencies is underway).

The larger objective was to retain the richness and texture of individual lives and, at the same time, simplify the variables into more parsimonious summaries. These procedures resulted in the differentiation of four life history pathways of resilience among the WLS women. Briefly summarized here, the first pathway (subgroup H_1) as composed of women with generally positive beginnings (e.g., high starting abilities, no alcoholism in childhood home) and subsequent experience of upward job mobility. They also perceived that their achievements in life compared favorably with their parents and siblings. Despite these advantages, all of these women had experienced the death of one parent, most had participated in caregiving for an ill person, and approximately half had two or more chronic conditions. Thus, their lives involved multiple difficulties of particular acute or chronic adversities that were offset by positive work experiences, good beginnings, and favorable self-evaluations.

The second subgroup, H_2, was composed of women for whom the primary early-life adversity was growing up with alcohol problems in the childhood home. All women in the subgroup met this condition. In addition, many (65%) of these women had experienced three or more major acute events (e.g., death of parent, child, spouse; divorce; job loss). However, the women had important advantages in social relationships and social participation, early employment with stable or upward occupational status, and positive social comparisons. The latter pluses are presumably part of why the women reported high psychological well-being, despite their early and later life adversities.

The third subgroup, H_3, showed primarily advantage in early life: all had parents who were both high school graduates, no alcohol problems existed in the childhood home, and the women had high starting abilities (high school grades, IQ). Later, however, they confronted various forms of adversity (e.g., poor social relationships, downward occupational mobility, job loss, divorce, single parenthood, caregiving). Thus, their lives were characterized by various forms of family adversity occurring largely in adulthood, but they began their life journeys with important strengths that likely facilitated their recovery from adverse experiences.

The final subgroup, H_4, were women whose early lives showed mixed advantages (intact families, no alcoholism) and disadvantage (all had one parent with less than a high school diploma). As life unfolded, these women confronted an array of adversities: job loss, downward mobility, living with alcohol problems in the home, divorce/single parenthood, and high profiles of major acute events. This array of negatives, combined with their less than uniformly positive beginnings, makes difficult the explanation for their resilience. As such, this subgroup underscores the need for additional information pertaining, for example, to their reactions to different life challenges or the quality of their significant social relationships.

Overall, the analyses underscore the diversity in what was bad and good in these women's lives: difficulties occurred across multiple life domains; some were chronic and enduring, others acute; some occurred early in life, others in adulthood. Their advantages and resources also varied across the life domains in which they occurred. From this variety emerged differing tales of why the women may have succumbed to depression as well as their routes out of it. Thus, rather than present a uniform characterization of the life histories of all 168 resilient women, our analysis clarified diverse pathways through adversity to high psychological well-being. The protective role of positive experiences or advantage (e.g., good starting resources), quality social relationships, advancements in work hierarchies, and favorable reactions (e.g., positive social comparisons) is central to the resilience story.

V. LINKING MENTAL AND PHYSICAL HEALTH: THE PHYSIOLOGICAL SUBSTRATES OF WELL-BEING

How the mind and body influence each other has been a long-standing human interest. Most scientific work has addressed negative influences of mind on body, or body on mind. An extensive literature on stress, for example, links negative mental perceptions and behavioral responses to stress with physiological and biochemical processes, and draws further connections with neuroendocrine, immune, and sympathetic nervous systems tied to disease outcomes. Our interest, in contrast, is to push forward an agenda that addresses the *positive interworkings* of mind and body. Much of this initiative is rethinking what is known about the negative spirals of mind–body interactions and asking how they unfold in salubrious, healthful ways. [*See* PSYCHONEUROIMMUNOLOGY; STRESS.]

In 1993 McEwen and Stellar proposed allostatic load—meaning the cumulative strain on multiple organs and tissues resulting from repeated fluctuations in physiological response to perceived threat—as a measure of organ-system breakdown and ultimately disease. There are two central features to the accumulation of allostatic load. One reflects wear and tear associated with acute shifts (generally elevations) in physiologic activity in response to specific stimuli. The second contributing feature to allostatic load is chronic elevations in physiologic activity outside of basal operating ranges.

Allostatic load has been operationalized with a number of indicators of physiological system impairment: high systolic and diastolic blood pressure are indices of cardiovascular activity; waist–hip ratio is an index of metabolism and adipose tissue deposition; serum HDL and total cholesterol are indices of atherosclerotic risk; blood plasma levels of glycosylated hemoglobin indicate glucose metabolism; 12-hour, integrated measure of urinary cortisol excretion is an indicator of HPA axis activity; and urinary epinephrine and norepinephrine excretion levels are indices of sympathetic nervous system (SNS) activity. In a study of elderly persons in the United States, those with higher allostatic load scores and no reported cardiovascular disease (meaning myocardial infarction, stroke, diabetes, or high blood pressure) at baseline in 1988 predicted 2.5 years later a subsequent decline in cognitive function, particularly memory decline, and also a decline in physical performance. As one would expect, allostatic load also predicted increased incidence of cardiovascular disease. [*See* HYPERTENSION; HEART DISEASE: PSYCHOLOGICAL PREDICTORS.]

Central to a positive health agenda is the question of *optimal allostasis*. That is, previous research has focused nearly exclusively on failures in the adaptation process rather than on how positive working of the physiologic system responds to stress. Dienstbier's formulation of "physiological toughness" is an exception to the prevailing concern for pathogenesis. This is a pattern of arousal (i.e., low SNS arousal base rates combined with strong, responsive challenge-induced SNS-adrenal-medullary arousal, with resistance to brain catecholamine depletion and suppression of pituitary-adrenal-cortical responses) that works in interaction with effective psychological coping to comprise positive physiological reactivity. Extrapolating over time, optimal allostasis then embodies the cumulative, long-term pattern of resistance to catecholamine depletion (SNS activity), rapid return of cortisol levels (HPA axis reactivity) to normal operating range after stress exposure, and maintenance within optimal operating ranges of the remaining markers (e.g., blood pressure, waist–hip ratio, cholesterol).

Across these formulations of optimal allostasis and physiological toughness, mind/body feedback processes are repeatedly emphasized—how events are construed or interpreted and how individuals cope with them have a major influence on how the physiological cascades unfold. And there are substantial individual differences in mental and physiological components of the stress response. We posit that psychological well-being and its variability can help to explain how and why these individual differences come about. A summary of the 30-year literature on the psychological modulation of immunity by Maier and colleagues underscores that the impact of stress on immunity cannot be explained in strictly physical or biological terms. Emotions and thoughts are central to understanding immune processes, but again, the examples compiled are all negative, for example, associations of depression with dysregulation of the pituitary-adrenal system and chronically elevated levels of glucocorticoids in the blood, or the effects of divorce and final exams on immune function.

On the positive side, it is important to consider how positive mental states contribute to *recovery* from health threats and to *enhancement or protection* of the organism. In 1988 Melnechuk summarized a literature on positive feelings, religious beliefs, and expression of goals and hopes as they relate to regression of cancers and other autoimmune disorders. Persons with positive life outlooks also show differences in wound healing and tissue repair. Quality relationships, another key dimension of being well, are implicated in survival time and breast cancer. Elderly nursing home residents who became involved in decision making and who received coping skills training showed cortisol responses to challenge resolution that were below pretraining baseline levels. Similarly, cortisol reactivity to naturalistic challenge in the elderly showed a sharp increase followed by rapid return to basal levels *only* for individuals with high self-esteem.

A central question for future mind–body research is how do positive experience and mental well-being serve *protective* roles? We propose that psychological well-being (deeply felt purposes, quality ties to others, self-regard, sense of mastery, etc.) provides a bedrock of mental resources that contribute to optimal allostasis and physiological toughness, and, hence, maintenance of positive physical health. That is, enduring experiences with personally meaningful life goals and love relationships facilitate optimal operating ranges for multiple biological systems and these, in turn, modulate immune factors and neuroendocrine response to challenge. Numerous autobiographical accounts, such as Victor Frankl's survival in Nazi concentration camps, Mark Mathabane's childhood under apartheid in South Africa, and Kay Jamison's successful struggle with manic-depressive illness, speak poignantly to the power of meaningful life pursuits and supportive love relationships. Furthermore, these accounts implicate physical health consequences and suggest underlying processes, such as immune function. The specification of the pathways from these protective factors to underlying physiological substrates is critical to the advancement of a positive mind–body health agenda.

Other avenues for explicating individual differences in protective factors follow from the vast literatures on how people react to, appraise, interpret, make sense of, and cope with their life experiences. Such meaning-giving activities are strongly implicated in mental health outcomes (e.g., attributional styles and depression), but again, the focus has been largely on *maladaptive* interpretations and coping mechanisms, rather than on *constructive* reactions. Moreover, connections between these higher-order cognitive activities and underlying neuroendocrine, immune, and sympathetic nervous systems remain a scientific frontier, particularly with regard to the positive, healthy, adaptive interworkings of these mind–body processes.

A final avenue for future work on protective mechanisms pertains to behavioral activities. Physical fitness through regular aerobic exercise is an important means for self-regulated toughening. A host of animal and human studies document the salubrious psychological and physiological consequences of exercise training. These benefits include those linked with the characterization of toughening: lower arousal base rates, including heart rate and blood pressure; quicker return to arousal base rate after stress; improved glucose utilization; and more circulating monocytes (active in resisting bacterial infection). We propose that physiological benefits of good health practices, ensuing from exercise as well as proper diet, adequate sleep, and so on, are more likely realized by those with high psychological well-being. That is, taking care of oneself presupposes a life worth taking care of, and in so doing, illustrates the fundamental connections between mental well-being, behavioral health practices, intervening physiological mechanisms, and physical health outcomes. [*See* EXERCISE AND MENTAL HEALTH; PHYSICAL ACTIVITY AND MENTAL HEALTH.]

Returning to the question of resilience—why some individuals prevail in the face of great difficulty and life challenge—we suggest that ultimate explanations will involve complex interworkings of the mind *and* the body. Thus, it is those who possess multiple protective factors (i.e., a solid foundation of psychological well-being, a positive lens through which problems are interpreted, positive behavioral practices) who will also show optimal allostasis, physiological toughness, and effective immune function. Such physiological benefits will, in turn, protect the body from disease, thereby feeding back to optimal mental states. Thus, what will be in active motion is a positive mind–body spiral of health.

ACKNOWLEDGMENTS

This research was supported by the John D. and Catherine T. MacArthur Foundation Research Network on Successful Midlife Development (Ryff), the Socioeconomic Status and Health Network (Singer), and grants from the National Institute on Aging (R01AG0879–Ryff & Essex, R01AG013613–Ryff & Singer) and the National Institute of Health Center for Research Resources to the University of Wisconsin Medical School (M01 RR03186).

BIBLIOGRAPHY

Antonovsky, A. (1987). *Unraveling the mystery of health*. San Francisco: Jossey-Bass.

Becker, L. C. (1992). Good lives: Prolegomena. *Social Philosophy and Policy, 9*, 15–37.

Bumpass, L. L., & Aquilino, W. S. (1994). A social map of midlife: Family and work over the middle life course. Vero Beach, FL: John D. and Catherine T. MacArthur Research Network on Successful Midlife Development.

Dienstbier, R. A. (1989). Arousal and physiological toughness: Implications for mental and physical health. *Psychological Review, 96*, 84–100.

Heidrich, S. M., & Ryff, C. D. (1993). Physical and mental health in later life: The self-system as mediator. *Psychology and Aging, 8*, 327–338.

Maier, S. F., Watkins, L. R., & Fleshner, M. (1994). Psychoneuroimmunology: The interface of behavior, brain, and immunity. *American Psychologist, 49*, 1004–1017.

McEwen, B. S., & Stellar, E. (1993). Stress and the individual. *Archives of Internal Medicine, 153*, 2093–2101.

Ryff, C. D. (1989a). Beyond Ponce de Leon and life satisfaction: New directions in quest of successful aging. *International Journal of Behavioral Development, 12*, 35–55.

Ryff, C. D. (1989b). Happiness is everything, or is it?: Explorations on the meaning of psychological well-being. *Journal of Personality and Social Psychology, 57*, 1069–1081.

Ryff, C. D., & Essex, M. J. (1992). The interpretation of experience and well-being: The sample case of relocation. *Psychology and Aging, 7*, 507–517.

Ryff, C. D., & Keyes, C. L. M. (1995). The structure of psychological well-being revisited. *Journal of Personality and Social Psychology, 69*, 719–727.

Ryff, C. D., Lee, Y. H., Essex, M. J., & Schmutte, P. S. (1994). My children and me: Midlife evaluations of grown children and of self. *Psychology and Aging, 9*, 195–205.

Ryff, C. D., & Magee, W. J. (1995). *Opportunity, achievement, and well-being: A midlife perspective*. Paper presented at the American Psychological Association Meetings, New York, NY.

Seeman, T. E., Singer, B. H., McEwen, B. S., Horwitz, R. J., & Rowe, J. W. (1997). The price of adaptation—allostatic load and its health consequences: MacArthur Studies of Successful Aging. *Archives for Internal Medicine, 157*, 2259–2268.

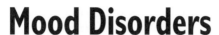

Mood Disorders

Charles DeBattista, H. Brent Solvason, and Alan F. Schatzberg

Stanford University School of Medicine

MOOD DISORDERS represent a common and heterogeneous group of disorders. According to the third edition of the *American Heritage Dictionary,* mood refers to "an emotional state," while affect is a verb that means "to act on one's emotions." The clinician tends to regard mood as a subjective state described by the patient, while affect is objective evidence of the mood state observed clinically. Mood disorders and affective disorders have been used synonymously to describe the four major mood disorders and their variations: major depressive disorder, bipolar disorder, Dysthymia, and Cyclothymia. However the current nosology, *DSM-IV,* uses the term "mood disorders" as a more encompassing class of psychopathology, since these disorders may not always be apparent as disorders of affect.

I. CLINICAL SYNDROMES

A. Major Depressive Episode

Major Depression represents a syndrome of both emotional and physical signs and symptoms lasting for at least two weeks (see Table I). Depression differs from sadness in its persistent quality, its physical manifestations, and by the fact that it significantly affects the ability of the patient to function normally. A major depressive episode can range from mild to incapacitating and life threatening. [*See* DEPRESSION.]

The symptom of depression most associated with depression is depressed mood. Depressed patients will often describe a gradually worsening sadness that becomes oppressive and unremitting. At times this dejection comes on abruptly after a significant stressor. However, some patients will develop depressive episodes that are cyclic in nature and seem to have little to do with external stressors. A few patients will not complain of depressed mood at all. They may describe other dysphoric states such as apathy, irritability, numbness, and so on. The description of mood states occurs within a specific social and cultural context. For instance, males in many cultures will be averse to endorsing depressed mood, but may describe other uncomfortable mood states.

Anhedonia, or loss of interest or pleasure in usual activities, is the other symptom that occurs in most patients with Major Depression. Activities that were previously enjoyed hold no or little interest in the patient. Recreational activities often cease, and work activities become a struggle. Libido, or sexual interest, tends to diminish along with other interests.

In addition to anhedonia and/or depressed mood, patients with Major Depression experience a variety of vegetative symptoms that affect energy, sleep, and appetite. Fatigue is experienced by most patients with Major Depression and is often the presenting symptom. The patient may feel that there is something physically wrong with them and seek advice from their general practitioner. Some patients describe a heaviness in the limbs and find that even small tasks are exhausting.

Sleep disturbance in Major Depression can take any form but is classically characterized by early morning

Table I   *DSM-IV* Criteria for Major Depressive Episode*

A. Five or more of the symptoms listed below have been present during the same 2-week period and represent a change from previous functioning; at least one of the symptoms is either depressed mood or loss of interest or pleasure.

(1) Depressed mood most of the day nearly every day, as indicated either by subjective report (e.g., feels sad or empty) or observations of others (e.g., appears tearful). Note: In children and adolescents, can be irritable mood.

(2) Markedly diminished interest or pleasure in all, or almost all, activities most of the day nearly every day, as indicated by subjective account or observations of others.

(3) Significant weight loss when not dieting or weight gain (e.g., a change of more than 5% body weight in one month or decrease or increase in appetite nearly every day. Note: In children, failure to achieve expected weight gains.

(4) Insomnia or hypersomnia nearly every day.

(5) Psychomotor agitation or retardation nearly every day, as indicated not merely by subjective feelings of restlessness or being slowed down but by observations of others.

(6) Fatigue or loss of energy nearly every day.

(7) Feelings of worthlessness or excessive or inappropriate guilt (which may be delusional) nearly every day, as indicated not merely by self-reproach or guilt about being sick.

(8) Diminished ability to think or concentrate or indecisiveness nearly every day, as indicated either by subjective account or observations of others.

(9) Recurrent thoughts of death (not just fear of dying), recurrent suicidal ideation without a specific plan, or a suicide attempt or a specific plan for committing suicide.

B. The symptoms do not meet criteria for a mixed episode.

C. The symptoms cause clinically significant distress or impairment in social, occupational, or other important areas of functioning.

D. The symptoms are not due to the direct physiological effects of a substance (e.g., an abused drug, a medication) or a general medical condition (e.g., hypothyroidism).

E. The symptoms are not better accounted for by bereavement (i.e., after the loss of a loved one) or the symptoms persist for longer than 2 months or are characterized by marked functional impairment, morbid preoccupation with worthlessness, suicidal ideation, psychotic symptoms, or psychomotor retardation.

*Reproduced with permission of APA Press.

awakenings with an inability to fall back asleep (terminal insomnia). These awakenings occur at least 2 hours before usual awakening. Patients typically feel at their worst in the early morning, but may feel somewhat better as the day progresses (diurnal variation of depression). Patients may have other types of sleep disturbance, including having trouble falling asleep (initial insomnia), trouble with waking up in the middle of the night (middle insomnia), or sleeping too much (hypersomnia). [*See* SLEEP.]

Appetite may be significantly impacted in depressed patients. Anorexia, or a loss of appetite, often occurs in depressed patients. The most severely depressed patients can require feeding tubes because they have lost all interest in food. Some loss of weight is common. However, other depressed patients gain weight when they are depressed and will find not overeating to be a significant struggle. [*See* ANOREXIA NERVOSA AND BULIMIA NERVOSA.]

Feelings of worthlessness, hopelessness, and guilt are also very common in Major Depression. Patients may dwell on previous indiscretions long ignored before the depressive episode, and decide that they are being punished for earlier sins. Sometimes, this guilt can take on delusional proportions and the patient is then said to have a psychotic depression. Those afflicted often feel hopeless that things will get any better and may feel they are a burden with nothing to contribute to their friends, family or society.

Most depressed patients will entertain thoughts of death at some point in their illness. These thoughts are often passive in nature: wishing they would die in their sleep or cease to exist. However, depressed patients commonly develop specific suicidal thoughts, and approximately 15% of untreated patients succeed in eventually killing themselves. [*See* SUICIDE.]

Patients with Major Depression often have their first episode in early adulthood, but 50% of patients experienced a first depressive episode after age 40. The mean age of onset for Major Depression is around age 40. An untreated episode tends to last from 6 to 12 months, but 20% of patients will have episodes that last for more than 2 years. Recurrences are expected in Major Depression, with at least 75% of patients having a second episode within 10 years of the first episode.

B. Bipolar Disorder

Along with Major Depression, bipolar, or manic depressive disorder, represents a major mood disorder. "Bipolar" refers to the fact that patients may experience two clinical poles: depression, and mania or hypomania. Most bipolar patients experience multiple cycles of depression interspersed with mania or hypomania. Less than 10% of bipolar patients tend to only experience manic-type episodes and not depression. However, any patient who experiences at least one hypomanic episode, that is not explained by another disorder, is conventionally described as bipolar.

A manic episode may be thought of as the flip side of a depressive episode. Instead of patients feeling depressed, they may feel euphoric and on top of the world. However, as the manic episode evolves, panic and dysphoria may be common features. Instead of feeling fatigued and lacking in energy, the manic patient has more energy than he can handle, and may need very little sleep or no sleep at all. Rather than feeling bad about himself like the patient in a depressive episode, the manic patient may be quite grandiose. Likewise, anhedonia in the depressed patient is replaced by an increase in goal-directed activity in which the patient may try to accomplish too much and have extremely unrealistic goals. There is often a certain impulsivity that may get manic patients into trouble in business and legal transactions as well as interpersonally. Their judgment tends to be impaired during manic states. For example, they may impulsively spend their life savings on a foolish business venture, or take a flight on the impulse that it would be nice to be in a different country. Manic patients may lose contact with reality, become floridly psychotic, and experience hallucinations as well as paranoid or grandiose delusions. A formal thought disorder characterized by disorganized, tangential, or circumstantial thought may be more common in mania than it is in schizophrenia. More rarely, impulsive criminal acts may occur during a manic state. Violent acts are sometimes carried out that are uncharacteristic of the patient. By convention, manic episodes must last at least 1 week but tend to average 8 to 16 weeks. Bipolar patients may have manic and depressive episodes that occur four or more times a year (rapid-cycling bipolar illness), but more commonly the episodes are separated by 6 months to a year as the illness progresses. Patients who experience full manic episodes as opposed to hypomanic periods are said to suffer from Bipolar I Disorder. About 10 manic episodes in a lifetime is the mean for bipolar I patients, but many patients suffer from more frequent episodes. (See Table II.)

Bipolar I Disorder may begin in childhood, but more commonly begins in early adulthood. The earlier the onset, the worse the prognosis tends to be. The mean age of onset is approximately 30 years old. The index or first mood disturbance in bipolar patients tends to be Major Depression. This depression can precede the advent of manic episodes by many years. Bipolar disorder is characterized by episodic cycles with a relative remission of symptoms between episodes.

Sometimes, bipolar patients will have episodes with features of depression and mania simultaneously. For example, they may describe high energy and decreased need for sleep, but complain of severe depression and suicidal thoughts. These episodes are referred to as mixed episodes and appear less common than manic, hypomanic, or depressed episodes.

A hypomanic episode, on the other hand is a grade below mania in its presentation. It may have a shorter duration than a typical manic episode (4 days or longer), is not characterized by psychosis, and is not of sufficient intensity that the patient requires hospitalization. The symptoms of hypomania are otherwise like the symptoms of mania including increased energy, hyperverbal speech, grandiosity, increase in goal directed activity, and so on, but of lower severity. Some bipolar disorders are characterized only by hypomanic episodes interspersed with Major Depression and are called Bipolar II Disorder, to distinguish them from classic or Bipolar I Disorder in which the patient has full blown manic episodes.

Bipolar II Disorder, like Bipolar I, often begins in early adulthood with a major depressive episode. The hypomanic episodes tend to be briefer than manic episodes, and rapid cycling appears to be more common than in Bipolar I Disorder. Cyclothymia often evolves into Bipolar II Disorder, and in turn, bipolar II sometimes evolves into bipolar I.

C. Dysthymic Disorder

Dysthymic Disorder is a low-grade depression lasting at least 2 years and often a lifetime. Like Major Depression, it is characterized by depressed mood. How-

Table II *DSM-IV* Criteria for Manic Episode *

A. A distinct period of abnormally and persistently elevated, expansive, or irritable mood, lasting at least one week (or any duration if hospitalization is necessary).

B. During the period of mood disturbance, three (or more) of the following symptoms have persisted (four if the mood is only irritable) and have been present to a significant degree:
  1. Inflated self-esteem or grandiosity;
  2. Decreased need for sleep (e.g., feels rested after only 3 hours of sleep);
  3. More talkative than usual or feels pressure to keep talking;
  4. Flight of ideas or subjective experience that thoughts are racing;
  5. Distractibility (i.e., attention to or easily drawn to unimportant or irrelevant external stimuli);
  6. Increase in goal-directed avtivity (socially, at work or school, or sexually) or psychomotor agitation;
  7. Excessive involvement in pleasurable activities that have a high potential for painful consequences (e.g., engaging in unrestrained buying sprees, sexual indiscretions, or foolish business investments).

C. The symptoms do not meet criteria from mixed episode.

D. The mood disturbance is sufficiently severe to cause marked impairment in occupational functioning in usual social activities or relationships with others or to necessitate hospitalization to prevent harm to self or others, or there are psychotic features.

E. The symptoms are not due to the direct physiological effects of a substance (e.g., an abused drug, a medication, or other treatment) or a general medical condition (e.g., hyperthyroidism). Note: Manic-like episodes that are clearly caused by somatic antidepressant treatment (e.g., medication, electroconvulsive therapy, light therapy) should not count toward a diagnosis of bipolar I disorder.

DSM-IV Criteria for Hypomanic Episode

A. A distinct period of persistently elevated, expansive, or irritable mood, lasting at least 4 days, that is clearly different from the usual nondepressed mood.

B. During the period of mood disturbance, three (or more) of the following symptoms have persisted (four if the mood is only irritable) and have been present to a significant degree:
  1. Inflated self-esteem or grandiosity;
  2. Decreased need for sleep (e.g., feels rested after only 3 hours of sleep);
  3. More talkative than usual or feels pressure to keep talking;
  4. Flight of ideas or subjective experience that thoughts are racing;
  5. Distractibility (i.e., attention too easily drawn to unimportant or irrelevant external stimuli);
  6. Increase in goal-directed activity (either socially, at work or school, or sexually) or psychomotor agitation;
  7. Excessive involvement in pleasurable activities that have a high potential for painful consequences (e.g., the person engages in unrestrained buying sprees, sexual indiscretions, or foolish business investments).

C. The episode is associated with an unequivocal change in functioning that is uncharacteristic of the person when not symptomatic.

D. The disturbance in mood and the change in functioning are observable by others.

E. The episode is not severe enough to cause marked impairment in social or occupational functioning or to necessitate hospitalization, and there are no psychotic features.

F. The symptoms are not due to the direct physiological effects of a substance (e.g., an abused drug, a medication, or other treatment) or a general medical condition (e.g., hyperthyroidism). Note: Hypomanic-like episodes that are clearly caused by somatic antidepressant treatment (e.g., medication, electroconvulsive therapy, light therapy) should not count toward a diagnosis of bipolar II disorder.

*Reproduced with permission of APA Press.

ever, the depressed mood need only be present more days than not, rather than most of the day every day as in Major Depression. Energy, appetite, and sleep disturbance may be present but not in the incapacitating way that is evident in Major Depression. Dysthymic Disorder tends to be more characterized by chronic, lifelong patterns of low self-esteem and pessimism, rather than discrete episodes of more severe depression. Thus, a mild depression pervades the personality of the dysthymic person to the extent that

such a person can often not recall not being depressed. (See Table III.)

Dysthymia usually begins gradually in adolescence or early adulthood. Patients often describe themselves as being depressed since birth. The disorder tends to define the person to some extent, and afflicted patients regard the Dysthymia as part of who they are. Dysthymic Disorder appears to be a risk factor for other mood disorders. For example, at least 20% of dysthymic patients go on to develop major depressive epi-

Table III *DSM-IV* Criteria for Dysthymia *

A. Depressed mood for most of the day more days than not for at least 2 years, as indicated either by subjective account or observations of others. Note: In children and adolescents, mood can be irritable, and duration must be at least 1 year.

B. Presence, while depressed, of two (or more) of the following:

    1. Poor appetite or overeating;

    2. Insomnia or hypersomnia;

    3. Low energy or fatigue;

    4. Low self-esteem;

    5. Poor concentration or difficulty making decisions;

    6. Feelings of hopelessness.

C. During the past 2-year period (one year for children or adolescents) of the disturbance, the person has never been without the symptoms in Criteria A and B for more than 2 months at a time.

D. No major depressive episode has been present during the first 2 years of the disturbance (1 year for children and adolescents), i.e., the disturbance is not better accounted for by chronic major depressive disorder or major depressive disorder in partial remission.

E. There has never been a manic episode, a mixed episode, or a hypomanic episode; and criteria has not been met for cyclothymic disorder.

F. The disturbance does not occur exclusively during the course of a chronic psychotic disorder, such as schizophrenia or delusional disorder.

G. The symptoms are not due to the direct psysiological effects of a substance (e.g., an abused drug or a medication) or a general medical condition (e.g., hypothyroidism).

H. The symptoms cause clinically significant distress or impairment in social, occupational, or other important areas of functioning.

*Reproduced with permission of APA Press.

sodes. Such patients may have Dysthymia interspersed with discrete, more severe, major depressive episodes in which they are incapacitated. This pattern of Dysthymia with superimposed Major Depression is referred to as "double depression" and appears to be a more difficult type of depression to treat. In addition, as many as 15% of dysthymic patients develop bipolar type I or II disorder.

D. Cyclothymic Disorder

Cyclothymic Disorder, like Dysthymic Disorder, is a chronic disorder of at least 2 years' duration in which the afflicted person has multiple episodes of hypomania interspersed with mild depressive periods. The cycles in cyclothymic patients tend to be neither as robust nor as long as they are in bipolar illness. However, the changes in cycles are often abrupt and disruptive. If the patient ever has a full manic episode or meets criteria for Major Depression along with hypomanic episodes, the patient would then have an established bipolar I or II disorder. Cyclothymic Disorder appears to be on a spectrum with bipolar illness.

In most cyclothymic patients, the disorder begins gradually in adolescence or early adulthood. Children who go on to be cyclothymic are sometimes described as irritable and moody. As one can imagine, the hypomanic and depressive periods in cyclothymic disorder may significantly interfere with interpersonal relationships, careers, and general well-being. During hypomanic episodes, the patient's judgment may be somewhat impaired and irritability may be a significant problem. On the other hand, the patient may be very productive during the hypomania and achieve significant success in their field. The depressive episodes tend to be disruptive but not disabling.

Cyclothymic Disorder tends to be lifelong, and may evolve into bipolar disorder. In some surveys, from 30 to 45% of cyclothymic patients will eventually meet criteria for bipolar disorder.

II. EPIDEMIOLOGY OF MOOD DISORDERS

Mood disorders are quite prevalent in the United States and represent among the most common reasons patients seek mental health treatment. For example, Major Depression may occur in up to 26% of women and 12% of men during their lives. At any point in time, as many as 6% of the American population suffer from Major Depression; this is upwards of 11 million people. In all cultures, depression appears to be about twice as common in women as it does in men. The prevalence of depression does not appear to be higher in any socioeconomic or racial group but is more common in single and divorced persons.

Dysthymic disorder is also fairly common with around 3% of the population suffering from this disorder. As with Major Depression, women are far more likely to be afflicted than men. Dysthymia also appears to be more common in lower socioeconomic groups and in unmarried adults.

Bipolar I Disorder is equally found in men and women. About 1% of the population suffers from Bipolar I Disorder, but the incidence of Bipolar II Disorder appears to be several times higher. There is some evidence that bipolar disorder may be more evident in higher socioeconomic groups. In contrast, bipolar disorder may occur at higher rates in populations who are not college educated, perhaps because the earlier onset of the illness may interfere with the ability to pursue higher education.

Cyclothymia may be somewhat more common in females than males. As in Bipolar I Disorder, the prevalence of Cyclothymia is estimated at about 1% of the population. [See EPIDEMIOLOGY: PSYCHIATRIC.]

III. ETIOLOGY

Mood disorders appear to have causes that defy simple explanations. In most cases there appears to be a complex interrelationship of biological, psychological, and social factors that contribute to the onset and maintenance of a mood disorder in a given person. The available data would suggest that Dysthymia is biologically related to Major Depression in many ways and the same is true for Cyclothymia and bipolar disorder.

The etiology of Major Depression and bipolar spectrum disorders has been the object of intense investigation over the past 50 years. Biological factors have been demonstrated to be significant in the cause of depression spectrum illness. Among the biological factors most studied are genetic contributions to the mood disorders. Depression and bipolar illness tend to run in families, although the evidence for familial transmission is greater in bipolar disorder. Perhaps the greatest risk factor for developing a major mood disorder is having a biologic parent who also suffers from a mood disorder. In bipolar disorder, for example, the rate of bipolar illness in first degree relatives is 10 to 20 times higher than it is in the general

population. Major depression is also more prevalent in the first-degree relatives of both bipolar patients and unipolar depressed patients. If one parent suffers from Bipolar I Disorder, the children have approximately a 1 in 4 chance of developing the illness. If both parents are afflicted, the rate increases to as much as 75% in some studies.

One could argue that having parents or siblings afflicted with a major mood disorder presents a significant environmental stressor that may account for the increased prevalence of the disorder in other family members. However, adoption and twin studies would argue that environmental factors only partially explain the higher rate of mood disorders among family members. For example, adoption studies indicate that the rate of Major Depression and bipolar illness is much higher in the biological children of patients with major mood disorders, even if the children are raised from birth by parents who are not afflicted. Monozygotic twin studies provide even more substantial evidence that some form of genetic transmission appears to increase the vulnerability of some patients to mood disorders. Identical twins, including those raised apart from birth, have a high concordance rate for both Major Depression and bipolar illness. If one twin develops Bipolar I Disorder, for example, there is a 30 to 90% chance the other twin will also develop the disorder. The concordance rate among monozygotic twins with Major Depression appears to be about 50%. Just what is being genetically transmitted is not at all clear. Attempts to find specific genes for the mood disorders have so far not yielded clear-cut nor reproducible results. [See GENETIC CONTRIBUTORS TO MENTAL HEALTH.]

Abnormalities with monoamine neurotransmitters such as serotonin, norepinephrine, and dopamine have been implicated in the etiology of mood disorders. The evidence that mood disorders may be related to monoamine abnormalities comes from several lines of evidence. The first is that drugs that deplete monoamines like reserpine appear to precipitate depression in some people. Likewise, in patients who respond to serotonergic antidepressants, depriving the diet of precursors necessary for the synthesis of serotonin quickly results in relapse of symptoms. Functional imaging studies suggest that there is a reduction in activity in ascending monoaminergic pathways in depressed patients and there is also some evidence of decreased activity of the monoamines from the evaluation of metabolites of monoamines in urine and cerebrospinal fluid. The strongest evidence for monoamine involvement in major depressive episodes comes from antidepressants. All known effective antidepressants appear to enhance neurotransmission of the monoamines, particularly serotonin and norepinephrine. During manic episodes, there is evidence of overactivity of dopamine and other monoamines. Dopaminergic antagonists such as typical antipsychotics, in addition to mood stabilizing agents, appear to be very helpful in treating acute mania. [See PSYCHOPHARMACOLOGY.]

Mood disorders are commonly associated with neuroendocrine abnormalities. Patients with Major Depression appear to have higher rates of abnormalities in the hypothalamic pituitary axis (HPA). For example, patients with Major Depression tend to have higher serum levels of the stress hormone cortisol. More severe depressions tend to be associated with higher levels of serum cortisol. Thus, depressed patients tend to show abnormalities in tests of the HPA axis such as the dexamethasone suppression test. This test is not specific nor sensitive enough, however, to make the diagnosis of Major Depression.

Abnormalities in the thyroid axis are also quite common in Major Depression and depressive spectrum illness. Hypothyroidism often presents with symptoms of depression. In addition, about 40% of depressed patients with normal thyroid levels will show blunting of the thyroid axis with provocative tests, such as the administration of thyroid stimulating hormone. It is unclear whether thyroid abnormalities are associated with an increased vulnerability for depression, or the presence of depression increases the likelihood of thyroid abnormalities.

Whatever biological vulnerability may be present in the etiology of mood disorders, psychosocial factors appear to be very important. Biological and psychological explanations need not be mutually exclusive. At least early in the natural course of a mood disorder, stresses and the social environment play a significant role. Major losses of various kinds, such as the death of loved one, the loss of a spouse through divorce, the loss of a career, and so on may precipitate either depression or mania in a susceptible patient. The loss of a parent before adolescence also appears to be a risk factor for developing Major Depression in adulthood. Real or imagined losses may be equally potent at precipitating mood disorders. [See STRESS.]

Even in the case of a significant stressor such as the loss of a loved one, both biological and psychological factors can be posited. Psychological explanations would include the Freudian concept of anger being associated with object loss. Freud suggested that object loss results in a patient trying to become like the lost person (introjection) as a way of possessing part of the lost person within themselves. However, the patient also feels angry at the lost person for abandoning them and since they have introjected the lost object, the anger is directed at themselves. The depressed patient starts hating himself, feels worthless, and may ultimately kill himself out of anger toward the lost object. In variations of this theory, the introjection is not necessarily a lost object but an ambivalently held love object such as parent. The part of the parent that is introjected is punitive, critical, and becomes part of the superego or conscience. The patient is always trying to achieve a parental standard that is idealized and unobtainable. As a result, the patient feels guilty and worthless. [See BEREAVEMENT.]

The biological theorist, on the other hand, would argue that losses, particularly early in life, may result in lifelong changes including higher cortisol responses to stress. These enhanced biological reactions to stress may result in long-term changes in noradrenergic and serotonergic neurotransmitters and their receptors. The psychoanalytic theories of depression may be way of describing the psychological machinery and personal experience associated with the biological changes that may occur secondary to object loss. Freud himself noted some forms of depression were biological in etiology.

In psychodynamic theory, mania and hypomania are considered a maladaptive defense to depression. As a way of defending against depression, a patient is occasionally able to throw off the shackles of an overly punitive superego. The neutralization of the superego may emerge from excessive denial or through the temporary merger of the ego with the superego. When this happens, self-criticism and self-loathing are replaced by euphoria and grandiosity. The patient believes that there is nothing he cannot accomplish and, with the absence or neutralization of the superego, guilt no longer is major factor. In this environment, sexual indiscretions, free spending, and other impulsive manic and hypomanic actions become possible. [See PSYCHOANALYSIS.]

Other more recent psychological theories include the cognitive behavioral theory of depression proposed by Aaron Beck. Beck and his colleagues conceptualize depression and Dysthymia as resulting from cognitive distortions. The problem, in this theoretical framework, is not loss or other stressors, but how these stressors are perceived. A depressed patient is likely to make cognitive errors in his perception of events that result in a negative mood and perhaps feelings of hopeless and worthlessness. For example, a patient prone to depression might perceive a work evaluation that shows a deficiency in some area, in a maladaptive way. The patient may magnify the significance of the evaluation and overgeneralize that he is incompetent at all aspects of his work instead of the narrow aspect defined the evaluation. Catastrophic thinking may ensue that the patient will lose his job, be out on the street, and never be able to find another job. The accumulation of cognitive errors such as these may result in the patient developing a major depressive episode or Dysthymia. [See BEHAVIOR THERAPY; COGNITIVE THERAPY.]

Social factors have also been implicated in the etiology of mood disorders. Early childhood deprivation in the form of grossly inadequate parenting or institutional care may be associated with developing depressive states in adulthood. While socioeconomic factors are not necessarily correlated with Major Depression, they are correlated with Dysthymia and bipolar illness. Lower socioeconomic status may be associated with Dysthymia and higher socioeconomic status with bipolar illness. These correlations may be the result of diagnostic bias, or may be a function of factors related to economic position. For example, economic success may be associated with increased motivation, perseverance, creativity and other factors. Some theorists have suggested that mania and hypomania may be the biological exaggeration of these traits and therefore would congregate in families in which these traits are present. There is little evidence for this theory but it remains an interesting idea. It is more intuitive that poverty can present a significant stressor that might be depressogenic in some people. [See SOCIOECONOMIC STATUS.]

IV. TREATMENT

A. Somatic Therapy

Once the diagnosis has been secured, and medical or substance-induced mood disturbances have been ruled out, the treatment of mood disorders will need to address the biological, interpersonal, and social dysfunction which cause such significant morbidity. Given our current knowledge of the biological basis for these disorders, a variety of somatic treatments are available.

For depressive spectrum disorders physicians and mental health practitioners currently employ six classes of antidepressants. These are the selective serotonin reuptake inhibitors (SSRIs) such as Prozac (fluoxetines); the serotonin and norepinephrine reuptake inhibitors (SNRIs) such as Effexor (venlafaxine); agents which act at postsynaptic receptors such as the 5HT2 receptor antagonists, such as Serzone (nefazodone) and Deseryl (trazodone); monoamine oxidase inhibitors (MAOIs) such as Nardil (phenelzine); the large class of tricyclic drugs (TCAs) that include Tofranil (imipramine) and Pamelor (nortriptyline); and atypical agents, such as Remeron (mirtazapine) and Bupropion (wellbutrin).

The available antidepressants differ in mechanism of action and side effects, but share a number of common features. For example, all of the antidepressants appear to work by enhancing the neurotransmission of monoamines in the brain. Overall, the antidepressants appear to be equally efficacious in the treatment of depression, but some subtypes may respond preferentially to one class over another. In general, a depressed patient has a 60 to 70% chance of responding to the first antidepressant they try, regardless of which agent that happens to be. The use of an antidepressant will double the likelihood that a patient will recover from an episode of Major Depression in the first 2 months. Therefore, atypical antidepressant trial is from 1 to 2 months, and patients who respond are kept on the medication for at least 6 months to reduce the risk of relapse. Patients who have had many recurrences of Major Depression may be kept on an antidepressant for many years or even a lifetime. Antidepressants do not carry the risk of tolerance and addiction that are common to mood-elevating street drugs, such as cocaine or amphetamine. Finally, none of the antidepressants work immediately. The maximum antidepressant effects may not be seen for 1 month or longer.

Given the many drug classes which may be used to treat depression, the choice of a particular antidepressant rests on considerations of safety, severity, a constellation of symptoms suggestive of Major Depression versus Dysthymia, the presence of a bipolar spectrum illness including Cyclothymia, tolerability, and the risk of toxicity. In this regard clinicians consider the age of the patient, and concurrent medical illness. In addition, a past history in the individual or in the family of a response to a particular class of drug may direct the selection of an antidepressant.

Patients with Major Depression who do not respond to an initial antidepressant trial have approximately an 80 to 90% chance of eventually responding to a subsequent trial of antidepressants. However, it may take several trials before an adequate medication is discovered. At least 10 to 20% of seriously depressed patients will fail to respond to all antidepressants. In such cases, approaches such as electroconvulsive therapy (ECT) are often considered. ECT is one of the oldest and most controversial procedures in psychiatry having been used since the 1930s. It involves passing small electric current through the cranium while a patient is under general anesthesia with their muscles relaxed. The stimulus results in a generalized seizure lasting for 30 to 120 seconds and a series of from 6 to 12 treatments given every other day often results in remission of the Major Depression. Compared to medications, ECT is probably more effective and faster acting. However, patients will typically have some problems with retrograde and anterograde memory that is typically short-lived, but may last for weeks or longer after a series of treatments.

When a patient suffers from recurrent seasonal depressions, light therapy (phototherapy) is sometimes employed. Winter depressions usually begin in the fall as days shorten, tend to be at their worst in the winter, and improve in the spring. The depression is thought to be related to the shorter periods of light in the winter that may result in some hormonal and neurochemical changes in susceptible patients, which leads to depression. Such patients may respond to exposure to a light box with full spectrum light at the beginning or end of the day during the winter months.

The pharmacological treatment of Dysthymia follows the treatment of Major Depression. Current strategies include SSRIs, MAOIIs, and TCAs. There are no "head-to-head" studies that define which treatments are more efficacious, but a first choice in treatment would be an SSRI, given its safety and ease of administration. Failure on one or more SSRIs may suggest trial of an MAOII, which in some studies show better improvement than TCAs. There is some

anecdotal evidence that response, for instance to an SSRI, may require a longer treatment window, up to 16 weeks. More aggressive treatment, such as ECT, does not appear to be useful in the treatment of Dysthymia.

In bipolar spectrum disorders, the depressive phase is treated with the agents described above, but concurrent with these agents, a mood stabilizer such as lithium, valproate, or carbamazepine will be used. There has recently been a surge of interest in valproate in the treatment of acute mania, with results suggesting it is more effective than the traditional agent lithium in patients with significant irritability and in mixed episodes. However, the data showing that valproate is also as effective as lithium in the prophylaxis of manic episodes has not yet been established.

Lithium has been the standard mood stabilizer in bipolar disorder for more than 25 years. It is an effective prophylactic agent in approximately two-thirds of patients for mania and possibly for depression. Responders to lithium are characterized by the presence of euphoric mood, infrequent episodes, a family history of bipolar disorder and response to lithium, and a profile of mood changes consisting of depression to mania to euthymic interval pattern. It is effective in treating 30% of rapid cyclers, and 40% in mixed or dysphoric manic states. In classic bipolar patients the response rate is as high as 60 to 80%, although including the mixed states the response overall is about 50% of patients.

All currently used mood stabilizers have the potential for significant toxicity. For example, the mood stabilizers have a potential for neurotoxicity ranging from a mild tremor at the therapeutic doses to delirium, coma, and death in overdose. The chronic use of lithium is sometimes associated with changes in kidney function, while valproate can be toxic to the liver. Carbamazepine is sometimes associated changes in blood cell and platelets that can sometimes be quite toxic.

The treatment of acute mania can include the use of a mood stabilizer, along with antipsychotic drugs and hypnotic agents such as diazepam (Valium) or lorezapam (Ativan). There is some suggestion that valproate alone can treat the acute manic symptoms as well as psychosis during the acute episode without an additional neuroleptic.

The treatment of the depressive phase (bipolar major depressive episodes) is characterized by treatment during the depressive phase only, and caution with agents with a history of inducing manic episodes. Tricyclic antidepressants have been most implicated in induced mania and induction of rapid cycling, but all antidepressants have the potential to induce mania. MAOIIs and Bupropion have some support for being less likely to induce mania or rapid cycling. Currently, the strategy recommended by some experts starts with a MAOII, followed by Bupropion or an SSRI, followed by a TCA. Light therapy may be useful when a seasonal variation is observed. Neuroleptics play an uncertain role in the absence of psychosis, although as noted above clozaril may act as a mood stabilizer and risperidone may act as an antidepressant.

Cyclothymia, a bipolar spectrum disorder, may be treated with lithium, valproate, or other mood stabilizer. There is some evidence that Cyclothymia responds at lower doses than those used to treat type I bipolar illness. Treatment with antidepressants risks a hypomanic or manic episode. About one-third of these patients become bipolar, and most often bipolar II. Therefore, in treatment of Cyclothymia, the presence of a developing bipolar disorder, and treatment strategies used in bipolar disorder, need to be considered.

B. Psychosocial Treatments

A number of psychotherapy strategies have been employed in the treatment of Major Depression, Dysthymia, and the depressive phase of bipolar illness. The most common of these are cognitive behavioral therapy, interpersonal psychotherapy and psychodynamic psychotherapy.

Cognitive Behavioral Therapy (CBT) is the best-studied psychotherapy for the treatment of depression. It appears to be as efficacious as medications in mild to moderate depression, and may have some prophylactic benefits as well. CBT is typically a time-limited psychotherapy of between 12 and 20 sessions.

As described earlier, the underlying premise of CBT is that depression is caused and maintained by cognitive distortions in a susceptible person. A number of cognitive errors have been described in depression. These include the tendency to catastrophic and all-or-nothing thinking. Depressed patients tend to amplify the negative aspects of their experience such that molehills are transformed into mountains. Depressed patients will dwell on minor events or flaws in their character to the extent that these take on undue importance in the patient's life. The emotional reaction to amplifying these negative events or traits is for the depressed patient to feel increasingly helpless, worthless, guilty, and depressed.

These cognitive errors are often of an automatic quality. They occur too rapidly for rational assessment and may be unconscious. For example, depressed patients will typically be quite self-critical in response to perceived shortcomings. But an assessment by the patient in response to a particular situation such as "I am so stupid" may be rapid and automatic that awareness of this assessment is lacking. However, the patient may be aware of the emotional reaction to this assessment: dysphoria.

The goal of CBT is to increase the awareness of these automatic thoughts and cognitive distortions so that they may be rationally challenged. The CBT therapist use a variety of techniques to this end. Patients undergoing CBT are assigned homework in which they may have to keep a diary after each session. The diary is a tool for the patient to track their cognitive process that is associated with negative states and allow the patient to focus on these. The diary is reviewed in the subsequent CBT session and cognitive errors are pointed out by the therapist. In time the patient becomes aware of the distortions as they occur and can effectively challenge them.

Behavioral techniques are also employed in CBT to mobilize the depressed patients. Social skills and assertiveness training are often used in CBT to help the depressed counter social isolation and feelings of inadequacy in interpersonal relationships. Patients are put on schedules of activities to further mobilize them. Patients are also assigned tasks in increasing order of complexity and challenge so that the depressed persons slowly develop a sense of mastery over tasks they felt they could not do.

Another type of psychotherapy that is well studied in the treatment of depressive states is interpersonal psychology (IPT). This therapy is based on the work of Gerald Klerman and Myrna Weissman and based on the theory that depression results from deficiencies in social functioning, dependency, intimacy, and social isolation. Like CBT, IPT is time-limited and typically lasts for 12 to 20 sessions.

The goals of IPT are to identify problem areas such as grief reactions, interpersonal disputes, and problems with interpersonal communication. IPT sessions revolve around clarifying the negative feeling associated with these problems and developing options for contending with these problems. Techniques used in

IPT include reassuring the patient, testing the patient's perceptions of what happened interpersonally, and teaching techniques for improving communication. IPT appears to be effective in mild to moderate depression alone. However, the best results often have been obtained when IPT is combined with pharmacotherapy.

Psychodynamic therapies are based on the work of Sigmund Freud and subsequent therapy, and has been used for almost 100 years in the treatment of depression. Psychodynamic therapy focuses on the childhood origins of depression as well as unconscious motives and defenses as they relate to current conflicts.

Dynamic therapy tend to be more open-ended and less directive than IPT or CBT. Sessions may occur up to several times a week and may last for years. The relationship of the patient to the therapist is evaluated as a way of correcting problems that may occur or have occurred in past relationships. Sessions may have the goal of obtaining insight into the roots of the depression so they can be effectively dealt with. However, dynamic therapy may also be supportive in nature and have the goals of encouraging rest, taking active steps to reduce stressors, and allowing the patient a safe place to vent emotions. While the efficacy of dynamic therapy is less well established than that of IPT or CBT, there are patients who clearly benefit from this approach over others.

Family and group therapies, as well as psychoeducation, are very important for patients with depression and bipolar spectrum illness. Depression does not occur in a vacuum, and tends to intimately affect family members. Families, in turn, can help buffer patients from stressors or increase their vulnerability.

Family therapy, then, can be used to educate families about the course of a mood disorder, facilitate communication, and limit the effects of isolation. [*See* FAMILY THERAPY.]

Group therapy allows patients with mood disorders to share their experiences with others who suffer from similar problems. Patients in group therapy derive considerable validation, support and insight from other group members as well as from the group therapist(s). Groups are very good settings for testing negative perceptions, comparing experiences about medications, and decreasing isolation. The group may help mobilize the patient to action, and most patients are tremendously comforted by knowing that they are not unique or alone in their suffering. Mood disorders groups tend to meet weekly and may be psychodynamic, supportive, or cognitively oriented among other forms. Group therapy usually lasts from 1 to 2 hours and may be time-limited or open-ended.

Whatever the form of therapy that is pursued, psychotherapy, pharmacotherapy or a combination of the two, education tends to play an important role in the treatment of mood disorders. Patients and their families derive considerable benefit from learning about the signs and symptoms of the illness, the disorder's course, and what can be expected from the treatments. Side effects of biological therapies tend to be reviewed in detail and the time it takes to respond is discussed. Likewise the rationale for pursuing a particular psychotherapy is discussed with patients as well as what can be expected from pursuing a given therapy. (See Table IV.)

We are currently in a period of rapid development for the treatment of mood disorders. Still, there is

Table IV   Comparison of Individual Psychotherapies of Depression *

Type:	Cognitive/Behavioral	Interpersonal	Psychodynamic
Premise	Depression secondary to cognitive distortion	Depression secondary to interpersonal problems	Depression secondary to unconscious conflict
Goal	Correct cognitive distortions	Enhance current social functioning	Resolve conflict over loss
Approach	Directive	Directive	Nondirective
Technique	Cognitive diary Homework assignments	Reassurance Improve interpersonal communication	Interpret unconscious material Graded tasks
	Assertiveness training	Role rehearse interpresonal solutions	Ventilation/catharsis
Duration	12 to 20 sessions	12 to 20 sessions	Brief (12 sessions)

* DeBattista C, Glick I: *Medical Management of Depression*, EMIS, 1996.

much to be learned about biological, psychological, and social approaches to the treatment of mood disorders. While most people with mood disorders can be significantly helped by the treatment options available, there continues to be a need for more efficacious, cost-effective, and less toxic treatments. Such treatments await further research.

BIBLIOGRAPHY

American Psychiatric Association (1994). *Diagnostic and statistical manual of mental disorders* (4th ed.). Washington, DC: Author.

Beck, A., Rush, A. J., Shaw, B. F., & Emery, G. (1979). *Cognitive therapy of depression.* New York: Guilford Press.

DeBattista, C., & Glick, I. D. (1996). *The medical management of depression.* Dallas, TX: Essential Medical Information Systems.

Goodwin, F., & Jamison, K. (1980). *Manic depressive illness.* New York: Oxford Press.

Kaplan, H. I., & Sadock, B. J. (1995). *Comprehensive textbook of psychiatry* (6th ed.). Baltimore: Williams & Wilkins.

Kessler, R. C., et al. (1994). Lifetime and 12 month prevalence of DSM III-R psychiatric disorders in the United States: Results from the national comorbidity survey. *Archives of General Psychiatry, 51,* 8–19.

Schatzberg, A. F., Cole, J. O., & DeBattista, C. (1996). *Manual of clinical psychopharmacology* (3rd ed.). Washington, DC: APA Press.

Moral Development

F. Clark Power

University of Notre Dame

Autonomy The capacity of self-governance according to reason.

Disequilibration The first part of the process of stage transition in which the equilibrium or balance achieved at a particular stage is disturbed.

Habituation Aristotle's approach to the learning of virtue through guided instruction and practice.

Heteronomy The subordination of the self to an external authority, law, or source of influence.

Intentionality The child's ability to take into account intentions or motives in making judgments of praise and blame.

Longitudinal Study A method that collects data on the same group of individuals over time.

Perspective or Role-Taking Stages Stages that describe the ability of children and adolescents to coordinate different viewpoints.

Structural Wholeness The assumption in cognitive developmental theory that a stage is an organized pattern of reasoning that underlies more particular content considerations of moral choice and values.

Transformational Model A model of stage development in which the lower stages are integrated by the higher stages.

MORAL DEVELOPMENT studies the acquisition of the attitudes, dispositions, sentiments, and cognitive competencies involved in the process of moral judgment and action. The nature and role of these components of the process depend on how morality is understood. Most contemporary moral psychologists distinguish morality from prudence or the pursuit of one's interests and from custom or etiquette. They generally agree that to be moral is to treat others fairly and with concern for their welfare without the anticipation of a reward or threat of punishment.

I. A HISTORICAL OVERVIEW

A. Introduction

How humans develop from impulse-governed infants to morally responsible adults has been a question of perennial concern and debate since the time of ancient Greece. Socrates, for example, believed that one's morality developed through rational inquiry into the nature of the good. He, therefore, challenged the youth of Athens to question popular views of morality and virtue, a practice that led to his being sentenced to death. Aristotle, on the other hand, emphasized the role of habituation over reasoning in moral upbringing. In his view, individuals learn how to be moral much the way apprentices learn their craft.

In the first half of the 20th century, the discussion of moral development took a more radical turn as psychoanalytic and behavioral psychologists called into question the very notions of universal morality, character, and virtue. The most significant of all the research at this time was Hartshorne and May's landmark study of deception, self-control, and service.

They indicated that moral behavior does not depend on an individual's character or virtue but is a function of influences operating in the situation. Following Hartshorne and May, the psychological study of morality, as it has traditionally been understood, practically ceased, until in the 1960s, the cognitive developmental approach of Piaget and Kohlberg emerged.

B. Psychoanalytic Theory

Psychoanalytic theorists take their definition of what is moral from the norms and values of the existing culture. They describe the operation of becoming moral as the internalization of those cultural norms and values in the superego through a process of parental identification, which according to Freud culminates the resolution of the Oedipal conflict at age 5 or 6. In their research they typically look for correlations between early childhood parenting and behavior, and between the arousal of guilt and behavior. This paradigm presents the essence of moral functioning as following one's conscience in order to avoid guilt. Given the irrational nature of the superego, psychoanalytic theorists are concerned not only that cultural standards are upheld but also that the superego does not become excessively punitive.

C. Social Learning Theory

Social learning theorists tend to equate morality with societal norms and more broadly with other-oriented or altruistic actions. Like the psychoanalytic theorists, they maintain that individuals become moral through the internalization of those societal norms. In place of processes of parental identification, however, social learning theorists attempt to demonstrate that these norms are acquired through rewards and punishments. Children are in this view initially motivated to satisfy their own needs and desires. They are then shaped or socialized by environmental mechanisms to find satisfaction in socially approved and other-oriented actions. The test of a person's morality is thus whether she or he will adhere to a social norm or perform an altruistic action without the expectation of reward or punishment or at some personal cost.

D. Cognitive Developmental Theory

Cognitive developmentalists reject the assumption shared by psychoanalytic and social learning theorists that morality can be equated with culturally relative standards. Taking an explicitly philosophic stance, they maintain that morality is a process of adjudicating conflicting claims on the basis of universally recognized principles of justice and benevolence. Cognitive developmentalists see moral development as occurring through a sequence of stages in which individuals reason about moral problems in progressively more adequate ways. In contrast to psychoanalytic and social learning theorists, who view the child as being passively formed by environmental forces, cognitive developmentalists picture the child (and later the adolescent and adult) as developing a personal "moral philosophy" through interacting with the environment.

In general, as White has noted, psychological approaches serve as windows on reality, bringing clarity to aspects of human experience that have been largely obscure. As windows, however, these approaches provide only partial views, framed by their guiding assumptions and research methods. The cognitive developmental approach has succeeded in providing a penetrating analysis of the way in which individuals reason about moral problems; but moral reasoning is, of course, only a part, although perhaps the key part, of moral functioning. The other approaches sketched here provide different windows on moral experience, windows aimed more directly on moral feelings and observable behaviors.

Because Piaget and Kohlberg pioneered the field of moral development as we know it today, this article will focus on the major features of their theories. It will also attend to some of the major criticisms of their work as well as to some of the more promising extensions of cognitive development theory, particularly insofar as it relates to the relationship between moral reasoning and action. [*See* COGNITIVE DEVELOPMENT.]

II. PIAGET'S THEORY

A. The Moral Judgment of the Child

The study of moral development as we know it today drew its initial inspiration from Jean Piaget's seminal study, *The Moral Judgment of the Child*; it is the fifth of a series of books that Piaget published at the beginning of a highly productive career. Developmentalists either have focused directly upon these studies to elaborate, refine, and confirm their conclusions or, like Kohlberg, have used Piaget's ideas and methods as a springboard for their own theories. *The Moral*

Judgment of the Child is subdivided into three empirical parts and a fourth theoretical part in which Piaget contrasts his views on moral development and education with those of other theorists, most notably the great French sociologist Emile Durkheim.

B. Heteronomy and Autonomy

In the first part of *The Moral Judgment of the Child,* Piaget examines the ways in which children from the ages of 3 to 12 understand and apply the rules of marbles and hopscotch, the most popular children's games in French-speaking Switzerland. Piaget believed that by studying children at play, he could penetrate into their own moral world, a world that they were attempting to understand and control on their own terms. Feigning that he had forgotten the rules of the game, he asked the children to teach him and let him play with them. He then proceeded to ask the children about the various shots in the game and how to determine the winner. All the while, he played the game as seriously as he could, letting the children beat him to sustain their sense of superiority but making an occasional good shot to avoid being dismissed as incompetent. Having determined children's "practice of the rules," Piaget proceeded to inquire into their consciousness of the origins of rules by asking such simple questions as "Can you make up a new rule?" "Would it be all right to play like that with your pals?" "Have people always played as they do today?"

Piaget found that young children (usually under the age of 8) typically believed that adults made the rules and the rules could not be changed. On the other hand, older children (usually over the age of 9) readily believed that they with their peers were authorized to make and change rules. Piaget theorized that children's belief in the creation of rules by adult authorities reflected a quasi-mystical, heteronomous respect for the rules, while older children's belief in their own power to make rules reflected a secular, autonomous respect. As is most evident in the final section of his book Piaget's perspective was deeply influenced by Durkheim, whose views on the sociology of religion and moral education were highly influential at that time. According to Durkheim, respect for rules could be generated only if the rules were regarded as emanating from a power superior to the individual. Durkheim's historical studies led him to postulate that religion and morality were originally undifferentiated and that all rules were regarded as sacred because of their divine origin.

With societal evolution rules became secularized, but, nevertheless, retained their power to elicit respect because of their transcendent, societal origin. In Durkheim's view, rules could only obligate if they were seen as issuing from a superior, quasi divine being. Individuals, therefore had to look beyond themselves to the collective being of society as the authority behind the rules.

Piaget's entire book may be regarded as an effort to respond to Durkheim by showing that children develop an alternative, autonomous morality through cooperative peer relationships. Unfortunately his preoccupation with Durkheim's view seems to have foreclosed his exploration of other types of moral reasoning, types later uncovered in Kohlberg's research. What Piaget's analysis loses in breadth, it gains, however, in depth by juxtaposing moral heteronomy with moral autonomy.

C. Egocentrism

Piaget found that children at the heteronomous stage flagrantly but unwittingly broke the very rules that they regarded as sacred and immutable. Piaget explained this paradox as a function of childhood egocentrism. This term should not be confused with egoism or selfishness; it simply connotes children's apparent inability to distinguish their subjective perspective from the perspective of others. As Piaget and others have noted, egocentrism is a salient characteristic of children's speech and play. For example, when telling stories or making requests young children typically fail to take the needs of their listeners into account. They seem to assume that their listeners know what they are talking about. Similarly when young children play with each other, they tend to parallel play or play as individuals in the company of others.

Although young children tend to behave in egocentric ways, there is considerable debate over whether their egocentrism should be regarded as a stage of cognitive immaturity. Some research indicates that very young children are capable of altering their speech and actions to meet the needs of others, and Piaget himself had noted that even adults can be egocentric in expressing their opinions. There are other studies, however, that have reconceptualized the egocentrism construct to consist of stages of perspective or role taking. These studies show that young children's conceptions of the self, friendship, groups, and morality are limited by their ability to coordinate the perspectives of others.

Overlooked in this debate, as Youniss has noted, is the relational dimension of the egocentrism construct. Piaget consistently maintained that the unequal relationship that children have with adults fosters egocentrism by encouraging children to submit to the adult authority. On the other hand, the equal relationship that exists among peers encourages children to consider their perspectives in making reasonable decisions through mutual agreement. Piaget's relational perspective on moral development leads to the radical conclusion, elaborated in a provocative study by Youniss, that peers, not parents, play the decisive role in promoting moral development.

D. Intentionality

In the next section of the book, Piaget examined children's modes of moral evaluations with a focus on the origin of children's awareness of intentionality. The best known of his queries asks who was the naughtiest, a child who knocked over 15 cups accidently or a child who broke 1 cup in an act of disobedience. Piaget found that children below 8 or 9 years old typically based their judgments of culpability on the extent of material damage. The older children, however, recognized the moral relevance of the intentions of the actors. Conceding that objective responsibility may largely be a function of the way in which parents respond to children's clumsiness, Piaget observed that his own young children made spontaneous judgments of objective responsibility even though he and his wife were careful not to punish or blame their children for unintentional damage. Furthermore, Piaget found that when considering cases of stealing and lying, younger children tended to make judgments of objective responsibility that their parents would be very unlikely to make. For example, the younger children regarded lying as saying something untrue, whether or not the misstatement was made intentionally. The mere violation of the moral rule was a sufficient determinant of guilt. As in his discussion of egocentrism, Piaget attributed young children's failure to differentiate moral from physical laws (moral realism) and intentions from consequences partly to their immature thinking and partly to authoritarian childrearing practices.

E. The Two Moralities of Childhood

In the third section of the book Piaget studied children's conception of punishment and distributive justice. Al-

though his data indicated that development generally proceeds from heteronomy to autonomy, the many exceptions to this pattern suggested that heteronomy and autonomy are not sequential stages but two irreducible types built on different relational foundations. For example, Piaget found that young children see expiatory punishment as fair only in the adult–child relationship, whereas, in the child–child relationship, children at all ages favor what Piaget called punishment by reciprocity, that is punishment aimed solely to make the transgressor aware of the undesirable consequences of his or her misdeed.

Post-Piagetian researchers, as indicated, have tended to view socio-moral development in a more cognitive and less relational framework than Piaget. Although this may have led many researchers to underestimate the effects of constraint and cooperation on socio-moral problem-solving, it also led to important breakthroughs in the study of such topics as perspective-taking and intentionality. Furthermore, in the case of moral development, the cognitive developmental focus has led away from the two-morality hypothesis to a unitary process of stage development.

III. KOHLBERG'S THEORY

A. The Moral Domain

When asked to give his views on moral development and education, Lawrence Kohlberg was fond of citing Socrates' response to a similar request at the beginning of Plato's *Meno*: "You must think I am very fortunate to know how virtue is acquired. The fact is, far from knowing whether it can be taught, I have know idea what virtue really is." Kohlberg, like Socrates, did not believe that one could address questions of moral psychology and education without first attempting to define in a philosophically justifiable way the nature of morality. Yet in the mid 1950s, when Kohlberg began his dissertation research on moral development, social scientists paid little if any attention to the philosophical presuppositions of their work.

Kohlberg was particularly distressed by the claim prevalent in social learning research and psychoanalytic theory that moral development reduces to the internalization of the rules and practices of one's society. Having become involved in the Hagganah's effort to smuggle European Jewish refugees into Israel following the Holocaust, Kohlberg was committed to an understanding of morality that transcends the status quo and provides a rational basis for responsible social criticism. He also questioned the assumption that morality can be reduced to culturally relative norms and values. Such an assumption, based on observed cultural differences, blurs an important distinction between morality and custom or social convention. Moral norms and values, such as prohibitions against causing physical injury, concern the rights and welfare of individuals in any societal arrangement. Customs or conventions (e.g., table manners), on the other hand, concern socially imposed rules that provide a certain order and decorum but are not recognized as obligatory in the same sense as moral norms.

In addition to differentiating morality from custom, Kohlberg also distinguished morality from personal and religious values or the right from the good. Underlying the distinction between the right and the good is a recognition that what is right or moral is obligatory, whereas what is good is left to individual choice, as long as it is in harmony with what is right. Kohlberg used this distinction to argue that moral education could be undertaken in the public schools without violating the separation between church and state or without indoctrinating personal values.

Following up on Kohlberg's philosophical attempt to delineate the moral sphere, Turiel and his colleagues have proposed that morality, convention, and personal values comprise three conceptual domains, each with its own developmental trajectory. Their research indicates that even very young children are capable of distinguishing moral violations from violations within the other domains. Such findings confirm the wisdom of Kohlberg's effort to base his research on a carefully defined conceptualization of morality, even as they call into question whether he consistently distinguished the moral from the conventional in some of his stage descriptions.

B. The Moral Judgment Interview

Kohlberg's definition of morality as justice, his emphasis on studying the development of moral reasoning, and his aim of charting moral development throughout the lifespan led him to construct a semiclinical moral judgment interview. His original interview posed 10 hypothetical moral dilemmas drawn, not from familiar episodes in the world of children (as were Piaget's) but from challenging problems in the world of adults. Kohlberg regarded the Heinz dilemma (slightly abbreviated here) as his best:

In Europe, a woman was near death from a special kind of cancer. There was a drug that could save her but the druggist was charging twice as much as the sick woman's husband, Heinz, could raise. Heinz pleaded with the druggist, but the druggist said, "No, I discovered the drug and I'm going to make money from it." Heinz has exhausted all other alternatives, should he steal the drug?

The Heinz dilemma puts subjects in the uncomfortable position of having to decide between his wife's claim to life and the druggist's legally sanctioned claim to property. The point of the interview is not to identify subjects' action choices but to examine the ways in which they justify their choices; therefore, interviewers are instructed to ask subjects to present, elaborate, and clarify their arguments.

C. Levels and Stages

Kohlberg's current theory describes a sequence of six stages grouped into three levels: The preconventional level (stages 1 and 2), the conventional level (stages 3 and 4), and the postconventional or principled level (stages 5 and 6). As the labels indicate, the levels are determined by the perspective taken on the moral expectations (rules, roles, norms, and values) of the conventional social order. The work "conventional" connotes simply what is commonly accepted and should not be confused with Turiel's use of the term to mean a normal custom. At the preconventional level, conventional expectations are seen as external to the self. The obligation to follow such expectations comes not from their intrinsic worth or their place within the social fabric but from the mere fact that they are commanded or that noncompliance is punished. At the conventional level, conventional expectations are internalized. Conventional expectations are respected because individuals value their membership in society and want to be regarded as upstanding members of their communities. At the postconventional level, conventional expectations are subordinated to general, foundational principles. Conventional expectations are critically appraised according to such principles from a prior to society perspective, that is from the perspective of a moral agent aware of basic rights and values that all societies should recognize.

Like the levels, the structural core of the stages depends upon what Kohlberg calls the socio-moral perspective of the subject. At stage one, subjects are, to use Piaget's term, egocentric: they fail to differentiate their perspective from others, particularly those in authority who are valued for their superior size and power. As a consequence, those at stage one believe that rules are to be obeyed for their own sake or for the avoidance of punishment, which is seen as inevitable. For example, children at this stage often state that Heinz should not steal the drug simply because stealing is wrong or because his theft will be punished. At stage two, subjects are aware that individuals have concrete wants and desires and that such wants and needs can come into conflict. It is right to pursue one's interests as long as others are not prevented from pursuing theirs. Subjects at this stage sometimes justify Heinz's stealing simply by appealing to his wife's need or to the presumption that anyone in Heinz's situation would not want their wife to die or would automatically do what was necessary. Subjects will likewise justify Heinz's not stealing by noting that the risk of punishment may not be worth it. Conflicts of interest are to be settled by making deals. For example, Heinz should steal the drug for his wife in return for what she has done for him or because he may need a favor from her sometime.

At stage three, subjects take a third person perspective and view themselves and others not only as individuals, but as members of relationships or small groups. They seek to uphold shared expectations for good behavior and value sympathetic and prosocial motives. For example, subjects will argue that Heinz should steal the drug because he loves her or because he is her husband. On the other hand, they will also argue that Heinz should not steal because stealing is selfish or takes advantage of the druggist who works hard. Subjects at the fourth stage take the perspective of the social system and respect its laws and legal processes as necessary for maintaining social order. Just as they see the need for consistency in society, they also see the need for developing individual character and respecting the dictates of conscience. Subjects at this stage sometimes maintain that Heinz should not take the law into his own hands by stealing. They will, however, also maintain that stealing may be justified in response to an idealized natural law that is higher than human law.

At stage five, subjects take a prior to society perspective and judge the moral worth of rules and values insofar as such rules and values are consistent with more fundamental considerations, such as liberty, the general welfare or utility, human rights, and contractual obligations. Subjects typically argue that Heinz should steal the drug because the right to life is more basic than the right to property. At stage six, subjects take a pro-

cedural or dialogical perspective on decision-making. What is right is what would be freely chosen by all interested parties who take each others' point of view into account and who respect others as equal and autonomous persons. Subjects at this stage make explicit appeals either to a procedure for adjudicating claims or to universal, regulative principles of justice.

The status of stage six is uncertain. Although stage six continues to be listed in the table of the stages, the current scoring manual provides only criterion judgments through stage five because no stage six examples were found in the longitudinal sample. The current formulation of stage six is embedded within the contractarian tradition in moral philosophy extending from Rousseau and Kant to Rawls and Habermas. Such a formulation and the fact that the few examples of stage six cited by Kohlberg come from individuals with philosophic training suggest that stage six may not be a psychological stage but a philosophical position.

D. Reliability and Validity

At the very heart of cognitive development theory are the assumptions of invariant stage sequence and structural wholeness. The test of invariant sequence is whether individuals develop through the stages in ascending order without skips or reversals. The test of structural wholeness is whether individuals respond to different kinds of moral dilemmas by using the same or adjacent stage reasoning. These assumptions have guided efforts over the years since Kohlberg's dissertation to refine the stage descriptions and methods for scoring interviews. The early definitions of and procedures for scoring were based on moral content, that is, the moral concerns and values typically associated with a particular stage. For example a simple statement of concern for law and order was scored as stage 4. At the 10th year of Kohlberg's longitudinal study, problems of regression and stage heterogeneity across the different dilemmas called the cognitive developmental assumptions of Kohlberg's theory into question. Case analysis indicated that regressions were occurring because content, like the law and order concern, was being coded as stage 4 regardless of its meaning in the larger context of the interview. Kohlberg thus revised both his stage definitions and scoring method to focus on structure rather than content. Because the structural scoring method required far greater interpretive judgment than the earlier method, inter-rater reliability suffered for a time, prompting critics to challenge the empirical foundation of the theory.

In response, Colby, Kohlberg, and their colleagues developed the present Standard Issue Scoring Manual, which supplements the structural scoring process by providing over 700 prototypes (criterion judgments) of common responses to nine dilemmas. Stage scores are assigned by matching arguments in the interview to these criterion judgments. This new method achieves high inter-rater reliability (from 88 to 100% agreement within a third of a stage) by eliminating much of the subjectivity in the structural coding method, while, nevertheless, providing guidance for distinguishing content from structure.

In addition to obtaining high inter-rater reliability, the new method also achieves substantial test–retest agreement over a 3- to 6-week interval (from 93 to 100% within a third of a stage), indicating the stability of the measure. A coefficient of internal consistency (Cronbach's alpha) in the 90s as well as factor analysis indicates that the interview taps a single, construct. Some critics have dismissed the moral judgment measure as simply another intelligence test, yet correlations with IQ are only moderate (.37 to .59), indicating that moral development is related but not reducible to general intelligence.

The case for the validity of the measure is based on how well longitudinal data support the major theoretical assumptions of invariant sequence and structural wholeness. Three major studies, of U.S. males, of Turkish mates from rural and urban areas, and of male and female adolescents from an Israeli kibbutz, were used to determine the validity of the construct. All of the studies show that development proceeds through an invariant sequence. There were no instances of stage skipping or stage reversal within the limits of measurement error (determined through test–retest instability). All of the studies also indicate that development proceeds as a structund whole. Individuals generally respond to different dilemmas using one or two adjacent stages (e.g., at stages 2 and 3). Cases in which three stages are used are infrequent (less than 10%). The data thus support Kohlberg's major theoretical claims as well the adequacy of the methodology.

E. Cross-Cultural Validity

Longitudinal studies in Turkey and Israel and cross-sectional studies in over 25 Western and non-Western countries, which include populations from both urban and traditional folk societies, generally support the universality of the moral stages. Although content differences were found, the interview responses were generally scorable with the new manual. The results displayed patterns of sequential stage development and structural wholeness similar to the United States longitudinal sample. Snarey and Keljo note, however, three discrepant cross-cultural findings of potential theoretical import. First, stage 5 was absent in traditional folk societies. Second, the rate of moral development was faster in urban than in traditional folk societies. Third, the current scoring manual does not have criterion judgments for responses typically found not only in traditional folk societies but in non-Western and communitarian societies. The first two of these findings do not necessarily indicate a problem with the theory. It is not surprising that individuals in small, relatively homogeneous traditional societies do not develop beyond the conventional stages and that the pace of their development is slower. The third finding, however, suggests at the very least that the scoring manual needs to be expanded. On the other hand, this finding may, as some critics have charged, be symptomatic of an underlying bias especially at the postconventional level in favor of the liberal, individualistic ideology of Western urban society.

IV. NEW DIRECTIONS

A. The Defining Issues Test

The Defining Issues Test (DIT) was developed by Rest as a practical alternative to the moral judgment interviewing and scoring procedures (for subjects at or above a 12-year-old reading level). It presents subjects with stage prototypic responses to six moral dilemmas and asks them to rate and then rank their preferences. Although the DIT has been widely and successfully used as a proxy for the clinical moral judgment method (it correlates moderately well with the Kohlberg measure), it is an important measure in its own right. The DIT measures individuals' comprehension of and preference for preformulated moral arguments, while the moral judgment interview measures individuals' ability to produce spontaneously moral arguments.

Finding considerable rating and ranking heterogeneity in the DIT and charging that Kohlberg's scoring procedures have tended to smooth over significant stage irregularities, Rest has suggested that an additive model of stage development may be more adequate than Piaget and Kohlberg's transformational or displacement model. Support for the additive model comes not only from DIT research but also from studies indicating considerable stage heterogeneity when comparisons are made between standard and certain nonstandard moral dilemmas and between hypothetical and real life dilemmas. Furthermore, most post-Piagetian psychologists, influenced by information processing, favor the additive model's more differentiated approach. The evidence favoring the holistic, transformational model comes from production tasks, like the moral judgment interview, which is designed to assess the moral reasoning competence and to facilitate the interpretation of discrete ideas into a more comprehensive framework. Perhaps both models (and others too) are necessary to elucidate different dimensions of the complex process of moral development.

B. Early Childhood Development

Kohlberg's longitudinal sample begins with 10-year-olds because the original intent of his research was to build upon Piaget's work. The nature of his moral dilemmas would have precluded his starting much earlier because they were specifically designed to describe how individuals develop the capacity to resolve moral problems in the adult world. Yet such dilemmas emphasize the limitations of children's thinking (as is evident in the punishment and obedience description of stage 1). Returning to Piaget's method of presenting children with familiar problems, Damon demonstrated that the socio-moral conceptions of young children (ages 4 to 9) in the areas of distributive justice, friendship, and authority develop through surprisingly varied and sophisticated developmental levels. For example, in describing the development of children's resolutions of distributive justice problems, Damon described a six-level scheme in which children based their judgments on the following sequence of considerations: their own desires, strict equality, merit, equity, and combinations of merit and equity that best serve the common good.

C. Gender and Development

Gilligan has since the mid-1970s charged that Kohlberg's stage theory is biased against women because it

describes the justice and rights orientation favored by males, while it neglects the care and responsibility orientation favored by females. She attributed the one-sidedness of Kohlberg's approach to his embeddedness in the Western male philosophical tradition, his all-male sample, and his use of hypothetical moral dilemmas, which were better suited to males, who preferred abstractions, than to females who preferred context. Originally support for Gilligan's critique came from several studies showing women's moral judgment scores were, on the average, lower than those of men. Yet reanalyses of those studies indicated that once adjustments were made for education and occupation, differences between men and women disappeared. Gilligan has, nevertheless, persisted in her claim that an alternative theory is needed to describe women's moral voice. She maintains that Kohlberg has overlooked the dynamics of relatedness and interdependence, dynamics that require a radically new approach to moral psychology.

Gilligan's criticisms of Kohlberg's position seem more applicable to some of his philosophical statements than to the organization of the scoring manual. The scoring manual puts concerns about building relationships on the same footing as concerns about justice and rights. Furthermore, although Kohlberg's moral stages were based on an all-male sample, they are similar to Loevinger's stages of ego development, which were originally developed from an all-female longitudinal sample. In sum, there is little evidence to support the view that men and women follow radically divergent developmental paths. On the other hand, Gilligan's analyses suggest that men and women may tend to have somewhat different moral concerns and sensitivities.

D. Moral Judgment and Moral Action

Gilligan's work is one of the many projects broadening the field of moral development to include a wide array of affective and personality variables influencing decision-making and action. In an effort to organize this literature and to integrate relevant research in other fields, Rest has proposed that the internal processes leading to moral action be divided into four sequential components or phases: (1) interpreting the moral situation; (2) formulating the moral ideal; (3) choosing a course of action in the light of one's moral and nonmoral values; and (4) executing one's choice.

The process of moral action begins with a perception that one is in a situation that will likely require a moral response. Feminist ethicists have pointed out that key to this perception is what Weil and Murdoch have called attentiveness and what Noddings has called engrossment, a sensitive openness to and focused awareness of the needs, thoughts, and feelings of others. Their analyses point to the critical role that empathy plays in motivating individuals to become involved and in providing information about the source of the other's distress and how it may be alleviated. Hoffman's research elaborates such notions from a psychological perspective by showing how empathy develops from the quasi-instinctual reactions of infants to the deliberative responses of older children.

The second phase involves the reasoning and decision-making process that result in a moral judgment or in the determination of a moral ideal. The cognitive developmental approach has dominated the research in this area; yet it has only identified deep structures of moral reasoning. Such structures do not directly predict to behavior or even to action choices, yet moral judgment stages have been shown to be related to delinquency, altruism, resistance to the temptation to cheat, the clinical performance of medical interns, participation in the Berkeley Free Speech Sit-in, and a willingness to disobey in the Milgram experiment. In most studies, the higher one's moral stage was, the greater the likelihood that one would perform the putatively moral action. In order to obtain a fuller picture of the moral judgment process, psychologists need to attend to how particular beliefs, values, and life commitments influence the choice of one course of action over another. Here recent narrative and hermeneutical approaches that look at moral judgment within the context of an individual's life story may prove helpful.

In the third phase, individuals ascertain the extent to which they feel personally responsible for acting on their moral choices at the second phase. For example, many of those who participated in the Milgram experiment admitted that it was wrong to administer painful shocks, but, nevertheless, believed that they did not have a responsibility to quit the experiment because they were following the instructions of the psychologist authority. Blasi's research indicates judgments of responsibility develop in stages that roughly parallel the moral judgment stages. As individuals develop to the higher stages, they experience themselves as more autonomous, that is, as more personally responsible for their values, decisions, and actions. Judgments of

responsibility, while related to cognitive moral development, appear rooted in processes of identity and development through which adolescents making the transition into adulthood must determine the centrality of moral commitments to their self-definition.

In the fourth phase, moral aims become moral deeds. Many personality variables may play a role at this phase. For example, research by Krebs and Kohlberg indicated that stage 4 subjects with high ego strength were better able to resist the temptation to cheat than stage 4 counterparts with low ego stage. More recently research by Haan has shown that defenses and coping and self-assertion strategies play an important role in the way in which individuals interact in game simulated moral situations.

E. Promoting Moral Development

Cognitive developmentalists generally explain stage change as the result of disequilibration brought about by experiences that are not readily assimilable within a person's existing cognitive structure. Such experiences are thought to lead to cognitive conflict, which in turn leads to the construction of a new stage. Experimental and educational research suggest that experiences fostering moral development provide at least one of the following conditions: (1) exposure to higher stage reasoning; (2) exposure to a conflicting opinion (at the same stage as one's own); and (3) perspective taking.

Relatively little attention has been paid to the role of families in promoting moral development. This is partly due to the research showing that moral development is not confined to early childhood as Freudians among others had posited but continues into adulthood. The lack of attention to the family may have also been influenced by Piaget's belief that the parent–child relationship tends to foster a heteronomous morality. Furthermore, the stages of parents and children are only modestly correlated and there is no evidence that parent's stage puts a ceiling on their children's development or that the children of higher stage parents necessarily develop to higher stages themselves. There is a growing body of research, however, that indicates that parenting style and the nature of family discussion play a significant role in stimulating moral development. Baumrind, for example, has found that the most effective parenting is neither authoritarian nor permissive, but authoritative. Authoritative parenting combines a high level of parent and child communication with control and realistic demands. Focusing on family discussions, Powers has identified that the patterns most conducive to moral development blend cognitive challenges with affective support. [*See* PARENTING.]

Considerable research has been conducted on educational applications of moral development theory. The most widely used approach based on cognitive developmental theory is the discussion of moral dilemmas. Hundreds of studies have found that moral discussions led by a teacher–facilitator employing Socratic questioning techniques promote modest (about a third of a stage) but significant stage change. Research by Berkowitz indicates that even leaderless discussion can promote stage change when the participants employ certain dialogical or transactional strategies, such as offering a countersuggestion, finding common ground, requesting a justification, and juxtaposing different arguments.

Kohlberg, Higgins, and Power have developed a more radical moral education strategy, the just community approach, which builds on Piaget's view that moral autonomy is fostered under conditions of equality and reciprocity. Just communities consist of a relatively small group of students (from 30 to 90) who take a core of courses together and who make and enforce their rules with their teachers in a direct participatory democracy. Research indicates that the just community approach not only promotes moral reasoning development but nurtures students' sense of responsibility and agency.

Key to the just community approach is an emphasis on building a positive moral culture. This culture has been described in terms of the extent to which norms and values expressive of a relatively high stage of fairness and group solidarity are shared and upheld by members of the program. A positive moral culture appears to provide both a motivating and a disequilibrating context for moral development. Students are attracted to a democratic group that they perceive as genuinely caring. At the same time, students are challenged by membership in a group with high expectations for responsible behavior.

V. CONCLUSION

The study of moral development emerged in the early 1960s as the seminal cognitive developmental studies of Jean Piaget and Lawrence Kohlberg captured the attention of developmental and social psychologists. The initial phase of cognitive developmental research focused on the description of stages of reasoning from childhood through adulthood. The current phase of research seeks to understand the relationship between moral reasoning and moral behavior by exploring dimensions of the self as well as the social environment.

This article has been reprinted from the *Encyclopedia of Human Behavior, Volume 3.*

BIBLIOGRAPHY

Damon, W. (1988). "The Moral Child: Nurturing the Children's Natural Moral Growth." Free Press, New York.
Garrod, A. (1993). "Approaches to Moral Development: New Research and Emerging Themes." Teachers College Press, New York.
Gilligan, C., Ward, J. V., & Taylor, J. (1988). "Remapping the Moral Domain: A Contribution of Women's Thinking to Psychological Theory and Education." Harvard University Press, Cambridge, MA.
Kuhmerker, L. (1991). "The Kohlberg Legacy for the Helping Professions." Religious Education Press, Birmingham, AL.
Kurtines, W. M., & Gewirtz, J. (Eds.) (1991). "Moral Behavior and Development," Vol. 1. Earlbaum, Hillsdale, NJ.
Kurtines, W. M. & Gerwirtz, J. (Eds.) (1991). "Moral Behavior and Development," Vol. II. Earlbaum, Hillsdale, NJ.
Power, F. C., Higgins, A., & Kohlberg, L. (1989). "Lawrence Kohlberg's Approach to Moral Education." Columbia University Press, New York.
Schrader, D. (1990). "The Legacy of Lawrence Kohlberg." Josey-Bass, San Francisco.

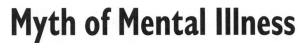

Myth of Mental Illness

Thomas Szasz

State University of New York, Syracuse Health Science Center

Diagnosis   The name of a condition considered to be an illness.

Literal Illness   Objectively demonstrable pathological alteration in cells, tissues, or organs.

Metaphorical Illness   Personal and interpersonal problems authoritatively defined and treated as diseases; the diagnosis-sounding name of disturbed or disturbing behavior.

Myth of Mental Illness   The thesis that because the mind is not a part of the body, mental illness is a mythological entity.

Therapeutic State   Political system characterized by social controls exercised in the name of health, largely by health professionals.

In 1960, I coined the phrase **"MYTH OF MENTAL ILLNESS"** to identify the intrinsically metaphoric nature of the idea of mental illness, to alert the public to the dangers of viewing distressed and distressing behaviors as diseases, and to undermine the moral legitimacy of psychiatric excuses and coercions. The claim that mental illnesses do not exist was not intended to imply that distressing personal experiences and deviant behaviors do not exist. Anxiety and depression, conflict and crime exist, and indeed are intrinsic to the human condition. But they are not diseases. We classify them as diseases in order to medicalize (mis)behaviors to our profit or at our peril.

I. THE CONCEPT OF DISEASE

The concept of illness, like all concepts, is a human construct whose meaning is culturally, and even personally, contingent. Because different individuals and institutions have different interests, conflicts concerning the definition of disease reflect their respective needs and desires. Thus, for the pathologist, disease is a demonstrable pathoananatomic or pathophysiologic condition of the human body; for the patient, it is a feeling of discomfort or the experience of disability; for the practicing physician, especially the psychiatrist, it is an undefinable mixture of bodily disease, personal distress, and violation of social rules; and for the mental patient, mental disease is likely to be a stigma (perhaps causing involuntary confinement in a mental hospital) or a special status (providing patients with excuses and/or economic support).

Similar considerations apply to other concepts, such as the concept of death. The traditional criterion of death is cessation of respiration, which terminates all bodily functions. The development of the mechanical respirator and the technology of organ transplantation rendered this criterion insufficient and led to the creation of the concept of brain death. When a machine can replace the function of the muscles of respiration, individuals unable to breathe on their own can be kept alive. Some persons on respirators are conscious and soon regain their power to breathe. Others are in a coma, never regain consciousness, and cannot be weaned from a respirator (without "killing" them). The need to identify clearly individuals who fall into the latter group led to the development of the concept of brain death, which supplements, rather than replaces, the concept of death as cessation of respiration. The former criterion is used to justify harvesting the brain-dead person's "live" organs. The latter criterion is still needed to justify burying the "dead" corpse.

Although the term "brain death" has a valid descriptive content, it also functions as a justification for harvesting "live" organs from human bodies. Expanding the category we call "disease"—by adding psychopathology to somatic pathology—must be understood as a similar process of accommodation to changing social conditions.

A. From the Humoral to the Cellular Theory of Disease

From the time of the ancient Greeks until the dawn of the modern age, disease was believed to be the manifestation of disequilibrium among the four humors—blood, phlegm, black bile, and yellow bile. This view, known as the humoral theory of disease, was intrinsically materialist, oriented solely to the body.

Hippocrates (fifth century BC) and Galen (second century AD) both viewed all diseases as malfunctions of the body. They considered madness, exemplified by melancholia, as much a bodily affliction as any other disease. Modern students of psychopathology seem to be unaware how closely the contemporary concept of mental illness as brain disease (amenable to drug treatment) resembles the old concept of (mental) illness as humoral disequilibrium (amenable to purging). At the same time, we must not lose sight of the fact that Greek and Roman poets and philosophers recognized the fundamental difference between bodily disease and personal distress: They regularly referred to the latter as "disease of the soul" and emphasized its metaphorical (nonmedical) character.

Although from the seventeenth century on, scientists view and study the human body as a machine, the humoral theory of disease was fully displaced only in the nineteenth century with the introduction of the concept of somatic pathology, that is, disease as a disturbance in the structure or function of cells, tissues, or organs.

B. Diagnosis of Disease

The scientific classification of disease, called nosology—aimed at distinguishing healthy tissue from unhealthy tissue, one illness from another illness—began at the autopsy table, with the dissection, examination, and identification of abnormalities of organs and tissues visible to the naked eye. This enterprise constituted the discipline of gross pathology. With the development of microscopy and tissue-staining techniques, the diagnostic process was refined and the discipline of microscopic pathology or histopathology was born. The invention of chemical and serological tests of blood and tissue fluids extended the process still further and the resulting discipline was called clinical pathology.

In the 1940s, the final arbiters of what constituted a bona fide illness were the pathologists. And they, too—not the patient's physicians—were the final arbiters of the correct name of the disease that ailed and killed the patient. In other words, the pathologist's findings at autopsy (called pathological diagnosis) always prevailed over the physician's findings at the bedside (the clinical diagnosis). This was the classic, somatic–pathologic criterion of disease in action.

It is important to mention here that the scientific diagnosis of live patients is, for the most part, a recent technological achievement. The medical measurement of body temperature dates from 1852. The sphygmomanometer (to measure blood pressure) was invented in 1896. Most of the sophisticated tests used today are post-World War II developments. Before World War II, there were still physicians who were famous and sought after because they were known as "great diagnosticians." Today, the great diagnosticians are not celebrated medical doctors but sophisticated medical machines.[7]

Before World War II, few disease were treatable. Nosology was then an honest, observation-oriented enterprise. Its aims were empirical validity and scientific respectability; treatment was not a relevant diagnostic consideration. Admittedly, this is an idealized and simplified version of the situation. There has always been a gray area in medicine, that is, an area characterized by physicians accepting certain behaviors or complaints—such as homosexuality, trigeminal neuralgia, chronic fatigue syndrome—as evidence of "disease" without demonstrable somatic pathology. This opened the door to equating (mis)behavior or complaint with disease, and psychiatry has marched right through.

The classic, objectively verifiable, pathological criteria of disease-as-lesion have thus been replaced with the new, socially correct economic and political criteria of disease-as-complaint-and-treatability. To maintain a semblance of similarity between the new criterion of disease as "treatability" (subjective response to medical intervention) and the old criterion of disease as somatic pathology, a new class of mental health professionals has arisen, whose function is to produce high-tech mind–brain correlates for mental disorders catalogued in the *Diagnostic and Statistical Manual* (DSM).

I maintain that our current psychiatric nosology does not encode the objectively verifiable condition of the patient's body at all; instead, it reflects the attitudes of family and society to his or her dependency and unproductivity and their justifications for the interventions they want politicians and physicians to provide for the patient (as therapy or, more precisely, interventions they want to impose on patients in the name of therapy).

When and from what source did the impetus arise to supplement the classic criterion of disease as somatic pathology with the new criterion of disease as psychopathology? It arose in the seventeenth century, from two interlocking sources. One was the desire to diminish the severity of criminal penalties (especially for suicide); the other was the desire to expand the scope of noncriminal social controls (to compensate for the inadequacy of criminal sanctions as a means of controlling distressing conduct, such as depression).

These dual pressures reached a critical level during the eighteenth century, when the desire for judicial mercy generated a huge increase in the use of the insanity defense, and the desire for effective social controls generated a huge increase in the use of involuntary mental hospitalization. Both of these practices rest squarely on the idea of insanity as an illness of the mind-as-brain. As the familiar bodily diseases were manifested by impaired functioning of the heart or kidneys, insanity was (said to be) manifested by impaired functioning of the will, causing a diminution or loss of the patients' responsibility for their actions. This medical–ideological perspective paved the way for the transformation of the person from citizen to madman. The result was that state authorities—in the main, jurists and psychiatrists working in concert—were permitted to treat individuals guilty of crimes as not guilty by reason of insanity, treat individuals innocent of legal wrongdoing as incompetent or dangerous, and incarcerate both groups in asylums or hospitals.

Not surprisingly, these uses of the idea of insanity as an illness quickly made it socially indispensable, illustrating the painful validity of Alexis de Tocqueville's observation, "To commit violent and unjust acts, it is not enough for a government to have the will or even the power; the habits, ideas, and passions of the time must lend themselves to their committal." The habits, ideas, and passions condensed into the idea of insanity led to the transformation of madness from melancholia and mania into mental disease, of the madhouse from insane asylum into mental hospital, and of the mad-doctor from alienist into psychiatrist. The concept of psychopathology was thus added to that of somatic pathology: Mental illness was defined as a brain disease, with "mental" rather than "bodily" manifestations. This materialist premise formed, and continues to form, the explanatory–justificatory basis of psychiatry. Two examples follow that illustrate this view.

In 1812, Benjamin Rush, the undisputed father of American psychiatry, asserted that "lying is a corporeal disease." Today, E. Fuller Torrey, a prominent research psychiatrist, asserts, "based on studies of gross pathology, neurochemistry, cerebral blood flow and metabolism, as well as electrical, neurological, and neuropsychological measures, schizophrenia has been clearly established to be a brain disease just as surely as multiple sclerosis, Parkinson's disease, and Alzheimer's disease are established as real brain diseases." Similar assertions abound in newspapers and magazines as well as in professional journals. Modern proponents of this conception of mental illness (as brain disease) no longer base their claims on adducing observable somatopathological findings; instead, they use the new criterion of biological markers, exemplified by identifying abnormalities in neurotransmitters or brain activities as revealed by positron emission tomography (PET) scanning techniques.

II. THE MYTH OF MENTAL ILLNESS

Most people who say or hear the term "mental illness" act as if they were unaware of the distinction between the literal and metaphoric uses of language. But of course they are not. No one believes that love sickness is a (literal) disease. Yet, (virtually) everyone believes that mental sickness is a (literal) disease; and (virtually) no one realizes that this proves the nonexistence, rather than the existence, of mental illness. For if mental illnesses are brain diseases (like Parkinsonism), then they are diseases of the body, not the mind; and if they are the names of behaviors (like substance abuse), then they are (mis)behaviors, not diseases. A screwdriver may be an alcoholic drink or a carpenter's implement. No amount of research on orange juice and vodka can establish that it is a hitherto unrecognized type of tool.

A. Conceptual Critique

Our contemporary mind set is so thoroughly medicalized (psychiatrized) that it is quite useless to demonstrate the logical–linguistic misconceptions inherent in the claim that "mental illness is like any other illness." Philosophers defending my views against those of my psychiatric critics have commented on the self-validating character of the fallacy of mental illness. For example, Ronald de Sousa, a professor of philosophy at the University of Toronto, wrote:

> [S]uppose we accept the claim that the manifestations referred to as 'mental illness' have biological causes, what would that entail about the existence of mental illness? The answer is *absolutely nothing*. For by exactly the same token the manifestations labelled 'sane behavior' have biological causes. So what is the difference? The obvious suggestion is that the causes of mental illness consist in biological malfunction or organic sickness . . . But actually, if we can show this we have done the opposite of what we intended: instead of vindicating the concept of mental illness we have rendered it otiose. For we now have an organic illness to worry about . . . But now either mental illness is *reduced* to physical illness, or it refers to *symptoms* of physical illness. Neither alternative vindicates the concept.

None of this matters. Unless a person is prepared to defy the combined forces of the state, science, medicine, law, and popular opinion, a person living in the United States today must believe, or at least pretend to believe, that mental illnesses are brain diseases, that scientists have identified the brain lesions that cause such illnesses, and that psychiatrists thus possess irrefutable proof that mental illnesses exist, are brain diseases, and hence are "like other illnesses." Conventional wisdom as well as political correctness preclude entertaining the possibility that mental illness, like spring fever, is a metaphor.

Everyday language is, of course, metaphoric through and through. There is not only nothing wrong with using evocative metaphors, but their use is the very essence of effective poetry and rhetoric. Hopefully, both speaker and listener remain aware of the distinction between literal and metaphorical language. "The greatest thing by far," declared Aristotle, "is to be a master of metaphor." Conversely, being a willing slave of metaphor constitutes an abuse of language, with grave consequences, typically for the speaker's intended victim, but in the end usually for the speaker as well.

If a person believes, or wants to believe, that mental diseases are brain diseases—perhaps because he or she wants to expand the category of illness by including medically managed life problems in it—then he or she will accept the view that "mental illness is like any other illness." However, if a person believes that mental diseases are not brain diseases—perhaps because he or she wants to restrict the category of illness to demonstrable bodily diseases—then he or she will reject the reality of mental illnesses.

Belief in the reality of a psychiatric fiction, such as mental illness, cannot be dispelled by reasoning any more than belief in the reality of a religious fiction, such as life after death, can be. The analogy between psychiatry and religion is more than a debating device; its power lies in the actual similarities between these two important social institutions. Religion provides, inter alia, an institutionalized denial of the human foundations of meaning and the finitude of life; this allows individuals to theologize life and entrust its management to clerical professionals. Similarly, psychiatry provides, inter alia, an institutionalized denial of the reality of free will and the tragic nature of life; this allows individuals to medicalize life and entrust its management to mental health professionals. In short, psychiatric metaphors play the same role in therapeutic societies as religious metaphors play in theological societies.

Linguistic clarification, such as I have just offered, is helpful to persons who want to think clearly, regardless of consequences. However, it is not helpful—in fact, it is harmful—to persons who want to respect social institutions whose integrity rests on the literal uses of a master metaphor, who want to have successful careers in those institutions, or, perhaps most importantly, who want to make use of the services offered by those institutions. Whenever someone invokes the term mental illness, we must immediately ask, *Cui bono?* (Who profits [from the stratagem]?).

In short, psychiatrists and their allies have succeeded in persuading the scientific community, the courts, the media, and the general public that the conditions they call mental disorders are diseases, that is, phenomena independent of human motivation or will. Because it is impossible to marshall empirical evidence to support this claim, the psychiatric profession relies on supporting it with a periodically revised version of its scientistic bible, the American Psychiatric Association's *Diagnostic and Statistical Manual of Mental Disorders*. The official view is that these manuals list the various "mental disorders" that afflict "patients." My view is that they are rosters of officially accredited psychiatric diagnoses, constructed by task forces appointed by officers of the American Psychiatric Association (APA). For more than 200 years, psychiatrists have thus constructed diagnoses, pretended that the terms they coined were morally neutral descriptions of brain diseases, and no one with political power has challenged their pretensions. [*See* DSM-IV.]

B. Consequentialist Critique

Because the idea of mental illness combines a faulty conceptualization (of nondisease as disease) with an immoral justification (of coercion as cure), its effect is two-pronged: it corrupts language and curtails freedom and responsibility. Accordingly, my critique of the concept has also been two-pronged, one conceptual or philosophical, the other consequentialist or political. My conceptual critique has focused on the distinction between the literal and metaphorical uses of language; my political critique has focused on the distinction between dealing with grown persons as adults (possessing free will and rights and responsibilities) and dealing with them as if they were infants or idiots (lacking free will and rights and responsibilities).

The differences between the descriptive and prescriptive modes of language merit a brief comment here. Saying that John's hair is brown is a description; saying that he should have it cut is a prescription. A purely descriptive sentence is the report of an observation that asks nothing of anyone; a purely prescriptive sentence is a request that asks for a specific response from the listener. However, the descriptive "is" or "has" is often used in the injunctive mode, in lieu of "must" or "should," making the difference between description and prescription a matter of context rather than vocabulary. For example, when a powerful First Lady says to a loyal subordinate that she is concerned about X, the message is that the subordinate should do to X what the First Lady wants done to X. Should the consequences of such an order be later scrutinized, the First Lady has "deniability": She can truthfully say that she did not order anyone to do anything to X.

Because the psychiatrist has power over patients (or over the person others designate as patients), the psychiatrist's seemingly descriptive statements also function as covert prescriptions. For example, a psychiatrist may describe a man who maintains that God's voice commands him to kill his wife because she is a witch as schizophrenic. However, this diagnostic description typically functions as a prescription, for example, to hospitalize the patient involuntarily (lest he kill his wife), or, after he has killed her, to acquit him as not guilty by reason of insanity and again hospitalize him against his will.

The essential feature of a claim is that it is a demand a person makes on others, typically for the recognition of an entitlement: to an excuse (as in criminal law), to money damages (as in civil law), to the historicity of an (alleged) past event (as in religion). For example, Muslims, Jews, and Christians agree that God created the world in six days and on the seventh He rested, but they disagree which day God had so consecrated. The adherents of each faith name—and, when they can, forcibly impose on others—a different day of the week as the Day of Rest.

Mutatis mutandis, certain persons assert that they hear voices, attribute the voices to God and believe that carrying out illegal acts commanded by the voices is morally and legally justified. Certain other persons assert that such claimants suffer from a disease called schizophrenia, attribute the disease to the brain and the diagnosis to science, and believe that excusing schizophrenics of crimes and incarcerating them in mental hospitals is morally and medically justified. These are the rationalizations of psychotics and psychiatrists to justify their respective recourse to violence. I reject the moral legitimacy of both parties' rationalizations. The psychotic who kills his wife and attributes his violence to "voices" knows right from wrong. The psychiatrist who incarcerates patients and attributes his or her violence to "treatment" knows that involuntary mental hospitalization entails the loss of liberty.

Ostensibly, what justifies the psychiatrists' use of force is the familiar dual claim of disease-and-treatment. Actually, what justifies it is an assumption, concealed in the idea of insanity but intrinsic to it—namely, that the mental patient is legally incompetent and that his or her coercion is a form of treatment. This presumption permits psychiatrists to pretend that coercion may, at any moment, be a necessary element in the conscientious and correct practice of their particular branch of medical healing. Indeed, because psychiatric coercion is defined as beneficial for the best interests of coerced patients, both law and psychiatry regard the principle of eschewing psychiatric coercion as synonymous with "withholding life-saving treatment" from patients who need it. As a result, when a person under the care of a psychiatrist kills himself (or someone else), his psychiatrist is likely to be held responsible for the patient's action.

The insistence of contemporary psychiatrists that all mental diseases are brain diseases has brought us full circle, in effect returning us to the days of the humoral theory. Ironically, in those days people recognized that problems in living—epitomized by grief—were metaphorical maladies. To repeat: If we define illness as a physicochemical disturbance of the body, then we can or must agree that diagnoses recognized by pathologists (using this criterion) are the names of diseases, and that diagnoses not so recognized by pathologists are the names of nondiseases. Because the mind is not a bodily organ, the foregoing definition precludes the existence of mental illnesses.

Similarly, if we restrict the concept of treatment to a voluntary relationship between a medical practitioner (physician) and an adult, competent client (patient), then involuntary medical interventions are disqualified from being bona fide treatments. It is important to keep in mind that in a free society, the physician's "right" to treat a person rests not on his or her diagnosis, but on the subject's consent to treatment. Psychiatry is a systematic violation of this legal–political principle, a violation especially odious because most persons treated against their will by psychiatrists are defined as legally competent: they can vote, marry and divorce, and so forth.

One of the crucial elements of my critique of the idea of mental illness is rejection of the view that once a person is categorized as a mental patient, that his or her status as a moral agent is at the mercy of the psychiatrist's say-so. I agree with Gilbert Chesterton's statement: "The madman is not a person who has lost his reason. The madman is a person who has lost everything but his reason." As a rule, the so-called mental patient is a conscious adult, possessing free will and responsibility, who has not been declared legally incompetent. Regardless of psychiatric diagnosis, he or she is entitled to liberty, unless convicted of a crime punishable by imprisonment; and if he or she breaks the law and is convicted of it, then he or she is guilty of a crime and ought to be punished for it. Under no circumstances should such a person profit from psychiatric excuses or suffer from psychiatric coercions.

III. DIAGNOSES ARE NOT DISEASES

The idea of illness implies a deviation from a norm. Despite the prevailing pretense that "mental illness is like any other illness," we typically use the term bodily illness to denote a deviation from the structural and functional integrity of the human body, and term mental illness to denote a deviation from a psychological, social, moral, political, or legal norm.

Every competent speaker of English understands that it is one thing to call "getting malaria" a disease, and another thing to call "getting marijuana" a disease. The person who gets malaria does not seek to acquire the parasite and is a passive victim of it. Whereas the person who "gets" marijuana seeks to acquire the plant and is an active consumer of it.

Diseases are bodily events—anatomical or physiological lesions, the results of natural processes or human actions—that "exist." People "have" malaria regardless of whether or not they know it or physicians diagnose it (recognize and name it). On the other hand, diagnoses are names that human beings invent and attach to "conditions" that they believe are diseases or that they want to treat as diseases. Because diagnoses are social constructs, they vary from time to time, and from culture to culture. In the past, physicians accepted focal infection and masturbatory insanity as diagnoses; now they regard them as diagnostic errors or medical fictions. Similarly, what counts as a diagnosis in one country, may not count as a diagnosis in another. In France, physicians diagnose "liver crises," in Germany, "low blood pressure," and in the United States, "substance abuse."

Human beings have a passion to name and classify everything in their environment. Constructing and deconstructing diagnoses is but one example of this propensity. Why do we make diagnoses? There are at least five important reasons:

1. Scientific. To identify the organs or tissues affected and perhaps the cause of the illness;
2. Medical-therapeutic—to reassure the patient that the physician knows what ails him or her and to aid the physician in selecting the appropriate treatment for the disease diagnosed;
3. Professional. To enlarge the scope, and thus the power and prestige, of a state-protected medical monopoly and the income of its practitioners;
4. Legal. To justify the state-sanctioned coercive interventions outside of the criminal justice system;
5. Political–economic. To justify enacting and enforcing measures aimed at promoting public health and providing funds for research and treatment on projects classified as medical
6. Personal. To enlist the support of public opinion, the media, and the legal system for bestowing special privileges, and imposing special hardships, on persons diagnosed as (mentally) ill.

One of the most important features of bodily diseases is that with the aid of modern diagnostic methods they can be identified without speaking with the subject, indeed without the subject being considered a patient—that is, without the subject having any complaints or seeking medical services. For example, diabetes or hypertension can be diagnosed without any information about the subject—say, in the context of examination for life insurance or military service—by testing body fluids and measuring physiological functions. In other words, it is possible to have a bodily illness and not know it; or, to put it more precisely, it is possible to have asymptomatic illnesses; indeed, in their early stages most illnesses fall into this class.

In contrast, it is not possible to have an asymptomatic mental illness; the term is an oxymoron. Panic disorder means that the subject complains of intense anxiety. Attention deficit disorder means that the teacher complains that the subject is inattentive. The observed or observable (mis)behavior is defined as

the disease. Strictly speaking, mental illness is not diagnosed. Instead, the role of mental patient is created, either by the subject assuming it voluntarily or by its being ascribed or imposed on the subject by force. Thus, when a man appears to be depressed and his wife and her physician believe that he is contemplating suicide, but he insists that he is fine, his illness is not considered to be asymptomatic and he is not regarded as being unaware of it; he is said to be "denying" his illness.

A. Diagnosing Illness and Mental Illness

How do we determine that a person is sick, in other words, that his or her organs misbehave? The penultimate proof of having a disease is objectively demonstrable physical disability, and its ultimate proof is death. Cancer of the pancreas disables and kills the person who has it. Because bodily disease is the name of a deviation from a biological norm, the "penalty" for it is biological (imposed by scientific laws).

How do we determine that a person is mentally ill? The penultimate proof of having a mental disease is subjectively experienced disability which the agent attributes to his or her mind, and its ultimate proof is involuntary confinement in a mental hospital. Because mental disease is the name of a deviation from an existential-behavioral norm, the "penalty" for it is existential social (self-imposed or socially imposed).

These differences between bodily illness and mental illness correspond to the familiar differences between nature and convention, science and law (e.g., the speed of light and the speed limit). The behavior of organs is subject to the laws of science, the behavior of persons, to the rules of society. The former are discovered by scientists, the latter are decreed by politicians and psychiatrists. The normal function of the pancreas is determined by nature, whereas the normal function of the person is determined by society. It makes no sense to talk about what the proper function of a bodily organ ought to be, but it makes eminently good sense to talk about what the proper function of a person ought to be. Because psychiatry deals with how people live, how they might live, and how they ought to live, it can be neither a science nor a therapy.

When and how did the modern diagnosis of mental illness arise? Like the modern diagnosis of bodily disease, it too arose during the latter part of the nineteenth century and was based on diagnostic advances in medicine. Many patients then confined in insane asylums suffered from some form of brain disease, often neurosyphilis. But many did not. The asylum directors were trained as neurologists and neuropathologists and were given the power to diagnose, treat, and incarcerate mental patients against their will. The fatal epistemological error of psychiatry was built into its very foundations: The theory of psychiatry (premised on the view of mental illness as neuropathology) was inconsistent with the empirical basis of the practice of psychiatry (as involuntary confinement).

The idea of mental illness as bodily illness was anchored in the identification of misbehaving brains, a type of misbehavior that typically could be detected only after the patient was dead. However, the practice of treating mental illness was anchored in the forcible incarceration of misbehaving persons, a type of misbehavior that by definition could be detected only in the living person (and then only in patients who were socially less powerful than their psychiatrists).

All the same, the die was cast. Once the focus of nosology had shifted from postmortem to antemortem diagnoses, it was a short step to turn so-called clinical attention from the behavior of the patient's body to the behavior of the patient's personality. The resulting medicalized political–economic atmosphere encouraged the constructing and deconstructing of psychiatric diagnoses, a practice with which we are now familiar. [*See* PERSONALITY.]

B. Constructing and Deconstructing Mental Diseases

Lawmakers do not discover prohibited categories of conduct called "crimes"; instead, they create them by decreeing legal rules that prohibit and punish conduct deemed undesirable, for example, unjustified killing or selling cocaine. Similarly, psychiatrists do not discover prohibited categories of conduct called "mental diseases"; instead, they create them by decreeing psychiatric rules that disapprove of and diagnose as diseases conduct deemed undesirable, for example, ingesting illegal drugs, called substance abuse, or feeling that life is not worth living, called clinical depression.

Enacting and repealing laws legitimizes politicians as benevolent legislators, who help people en-masse to remedy social problems. Constructing and decon-

structing diagnoses legitimizes psychiatrists as benevolent physicians who help people as individuals to remedy mental diseases. This self-aggrandizing and self-legitimizing urge led the early alienists to create masturbatory insanity; Emil Kraepelin to create *dementia praecox*, Eugen Bleuler to create schizophrenia, and Sigmund Freud to create transference neurosis; and now leads task forces of the APA to construct periodically new versions of the *Diagnostic and Statistical Manual*.

Thus, psychiatric nosologists busy themselves not only with discovering the existence of new mental diseases, but also with discovering the nonexistence of old ones. For example, homosexuality, long a favorite psychiatric diagnosis, ceased to be a disease in 1980, unless it was ego-dystonic, in which case it was still an illness. In 1994, the diagnosis of neurosis was deleted from the roster, but body dysmorphic disorder was added to it.

I am not saying that making rules to govern personal conduct is not important. On the contrary. Breakdown in the just enforcement of just laws is far more destructive of the social order than the absence of accurate medical diagnoses or effective methods of medical treatment. What I am saying is that our old social order, based on the Rule of Law, is on a collision course with our new social order, based increasingly on allegedly therapeutic coercions justified by "mental illness."

IV. MENTAL ILLNESS AND THE "MEDICAL MODEL"

Since the end of World War II, the word *medical* has become virtually synonymous with *true, scientific,* and *good*. In this milieu, opposing something labeled "medical" is like opposing the proverbial motherhood. Hence, when I asserted that mental illnesses are not diseases and therefore fall outside the scope and authority of medicine, my writings were interpreted as not only advancing certain observations and opinions, but as also impugning the authority and legitimacy of both medicine and psychiatry. As I see it, then, the term medical model—and related phrases, such as "biological psychiatry" and "remedicalization"— arose in dialectical opposition to the sustained argument that mental illnesses are nondiseases.

The defenders of conventional psychiatric excuses and coercions identify themselves as supporters of the medical model and deploy the phrase, "rejecting the medical model," as an epithet. Identifying a speaker as one who rejects the medical model does the same sort of semantic work as calling him or her a racist: It proves, without need for argument or evidence, that he or she is an uninformed charlatan who denies the advances of modern psychiatry, who wants to deprive suffering people of the treatment they need, and who is probably also mad.

In short, supporters of the medical model behave as if they believe that if they could convince politicians and the families of mental patients that persons diagnosed mentally ill are sick, then they could treat them, regardless of whether or not the patients want to be treated. This belief is fallacious. As noted earlier, in ordinary medical practice, the doctor's "right" to treat a patient depends on, and is (legally) legitimized by, not the patient's illness, but by the patient's consent. The patient with hypertension takes medication not (only) because he or she is ill, but because he or she agrees to take it. The physician cannot force a noncompliant patient to ingest an antihypertensive drug. It follows that if depression were a bodily disease, the psychiatrist, as a medical (model) practitioner, would lose, not gain, the right to coerce his or her patient (to ingest a drug or to hospitalize the patient against his or her will).

Opponents of the medical model often use the same fallacious argument. Most antipsychiatrists and other critics of psychiatry uncritically embrace the role of opposing the so-called medical model. They too behave as if they believe that if they could convince politicians and the families of mental patients that persons diagnosed mentally ill are not sick, then they could prevent psychiatrists from treating them, regardless of whether or not the patients want to be treated. Thus, they fail to oppose therapeutic statism on principle. On the contrary, many critics of psychiatry actually curry the favor of the Therapeutic State, hoping to enlist its power to impose their beliefs and practices on others. Sad to say, psychiatrists and (most of) their critics alike embrace "therapeutic" coercion: the former, to forcibly impose on nonconsenting subjects interventions officially defined as helpful; the latter, to forcibly prevent consenting subjects from availing themselves of interventions officially defined as harmful.

V. INCOMPETENCE, COERCION, AND THE "PEDIATRIC MODEL"

Both groups use the sloppy phrase "medical model" to refer to what ought to be called the "pediatric model" or, more precisely, the "coercive model." To treat the child patient, the pediatrician must convince the child's parents (or guardian) that the child is sick, would benefit from treatment, and obtain their permission to treat the child. By definition, all pediatric treatment (of the very young child) is involuntary; legally, all such treatment rests on viewing the child as (mentally) incompetent to consent to, or refuse, treatment, and the parent (or guardian) as representing the child's best interests. Actually or potentially, all psychiatric treatment is similarly involuntary or coercive.

This author stands for strict adherence to a contractual, noncoercive model for interventions denominated as therapeutic. I support the rights of physicians to engage in mutually consenting psychiatric acts with other adults, regardless of whether I approve or disapprove of their choice of diagnoses and treatments. By the same token, I object to involuntary psychiatric interventions, regardless of the nature of the intervention. I recognize, of course, the practical necessity for, and moral legitimacy of, certain involuntary interventions vis-a-vis individuals declared to be legally incompetent. A comatose person cannot discharge his or her duties or represent his or her desires (except by means of a health proxy or power of attorney). Accordingly, the law provides appropriate procedures for relieving such a person of his or her rights and responsibilities as a moral agent. Although persons entrusted with the responsibility of reclassifying patients from competent adults to incompetent wards of the state might make use of medical information, they should be lay persons (jurors) and judges, not physicians or mental health specialists. Most importantly, their determination should be viewed as a legal and political procedure, not as a medical or therapeutic intervention.

VI. SUMMARY

In the early 1960s, I proposed the terms "the myth of mental illness" and "Therapeutic State" to alert the professions as well as the public to the dangers lurking in the tendency of modern states to classify deviant behaviors as mental diseases, deviant actors as mental patients, and interventions aimed at relieving personal dissatisfaction and social deviance as mental treatments. Listed below are the dangers I claim to be lurking in these fashionable ideas and interventions.

They are, briefly, the following: (1) legitimizing the belief, and habituating Americans to the idea, that it is the duty of the government to protect competent adults from themselves; (2) destroying peoples' attachment to, indeed their very understanding of, limited government; (3) confusing the medical criteria of disease and treatment (by defining certain "bad" choices as diseases, and certain "good" coercions as treatments); (4) undermining personal self-discipline and respect for responsibility by excusing persons as not responsible for their actions (because of mental illness), and undermining the Rule of Law by replacing penal sanctions with (so-called) psychiatric treatments; (5) converting the relationship between doctor and patient from a contract between two responsible adults into a domination–dependence relationship; (6) turning doctors into monopolists of diagnoses, drugs, and treatments; (7) aiding and abetting the conversion of tort law into an instrument of economic redistribution and the principle of caveat emptor into that of caveat vendor. The ideology of mental illness is making Americans increasingly dependent on a capricious and paternalistic state.

It is a truism that the interests of the individual, his or her family, and the state often conflict. Medicalizing personal problems, domestic disputes, and conflicts between the citizen and the state threatens to destroy respect not only for persons as responsible moral agents, but also for the state as an arbiter and dispenser of justice. We must never forget that the state is an organ of coercion with a monopoly on force, for good or ill. The more the state empowers physicians, the more physicians will strengthen the state (by authenticating political preferences as health values), and the more the resulting union of medicine and the state will enfeeble the individual (by depriving him or her of the right to reject interventions classified as therapeutic). "We are all here to help someone else," declares Hillary Rodham Clinton. W. H. Auden satirized this sort of solicitude by putting these words in the mouth of the therapeutic tyrant: "We are all here on earth to help others; what on earth the others are here for, I don't know."

In his great work on ancient law, Sir Henry Maine articulated his famous general proposition: "The movement of the progressive societies has hitherto been a movement from Status to Contract." The ideology of mental illness is perhaps the single most important manifestation of a radical reversal of this movement. Slowly but surely, the American polity has been transformed from a limited government based on contractual relations between adults, into an unlimited Therapeutic State based on status relations between helpers and helped.

BIBLIOGRAPHY

Macalpine, I., & Hunter, R. (1963). *Three hundred years of psychiatry, 1535–1860: A history presented in selected texts.* New York: Oxford University Press.

Maine, H. S. (1986). *Ancient law: Its connection with the early history of society, and its relation to modern ideas.* Tucson, Az: University of Arizona Press. (Original work published in 1864.)

de Sousa, R. (1972). The politics of mental illness. *Inquiry, 15,* 187–202.

Szasz, T. (1970). *The manufacture of madness: A comparative study of the inquisition and the mental health movement.* New York: Harper & Row.

Szasz, T. (1974). *The myth mental illness: Foundations of a theory of personal conduct* (rev. ed.). New York: Harper & Row. (Original work published in 1916.)

Szasz, T. (1987). *Insanity: The idea and its consequences.* New York: John Wiley.

Szasz, T. (1994). *Cruel compassion: Psychiatric control of society's unwanted.* New York: John Wiley.

Narcissistic Personality Disorder

Salman Akhtar

Jefferson Medical College

I. Manifestations
II. Distinction from Related Conditions
III. Intrinsic Nature
IV. Treatment

Narcissism Emotional investment into the self. When normal, it leads to sustained self-regard and mature aspirations. When pathological, it is accompanied by inordinate demands upon the self, excessive dependence upon acclaim from others, and deteriorated capacity for interpersonal relations.

Personality Disorder A pervasive pattern of chronically maladaptive behavior which is a source of constant interpersonal problems. Personality disorders are ego-syntonic, i.e., such individuals are not aware of their own personalities as being deviant or abnormal. They suffer from the interpersonal consequences of their behavior but they do not recognize their own role in the origin and perpetuation of these problems. Such individuals are therefore unlikely to seek professional advice although they may consent to it if this is urged by others or forced by social repercussions of their behavior.

NARCISSISTIC PERSONALITY DISORDER is a newly recognized diagnostic entity in clinical psychiatry. It was introduced into "official" psychiatric nomenclature in 1980 with the publication of the third edition of the American Psychiatric Association's *Diagnostic and Statistical Manual of Mental Disorders* (*DSM-III*). There is, however, evidence that the concept had been evolving since the turn of the century

beginning with Sigmund Freud's elucidation of the concept of narcissism.

Freud published his seminal paper "On Narcissism" in 1914. He defined narcissism as the concentration of libidinal interest upon one's ego and distinguished primary from secondary narcissism. The former was a normal phenomenon of infancy, the latter a result of withdrawal of interest from the outer world. Freud noted that human attachments are of two types: anaclitic and narcissistic. The former are evident when we are involved with those who nourish and protect us and the latter when we are involved with those who merely reflect us (the way we are, or were, or will be). In essence, the narcissistic relationship is nothing but thinly veiled self-affirmation. While avoiding character typology in this paper, Freud did refer to individuals who compel our interest by the narcissistic consistency with which they manage to keep away from their ego anything that would diminish it." However, it was not until 1931 that he described the "narcissistic character type."

> The subject's main interest is directed to self-preservation: he is independent and not open to intimidation. His ego has a large amount of aggressiveness at its disposal, which also manifests itself in readiness for activity. In his erotic life loving is preferred above being loved. People belonging to this type impress others as being "personalities"; they are especially suited to act as a support for others, to take on the role of leaders and to give a fresh stimulus to cultural development or to damage the established state of affairs.

This description is generally viewed as the pioneering portrayal of narcissistic personality disorder. The fact, however, is that a 1913 paper by Ernest Jones, one of Freud's distinguished pupils, also contained significant details regarding the phenomenology of this condition. Using the term "God Complex" for their condition, Jones portrayed such individuals as excessively admiring of themselves, having omnipotent fantasies, being exhibitionistic, and scornful of others. Such grandiosity is, at times, masked by caricatured modesty, pseudohumility, and a pretended contempt for materialistic aspects of life.

Over the subsequent decades, many other psychoanalysts contributed to the study of narcissistic personality. Prominent among these were Robert Waelder, Wilhem Reich, Christine Olden, Helen Tartakoff, and John Nemiah. These authors clearly recognized this condition though often without designating it as such. They noted that the central feature of this condition, grandiosity, is a defensive maneuver against feelings of inferiority which they traced to severe frustrations during early childhood.

In the 1970s the publication of two psychoanalytic books breathed new life in the study of narcissistic personality disorder: *The Analysis of the Self* (1971) by Heinz Kohut and *Borderline Conditions and Pathological Narcissism* (1975) by Otto Kernberg. The views of Kohut and Kernberg are summarized below. Suffice it to say here that their works stirred up considerable controversy and mobilized further interest in investigating the true nature of narcissistic personality disorder. Among those who made subsequent major contributions are Sheldon Bach, Ben Bursten, Mardi Horowitz, Arnold Modell, Arnold Rothstein, and Vamik Volkan.

Finally, when in 1980 the *DSM-III* included narcissistic personality disorder as a separate diagnostic entity, an official imprimatur was added to the evolving concept. The *DSM-IV* retained the condition with only minor modifications of its diagnostic criteria.

I. MANIFESTATIONS

The cardinal feature of narcissistic personality disorder is heightened narcissism. Individuals with this disorder display grandiosity, intense ambition, and an insatiable craving for admiration. Their consuming self-interest renders them incapable of appreciating and understanding the independent motivations and needs of others. Consequently, they come across as cold, unempathic, exploitative, and having little concern for those around them.

The clinical features of narcissistic personality disorder involve six areas of psychosocial functioning: (i) self-concept, (ii) interpersonal relations, (iii) social adaptation, (iv) ethics, standards, and ideals, (v) love and sexuality, and (vi) cognitive style. In each of these areas there are "overt" and "covert" manifestations. These designations do not necessarily imply their conscious or unconscious existence although such topographical distribution might also exist. In general, however, the "overt" and "covert" designations denote seemingly contradictory phenomenological aspects that are more or less easily discernible. Moreover, these contradictions are not restricted to the individual's self-concept but permeate his interpersonal relations, social adaptation, love life, morality, and cognitive style.

Narcissistic individuals have a grandiose *self-concept*. They give an appearance of self-sufficiency and are preoccupied with achieving outstanding success. Covertly, however, they are fragile, vulnerable to shame, sensitive to criticism, and filled with morose self-doubts and feelings of inferiority.

Their *interpersonal relations* are extensive but exploitative and driven by an intense need for tribute from others. They are unable to genuinely participate in group activities and, in family life, value children over the spouse. Inwardly, they are deeply envious of others' capacity for meaningful engagement with life. They attempt to hide such envy by scorn for others; this may, in turn, be masked by pseudo-humility.

Capable of consistent hard work, narcissistic individuals often achieve professional success and high levels of *social adaptation*. However, they are preoccupied with appearances and their work is done mainly to seek admiration. The overly zealous vocational commitment masks a dilettante-like attitude, chronic boredom, and gnawing aimlessness.

Their *ethics, standards, and ideals* display an apparent enthusiasm for sociopolitical affairs, a caricatured modesty, and pretended contempt for money in real life. At the same time, they are often quite materialistic, ready to shift values to gain favor, irreverent toward authority, and prone to pathologic lying and cutting ethical corners.

A similar contradiction is evident in the realm of *love and sexuality*. Overtly, narcissistic individuals are charming, seductive, and given to extramarital affairs, even promiscuity. Covertly, however, they draw little gratification beyond physical pleasure from sexuality and are unable to have deep and sustained romantic relations. Moreover, they seem unable to genuinely accept the incest taboo and are vulnerable to sexual perversions. [*See* LOVE AND INTIMACY.].

Superficially, their *cognitive style* suggests a decisive, opinionated, and strikingly supple intellect. However, their knowledge is often limited to trivia ("headline intelligence") and they are forgetful of details. Their capacity for learning is also compromised since learning forces one to acknowledge one's ignorance and they find this unacceptable. They are articulate but tend to use language and speaking for regulating self-esteem rather than communicating. [*See* SELF-ESTEEM.]

In sum, narcissistic personality disorder is characterized by a defensively inflated self-concept which is fueled by fantasies of glory, protected by being constantly admired for social success, and buttressed by scornful devaluation of those who stir up envy. Underneath this grandiose self-concept (not infrequently built around some real talent or special aptitude) lie disturbing feelings of inferiority, self-doubt, boredom, alienation, and aimlessness.

II. DISTINCTION FROM RELATED CONDITIONS

Individuals with narcissistic personality disorder have superficial resemblances to those with compulsive personality disorder. Both types of individuals display high ideals, great need for control, perfectionism, and a driven quality to their work. However, the compulsive seeks perfection while the narcissistic claims it. Consequently, the compulsive is modest, the narcissist haughty. The compulsive loves details that the narcissist casually disregards. The compulsive has a high regard for authority and strict inner morality, while the narcissist is often rebellious and prone to cutting ethical corners. [*See* OBSESSIVE–COMPULSIVE DISORDER.]

Three other characterological constellations need to be distinguished from narcissistic personality disorder: borderline, antisocial, and paranoid personality disorders.

Both borderline and narcissistic individuals are self-absorbed and vacillating in their relationships. Borderline individuals, however, show a greater propensity for disorganization into really regressed mental states. They are less tolerant of aloneness, more angry, and have a poorer capacity for sustained work than narcissistic individuals. [*See* BORDERLINE PERSONALITY DISORDER.]

Both antisocial and narcissistic individuals dream of glory and can lie, cheat, and indulge in ethically dubious acts to achieve success. However, in narcissistic personality such disregard of conventional morality is hidden, occasional, and cautious whereas in antisocial personality it is open, frequent, ruthless and calculated. [*See* ANTISOCIAL PERSONALITY DISORDER.]

Both paranoid and narcissistic individuals are grandiose, emotionally stilted, envious, sensitive to criticism, and highly entitled. However, the paranoid individual is pervasively mistrustful and lacks the attention-seeking charm and seductiveness of the narcissist. The cognitive style of the two types of individuals differs in a striking way. The narcissist is inattentive to real events and forgetful of details. The paranoid, in contrast, has a biased but acutely vigilant cognition. [*See* PARANOIA.]

III. INTRINSIC NATURE

In the realm of probable causes and the intrinsic nature of narcissistic personality disorder the views of Heinz Kohut and Otto Kernberg form the two major, if sharply divergent, contemporary perspectives. According to Kohut, the origin of narcissistic personality disorder resides in faulty parental empathy with the child. Kohut posits that a growing child needs an enthusiastically responsive audience ("mirroring") for his or her activities and achievements. When such mirroring is deficient, the child's ordinary pride and associated healthy need to be affirmed take on an insistent and unhealthy exhibitionistic quality (the "grandiose self Kohut also proposes that, in addition to mirroring, the child needs the opportunity to idealize the parents and draw strength from this borrowed sense of importance. When parents either are truly not admirable or their weaknesses are prematurely or shockingly revealed to the child, the hunger for powerful figures goes unsatisfied and becomes a persistent feature of later, adult life. It is this paradoxical mixture of grandiosity and hunger to belong to prestigious others that forms the nucleus of narcissistic character. Inner fragility of self-esteem is hidden by these compensatory structures. Any threat to such self-regulation mobilizes shameful sense of imperfection and intense, vengeful anger ("narcissistic rage").

In contrast to Kohut, Kernberg regards narcissistic personality not as a developmental arrest but a specific pathological formation to begin with. Kernberg differentiates the normal narcissism of children (which retains a realistic quality and does not affect the capacity for mutuality) from the early development of pathological narcissism (which creates fantastically grandiose fantasies and impairs the capacity for mutuality). Kernberg agrees that narcissistic individuals were treated by their parents in a cold, even spiteful manner. However, he adds that they were also viewed as special since they possessed some outstanding attribute, e.g., talent, beauty, superior intelligence, etc. Using Kohut's term with a different formulation, Kernberg proposes that "grandiose self" is formed by the fusion of a highly idealized view of oneself (built around some truly good aspect of oneself) and a fantastically indulgent and admiring inner audience of imagined others. Such grandiose self is a defensive structure against the anger directed at the frustrating parents of childhood. Rage in narcissistic personality is therefore the inciting agent, not merely an epiphenomenon.

The views of Kohut and Kernberg differ in many other ways but their most important differences involve (i) a developmental arrest versus a pathological formation view of grandiosity, and (ii) the reactive versus the fundamental view of aggression in narcissistic personality disorder. These differences affect the techniques which the two theoreticians propose as being suitable to treat this condition.

IV. TREATMENT

The treatment of choice for narcissistic personality disorder is psychoanalysis, provided the patient is psychologically minded, has verbal facility, and is earnestly motivated for change. Within the psychoanalytic framework, however, the approaches outlined by Kohut and Kernberg (and developed further by their proponents) differ considerably. Kohut's approach aims at a full-blown reactivation, in vivo, of the frustrated childhood mirroring and idealizing needs. The analyst accepts the validity of such needs and helps the patient see their persistence as emanating from childhood deprivations. The patient's rage, if it erupts in treatment, is interpreted as an understandable response to the inevitable empathic failures of the analyst. Such an experience is then shown to have connections with similar experiences caused by faulty parental empathy during childhood. Countless repetitions of feeling understood and seeing the present in the light of past gradually facilitate the relinquishment of grandiosity and idealizations.

Kernberg's approach differs. He emphasizes that the experiences of narcissistic patients in analysis are not readily traceable to the actuality of their childhoods. Instead, these are multilayered and include in them early wishes, defenses against those wishes, real experiences, and unconscious distortions of them. Kernberg notes that the patient's disappointments in the analyst not only reveal his or her real or fantasied frustrations of childhood, now being repeated in the treatment situation, but also dramatically reveal the patient's psychic readiness for hate and total devaluation of others. Kernberg does not view the patient's rage as a reaction to the analyst's failures but as an inevitable manifestation of the patient's pathology. At its core, this involves seething rage against real and imagined hurts from parents, a rage that is also used defensively to ward-off dependent longings. Empathy, for Kernberg, is not a therapeutic measure but a technical necessity. The mainstay of treatment is working through the patient's rage and mistrust, anxiety about dependence, and, in later phases of treatment, the guilt over having exploited, devalued, and hurt others including the analyst. With diminution of rage and dread of true attachment, there emerges a capacity to empathize with others, a reduction in self-centeredness, an ability to give, and a dawning awareness of life's complex emotional offerings in the context of genuine affective involvement with fellow human beings. [See PSYCHOANALYSIS.]

This article has been reprinted from the *Encyclopedia of Human Behavior, Volume 3.*

BIBLIOGRAPHY

Akhtar, S. (1992). "Broken Structures: Severe Personality Disorders and Their Treatment." Jason Aronson, Northvale, NJ. Akhtar, S. (1989). Narcissistic personality disorder: Descriptive features and differential diagnosis. *Psychiatric Clinics of North America* **12**, 505–529.

Bach, S. (1977). On the narcissistic state of consciousness. In "Narcissistic States and the Therapeutic Process." Jason Aronson, New York.

Kernberg, O. F. (1975). "Borderline Conditions and Pathological Narcissism." Jason Aronson, New York.

Kernberg, O. F. (Ed.) (1989). Narcissistic personality disorder. *The Psychiatric Clinics of North America,* **xii** (3).

Kohut, H. (1971). "The Analysis of the Self." International Universities Press, New York.

Kohut, H. (1977). "The Restoration of the Self." International Universities Press, New York.

Mahler, M. S., & Kaplan, L. (1977). Developmental aspects in the assessment of narcissistic and so-called borderline personalities. In "Borderline Personality Disorders: (P. Hartocolis, Ed). International Universities Press, New York.

Modell, A. (1984). "Psychoanalysis in a New Context." International Universities Press, New York.

Volkan, V. D. (1982). Narcissistic personality disorder. In "Clinical Problems in Psychiatry" (J. O. Cavenar, and H. K. H. Brodie, Eds.). Lippincott, Philadelphia, PA.

Negotiation and Conflict Resolution

Leonard Greenhalgh

Dartmouth College

Roxanne L. Okun

Personnel Decisions International

Agreement Commitment to a course of action that concludes a negotiation.

Conflict An anger-induced strain in an interpersonal relationship that is experienced at the individual level and has emotional and behavioral dimensions.

Conflict Resolution 1. A process aimed at reducing the anger-induced strain and managing the divisiveness and violence of the tactics used by the parties in conflict. 2. The conclusion of a dispute in which both parties in conflict experience a satisfactory reduction in anger-induced strain.

Negotiation A process by which the parties in conflict engage in discussion to reach an agreement (i.e., a commitment by both parties) on a course of action that meets at least some of their needs in the dispute.

Power The ability to induce compliance in the other party.

Conflict, as a sociopsychological phenomenon, is a strain in an interpersonal relationship. It is experienced at the individual level and involves thoughts, feelings, and behaviors. The thoughts define the issues (an issue is what people would say in response to the question, What is this conflict about?) and frame the dispute (e.g., is the dispute a struggle over scarce resource allocation, an interpersonal problem that must be solved, or a situation that calls for contrition and apology by one or both parties?). The feelings (e.g., anger, hurt, resentment) arise from these thoughts but, in turn, shape thought patterns. The thoughts and feelings combine to influence the individual's behavioral response to the conflict. The term **CONFLICT RESOLUTION** refers to a set of processes for reducing the strain in a relationship caused by anger and managing the divisiveness and violence of the tactics used by the parties in conflict. **NEGOTIATION** is one process within the set, but it is the primary means by which individuals address conflicts in their daily lives. When negotiating, the parties engage in discussion to reach an agreement (i.e., a commitment by both parties) on a course of action that meets at least some of their needs in the dispute. Effectiveness in negotiation and conflict resolution depends on personality predispositions as well as tactical choices.

I. CONFLICT

Conflict has been studied at several levels of analysis. At the most micro level, clinical psychologists study intrapsychic conflicts (such as the simultaneous motivation to resist being controlled and thereby gain autonomy, and to submit to control and thereby gain approval); at the most macro level, political scientists study global conflicts (such as the decades-long cold war between capitalist and communist regimes). This entry concerns interpersonal conflicts, and for clarity, we will focus on the simplest case—the dyad, in which the two people involved are referred to as the two "parties" to the conflict. Despite this focus, the analysis is generally applicable to conflicts involving more than two people.

Conflicts are endemic to relationships. People are never identical in their values, preferences, habits, schedules, and personalities. Therefore, differences of opinion arise whenever people are interdependent rather than completely independent. The most common conflict occurs in an ongoing relationship—between people at work, in a family, or within a couple, for example—because such people have the most interaction, and therefore the most opportunity for strains to arise. Much less frequent are conflicts involving a single, isolated interaction, such as when two strangers, arriving in a parking lot at the same time, get into a confrontation over who will take the last available parking space. Rarer still are terminal conflicts, where the person who loses a dispute is eliminated from the dispute context (such as when a boss fires a subordinate over a disagreement). In ongoing relationships, a particular conflict can be identified in terms of an issue or an interrelated set of issues, and several such conflicts can occur simultaneously. The relationship remains strained as long as a conflict goes unaddressed, although the parties have some control over how the conflict is expressed (e.g., they can suppress angry thoughts and the impulse to retaliate).

Conflicts sometimes involve a simple, easily defined issue, such as the price at which an object will be sold. More often, there is complexity because of the meanings each party attaches to the issues in dispute, the process by which the conflict is being addressed, the relationship between the parties, and the fairness of alternative outcomes. Each party's level of awareness of these complexities may be limited because relationship strains cause anxiety, and the individual may be using one or more coping mechanisms—such as denial, avoidance, or displacement—to escape from that anxiety.

It is useful to distinguish two dimensions along which conflict can be assessed: the intensity of conflictual feelings, and the severity of conflictual behaviors. These are shown in Figure 1. The vertical axis indicates varying degrees of anger, the core emotion in a conflict. Anger can be directed toward a person, as in the case of resentment or hostility, or toward a situation, as in the case of envy or feeling slighted. When the anger is mild, it is experienced as annoyance; when it is intense, it can involve a rage so strong that other thoughts and feelings are blocked out. The horizontal axis indicates varying degrees of severity of the behavioral response. This can range from not expressing any reaction at all to extreme violence. It is logical to expect a correlation between feelings and behaviors. A relatively trivial conflict will give rise to mild anger, experienced as annoyance, and the individual is likely to do no more than show displeasure. If the conflict is very serious and the anger intense, one would expect a much stronger retaliatory reaction, perhaps involving violence. Degrees of anger falling between these extremes would be expected to engender a commensurate response on a diagonal line between showing displeasure and malicious retaliation. [See ANGER.]

Drive theory provides the basis for understanding

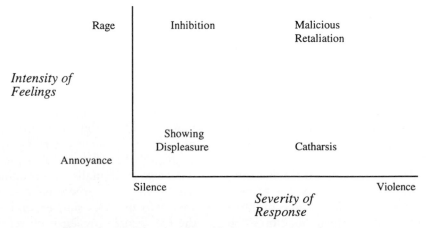

Figure I   Intensity of conflictual feelings and severity of response.

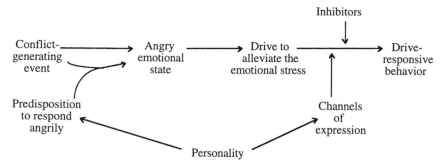

Figure 2 Drive theory as it applies to conflict.

the link between the intensity of feelings and the severity of response. Figure 2 depicts the causal linkage. The angry emotional state is stressful to the person experiencing these emotions. This sets up a drive to alleviate the stress, which motivates the individual to take action. Personality can predispose an individual to respond angrily (as in the case of someone with an early history of abuse) and can influence the choice of channels of expression (e.g., one person may openly confront the situation; another may respond passive–aggressively).

There are cases where the intensity of feelings does not match the severity of response. When there is intense anger, but only a mild response (see upper left quadrant of Figure 1), we can presume an inhibitor to be shaping drive-responsive behavior. Perhaps the angry person is afraid of the person who provoked the anger (e.g., the anger-provoker might be a boss or a mugger with a weapon), or the situation precludes retaliation (e.g., it involves a police officer or an anonymous telephone caller), or expression of anger is proscribed (e.g., by cultural or organizational norms). When there is inhibition, the conflict is unmanaged: it continues unresolved as long as there is intensity of feelings.

When there is a severe response in the presence of mild anger (see lower right quadrant of Figure 1), we can assume that the aggressive display produces some sort of catharsis in the aggressor. Extremely violent episodes can be observed in hockey games, for example, but these are seldom expressions of enmity. The violence is an integral aspect of the sport, and presumably, one of the features that attract certain personalities to hockey rather than to speed skating or figure skating.

Conflict can be approached through direct or tacit behaviors. Direct approaches include conversations in which differences are aired, each party gives an account of what he or she has experienced, empathy is induced, apologies are expressed, solutions are offered, and agreement is sought. Tacit approaches include symbolic acts that may signal the existence of relationship strains, a desire to restore the relationship, contrition, submission, or dominance. Tacit approaches are typically chosen to allow face-saving, to reduce the risk of a vindictive response by a defensive or more powerful adversary, or to allow discussion of issues that are uncomfortable to address candidly. It is typical for the parties to use direct and tacit approaches in combination, and to make adjustments in response to cultural norms (e.g., face-saving is more important to many Asians, so tacit approaches are prevalent). Such cultural norms function as inhibitors.

Thus far, we have considered conflict from the perspective of only one party, without looking at how interaction with the other party shapes how the conflict unfolds. We have also portrayed conflict as a static phenomenon, a stable state resulting from a given level of provocation that will remain at that level until the angry person takes actions that reduce the conflictual drive. In practice, conflicts are rarely stable and are prone to escalation. Escalation arises from emotional exacerbation or tactical retaliation. Figure 3 shows how escalation occurs as a result of emotional exacerbation.

This type of escalation occurs when an angry focal party attempts drive-responsive behavior to no avail (e.g., an apology is rebuffed, the other party refuses to discuss the conflict, or the focal party's show of contrition and vulnerability is not reciprocated and the focal party is left feeling ashamed and embarrassed). This lack of efficacy frustrates the focal party, which in turn motivates aggression. The aggressive act provokes a

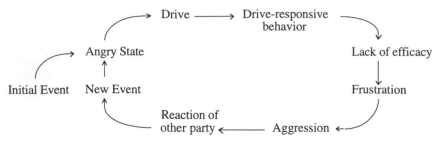

Figure 3 Emotional conflict escalation.

reaction by the other party; this is experienced as a new event that adds to the focal party's angry state, completing the positive feedback loop to create a self-escalating process.

Figure 4 shows a different escalation dynamic resulting from the inherent difficulty in achieving perceived parity when using reciprocal retaliation tactics. We will use an example to illustrate the dynamic. A boy teases a girl in a kindergarten school yard. The girl gets angry at the affront and kicks the boy. In her mind, she has "evened the score": the kick was a fitting punishment for the public insult. The boy is surprised that she got angry at what he considered good-natured teasing, makes the judgment that she overreacted and hurt him more than he hurt her, and slaps her to "even the score." From her perspective, the score is anything but even: she has been insulted and slapped, and he has only been kicked, so she bites him to "even the score." He responds to her apparent further escalation by punching her in the nose. With a bleeding nose and a crowd of sympathetic classmates joining her in vowing never again to speak to this "school-yard bully," we have a conflict that has within a minute escalated beyond manageability by the parties involved.

The scenario seems simplistic but has strong parallels in family feuds, Mafia wars, fights between couples, enemy-making in corporations, and even wars between countries. The key dynamic is how the tactic used by one party is assessed by the other. Often, the other party is totally unaware of what he or she did that created the anger and thus decides that the focal party's behavior is unjustified and deserves a punitive response. Alternatively, the other party realizes the affront to the focal party, but then assesses the equity of the response and decides whether it was unjust retaliation. As a participant in the conflict, both parties have perceptual and cognitive biases that make them more aware of the impact of the other's behavior on them than of the impact of their own behavior on the other. Furthermore, both parties are more likely to have self-justification tendencies that are stronger than their self-blame (as predicted by attribution theory). Thus, the individual is predisposed to judge the other party to have overreacted. The conflict escalates in this manner even though both parties believe, with every action, that they are simply achieving parity of harm done. The dynamic, however, takes them up the diagonal line in Figure 1 toward a very severe conflict, perhaps even a feud, that started as a minor annoyance.

II. CONFLICT RESOLUTION

An understanding of the central processes that energize and maintain conflicts sets the stage for understanding how individuals engaged in conflicts—and

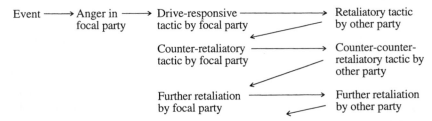

Figure 4 Tactical conflict escalation.

Table I Some Alternative Conflict Resolution Intervention Behaviors

Intervention process	Emphasis of intervention	Party involved in intervention		
		Focal party	*Other party*	*Third party*
Two-party strategies				
Negotiation	Issues, process	x	x	
Argument	Issues, catharsis	x	x	
Delegation to agents	Issues	(By proxy)	(By proxy)	
Third party strategies				
Adjudication	Issues	x	x	x
Mediation	Issues, meanings, emotions, process	x	x	x
Psychotherapeutic interventions				
Individual therapy	Issues, meanings, emotions	x		x
Conjoint therapy	Issues, meanings, emotions	x	x	x
Psychoeducation	Process	x		x

professionals who might wish to help them—can effectively intervene. Conflict resolution is a process for reducing the anger-induced strain and managing the divisiveness and violence of the tactics used by the parties in conflict. Table I summarizes the principal conflict resolution intervention behaviors. Our choice of the term intervention reflects the assumption that without intervention, the conflict will persist. The intervention may involve actions by the focal party, the other party, or someone who is not a disputant (a third party). The third party may be a dispute resolution professional (who can mediate or arbitrate) or a psychotherapist (who can provide individual or conjoint therapy or psychoeducation). The emphasis of the intervention may be the issues (what is in dispute), the process (how the parties deal with one another), the meanings and emotions that energize the conflict, or the catharsis that may result from participation in the conflict.

A. Two-Party Intervention Strategies

Negotiation is the first intervention strategy in the set. It is discussed at length in the next section because it is the most frequently used intervention strategy. Negotiation involves engagement by both parties in issue-focused discussion to reach an agreement on a course

of action that meets at least some of their needs in the dispute. It is different from argument in that the objective of an argument is to dominate the other verbally, not to reach agreement. The most frequent outcome of an argument is catharsis for the winner and resentment by the loser, so it is seldom an effective means of conflict resolution. Occasionally, the outcome of an argument is for one party to convince the other to alter his or her stance on the issue at hand, but this is unlikely because losing an argument incurs loss of social face, as well as humiliation when conceding that one has taken an erroneous stance. Closely related to negotiating and arguing is delegation to agents. This can be done with constructive intent, such as when the parties turn the issues over to professional negotiators who are skilled in problem solving and seeking out creative options that generate value for the client; it can also be done with destructive intent, such as when an angry disputant hires a particularly nasty lawyer to deal with the other party.

B. Third-Party Intervention Strategies

Third-party strategies involve enlisting the help of someone who is not a party to the dispute. Adjudication is characterized by the third party making a judgment intended to settle the dispute. Such judgments are made when the parties litigate the dispute and the issue is settled in court. An arbitrator may also pronounce such a judgment, but is not constrained by the same rules of law that a judge must observe: the arbitrator can use considerable discretion in trying to discover the facts of the case and the needs of the parties, and will try to decide on a fair settlement. In binding arbitration, the arbitrator's decision must be accepted, just like a judge's decision in court. In nonbinding arbitration, the decision is advice from an impartial but knowledgeable observer about what would be a fair settlement.

In mediation, the third party has no decision-making role at all and instead focuses on the process by which the parties interact. The mediator must pass the test of neutrality: to be totally indifferent as to what the settlement is and whether it favors one party or the other. The mediator's role is simply to help the parties negotiate a settlement to which they will both commit. Mediation often is effective simply because the parties are too angry to talk to each other, but have no trouble discussing issues and settlements with the mediator: the mediator can stem escalation by using "shuttle diplomacy" to preclude face-to-face contact when anger is strong. The mediator, as an empathic listener, also facilitates emotional discharge, which can reduce the level of anger that is energizing the conflict and aid in emotional de-escalation. A mediator who is respected also constrains the severity of the tactics used, because the parties are now carrying on the conflict in front of an audience whose opinion of them is important and this dynamic can prevent further retaliatory escalation. Mediation services can be provided by dispute resolution professionals, couples therapists, and sometimes mutual friends (although a well-meaning but untrained friend can easily get drawn into the conflict as a disputant).

C. Psychotherapeutic Intervention Strategies

Two conflict resolution interventions shown in Table I are individual and conjoint therapy. In individual therapy, the focal party explores the meanings and emotions that energize the dispute, discharges his or her emotional energy, and constructively plans interactions with the other party. The two most useful contributions of individual therapy in conflict resolution are helping the focal party identify trait anger and creating awareness of transferences.

Trait anger is the predisposition to respond angrily across conflict–stimulus situations. The therapist explores with the focal party the level of anger and conflictual cognitions generated by a range of stimuli to see whether there is a general tendency to overreact. If there is such a tendency, then a personality trait may be adding to the state anger that would be expected in a given situation. Trait anger is usually the result of anger that was not discharged in earlier life, perhaps dating back to childhood. Nontherapists recognize this trait and describe such individuals as irascible or as "having a bad temper." The therapist can usefully intervene with the client through anger-management training, which may be particularly important if conflict escalation is leading to violence against a less powerful other party (as in spouse abuse and child abuse). Conversely, therapy is also useful in helping individuals recognize patterns of submission in conflict, passive-aggressive responses, and maladaptive responses to others who have anger-management difficulties.

Transferences involve patterns of responses to certain stimulus–situation characteristics. The situation, in effect, reminds the focal party of an earlier event that created intense anger which was never fully resolved. The trigger for the anger "overreaction" may be the other party, or it may be characteristics of the situation. Nontherapists sometimes refer to the former type of transference as "a personality conflict," and to the latter as a situation that "pushes his/her hot buttons." If the focal party can recognize transferences, he or she can either avoid such situations or people, or cognitively override the escalation tendency.

There are additional ways in which psychotherapeutic intervention may be helpful to individuals with conflict-management problems: (1) therapists can coach their clients in constructive ways to approach interactions; (2) therapists generally offer a safe place for individuals to get in touch with and express negative feelings (e.g., anger, resentment, jealousy, disappointment) and to understand the origins of these emotions; and (3) therapists may be helpful in facilitating an understanding of individual wants and needs, defining issues and underlying emotions, and how to communicate interests and desires effectively.

Conjoint therapies involve two or more individuals in treatment with a single therapist (e.g., couples therapy, family therapy). Conjoint therapy is particularly useful in helping individuals learn to manage interpersonal conflict because the therapist can directly observe maladaptive behaviors and interactions between the parties in sessions, enabling a more accurate diagnosis of group or couple dynamics. The conjoint therapist may take the role of a neutral third party in the management of conflict. The therapist allows the parties to express their views safely without fear of immediate retaliation and discourages harmful forms of aggression. Conjoint therapists may also help the couple or family to recognize patterns and roles in conflict and facilitate the adoption of new roles and behaviors. [*See* COUPLES THERAPY; FAMILY THERAPY.]

There has been increasing interest in using psychoeducational classes to teach basic interpersonal skills that are useful in dispute resolution (such as anger-management skills, couples communication, assertiveness training, and parent education). Information can be communicated more efficiently in classes and seminars than one-on-one during a therapy hour. Furthermore, classes and seminars are often perceived as less threatening than individual or conjoint psychotherapy: an educational program may be considered acceptable to many who struggle with interpersonal problems, but who resist participating in more traditional therapies. Psychoeducation may be used preventively to provide individuals with self-help tools to manage everyday interpersonal conflict, or it may be used as an adjunct to more intensive individual therapy.

III. NEGOTIATION

Negotiation is the most common form of conflict resolution. The objective in negotiating is to achieve an agreement (i.e., a commitment by both parties) to a course of action that meets at least some of each party's needs in the dispute. At a minimum, negotiation involves the parties presenting their perspectives, expressing their preferences, and indicating the acceptability of proposed settlements.

A. Distributive Bargaining

Scholars have focused their investigations on two primary negotiation processes. Walton and McKersie (1965), in their celebrated work, *A Behavioral Theory of Labor Negotiations,* distinguish these processes as distributive and integrative bargaining. *Distributive bargaining* involves contending for the maximum attainable share of something that is scarce. There is zero-sum interdependence between the parties in the

sense that one party's gain is the other's loss. In the case of a used car transaction, for example, the lower the selling price, the greater the buyer's gain and the greater the seller's loss. The negotiation concerns how value (i.e., what economists call utility) will be distributed in the transaction, hence the term "distributive" bargaining.

B. Integrative Bargaining

Integrative bargaining occurs when the negotiation is approached as an opportunity to achieve joint gain rather than to gain at the other party's expense. The term comes from the concept of integrating one party's interests with the other's. In integrative bargaining, the parties see as a problem that a conflict is straining the relationship and construe the negotiation as a means of addressing this problem. The parties join in the shared objective to find solutions that meet both parties' needs. An example of integrative bargaining is when two siblings are arguing about who is the owner of a teddy bear. One wants to play with it during the day, the other wants to sleep with it at night. A very obvious integrative agreement is to de-emphasize ownership and focus on needs being met. Another example is a couple negotiating over vacation. The wife is burned out on her job and wants to go to the mountains for alpine skiing as soon as possible; the husband has experienced too much winter weather and wants to go water-skiing in the tropics and has a mild preference for taking the vacation in 2 months. An integrative solution would be to accede to each party's stronger preference (immediacy for the wife and warm weather for the husband) and take the tropical vacation soon.

Negotiation theorists are fond of the metaphor of dividing up a pie to convey the difference between these two kinds of bargaining. In distributive bargaining, the parties contend for as big a slice of the pie as possible; in integrative bargaining, they seek ways to make the pie bigger, so both will come out with more. Yet both distributive and integrative bargaining are ideal types, and many situations in practice call for a combination of the two. For example, in the modern auto industry, manufacturers negotiate both price and quality standards with parts suppliers. Both parties have a joint interest in maximizing parts quality, and engage in problem solving to address this. At the same time, both companies have a responsibility to generate wealth for their shareholders, so the supplier will want to charge high prices and the auto manufacturer will want to

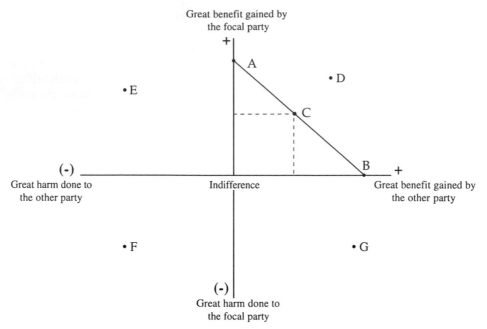

Figure 5 The utility of various negotiated outcomes for the two parties.

keep costs low. Negotiation involves simultaneously dealing with collaborating for efficiency and quality, and competing over profitability.

Figure 5 shows the utility (i.e., value or benefit) to each party that accrues from various negotiated outcomes. The vertical axis shows the degree to which the focal party likes or dislikes a particular outcome, with desirable outcomes above the horizontal axis and undesirable outcomes below. The horizontal axis shows the degree to which the other party likes or dislikes a particular outcome, with desirable outcomes to the right of the vertical axis and undesirable outcomes to the left.

The upper right quadrant shows the feasible range of settlements when negotiations are undertaken constructively. In distributive bargaining, the parties contend for an outcome along the line connecting points A and B that maximizes their gain. Point A is a perfect victory for the focal party, because it is the most beneficial outcome that the other party will agree to (settlements to the left of point A have higher utility for the focal party but the other party will not willingly agree to these because they involve a sacrifice). Similarly, point B is a perfect victory for the other party. Point C is a compromise that has substantial but not maximum utility to both parties (the dotted lines show the utility to each party on the respective axes). In integrative bargaining, the parties seek mutual-gain outcomes that improve on distributive compromises: Point D depicts such an outcome.

The discussion thus far has focused on the interaction of equals. In practice, however, the parties are never equals, and the aspect of inequality that is most salient to conflict resolution is power. Power is the ability to induce compliance. It can come from a variety of sources (e.g., coercion, authority, guilt-inducement, charisma, guile, or rewards and punishments) and can be used to bias the outcome in one party's favor. For example, by using power exploitatively, the focal party can get the other party to agree to settlements that are closer to point A than to point B in Figure 5, or even force the other party to accede to point E. (Point G may be the result of exploitative power use by the other party, or it may result from the focal party's ingratiating, self-defeating, or relationship-enhancing behavior.) Both parties can use power malevolently to harm the other party, which might result in the outcome shown as point F.

Negotiation is widely recognized as the most common strategy for addressing disputes. Scholars have devoted a lot of attention to the study of negotiations, but little of their writing is useful to people who want to learn how to manage the conflicts that arise in their daily lives. Scholars have been overly influenced—and therefore constrained—by how economists (particularly game theorists) define and study negotiation, and as a result have primarily investigated the outcomes of strangers negotiating for purely economic benefit in isolated transactions. In real life, conflicts usually occur in the context of an ongoing relationship, and the parties care about the process by which the conflict is addressed and its impact on the relationship, as well as economic benefit. Typically, they do not have the option of dealing with someone else instead if they should hit an impasse. As a result of this unfortunate conceptual bias, much of what has been written is in fact bad advice for the majority of negotiation situations.

IV. INDIVIDUAL EFFECTIVENESS IN ADDRESSING DISPUTES

Conflicts can be dealt with effectively or ineffectively. The approach an individual uses is the result of predispositions arising from personality as well as the tactical choice of one approach over another. In this section, we look at how broad patterns of response that result from personality traits impact individual effectiveness, and then look at tactical choices in conflicts that tend to be ineffective and effective.

A. Effect of Personality

Personality structure is shaped by childhood experiences and affects the way individuals relate to others in the world. Personality traits can either impede or enhance one's ability to deal with interpersonal conflict in a healthy fashion. This section outlines the impact of reinforced early history, narcissism, borderline tendencies, passive–aggressive personality, and gender on the ability to manage appropriately anger and conflict.

1. Reinforced Early History

From an early age, children observe and experience interpersonal conflicts, both in their families of origin and in their peer relationships. During these formative years, children struggle with anger and its meaning, learn how to identify and label angry feelings, observe role models experiencing and dealing with anger, and discover how to control their own angry impulses.

As a result of copying role models, engaging in trial-and-error experimentation, and having their behavior shaped by adults, children develop their characteristic style of handling interpersonal disputes.

Operant conditioning is one explanation of the development of an individual conflict management style that originates in childhood and persists through adulthood. This model suggests that children will learn and repeat behaviors that yield successful outcomes in reducing frustration and anger, and they will tend to avoid behaviors that exacerbate anger or produce other aversive reactions. For example, a child in a chaotic household may learn that the only way to gain the attention of his or her parents is to throw a tantrum; this approach may evolve into a sophisticated form in adulthood—"creating an uproar"—yet it may still be recognizable as a tantrum. Or, children who are constantly teased by their peers may learn to defend themselves through verbal or physical assault in some situations, and to run and hide in others; as adults, they may experience a "fight or flight" dichotomous impulse, with choices between these extremes overlooked. Another child's aggressive behavior toward his sister may decrease after he is punished; but this may result in a "shaping" effect, where the adult is aggressive toward men but not toward women. In each of these instances, the adult repeats conflict management behaviors that were reinforced during early childhood experiences.

Modeling is an additional mechanism that could explain the development of conflict management style. Modeling involves copying the responses of others to stimulus situations. Thus, children who witness continued physical or verbal conflict between their parents may come to believe that unmodulated aggression (in which the angry person acts on whatever aggressive impulses arise) is the appropriate way to handle interpersonal conflict. In contrast, children raised in households where conflict is suppressed may copy a repertoire of passive–aggressive responses. Modeling may result in the acquisition of cultural norms and styles as well as patterns that are idiosyncratic in their family of origin. For example, open expression of conflict is absent from many Asian cultures, and the child may copy the pervasive cultural pattern even when brought up in a family environment that is inconsistent with the culture.

An even broader influence of culture is the need to handle conflict according to societal rules. As children learn to identify and understand angry impulses, they must also learn to control their behavior and to channel the anger into socially acceptable outlets. Failure to do so can result in some degree of societal rejection, as in the case of a child who is suspended from school after punching a classmate. These rules of civilized society exist as a deterrent to the impulsive expression of aggression that is not tolerated beyond early childhood. Societies generally hold parents responsible for indoctrinating their children with social values and mores; in the process of early superego (conscience) development, societal expectations and values become internalized as the child gains appropriate understanding of what is considered acceptable behavior.

2. Narcissism and the Capacity for Empathy

Narcissism is a deep-seated character dimension that results from failure to achieve robust self-esteem during the critical formative years. Symptoms of narcissistic impairment include pervasive self-importance, a sense of entitlement, and disregard for the feelings and needs of others. Such individuals are often interpersonally exploitative, a trait which may be beneficial in business and athletic situations but harmful in interpersonal relationships. Narcissistic individuals typically view "winning" as the ultimate goal of any negotiation; this orientation limits the person's adaptability across conflict situations.

Narcissistically impaired individuals are less effective in negotiation and conflict management because (1) their difficulty in empathizing hurts their ability to accommodate the needs of the other party; (2) they ignore or sacrifice relationships when striving for advantage; (3) they are inflexible, inequitable, and uncreative in their negotiation styles; (4) they tend toward a distributive (win or lose) orientation, placing little value on achieving mutual gain through integrative bargaining; and (5) their sense of entitlement interferes with their ability to achieve collaborative solutions—the other party is viewed simply as an obstacle to claiming their rightful outcome.

In terms of the emotional conflict model shown in Figure 3, the narcissist's inflexibility and refusal to accommodate energizes the cycle of escalation with greater speed and intensity than one normally expects. As the conflictual drive increases, the narcissists' self-oriented initiatives toward drive reduction are unsuccessful (i.e., they are unable to get their way). This leads to frustration and anger (a response to narcissistic in-

jury), which often results in aggression (an expression of narcissistic rage). The narcissist's behaviors are experienced by the other party as grandiose (i.e., haughty), unempathic, and self-centered, leaving room for only two possible responses: capitulate or counter with a similarly inflexible posture. With either alternative, the other party's angry state leads to reactive behavior, and this response is the new event that begins the cycle again for the narcissist, now with more intensity.

3. Borderline Personality

The borderline personality can be equally disruptive in conflict situations. The symptoms of borderline personality include intense and unstable interpersonal relationships, fear of abandonment, chronic dysphoric affect (i.e., unhappiness), cognitive distortion characterized by black or white thinking, and self-destructive behaviors. These symptoms combine to create a syndrome that can make conflict resolution very difficult.

Borderlines' characteristic approaches to resolving strains in relationships are heavily influenced by their fear of abandonment. They become hypervigilant about relationship instability, and often reject the other party preemptively (e.g., they may walk out of the negotiation precipitously so that the other party cannot be the one to walk out). Trust and loyalty are therefore of the utmost importance to these individuals, and their relationship partners are likely to be repeatedly tested—subtly or unsubtly—to gain reassurances about their continued loyalty. The chronic unhappiness of borderlines makes them less appealing relationship partners to many people, which adds to the relationship instability they create by their own behavior.

Turbulence in relationships also results from borderlines' cognitive distortions, particularly their tendency to experience others as all good or all bad. Some theorists attribute this splitting defense to borderlines' inability to integrate good and bad aspects of themselves and their mothers during early development. By the age of 3, most children develop the capacity to attain an internal representation of another as a whole person with good and bad characteristics, and they are able to maintain an image of the good characteristics even when that person behaves in some way that is disappointing or anger inducing (e.g., most children come to understand that their mother loves them even if she does not immediately buy the toy they want). In contrast, borderline-prone children keep contradictory images of good and bad separate, and view others through a lens of either extreme idealization or devaluation. The change from idealization to devaluation can be sudden: once the idealized other makes a mistake or does something the borderline perceives as a slight, the other is seen to be malicious. Borderlines' black-or-white thinking also impedes their ability to arrive at integrative solutions: they tend to see situations—as well as people—in all-good or all-bad terms, thus they have trouble crafting solutions that have the optimum combination of advantages and disadvantages to each party.

Conflict management is made even more difficult because of borderlines' impulsivity and willingness to endure self-destructive behavior. Borderlines can be extremely vindictive, which makes mutually destructive conflict outcomes, such as point F in Figure 5 tolerable, but they also are willing to inflict pain and suffering on themselves, which makes point G in Figure 5 acceptable, and sometimes even appealing. Borderlines' self-destructive behavior is often motivated by a need to "drown out" deeper psychic pain with a more immediate stimulus, but the manifest behavior is baffling and disturbing to the other party and utterly incomprehensible to economics-oriented scholars who have an "economic man" theory of human motivation (i.e., people want to maximize utility and minimize disutility).

A final problem is that conflicts escalate quickly for such individuals. The borderline is extremely volatile, and even small events can trigger raw emotion—an anger state that is disproportionate to the issue in dispute. In an uncontrollable anger state, borderlines' initiatives toward drive reduction are often unsuccessful, building frustration which results in aggression (see Figure 3). This phenomenon of borderline rage is often so forceful that it drives the other party away or provokes primal, irrational combat, leaving borderlines facing the predicament they feared most: abandonment. [*See* BORDERLINE PERSONALITY DISORDER.]

4. Passive–Aggressive Personality

Passive–aggressives avoid overtly expressing their anger and instead choose to express it indirectly, usually in the form of passive resistance to the other party's demands. Passive–aggressive personality traits may develop as a result of chronic suppressed anger during formative years. Often, these individuals have felt powerless to face up to a domineering sibling or par-

ent, or have endured situations in which direct expression of anger was perceived as extremely risky. As we noted earlier, suppressed anger does not abate, but rather festers until an opportunity arises where it can be expressed with low risk of reprisal. Thus, passive–aggressives are unlikely to confront authority figures; instead, they will "forget" to carry out directives or ensure that situational factors will preclude compliance. These techniques are aggressive in that they cause harm to the authority figure and passive in that the focal party is not the obvious or willful cause of the harm. By design, passive–aggressive responses are more difficult to address than overt conflictual behaviors, and eventually will infuriate the other party.

Individuals with a passive–aggressive style have difficulty in negotiation because their feelings and needs do not get expressed and therefore do not get addressed. Furthermore, their manner of handling conflict engenders rage in the other, without providing opportunities to reduce the drive through communication and problem solving. Frustrated, the authority figure is likely to take a stronger stance, presenting a greater challenge to which the passive–aggressive responds with relish: their behavior is reinforced when the authority figure becomes frustrated but has no grounds for directing hostility toward them. In fact, the reinforcement is potent enough that passive–aggressives often seek out relationships with strong authority figures so they can gain the catharsis from defying these chosen oppressors. Passive-aggressiveness is an unhealthy pattern of dealing with conflict because the positive feedback loop that locks both parties into a conflict spiral contains no pathway toward resolution.

5. Gender Differences

In Western countries, boys and girls undergo different socialization experiences. Boys are typically brought up playing competitive games where the objective is to beat the opponent. Girls play different games: their typical objective is a mutually positive experience and reinforcement of the friendship bonds, and they are likely to stop the game or change the rules if the other person is not enjoying the experience.

Many years of immersion in this strong learning environment produce tendencies that last into adulthood. Men tend to see conflicts as occasions to compete. Disputes are considered to be discrete episodes in a series of "games" to be won or lost, each of which is disconnected from past and anticipated future interactions. Negotiations are seen as opportunities to beat the opponent using any tactics within the "rules" of engagement. Women tend to see conflict as threats to the relationship, and are motivated to take conciliatory actions to prevent further damage. This may involve making concessions when the relationship is valued more highly than the issues in conflict.

Problems frequently arise when a man and a woman negotiate to resolve conflicts. In the stereotypical case, the competition-oriented man makes the first move by taking a strong position. The relationship-oriented woman, realizing the potential for conflict escalation, expresses concern that the dispute has arisen and reiterates her commitment to the relationship. The man becomes frustrated by her response—which he sees as irrelevant and illogical—and demands that she address the issues *as he has defined them*. She, however, does not define the issues the same way, and tries to explain her perspective, but he uses whatever power he has available to resist her perceived ploy to "switch to a different playing field." As she reluctantly addresses the conflict on his terms, she deals with his intransigence by making concessions that are intended to signal her desire to settle the dispute amicably. Her conception of fairness leads her to believe that her generosity will be reciprocated in the next dispute, but he interprets her concession as weakness and as acknowledgment that his position is justified. When the next dispute arises, he feels no obligation to reciprocate because, he reasons, "this is a new ball game." She feels betrayed, exploited, and disappointed, and instead of blaming him for being insensitive, blames herself for being unassertive.

Despite her self-assessment as being ineffective, objectively, the woman has the stronger skills in handling everyday conflicts. Most conflicts occur in an ongoing relationship that has a history and a future; she excels in this context because the primary objective should be relationship preservation. The man's approach is more suited to one-time transactions between strangers. Nevertheless, the masculine style is normatively assessed as superior, reflecting gender biases in the field of negotiation and conflict resolution. Examples of gender bias are that women's approaches are viewed—and judged—as deviations from the male approach; game theory is a central organizing principle in the discipline; virtually all of the research focuses on success in transactions; and schol-

ars in the field seem unable to escape the masculine-oriented imagery of winning—even when it is illogical, as in the case of a win–win outcome.

B. Ineffective Behaviors in Conflict Management

The previous section discussed predispositions to respond to conflict situations. The next two sections examine ineffective and effective drive-responsive behavior (see Figure 2). The paragraphs which follow focus on five behavior patterns that are frequently associated with ineffectiveness: conflict avoidance, intellectualization, domination, disinhibition, and conflict-seeking behaviors.

1. Conflict Avoidance

Some individuals choose to avoid confrontation rather than face the interpersonal strain inherent in conflict resolution. One form of this is unconscious denial, a psychological defense against feelings of anxiety. Denial results in the individual remaining unaware of all or part of the conflict, or not interpreting the anger-induced situation as a conflict.

Other individuals consciously avoid conflict through self-sacrifice: they are willing to ignore their own interests to avoid the stress or consequences of conflict. Such individuals may be in oppressed situations (as in the case of members of minority groups who are afraid police officers might abuse their authority) or may be seeking the approval of others at high personal cost (as in the case of a teenage girl who sacrifices her own views to gain peer acceptance).

Some techniques used by conflict-avoiders give the appearance of dealing with the conflict when actually they are avoiding it. For example, providing an ultimatum may have the appearance of domination when the individual actually may be avoiding the difficult interpersonal issues that energized the conflict. Another example of subtle conflict avoidance is when people remove themselves from the dispute by assuming the relatively neutral role of mediator or peacekeeper: this is designed to spare them from confronting the issues in dispute.

Avoidance obviously interferes with the individual's capacity to manage the conflict effectively and generates anger and frustration if the other party is trying to address the conflict. If both parties avoid dealing with the anger-induced strain in the relationship, neither is frustrated, but the anger will build cumulatively. The anger may eventually erupt outwardly as sudden rage, or the anger may be directed inwardly resulting in symptoms of depression or somatic complaints (such as ulcers and high blood pressure).

2. Intellectualization

The process of intellectualization occurs when conflicts are handled in a detached, factual, and rational manner. This defense mechanism is related to denial in that it allows the individual to avoid dealing with the emotional component of conflict. Intellectualization often leads to unsatisfactory outcomes because it ignores powerful emotions that make the conflict intense (see the vertical axis of Figure 1). For example, a husband and wife may enter a dispute over financial matters. Whereas the husband focuses rationally on the actual amount of money she is spending, the wife may be preoccupied with resentment of his control, the unfairness of their differential earning power, and his selfish, lavish spending on a country club membership which results in his abandoning her and the children to play golf. His intellectualization dooms conflict resolution to failure because it precludes addressing her issues.

3. Power and Domination

Power is the ability to induce compliance in the other party. When power is used in a conflict, it typically yields unsatisfactory outcomes because the other party has been coerced to accede to an unfair agreement. Even when the outcome is fair, the process is unfair because the use of power denies the other party a fair say in deciding on the settlement terms. Thus domination generates resentment. Because dominated individuals fear retaliation, they have no outlet for their resentment, which builds over time and erupts as uncontrolled anger and aggression. Thus, for example, racial tension explodes into race riots.

4. Disinhibition and the Loss of Control

As anger-induced strain builds in a relationship, the anger must eventually be released (resulting in a feeling of catharsis) or reduced, preferably through appropriate, safe channels (such as discussion or venting). Societal norms and laws restrict the use of extreme aggression as a means of anger release, and internal mechanisms of control in most individuals will enable

them to suppress intensely hostile or violent urges. However, some individuals have a very low tolerance for anger or have inadequately developed capacities for restraining aggressive behaviors, and even less aggressive personalities may find themselves in situations where suppressed anger can no longer be controlled. In such cases, anger can become overwhelming, suspending rational thought, and often leading to disinhibited actions. In its mildest form, the individual's disinhibited, irrational behaviors act as an impediment to the individual's ability to facilitate satisfactory conflict resolution (e.g., an exasperated mother may be too angry to say anything coherent to her teenage son). In its most extreme form, the anger becomes so out of control that the individual may commit illegal and violent acts with devastating outcomes (e.g., a teenage girl may kill her father after years of sexual abuse).

5. Conflict-Seeking Behaviors

In contrast to conflict-avoiders, some individuals *seek* conflict in their daily lives, experiencing pleasure or excitement from engaging in the dispute. The pleasure may result from using power to dominate others (which can produce a feeling of self-efficacy), from "winning" a confrontation (e.g., gaining feeling of self-worth from beating an opponent in an argument), or from gaining the stimulation of tension and discord (when other stimuli are too mild for that individual). Others may seek conflict as a means of discharging pent-up anger or aggression, such as when anger is displaced onto another target person (e.g., a worker suppresses anger toward his boss but later gets into a fight with his neighbor). Some individuals are consumed by "free-floating" rage, and, as a result of this trait, continually engage in disputes as a means of discharging emotion (as in the case of chronically violent felons).

C. Effective Conflict Management Behaviors

The goal of effective conflict management is to reduce the relationship strain caused by anger. This section describes drive-responsive behaviors that increase disputants' control over angry impulses and lead to mutually agreeable outcomes. We focus on three behavior patterns that are most likely to be effective: drive reduction, relationship preservation, and constructive communication.

I. Drive Reduction

Effective conflict management practices require reduction of the anger drive in a nonharmful and socially acceptable manner. Socially acceptable means that the focal party maintains control of his or her response and does not resort to exploitation, verbal abuse, or violence. Effective individuals are able to express their anger in constructive ways. They address the problem candidly rather than tacitly (unless candor is culturally proscribed) and develop ways of modulating the intensity of emotion (venting the anger by telling a friend, using a therapist as a sounding board, managing the stress through physical exercise, rechanneling destructive energy into constructive activities, or taking "time-out" when anger levels pose the risk of loss of control). These methods prevent anger and resentment from building or festering, and foster constructive conflict management.

2. Relationship Preservation

Virtually all conflicts occur in the context of ongoing relationships. Effective negotiators are motivated to preserve those relationships and conceptualize the current dispute as a difficult episode within the parties' long-term interaction. The focus on relationship includes a willingness to compromise where appropriate, an emphasis on fairness, empathy for the needs of the other, and the quest for mutual gain. This pattern of conflict management (which is, in effect, a personality trait) has been characterized as relationship-orientation. Research by Greenhalgh and Gilkey shows that relationship-oriented negotiators (often, women) tend to share information and to avoid the use of coercive tactics; this creates a process that has a high likelihood of achieving mutually satisfying integrative outcomes.

3. Constructive Communication

Effective negotiators have a clear understanding of their own needs and feelings and can communicate their desires constructively. Constructive communication of cognitive issues and emotional states has two properties: candor (being unambiguous and direct) and supportiveness (tempering criticism with positive messages). Such communication increases the likelihood that each party will feel understood by the other and facilitates the discovery or design of mutually satisfying and equitable solutions. Constructive communication also creates a means of reducing the anger drive before it builds to an unmanageable state. It is an ongoing process in relationships, so that issues and feelings are discussed as they arise, rather than after they have built and festered.

Constructive communication requires enough trust to allow the parties to reveal their vulnerabilities. It is important to note that constructive communication in relationships does not mean that the negotiators must be brutally honest (which is indistinguishable from unmodulated expression of aggression); rather, the parties must maintain tact and sensitivity to the feelings of the other while conveying their own interest in restoring the relationship.

V. CONCLUDING THOUGHTS

Conflict is a crucial phenomenon to understand, in that it touches everyone's lives and determines the quality of relationships both at work and at home. Yet it remains poorly understood, largely as a result of the masculine, economics-oriented biases that have pervaded its study. These biases have distorted normative thinking, with the result that even healthy personalities have trouble figuring out what ought to be done in conflict situations. Normative thinking tells them how to "win" the encounter, but this advice may lead them to lose the relationship. This article has outlined some of the major factors that determine healthy functioning; effectiveness in dealing with disputes depends on managing emotions and attributed meanings as well as addressing surface issues, and giving as much attention to the process of dispute resolution as to securing beneficial outcomes. The research and theory may be adequate to explain contrived laboratory interactions, but for the most part, scholars would do well to study what highly effective people are doing in real-world situations and then build a theory of conflict resolution within relationships.

ACKNOWLEDGMENTS

The authors are grateful to Deborah I. Chapman and Roy J. Lewicki for their comments on an earlier version of this article.

BIBLIOGRAPHY

Bazerman, M. H., & Neale, M. A. (1992). *Negotiating rationally.* New York: Free Press.

Greenhalgh, L. (1986). Managing conflict. *Sloan Management Review, 27*(4), 45–52.

Greenhalgh, L. (1987). Relationships in negotiations. *Negotiation Journal, 3,* 235–243.

Greenhalgh, L., & Gilkey, R. W. (1993). Effects of relationship-orientation on negotiators' cognitions and tactics. *Group Decision and Negotiation, 2,* 167–178.

Kolb, D. M., & Bartunek, J. M. (Eds.). (1992). *Hidden conflict in organizations.* Newbury Park, CA: Sage.

Lewicki, R. J., Litterer, J. A., Minton, J. M., & Saunders, D. M. (1994). *Negotiation.* Burr Ridge, IL: Irwin.

Rubin, J. Z., & Brown, B. R. (1975). *The social psychology of bargaining and negotiation.* New York: Academic Press.

Walton, R. E., & McKersie, R. B. (1965). *A behavioral theory of labor negotiations.* New York: McGraw-Hill.

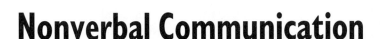

Nonverbal Communication

Nalini Ambady and Robert Rosenthal

Harvard University

Channel A specific source of nonverbal behaviors: for example, the face, the body, or tone of voice.
Decoding Detection of true feelings, states, or messages from observed nonverbal behavior.
Empathy Process of understanding another's feelings or thoughts, and experiencing those feelings or thoughts to some degree.
Encoding Display of nonverbal behavior that may be decoded by others.
Leakage Nonverbal behavior displayed without intention or awareness, revealing true feelings or affective states.
Rapport A relationship between individuals characterized by mutual attentiveness or involvement, high positivity or warmth, and high levels of behavioral coordination.
Social Influence Process of one person's behavior affecting the behavior of another.
Synchrony A high level of behavioral coordination between individuals characterized by interaction rhythm, simultaneous movement, and behavioral meshing.

NONVERBAL COMMUNICATION refers to the communication and interpretation of information by any means other than language. Nonverbal communication includes communication through any behavioral or expressive channel of communication such as facial expression, bodily movements, vocal tone and pitch, and many other channels. Nonverbal communication involves cues related to the communication (also referred to as the encoding or sending) of information as well as the interpretation (or the decoding or receiving) of information. The communication and interpretation of nonverbal behavior draws on tacit, implicit knowledge that all human beings possess. Such communication is often subtle, uncontrollable, spontaneous, rapidly and unconsciously communicated and interpreted, and provides a great deal of information regarding affective states. Although nonverbal communication can be controlled to adhere to cultural display rules (norms that regulate the expression of emotion) and to meet certain personal goals such as impression management or deception, such communication is generally a more automatic rather than controlled process. In this article, nonverbal communication refers to facial expressions, gaze, body movements, gestures, and tone of voice, as well as quasiverbal vocal behaviors such as interruptions, hesitations, and speech errors. We discuss the role of nonverbal communication in health care settings. These settings encompass the contact between medical providers, psychotherapists, physical therapists, occupational therapists, counselors, and other health care providers, and their clients.

I. IMPORTANCE OF NONVERBAL COMMUNICATION IN HEALTH CARE SETTINGS

Nonverbal communication is used to express and communicate thoughts, feelings, and emotions, to establish and maintain relationships, and to influence others. In health care settings, nonverbal communication is particularly important in establishing and maintaining the provider–client relationship and in influencing the client to comply with the treatment regimen. Nonverbal communication affects the provider, the client, and the relationship in the provider–client dyad.

The nonverbal communication of the provider is important for the client. Such communication can affect several important health-related outcomes, such as the client's adherence to treatment regimens, the client's recovery, and, ultimately, the client's survival. Clients are particularly sensitive to providers' nonverbal behaviors because they are often nervous and insecure and want to discern the true feelings of the provider. In seeking information about their health and prognosis, clients pay close attention not only to the information given by the provider, but also to the manner in which the information is communicated. A subtle gesture, a change in vocal tone, or too little or too much eye contact may result in a very different interpretation of a message by a client. Thus, often it is not what providers say but the manner in which they say it that leads a client to trust or mistrust or like or dislike them. Providers' nonverbal behaviors also contribute to provider expectancy effects. When providers communicate their expectations, they are often quite unaware that they are doing so in very subtle ways. These expectations are sensed and interpreted by the client and have important implications for recovery and healing.

The nonverbal communication of the client is also very important for the provider. Providers gather information about clients' physical as well as mental states from clients' nonverbal cues: clients may not always say what they really feel, but their nonverbal cues might convey their true underlying feelings. For example, a client may deny being anxious, but the provider may sense anxiety from nonverbal cues.

Nonverbal communication in the provider–client dyad is important for establishing and maintaining the relationship. Positive communication in the dyad is related to greater mutual liking, empathy, rapport, and trust. These processes, in turn, are related to client compliance and to more positive outcomes for the client.

II. CHANNELS OF COMMUNICATION

A. Basic Channels

Typical channels of communication include facial expressions, eye gaze, bodily movements, gestures, and vocal cues, such as pitch, speech rate, and intonation.

1. Face

The face is one of the most expressive channels of communication, particularly for expressing emotions. Emotional expression occurs primarily through changes in the mouth, eyebrows, cheek and eye muscles, pupil dilation, and the amount and direction of gaze. Specific facial expressions for specific emotions have been observed in a variety of different cultures, suggesting that facial expressions of emotion may be universal. Facial expressions of happiness, anger, disgust, sadness, and combined fear and surprise are readily communicated across cultures.

2. Body

Bodily expression occurs through arm and hand gesturing, positioning of the trunk (leaning), positioning of the arms and legs, posture, and the angle of the body. The study of body orientation and positioning in relation to other people or the physical environment is called *proxemics*.

3. Gestures

Gestures that clarify or supplement speech are called *illustrators*. They help in communicating messages by giving a visual clarification—for example, pointing to an object. Gestures that can replace speech and have direct verbal meanings are called *emblems*. An example of a North American emblem would be the thumbs-up sign. Emblems vary considerably across cultures.

4. Voice

The voice, also known as the paralinguistic channel, expresses feelings and emotions through pitch, intonation, speed, rhythm, pitch range, and volume.

Although the channels are described here separately, information from these channels is rapidly integrated to form and convey distinct impressions. For example, a smile, direct gaze, a forward lean, and a warm vocal tone all taken together convey interest and liking. However, direct gaze and a forward lean, without the smile and warm tone, taken together might convey dominance or intimidation.

B. Leakage Hierarchy

Nonverbal channels of communication can be ranked in terms of volitional controllability. The face is the channel that is most easily controlled, bodily movements are less controllable, and the voice is the least controllable of these three channels of communication. Lack of controllability in the channels of expression is associated with leakage of "true" emotions and attitudes. Thus, the most leaky of these three channels is the voice, followed by the body, and then the face. By paying careful attention to clients' bodily and vocal cues, providers may be able to detect underlying feelings and affect.

C. Deception

Deception is the expression of behavior that is inconsistent with the true thoughts and feelings of the encoder, sender, or actor. In certain situations, such as for the purposes of self-presentation, deceptive behavior is considered socially acceptable. For example, it is acceptable, or indeed expected, for employment interviewees to appear confident although they might actually feel quite nonconfident. In other situations, such as when people tell self-serving lies, deception is widely held to be unacceptable.

When lying, people tend to direct more attention to managing their facial expressions than to managing their bodily or vocal behaviors; they tend to move their face, head, and body less than when not lying. Moreover, when lying, people show more mis-

match between channels and more micromomentary facial expressions, lasting less than a quarter of a second. Deception is typically detected at rates only slightly higher than chance, although situational factors such as the relationship between the person lying and the target and the motivation of the person lying can increase the accuracy of detecting deception. [*See* DECEPTION.]

III. NONVERBAL SKILLS

Nonverbal skill is the term used to describe individuals' abilities to use nonverbal communication effectively and accurately. Nonverbal skills tend to be associated with enduring characteristics of people such as gender, personality, and culture. Generally, nonverbal skills are conceptualized in terms of two separate subskills: encoding skills and decoding skills.

A. Encoding Skills

Encoding skills (also called expressivity or legibility) refer to the ability to communicate emotions, attitudes, or other messages through nonverbal cues so that the observer can interpret the meaning of the message as the encoder intended. For example, a person scoring high on this skill would be able to convey emotions, such as empathy, accurately from nonverbal channels alone. Thus, more skilled encoders tend to be judged as more empathic when they are being empathic, and judged so purely from nonverbal channels such as the face or the voice. More-skilled encoders tend to be more popular, dominant, and extraverted than less-skilled encoders.

B. Decoding Skills

Decoding skills refer to individuals' abilities to interpret the nonverbal communication of other people. Good decoders are more accurate judges of nonverbal behavior. They tend to be better adjusted, more interpersonally democratic, more popular, less dogmatic, and are judged by others to be more interpersonally sensitive than poor decoders.

Both encoding and decoding skills vary considerably among people. Encoding and decoding skills are not very highly correlated; that is, a person can be good at one skill and not the other. In general, women are more accurate encoders as well as decoders of non-verbal communication than men.

IV. NONVERBAL COMMUNICATION AND SOCIAL INFLUENCE

In any interpersonal relationship, people influence each other in multiple ways. This influence process, in which the behavior of one person affects the behavior of another person, is called social influence. In health care settings, social influence is related to important client outcomes. Health care providers can influence their clients in many ways. Moreover, because of the reciprocative nature of the relationship, clients can also influence the behavior of their providers, albeit in more subtle ways. Important sources of social influence include interpersonal expectations, power, gender, physical appearance, and culture.

A. Interpersonal Expectations

Individuals' expectations about each other's behavior can bring about actual changes in behavior. Thus, merely by expecting another person to fail or to succeed, an individual can facilitate the success or failure of that person. Expectations are conveyed through subtle nonverbal behaviors such as smiling, head nodding, leaning forward, and subtle changes in vocal tone. When individuals hold high expectations of others, they tend to behave more warmly and approvingly. When they have low expectations of others, individuals tend to behave more coldly and distantly. In health care settings, both providers and clients may facilitate or inhibit the behavior of the other. Because of their relative lack of power and control, clients are particularly sensitive to providers' subtle cues that indicate their expectations about a client's prognosis.

B. Power

Higher status generally allows for more flexibility and for more initiation of nonverbal behavior. Higher-status individuals tend to initiate more nonverbal behavior, including touch and gaze. Nonverbal behavior can be used strategically to gain compliance. A carefully timed smile, touch, or vocal inflection can help in gaining compliance with requests. In health care settings, providers have control over expertise, infor-mation, and resources, and thus their behaviors have a great deal of influence on the relationship. Although clients are relatively less powerful, they can nevertheless exert power by disclosing or withholding information and by choosing whether or not to comply with treatment plans.

C. Gender

Females are more accurate decoders of most nonverbal cues. The overall superiority of females as decoders has been found in many different cultures. Females also tend to be more accurate encoders of emotional cues than males. Females are more nonverbally expressive; they smile, laugh, and gaze more at others than do males. They also stand closer to others, touch themselves more, and use their hands more expressively.

In dyadic interactions, particularly same-sex interactions, females exhibit more nonverbal involvement (closer distance, direct gaze, touch, direct body orientation, facial expressiveness, nods, and positive vocal cues) than do males. Females both initiate as well as receive higher levels of involvement.

Female clients tend to be given more information than male clients in medical visits, perhaps because they tend to ask more questions in general. Female clients also provide more information to physicians. In addition, female clients tend to be more expressive, and both male and female physicians tend to be more expressive with female clients. Female physicians are judged as more empathic than male physicians, especially with female clients. Female physician–female client dyads express the highest levels of eye contact and touching, and the closest interpersonal distances, whereas male–male dyads express the lowest levels of these behaviors.

D. Physical Appearance

Appearance and dress have considerable influence on interpersonal behavior and are likely to influence providers' and clients' impressions of and behavior toward each other. Attractive people are more popular and can exert more social influence. For example, physicians make more eye contact and orient their body more toward clients who are well groomed compared with disheveled clients. Attractive clients are also interrupted less by physicians.

Although physical attractiveness is a highly desirable quality, other factors such as situational factors, personality, and other communicative behavior also determine the impression, behavior, and influence of others.

E. Culture

Although facial expressions are universally encoded and decoded, there are considerable cultural differences in the usage of nonverbal cues. Hand gestures, with specific meanings (emblems), vary widely from culture to culture and serious misunderstandings can occur between people from different cultures in interpreting these gestures. Furthermore, there are cultural differences in the display rules for specific emotions. Thus, people from certain cultures are more likely to control their display of emotions to other people. People from cultures characterized as "high-contact cultures" stand closer to each other, gaze at each other more, touch each other more, and use a more direct body orientation toward each other than people from low-contact cultures. High-contact cultures include Latin American, Middle Eastern, and Southern European cultures, and low-contact cultures include Northern European, North American, and Asian cultures, although there are some exceptions. Because of familiarity with the appropriate cues, both the encoding and decoding of nonverbal cues seem to be more accurate within rather than between cultures.

Of particular importance to health care settings are cultural differences in the expression of pain. Providers should be aware that certain cultural and ethnic groups, such as high-contact cultures, express pain more readily than other more stoic, less-expressive groups. Sensitivity to cultural norms in the expression of pain as well as other negative states is, therefore, extremely important. [*See* PAIN.]

V. NONVERBAL COMMUNICATION IN DYADIC INTERACTIONS

In any interpersonal dyadic relationship, three theoretical concepts relating to nonverbal behavior are extremely important to successful communication and interaction of the participants. These three concepts— empathy, synchrony, and rapport—are particularly relevant to health care settings.

A. Empathy

Empathy refers to the process of understanding another person's feelings and thoughts and actually experiencing those feelings and thoughts to some degree. Clinicians' empathy is revealed through their nonverbal behavior. Empathic clinicians communicate positive affect through nonverbal behaviors such as head nodding and smiling, making more eye contact, leaning forward, and using a serious, warm, and relaxed tone of voice in communicating with clients.

B. Interactional Synchrony

Interactional synchrony in a dyad is characterized by simultaneous movement, interaction rhythm, and behavioral meshing of both members of the dyad. Synchrony is characterized by mutuality; whereas empathy is a phenomenon that occurs at the level of the individual, synchrony occurs at the level of the dyad. Postural mirroring between clients and therapists has been found to be positively related to empathy in counseling sessions.

C. Rapport

Rapport, like synchrony, is characterized by mutuality between the members of the dyad. Dyads high in rapport show mutual positivity or warmth, mutual attentiveness or involvement, and behavioral coordination between the members of the dyad. Behavioral coordination is reflected in posture similarity and in interaction synchrony. Members of high-rapport dyads show more "immediacy": they smile at each other, nod their heads, lean forward, gaze directly at each other, display a direct body orientation, have an open posture with uncrossed arms, and mirror each other's posture.

VI. CLIENT NONVERBAL COMMUNICATION: CLUES TO PERSONALITY AND PSYCHOPATHOLOGY

A. Personality and Nonverbal Behavior

Certain personality traits are related to stylistic differences in nonverbal communication. Three personality traits that show strong relationships to nonverbal communication are extraversion, self-monitoring, and the Type A personality. Individuals possessing these personality traits display certain distinctive styles of nonverbal behavior. [*See* PERSONALITY.]

I. Extraversion

Extraverted people are more nonverbally expressive, are more skilled encoders of nonverbal behavior, and gaze more at others during conversations than do introverts. In contrast, introverted people are less expressive and tend to be better decoders rather than encoders of nonverbal behavior than extraverts.

2. Self-Monitoring

High self-monitoring is the tendency to monitor one's behavior in relation to others and to attend to the social appropriateness of one's actions. High self-monitoring is related to better nonverbal encoding as well as to better nonverbal decoding ability. High self-monitors tend to be more socially skilled in general and tend to pay more attention to social cues than do low self-monitors.

3. Type A/B Personality

Type A or "coronary prone" (prone to coronary heart disease or CHD) individuals tend to possess a distinctive nonverbal behavioral style. Such individuals have loud, dominant voices and tend to be more restless, impatient, aggressive, and hostile than Type B individuals, who are less prone to CHD. Type A individuals tend to make rapid facial and bodily movements, display loud, rapid, and explosive speech with short speech latencies, interrupt others, and express hostility and aggression nonverbally. Type A people tend to glare more at others and also tend to express more disgust than Type B people. An observational study revealed that individuals who were labeled Type A, based on a standard interview, showed more arm movements and were more restless during a relaxation period than non-Type A people. Thus, the behavior of Type A people carries over to nonstressful experiences, and providers should be sensitive to such behavior.

B. Psychopathology and Nonverbal Behavior

Certain specific combinations of nonverbal behaviors are related to different types of psychopathology. De-

pressed and schizophrenic patients, in particular, exhibit distinctive nonverbal behaviors.

I. Depression

Mentally ill individuals generally are less able to decode and encode nonverbal cues. For example, depressed people use fewer hand gestures, speak more slowly, show less pitch variation, and gaze less at their interactional partner both while listening and while speaking. Depressed people also show less facial activity and smiling. This slowed-down behavioral style characterizes depressed people across age, gender, and culture. As people become less depressed, eye contact, general movement, speech rate, and smiling increase.

Depressed individuals are also less sensitive to the nonverbal cues of others. They show poor discrimination among facial expressions of emotions and exhibit a negative bias when identifying emotions. There is some evidence, however, that depressed people are more accurate judges of real interactions between two other people. Depressed people tend to elicit a similar style of behavior from their partners. For example, infants of depressed mothers tend to show behaviors related to depression that are similar to those of their mothers. When paired with caregivers who are not depressed, however, these same infants do not show behaviors that are associated with depression. [*See* DEPRESSION.]

2. Schizophrenia

Nonverbal behaviors have been studied as indicators of other forms of psychopathology as well. Schizophrenic clients show stereotypic behaviors (such as rocking and grimacing), decreased hand gestures, less facial activity, less direct gaze, and a lack of coordination between their speech and their movements. Schizophrenic clients also tend to be poor decoders of affect, but this decrement is related to the chronicity and duration of the illness. [*See* SCHIZOPHRENIA.]

3. Other Psychopathology

Highly anxious clients tend to display behaviors such as hand-wringing, pacing, frequent posture shifts, uncoordinated speech, and decreased eye contact. Psychopaths tend to use more hand gestures, lean forward more, make more eye contact but smile less at their therapists than nonpsychopaths. People under the influence of alcohol are less able to decode affect and nonverbal behaviors. Violent individuals require a greater distance from others to feel comfortable in interpersonal situations compared with nonviolent controls. Although these findings are promising, a great deal of work still needs to be done to systematically identify nonverbal indicators of psychopathology.

VII. PROVIDER NONVERBAL COMMUNICATION AND CLIENT OUTCOMES

A. Providers' Skills

Physicians' nonverbal skills have been found to predict client satisfaction and compliance. Physicians who are more accurate at judging interpersonal cues expressed by the body tend to have the most satisfied clients. Furthermore, physicians who are better at encoding nonverbal emotion cues have more satisfied clients who show better treatment compliance. In addition, physicians who are better encoders have a larger workload than do poorer encoders. Thus, the nonverbal encoding and decoding skills of treatment providers seem to be quite important in predicting client satisfaction and compliance.

B. Providers' Nonverbal Behaviors

The majority of studies that have examined the relationship between nonverbal behavior and therapeutic or health-related outcomes have been analogue studies rather than studies of actual treatment sessions, thereby limiting the generalizability of the findings. The summary provided in this section relies mostly on analogue studies that have examined behaviors of counselors and clients.

Studies reveal that affiliative behaviors such as smiling and head nodding that indicate positive affect are related to more positive judgments of counselor empathy and competence. In addition, high immediacy behaviors such as close proximity between the client and therapist, forward lean, open arm and leg postures, facing one another, and direct eye contact are related to the creation of an open, warm environment and a positive, involved relationship between the therapist and the client. Eye contact has also been found to be positively related to ratings of respect and genuineness on the part of the therapist. But either too much or too little of these behaviors can have negative consequences; there seems to be a curvilinear relationship between nonverbal cues and client–therapist affect.

Besides posture and eye contact, therapists' frequency of movement influences judgments about their competency. Therapists who were more active were judged as more warm, energetic, trustworthy, responsive, and agreeable. Furthermore, clients of therapists who nodded more expressed more satisfaction with the therapeutic work. Interestingly, very little information is needed to judge therapist empathy: accurate evaluations of therapists' empathy and warmth have been obtained from photographs of the therapists' faces while interacting with clients.

Tone of voice is an extremely important channel in health care settings. The voice is closely attended to because it is thought to convey true feelings in addition to carrying verbal messages. Auditory cues such as vocal intensity and pitch level distinguish between therapists' exceptionally good (peak) and poor hours. During poor hours, therapists sound uninvolved and dull, whereas during peak hours, they sound relaxed and warm. Furthermore, physicians who sounded more anxious were more successful at treating alcoholic clients than physicians who sounded less anxious.

Sometimes combined cues from different channels convey important messages. For example, clients in one study expressed the most satisfaction when doctors conveyed a positive verbal message in a negative tone of voice, thus simultaneously communicating concern and acceptance.

VIII. CONCLUSIONS

Nonverbal communication is extremely important in affecting client outcomes in health care settings. Nonverbal communication in the client–provider relationship is dynamic, interactive, and reciprocal. Providers' nonverbal behaviors affect client behaviors and vice versa. This social influence process often occurs through subtle and unconscious cues and can have profound consequences for the provider–client relationship and client outcomes.

ACKNOWLEDGMENTS

Work on this manuscript was supported by grants from the Bayer Institute for Health Care Communication and the National Science Foundation.

BIBLIOGRAPHY

Blanck, P. D., Buck, R., & Rosenthal, R. (Eds.). (1986). *Nonverbal communication in the clinical context*. University Park, PA: Pennsylvania State University Press.

Hall, J. A., Harrigan, J. A., & Rosenthal, R. (1995). Nonverbal behavior in clinician–client interaction. *Applied and Preventive Psychology, 4*, 21–37.

Knapp, M. L., & Hall, J. A. (1992). *Nonverbal communication in human interaction* (3rd ed.). New York: Harcourt Brace Jovanovich.

Roter, D. L., & Hall, J. A. (1992). *Doctors talking with clients/clients talking with doctors: Improving communication in medical visits*. Westport, CT: Auburn House.

Wiener, M., Budney, S., Wood, L., & Russell, R. L. (1989). Nonverbal events in psychotherapy. *Clinical Psychology Review, 9*, 487–504.